IAN Textbook of

Neurology

IAN Textbook of
Neurology

SECOND EDITION

VOLUME 2

Editors

Satish V Khadilkar MD DM DNB FIAN FICP FAMS FRCP (London)
Dean
Bombay Hospital Institute of Medical Sciences
Mumbai, Maharashtra, India

Gagandeep Singh MD DM (Neurology) FAMS FRCP (London) FIAN FICP
Professor and Head
Department of Neurology
Dayanand Medical College and Hospital
Ludhiana, Punjab, India
and
Honorary Senior Research Fellow
Department of Clinical and Experimental Epilepsy
Institute of Neurology
Queen Square
London, United Kingdom

Foreword

Wolfgang Grisold

JAYPEE BROTHERS MEDICAL PUBLISHERS
The Health Sciences Publisher
New Delhi | London

Jaypee Brothers Medical Publishers (P) Ltd

Headquarters
EMCA House
23/23-B, Ansari Road, Daryaganj
New Delhi 110 002, India
Landline: +91-11-23272143, +91-11-23272703
+91-11-23282021, +91-11-23245672
E-mail: jaypee@jaypeebrothers.com

Corporate Office
4838/24, Ansari Road, Daryaganj
New Delhi 110 002, India
Phone: +91-11-43574357
Fax: +91-11-43574314
E-mail: jaypee@jaypeebrothers.com

Overseas Office
J.P. Medical Ltd
83 Victoria Street, London
SW1H 0HW (UK)
Phone: +44 20 3170 8910
E-mail: info@jpmedpub.com

EU GPSR Authorised Representative
Logos Europe, 9 rue Nicolas Poussin
17000, La Rochelle, France
Phone: +33 (0) 6 67 93 73 78
E-mail: contact@logoseurope.eu

Website: www.jaypeebrothers.com
Website: www.jaypeedigital.com

Inquiries for bulk sales may be solicited at: jaypee@jaypeebrothers.com

IAN Textbook of Neurology (Volume 2) / Satish V Khadilkar, Gagandeep Singh

First Edition: 2018

Second Edition: 2024

Reprint: 2026

ISBN: 978-93-5465-682-8

Printed in India

FOREWORD

The "*IAN Textbook of Neurology*" edited by Satish V Khadilkar and Gagandeep Singh is based on classical neurological principles, which takes into account the history and neurological examinations, finds the correlates in anatomy, neurophysiology, and molecular levels, and is a large compendium on common neurological symptoms and signs.

The book contains a list of diseases of the brain that start from frequent types, such as stroke, toward rare diseases, such as diseases of the spinal cord as well as functional disorders.

The chapter on investigations explains the importance of imaging, neurophysiology, and testing with various other methods including genetics. Drug therapies are increasingly important and equally important to counselling and doctor–patient relationship.

The *IAN Textbook of Neurology* is a comprehensive textbook and will be useful for all physicians concerned in the treatment of neurology from trainees to practicing neurologists. In one of the countries with the world's second largest population, the impact will be meaningful.

The ongoing development of electronic media, availability of easy-access knowledge, and recent research as well as other electronic apps as libraries, blended learning apps have instigated an ongoing discussion of the value of textbooks.

Textbooks in neurology are essential and often the basis for training curricula and also individual studies and therapies. They are used in many scientific fields, and not only medicine, and are considered to be a legitimized and institutional knowledge. Textbooks are based on a broad width of knowledge, which cannot be provided in a single article, which is usually topic specific.

They thus have an impact on summarizing the current knowledge and at present remain the best expert platform, which must receive timely additional update from easily available media, and definitely case- and problem-specific additional research is necessary to be updated on the latest developments.

I hope that this tremendous work will be used for the care of patients and once a book of this dimension is released, the editors will start planning the next edition. The effort of the editors to collect such a large spectrum of sections and chapters is enormous and will benefit trainees and practicing neurologists. On behalf of the World Federation of Neurology whose mission is to foster neurology and education, this will be an important contribution.

Wolfgang Grisold MD FAAN
Professor
Department of Neurology
Ludwig Boltzmann Institute for
Experimental and Clinical Traumatology
Vienna, Austria, Europe
President, World Federation of Neurology

PREFACE TO THE SECOND EDITION

The second edition of the "*IAN Textbook of Neurology*" has been prepared for clinicians who participate in the care of neurological patients, including those who are in training to become neurologists, internists, neurosurgeons, and neuroscientists.

The basic structure of this second edition has changed. The book is divided into seven parts. Section 1 discusses the History-taking and the Neurological Examination, inclusive of the systemic examination that helps the neurological diagnoses. Section 2 covers the Applied Neuroanatomy and Neurophysiology aspects that are important to clinicians. Section 3 discusses the clinical Approach to various Common Neurological Symptoms. Section 4 describes Diseases of the Nervous System. Section 5 discusses Investigations, Section 6 the Principles of Management, and Section 7 is about the Counseling and Doctor–Patient Relationship.

Thus, in some ways, this edition has tried to make the book comprehensive. Conventionally, textbooks carrying information regarding neurological examination have been separate from those that discuss diseases of the nervous system. This book covers both aspects. In the section on diseases of the nervous system, peculiarities and points relevant to the Indian setting have been highlighted for the practitioners working with Indian patients. Diagrams and flowcharts have been used for the ease of assimilation and chapters are extensively referenced.

The hard copy of the book will have access to online materials like multiple-choice questions which can be utilized for self-assessment and illustrative videos.

The chapters are written by authorities in their field, mainly from India and some overseas. Their expositions of the subjects reflect the ever-expanding extent of accumulated information and how it applies directly to the clinicians caring for their patients. The standard templates have ensured uniformity of the style and content. As many of the authors for this edition are newly inducted to this edition, the coordination was challenging to an extent, but all the authors responded with precision and we would like to thank them.

Collaboration with many individuals has been the backbone of the preparation of this edition. Jaypee Brothers Medical Publishers, Shri Jitendar P Vij (Group Chairman), and his team, namely, Ms Chetna Malhotra (Senior Director—Professional Publishing, Marketing and Business Development), Ms Nedup Bhutia Pillai (Team Leader—Print Publishing) and entire production team have worked systematically for many months and we thank them. Deepak Sharma from the office of Dr Gagandeep Singh has been instrumental in the early and continuing electronic communication with the authors for the past whole year and we thank him.

Medicine is an ever-changing science and the information pool changes at a phenomenal speed. We do hope that the readers keep themselves updated with the emerging information, using the base that this edition provides.

Satish V Khadilkar
Gagandeep Singh

PREFACE TO THE FIRST EDITION

Neurology is a field in medical sciences which has made phenomenal progress over the last two decades. Advancement in technology has changed our understanding of many diseases leading to improvement of patient care. Textbooks provide rapid access to the current status of the diseases and serve as ready reference for the physicians. There are many textbooks in neurology available in print and electronic versions. They are comprehensive, well-written, and serve as important source of information to the practicing and trainee neurologists. However, majority of them are contributed by authors from the Western world and are based on their research and clinical experience in Western countries. It is well documented that prevalence, presentations, genetics, and treatment response of various neurological diseases have significant regional variation. In order to overcome this, Indian Academy of Neurology envisaged bringing out a textbook of neurology to be planned and written by neurologists and neuroscientists who are researching, teaching, and practicing in India. It is impossible to capture the entire spectrum of neurological disorders in one volume of a textbook. In fact, literature concerning each subspecialty of neurology would constitute an enormous compendium of information. The chapters are, therefore, designed to give broad overview with recent advances in the designated field.

The book has 12 sections. Each section is dedicated to one subspecialty of neurology. Each section is edited by a senior member of the society with special interest in the specialty. The authors are chosen based on their experience and contributions in the specialized areas. The book chapters are comprehensive, well-written, and carry information with special emphasis on Indian scenario. The references quoted are extensive and will guide interested readers for further reading.

Thus, the book will be an important addition to already existing books in neurology with the unique feature of being contributed by neuroscientists of India who have extensive experience in the field of neurological diseases prevalent in India.

Arabinda Mukherjee

CONTENTS

VOLUME 1

Section 1: History and Clinical Neurological Examination

Section 2: Applied Neuroanatomy and Neurophysiology

Section 3: Approach to Common Neurological Symptoms

Section 4: Diseases of the Nervous System

Part 4A: Vascular Diseases

Part 4B: Infections

VOLUME 2

Part 4F: Cognitive Decline

Part 4G: Diseases of the Lower Motor Neuron

Part 4H: Ataxias

Part 4I: Miscellaneous

VIDEO CONTENT

Chapter 66: Psychogenic Nonepileptic Seizures

Video 1: Swoon. This nonepileptic attack disorder (NEAD) video shows the neurologist giving a "suggestion" to the patient using the tuning fork as an induction protocol. This is a swoon as described in our text. This patient had no postictal confusion and a very rapid recovery.

Video 2: This nonepileptic attack disorder (NEAD) video shows the posturing of opisthotonus, also called "arc de cercle" as seen in NEAD. This nonepileptic spell also stopped when suggested to the patient.

Video 3: This nonepileptic attack disorder (NEAD) episode shows ictal biting, bipedaling movements, side-to-side head movements. His electroencephalogram (EEG) during this record was also without any epileptiform discharges. The patient's ictus stopped on giving suggestion.

Chapter 71: Parkinson's Disease

Video 1: Bradykinesia: Video demonstrates bradykinesia in the form of an asymmetric reduction (right>left) in amplitude of finger tapping, hand movement, rapid alternating movement and leg agility. The patient also has a stooped posture with reduced arm swing while walking, slowness of gait with freezing and a positive pull test.

Video 2: Tremor dominant Parkinson's disease (PD): Video demonstrates the tremor dominant phenotype of PD wherein the patient has a severe rest and action tremor of bilateral upper and lower limbs (left>right).

Video 3: Choreiform peak dose dyskinesia occurring post comsumption of dopaminergic medication (levodopa–carbidopa). Segment 1: Mild choreiform dyskinesia. Segment 2: Severe choreiform dyskinesia.

Video 4: Freezing of gait: The patient has significant gait freezing with improves significantly with visual cues.

Video 5: Effect of bilateral STN DBS in a patient with akinetic rigid variant of PD: In the Pre DBS, OFF state, the patient has significant bradykinesia and freezing of gait. In the post DBS. OFF state, the patient has no evident bradykinesia and gait is normal.

Chapter 109: Functional Neurological Disorders

Video 1: A boy with functional imbalance falls to either side when doing the Romberg test with his feet close and eyes closed.

Video 2: Now when the boy is asked to stand the same way with feet close, but instructed to focus on doing rapid alternating movements with the hands (dysdiadochokinesia), he no longer loses balance, even when his eyes are closed as in the earlier Romberg test. This shows the effect of distraction on the Romberg test.

Video 3: La belle indifference seen in a lady with focal "dystonic" movements of the left lower face.

Video 4: A man with functional tremor first affecting the whole hand. When the thumb is plugged into the ear, preventing it from moving, only the hand moves. When the thumb is removed, only the thumb moves. When the hands are placed on a pillow the hands tremble again, and finally when the feet are placed against each other they get the same tremor immediately. This is the whack-a-mole sign where movement (tremor) suppression of one body part is followed by immediate reemergence of movement (tremor) in another.

Video 5: An irregular tremor in the outstretched left hand, which slows down and almost stops when the person is asked to do tapping movements with the normal right thumb and finger.

Video 6: This video shows how suggestion using a tuning fork could induce the dystonia of the lips and jaw that the patient came for. On reminding, even her eyes close, like in her "spontaneous attacks." In the later part of the video, just pressing on the cheeks abruptly ends this dystonia.

Video 7: A lady showing functional hemifacial movements of the left face involving only the left lower face, with rhythmic movements unlike the irregular jerks of hemifacial spasm. The movements abruptly cease when she is asked to show her teeth. When she holds her hands outstretched, there emerges the tremor of the right hand on suggestion.

Video 8: A person with functional imbalance of gait demonstrates exquisite balance when doing tandem walking. The wild, flailing movements actually show excellent balance.

Video 9: A boy with functional ataxic gait suddenly veers and takes support of the wall, both when walking toward us and walking away from us and also when standing.

Video 10: A girl with functional hemiplegia dragging the right leg like a stick without circumduction, as would be expected in hemiplegic gait.

Video 11: A man with functional hemiplegia dragging the right leg very slowly like a stick without circumduction.

Video 12: This lady with shrug-like jerking of her shoulders while walking and standing later starts getting a tremor of her feet when she lies down in bed. This is also akin to whack-a-mole sign.

Video 13: A lady with a functional gait disorder shows her suddenly coming backward without losing balance, every time she takes a few steps ahead.

Video 14: A lady with a functional gait disorder shows wild swinging and swaying, as well as giving way at the knees without actually losing balance or falling.

Video 15: This girl with functional drop attacks shows how she walks quite normally, and then gets some sort of warning in her head and falls down without any injury.

Video 16: A girl with functional seizures shows a dystonic posture of the right hand, neck, face, and body as she holds her breath and keeps her eyes clenched tightly and resists opening. The attack stops suddenly when the doctor speaks to her, and she takes a breath again without any postictal confusion.

Video 17: This boy with functional seizure shows the gradual buildup of asynchronous limb and body movements. The video also demonstrates preserved consciousness as shown by him showing the tongue when asked to.

Video 18: A boy with a functional seizure, which is induced by suggestion with the use of a tuning fork. The attack shows typical asynchronous limb movements as well as arching of the back. It also shows how suggestion abruptly stops the attack, and there is no postictal confusion.

Video 19: A girl with functional loss of vision who also shows convergence spasm.

Video 20: Preserved optokinetic nystagmus in a lady who is functionally blind.

Video 21A: A lady able to touch her fingers to each other accurately when the "blind eye" is patched and she can see with the other one.

Video 21B: The same lady with functional blindness missing her fingers, when asked to touch both her index fingers to each other, when her seeing eye is patched. The ability to touch fingers to each other is not dependent on vision but on proprioception.

Video 22: Radio tactical shows a boy with functional voice order showing irregular stammering speech with hyperventilation and tremor of the body toward the end of the video.

Video 23: A person with an acute onset of whispering voice. He can make a sound when coughing though.

Free Online Resources

You can access following content on https://learn.ejaypee.com/login/ by redeeming the scratch code given on the front-in of the cover.

1. **E-version of the book:** All the chapters in the printed version can be accessed online.
2. **MCQs:** Each section is followed by 5–10 MCQs. These MCQs have 4–5 options and one correct answer. They are from the contents of the chapter. You are advised to solve these after reading the whole chapter.
3. **Videos:** Some of the chapters have videos and these videos can be accessed online.

4

SECTION

Diseases of the Nervous System

Part 4F: Cognitive Decline

76

CHAPTER

Alzheimer's Disease

Faheem Arshad, Sandeep Kumar, Priya Thomas, Suvarna Alladi

INTRODUCTION

Alzheimer's disease (AD) is a progressive neurodegenerative disorder characterized by cognitive disturbances, gradual impairment of daily activities of living, and a wide range of neuropsychiatric symptoms. It is the most common form of dementia in the elderly, accounting for 60–80% of cases.[1] Mixed pathologies are however common, and about 13–17% of AD are associated with intracerebral vascular disease.[2,3] The main risk factor for AD and related dementias is advanced age. While dementia overall is the fifth leading cause of death,[4] AD is the fourth leading cause of disability-adjusted life years (DALYs) lost in persons aged 75 years and older,[5] having a considerable impact on caregivers.[6]

EPIDEMIOLOGY

Globally, the number of people with dementia is projected to rise from 57.4 million cases in 2019 to 152.8 million cases in 2050.[7] The overall burden of AD is substantial, and it remains the leading neurodegenerative cause of dementia worldwide. The prevalence of AD rises with advancing age,[8] and estimates suggest that there are 30 million persons with AD and related dementias worldwide.

Prevalence of Dementia in India

The Global Burden of Disease Study recorded that in 2016, 3.74 million people in South Asia had dementia, including 2.93 million people from India.[4] There have been regional differences in dementia prevalence in India, according to studies conducted between 1996 and 2017. According to these studies, the overall prevalence of dementia in India may range from 10.6% across different states[9,10] as well as within the same region.[9-11] While this variation could be attributed to the wide variation in demography, this could also be due to different sampling techniques and diagnostic tools used, particularly given how these tools were adapted to the local sociocultural context. According to the Dementia India Report, the number of people with dementia is estimated to be 5.3 million and is expected to increase to 14.32 million in the year 2050.[12] In a memory clinic study among the subtypes of dementia in India, AD was the most common subtype (38.3%), followed by a high proportion of vascular dementia (25.4%).[13] According to a recent meta-analysis of 20 epidemiological studies, the prevalence of dementia in India is 20 per 1,000. The prevalence rates were similar for males and females, and rural and urban populations.[14] Due to the heterogeneity in individual studies based on their methodology, there is still a need for multicentric epidemiological studies on dementia prevalence in India, using harmonized protocols, an effort being made by the Dementia Science Program supported by the Department of Biotechnology (DBT).[15]

PATHOLOGY AND PATHOPHYSIOLOGY

The neuropathologic hallmarks of AD are extracellular β-amyloid deposits as neuritic plaques and intracellular hyperphosphorylated tau as neurofibrillary tangles. In addition to these features, several other pathologic changes are commonly observed in association with AD. Cerebral amyloid angiopathy is often seen in cases with parenchymal amyloid deposits.[16] Accumulation of abnormal α-synuclein inclusions is also commonly observed in intermediate-to-high levels of AD neuropathologic change.[17] Increasing evidence indicates that AD pathophysiology extends beyond the "hallmark" amyloid and tau accumulation. A complex cascade of the cellular phase of AD comprised of dysfunctional neuronal, glial, and endothelial mechanisms contributes to irreversible damage.[18] This intricate cell-mediated pathophysiology is poorly reflected by core AD biomarkers.

Growing evidence supports that the neurovascular unit is altered in AD and the disease is mediated by vascular pathogenesis.[19-21] It is becoming more evident that vascular risk factors and neurovascular dysfunction, including the risk factor apolipoprotein E ε4 allele (APOE 4), are crucial in the pathogenesis of AD. These risk factors include hypotension, hypertension, cholesterol levels, type 2 diabetes mellitus, smoking, oxidative stress, and iron overload.[21,22] Vascular dysfunction is becoming more widely recognized as a pathological hallmark underlying AD pathogenesis, but the underlying mechanism has only been recently understood.[22] Blood-brain barrier (BBB) tight junction disruption and vessel wall leakage appear to be a compensatory response to impaired cerebral blood flow (CBF) in AD mice models.[23] These findings suggest an alternative hypothesis where cerebrovascular neoangiogenesis secondary to amyloidogenesis and underlying CBF impairment leads to defective neurovasculature, thereby disrupting the BBB, further impairing CBF, and thus compromising the clearance of amyloid from the brain.[24,25]

Neuroinflammation is an evolving hallmark in the pathogenesis of AD, which manifests as gliosis, proliferation, and activation of microglia and astrocytes, the two major cell types in the brain. Many recently identified AD risk genes such as triggering receptors expressed on myeloid cells-2 (*TREM2*) are highly expressed on glial cells. This potential involvement of glia in AD pathogenesis has been a focus of attention as inhibition of glial response as well as blockade of proinflammatory cytokine release may impede AD pathogenesis.[26-28] There is emerging evidence to suggest the role of immune system activation and gut-brain axis interaction in the pathophysiology of AD.[29,30] These novel mechanisms in modulating AD pathology are currently under active investigation.

CLINICAL PRESENTATIONS

Alzheimer's disease is characterized by slowly progressive neurodegeneration with synaptic and neuronal loss. The symptomatic phase represents an advanced stage of this process that progresses for 1-2 decades. The average time between the onset of symptoms and the time of death is 7-10 years.[31] Patients with typical AD present with episodic memory impairment, which is memory related to events occurring at a particular time and event, characterized by frequent misplacing of objects, forgetting appointments, repeating questions, getting lost, and forgetting to pay bills. Early involvement of episodic memory reflects the selective vulnerability of the medial temporal lobe to AD pathology. Early in the course of the disease, patients may also manifest executive dysfunction (problems in planning, organization, problem solving, set switching), but the symptoms are mild until the late stage.[32] In mild-to-moderate stages patients also develop visuospatial impairment in the form of wayfinding difficulty in unfamiliar places, and language disturbances such as word finding or naming difficulty. In later stages of the disease, some patients have difficulty in performing learned motor tasks that further contribute to an increase in dependency on caregivers **(Table 1)**.[33]

Patients with AD can also present with a wide variety of symptoms, clinical signs, and syndromes that do not always resemble the typical amnestic syndrome. Nonamnestic (i.e., atypical) presentations of AD are associated with less salient memory deficits and a greater likelihood of impairment of other cognitive domains including language, visuospatial, executive and motor functions, and behavioral disturbances. This clinical heterogeneity is partly responsible for the misdiagnosis and delay in diagnosis. These presentations form a clinical spectrum of AD and fulfill the criteria for specific nonamnestic syndromes, also referred to as focal cortical presentations.[34] These presentations are typically associated with insidious onset (typically before 65 years of age) and gradual progression of clinical deficits **(Table 2)**.

The most commonly studied nonamnestic phenotype is posterior cortical atrophy (PCA), which is characterized by impaired space and object perception; Balint syndrome (simultanagnosia, optic ataxia, oculomotor apraxia); Gerstmann syndrome (dyscalculia, dysgraphia, left-right confusion, finger agnosia); constructional, dressing, or limb apraxia; and environmental agnosia alexia, with relative sparing of other functions. While the majority of PCA cases have underlying AD neuropathology, other degenerative

TABLE 1: Clinical features of mild, moderate, and severe Alzheimer's disease (AD).

Mild AD	Moderate AD	Severe AD
• Complaints related to episodic memory impairments such as misplacement of items, skipping of medication dosages, forgetting payment of bills, and inability to keep track of appointments • Confusing ways in new areas and localities • Mild anxiety, depression, and irritability • Sleep disturbances	• Symptoms due to executive dysfunctions and poor judgement, i.e., difficulty in planning activities, managing finances, problems with calculations and daily chores • Word finding and naming difficulties • Disorientation to time and place • Mild apraxia • Behavioral abnormalities such as mood lability, aggressive behaviors, delusions, and increased anxiety • Decreased food intake, leading to weight loss • Rarely mild extrapyramidal symptoms such as bradykinesia and myoclonus • Wayfinding difficulties in known areas and places	• Apraxia • Global aphasia • Impaired recognition of familiar peoples • Hallucinations and apathy • Urinary incontinence, gait difficulty, and impaired balances • Rarely seizures

TABLE 2: Clinical features of nonamnestic variants of Alzheimer's disease (AD).

Posterior cortical atrophy variant of AD	Logopenic variant of AD	Frontal variant of AD
• Second most common variant of AD • Visuospatial and visuoperceptual impairment • Balint syndrome (simultanagnosia, optic ataxia, oculomotor apraxia) • Gerstmann syndrome (dyscalculia, dysgraphia, left–right confusion, finger agnosia) • Limb-kinetic and dressing apraxia and constructional apraxia • Impaired space and object perception • Environmental agnosia • Homonymous visual field defect	• Most common variant of AD • Word finding difficulty with frequent pauses • Decrease in verbal output • Word retrieval difficulty with phonological paraphasias • Impairment of repetition of sentences • Preservation of grammar and motor articulation	• Features suggestive of frontolobar degeneration • Apathy, with decrease in motivation • Dysexecutive features such as impaired planning and organization • Differ from bvFTD by presence of prominent episodic memory impairment

(bvFTD: behavioral variant frontotemporal dementia)

etiologies including Lewy body disease, corticobasal degeneration, and prion disease have also been observed.[34,35] The language presentation of AD is the logopenic variant of a primary progressive aphasia (lvPPA), with predominant impairment of single-word retrieval in spontaneous speech and naming, phonological errors, and difficulty in repeating phrases and sentences.[36]

Other manifestations of AD have been described, mainly involving executive function and behavior. These phenotypes, sometimes referred to as frontal AD, may be challenging to diagnose because their features overlap with the behavioral variant frontotemporal dementia (bvFTD).[37,38] Corticobasal syndrome (CBS) can be a manifestation of patients with AD, characterized by predominant motor and sensory symptoms including limb rigidity, bradykinesia, apraxia, myoclonus, dystonia, and alien limb phenomenon. Unlike PCA and lvPPA, CBS is not highly predictive of underlying AD pathology; less than a third of patients with CBS have AD.[34,39]

Neuropsychiatric symptoms such as mild irritability and mood changes are common in the initial stages of AD with a gradual increase in frequency and severity during moderate stages. The most common neuropsychiatric symptoms associated with AD are apathy, agitation, and anxiety. Frequency of psychotic symptoms such as delusions and hallucinations increases with progressive decline in cognition.[40] Noncognitive symptoms like psychiatric symptoms are common in moderate-to-severe stages of disease, leading to significant functional impairment. These symptoms include sleep disturbances, mild tremor, myoclonus, clinical seizures, and rarely extrapyramidal symptoms.[41,42]

DIAGNOSIS

The diagnostic criteria of AD have undergone multiple revisions during the past 3 decades as the understanding of the disease has improved. These include: (1) The National Institute of Neurological and Communicative Disorders and Stroke, and the Alzheimer's Disease and Related Disorders Association (NINCDS-ADRDA) (1984),[43] (2) International Classification of Diseases, 10th edition (1993) (ICD-10),[44] (3) International Working Group for New Research Criteria for Diagnosis of AD (2010, 2014),[45,46] and (4) American Psychiatric Association's Diagnostic and Statistical Manual of Mental Disorders-5 (2013) (DSM-5).[47] In practice, the criteria used to make a diagnosis of AD include the DSM-5 criteria and the National Institute on Aging and the Alzheimer's Association (NIA-AA) criteria for probable AD updated in 2011. The DSM-5 recognizes two cognitive syndromes—major and mild neurocognitive disorders (NCDs). The diagnosis of the former requires objective cognitive decline that is severe enough to interfere with activities of daily living, and not caused by delirium or another neurologic, medical, or psychiatric disorder, while the latter has milder cognitive decline from previous level of performance without any interference with daily activities of living.[47] Similar to DSM-5, the NIA-AA criteria for AD span all three stages of AD [preclinical, mild cognitive impairment (MCI), and Alzheimer's dementia]. It further classifies AD clinically into probable AD and possible AD. This criteria recognizes the potential use of biomarkers [cerebrospinal fluid (CSF) and neuroimaging] to diagnose AD, especially the preclinical stage of AD, and classifies dementia due to AD into three subgroups of uncertain, intermediate, and high likelihood to have an underlying AD pathology **(Box 1)**.[48] The NIA-AA 2018 research framework defined AD biologically by the presence of biomarkers, i.e., (1) amyloid beta (Aβ), (2) pathological tau, and (3) neurodegeneration [AT(N)] independent of clinical syndrome. The advantage of this criteria is its ability to classify individuals' earlier stages of the disease process and also helps to prevent classifying all amnestic dementia as AD **(Table 3)**.[49]

Formal neuropsychological assessment is essential in evaluating individuals with dementia. It can be useful as it provides a better understanding of the cognitive construct of the patient, thereby allowing identification of what cognitive functions are preserved or deficient. It is also helpful in establishing a baseline in order to follow the patient over time. The pattern of abnormalities in the assessment can help predict underlying anatomical basis of the impairment and also in establishing the differential diagnosis of

BOX 1 NIA-AA 2011 criteria for AD.

NIA-AA criteria 2011

1. *Preclinical AD*: Stage where subjects are cognitively and functionally normal in spite of harboring pathophysiological markers of AD such as amyloid deposition
   - *Stage 0*: Normal AD biomarkers
   - *Stage 1*: Asymptomatic amyloidosis
   - *Stage 2*: Amyloidosis with evidence of neuronal degeneration
   - *Stage 3*: Amyloidosis, neurodegeneration, and subtle cognitive impairment
   - *sNAP*: Presence of neurodegeneration but without evidence of amyloidosis, also known as suspected non-Alzheimer pathophysiology
2. *MCI due to AD*:
   - *Core clinical criteria:*
     - Concern about change in cognition, reported by the patient/informant/clinician
     - Objective evidence of impairment in one or more cognitive domains typically including memory
     - Preservation of independence of daily activities
     - Not demented
     - Other causes of cognitive impairment such as head injury and medical causes are ruled out
     - Presence of AD genetic factors
   - *Criteria after incorporating biomarkers:*
     - *MCI core clinical criteria*: Without evidence of biomarkers
     - *MCI due to AD intermediate likelihood*: Positive for amyloid beta (PET/CSF); untested for neuronal injury (tau/FDG PET)
     - *MCI due to AD high likelihood*: Positive for both the AD biomarkers
     - *MCI unlikely due to AD*: Negative for both the biomarkers
3. *Probable AD*:
   - *Core clinical criteria:*
     - Insidious onset
     - History of worsening
     - Initial and prominent cognitive domains affected are: (1) amnestic, i.e., impairment in learning and recall of recently learned information, (2) nonamnestic presentation, i.e., language (word finding difficulty), visuospatial, and dysexecutive presentation
     - No evidence of substantial concomitant of cerebrovascular disease, core features of dementia of Lewy body, bvFTD, semantic or nonfluent PPA nor any evidence of other active neurological and non-neurological diseases or any medication use

   Possible AD:
   - *Core clinical criteria*:
     - *Atypical course*: Core clinical criteria are met in terms of cognitive deficits, but there is either sudden onset of impairment or insufficient historical detail or objective documentation of the progressive decline
     - *Etiologically mixed presentation*: Core clinical criteria plus evidence of concomitant cerebrovascular disease, features of DLB, or evidence of other neurological or non-neurological disease or medical comorbidity as well as evidence of medication use that may affect cognition

Continued

Continued

- *Criteria after incorporating biomarkers:*

  A. *Probable AD*:
  - *Based on clinical criteria*: Unavailable/conflicting/indeterminate evidence of AD biomarker
  - *Intermediate*: If any of the biomarker is positive and other is indeterminate or unavailable
  - *High*: If both the biomarker, i.e., amyloid (PET/CSF) and neuronal injury (tau/FDG PET) are positive

  B. *Possible AD*:
  - *Based on clinical criteria*: Unavailable/conflicting/indeterminate evidence of AD biomarker
  - *Evidence of AD pathophysiological process*: Biomarker probability of AD is high (positive AD biomarker) but secondary cause to be ruled out
  - *Dementia unlikely due to AD*: Negative AD biomarkers

(AD: Alzheimer's disease; bvFTD: behavioral variant frontotemporal dementia; CSF: cerebrospinal fluid; DLB: dementia with Lewy bodies; FDG: 18-fluorodeoxyglucose; MCI: mild cognitive impairment; NIA-AA: National Institute on Aging and the Alzheimer's Association; PET: positron emission tomography; PPA: primary progressive aphasia; sNAP: suspected non-AD pathophysiology)

TABLE 3: NIA-AA 2018 research framework biomarker profiles and categories with cognitive staging.

AT(N) profiles	Biomarker category and cognitive staging
A-T-(N)-	**Normal AD biomarkers** • Cognitively unimpaired • MCI • Dementia
A+T-(N)-	**Alzheimer's continuum** • *Alzheimer's pathologic changes:* ○ Preclinical Alzheimer's pathological changes (cognitively unimpaired) ○ Alzheimer's pathological changes with MCI ○ Alzheimer's pathological changes with dementia
A+T+(N)- A+T+(N)+	*Alzheimer's disease (AD):* • Preclinical AD • AD with MCI (prodromal AD) • AD with dementia
A+T-(N)+	*AD and concomitant non-Alzheimer's pathologic changes:* • Cognitively unimpaired • MCI • Dementia
• A-T+(N)- • A-T-(N)+ • A-T+(N)+	*Non-AD pathologic changes:* • Cognitively unimpaired • MCI • Dementia

Note: A: amyloid beta biomarker presence or absence of which determines whether an individual is in the Alzheimer's continuum; T: pathological biomarkers to determine whether the individual who is in Alzheimer's continuum has disease or not; N: neurodegenerative or neuronal injury biomarker.

(MCI: mild cognitive impairment; NIA-AA: National Institute on Aging and the Alzheimer's Association) dementia. In addition, it would also assist in identifying opportunities for compensatory and rehabilitative treatment strategies. Neuropsychological assessment of AD shows deficits in poor learning and consolidation of memory, defect in category fluency with relatively preserved letter fluency reflecting temporal lobe involvement in AD. Confrontation naming and executive function tasks may be impaired in early AD.[32] Validated scales and questionnaires should be used in the local language and cultural context to assess the cognitive domains in patients with dementia.[50,51]

DIFFERENTIAL DIAGNOSIS

Vascular dementia and other neurodegenerative dementias are considered as the most common differential diagnosis of AD. The most common degenerative dementias after AD are dementia with Lewy bodies (DLB) and frontotemporal dementia (FTD).

Vascular dementia is caused by either ischemic or hemorrhagic strokes or small vessel cerebrovascular disease. The presence of a stroke-like course of illness, neurological signs of strokes on examination, and imaging evidence of cerebrovascular disease help in differentiating vascular dementia from AD.[52,53] DLB is the second most common degenerative dementia after AD. The presence of prominent visual hallucination, along with parkinsonism, cognitive fluctuation, dysautonomia, rapid eye movement disorder, and neuroleptic sensitivity helps in differentiating from AD.[54] FTD is a clinically and pathologically heterogenous disorder characterized by atrophy of frontal and temporal lobes. The presence of early and prominent alteration in personality, social and emotional behaviors, and executive function helps in differentiating bvFTD from AD.[55] Primary progressive aphasia, which is a form of frontotemporal lobar degeneration (FTLD), is characterized by progressive language impairment as core features with or without the involvement of other cognitive domains.[36] Other potentially treatable causes of cognitive impairment such as subdural hematoma, normal pressure hydrocephalus (NPH), or intracranial neoplasms should also be considered as differential diagnosis.

INVESTIGATIONS

A standard medical workup for AD often includes blood investigations, neuroimaging, fluid biomarkers, and genetics.

Laboratory Investigations

The American Academy of Neurology (AAN) practice parameter recommends routine assessment of vitamin B12 deficiency and thyroid hormone abnormalities as they are known to be associated with cognitive impairment. Other routine investigations include complete blood count, electrolyte panel, glucose, liver function test, and creatinine, and screening for syphilis should be done based on clinical suspicion. These laboratory tests are not useful in the diagnosis of AD but help exclude secondary causes or conditions that may exacerbate the cognitive impairment.[56]

Neuroimaging

As per the AAN practice parameter[56] all patients with suspected dementia should be evaluated with brain imaging, preferably with magnetic resonance imaging (MRI). Structural brain MRI can be useful in identifying alternating and potentially reversible causes of dementia such as subdural hematoma, hydrocephalus, and intracranial neoplasm **(Figs. 1A to F)**.

Structural Magnetic Resonance Imaging

The most characteristic MRI finding in early AD dementia is medial temporal lobe atrophy of the hippocampus and entorhinal cortex with concomitant dilatation of the temporal horn. Hippocampal volume reduction also correlates with neurofibrillary tangle pathology at autopsy and also with cognitive decline.[57] It can also predict conversion from normal cognition to MCI and from MCI to AD dementia. The extent of atrophy also correlates with the stage of the disease. In MCI, atrophy is limited to the medial temporal lobe whereas with AD onset, atrophy spreads to lateral temporal and parietal cortices, which corresponds with Braak staging.[58] Hence, structural MRI can be used as a neurodegeneration biomarker.

Functional Imaging

Functional brain imaging such as single-photon emission computed tomography (SPECT) and F18-fluorodeoxyglucose positron emission tomography (FDG-PET) helps detect disease-specific patterns of hypoperfusion and hypometabolism. It can be useful in diagnosing AD and also differentiating AD from FTD.[59] AD-specific regions which show hypoperfusion and hypometabolism in SPECT and FDG-PET, respectively, are the hippocampus, precuneus (mesial parietal lobes), and lateral parietal and posterior temporal cortices.

Amyloid and Tau Imaging

As the core pathologies of AD are extracellular aggregates of Aβ plaques and intracellular neurofibrillary tangles, demonstration of these two with appropriate PET tracers will be useful in diagnosing as well as differentiating AD from other non-AD dementias. Amyloid tracers such as Pittsburgh compound B (PiB-PET) and several F18 analog tracers such as florbetapir, flutemetamol, and florbetaben help detect amyloid burden in patients with AD. Imaging is considered negative if the tracers are confined to white matter and positive if there is extension into cortical gray matter. Similar to the amyloid tracer, tau tracer PET can be helpful in the evaluation of patients with AD. Recently

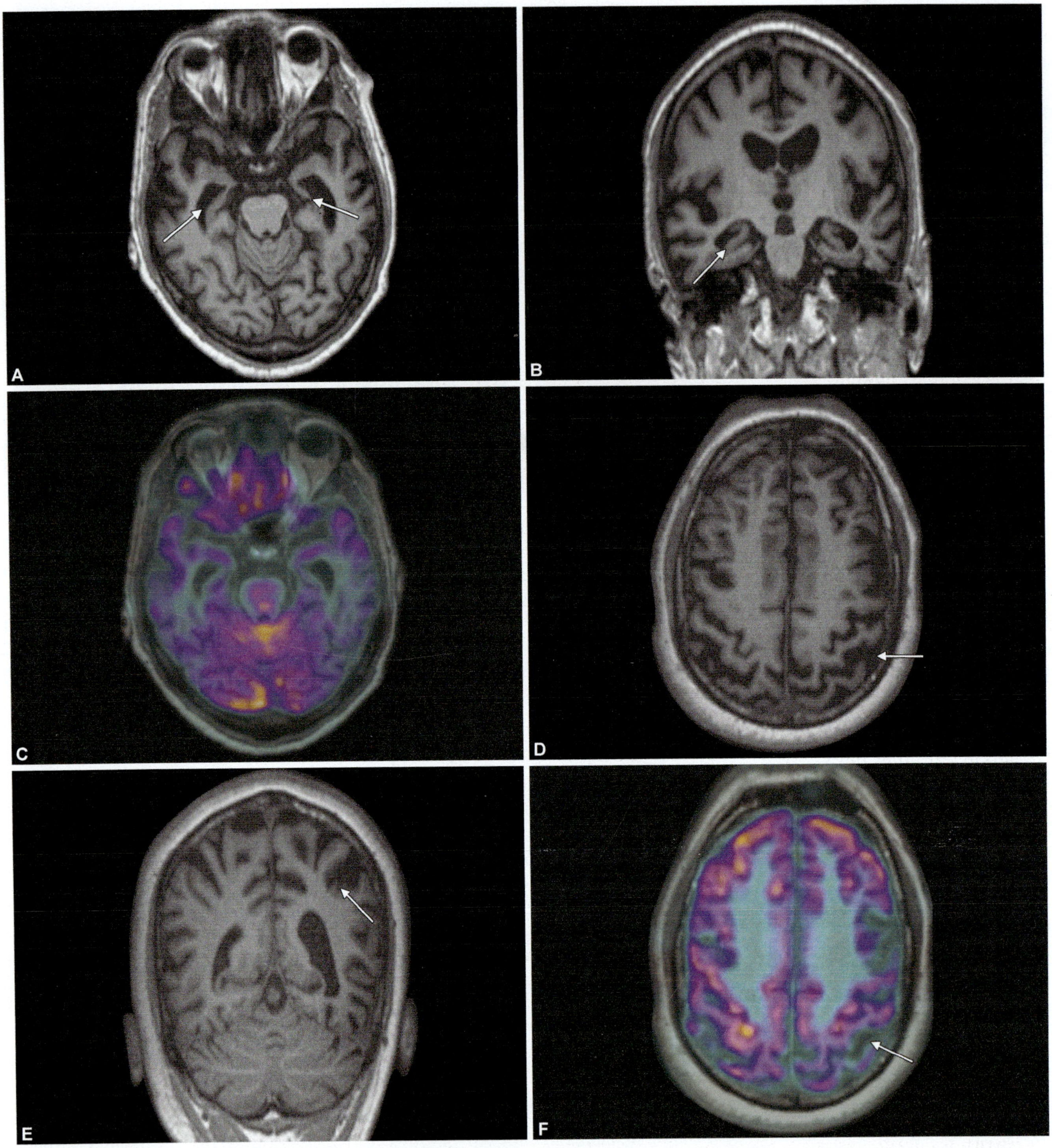

FIGS. 1A TO F: (A) T1-weighted axial image showing medial temporal lobe atrophy in a patient with AD; (B) T1-weighted coronal image showing hippocampal atrophy in the same patient; (C) FDG-PET axial image of the same patient showing medial temporal lobe hypometabolism; (D) T1-weighted axial image showing parieto-occipital lobe atrophy in patients with posterior cortical atrophy variant of AD; (E) T1-weighted coronal image showing parieto-occipital lobe atrophy; (F) FDG-PET axial image of same patient's showing parieto-occipital hypometabolism.

(AD: Alzheimer's disease; FDG-PET: F18-fluorodeoxyglucose positron emission tomography) flortaucipir has been approved by the Food and Drug Administration (FDA) for determining neurofibrillary tangle burden in patients evaluated for AD.[60]

Task-free Functional Magnetic Resonance Imaging

Neuronal activation in a region of the brain is associated with an increase in blood flow in that region and this is the basis of functional MRI (fMRI), which measures the blood oxygen level-dependent (BOLD) signal. Disruption of specific large-scale networks in the brain caused by neurodegeneration is responsible for dementia. fMRI is helpful to study these networks. The default mode network which is active when an individual is at rest or not focused on the external environment is targeted in AD.[61] The default mode network consists of medial prefrontal cortex, inferior parietal lobule, posterior cingulate gyrus, hippocampal formation, and lateral temporal cortex. These changes are detected in fMRI early in the disease process, even earlier than amyloid deposition in the brain as detected by PET scan and CSF Aβ42 level. Hence, it could be a very early marker of the pathophysiology of AD.

Fluid Biomarkers

Cerebrospinal Fluid Biomarkers

The most established fluid-based biomarker for detection of core AD neuropathology is a combination of reduction of Aβ 42 levels and elevation of phosphorylated and total tau (t-tau) in CSF. They have a sensitivity of 85% and specificity of 86% for the diagnosis of AD.[62] Aβ42 and p-tau correspond to amyloid plaques and neurofibrillary tangles deposition in the brain, whereas t-tau is indicative of neurodegeneration and can be seen in other conditions associated with rapid neuronal loss such as Creutzfeldt–Jakob disease (CJD), acute ischemia, and traumatic brain injury.

Blood-based Biomarkers

Although serum biomarkers are more feasible and minimally invasive than CSF biomarkers, the role of blood-based biomarkers including serum Aβ, t-tau, and phosphorylated tau (p-tau) in the diagnosis of AD, and differentiating AD from other non-AD dementias is still evolving but promising.[63,64] Plasma levels of p-tau, especially that of p-tau181, p-tau217, and p-tau231, are increased in patients with AD compared to healthy controls and patients with non-AD dementia.[65] Plasma neurofilament (NfL) level is a marker for neurodegeneration and neuroaxonal injury. Increased levels of plasma NfL have been suggested as a biomarker to monitor neurodegeneration in AD.[66]

Genetic Testing

Routine genetic testing is not recommended for the evaluation of individuals with AD dementia. Genetic testing should be reserved for individuals who have early onset AD and those with a family history of AD. Genetic tests for genes that are responsible for early onset AD (*APP, PSEN1, PSEN2*) are commercially available. There are two forms of genetic testing—symptomatic (person with early onset AD with a family history suggestive of autosomal dominant inheritance) and predictive (presymptomatic person with a known mutation in the family). For late-onset AD, apolipoprotein is the most important genetic determinant. Among the three variants of APOE, APOE4 is associated with maximum risk, whereas APOE2 is protective for the development of AD. Genetic testing usually has significant implication on patients as well as their family members mostly in terms of family planning, financial costs, and depression risk. There is no change in the treatment plan of the patient on the basis results of genetic testing, but it provides an opportunity to participate in future research studies.[67]

MANAGEMENT

The management of AD requires a comprehensive pharmacological and nonpharmacological approach that evolves according to disease progression and targets both cognitive and noncognitive symptoms. Any secondary causes of the symptoms such as undiagnosed infections, hyponatremia, significant change in environment, and side effects of medications should be identified and treated.

Pharmacological Therapy

Acetylcholinesterase Inhibitors

Alzheimer's disease is associated with cholinergic neuron loss in the basal forebrain, and acetylcholinesterase inhibitors (AChEIs) by inhibiting hydrolysis of acetylcholine increase neurotransmission by an increase in acetylcholine concentration in the synaptic cleft. Three AChEIs are approved by the US FDA for clinical use: donepezil, rivastigmine, and galantamine. Maximum clinical benefit is seen in mild-to-moderate stages of AD,[68] which is typically modest with a small improvement in cognition and neuropsychiatric symptoms, and activities of daily living. Common adverse effects include gastrointestinal disturbance such as diarrhea, nausea, vivid dreaming, muscle cramps, and serious side effects such as bradycardia and heart block in patients with the cardiac conductive disorder.

N-methyl-D-aspartate Receptor Antagonist

Memantine is a noncompetitive N-methyl-D-aspartate (NMDA) receptor antagonist and also a 5-hydroxytryptamine-3 receptor blocker. It has been approved for the treatment of moderate-to-severe AD but does not have any effect on mild AD or MCI. Benefits due to memantine are modest in a patient with moderate-to-severe AD. Adverse effects are rare with dizziness being the most common side effect reported along with confusion and hallucination in some cases. Memantine should be started with 5 mg/day and can be increased by 5 mg weekly to a maximum tolerated dose of 20 mg/day usually in a divided dosage.[69]

Antipsychotic Medications

Behavioral and neuropsychiatric symptoms are the most challenging manifestation of the disease, and they are also important prognostic markers associated with the rapid progression of the disease. These symptoms can be difficult to treat. Whenever possible, nonpharmacological approach should be preferred over pharmacotherapy to avoid undesirable side effects. Selective serotonin reuptake inhibitors (SSRIs) and related compounds can be considered as the next class of therapy for the treatment of behavioral symptoms, especially citalopram (up to a maximum dosage of 30 mg/day) as they have no or minimal anticholinergic properties as tricyclic antidepressants that can exacerbate the cognitive decline.[70] The last class of medication that can be used to treat behavioral symptoms includes atypical antipsychotics, and they should also be used at the lowest possible dosage as they are associated with an increased mortality rate.[71] The strongest evidence for the treatment of behavioral symptoms is for risperidone (maximum 1 mg/day) followed by aripiprazole (5–10 mg/day).[72,73] If nonpharmacological approaches are not effective, then pharmacotherapy can be considered. AChEIs and memantine have a modest effect on behavioral symptoms and can be considered as first-line therapy.

Vascular Risk Factor Management

Hypertension, hyperlipidemia, and other vascular risk factors are important and modifiable for the development and progression of AD. Hence, identification and treatment of vascular risk factors represent an important strategy to slow the progression of cognitive decline.

Nonpharmacological Approach

The aim of nonpharmacological management is maintenance and improvement of cognitive function, addressing patient behavioral and psychiatric disturbances that accompany dementia, so that patients can continue to do their activities of daily living independently and caregiver distress can be reduced. As this approach is effective, and avoids the use of medications and their side effects caused, it has attracted rising support for the management of dementia. Nonpharmacological interventions include approaches such as:

- *Reminiscence therapy*: This form of therapy includes recalling past memories of events and activities with the help of aids such as photographs, movies, and other familiar items related to the past. It can be administered in a group setting or on an individual basis. It helps in improving mood in persons with dementia.[74]
- *Validation therapy*: It is a form of therapeutic communication in persons with AD and related dementia.[75] This method includes validation of the feelings and views of the person with dementia, hence it is useful in preventing argumentative and agitated behavior, promoting contentment, and also helping to alleviate stress in the person with dementia.[76] Benefit of this therapy is limited to the person with mild-to-moderate forms of dementia.
- *Reality orientation*: Main aim of this method of therapy is to alleviate confusion and behavioral symptoms by promoting the orientation of a person with dementia to time and place. This method includes classroom-like group sessions where the facilitators present personal and current information to the participants by using games, puzzles, and calendars as aids.[77]
- *Cognitive stimulation therapy (CST)*: Like reality orientation, it is also a psychosocial individual or group intervention for a person with mild-to-moderate dementia. It helps improve confidence, cognition, social interaction, and quality of life in a person with dementia. CST offers activities that are fun, patient centric, and mentally stimulating, thereby helping persons with dementia to enhance memory, language, and reasoning.[78,79] Currently it is the only nonpharmacological intervention that is recommended by the UK government guidelines.

Other nonpharmacological interventions that are helpful in a person with dementia include:

- *Nutrition*: Decreased food intake is common in patients with advanced dementia, and inadequate nutrition is associated with an increase in morbidity and mortality. So interventions such as assisted feeding and oral nutritional supplementation may improve weight and fat-free mass.
- *Occupational therapy*: The focus of the therapy is to train persons with dementia and their caregivers in the use of aids, coping behaviors, and other strategies that could help them to compensate for the deficits that a person with dementia develops due to the disease process. It helps improve daily functioning, well-being, and social participation in people with dementia.
- *Exercise programs*: These include aerobic exercise and regular. Exercise programs not only improve physical functioning but also slow the progressive functional decline in AD patients.[80]
- *Caregiver counseling*: Counseling is required for all the caregivers on how to deal with the symptoms and overall management of the disease. In addition, a caregiver can be trained regarding avoidance and identification of possible stressors by avoiding prior triggers, limiting the change in environment, and ensuring compliance with all instructions.

Recent Advances in Management

Aducanumab, anti-Aβ immunotherapy which has shown to have a strong effect on Aβ reduction as measured by amyloid PET,[81] has been approved by the FDA in June

2021.[82] It has been approved for the treatment of MCI due to AD and mild AD dementia, and in those patients with a positive amyloid biomarker (by PET or CSF). About 40% of the patients on active treatment have shown the presence of amyloid-related imaging abnormalities (ARIA), i.e., brain edema and microhemorrhages on MRI. Major risk factors for the development of ARIA are the presence of the APOE4 allele and prior evidence of microhemorrhages. Hence, it is recommended to do MRI within 1 year of starting therapy, before starting the highest dosage (6 months after starting), and before the 12th dose (1 year after starting).[83]

Other drugs that are in the pipeline for the management of AD target various proteins, and pathological processes that are responsible for the disease pathogenesis include (1) antiamyloid agents: donanemab, lecanemab, and gantenerumab; (2) antitau agents: bepranemab, ACI-35, E2814 are in phase 2 of clinical trials, and other anti tau agents such as semorinemab, zagotenemab, gosuranemab have failed to establish drug–placebo difference in AD trails. Other targets for which monoclonal antibodies for AD are in pipeline are TREM2, CD38, semaphorin 4D, and galactin 3.[84]

SPECIAL FEATURES IN THE INDIAN CONTEXT

According to the Global Burden of Disease Study, 2.93 million people from India had dementia in 2016. However, this data was extrapolated from the sparse available data.[4] Thus, large-scale robust epidemiological studies on dementia prevalence in India are still required. With a rich sociocultural, language, and economic diversity, dementia research in India poses unique challenges such as low awareness, stigma, and inadequate healthcare systems and professionals to diagnose, treat, and manage persons living with dementia and their caregivers. To improve diagnosis, there is a need to adapt cognitive tests to its linguistically, educationally, and culturally diverse population. With this background many cognitive assessment tests have been validated in the Indian context. These include the Hindi Mental State Examination (HMSE),[85] and Addenbrookes Cognitive Examination (ACE-III) scale,[51] which is adapted in seven Indian languages to screen for dementia. A comprehensive neurocognitive battery called the Indian Council of Medical Research-Neurocognitive Tool Box (ICMR-NCTB)[50] has been developed for use among literate and illiterate patients with dementia in six languages, picture naming,[86] and semantic association task[87] for assessing executive functions, language, and visuospatial and semantic memory, respectively, in the Indian context.

Lifestyle factors are important for the prevention of dementia. The Lancet commission on dementia identified 12 modifiable risk factors, including low education, hearing impairment, physical inactivity, obesity, hypertension, diabetes, smoking, depression, low social contact, air pollution, excessive alcohol consumption, and traumatic brain injury, that may account for 40% of dementias.[88] Factors such as education, exercise, diet, occupation, good social networking, and cognitively stimulating activities have been recognized to provide resilience against brain pathology. Countries like India are characterized by a rich diversity of experiential factors, but the role of life-course experiences in such diverse contexts remains unknown. This will provide an important research avenue to facilitate understanding of the concept of cognitive reserve. Thus, the potential for the prevention of dementia is high in the Indian context.

Dementia management and care in India are influenced by the existing sociocultural and healthcare systemic context.[89] The health system support available at present is predominantly urban, clinic-based, and focuses on the diagnosis and ensuring optimal pharmacological and nonpharmacological management. Subsequent care is provided at home, and often by primary caregivers who are immediate family members. As a collectivistic society that is guided by filial obligations and social sanctions that influence the behavior of people, dementia caregiving in India continues to be home based, with limited institutional support.[90,91] Despite the social change that has resulted in dual earning families, the caregiving roles continue to be the forte of women in the family, who often report poor mental health. High gender inequality also continues to influence the access to healthcare and the type of care that women in the society receive. Families that provide care need to be supported to do so that the optimum care can be provided at lesser direct and indirect costs to the family, and to society. Long-term care support, in this context, needs to be linked with existing health programs. Advanced care for dementia requires a multidisciplinary and intersectoral approach involving the public health and nongovernmental organizations in the country.[91]

CONCLUSION

Alzheimer's disease is the most common cause of degenerative dementia globally. The prevalence of dementia is rising more in low-income countries like India than in high-income countries because of aging and the higher frequency of potentially modifiable risk factors. The etiology of dementia can be diagnosed by history, clinical, and cognitive examinations, supported by laboratory testing, brain imaging, and fluid biomarkers. While the development of disease-modifying therapies to slow or end the progression of dementia is an ongoing process, prevention intervention strategies might yield the largest dementia reductions in low-and middle-income countries (LMICs) like India. A comprehensive, multimodal approach inclusive of pharmacotherapy, cognitive rehabilitation, exercise program and occupational therapy, and proper counseling of caregivers remains the cornerstone for the management of patients with AD.

REFERENCES

1. Alzheimer's Association. (2020). 2020 Alzheimer's disease facts and figures. [online]. Available from https://alz-journals.onlinelibrary.wiley.com/doi/full/10.1002/alz.12068. [Last accessed January, 2023].
2. Olichney JM, Ellis RJ, Katzman R, Sabbagh MN, Hansen L. Types of cerebrovascular lesions associated with severe cerebral amyloid angiopathy in Alzheimer's disease. Ann N Y Acad Sci. 1997;826: 493-7.
3. Knopman DS, Parisi JE, Boeve BF, Cha RH, Apaydin H, Salviati A, et al. Vascular dementia in a population-based autopsy study. Arch Neurol. 2003;60(4):569-75.
4. GBD 2016 Dementia Collaborators. Global, regional, and national burden of Alzheimer's disease and other dementias, 1990-2016: a systematic analysis for the Global Burden of Disease Study 2016. Lancet Neurol. 2019;18(1):88-106.
5. GBD 2019 Diseases and Injuries Collaborators. Global burden of 369 diseases and injuries in 204 countries and territories, 1990-2019: a systematic analysis for the Global Burden of Disease Study 2019. Lancet. 2020;396(10258):1204-22.
6. Prince MJ, Wimo A, Guerchet MM, Ali GC, Wu YT, Prina M. (2015). World Alzheimer Report 2015—the global impact of dementia: an analysis of prevalence, incidence, cost and trends. [online] Available from https://kclpure.kcl.ac.uk/portal/en/publications/world-alzheimer-report-2015--the-global-impact-of-dementia(ae525fda-1938-4892-8daa-a2222a672254).html. [Last accessed January, 2023].
7. GBD 2019 Dementia Forecasting Collaborators. Estimation of the global prevalence of dementia in 2019 and forecasted prevalence in 2050: an analysis for the Global Burden of Disease Study 2019. Lancet Public Health. 2022;7(2):e105-25.
8. Jellinger KA, Attems J. Prevalence of dementia disorders in the oldest-old: an autopsy study. Acta Neuropathol (Berl). 2010;119(4): 421-33.
9. Chandra V, Ganguli M, Pandav R, Johnston J, Belle S, DeKosky ST. Prevalence of Alzheimer's disease and other dementias in rural India: the Indo-US study. Neurology. 1998;51(4):1000-8.
10. Rodriguez JJL, Ferri CP, Acosta D, Guerra M, Huang Y, Jacob KS, et al. Prevalence of dementia in Latin America, India, and China: a population-based cross-sectional survey. Lancet. 2008; 372(9637):464-74.
11. Rajkumar S, Kumar S. (1996). Prevalence of dementia in the community: a rural–urban comparison from Madras, India. [online]. Available from https://onlinelibrary.wiley.com/doi/abs/10.1111/j.1741-6612.1996.tb00204.x. [Last accessed January, 2023].
12. Kumar CTS, Shaji KS, Varghese M, Nair MKC. (2019). Dementia in India 2020. [online]. Available from https://dementiacarenotes.in/dcnfiles/Dementia-in-India-2020.pdf. [Last accessed January, 2023].
13. Alladi S, Mekala S, Chadalawada SK, Jala S, Mridula R, Kaul S. Subtypes of dementia: a study from a memory clinic in India. Dement Geriatr Cogn Disord. 2011;32(1):32-8.
14. Choudhary A, Ranjan JK, Asthana HS. Prevalence of dementia in India: a systematic review and meta-analysis. Indian J Public Health. 2021;65(2):152.
15. Alladi S, AADAR Dementia Science Program Research Group I. AADAR Dementia Science Program: methodology of a longitudinal multicentric and multidisciplinary commitment from India for epidemiology, clinical case registry and basic science research on dementia and related disorders. Alzheimers Dement J Alzheimers Assoc. 2019;15(7):P818-9.
16. Thal DR, Griffin WST, de Vos RAI, Ghebremedhin E. Cerebral amyloid angiopathy and its relationship to Alzheimer's disease. Acta Neuropathol (Berl). 2008;115(6):599-609.
17. Hamilton RL. Lewy bodies in Alzheimer's disease: a neuropathological review of 145 cases using α-synuclein immunohistochemistry. Brain Pathol. 2006;10(3):378-84.
18. De Strooper B, Karran E. The cellular phase of Alzheimer's disease. Cell. 2016;164(4):603-15.
19. Biron KE, Dickstein DL, Gopaul R, Jefferies WA. Amyloid triggers extensive cerebral angiogenesis causing blood brain barrier permeability and hypervascularity in Alzheimer's disease. PLoS One. 2011;6(8):e23789.
20. Dickie BR, Vandesquille M, Ulloa J, Boutin H, Parkes LM, Parker GJM. Water-exchange MRI detects subtle blood–brain barrier breakdown in Alzheimer's disease rats. Neuroimage. 2019;184:349-58.
21. Dickstein DL, Walsh J, Brautigam H, Stockton Jr SD, Gandy S, Hof PR. Role of vascular risk factors and vascular dysfunction in Alzheimer's disease. Mt Sinai J Med J Transl Pers Med. 2010;77(1):82-102.
22. Sweeney MD, Montagne A, Sagare AP, Nation DA, Schneider LS, Chui HC, et al. Vascular dysfunction: the disregarded partner of Alzheimer's disease. Alzheimers Dement J Alzheimers Assoc. 2019;15(1):158-67.
23. Kara F, van Dongen ES, Schliebs R, van Buchem MA, de Groot HJM, Alia A. Monitoring blood flow alterations in the Tg2576 mouse model of Alzheimer's disease by in vivo magnetic resonance angiography at 17.6T. Neuroimage. 2012;60(2):958-66.
24. Zlokovic BV. Neurovascular pathways to neurodegeneration in Alzheimer's disease and other disorders. Nat Rev Neurosci. 2011;12(12):723-38.
25. Ruitenberg A, den Heijer T, Bakker SL, van Swieten JC, Koudstaal PJ, Hofman A, et al. Cerebral hypoperfusion and clinical onset of dementia: the Rotterdam Study. Ann Neurol. 2005;57(6):789-94.
26. Sofroniew MV. Astrocyte barriers to neurotoxic inflammation. Nat Rev Neurosci. 2015;16(5):249-63.
27. Parpura V, Heneka MT, Montana V, Oliet SHR, Schousboe A, Haydon PG, et al. Glial cells in (patho)physiology. J Neurochem. 2012;121(1):4-27.
28. Gratuze M, Leyns CEG, Holtzman DM. New insights into the role of TREM2 in Alzheimer's disease. Mol Neurodegener. 2018;13(1):66.
29. Arshad F, Varghese F, Paplikar A, Gangadhar Y, Ramakrishnan S, Chaudhuri JR, et al. Role of autoantibodies in neurodegenerative dementia: an emerging association. Dement Geriatr Cogn Disord. 2021;50(2):153-60.
30. Abdel-Haq R, Schlachetzki JCM, Glass CK, Mazmanian SK. Microbiome-microglia connections via the gut–brain axis. J Exp Med. 2019;216(1):41-59.
31. Brodaty H, Seeher K, Gibson L. Dementia time to death: a systematic literature review on survival time and years of life lost in people with dementia. Int Psychogeriatr. 2012;24(7):1034-45.
32. Peterson R, Graff-Radford J. Alzheimer disease and other dementias. In: Bradley and Daroff's Neurology in Clinical Practice, 8th edition. Philadelphia: Elsevier; 2022.
33. Sarazin M, Stern Y, Berr C, Riba A, Albert M, Brandt J, et al. Neuropsychological predictors of dependency in patients with Alzheimer disease. Neurology. 2005;64(6):1027-31.
34. Alladi S, Xuereb J, Bak T, Nestor P, Knibb J, Patterson K, et al. Focal cortical presentations of Alzheimer's disease. Brain. 2007;130(10):2636-45.
35. Crutch SJ, Schott JM, Rabinovici GD, Murray M, Snowden JS, van der Flier WM, et al. Consensus classification of posterior cortical atrophy. Alzheimers Dement J Alzheimers Assoc. 2017;13(8):870-84.
36. Gorno-Tempini ML, Hillis AE, Weintraub S, Kertesz A, Mendez M, Cappa SF, et al. Classification of primary progressive aphasia and its variants. Neurology. 2011;76(11):1006-14.
37. Johnson JK, Head E, Kim R, Starr A, Cotman CW. Clinical and pathological evidence for a frontal variant of Alzheimer disease. Arch Neurol. 1999;56(10):1233-9.

38. Sawyer RP, Rodriguez-Porcel F, Hagen M, Shatz R, Espay AJ. Diagnosing the frontal variant of Alzheimer's disease: a clinician's yellow brick road. J Clin Mov Disord. 2017;4(1):2.
39. Lee SE, Rabinovici GD, Mayo MC, Wilson SM, Seeley WW, DeArmond SJ, et al. Clinicopathological correlations in corticobasal degeneration. Ann Neurol. 2011;70(2):327-40.
40. Scarmeas N, Brandt J, Albert M, Hadjigeorgiou G, Papadimitriou A, Dubois B, et al. Delusions and hallucinations are associated with worse outcome in Alzheimer disease. Arch Neurol. 2005;62(10):1601-8.
41. Scarmeas N, Honig LS, Choi H, Cantero J, Brandt J, Blacker D, et al. Seizures in Alzheimer disease: who, when, and how common? Arch Neurol. 2009;66(8):992-7.
42. Scarmeas N, Hadjigeorgiou GM, Papadimitriou A, Dubois B, Sarazin M, Brandt J, et al. Motor signs during the course of Alzheimer disease. Neurology. 2004;63(6):975-82.
43. McKhann G, Drachman D, Folstein M, Katzman R, Price D, Stadlan EM. Clinical diagnosis of Alzheimer's disease: report of the NINCDS-ADRDA work group under the auspices of Department of Health and Human Services Task Force on Alzheimer's disease. Neurology. 1984;34(7):939-44.
44. World Health Organization. (1992). The ICD-10 classification of mental and behavioral disorders: clinical descriptions and diagnostic guidelines. [online]. Available from https://apps.who.int/iris/handle/10665/37958. [Last accessed January, 2023].
45. Dubois B, Feldman HH, Jacova C, Cummings JL, Dekosky ST, Barberger-Gateau P, et al. Revising the definition of Alzheimer's disease: a new lexicon. Lancet Neurol. 2010;9(11):1118-27.
46. Dubois B, Feldman HH, Jacova C, Hampel H, Molinuevo JL, Blennow K, et al. Advancing research diagnostic criteria for Alzheimer's disease: the IWG-2 criteria. Lancet Neurol. 2014;13(6):614-29.
47. American Psychiatric Association, American Psychiatric Association, editors. Diagnostic and statistical manual of mental disorders: DSM-5. 5th ed. Washington, D.C: American Psychiatric Association; 2013. 947 p.
48. McKhann GM, Jack CR Jr, Albert MS, Knopman DS, Sperling RA, Carrillo MC, et al. Introduction to the recommendations from the National Institute on Aging-Alzheimer's Association workgroups on diagnostic guidelines for Alzheimer's disease. Alzheimers Dement. 2011;7:257-62.
49. Jack CR, Bennett DA, Blennow K, Carrillo MC, Dunn B, Haeberlein SB, et al. NIA-AA research framework: toward a biological definition of Alzheimer's disease. Alzheimers Dement J Alzheimers Assoc. 2018;14(4):535-62.
50. Verma M, Tripathi M, Nehra A, Paplikar A, Varghese F, Alladi S, et al. Validation of ICMR neurocognitive toolbox for dementia in the linguistically diverse context of India. Front Neurol. 2021;12:661269.
51. Mekala S, Paplikar A, Mioshi E, Kaul S, Divyaraj G, Coughlan G, et al. Dementia diagnosis in seven languages: the Addenbrooke's cognitive examination-III in India. Arch Clin Neuropsychol. 2020;35(5):528-38.
52. Arshad F, Mm S, Paplikar A, Rajendran S, Kalkonde Y, Alladi S. Vascular cognitive impairment in India: challenges and opportunities for prevention and treatment. Cereb Circ Cogn Behav. 2022;3:100034.
53. Alladi S, Arshad F, Paplikar A. Vascular dementia. In: Reference Module in Neuroscience and Biobehavioral Psychology. Philadelphia: Elsevier; 2021.
54. McKeith IG, Boeve BF, Dickson DW, Halliday G, Taylor JP, Weintraub D, et al. Diagnosis and management of dementia with Lewy bodies. Neurology. 2017;89(1):88-100.
55. Rascovsky K, Hodges JR, Knopman D, Mendez MF, Kramer JH, Neuhaus J, et al. Sensitivity of revised diagnostic criteria for the behavioral variant of frontotemporal dementia. Brain. 2011;134(9):2456-77.
56. Knopman DS, DeKosky ST, Cummings JL, Chui H, Corey–Bloom J, Relkin N, et al. Practice parameter: diagnosis of dementia (an evidence-based review): report of the Quality Standards Subcommittee of the American Academy of Neurology. Neurology. 2001;56(9):1143-53.
57. Jack CR, Dickson DW, Parisi JE, Xu YC, Cha RH, O'Brien PC, et al. Antemortem MRI findings correlate with hippocampal neuropathology in typical aging and dementia. Neurology. 2002;58(5):750-7.
58. Braak H, Braak E. Neuropathological staging of Alzheimer-related changes. Acta Neuropathol (Berl). 1991;82(4):239-59.
59. Rabinovici GD, Rosen HJ, Alkalay A, Kornak J, Furst AJ, Agarwal N, et al. Amyloid vs FDG-PET in the differential diagnosis of AD and FTLD. Neurology. 2011;77(23):2034-42.
60. Jie CVML, Treyer V, Schibli R, Mu L. TauvidTM: The First FDA-approved PET tracer for imaging tau pathology in Alzheimer's disease. Pharmaceuticals. 2021;14(2):110.
61. Raichle ME, MacLeod AM, Snyder AZ, Powers WJ, Gusnard DA, Shulman GL. (2001). A default mode of brain function. [online]. Available from https://www.pnas.org/doi/10.1073/pnas.98.2.676?url_ver=Z39.88-2003&rfr_id=ori:rid:crossref.org&rfr_dat=cr_pub%20%200pubmed. [Last accessed January 2023].
62. Hampel H, Blennow K. CSF tau and β-amyloid as biomarkers for mild cognitive impairment. Dialogues Clin Neurosci. 2004;6(4):379-90.
63. Keshavan A, Pannee J, Karikari TK, Rodriguez JL, Ashton NJ, Nicholas JM, et al. Population-based blood screening for preclinical Alzheimer's disease in a British birth cohort at age 70. Brain J Neurol. 2021;144(2):434-49.
64. Stockmann J, Verberk IMW, Timmesfeld N, Denz R, Budde B, Lange-Leifhelm J, et al. Amyloid-β misfolding as a plasma biomarker indicates risk for future clinical Alzheimer's disease in individuals with subjective cognitive decline. Alzheimers Res Ther. 2020;12(1):169.
65. Brickman AM, Manly JJ, Honig LS, Sanchez D, Reyes-Dumeyer D, Lantigua RA, et al. Plasma p-tau181, p-tau217, and other blood-based Alzheimer's disease biomarkers in a multiethnic, community study. Alzheimers Dement J Alzheimers Assoc. 2021;17(8):1353-64.
66. Mattsson N, Cullen NC, Andreasson U, Zetterberg H, Blennow K. Association between longitudinal plasma neurofilament light and neurodegeneration in patients with Alzheimer disease. JAMA Neurol. 2019;76(7):791-9.
67. Goldman JS, Hahn SE, Catania JW, LaRusse-Eckert S, Butson MB, Rumbaugh M, et al. Genetic counseling and testing for Alzheimer disease: joint practice guidelines of the American College of Medical Genetics and the National Society of Genetic Counselors. Genet Med. 2011;13(6):597-605.
68. Aisen PS, Cummings J, Schneider LS. Symptomatic and nonamyloid/tau based pharmacologic treatment for Alzheimer disease. Cold Spring Harb Perspect Med. 2012;2(3):a006395.
69. Arvanitakis Z, Shah RC, Bennett DA. Diagnosis and management of dementia: a review. JAMA. 2019;322(16):1589-99.
70. Leonpacher AK, Peters ME, Drye LT, Makino KM, Newell JA, Devanand D, et al. Effects of citalopram on neuropsychiatric symptoms in Alzheimer's dementia: evidence from the CitAD study. Am J Psychiatry. 2016;173(5):473-80.
71. American Geriatrics Society 2015 Beers Criteria Update Expert Panel. American Geriatrics Society 2015 updated Beers criteria for potentially inappropriate medication use in older adults. J Am Geriatr Soc. 2015;63(11):2227-46.
72. Mintzer JE, Tune LE, Breder CD, Swanink R, Marcus RN, McQuade RD, et al. Aripiprazole for the treatment of psychoses in institutionalized patients with Alzheimer dementia: a multicenter, randomized, double-blind, placebo-controlled assessment of three fixed doses. Am J Geriatr Psychiatry. 2007;15(11):918-31.

73. Kales HC, Lyketsos CG, Miller EM, Ballard C. Management of behavioral and psychological symptoms in people with Alzheimer's disease: an international Delphi consensus. Int Psychogeriatr. 2019;31(1):83-90.
74. Huang HC, Chen YT, Chen PY, Huey-Lan Hu S, Liu F, Kuo YL, et al. Reminiscence therapy improves cognitive functions and reduces depressive symptoms in elderly people with dementia: a meta-analysis of randomized controlled trials. J Am Med Dir Assoc. 2015;16(12):1087-94.
75. Wingbermuehle C, Bryer D, Berg-Weger M, Tumosa N, McGillick J, Rodriguez C, et al. Baseball Reminiscence League: a model for supporting persons with dementia. J Am Med Dir Assoc. 2014;15(2):85-9.
76. Hitch S. Cognitive therapy as a tool for caring for the elderly confused person. J Clin Nurs. 1994;3(1):49-55.
77. Berg-Weger M, Stewart DB. Nonpharmacologic interventions for persons with dementia. Mo Med. 2017;114(2):116-9.
78. Stewart DB, Berg-Weger M, Tebb S, Sakamoto M, Roselle K, Downing L, et al. Making a difference: a study of cognitive stimulation therapy for persons with dementia. J Gerontol Soc Work. 2017;60(4):300-12.
79. McAulay J, Streater A. Delivery of cognitive stimulation therapy for people with dementia in an inpatient setting (innovative practice). Dementia. 2020;19(7):2513-20.
80. Forbes D, Forbes SC, Blake CM, Thiessen EJ, Forbes S. Exercise programs for people with dementia. Cochrane Database Syst Rev. 2015;2015(4):CD006489.
81. Sevigny J, Chiao P, Bussière T, Weinreb PH, Williams L, Maier M, et al. The antibody aducanumab reduces Aβ plaques in Alzheimer's disease. Nature. 2016;537(7618):50-6.
82. Cavazzoni P. (2021). FDA's decision to approve new treatment for Alzheimer's disease. [online]. Available from https://www.fda.gov/drugs/news-events-human-drugs/fdas-decision-approve-new-treatment-alzheimers-disease. [Last accessed January, 2023].
83. Cummings J, Aisen P, Apostolova LG, Atri A, Salloway S, Weiner M. Aducanumab: appropriate use recommendations. J Prev Alzheimers Dis. 2021;8(4):398-410.
84. Cummings J, Lee G, Nahed P, Kambar MEZN, Zhong K, Fonseca J, et al. Alzheimer's disease drug development pipeline: 2022. Alzheimers Dement Transl Res Clin Interv. 2022;8(1):e12295.
85. Ganguli M, Ratcliff G, Chandra V, Sharma S, Gilby J, Pandav R, et al. A Hindi version of the MMSE: the development of a cognitive screening instrument for a largely illiterate rural elderly population in India. Int J Geriatr Psychiatry. 1995;10(5):367-77.
86. Paplikar A, Varghese F, Alladi S, Vandana VP, Darshini KJ, Iyer GK, et al. Picture-naming test for a linguistically diverse population with cognitive impairment and dementia. Int J Lang Commun Disord. 2022;57(4):881-94.
87. Paplikar A, Vandana VP, Mekala S, Darshini KJ, Arshad F, Iyer GK, et al. Semantic memory impairment in dementia: a cross-cultural adaptation study. Neurol Sci. 2022;43(1):265-73.
88. Mukadam N, Sommerlad A, Huntley J, Livingston G. Population attributable fractions for risk factors for dementia in low-income and middle-income countries: an analysis using cross-sectional survey data. Lancet Glob Health. 2019;7(5):e596-603.
89. Hurzuk S, Farina N, Pattabiraman M, Ramasamy N, Alladi S, Rajagopalan J, et al. Understanding, experiences, and attitudes of dementia in India: a qualitative study. Dementia (London). 2022;21(7):2288-306.
90. Kumar CS, George S, Kallivayalil RA. Towards a dementia-friendly India. Indian J Psychol Med. 2019;41(5):476-81.
91. Brinda EM, Rajkumar AP, Enemark U, Attermann J, Jacob KS. Cost and burden of informal caregiving of dependent older people in a rural Indian community. BMC Health Serv Res. 2014;14:207.

77

CHAPTER

Frontotemporal Dementia

Suman Kushwaha, Puneet Talwar

INTRODUCTION

Frontotemporal dementia (FTD) is second most common cause of degenerative dementia. It is clinically characterized by progressive changes in behavior, executive function, or language caused by an underlying neurodegenerative pathology causing degeneration of the frontotemporal network. It is defined as a genetically and pathologically heterogeneous group of neurodegenerative disorder with predominant degeneration of the frontal and/or temporal lobes, in which the main neuropathological hallmarks are characterized by tau, TAR DNA-binding protein 43 (TDP-43), or fused in sarcoma (FUS) inclusions.[1,2] The early diagnosis of FTD is important for clinical subphenotype categorization and for developing management strategies as well as interventions for these patients.

EPIDEMIOLOGY

Historically, Arnold Pick in 1892 was the first to report frontotemporal-associated clinical syndromes. The term "Picks disease" was coined by Onari and Hugo Spatz in 1926 for frontotemporal lobe atrophy with the presence of cytoplasmic inclusion bodies known as Pick bodies. The term FTD was assigned by a research group from the United Kingdom and Sweden in 1994 based on distinct clinical and histopathological criteria.[3]

Frontotemporal dementia classically affects adults in their fifth to sixth decade. Both the genders are equally affected. Prevalence of FTD is highest in the 45–64-year age group and ranges from 15 to 22 per 100,000 persons age from 45 to 64, with 10% of FTD occurring in patients <45 years of age and approximately 30% occurring in patients >65.[4] Among the clinical phenotypes, the behavior variant is the most common type of FTD reported.[5] The genetic association is seen in approximately 40% of FTD cases with an autosomal dominant pattern of inheritance.

CLINICAL EVALUATION AND DIAGNOSIS

The diagnosis of FTD is challenging. A patient with FTD should be evaluated by taking detailed and thorough clinical history with the goal of identifying the brain region where the disease begins followed by extensive cognitive and neurological examination. Detailed family history of first- and second-degree relatives for neurological and psychiatric disorders [with particular attention to dementia, amyotrophic lateral sclerosis (ALS), and Parkinsonism] is a crucial component of the evaluation. The investigations are planned accordingly involving laboratory testing, neuropsychological testing, and neuroimaging (both structural and functional are recommended).

On evaluating the clinical history if clinical suspicion for FTD is high, the bedside neurocognitive tests for frontal and temporal dysfunctions should be performed. The below-mentioned tests are validated for evaluating the frontal and temporal lobes:

- *Frontal lobe tests*: The Frontal Assessment Battery (FAB) with the following components should be applied for knowing the extent of frontal lobe involvement.
- *Go-no-go test*: The patient is asked to perform an action in response to a particular stimulus and inhibit that action in response to different stimuli.
- *Attention test*: To evaluate the attention span. It is done either by serial seven subtractions from 100 or spells the word "world" backward.
- *Letter fluency test*: In this test, the patient is asked to say as many words (except proper nouns), starting with a single letter in 1 minute.
- *Similarities and differences*: It is done to evaluate abstract thinking. The patient is instructed to compare items (table and chair, apple, and orange).

Behavioral changes can be assessed by standardized questionnaires such as the Frontal Behavioral Inventory. FTD rating scale is also used in clinical practice.[6]

Alzheimer's disease (AD) is the main differential diagnosis. The validated cerebrospinal fluid (CSF) biomarkers help to distinguish between FTD and AD; however, presently there are no validated blood biomarkers that can reliably distinguish patients with FTD from controls or other non-AD dementias. The reduced level of amyloid beta and increased tau/phosphorylated tau can distinguish AD from FTD (sensitivity of ~80%, specificity of ~80%), in which tau levels are normal or low and amyloid beta levels are higher than in AD.[7]

The phenotypes of the FTD have been defined based on clinical presentation, anatomic, genetic, and neuropathologic categorization includes:[8] (1) behavioral variant of FTD (bvFTD) with early behavior and personality changes; (2) the primary progressive aphasia (PPA) phenotype is divided into—the nonfluent or agrammatic variant of primary progressive aphasia (nfvPPA) with progressive deficits in speech, grammar, and word output and the semantic variant of PPA (svPPA), a progressive disorder of semantic knowledge and naming; (3) the overlap syndromes with extrapyramidal system are classified as progressive supranuclear palsy (PSP), corticobasal syndromes (CBS); (4) FTD associated with motor neuron disease (FTD-MND). These clinical phenotypes are described briefly.

Behavior Variant of Frontotemporal Dementia

It is defined by the gradual onset and progression of changes in behavior, including disinhibition, loss of empathy, apathy, and may include hyperorality and perseverative or compulsive behavior. Patients may exhibit psychotic features early in the disease course, including visual or auditory hallucinations and bizarre or somatic delusions and usually report to psychiatrist. Bizarre delusions and/or hallucinations are rare in bvFTD but, when it present, raise suspicion for *C9orf72*-associated bvFTD.[9] Majority of patients with bvFTD are sporadic and have no relevant family history of neurodegenerative disease and no identifiable mutation in any of the known frontotemporal lobar degeneration (FTLD)-associated genes, an apparently sporadic disorder. There is considerable overlap in the clinical and associated features of bvFTD with AD.

It is important to consider the patient's baseline personality, life events, and relationship factors that may influence behavior, and the caregiver's perspective on behaviors is necessary for accurate diagnosis of behavioral variant FTD. The patients are usually socially disinhibited and loss of social behavior such as telling off colored jokes, using abusive language, and rudeness with lack of embarrassment is common in bvFTD with main presenting complaints. Changes in food habits and craving for sweet food and carbohydrates are common and lead to weight gain. Hyperorality, overeating, and stuffing the food in mouth can also manifest in bvFTD.[10]

The challenge would be to disentangle cognitive impairment that can be explained by an acute mental illness. During acute episodes of depression, mania, psychosis, or delirium, attentional disturbances often severely interfere with cognitive performance for a temporary period.[11]

The subsets of the patients with FTD phenocopy or slowly progressive bvFTD meet the clinical criteria of possible bvFTD.[12] Recently, at the University of California, San Francisco (UCSF), a new subgroup was identified with slow progression associated with minimal cortical atrophy but with subcortical atrophy, of which 88% carry the *C9orf72* repeat.[12,13]

The diagnosis is made by using the updated International Consensus Criteria for bvFTD, which have been commonly used in clinical practice and research programs because of their relative simplicity and applicability.[5] A Diagnostic and Statistical Manual of Mental Disorders, Fifth Edition (DSM-5) diagnosis of bvFTD requires the insidious onset and gradual progression of a neurocognitive disorder combined with at least three behavioral symptoms and a prominent decline in social cognition and/or executive abilities. The presence of the one or more core clinical symptoms—behavioral disinhibition; apathy or inertia; loss of sympathy or empathy; perseverative, stereotyped, or compulsive/ritualistic behavior; or hyperorality and dietary changes—in any patient should be considered as possibly having bvFTD. The social cognition (i.e., emotion recognition, empathy, and mentalizing) is impaired or lost in bvFTD. The paralimbic regions including medial frontal, orbital frontal, anterior cingulate, and frontoinsular cortices are the neurological substrate for behavioral dysfunction.[14]

Neuropsychological assessment shows that the primary cognitive domains mainly attention, executive dysfunction, and language functioning are impaired in bvFTD. However, memory and visuospatial functions are relatively spared. This can help in differentiating it with AD where the memory and the visuospatial impairment are seen early in course.[15] There are no specific findings on laboratory testing of blood, urine, or CSF that have yet been identified as characteristic of FTLD, while the plasma and CSF biomarkers that are sensitive and specific for AD may aid in differentiating between AD and FTLD.[7] Structural imaging with CT or magnetic resonance imaging (MRI) and nuclear imaging with positron emission tomography (PET), done with coronal and sagittal images, show the hallmark atrophy or hypometabolism of the right frontal or right temporal lobe in bvFTD, respectively. The frontal or anterior temporal pattern of hypoperfusion with preserved parietal signal on single-photon emission computed tomography (SPECT) can distinguish FTD from AD with a sensitivity and specificity of approximately 80%.[16] PET tau ligands are currently under investigation in FTD but are not validated to date.

Primary Progressive Aphasia

Mesulam, in 1982, described the neurodegenerative syndrome PPA with characteristic language dysfunction. The recent clinical research criteria for PPAs include svPPA, nfvPPA, and logopenic variant of PPA.[17]

Semantic Variant of Primary Progressive Aphasia

A variant of PPA, semantic dementia, is characterized primarily by loss of word meaning. The left temporal lobe is primarily involved. Initially, the patient develops deficits in single word comprehension for low-frequency words; later, the meaning of the word is lost. Phonemic and semantic cues may improve this deficit. Neuropsychological examination on Boston naming test is diagnostic in svPPA. Repetition is spared, speech apraxia is not present, and syntax and grammar remain intact.

The diagnostic criterion given by Gorno-Tempini et al. in 2011 is extensively used in clinical practice and research.[17] The neuroimaging demonstrating the anterior temporal pole atrophy on structural imaging or hypoperfusion on functional imaging further supports a diagnosis of svPPA. Patients with svPPA tend to have slow progression and can live a decade or more after symptom onset.[18]

Nonfluent/Agrammatic Primary Progressive Aphasia

Clinically, the patients with nfvPPA present with effortful speech, which is slow, slurred, and disrupted. Word-finding difficulties are often present. Grammatical mistakes are evident in speech. Comprehension remains intact, except for longer complex sentences. Mild executive dysfunction is seen, but memory and visuospatial skills remain relatively spared early in the disease course.

The diagnostic criterion for the svPPA and classification of PPA and its variant are given by Gorno-Tempini et al.[19] Broadmann's areas 44 and 45 (Broca's area) in the left inferior frontal gyrus and the anterior insula are the neuroanatomical correlate of nfvPPA.[19] The neuroimaging shows atrophy on MRI or hypometabolism on PET or SPECT in left inferior frontal gyrus, near perisylvian area and involving Broca's area.

Frontotemporal Dementia Overlap Syndromes with Extrapyramidal System

Corticobasal Degeneration

Corticobasal degeneration (CBD) is a progressive neurodegenerative disorder affecting the frontal and parietal cortices and basal ganglia associated with abnormal 4-repeat tau isoform. In the current literature, the term CBS is used to describe the "canonical" clinical entity associated with CBD, understanding that many cases of CBS are not associated with CBD neuropathology and vice versa. CBS presentations may be associated with a variety of underlying neuropathologies including AD, FTD, and CBD.

The classic clinical features of CBS include apraxia and alien limb phenomenon, frontal deficits, and extrapyramidal motor symptoms as dystonia and limb rigidity and myoclonus. These symptoms are usually asymmetrical. Approximately, 25% of the patients show cortical sensory deficits and 30% of the patients will develop alien limb syndrome. The diagnostic criterion given by Armstrong et al. is used widely for diagnosis of the CBS.[20]

No specific biomarkers for the prediction of CBD pathology exist. Neuroimaging in patients with CBS may show asymmetric frontal and parietal lobe atrophy.

Progressive Supranuclear Palsy

Progressive supranuclear palsy, a Parkinson's plus syndrome, is also included as an FTD-related disorder based on the presence of frontal lobe involvement and tau pathology. Executive dysfunction, personality changes, reduced mental speed, and attention deficits causing frontal behavior syndrome are the main presenting complaints of PSP patients. Apathy is the most common behavioral problem. PSP patients presenting with apraxia of speech show atrophy or hypometabolism in the superior premotor cortex and supplementary motor area.[21]

The subtype of clinical presentation of PSP includes:

- Richardson syndrome with early falls, cognitive dysfunction, vertical gaze abnormalities, axial rigidity, postural instability, symmetric bradykinesia, and little or no response to levodopa
- Progressive supranuclear palsy Parkinsonism (early asymmetric bradykinesia and some response to levodopa)
- Corticobasal syndrome
- Pure akinesia with freezing of gait
- Primary progressive apraxia of speech
- Progressive nonfluent aphasia
- Behavioral variant of FTD
- Cerebellar ataxia

The structural neuroimaging in PSP may reveal midbrain atrophy called as the hummingbird sign on sagittal images while FDG-PET shows hypometabolism in frontal, caudate, midbrain, and thalamic regions.[22,23]

Neuroimaging in Frontotemporal Dementia

The structural neuroimaging plays an important role in subtyping of FTD. It quantifies the atrophy from volumetric MRI. The pattern of the volume loss in different subtypes has been summarized in **Figure 1**. Neuroimaging in FTD has made significant advances in last decade. The advances in novel imaging modalities including diffusion tensor imaging, resting-state functional MRI, and molecular PET imaging allow the possibility of understanding the alterations in structural and functional connectivity.

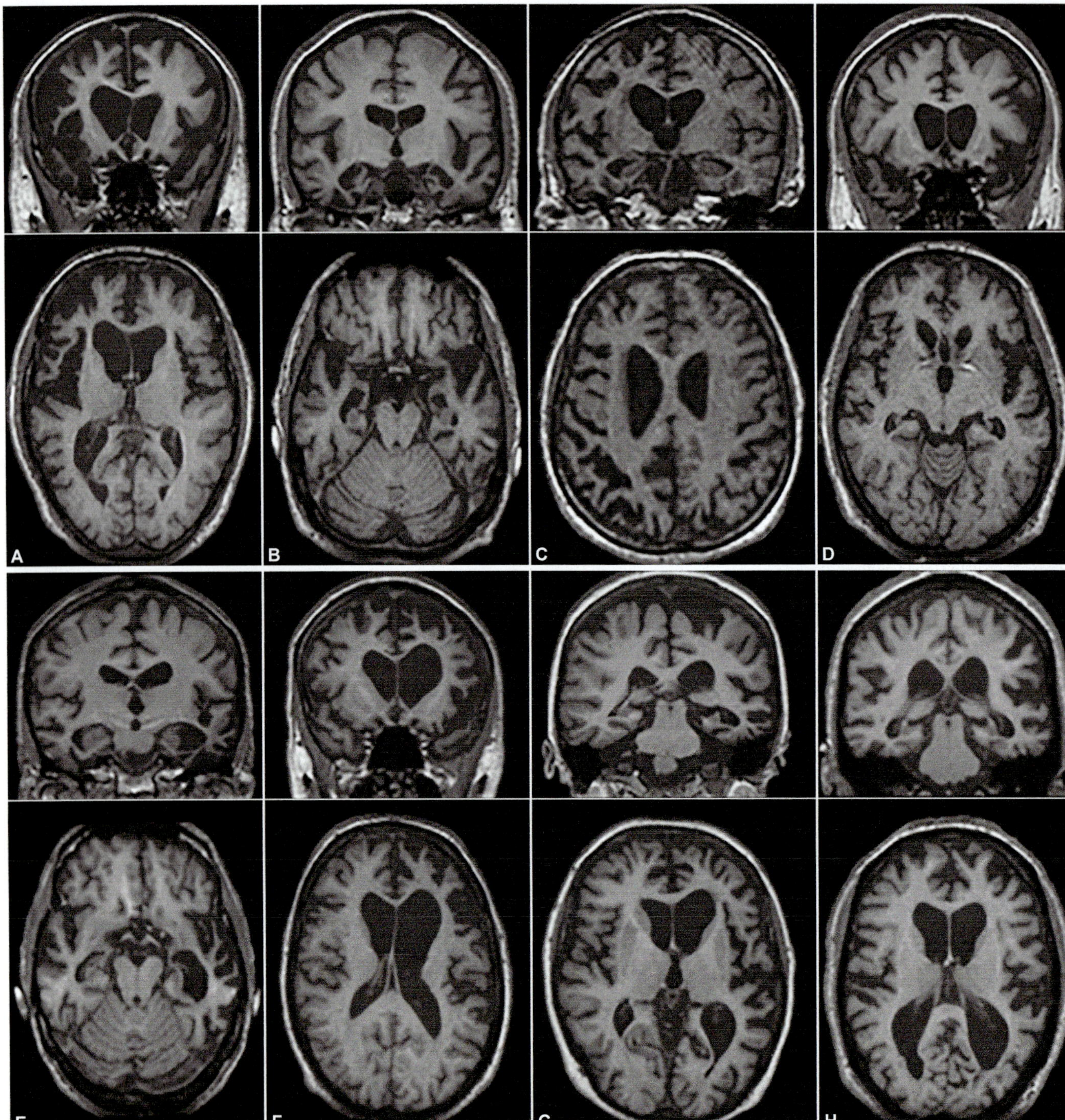

FIGS. 1A TO H: MRI images—each show coronal (top) and axial (bottom) sections for bvFTD: (A) FTLD-tau Pick's disease; (B) FTLD-tau MAPT mutation; (C) FTLD-TDP type A with GRN mutation; (D) FTLD-FUS (aFTLD-U), SD; (E) FTLD-TDP type C, PNFA; (F) FTLD-tau Pick's disease; (G) GRN mutation and LPA; (H) Alzheimer's disease.

(FTLD: frontotemporal lobar degeneration; FUS: fused in sarcoma; GRN: granulin; LPA: logopenic progressive aphasia; MAPT: microtubule-associated protein tau gene; TDP: TAR DNA-binding protein 43)

Frontotemporal Dementia with Motor Neuron Disease

This is an overlap syndrome where up to 15% of FTD patients and up to 30% of patients with MND experience overlap between the two syndromes. FTD–MND genetic linkage was discovered in 2000 and found on chromosome 9q21-q22.[24]

Fasciculation, hyperreflexia, and emotional incontinence are observed in patients of FTD. Electrophysiological

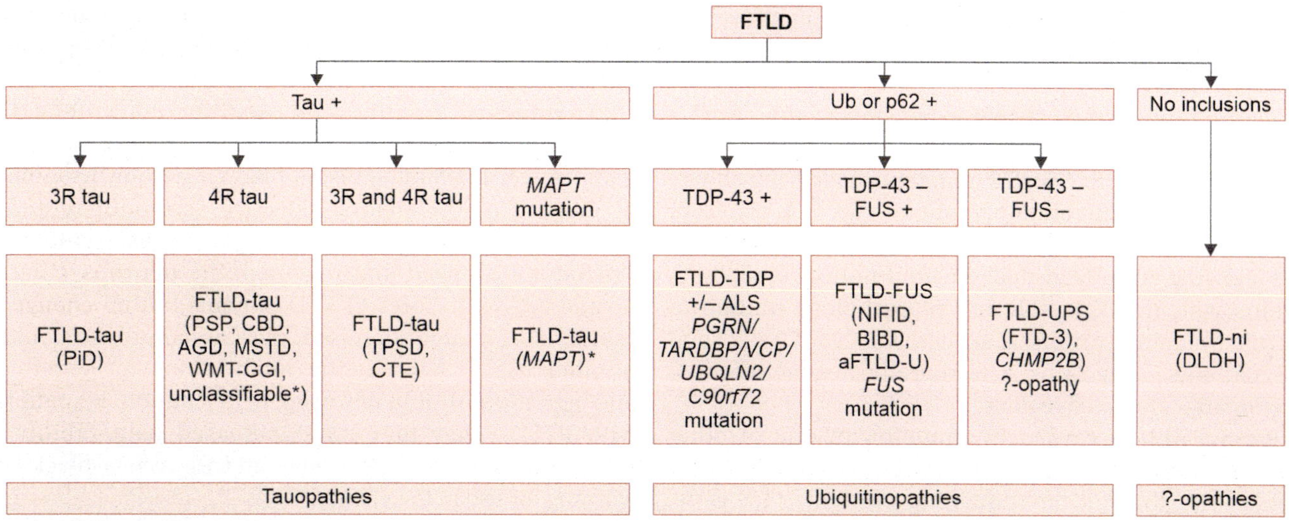

*Unclassifiable and MAPT related 3R, 4R or both.

FLOWCHART 1: Graphic representation of frontotemporal dementia (FTD) neuropathologic classification.

(aFTLD-U: atypical frontotemporal lobar degeneration with ubiquitin-positive inclusions; AGD: argyrophilic grain disease; ALS: amyotrophic lateral sclerosis; BIBD: basophilic inclusion body disease; CBD: corticobasal degeneration; CTE: chronic traumatic encephalopathy; DLDH: dementia lacking distinctive histology; FTD-3: frontotemporal dementia associated with chromosome 3; FTLD-FUS: frontotemporal lobar degeneration with fused in sarcoma proteinopathy; FTLD-ni: frontotemporal lobar degeneration with no inclusions; FTLD-tau: frontotemporal lobar degeneration with tauopathy; FTLD-TDP: frontotemporal lobar degeneration with TDP-43 proteinopathy; FTLD-UPS: frontotemporal lobar degeneration with involvement of the ubiquitin proteasome system; FUS: fused in sarcoma protein; MSTD: multiple system tauopathy with dementia; NIFID: neuronal intermediate filament inclusion dementia; PiD: Pick disease; PSP: progressive supranuclear palsy; TDP-43: transactive response deoxyribose nucleic acid binding protein of 43 kDa; TPSD: tangle predominant senile dementia; Ub: ubiquitin; WMT-GGI: white matter tauopathy with globular glial inclusions; 3R: 3 microtubule-binding repeats; 4R: 4 microtubule-binding repeats)

Source: Reprinted with permission from College of American Pathologists, Bigio EH. Making the diagnosis of frontotemporal lobar degeneration. Arch Pathol Lab Med. 2013;137(3):314-25.

evaluation to confirm MND should be done in all patients. In FTD–ALS patients with chromosome 9 open reading frame 72 (*C9orf72*) expanded repeat genetic mutations, the psychotic symptoms such as hallucinations and delusions are more often seen. The survival is shorter, average 2–3 years in patients with both FTD and MND.[25]

NEUROPATHOLOGY OF FRONTOTEMPORAL DEMENTIA

The abnormal tau and TDP-43 accumulation are seen in pathologically confirmed cases of FTD with FUS inclusions. FUS pathology is associated with an earlier age of onset of FTD, prominent neuropsychiatric features, and a more rapid course. TDP-43 pathology is characterized by four patterns that show associations with FTD clinical phenotypes.[25-27] The summary of the neuropathology of FTD is given in **Flowchart 1**.

GENETICS OF FRONTOTEMPORAL DEMENTIA

As per the current estimate, around 20–40% of all FTD cases are genetic with positive family history in a first-degree relative. The most common mode of inheritance for familial monogenic FTD is by autosomal dominant mutations mainly in three genes namely: progranulin (*GRN*), *C9orf72*, and microtubule-associated protein tau *(MAPT)*.[28] Pathogenetic variants in *MAPT* lead to abnormal tau deposition, while pathogenic variations in *GRN* or a pathogenic expansion in the *C9orf72* is associated with TDP-43 deposition. Following family members carrying any of these pathogenic mutations provides window to preclinical and prodromal stages of the disease. Carriers with loss-of-function *GRN* and *C9orf72* mutations show variable age at onset along with variability in clinical presentation in a dosage-dependent manner.[8]

The *MAPT* gene mutations have been associated with several neurodegenerative disorders such as AD, FTD, CBD, and PSP. Almost 80 diseases caused by missense mutations and intronic mutations in the tau gene have been found in familial cases of FTD.[29] Structural brain changes on MRI in preclinical FTD *MAPT* mutation carriers have found temporal lobe, cingulate cortex, and the lingual gyrus to be early predictive biomarkers for FTD.[30]

Progranulin (PGRN), a secreted glycoprotein, is encoded by the *GRN* gene in humans. It is an immune regulatory protein that plays an important role in regulating neuronal and microglial development, function, and survival in the central nervous system (CNS).[31,32] Recent systematic review encompassing neuroimaging evidence in *GRN* carriers revealed that measurable structural changes in the brain are observed in few mutation carriers 20–25 years prior to clinical disease onset but less consistently over time than metabolic changes. Further, the topographic pattern is anterior to posterior, not always asymmetric, and maps onto known functional networks.[33] Further, high levels of CSF neurofilament light chain were found in patients with *GRN*-associated FTD.[34]

The hexanucleotide repeat expansion in the *C9orf72* gene was identified as main cause of FTD and ALS in 2011. Human subjects with *C9orf72* mutations have been shown to exhibit neuroinflammatory phenotype.[35] Apart from expected atrophy in the prefrontal and temporal subregion, MRI showing atrophy in thalamus but not in cerebellum, regions with the dipeptide repeat pathology unique to *C9orf72* mutation carriers, is specific for *C9orf72* FTD and ALS patients, suggesting a retrograde degeneration of functionally connected regions.[36]

Rarely, FTD is caused by mutation in one of other genes: *TARDBP* (the TARDNA-binding protein 43 encoding gene), *VCP* (the valosin-containing protein), *FUS* gene, *CHMP2B* (the chromatin-modifying 2B), *SQSTM1* (sequestosome-1), *UBQLN1* (ubiquilin-1) or *TBK1* (the TANK-binding kinase 1), *CTSF* (cathepsin F), and *ABCA7* (ATP-binding cassette subfamily A member 7)[34,37] (*https://omim.org/entry/600274*). Further, genetic variants in other genes such as *APOE* can help with identification of misdiagnosed FTD cases as the *APOE* locus may comprise "hidden" "frontal variants" of Alzheimer's disease (fvAD) cases within an FTD sample.[38] Currently, large studies of presymptomatic genetic FTD are being carried out in Europe/Canada under the GENFI—the Genetic FTD Initiative and also in the US (ARTFL/LEFFTDS study), both collaborating together under the FTD Prevention Initiative (FPI).

MANAGEMENT OF FRONTOTEMPORAL DEMENTIA

Currently, there are no FDA-approved treatments for FTD. Only supportive and symptomatic treatment is available for the management of FTD patients. Follow-up is advised to monitor the cognitive and behavior symptoms and treat accordingly. Screening of speech difficulties and swallowing assessments should be done regularly to optimize communication strategies and maintenance of nutrition. Caregivers should be educated and counseled regarding all the legal matters to be executed timely. Occupational therapy, physiotherapy, and social support are the integral parts of neurorehabilitation and facilitate the improved quality of life.

Therapeutic options are used for controlling the symptoms of the patients. Behavioral symptoms are the main concern including disinhibition, agitation/irritability, or compulsive behaviors; selective serotonin reuptake inhibitors (SSRIs) are used to improve these symptoms. Trazodone showed improvement in neuropsychiatric inventory (NPI) scores of FTD patients but no change in MMSE in a small randomized, placebo-controlled double-blinded trial.[39] Neuroleptic medications for psychosis and agitation should be used with caution in patients with FTLD. They may have increased vulnerability to the extrapyramidal side effects and there is a black box warning for use in the elderly.[40]

The research continues for the novel compound for treatment of FTD. The current trials are targeted at tau pathology with therapeutics aimed at preventing tau aggregation, tau microtubule stabilization, and removal of tau with tau-targeted antibodies. The antisense oligonucleotide (ASO) therapy is being developed to target the toxin gain of function in the *C9orf72* gene.[41]

CONCLUSION

Frontotemporal dementia is a second most common complex progressive neurodegenerative disease. However, significant improvement has occurred in clinical understanding of its variants along with cognitive, genetic, CSF, and neuroimaging-based detection of subtle abnormalities.

Although currently no disease-modifying treatments exist, an early diagnosis and subtype classification especially bvFTD might help clinicians in better patient management as well as families to prepare for this devastating disease. Although the majority of autosomal dominant FTD has now been accounted for, radiogenomics can play a significant role in early FTD diagnosis. Further, newer developments in quantitative MRI, FDG-PET, tau-PET ligands, and CSF biomarkers will also lead to much-needed improvement in the early diagnosis and better management.

REFERENCES

1. Neumann M, Mackenzie IRA. Review: Neuropathology of non-tau frontotemporal lobar degeneration. Neuropathol Appl Neurobiol. 2019;45(1):19-40.
2. Spillantini MG, Goedert M. Tau pathology and neurodegeneration. Lancet Neurol. 2013;12(6):609-22.
3. The Lund and Manchester Groups. Clinical and neuropathological criteria for frontotemporal dementia. J Neurol Neurosurg Psychiatry. 1994;57(4):416-8.
4. Knopman DS, Roberts RO. Estimating the number of persons with frontotemporal lobar degeneration in the US population. J Mol Neurosci. 2011;45(3):330-5.
5. Rascovsky K, Hodges JR, Knopman D, Mendez MF, Kramer JH, Neuhaus J, et al. Sensitivity of revised diagnostic criteria for the behavioural variant of frontotemporal dementia. Brain. 2011; 134(Pt 9):2456-77.

6. Kertesz A, Davidson W, Fox H. Frontal behavioral inventory: diagnostic criteria for frontal lobe dementia. Can J Neurol Sci. 1997;24(1):29-36.
7. Grossman M, Farmer J, Leight S, Work M, Moore P, Van Deerlin V, et al. Cerebrospinal fluid profile in frontotemporal dementia and Alzheimer's disease. Ann Neurol. 2005;57(5):721-9.
8. Benussi A, Alberici A, Samra K, Russell LL, Greaves CV, Bocchetta M, et al. Conceptual framework for the definition of preclinical and prodromal frontotemporal dementia. Alzheimers Dementi. 2022;18(7):1408-23.
9. Snowden JS, Rollinson S, Thompson JC, Harris JM, Stopford CL, Richardson AM, et al. Distinct clinical and pathological characteristics of frontotemporal dementia associated with C9ORF72 mutations. Brain. 2012;135(Pt 3):693-708.
10. Woolley JD, Gorno-Tempini ML, Seeley WW, Rankin K, Lee SS, Matthews BR, et al. Binge eating is associated with right orbitofrontal-insular-striatal atrophy in frontotemporal dementia. Neurology. 2007;69(14):1424-33.
11. Ducharme S, Price BH, Larvie M, Dougherty DD, Dickerson BC. Clinical approach to the differential diagnosis between behavioral variant frontotemporal dementia and primary psychiatric disorders. Am J Psychiatry. 2015;172(9):827-37.
12. Hornberger M, Shelley BP, Kipps CM, Piguet O, Hodges JR. Can progressive and non-progressive behavioural variant frontotemporal dementia be distinguished at presentation? J Neurol Neurosurg Psychiatry. 2009;80(6):591-3.
13. Ranasinghe KG, Rankin KP, Lobach IV, Kramer JH, Sturm VE, Bettcher BM, et al. Cognition and neuropsychiatry in behavioral variant frontotemporal dementia by disease stage. Neurology. 2016;86(7):600-10.
14. Rosen HJ, Allison SC, Schauer GF, Gorno-Tempini ML, Weiner MW, Miller BL. Neuroanatomical correlates of behavioural disorders in dementia. Brain. 2005;128(Pt 11):2612-25.
15. Kramer JH, Jurik J, Sha SJ, Rankin KP, Rosen HJ, Johnson JK, et al. Distinctive neuropsychological patterns in frontotemporal dementia, semantic dementia, and Alzheimer disease. Cogn Behav Neurol. 2003;16(4):211-8.
16. McNeill R, Sare GM, Manoharan M, Testa HJ, Mann DM, Neary D, et al. Accuracy of single-photon emission computed tomography in differentiating frontotemporal dementia from Alzheimer's disease. J Neurol Neurosurg Psychiatry. 2007;78(4):350-5.
17. Gorno-Tempini ML, Hillis AE, Weintraub S, Kertesz A, Mendez M, Cappa SF, et al. Classification of primary progressive aphasia and its variants. Neurology. 2011;76(11):1006-14.
18. Hodges JR, Mitchell J, Dawson K, Spillantini MG, Xuereb JH, McMonagle P, et al. Semantic dementia: demography, familial factors and survival in a consecutive series of 100 cases. Brain. 2010;133(Pt 1):300-6.
19. Gorno-Tempini ML, Dronkers NF, Rankin KP, Ogar JM, Phengrasamy L, Rosen HJ, et al. Cognition and anatomy in three variants of primary progressive aphasia. Ann Neurol. 2004;55(3):335-46.
20. Armstrong MJ, Litvan I, Lang AE, Bak TH, Bhatia KP, Borroni B, et al. Criteria for the diagnosis of corticobasal degeneration. Neurology. 2013;80(5):496-503.
21. Josephs KA, Duffy JR, Strand EA, Machulda MM, Senjem ML, Master AV, et al. Characterizing a neurodegenerative syndrome: primary progressive apraxia of speech. Brain. 2012;135(Pt 5): 1522-36.
22. Boeve BF. Progressive supranuclear palsy. Parkinsonism Relat Disord. 2012;18(Suppl 1):S192-4.
23. Zalewski N, Botha H, Whitwell JL, Lowe V, Dickson DW, Josephs KA. FDG-PET in pathologically confirmed spontaneous 4R-tauopathy variants. J Neurol. 2014;261(4):710-6.
24. Hosler BA, Siddique T, Sapp PC, Sailor W, Huang MC, Hossain A, et al. Linkage of familial amyotrophic lateral sclerosis with frontotemporal dementia to chromosome 9q21-q22. JAMA. 2000; 284(13):1664-9.
25. Olney RK, Murphy J, Forshew D, Garwood E, Miller BL, Langmore S, et al. The effects of executive and behavioral dysfunction on the course of ALS. Neurology. 2005;65(11):1774-7.
26. Rademakers R, Neumann M, Mackenzie IR. Advances in understanding the molecular basis of frontotemporal dementia. Nat Rev Neurol. 2012;8(8):423-34.
27. Neumann M, Tolnay M, Mackenzie IR. The molecular basis of frontotemporal dementia. Expert Rev Mol Med. 2009;11:e23.
28. Peakman G, Russell LL, Convery RS, Nicholas JM, Van Swieten JC, Jiskoot LC, et al. Comparison of clinical rating scales in genetic frontotemporal dementia within the GENFI cohort. J Neurol Neurosurg Psychiatry. 2022;93(2):158-68.
29. Pîrşcoveanu DFV, Pirici I, Tudorică V, Bălşeanu TA, Albu VC, Bondari S, et al. Tau protein in neurodegenerative diseases - a review. Rom J Morphol Embryol. 2017;58(4):1141-50.
30. Domínguez-Vivero C, Wu L, Lee S, Manoochehri M, Cines S, Brickman AM, et al. Structural Brain Changes in Pre-Clinical FTD MAPT Mutation Carriers. J Alzheimer's Dis. 2020;75(2):595-606.
31. Rhinn H, Tatton N, McCaughey S, Kurnellas M, Rosenthal A. Progranulin as a therapeutic target in neurodegenerative diseases. Trends Pharmacol Sci. 2022;43(8):641-52.
32. Kao AW, McKay A, Singh PP, Brunet A, Huang EJ. Progranulin, lysosomal regulation and neurodegenerative disease. Nat Rev Neurosci. 2017;18(6):325-33.
33. Alexander C, Pisner D, Jacova C. Predementia brain changes in progranulin mutation: A systematic review of neuroimaging evidence. Dement Geriatr Cogn Disord. 2019;47(1-2):1-18.
34. Wagner M, Lorenz G, Volk AE, Brunet T, Edbauer D, Berutti R, et al. Clinico-genetic findings in 509 frontotemporal dementia patients. Mol Psychiatry. 2021;26(10):5824-32.
35. Pang W, Hu F. Cellular and physiological functions of C9ORF72 and implications for ALS/FTD. J Neurochem. 2021;157(3):334-50.
36. Schönecker S, Neuhofer C, Otto M, Ludolph A, Kassubek J, Landwehrmeyer B, et al. Atrophy in the thalamus but not cerebellum is specific for C9orf72 FTD and ALS patients - An atlas-based volumetric MRI Study. Front Aging Neurosci. 2018;10:45.
37. Olszewska DA, Lonergan R, Fallon EM, Lynch T. Genetics of frontotemporal dementia. Curr Neurol Neurosci Rep. 2016;16(12): 107.
38. Hernández I, Mauleón A, Rosense-Roca M, Alegret M, Vinyes G, Espinosa A, et al. Identification of misdiagnosed fronto-temporal dementia using APOE genotype and phenotype-genotype correlation analyses. Curr Alzheimer Res. 2014;11(2):182-91.
39. Lebert F, Stekke W, Hasenbroekx C, Pasquier F. Frontotemporal dementia: a randomised, controlled trial with trazodone. Dement Geriatr Cogn Disord. 2004;17(4):355-9.
40. Pijnenburg YA, Sampson EL, Harvey RJ, Fox NC, Rossor MN. Vulnerability to neuroleptic side effects in frontotemporal lobar degeneration. Int J Geriatr Psychiatry. 2003;18(1):67-72.
41. Lagier-Tourenne C, Baughn M, Rigo F, Sun S, Liu P, Li HR, et al. Targeted degradation of sense and antisense C9orf72 RNA foci as therapy for ALS and frontotemporal degeneration. Proc Natl Acad Sci U S A. 2013;110(47):E4530-9.

78
CHAPTER

Lewy Body Disease

Sinjan Ghosh, Morris Freedman

INTRODUCTION

Dementia with Lewy bodies (DLB) is a progressive neurodegenerative disorder that has been classified as a synucleinopathy. Shared neuropathological features and phenotypic similarities with Parkinson's disease dementia (PDD) led to the broader term Lewy body dementia which encompasses DLB and PDD. In contrast to the clinical syndrome, the term Lewy body disease signifies a pathological diagnosis associated with the detection of Lewy bodies that are aggregated α-synuclein inclusions in neurons.[1] With the development of immunostains targeted to detect Lewy bodies and thus more cases being identified as having this pathology, Lewy body disease has become recognized as the second most common cause of neurodegenerative dementia after Alzheimer's disease (AD).[2]

In 1912, Fritz Jakob Heinrich Lewy described eosinophilic intraneuronal inclusion bodies while studying the neuropathology of Parkinson's disease (PD) at the Alois Alzheimer's laboratory in Munich, Germany. These inclusion bodies were later named after him by Konstantin Tretiakoff in 1919. In 1997, α-synuclein was identified as the main component of Lewy bodies and Lewy neurites.[3] It then became clear that the prevalence of Lewy bodies was not uncommon. Kenji Kosaka and colleagues from Japan reported autopsies of patients who presented with cognitive impairment, as well as neuropsychiatric and motor symptoms. In 1980, they proposed the term Lewy body disease based on autopsy findings in 20 cases.[4]

The clinical spectrum of DLB includes dementia, fluctuations in cognition, arousal and attention, parkinsonism, neuropsychiatric symptoms such as hallucinations and delusions, rapid eye movement (REM) sleep behavior disorder, and autonomic dysfunction. In this chapter, we shall review the clinical features of DLB, as well as diagnosis and management. We shall also discuss the controversy around the 1-year rule which is generally used to differentiate PDD from DLB.

EPIDEMIOLOGY

About 0.4% of those over the age of 65 years are affected by DLB. Symptoms usually appear between the ages of 50 and 80 years. There is a slight male predominance.[5] Moreover, DLB accounts for 0.3–24.4% of all cases of dementia.[6] Incidence is 1.4 per 1,000 annually.[7]

PATHOLOGY AND PATHOPHYSIOLOGY

Lewy bodies in both cortical and subcortical neurons are round intraneuronal eosinophilic cytoplasmic inclusions that contain phosphorylated α-synuclein protein. DLB may be classified into the following types, according to the Lewy pathology consensus criteria:[8]

- Olfactory bulb only
- Amygdala predominant
- Brainstem predominant
- Limbic (transitional)
- Neocortical (diffuse)

The clinical presentation may be associated with the sequential involvement of the olfactory bulb, the dorsal motor nucleus of the vagus nerve in the medulla, substantia nigra, amygdala, medial-temporal cortex, cingulate cortex, and frontal or parietal cortices. Individuals with limbic Lewy body disease have a better prognosis and survival than those with neocortical (diffuse) Lewy body disease.[1] The brains of patients with neurodegenerative dementia typically include multiple pathologies which may combine to contribute to the clinical presentation, e.g., Lewy body pathology, AD neuropathological change, transactive response DNA-binding protein-43 (TDP-43) pathology, and cerebrovascular disease.

Individuals with AD can have co-existing Lewy bodies resulting in a dual pathological diagnosis (AD + Lewy body disease) or AD with Lewy bodies insufficient to meet formal DLB pathological consensus criteria.[8] The presence of AD pathology may also potentiate the manifestation of depression and dysphoria in DLB.[9] Up to 80% of clinical cases with DLB demonstrating AD pathology have been detected at autopsy and approximately 30% of cases with PD dementia have AD co-pathology.[10] The presence of α-synuclein along with tau and β-amyloid can be additive and may result in more aggressive pathology.[11]

The neural underpinnings for the generation of complex visual images are the parahippocampus, inferior temporal lobe, and amygdala. Increased Lewy body burden in the parahippocampal and inferior temporal regions has been associated with the early onset of visual hallucinations. Reduced cerebral perfusion in areas corresponding to the primary visual cortices in the occipital lobe also contributes to hallucinations.[12] Cholinergic deficiency has been implicated as a potential mechanism for visual hallucinations in DLB.[13] There is a profound depletion of neocortical choline acetyltransferase and corresponding basal forebrain cholinergic neuronal loss in DLB compared with AD. The limited binding to the nicotinic acetylcholine receptors (nAchR), because of the predominant depletion of α7nAchR in DLB, has been associated with hallucinations and delusional misidentification.[14]

Fluctuating cognition and alertness are a key feature of DLB. Segregation and integration are two brain information-processing modes. Segregation is the degree of within-community or intranetwork functional connectivity and integration is the diversity of cross-community or internetwork functional connectivity. The balance of integration and segregation is related to the neuromodulatory roles of noradrenaline from locus coeruleus and acetylcholine from the basal forebrain, respectively. These neurotransmitters are important components of the ascending arousal system. An imbalance between these two neurotransmitter systems may result in fluctuation of attention.[15,16]

CLINICAL PRESENTATIONS

Dementia is essential for diagnosing DLB. The core clinical features within the diagnostic criteria are fluctuating cognition, alertness or attention, REM sleep behavior disorder (RBD), spontaneous parkinsonism, and recurrent visual hallucinations. The diagnostic criteria previously had a lower sensitivity which improved from 85 to 88% following the inclusion of RBD in the core clinical feature. Specificity remained unaltered at 73%.[17]

■ REM Sleep Behavior Disorder[18]

RBD is usually associated with synucleinopathies, i.e., idiopathic PD, multiple system atrophy, and DLB. RBD occurs in 76% of autopsy-confirmed cases with DLB.[17] Patients with DLB can manifest RBD decades prior to the onset of motor or cognitive features. The history can be obtained from the bed partner of the patient and can range from very mild loss of REM sleep atonia to severe dream enactment behavior and violent limb movements. The consequences of RBD can be serious and may result in self-injury or physical harm to the bed partner. Conditions masquerading as RBD include sleep apnea and non-REM parasomnias (e.g., sleep talking and sleepwalking). RBD meets one of the core clinical criteria for diagnosing DLB. If the history is unclear, a sleep study (polysomnography) may be helpful.

■ Spontaneous Parkinsonism

Psychomotor retardation such as slowed speech, thinking, body movements, and gait may occur in DLB. To qualify as a core clinical feature of DLB, Parkinsonism should be spontaneous, i.e., not due to medications or stroke. Parkinsonism in DLB usually has a poor response to levodopa. In addition, patients with DLB are susceptible to the development of significant extrapyramidal side effects following the administration of antipsychotics due to neuroleptic sensitivity.

■ Fluctuating Cognition, Attention, and Alertness

Fluctuations comprise a core clinical criterion for DLB. The descriptions of fluctuations in DLB suggest an interruption in the flow of attention or awareness. This is frequently associated with transient episodes of confusion and a reduction in the ability to engage in meaningful cognitive activity that may be followed by an almost normal level of functioning. The Clinician Assessment of Fluctuation, the One Day Fluctuation Assessment Scale,[19] and the Dementia Cognitive Fluctuations Scale[20] may be helpful for identifying clinical fluctuations.

Ferman et al.[21] studied cognitively normal elderly individuals and patients with AD and DLB.

The following four characteristics of fluctuations significantly differentiated DLB from AD:

1. Daytime drowsiness and lethargy, despite getting enough sleep the night before
2. Daytime sleep of 2 or more hours (before 7 PM)
3. Staring into space for long periods
4. Episodes of disorganized speech

The presence of three or four of these features occurred in 63% of patients with DLB compared with 12% of patients with AD patients and 0.5% of normal elderly individuals and yielded a positive predictive value of 83% for the clinical diagnosis of DLB.[21]

■ Cardiovascular Dysfunction and Dysautonomia

Cardiovascular impairment and dysautonomia are other important associations, attributable to Lewy body deposition in cardiac muscles, blood vessels, and the peripheral autonomic nervous system. Cardiovascular impairment may manifest as sinoatrial node dysfunction, baroreceptor reflex dysfunction, and impaired blood pressure regulation.[22]

Extracardiac autonomic dysfunctions include orthostatic hypotension, supine hypertension, constipation, urinary incontinence or retention, and sexual dysfunction. The significantly reduced cardiac metaiodobenzylguanidine (MIBG) uptake in DLB relative to that in PD is due to greater postganglionic cardiac sympathetic denervation and depletion of cardiac nerves caused by Lewy body deposition in the sympathetic ganglia. Carotid baroreceptor reflex dysfunction is also more predominant in DLB than in PD.

Prodromal Phenotypes[18]

Three prodromal phenotypes of DLB have been described based upon research criteria:

1. Mild cognitive impairment (MCI)
2. Delirium onset
3. Psychiatric onset

MCI with Lewy Bodies

Mild cognitive impairment may be either amnestic or nonamnestic with single or multiple domain involvement. Prodromal stages of DLB can be referred to as mild cognitive impairment with Lewy bodies (MCI-LB), a stage when there is minimal disruption in day-to-day function. Attention, processing speed, and verbal fluency are typically disproportionately affected with memory and object naming being relatively preserved **(Box 1)**. MCI-LB is usually characterized by a single or multiple domain nonamnestic or multiple domain amnestic profile. In contrast, single domain amnestic MCI is more typical of MCI due to AD.

Delirium Onset[18]

Recurrent delirium may be an early feature of DLB. However, it is unclear whether these episodes represent severe fluctuations with clouded consciousness or delirium.

BOX 1 Research criteria for the diagnosis of mild cognitive impairment with Lewy bodies.[18]

Core clinical features:

- Fluctuating cognition with variations in alertness and attention
- Recurrent visual hallucinations
- REM sleep behavior disorder
- Parkinsonism (presence of one or more of bradykinesia, rest tremor, and rigidity)

Proposed biomarkers:

- Reduced basal ganglia dopamine transporter uptake (SPECT or PET)
- Abnormal (low uptake) ^{123}iodine-MIBG on myocardial scintigraphy
- Polysomnographic confirmation of REM sleep without atonia

Probable MCI-LB:

- Required criterion: Mild cognitive impairment as defined by the presence of: (i) subjective cognitive complaint (from patient, informant, or clinician), (ii) impairment in 1 or more domains (typically attention-executive and/or visual processing), and (iii) preserved or minimally affected independence in functional abilities which do not meet the criteria for dementia.
- Presence of ≥2 core clinical features (± proposed biomarker) or 1 core clinical feature + ≥1 proposed biomarker(s)

Possible MCI-LB:

- Required criterion: Mild cognitive impairment as defined by the presence of: (i) subjective cognitive complaint (from patient, informant, or clinician), (ii) impairment in 1 or more domains (typically attention executive or visual processing), and (iii) preserved or minimally affected independence in functional abilities which do not meet the criteria for dementia.
- Presence of 1 core clinical feature (no proposed biomarker) or ≥1 proposed biomarker (no core clinical features)

Supportive clinical features:

- Severe sensitivity to antipsychotic agents; postural instability; repeated falls; syncope or other transient episodes of unresponsiveness; prolonged or recurrent delirium; autonomic dysfunction, e.g., constipation, orthostatic hypotension, and urinary incontinence; hypersomnia; hyposmia; hallucinations in other modalities including passage and sense of presence phenomena; systematized delusions; apathy; anxiety; and depression.

Potential biomarkers of MCI-LB:

- Quantitative EEG showing slowing and dominant frequency variability
- Relative preservation of medial temporal lobe structures on structural imaging
- Insular thinning and gray matter volume loss on MRI
- Low occipital uptake on perfusion/metabolism scan
- MCI plus supportive clinical features or potential biomarkers are insufficient to diagnose MCI-LB but may raise suspicion of it and prompt biomarker investigation and may add weight to an existing MCI-LB diagnosis

MCI-LB is less likely in the presence of any other physical illness or brain disease including cerebrovascular disease, sufficient to account in part or in total for the clinical picture, although these do not exclude an MCI-LB diagnosis and may serve to indicate mixed or multiple pathologies contributing to the clinical presentation

(MCI-LB: mild cognitive impairment with Lewy bodies; MIBG: metaiodobenzylguanidine; PET: positron emission tomography; REM: rapid eye movement; SPECT: single-photon emission computed tomography)

Source: With permission from McKeith IG, et al (2020).[18]

Delirium should be treated with the consideration that DLB might be a possibility. This is particularly relevant with respect to caution regarding the use of antipsychotics to treat delirium in DLB. The reason is that patients with DLB may have neuroleptic sensitivity which can lead to severe adverse effects with the use of antipsychotics.

Psychiatric Onset[18]

Patients may present with late-onset psychosis in the form of hallucinations and delusions. Hallucinations are predominantly visual. Patients usually complain of formed or unformed hallucinations. There may be illusions and misperceptions as well. Visual hallucinations are associated with greater deficits in cortical acetylcholine and may predict a good response to cholinergic therapy.[13] Auditory, tactile, and olfactory hallucinations may also be a part of the presentation. Delusions of paranoia, infidelity, abandonment, and Capgras syndrome may be seen in DLB. Late-onset anxiety and depression may also raise suspicion of DLB.

DIAGNOSIS

The most recent consensus criteria for DLB were published in 2017 **(Box 2)**.[23] Updates were based on interim research and included distinguishing between clinical features and

BOX 2 Criteria for the clinical diagnosis of DLB from the fourth consensus report of the DLB consortium.[23]

Essential for diagnosis of DLB is dementia, defined as a progressive cognitive decline of sufficient magnitude to interfere with normal social or occupational functions, or with usual daily activities. Prominent or persistent memory impairment may not necessarily occur in the early stages but is usually evident with progression. Deficits on tests of attention, executive function, and visuoperceptual ability may be especially prominent and occur early.

Core clinical features (The first 3 typically occur early and may persist throughout the course):
- Fluctuating cognition with pronounced variations in alertness and attention
- Recurrent visual hallucinations that are typically well formed and detailed
- REM sleep behavior disorder, which may precede cognitive decline
- One or more spontaneous cardinal features of parkinsonism: These are bradykinesia (defined as slowness of movement and decrement in amplitude or speed), rest tremor, or rigidity

Indicative biomarkers:
- Reduced basal ganglia dopamine transporter uptake by SPECT or PET
- Abnormal (low uptake) ^{123}iodine-MIBG myocardial scintigraphy
- Polysomnographic confirmation of REM sleep without atonia

Probable DLB:
- Presence of ≥2 core clinical features (± indicative biomarker) or 1 core clinical feature + ≥1 indicative biomarker(s)
- Probable DLB should not be diagnosed based on biomarkers alone

Possible DLB:
- Presence of 1 core clinical feature (no indicative biomarker) or ≥1 indicative biomarker(s) (no core clinical features)

The supportive features include:
- Severe sensitivity to antipsychotic agents
- Postural instability, repeated falls, syncope, or other transient episodes of unresponsiveness
- Severe autonomic dysfunction (e.g., constipation, orthostatic hypotension, and urinary incontinence)
- Excessive daytime sleepiness
- Hyposmia
- Hallucinations in nonvisual modalities
- Systematized delusions, apathy, anxiety, and depression

Supportive biomarkers:
- Relative preservation of medial temporal lobe structures on computed tomography (CT) or magnetic resonance imaging (MRI) (i.e., findings suggesting that AD is less likely)
- Generalized low uptake on single-photon emission computed tomography (SPECT) or positron emission tomography (PET) perfusion or metabolism scans with reduced occipital activity and/or the "cingulate island sign", on FDG (fluorodeoxyglucose)-PET imaging
- Prominent posterior slow-wave activity on electroencephalogram (EEG) with periodic fluctuations in the pre-alpha or theta range

DLB is less likely if:
- In the presence of any other physical illness or brain disorder including cerebrovascular disease, sufficient to account in part or in total for the clinical picture, although these do not exclude a DLB diagnosis and may serve to indicate mixed or multiple pathologies contributing to the clinical presentation
- If parkinsonian features are the only core clinical feature and appear for the first time at a stage of severe dementia.

(DLB: dementia with Lewy bodies; MIBG: metaiodobenzylguanidine; REM: rapid eye movement)

Source: With permission from McKeith IG, et al (2017).[23]

biomarkers, removing the "suggestive feature" category, changing RBD to a core clinical feature, and moving the antipsychotic (neuroleptic) hypersensitivity to a supportive feature. Clinicians make the diagnosis of possible or probable DLB based on the presence of core clinical features and indicative biomarkers **(Box 2)**. However, additional "supportive" clinical features strengthen a diagnosis of DLB.

DIFFERENTIAL DIAGNOSIS

Classically, DLB is distinguished from PDD by the temporal course of appearance of parkinsonian features and dementia. If dementia was present at symptom onset or within 1 year of onset of parkinsonism, then a diagnosis of DLB is made rather than PDD. If an individual had a diagnosis of PD for at least 1 year prior to the onset of dementia, the diagnosis is PDD. Dementia at onset was an exclusion criterion for the diagnosis of PD in most PD criteria prior to 2014.

In 2014, the International Parkinson and Movement Disorder Society (MDS) published new criteria for the diagnosis of PD (MDS-PD Criteria). The task force proposed omitting the prior exclusion criterion of dementia at onset when diagnosing PD, as well as the "one-year rule". It proposed that individuals meeting the criteria for PD but with dementia at onset and sufficient features to also meet DLB criteria be diagnosed as "PD (DLB subtype)". The rationale for this change was based on citing similarities in prodromal features, dementia presentations, neuropsychological findings, nonmotor features (anosmia, RBD, and constipation), imaging, genetics, and pathology.[24] Members of the Lewy Body Dementia Association Scientific Advisory Council objected to this change, noting that despite important overlaps between DLB, PD, and PDD, there remained key differences. They argued that some individuals with DLB never develop parkinsonism and that those with parkinsonism may not have enough features for a diagnosis of PD. The dichotomy also lies in the frequency of amyloid co-pathology, including neuroimaging. Amyloid burden imaged with PET is higher in DLB when compared with PD and PDD. Other differences in neuroimaging parameters also exist. For example, PDD has less gray matter atrophy on structural MRI as compared with DLB. The clinical course varies in DLB compared with PD/PDD as well. Some genetic differences between DLB and PDD have also been identified. PDD has been associated with single nucleotide polymorphisms in the gene encoding mitochondrial transcription factor A. This is not associated with DLB. There is an increased frequency of apolipoprotein E ε4 allele (ApoE-ε4) in pure DLB (i.e., without concomitant AD pathology) than in PDD. While acknowledging that the 1-year rule remains arbitrary, they argued that maintaining DLB and PDD as separate phenotypes has important implications for patient care in terms of prognosis and research related to genetics, pathophysiology, prodromal states, and treatment.[25]

Table 1 shows key features differentiating DLB from AD and PDD.[10]

INVESTIGATIONS

Investigations may be helpful in complementing a clinical diagnosis of DLB.

Polysomnography

A sleep study may help in confirming a diagnosis of RBD, especially in the absence of a clear history of loss of REM sleep atonia. It may also help in detecting other sleep-related disorders.

^{123}Iodine-MIBG Myocardial Scintigraphy

A lower cardiac tracer uptake of ^{123}I-labeled MIBG suggests cardiac autonomic dysfunction related to postganglionic sympathetic innervation. The result should be carefully interpreted in the setting of comorbid conditions such as diabetes mellitus and underlying cardiac diseases which can produce cardiac autonomic dysfunction irrespective of Lewy pathology. The confounding effects of drugs such as beta-blockers and tricyclic antidepressants also need to be considered. In a multicenter study from Japan, this test had a high antemortem diagnostic value in differentiating between DLB and AD, with a lower tracer uptake detected in DLB compared to AD. The test had 68.9% sensitivity and 89.1% specificity by automated system, whereas a sensitivity of 68.9% and specificity of 87% were noted using visual assessment.[26]

Genetic Testing

This is not routinely recommended because hereditary DLB is very rare. Genes reported to be associated with DLB are *SNCA, LRRK2, PSEN1, PSEN2, APP, SNCB, MAPT, SCARB2, GBA*, and *APOE*. Patients with a DLB phenotype are eight times more likely to be carriers of *GBA* mutations than controls and have a younger age of onset and more severe phenotype. The *GBA* gene encodes a lysosomal enzyme involved in the formation of glucocerebrosidase. Double mutation of the *GBA* gene results in Gaucher's disease and single mutation results in DLB.[27]

MRI Scan of the Brain

Hippocampal atrophy is less marked in DLB as compared to AD. However, the presence of medial temporal atrophy does not rule out DLB. It may signify the coexistence of AD pathology along with DLB.

SPECT/FDG-PET Scan of Brain[18]

Occipital hypoperfusion on single-photon emission computed tomography (SPECT) scan, or occipital hypometabolism on fluorodeoxyglucose-positron emission

TABLE 1: Key differentiating features between PDD, DLB, and AD.[10]

Parameters	Parkinson's disease dementia	Dementia with Lewy bodies	Alzheimer's disease dementia
Onset of dementia	Usually later, >1 year after the onset of motor features	Earlier, <1 year after motor symptoms or prior	Early
Prominent cognitive symptoms	Attention, executive function, and visuospatial function	Attention, executive function, and visuospatial function	Memory and language
Parkinsonism	Yes	Maybe, resting tremor less frequent	Rarely
Fluctuation of cognitive impairment	Possible	Common	Rarely
Visual hallucinations	Possible	Common	Rarely
REM sleep behavior disorder	Common	Common	Rarely
Structural neuroimaging (CT/MRI scan of brain)	Can be normal with relative preservation of medial temporal lobe volumes	Diffuse cortical atrophy, white matter hyperintensities in temporal lobes with preservation of medial temporal lobe volumes	Medial temporal and parietal lobar atrophy
Fluorodeoxyglucose–positron emission tomography (FDG-PET) scan	Posterior hypometabolism	• Posterior cerebral hypometabolism including occipital lobes • "Cingulate island sparing" sign present	Temporal and parietal hypometabolism
Dopamine transporter (DAT) scan	Abnormal	Abnormal	Normal
Average duration from cognitive symptom onset to death	5–7 years	5–7 years	7–10 years
Neuropathology	Lewy body/α-synuclein pathology in cortex, brainstem, and limbic region. More severe nigral cell loss with around 30% AD co-pathology	Lewy body/α-synuclein pathology in cortex and limbic region with more severe hippocampal affection. About 80% AD co-pathology with higher amyloid-β and tau load in cortex and striatum relative to PD dementia	Granulovacuolar degeneration, vascular amyloid deposition, extracellular amyloid β42 plaques, and intracellular hyperphosphorylated tau neurofibrillary tangles

(AD: Alzheimer's disease; DLB: dementia with Lewy bodies; PDD: Parkinson's disease dementia; REM: rapid eye movement)

Source: With permission from Goldman JG, et al (2022).[10]

tomography (FDG-PET) scan, is associated with DLB. In addition, preservation of posterior cingulate metabolism (the cingulate island sign) on FDG-PET scan relative to the precuneus and cuneus is an important supportive feature for the diagnosis.

Dopamine Transporter Scan

Reduced striatal dopamine transporter (DAT) uptake is suggestive of prodromal DLB in a person with MCI. However, a normal striatal DAT uptake in the early stages does not exclude it.

Fluid Biomarkers

Cerebrospinal fluid (CSF) α-synuclein RT-QuIC (real-time quaking-induced conversion) is an innovative biomarker for confirming synucleinopathies. The measurement of CSF α-synuclein aggregates using seeding aggregation assays such as protein misfolding cyclic amplification and RT-QuIC is showing positive preliminary results in diagnosing synucleinopathies and may be extended to more accessible biofluids including saliva, plasma, serum, or urine.[18,28]

Electroencephalography

Prominent posterior slow-wave activity with periodic fluctuations in pre-alpha and theta range is supportive of DLB. Quantitative electroencephalography (EEG) methods show that a dominant frequency <8 Hz and dominant frequency variability >1.5 Hz are typical of DLB. In a 3-year, follow-up study, 83.3% of participants with MCI with this pattern at presentation converted to DLB.[29]

Skin Biopsy[1]

Proximal (cervical) and distal (thigh and leg) region skin biopsy may reveal phosphorylated α-synuclein in cutaneous nerves of individuals with DLB. Immunofluorescence and RT-QuIC approaches can have comparable and similar diagnostic accuracy to CSF RT-QuIC samples.

MANAGEMENT

The challenges of managing DLB include its broad spectrum of clinical features. Treating one symptom may worsen or unmask another problem. For example, treating parkinsonism with levodopa may worsen psychosis and orthostatic hypotension while antipsychotics for hallucinations or delirium may be detrimental in terms of the motor symptoms of parkinsonism. The pharmacological and nonpharmacological approaches are aimed at alleviating cognitive dysfunction, neuropsychiatric features, motor impairments, sleep disorders, and dysautonomia. The management goal is to maximize the efficacy of treatment and limit adverse effects.

Pharmacological Management[1,23]

Cognitive Symptoms

Cholinesterase inhibitors are used for the management of cognitive dysfunction. McKeith et al.[30] showed significant improvement in objective measures of cognitive functioning with rivastigmine, especially attention and memory. There was no deterioration in the Unified Parkinson's Disease Rating Scale (UPDRS). Studies show less overall deterioration in cognitive impairment with the use of cholinesterase inhibitors. The added advantage of this class of medication is that it has an antipsychotic effect, which might be beneficial in DLB patients presenting with psychosis. There is limited evidence in favor of memantine as an option.

Neuropsychiatric Symptoms

To manage psychosis, especially hallucinations, clinicians should evaluate the patient's existing medications before adding any new drug. If a patient is on dopaminergic agents, then consideration should be given to a slow reduction in dosage. Tricyclic antidepressants, anticholinergics, benzodiazepines, and opioid drug dosages should be minimized. McKeith et al.[30] found that rivastigmine at daily doses of 6–12 mg produced statistically significant improvement in terms of behavioral effects in Lewy body dementia. Psychiatric features such as apathy, indifference, anxiety, delusions, and hallucinations improved noticeably in rivastigmine-treated patients, without any worsening of motor symptoms of parkinsonism.[30] Antipsychotics to treat hallucinations in patients with DLB may have life-threatening consequences and motor deterioration, given the commonly noted neuroleptic sensitivity. If an antipsychotic is needed, quetiapine and clozapine should be considered, since these drugs have the least extrapyramidal adverse effects compared to other antipsychotics. Regular laboratory monitoring is required for clozapine to detect agranulocytosis, which is a serious adverse effect of the drug.

Pimavanserin is currently approved by the United States Food and drug administration (US-FDA) for the indication of PD psychosis. However, it is not approved in India. It acts as an inverse agonist and antagonist at the serotonin 2A receptors (5-HT2A) and, to a lesser extent, at the 5-HT2C receptors. It does not have antidopaminergic action like other antipsychotics, which makes it a preferable agent in parkinsonism. The HARMONY trial, published in 2021, was a phase III, double-blind, randomized, placebo-controlled pimavanserin discontinuation trial. It recruited individuals with dementia-related psychosis in AD, PDD, DLB, frontotemporal dementia (FTD), and vascular dementia.[31] The study was terminated early due to a clear benefit noted during interim analysis.

Sleep Disorders

The most important sleep disorder associated with DLB is RBD. The first-line agent for the treatment of RBD is melatonin, followed by clonazepam. Melatonin is safer and the preferred agent over clonazepam, as the latter may worsen cognition, sleep apnea, and gait. It should be kept in mind that antidepressants, cholinesterase inhibitors, beta-blockers, caffeine, and tramadol may worsen symptoms of RBD.

Parkinsonism

Parkinsonism in DLB usually has a poor response to levodopa. In the early stages of DLB, there might be some positive response to dopaminergic agents, but the dose titration should be done slowly and cautiously. Levodopa responsiveness is poor, possibly because of intrinsic striatal degeneration, and a significant proportion of the parkinsonian symptoms may have a nondopaminergic origin.[32]

Dysautonomia

To address the symptoms related to orthostatic hypotension, a medication review is essential to check if there are drugs that might be partly responsible for postural changes in blood pressure. Diuretics, α-blockers, dopaminergic agents, and antipsychotic medications should be reduced or replaced if possible. Fludrocortisone and midodrine may be administered for orthostatic hypotension. An increase in dietary salt intake might be helpful; however, caution must be exercised in patients with hypertension or renal impairment. Regular blood pressure monitoring is suggested as fludrocortisone or midodrine can produce supine hypertension. Fludrocortisone can also cause electrolyte imbalance and edema.

For constipation, stool softeners and laxatives may be helpful. If a patient is on anticholinergic agent, which can cause drug-induced constipation, then it should be stopped if possible. Urinary incontinence can be managed with mirabegron, which is a β3-adrenoceptor agonist and is effective in controlling overactive bladder-related symptoms. It does not have a negative effect on cognition.

Nonpharmacological Management

A creative and individualized nonpharmacological approach should be formulated considering the patient's cognitive status, present physical capabilities, and premorbid personality. A multidisciplinary team including a psychologist, dietician, nurses, occupational therapist, recreational therapist, music therapist, speech-language pathologist, and physiotherapist is ideal for rendering an individualized management plan. Nonpharmacological approaches are complementary to pharmacological measures.

Implementing the following measures may have promising outcomes. Patients with orthostatic hypotension may benefit from increasing dietary salt and fluid intake. Postprandial hypotension may be kept under control by taking smaller portions and frequent meals. Elevating the head end of the bed is helpful in managing supine hypertension. Post-meal walks and increased consumption of dietary fibers may help to improve constipation. Sleep disorders and parasomnias including RBD can have significant consequences. Bed safety involves the use of bed rails and the removal of sharp objects around the bed to reduce the chances of major injuries. Good sleep hygiene, such as maintaining a sleep routine, avoiding caffeine within a few hours before going to bed, and darkening the room at night, may help with insomnia. Continuous positive airway pressure (CPAP) may be beneficial in patients with sleep apnea in alleviating daytime somnolence and cognitive impairment associated with sleep apnea.

Patients with DLB may develop neuropsychiatric symptoms such as agitation, physical or verbal aggression, and disinhibition. These symptoms may reflect the patient's attempt to convey unmet needs to the caregiver, such as physical discomfort and hunger. Addressing these needs may improve neuropsychiatric symptoms. Structured group or individual exercise programs or supervised walking can be helpful. Social interactions with people, visits from family and friends, or one-on-one conversations with healthcare staff may also have positive outcomes. Simulated presence therapy by pre-recorded videos made by friends or family may sometimes have a calming effect. Engaging in meaningful activities such as ball toss, cards, jigsaw puzzles, and crossword puzzles may also have a positive impact. Environmental design strategically planned to designate areas for wandering or pacing can be useful.

When patients refuse food and medications, consideration should be given to simplify the drug regimen by limiting the frequency of dosing. An alternate strategy is to mix medications with food or drink. To address hypersexuality, it may be useful to provide appropriate outlets for showing affection and facilitating privacy either alone or with the patient's spouse. For hyperoral behaviors, dangerous objects should be removed. It may also be beneficial to keep the patient away from the dining area during meals to stop them from taking food from others.[33]

SPECIAL FEATURES IN THE INDIAN CONTEXT

Dementia with Lewy bodies was reported in 1.6% in a cohort by Nair et al.,[34] whereas Alladi et al.[35] detected 8.9% cases of DLB with male predominance and older age at presentation (70.2 ± 8.0 years) compared to AD, FTD, and vascular dementia. Chandra and Mehta[36] found that 24.4% of cases in their cohort had DLB compared to 5.8% of cases with AD. Implementation of different dementia-screening tools and diagnostic methods is responsible for regional variability in dementia prevalence reported from different parts of India. However, in recent years, progress has been made toward addressing this issue. Uniformity in evaluation will be guided by the European DLB (E-DLB) protocol. The assessment includes the Indian Council of Medical Research Neurocognitive Tool Box (ICMR-NCTB), which is available in five languages. It has been standardized with a focus on a multicultural and diverse Indian population belonging to different language backgrounds.[37,38]

CONCLUSION

Dementia with Lewy bodies is now recognized as the second most common neurodegenerative cause of dementia and may co-exist with AD which is the most common cause of dementia. The growing development of global DLB consortia represents an important step toward international collaboration to create a better understanding of this disorder, as well as to develop effective treatment.[38]

ACKNOWLEDGMENTS

Morris Freedman receives support from the Saul A Silverman Family Foundation as a Canada International Scientific Exchange Program and Morris Kerzner Memorial Fund.

REFERENCES

1. Armstrong MJ. Advances in dementia with Lewy bodies. Ther Adv Neurol Disord. 2021;14:17562864211057666.
2. Barker WW, Luis CA, Kashuba A, Luis M, Harwood DG, Loewenstein D, et al. Relative frequencies of Alzheimer disease, Lewy body, vascular and frontotemporal dementia, and hippocampal sclerosis in the State of Florida Brain Bank. Alzheimer Dis Assoc Disord. 2002;16:203-12.
3. Goedert M, Spillantini MG, Del Tredici K, Braak H. 100 years of Lewy pathology. Nat Rev Neurol. 2013;9:13-24.
4. Kosaka K. Latest concept of Lewy body disease. Psychiatry Clin Neurosci. 2014;68:391-4.
5. Levin J, Kurz A, Arzberger T, Giese A, Hoglinger GU. The differential diagnosis and treatment of atypical parkinsonism. Dtsch Arztebl Int. 2016;113:61-9.
6. Hogan DB, Fiest KM, Roberts JI, Maxwell CJ, Dykeman J, Pringsheim T, et al. The prevalence and incidence of dementia with Lewy bodies: a systematic review. Can J Neurol Sci. 2016;43(Suppl 1): S83-95.
7. Mizuno Y. Parkinson symptoms in dementia with Lewy bodies. In: Kosaka K (Ed). Dementia with Lewy Bodies: Clinical and Biological Aspects, 1 edition. Japan: Springer, Japan KK; 2017. pp. 93-109.
8. Attems J, Toledo JB, Walker L, Gelpi E, Gentleman S, Halliday G, et al. Neuropathological consensus criteria for the evaluation of Lewy pathology in post-mortem brains: a multi-centre study. Acta Neuropathol. 2021;141:159-72.
9. de Oliveira FF, Miraldo MC, de Castro-Neto EF, de Almeida SS, Matas SLA, Bertolucci PHF, et al. Associations of neuropsychiatric features with cerebrospinal fluid biomarkers of amyloidogenesis and neurodegeneration in dementia with Lewy bodies compared with Alzheimer's disease and cognitively healthy people. J Alzheimer's Dis. 2021;81:1295-309.
10. Goldman JG, Holden SK. Cognitive syndromes associated with movement disorders. Continuum (Minneapolis, Minn). 2022;28:726-49.
11. Moussaud S, Jones DR, Moussaud-Lamodiere EL, Delenclos M, Ross OA, McLean PJ. Alpha-synuclein and tau: teammates in neurodegeneration? Mol Neurodegener. 2014;9:43.
12. Harding AJ, Broe GA, Halliday GM. Visual hallucinations in Lewy body disease relate to Lewy bodies in the temporal lobe. Brain. 2002;125(Pt 2):391-403.
13. McKeith IG, Wesnes KA, Perry E, Ferrara R. Hallucinations predict attentional improvements with rivastigmine in dementia with Lewy bodies. Dement Geriatr Cogn Disord 2004;18:94-100.
14. Gamage R, Wagnon I, Rossetti I, Childs R, Niedermayer G, Chesworth R, et al. Cholinergic modulation of glial function during aging and chronic neuroinflammation. Front Cell Neurosci. 2020;14:577912.
15. Zuberer A, Kucyi A, Yamashita A, Wu CM, Walter M, Valera EM, et al. Integration and segregation across large-scale intrinsic brain networks as a marker of sustained attention and task-unrelated thought. Neuroimage. 2021;229:117610.
16. Matar E, Ehgoetz Martens KA, Phillips JR, Wainstein G, Halliday GM, Lewis SJG, et al. Dynamic network impairments underlie cognitive fluctuations in Lewy body dementia. NPJ Parkinsons Dis. 2022;8:16.
17. Ferman TJ, Boeve BF, Smith GE, Lin SC, Silber MH, Pedraza O, et al. Inclusion of RBD improves the diagnostic classification of dementia with Lewy bodies. Neurology. 2011;77:875-82.
18. McKeith IG, Ferman TJ, Thomas AJ, Blanc F, Boeve BF, Fujishiro H, et al. Research criteria for the diagnosis of prodromal dementia with Lewy bodies. Neurology. 2020;94:743-55.
19. Walker MP, Ayre GA, Cummings JL, Wesnes K, McKeith IG, O'Brien JT, et al. The clinician assessment of fluctuation and the one day fluctuation assessment scale. Two methods to assess fluctuating confusion in dementia. Br J Psychiatry. 2000;177:252-6.
20. Lee DR, McKeith I, Mosimann U, Ghosh-Nodial A, Grayson L, Wilson B, et al. The dementia cognitive fluctuation scale, a new psychometric test for clinicians to identify cognitive fluctuations in people with dementia. Am J Geriatr Psychiatry. 2014;22:926-35.
21. Ferman TJ, Smith GE, Boeve BF, Ivnik RJ, Petersen RC, Knopman D, et al. DLB fluctuations: specific features that reliably differentiate DLB from AD and normal aging. Neurology. 2004;62(2):181-7.
22. Oka H, Morita M, Onouchi K, Yoshioka M, Mochio S, Inoue K. Cardiovascular autonomic dysfunction in dementia with Lewy bodies and Parkinson's disease. J Neurol Sci. 2007;254:72-7.
23. McKeith IG, Boeve BF, Dickson DW, Halliday G, Taylor JP, Weintraub D, et al. Diagnosis and management of dementia with Lewy bodies: Fourth consensus report of the DLB Consortium. Neurology. 2017;89:88-100.
24. Berg D, Postuma RB, Bloem B, Chan P, Dubois B, Gasser T, et al. Time to redefine PD? Introductory statement of the MDS Task Force on the definition of Parkinson's disease. Mov Disord. 2014;29:454-62.
25. Boeve BF, Dickson DW, Duda JE, Ferman TJ, Galasko DR, Galvin JE, et al. Arguing against the proposed definition changes of PD. Mov Disord. 2016;31:1619-22.
26. Yoshita M, Arai H, Arai H, Arai T, Asada T, Fujishiro H, et al. Diagnostic accuracy of ^{123}I-meta-iodobenzylguanidine myocardial scintigraphy in dementia with Lewy bodies: a multicenter study. PLoS One. 2015;10:e0120540.
27. Outeiro TF, Koss DJ, Erskine D, Walker L, Kurzawa-Akanbi M, Burn D, et al. Dementia with Lewy bodies: an update and outlook. Mol Neurodegener. 2019;14:5.
28. Schindler SE. Fluid biomarkers in dementia diagnosis. Continuum (Minneapolis, Minn). 2022;28:822-33.
29. Bonanni L, Perfetti B, Bifolchetti S, Taylor JP, Franciotti R, Parnetti L, et al. Quantitative electroencephalogram utility in predicting conversion of mild cognitive impairment to dementia with Lewy bodies. Neurobiol Aging. 2015;36:434-45.
30. McKeith I, Del Ser T, Spano P, Emre M, Wesnes K, Anand R, et al. Efficacy of rivastigmine in dementia with Lewy bodies: a randomised, double-blind, placebo-controlled international study. Lancet. 2000;356:2031-36.
31. Tariot PN, Cummings JL, Soto-Martin ME, Ballard C, Erten-Lyons D, Sultzer DL, et al. Trial of pimavanserin in dementia-related psychosis. N Engl J Med. 2021;385:309-19.
32. Bonnet AM. Involvement of non-dopaminergic pathways in Parkinson's disease. CNS Drugs. 2000;13:351-64.
33. Wolf MU, Goldberg Y, Freedman M. Aggression and agitation in dementia. Continuum. 2018;24:783-803.
34. Nair G, Van Dyk K, Shah U, Purohit DP, Pinto C, Shah AB, et al. Characterizing cognitive deficits and dementia in an aging urban population in India. Int J Alzheimers Dis. 2012;2012:673849.
35. Alladi S, Mekala S, Chadalawada SK, Jala S, Mridula R, Kaul S. Subtypes of dementia: a study from a memory clinic in India. Dement Geriatr Cogn Disord. 2011;32:32-8.
36. Chandra V, Mehta VS. Five hundred patients with memory loss in one clinic in India: Does the prevalence vary between communities? J Alzheimer's Dis Rep. 2019;3:313-7.
37. Iyer GK, Paplikar A, Alladi S, Dutt A, Sharma M, Mekala S, et al. Standardising dementia diagnosis across linguistic and educational diversity: Study design of the Indian Council of Medical Research-Neurocognitive Tool Box (ICMR-NCTB). J Int Neuropsychol Soc. 2020;26:172-86.
38. D'Antonio F, Kane JPM, Ibanez A, Lewis SJG, Camicioli R, Wang H, et al. Dementia with Lewy bodies research consortia: A global perspective from the ISTAART Lewy Body Dementias Professional Interest Area working group. Alzheimers Dement (Amst). 2021;13:e12235.

79

CHAPTER

Rapidly Progressive Dementia

Man Mohan Mehndiratta, Divyani Garg

INTRODUCTION

Rapidly progressive dementia (RPD) refers to the development of dementia, defined as cognitive impairment in at least two cognitive domains with functional impairment, over a short span of time, compared to that expected typically for a neurodegenerative process. The time frame used to define RPD is variable in the literature, but by convention, the term is used to denote a time period from onset to development of dementia as 1–2 years.[1] This definition emanates from the definition of dementia used in Creutzfeldt–Jakob disease (CJD), an important cause of RPD.[1] However, the usual duration is usually over a few days to weeks.[2] It is crucial to define this syndrome as the disease entities associated with RPD differ from the usual dementia syndromes, and several of them are treatable. Hence, a meticulous effort is warranted to uncover a potentially reversible etiology in all patients who present with RPD.

Various approaches may be utilized as diagnostic paradigms in RPD. One approach may be to consider reversible and nonreversible causes. The former may include entities such as autoimmune encephalitis, severe vitamin B12 deficiency, hepatic encephalopathy, and normal pressure hydrocephalus. Another approach may be to consider medical versus surgical conditions. The latter may include strategically located tumors, normal pressure hydrocephalus, subdural hematoma (SDH), etc. Another consideration may be to consider broad etiological categories, such as infective, immune-mediated, vascular, metabolic-toxic, neoplastic, degenerative, and the like.

Rapidly progressive forms of degenerative conditions have also been recognized.[3] For example, rapidly progressive Alzheimer's disease (AD) is defined in patients with probable AD as a loss of at least six points on the Mini-Mental State Examination (MMSE) score.[4] Similarly, a rapidly progressive form of dementia with Lewy bodies and frontotemporal dementia has also been reported.[5,6]

In this chapter, we will illustrate the disease conditions associated with RPD through various case vignettes and summarize an approach to the diagnosis and management of RPD.

EPIDEMIOLOGY

Of the myriad causes of RPD, the most common ones, based on published cohorts of RPD, include degenerative and immune-mediated causes.[1,7,8] These are depicted in **Figure 1** below.

ETIOLOGY

A convenient acronym to remember the causes of RPD is "VITAMINS" [V = vascular, I = infectious, T = toxic-metabolic, A = autoimmune, M = malignancy, I = iatrogenic, N = neurodegenerative, S = structural].[1] These are further expanded in **Table 1**.[9,10]

It is also important to remember the "reversible" causes of RPD **(Box 1)**.

Vascular

Vascular causes of RPD include stroke (multiple infarcts or strategic location), dural arteriovenous fistula (dAVF), cerebral amyloid angiopathy, amyloid-beta-related angiitis,[11] central nervous system (CNS) vasculitis, and intravascular lymphoma.[12] Thalamus is a strategic location, and its involvement, especially bilateral, in vascular problems can lead to dementia. Bilateral thalamic involvement may occur in artery of Percheron infarction or deep cerebral venous thrombosis. Another important consideration is dural AVF, which presents as RPD developing over days to weeks.[13] Seizures and headache may be associated. Magnetic resonance imaging (MRI) may show cerebral or cerebellar white matter involvement, and the diagnosis is made by angiography.

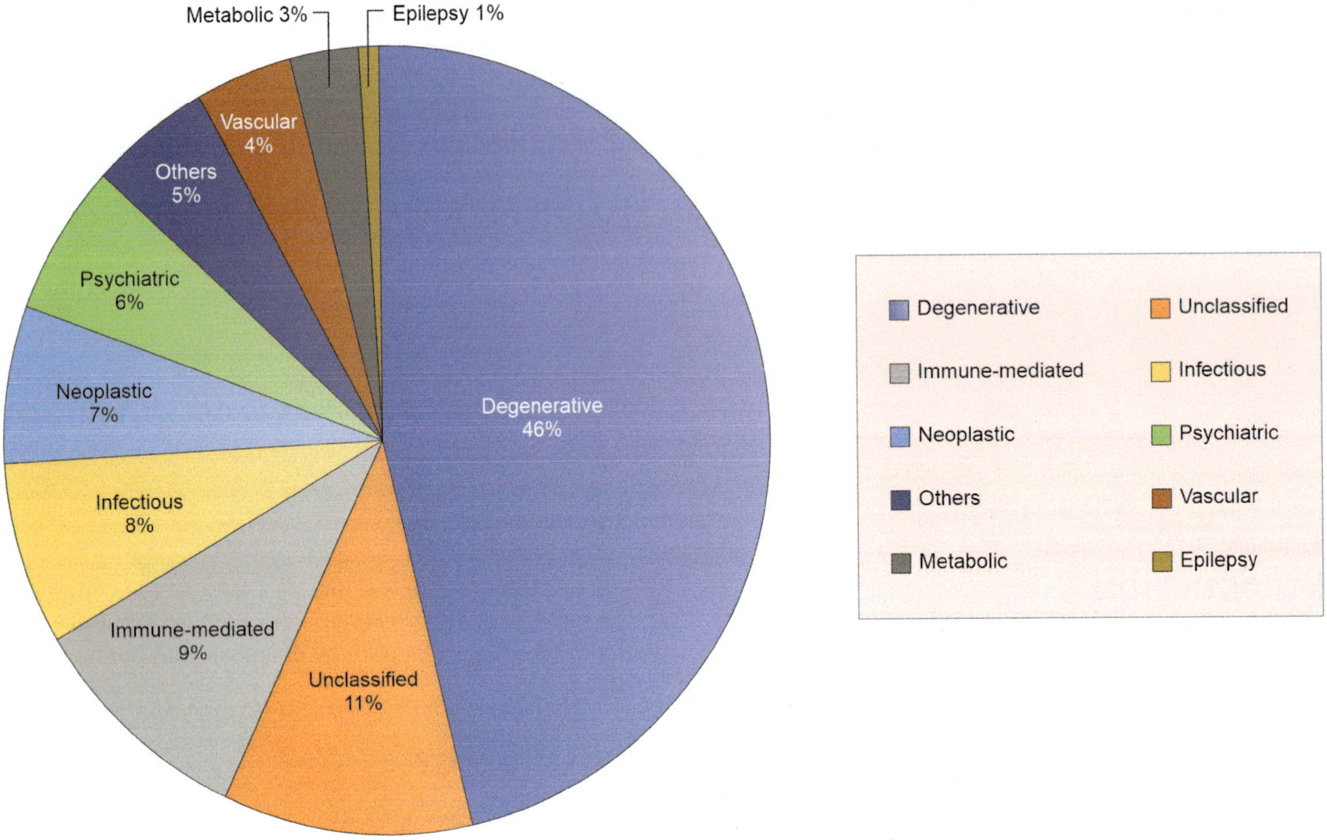

FIG. 1: Distribution of etiological categories of rapidly progressive dementia.

Infectious

Infectious agents as a cause of RPD must be considered in patients who present with associated fever (Case vignette 1). The presence of systemic or cerebrospinal fluid (CSF) pleocytosis also offers a clue toward the presence of infection. Herpes simplex encephalitis presents with seizures and headache, in association with cognitive decline. Two important considerations in our setting are chronic meningitis due to tuberculosis and multiple intraparenchymal neurocysticercosis. Fungal meningitis is an important consideration in immunocompromised individuals, including diabetics and persons with human immunodeficiency virus (HIV), but may also occur in immunocompetent persons. In persons with HIV, opportunistic infections such as cryptococcosis, toxoplasmosis, and progressive multifocal leukoencephalopathy must be considered. HIV-associated neurocognitive disorder (HAND) is a cause of RPD in advanced HIV.[14,15] Neurosyphilis and Whipple's disease have also been reported to lead to RPD.[16-18]

Case Vignette 1

A 24-year-old male presented with 3 weeks' history of fever, associated with confusion, irrelevant talk, and generalized recurrent seizures. His family reported that he had complained of a headache in the initial few days of the onset of the illness.

On examination, he was disoriented to time, place, and person. He had no focal deficits. There were no signs of meningeal irritation.

He was admitted to the hospital. MRI brain was done, which showed T2/fluid-attenuated inversion recovery (FLAIR) hyperintensities in bilateral caudate nucleus, putamen, and thalamus **(Fig. 2)**. Electroencephalography (EEG) demonstrated diffuse slowing. A diagnostic lumbar puncture was performed. This showed 10 cells (lymphocytes), protein 104 mg/dL (elevated), and sugar of 78 mg/dL (concomitant blood glucose was 112 mg/dL). CSF was evaluated for neurotropic viruses and showed elevated titers of Japanese B encephalitis. A diagnosis of viral encephalitis due to Japanese B encephalitis was made. The patient was initiated on injection acyclovir and antiseizure medications. With these measures, seizures were controlled. The patient showed gradual improvement in confusion. He continued to improve over the next 12 months but did not return to independent living.

Toxic and Metabolic

Rapidly progressive dementia may be associated with exposure to toxins such as lead and mercury. High bismuth

TABLE 1: Causes of rapidly progressive dementia.

Category	Etiological entities
Vascular	• *Stroke*: Arterial, ischemic/hemorrhagic (strategic location or multiple) • *Stroke*: Venous, cerebral venous thrombosis • Subdural hematoma • *Angiopathy*: Cerebral amyloid angiopathy (inflammatory/noninflammatory) • CNS vasculitis • CADASIL • MELAS • Intravascular lymphoma
Infectious	• Meningitis/encephalitis (bacterial/viral/ fungal/parasitic) • SSPE[9] • HAND
Toxic-metabolic	• Hepatic encephalopathy • Uremic encephalopathy • Hypo/hyperthyroidism • Hypo/hyperparathyroidism • Hypo/hypercalcemia • Hypo/hypernatremia • Hypoxia • Hypercarbia • *Vitamin deficiency*: B1, B12, B3 • *Toxins*: Lead, mercury, arsenic, etc. • Wilson's disease • *Drugs*: Lithium, anticholinergics
Immune-mediated	• Autoimmune encephalitis • Hashimoto encephalitis • *Demyelination*: MS, NMOSD, MOGAD • Vasculitis (primary/secondary) • Sarcoidosis
Malignancy/ neoplasm	• Metastases • Primary CNS tumors • Lymphomatous or carcinomatous meningitis • Paraneoplastic encephalitis
Iatrogenic	• Polypharmacy • *Drugs*: Anticholinergic agents, lithium • Extrapontine myelinolysis • Radiation induced
Neurodegenerative	• Prion disease • Alzheimer's disease • Frontotemporal lobar degeneration • Huntington disease
Structural/seizure	• Nonconvulsive status epilepticus • Hydrocephalus

(CADASIL: cerebral autosomal dominant arteriopathy with subcortical infarcts and leukoencephalopathy; CNS: central nervous system; HAND: human immunodeficiency virus-associated neurological disorder; MELAS: mitochondrial encephalomyopathy, lactic acidosis, and stroke-like episodes; MOGAD: myelin oligodendrocyte glycoprotein antibody-associated disease; MS: multiple sclerosis; NMOSD: neuromyelitis optica spectrum disorder)

Source: Adapted from Day GS (2022).[10]

BOX 1 Reversible causes of rapidly progressive dementia.

- *Immune mediated*: Autoimmune encephalitis, paraneoplastic encephalitis, Hashimoto's encephalitis
- *Toxic-metabolic*: Vitamin B12 deficiency, thiamine deficiency, pellagra, dyselectrolytemia, hypoxia/hypercarbia, hepatic encephalopathy, uremic encephalopathy
- *Infectious*: Meningitis/encephalitis, neurosyphilis, HIV
- *Neoplastic*: CNS tumor, single metastases
- *Vascular*: Subdural hematoma, vasculitis
- *Seizure*: Nonconvulsive status epilepticus
- *Drug induced*: Lithium, anticholinergics
- *Structural*: Hydrocephalus

(CNS: central nervous system; HIV: human immunodeficiency virus)

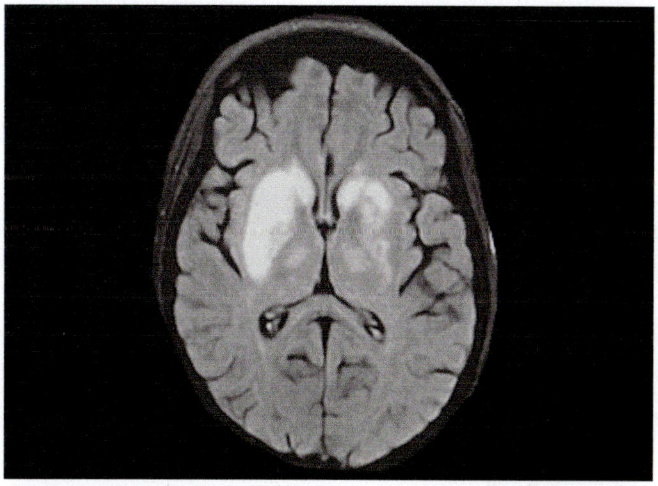

FIG. 2: T2/fluid-attenuated inversion recovery (FLAIR) axial images of the brain showing bilateral caudate, putamen, and thalamic hyperintensity, suggestive of Japanese B encephalitis.

intake is also known to mimic CJD.[19] Several vitamin-related deficiencies can cause RPD, including niacin, B12, and thiamine.[20,21] Niacin deficiency leads to pellagra, associated with the three D's: *d*iarrhea, *d*ermatitis, and *d*ementia. Thiamine deficiency leads to Wernicke's encephalopathy, characterized by cognitive impairment, ophthalmoparesis, and ataxia. Both niacin and thiamine deficiencies occur among individuals who are malnourished, alcoholics, and diabetics. Prompt administration of these vitamins will remedy the associated rapid cognitive decline.

A host of metabolic abnormalities is associated with RPD. Rapid correction of sodium abnormalities may lead to extrapontine myelinolysis, which mimics CJD. Endocrine dysfunction, including thyroid disorders, must also be assessed, as the latter are well known to cause cognitive impairment. Hepatic and uremic encephalopathies are additional causes of RPD that must be considered in the clinically relevant scenario (Case vignette 2). Portosystemic shunting is another cause of metabolic RPD.[22]

Drug-induced RPD may occur due to lithium neurotoxicity[23] or certain agents such as anticholinergics.

Case Vignette 2

A 50-year-old male presented with history of disorientation and bizarre behavior for 3 months. He had no history of fever, headache, seizures, weight loss, or other systemic features. There was no history of alcohol or any other drug use. He had developed one episode of abdominal distension 1 year back, which was managed at an outside hospital. No records of the evaluation or treatment done at that time were available. He also had history of a road traffic accident 5 years previously with significant blood loss necessitating transfusions. On examination, the patient appeared confused and inattentive. Other neurological and systemic examinations were normal. Neuroimaging was done, which was normal. EEG showed generalized slowing with the occurrence of triphasic waves, suggestive of metabolic encephalopathy **(Fig. 3)**. Further workup showed mildly deranged liver function test, low albumin, prolonged prothrombin time, and low platelet count. Ultrasound abdomen showed features of liver cirrhosis. Viral markers showed hepatitis C positivity. A diagnosis of chronic hepatic encephalopathy secondary to hepatitis C infection-related liver cirrhosis was made. The patient was managed along those lines, and he showed improvement in sensorium gradually over the next 2–3 weeks.

Immune Mediated

Rapidly progressive dementia may be a manifestation of both paraneoplastic and nonparaneoplastic encephalitis.[24] Paraneoplastic encephalitis is a paraneoplastic neurological syndrome that frequently affects the neurological axis at multiple levels, manifesting as encephalomyelitis, cerebellar ataxia, peripheral neuropathy, and opsoclonus-myoclonus, and are associated with the development of cancer within 5 years.[25] Nonparaneoplastic encephalitis, or autoimmune encephalitis, is associated with a host of antibodies that targets extracellular epitopes, and is increasingly recognized as a cause of RPD.[26] These are summarized in **Table 2**. Another important cause is Hashimoto's encephalitis, or steroid-responsive encephalopathy associated with autoimmune thyroiditis (SREAT).

Case Vignette 3

A 32-year-old female, on treatment for hypothyroidism, presented with 4 months' history of fluctuation in alertness, with periods of confusion and memory impairment. Her family reported that she had developed paranoid delusions for the past 2 months. On examination, the patient had severely impaired attention. She had no focal neurological deficits, but intermittent orofacial dyskinesias were observed. She had also experienced three-to-four episodes of seizures.

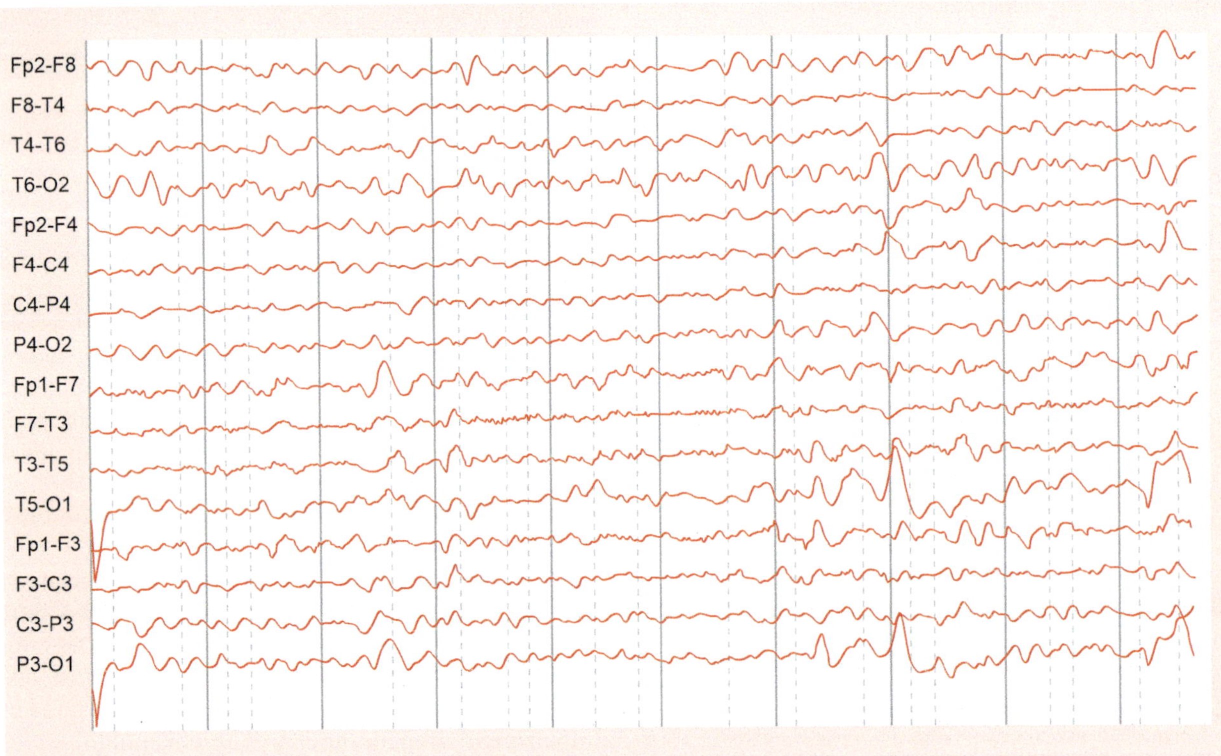

FIG. 3: Electroencephalography (EEG) showing generalized slowing and triphasic waves.

TABLE 2: Autoimmune encephalitis causing rapidly progressive dementia.

Antibody	Clinical syndrome	Associated neoplasm
Anti-NMDAR	Limbic encephalitis	Ovarian teratoma
Anti-LGI1	Limbic encephalitis	–
Anti-Caspr	Limbic encephalitis	Thymoma
Anti-GAD	Stiff person syndrome, ataxia	–
Anti-$GABA_A$ receptor	Stiff person syndrome, limbic encephalitis	Thymoma
Anti-$GABA_B$ receptor	Limbic encephalitis	Small cell lung cancer
Anti-DPPX	Limbic encephalitis	–
Anti-mGluR5	Limbic encephalitis	Hodgkin's lymphoma
Anti-Gly receptor	Limbic encephalitis, stiff person syndrome	Thymoma, lymphoma
Anti-D2 receptor	Basal ganglia encephalitis	–
Paraneoplastic antibodies		
Anti-Hu	Encephalomyelitis, sensory neuropathy	Small cell lung cancer
Anti-Yo	PCD	Breast cancer, ovarian cancer
Anti-Ri	Limbic encephalitis, PCD, opsoclonus	Breast cancer
Anti-Tr	PCD	Hodgkin's lymphoma
Anti-Ma1	Brainstem encephalitis, PCD	Small cell lung cancer
Anti-Ma2	Encephalomyelitis, PCD	Germ cell tumors
Anti-Zic4	Cerebellar ataxia	Small cell lung cancer
Anti-P/Q VGCC	LEMS, cerebellar ataxia	Small cell lung cancer
Anti-amphiphysin	Limbic encephalitis, stiff person syndrome	Small cell lung cancer, breast cancer
Anti-CRMP5	Encephalomyelitis, peripheral neuropathy, optic neuritis	Small cell lung cancer, thymoma

(CRMP5: collapsin response mediator protein 5; D2: dopamine-2; DPPX: dipeptidyl-peptidase-like protein 6; GABA: gamma aminobutyric acid; GAD: glutamic acid decarboxylase; Gly: glycine; LEMS: Lambert–Eaton myasthenic syndrome; LGI1: leucine-rich glioma-inactivated 1; mGluR5: metabotropic glutamate receptor 5; NMDAR: N-methyl-D-aspartate receptor; PCD: paraneoplastic cerebellar degeneration; VGCC: voltage-gated calcium channel)

Source: Adapted from Zerr, et al (2018).[2]

An urgent MRI was done, which showed bilateral T2/FLAIR mesial temporal lobe hyperintensities **(Fig. 4)**. EEG showed polymorphic delta slowing. Lumbar puncture showed seven cells (lymphocytes), protein 90 mg/dL, and sugar 89 mg/dL (concomitant blood sugar 118 mg/dL). Acyclovir and intravenous (IV) methylprednisolone, along with antiseizure medications, were initiated. Autoimmune panel and neurotropic virus panel in CSF were sent.

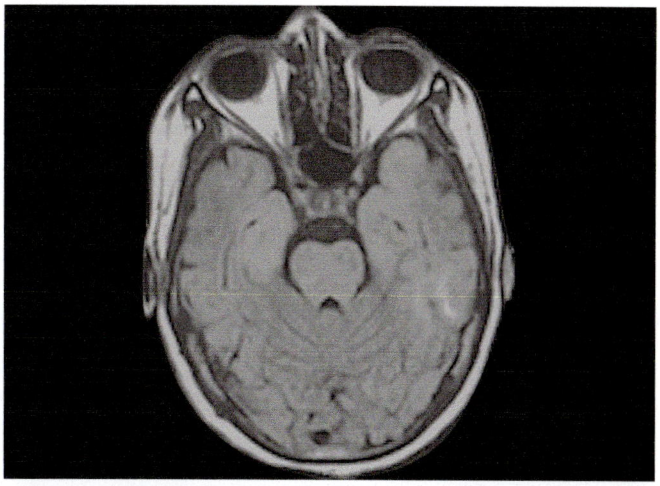

FIG. 4: T2/fluid-attenuated inversion recovery (FLAIR) axial image showing bilateral mesial temporal and left lateral temporal lobe hyperintensities.

Virus panel was negative. Autoimmune panel showed the presence of anti-N-methyl-D-aspartate (NMDA) receptor antibodies. A diagnosis of NMDA receptor encephalitis (NMDARE) was established. The patient was initiated on high dose methylprednisolone together with plasma exchange.

Mild improvement was noted in the patient's sensorium. However, she continued to have intermittent seizures and fluctuations in the sensorium. After 2 weeks, an injection rituximab was administered (1,000 mg IV) followed by a repeat dose 2 weeks later. At 3 months of follow-up, the patient had improved significantly, and seizures had not recurred.

Case Vignette 4

A 60-year-old teacher presented with 3 months' history of difficulty in driving, and language problems with paraphasias while speaking. She has also developed delusions of paranoia, and mild tremors. Occasional myoclonic jerks had been noted by her husband. She had also developed significant weight loss of around 8 kg over the past 3 months. She had also developed one episode of seizure during the course of her illness, for which antiseizure medication (carbamazepine) had been initiated.

She was evaluated for these complaints. MRI brain was unremarkable. CSF showed mildly elevated protein and normal sugar, and was acellular. Autoimmune and paraneoplastic profile was normal. Routine blood tests, including renal, hepatic, and thyroid function tests, were normal. EEG was done, which showed generalized periodic discharges **(Figs. 5A and B)**. Antithyroid peroxidase antibodies were highly elevated (1,050 IU/mL). A diagnosis of SREAT was made, and the patient was initiated on pulse methylprednisolone 1,000 mg intravenously once daily for 5 days, followed by oral prednisolone (1 mg/kg). The patient showed significant improvement.

Degenerative

An important cause of RPD is a human prion disease, of which sporadic CJD is the most common.[27] CJD is characterized by the rapid development of cognitive impairment, in association with the involvement of two other neurological systems (visual/extrapyramidal/pyramidal/myoclonus/cerebellar ataxia). MRI in sporadic CJD shows the presence of hyperintense basal ganglia and cortical ribboning, seen better on diffusion-weighted imaging compared to T2/FLAIR. CSF may show elevated

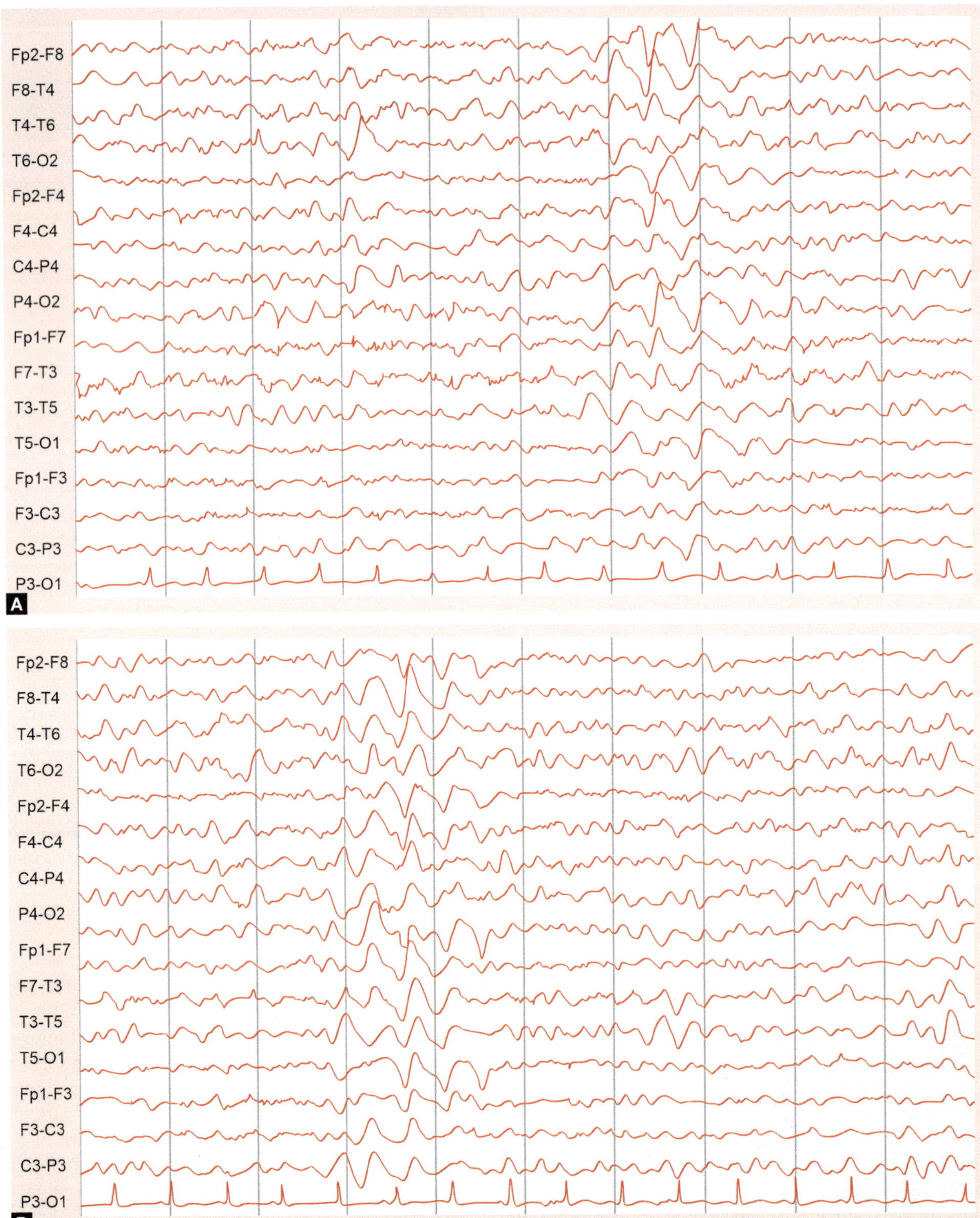

FIGS. 5A AND B: Electroencephalography (EEG) showing generalized slowing and generalized discharges.

CSF 14-3-3, which is not specific, and may also be seen in other conditions that cause neuronal injury including encephalitis, ischemia, etc. CSF real-time quaking-induced conversion (RT-QuiC) has high sensitivity and specificity. Variant CJD presents usually with psychiatric symptoms. MRI may show bilateral pulvinar hyperintensities. Familial forms include Gerstmann–Straussler–Scheinker syndrome, familial CJD, and fatal familial insomnia.[28]

Rapidly progressive forms of AD have been established as a distinct subtype. Clinical features that differentiate typical AD from rapidly progressive forms include the presence of myoclonus, rigidity, hallucinations, and aphasia.[29] Various definitions exist to delineate RPD, and include loss of six or more MMSE points per year, or three or more points over 6 months.[30] Another definition emphasizes shortened survival time, less than 4 years.[31]

Case Vignette 5

A 68-year-old female presented with a history of progressive memory impairment, apathy, and hallucinations for 2 months. These events were noted by the family after the demise of the patient's husband. The patient's family also reported sleep issues, and occasional jerks of the body. The patient had developed disinhibited behavior, and poor appetite for 1 month.

On examination, the patient was found to have severe dementia, with an MMSE score of 11/30, and a detailed cognitive assessment revealed deficits involving all lobes. There were no focal deficits. Occasional myoclonic jerks were observed during the course of the examination.

Further evaluation was done. MRI brain showed symmetrical bilateral basal ganglia hyperintensities, better seen on diffusion-weighted image than T2/FLAIR **(Figs. 6A and B)**. EEG showed short-interval periodic discharges **(Fig. 7)**. CSF analysis showed no cells, protein of 58 mg/dL, and normal sugar. Based on the above constellation of findings, the patient fulfilled the diagnostic criteria of sporadic CJD.

The patient's family was counseled about the prognosis. The patient was managed symptomatically for behavioral issues.

Structural

Certain structural causes may lead to RPD, including CNS tumors (primary/secondary). Among tumors, primary CNS lymphoma is an important consideration.[32-34] Among immunocompetent patients, CNS lymphoma presents as single or multiple contrast-enhancing lesions, whereas in immunocompromised individuals, it is usually multifocal. Large-volume CSF studies are required for the detection of atypical cells. Normal pressure hydrocephalus is another important cause in which ventriculomegaly occurs out of proportion to cerebral atrophy and presents with the triad of clinical features of urinary issues, gait abnormalities, and dementia.[35] SDH must always be considered in the setting of a geriatric or alcoholic patient, in whom even trivial trauma may precipitate SDH. The presence of focal features and raised intracranial pressure are other clues, but these may not be apparent in chronic cases (Case vignette 6).

Case Vignette 6

A 75-year-old male with known case of nonvalvular atrial fibrillation on anticoagulation (apixaban 5 mg twice daily) presented with a headache associated with giddiness, vomiting, and confusion, following a trivial fall in the washroom 2 weeks back. On examination, he appeared irritable and confused. There were no focal neurological deficits.

Magnetic resonance imaging of the brain showed a left SDH with a midline shift **(Fig. 8)**. He underwent burr hole

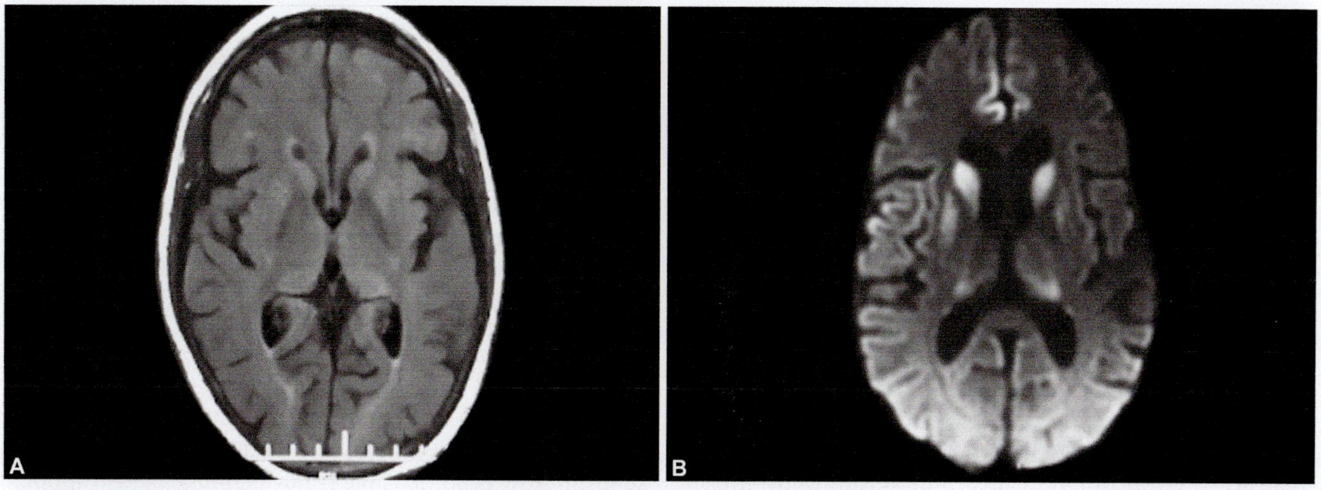

FIGS. 6A AND B: (A) FLAIR and (B) DWI show bilateral basal ganglia hyperintensities and bifrontal cortical ribboning.
(DWI: diffusion-weighted imaging; FLAIR: fluid-attenuated inversion recovery)

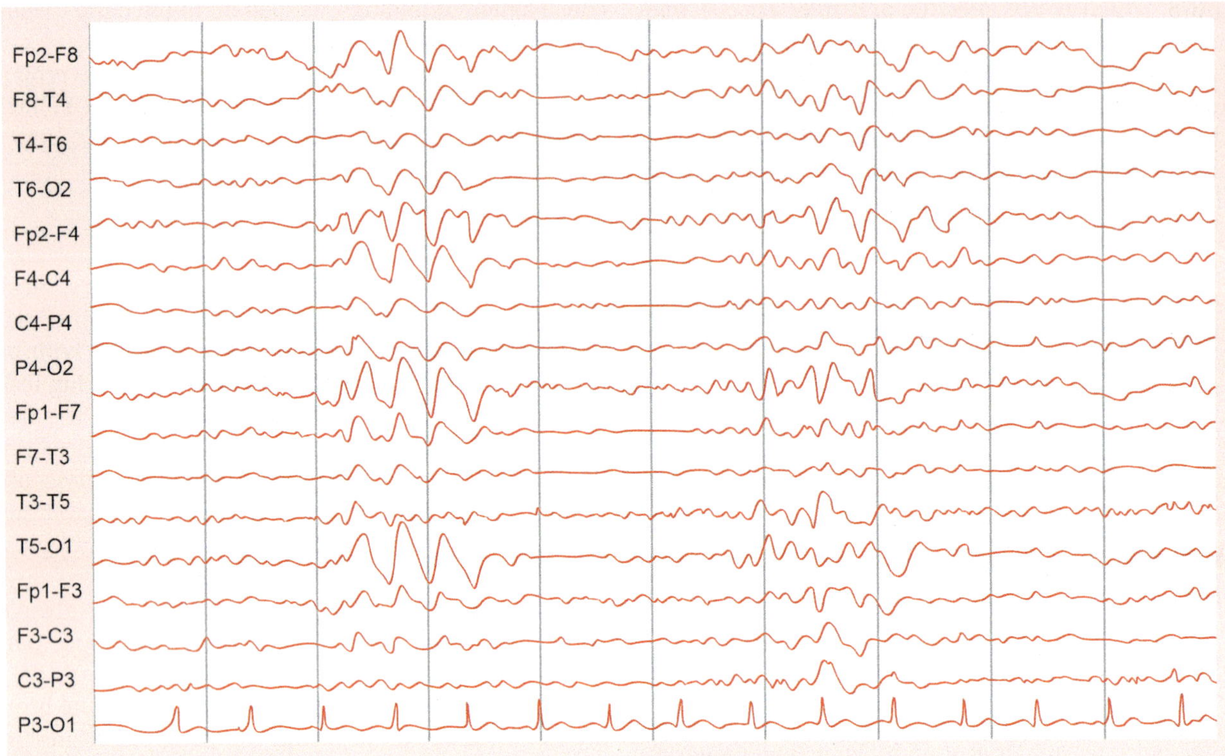

FIG. 7: Electroencephalography (EEG) showing short-interval periodic discharges.

evacuation of the SDH, following which he made a complete recovery.

Others

Nonconvulsive status epilepticus may mimic RPD.[36] It should be suspected in patients with a history of epilepsy but may also arise as new-onset status epilepticus.

EVALUATION OF RAPIDLY PROGRESSIVE DEMENTIA

Evaluation of RPD is dictated by the clinical syndrome with which the patient presents.[37,38] Clinical history may yield certain vital clues, such as the use of incriminating drugs. However, certain core tests must be performed on all patients, as soon as possible. Further testing is determined by the list of differential diagnoses considered in each patient. This is a hybrid approach, which is practiced by consensus.[9] The utility of diagnostic tests is further discussed below.

Screening Studies

Biochemical analysis aids in assessing the presence of metabolic abnormalities, and must include a hepatic function test, renal function test, electrolytes (sodium, calcium), thyroid function test, and serum ammonia. A complete blood count may provide clues about a systemic infection (leukocytosis) or chronic disease (anemia). Urine analysis and chest X-ray must also be done to look for a focus of infection in the urinary tract.

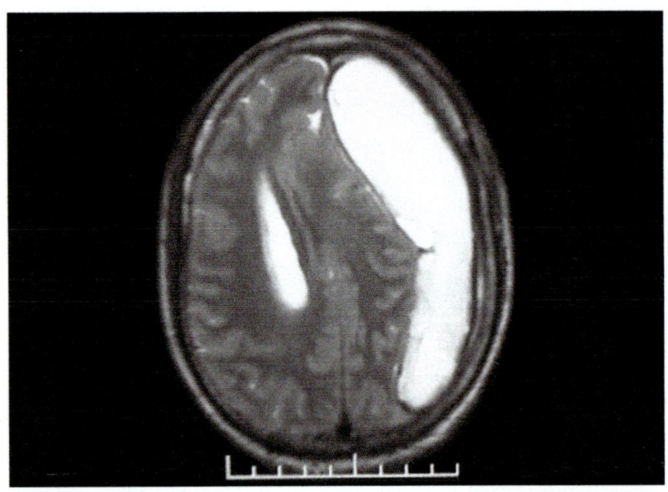

FIG. 8: Magnetic resonance imaging (MRI) showing left subdural hematoma.

Neuroimaging

Structural neuroimaging may provide essential clues, if present, toward the diagnosis in specific disease conditions **(Table 3)**. MRI is preferred to computed tomography (CT), and contrast studies are preferable to noncontrast scans. If MRI is not feasible (unavailability, claustrophobia, pacemaker implant, etc.), a CT scan should be done to rule out a space-occupying lesion, SDH, or infarct. Most of the time, however, in RPD, the MRI findings may be nonspecific.

Electroencephalography

Similar to MRI, EEG findings in patients with RPD may be nonspecific. However, the presence of specific patterns may enable the recognition of specific diseases. 1-Hz periodic complexes are seen in CJD.[39] Long-interval generalized high-amplitude periodic discharges may be seen in subacute sclerosing panencephalitis (SSPE).[40] The presence of extreme delta with brush pattern is a feature of anti-NMDARE.[41] The presence of musicogenic epilepsy is an indicator of anti-glutamic acid decarboxylase 65 (GAD65)-related encephalitis.[42]

TABLE 3: MRI findings in various causes of rapidly progressive dementia.

Disease entity	MRI findings
Creutzfeldt–Jakob disease	Cortical ribboning and involvement of deep gray nuclei are seen better on diffusion than on T2/FLAIR
Autoimmune encephalitis	Asymmetrical T2/FLAIR hyperintensity involving mesial temporal lobes, deep gray nuclei (anti-LGI1 encephalitis)
Wernicke's encephalopathy	Symmetrical increase in T2/FLAIR signal in bilateral mammillary bodies, dorsomedial thalamus, periaqueductal gray, around the third ventricle
SSPE	Bilateral parieto-occipital T2/FLAIR white matter hyperintensities may be seen, along with generalized cortical atrophy; MRI may be normal in the early stages
CNS vasculitis	Presence of cerebral microbleeds, beading of vessels on angiography
Normal pressure hydrocephalus	Evans' index > 0.3, acute narrowing of callosal angle, enlarged third ventricle, disproportionate enlargement of subarachnoid space hydrocephalus

(CNS: central nervous system; FLAIR: fluid-attenuated inversion recovery; LGI1: leucine-rich glioma-inactivated 1; MRI: magnetic resonance imaging; SSPE: subacute sclerosing panencephalitis)

Cerebrospinal Fluid Analysis

Cerebrospinal fluid analysis should be performed in all patients with RPD, if there are no contraindications. The presence of CSF pleocytosis (>5 cells/mm^3) indicates the presence of infection or inflammation.

Additional Tests

Additional tests must be considered based on the clinical scenario. In patients with suspected autoimmune encephalitis, CSF and/or serum panel for autoimmune antibodies may be done. Suspected paraneoplastic etiology necessitates paraneoplastic antibody panel and tumor markers. Malignancy screening may also require a positron emission tomography (PET) scan of the body to look for increased metabolic uptake in lesions. For suspected CJD, CSF 14-3-3 and RT-QuiC may be done. Invasive testing, such as brain biopsy, may be necessary sometimes, in patients with suspected tumors and CNS vasculitis.

APPROACH

An approach to the evaluation of RPD is summarized in the algorithm represented in **Flowchart 1**.

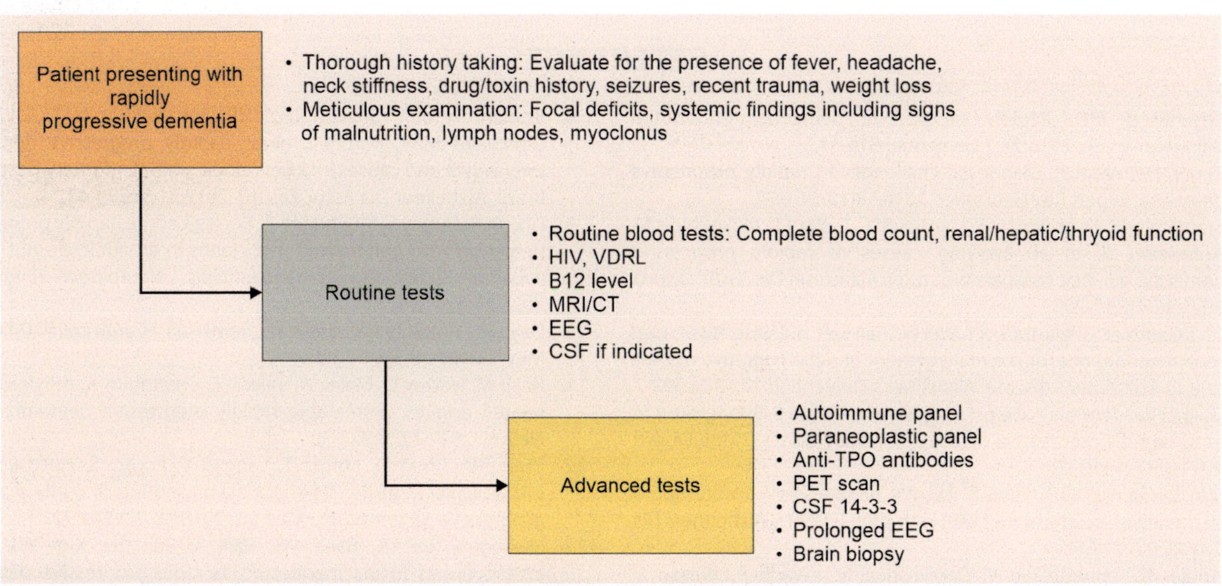

FLOWCHART 1: Stepwise approach to the evaluation of rapidly progressive dementia.

(CSF: cerebrospinal fluid; CT: computed tomography; EEG: electroencephalography; HIV: human immunodeficiency virus; MRI: magnetic resonance imaging; PET: positron emission tomography; TPO: thyroid peroxidase; VDRL: venereal disease research laboratory)

TABLE 4: Treatment of reversible causes of RPD.

Disease condition	Treatment
Vasculitis	*Immunomodulation*: Intravenous pulse methylprednisolone, followed by cyclophosphamide, rituximab
Autoimmune encephalitis	*Immunomodulation*: Intravenous pulse methylprednisolone/IVIg/PLEX, followed by oral steroids/ azathioprine/mycophenolate. In case of poor response, consider rituximab/cyclophosphamide
Paraneoplastic encephalitis	Treatment of the underlying tumor, if found. If the tumor is not detected, regular screening for malignancy for 5 years. Treat with immunomodulation in addition
Infections: • Bacterial meningitis • Viral meningoencephalitis/encephalitis • Fungal meningitis • SSPE • HAND	 • Intravenous antibiotics • Intravenous acyclovir • Intravenous antifungals • Interferon, Isoprinosine • Institution of antiretroviral therapy
Structural lesion: • Tumor • Normal pressure hydrocephalus	 • Removal of tumor • CSF diversion procedures
Metabolic abnormalities	Correction of the underlying metabolic abnormality
Toxin/drug	Removal of the offending toxin/drug

(CSF: cerebrospinal fluid; HAND: human immunodeficiency virus-associated neurocognitive disorder; IVIg: intravenous immunoglobulin; PLEX: plasma exchange; RPD: rapidly progressive dementia; SSPE: subacute sclerosing panencephalitis)

TREATMENT

A large amount of focus in the evaluation of RPD is directed toward unearthing a reversible cause. Treatment of reversible causes is outlined in **Table 4**.

CONCLUSION

Rapidly progressive dementia is a unique entity, which refers to the rapid development of dementia over weeks to months but may develop over up to 1–2 years. RPD may occur due to a heterogeneous range of causes, which span vascular, infectious, immune-mediated, toxic, metabolic, structural, and neoplasm-related conditions. In all these conditions, it is imperative to evaluate for reversible entities. The evaluation must not only be comprehensive but also expeditious, as long-term outcomes may worsen with a delay in the institution of treatment, due to neurodegeneration setting in.

REFERENCES

1. Geschwind MD. Rapidly progressive dementia. Continuum (Minneap Minn). 2016;22(2 Dementia):510-37.
2. Zerr I, Hermann P. Diagnostic challenges in rapidly progressive dementia. Expert Rev Neurother. 2018;18(10):761-72.
3. Stamatelos P, Kontokostas K, Liantinioti C, Giavasi C, Ioakeimidis M, Antonelou R, et al. Evolving causes of rapidly progressive dementia: a 5-year comparative study. Alzheimer Dis Assoc Disord. 2021;35(4):315-20.
4. Jia J, Gauthier S, Pallotta S, Ji Y, Wei W, Xiao S, et al. Consensus-based recommendations for the management of rapid cognitive decline due to Alzheimer's disease. Alzheimer's Dement. 2017;13(5):592-7.
5. Gaig C, Valldeoriola F, Gelpi E, Ezquerra M, Llufriu S, Buongiorno M, et al. Rapidly progressive diffuse Lewy body disease. Mov Disord. 2011;26(7):1316-23.
6. Sun L, Chen K, Li X, Xiao S. Rapidly progressive frontotemporal dementia associated with MAPT mutation G389R. J Alzheimers Dis. 2017;55(2):777-85.
7. Anuja P, Venugopalan V, Darakhshan N, Awadh P, Wilson V, Manoj G, et al. Rapidly progressive dementia: an eight year (2008–2016) retrospective study. PLoS One. 2018;13(1):e0189832.
8. Studart Neto A, Soares Neto HR, Simabukuro MM, Solla DJF, Gonçalves MRR, Fortini I, et al. Rapidly progressive dementia: prevalence and causes in a neurologic unit of a tertiary hospital in Brazil. Alzheimer Dis Assoc Disord. 2017;31(3):239-43.
9. Ghosh R, Dubey S, Mukherjee A, Benito-León J. Rapidly progressive dementia with generalized myoclonus in an adult: do not forget subacute sclerosing panencephalitis. Neurologia (Engl Ed). 2022;37(5):415-8.
10. Day GS. Rapidly progressive dementia. Continuum (Minneap Minn). 2022;28(3):901-36.
11. Nasir M, Nortey D, Malek N, Valerio F, Chaudhuri A. Amyloid-beta-related angiitis: a treatable rapidly progressive dementia. Pract Neurol. 2022;22(3):228-30.
12. Brett FM, Chen D, Loftus T, Langan Y, Looby S, Hutchinson S. Intravascular large B-cell lymphoma presenting clinically as rapidly progressive dementia. Ir J Med Sci. 2018;187(2):319-22.
13. Hwang H, La YK, Baek MS, Baik K, Suh SH, Kim WJ. Dural arteriovenous fistula manifested as rapid progressive dementia successfully treated by endovascular embolization only. Neurointervention. 2017;12(1):50-3.

14. Eggers C, Arendt G, Hahn K, Husstedt IW, Maschke M, Neuen-Jacob E, et al. HIV-1-associated neurocognitive disorder: epidemiology, pathogenesis, diagnosis, and treatment. J Neurol. 2017;264(8):1715-27.
15. McArthur JC. HIV dementia: an evolving disease. J Neuroimmunol. 2004;157(1-2):3-10.
16. Paviolo JP, Imbach MC, Nocenti ZA, Durand BL. [Rapidly progressive dementia due to neurosyphilis (general paralysis). A treatable case of dementia]. Medicina (B Aires). 2020;80(4):401-4.
17. Manini A, Querzola G, Lovati C, Pantoni L. Rapidly progressive dementia and intractable diarrhea: a teaching case report and a systematic review of cognitive impairment in Whipple's disease. Neurol Sci. 2022;43(2):907-26.
18. Stefani A, Riello M, Rossini F, Mariotto S, Fenzi F, Gambina G, et al. Neurosyphilis manifesting with rapidly progressive dementia: report of three cases. Neurol Sci. 2013;34(11):2027-30.
19. Teepker M, Hamer HM, Knake S, Bandmann O, Oertel WH, Rosenow F. Myoclonic encephalopathy caused by chronic bismuth abuse. Epileptic Disord. 2002;4(4):229-33.
20. Gibson GE, Hirsch JA, Fonzetti P, Jordan BD, Cirio RT, Elder J. Vitamin B1 (thiamine) and dementia. Ann N Y Acad Sci. 2016;1367(1): 21-30.
21. Moore E, Mander A, Ames D, Carne R, Sanders K, Watters D. Cognitive impairment and vitamin B12: a review. Int Psychogeriatr. 2012;24(4):541-56.
22. Paul WB, Aggarwall V, Kurian S, Mathews KP, Viggeswarpu S. Portosystemic shunt presenting as rapidly progressive dementia. J Assoc Physicians India. 2015;63(5):82-3.
23. Mignarri A, Chini E, Rufa A, Rocchi R, Federico A, Dotti MT. Lithium neurotoxicity mimicking rapidly progressive dementia. J Neurol. 2013;260(4):1152-4.
24. Dalmau J, Graus F. Antibody-mediated encephalitis. N Engl J Med. 2018;378(9):840-51.
25. Tirthani E, Said MS, Smith RG, Jadhav N, Shanina E. Paraneoplastic Encephalomyelitis. In: StatPearls. StatPearls Publishing; 2022.
26. Wesley SF, Ferguson D. Autoimmune encephalitides and rapidly progressive dementias. Semin Neurol. 2019;39(2):283-92.
27. de Villemeur TB. Creutzfeldt–Jakob disease. Handb Clin Neurol. 2013;112:1191-3.
28. Capellari S, Strammiello R, Saverioni D, Kretzschmar H, Parchi P. Genetic Creutzfeldt–Jakob disease and fatal familial insomnia: insights into phenotypic variability and disease pathogenesis. Acta Neuropathol. 2011;121(1):21-37.
29. Schmidt C, Redyk K, Meissner B, Krack L, von Ahsen N, Roeber S, et al. Clinical features of rapidly progressive Alzheimer's disease. Dement Geriatr Cogn Disord. 2010;29(4):371-8.
30. Schmidt C, Wolff M, Weitz M, Bartlau T, Korth C, Zerr I. Rapidly progressive Alzheimer disease. Arch Neurol. 2011;68(9):1124-30.
31. Josephs KA, Ahlskog JE, Parisi JE, Boeve BF, Crum BA, Giannini C, et al. Rapidly progressive neurodegenerative dementias. Arch Neurol. 2009;66(2):201-7.
32. Yamada SM, Tomita Y, Takahashi M, Kawamoto M. A case of lymphomatosis cerebri presenting with rapid progression of dementia: a literature review. NMC Case Rep J. 2022;9:83-8.
33. Samani A, Davagnanam I, Cockerell OC, Ramsay A, Patani R, Chataway J. Lymphomatosis cerebri: a treatable cause of rapidly progressive dementia. J Neurol Neurosurg Psychiatry. 2015;86(2):238-40.
34. Rivero Sanz E, Torralba Cabeza MÁ, Sanjuán Portugal F, García-Bragado F. Lymphomatosis cerebri mimicking iatrogenic Creutzfeldt–Jakob disease. BMJ Case Rep. 2014;2014: bcr2013201246.
35. Kuruppu DK, Matthews BR. Young-onset dementia. Semin Neurol. 2013;33(4):365-85.
36. Zhao Q, Sun L, Hu B, Lin W. Nonconvulsive status epilepticus manifesting as rapidly progressive dementia and infarction in the splenium of the corpus callosum: a case report. Medicine (Baltimore). 2021;100(15):e25263.
37. Rosenbloom MH, Atri A. The evaluation of rapidly progressive dementia. Neurologist. 2011;17(2):67-74.
38. Mahajan S, Appleby BS. Comprehensive and methodical: diagnostic and management approaches to rapidly progressive dementia. Curr Treat Options Neurol. 2017;19(11):40.
39. Neufeld MY, Korczyn AD. Topographic distribution of the periodic discharges in Creutzfeldt–Jakob disease (CJD). Brain Topogr. 1992;4(3):201-6.
40. Garg RK, Mahadevan A, Malhotra HS, Rizvi I, Kumar N, Uniyal R. Subacute sclerosing panencephalitis. Rev Med Virol. 2019;29(5):e2058.
41. Schmitt SE, Pargeon K, Frechette ES, Hirsch LJ, Dalmau J, Friedman D. Extreme delta brush: a unique EEG pattern in adults with anti-NMDA receptor encephalitis. Neurology. 2012;79(11):1094-100.
42. Smith KM, Zalewski NL, Budhram A, Britton JW, So E, Cascino GD, et al. Musicogenic epilepsy: expanding the spectrum of glutamic acid decarboxylase 65 neurological autoimmunity. Epilepsia. 2021;62(5):e76-81.

Part 4G: Diseases of the Lower Motor Neuron

80

CHAPTER

Amyotrophic Lateral Sclerosis

Idha Sood, Vineeth Jaison, Ashok Verma

INTRODUCTION

Jean-Martin Charcot in a series of lectures, pathological findings, and articles in the 1860s first described amyotrophic lateral sclerosis (ALS) as a degenerative condition of anterior horns and lateral columns of the spinal cord causing purely motor symptoms. It is also called Charcot's disease, motor neuron disease, or Lou Gehrig's disease, named after a famous baseball player who was afflicted with the illness. It is now recognized to affect certain other neuronal systems and can have varying clinical, genetic, and neuropathological presentations. The most common and typical manifestation involves both upper motor neurons (UMNs) and lower motor neurons (LMNs), spreading from one neuroaxis to the next. The disease is relentlessly progressive in course, eventually causing death from respiratory failure in 3–5 years in most cases. The World Federation of Neurology Research Group on Neuromuscular Diseases clubbed four clinical phenotypes, namely ALS, progressive muscular atrophy (PMA), primary lateral sclerosis (PLS), and progressive bulbar palsy, as motor neuron diseases.

EPIDEMIOLOGY

The prevalence of ALS is 4–8 per 100,000 people, and the incidence rate ranges between 0.6 and 3.8 per 100,000 person-years, with some variations in populations of different regions.[1] Divided by subcontinents and economic levels, the highest incidence and prevalence are reported in Europe [prevalence 9.62, 95% confidence interval (CI) 4.80–16.10; incidence 2.76, 95% CI 2.00–3.64] and lowest in South Asia (prevalence 1.57, 95% CI 0.17–4.39; incidence 0.42, 95% CI 0.06–1.11).[1] The estimated number of people living with ALS in India in 2019 was ~25,000 (accounting for 0.1% of total neurological disorder disability-adjusted life years).[2]

The single most important risk factor for patients with ALS is age, with mortality increasing up until the eighth decade. While the global median age of onset is 51–66 years, it is reported to occur a decade earlier in India and China.[1] The median age at diagnosis varies from 54 to 69 years, with higher values for women and patients with cognitive impairment.[1] Men have a slightly higher rate of developing ALS, with male-to-female ratio (M:F) of approximately 1.5:1. Patients with cognitive impairment, the elderly, and women have a higher prevalence of bulbar onset ALS, i.e., manifesting with early difficulty in speaking or swallowing. In contrast, patients without cognitive impairment, relatively young individuals, and men have a higher prevalence of spinal onset ALS, i.e., manifesting early as weakness in limbs.[1]

PATHOLOGY AND PATHOPHYSIOLOGY

Approximately 92% of ALS is sporadic (sALS), and the rest is familial (monogenic, fALS). The cause of sALS is unknown but appears to be multifactorial, with environmental factors interacting with susceptibility genes to finally lead to motor neuron degeneration. Risk factors causing neuronal injury can be related to certain occupations, activity levels, exposure to toxins, and possible geographical influences **(Table 1)**. These elements can produce multiple "hits" causing changes at the molecular level, thus making ALS pathogenesis to be a multistep process. Studies have shown that fewer steps are required in individuals already carrying a large-effect mutation.[3]

Multiple genes are associated with different mechanisms of injury in patients with ALS, the most common being *C9orf72* (chromosome 9 open reading frame 72), *SOD1* (superoxide dismutase 1), *TDP43* (TAR DNA-binding protein 43), *FUS* (fused in sarcoma), etc. These pathways of injury likely converge to cause neurodegeneration at the molecular level by inducing oxidative stress, glutamate

TABLE 1: Risk factors attributed to ALS.

Toxins	Heavy metals (lead and mercury), smoking, pesticides, solvents, silica, organic dust, diesel exhaust
Occupation	Hunting, agriculture, fishing, construction work, forestry, laboratory technicians
Activity	Lower BMI, high muscle mass, exercise, athletes, head injury, or trauma
Geographical and environmental factors	Rural areas, Kii Peninsula Japan (50–100% higher), extremely low magnetic fields, electric shocks
Infections	*Enterovirus*, herpesvirus, and retrovirus

(ALS: amyotrophic lateral sclerosis; BMI: body mass index)

TABLE 2: Pathogenic mechanisms of ALS.

Biological stress	Gene association
Mitochondrial dysfunction	*SOD1, CHCHD10, TARDBP*
Oxidative stress	*SOD1, ALS2, TARDBP*
Impaired protein homeostasis	*SIGMAR1, CHMP2B, C9orf72, SQSTM1, UBQLN2, SOD1, ALS2, VAPB, OPTN, VCP, TBK1*
Hyperexcitability	*SOD1*
Glial dysfunction	*SOD1, C9orf72*
Aberrant RNA metabolism	*SETX, FUS, ANG, TARDBP, TAF15, EWSR1, ATXN2, hnRNPA1, C9orf72, hnRNPA2B1, MATR3*
Axonopathy	*SOD1, SGP11, TUBA4A, PFN1, DCTN, PRHPH, NEFH*
Nuclear export	*C9orf72*
Impaired DNA repair	*NEK1, C21orf2, SGP11, FUS*
Dysregulated vesicle transport	*SOD1, ALS2, FIG4, VAPB, OPTN, UNC13A, CHMP2B*

(ALS: amyotrophic lateral sclerosis; ALS2: alsin; ANG: angiogenin; ATXN2: ataxin 2; C9orf72: chromosome 9 open reading frame 72; CHCH10: coiled-coil-helix-coiled-coil-helix domain-containing 10; CHMP2B: charged multivesicular body protein 2B; DCTN1: dynactin 1; DNA: deoxyribonucleic acid; EWSR1: RNA-binding protein EWS; FIG4: factor-induced gene 4; FUS: fused in sarcoma; hnRNPA1: heterogeneous nuclear ribonucleoprotein A1; hnRNPA2B1: heterogeneous nuclear ribonucleoprotein A2B1; KIF5A: kinesin heavy chain isoform 5A; MATR3: matrin 3; NEFH: neurofilament heavy polypeptide; NEK1: NIMA-related kinase 1; OPTN: optineurin; PFN1: profilin 1; PRHPH: peripherin; RNA: ribonucleic acid; SETX: senataxin; SGP11: spastic paraplegia 11; SIGMAR1: sigma nonopioid intracellular receptor 1; SOD: superoxide dismutase; SQSTM1: sequestosome 1; TAF15: TATA-binding protein-associated factor 2N; TBK1: TANK binding kinase 1; TDP43: TAR DNA binding protein 43; TUBA4A: tubulin alpha 4a; UBQLN2: ubiquilin 2; UNC13A: UNC-13 homologue A; VCP: valosin-containing protein)

excitotoxicity, mitochondrial dysfunction, neurofilament accumulation, etc.,[4,5] as enumerated in **Table 2**. In SOD1 ALS patients, a recent study showed that a particular genotype might have a more clinical effect on the age of onset while a different variant affects the disease progression. Hence, the age of symptom onset and survival after symptom onset appear to be uncoupled, which suggests that separate mechanisms may be at play in the majority of variations for the initiation of neurodegeneration versus its progression.[6]

Gross Pathology

The primary gross pathological characteristics of ALS include skeletal muscle and motor cortex atrophy, pallor and sclerosis of the pyramidal (corticospinal and corticobulbar) tracts, and thinning of the hypoglossal nerves and ventral roots of the spinal cord.

Microscopic Pathology

The gray and white matter of the spinal cord typically exhibit microglial infiltration, extensive astrocytic gliosis, and depletion of ≥50% of spinal motor neurons. The corticospinal pathways exhibit axonal loss, gliosis, and myelin pallor, while the motor cortex typically exhibits astrocytic gliosis along with a varied depletion of UMNs. Skeletal muscles show clustering of atrophic angulated fibers and fiber-type grouping, thus demonstrating features of both denervation and reinnervation.[5]

CLINICAL PRESENTATIONS

Typical ALS manifests itself with UMN and LMN syndromes by affecting motor neurons in the brain, brainstem, and spinal cord. UMN and LMN signs present in classic ALS are summarized in **Table 3**. **Figures 1A and B** show disproportionate wasting of thenar eminence (split hand sign) in an individual with ALS. **Figures 2A and B** show the atrophied tongue of a patient with ALS.

Typical Features

Weakness

Amyotrophic lateral sclerosis presents most commonly with weakness. Typically, it begins focally and then spreads to neighboring myotomes in the same limb before involving the contralateral side, later spreading to other segments. While there is no difference in the lower limbs, the dominant upper limb is slightly more affected than the nondominant one. If a deep tendon reflex is easily elicited in a weak, atrophied, and flaccid limb, it should be considered a UMN sign. Painless, involuntary, rapid twitches in muscles of the limb and trunk are fasciculations that should be seen as an important sign. Since these are rarely noticeable to the patient, they should be carefully searched on clinical examination. If absent, the clinician should rethink the ALS diagnosis.

Bulbar Involvement

Amyotrophic lateral sclerosis patients with bulbar onset present most commonly with difficulty in speaking and swallowing. Impaired oral secretion clearance and automatic swallowing made worse with weak neck extensors can cause sialorrhea and silent and symptomatic aspirations.

TABLE 3: Clinical manifestations of ALS.

Area		UMN	LMN
Trunk and extremity	Symptoms	Loss of dexterity, weakness, spasms, fatigue, stiffness, slowness	More pronounced weakness, wasting of muscles, split hand, pain due to pericapsulitis, buckling of knees, and painful contractures
	Signs	Spasticity, hyperreflexia, clonus, positive Babinski's sign	Decreased motor power, bulk, diminished reflexes, fasciculations, cramps, pseudoneuritic pattern (foot drop, wrist drop, and claw hand), camptocormia, and head drop
Bulbar	Symptoms	Forced speech, choking on liquids, slowed chewing, and inappropriate or spontaneous crying, laughing, or yawning	Greater degrees of weakness of the face, palate, and tongue
	Signs	Spastic tongue and speech, hyperactive gag, brisk cough, and jaw jerk	Asymmetrical wasting of the tongue, fasciculations, hypoactive gag, weak cough, and jaw jerk

(ALS: amyotrophic lateral sclerosis; LMN: lower motor neuron; UMN: upper motor neuron)

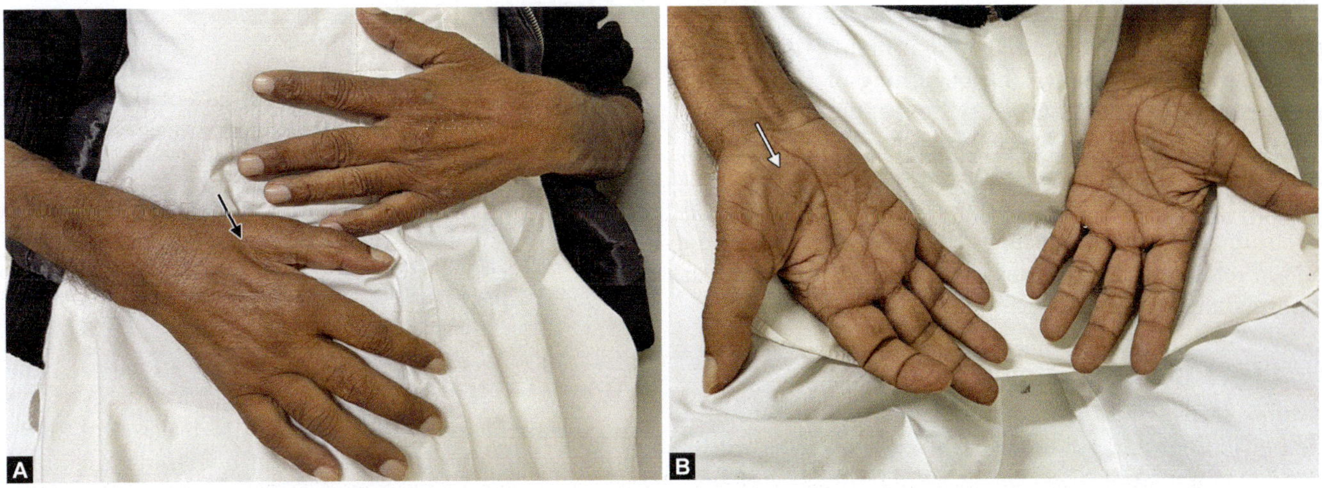

FIGS. 1A AND B: Disproportionate wasting of thenar eminence in an individual with amyotrophic lateral sclerosis (split hand sign). (A) Dorsal aspect (black arrow); (B) Ventral aspect (white arrow).

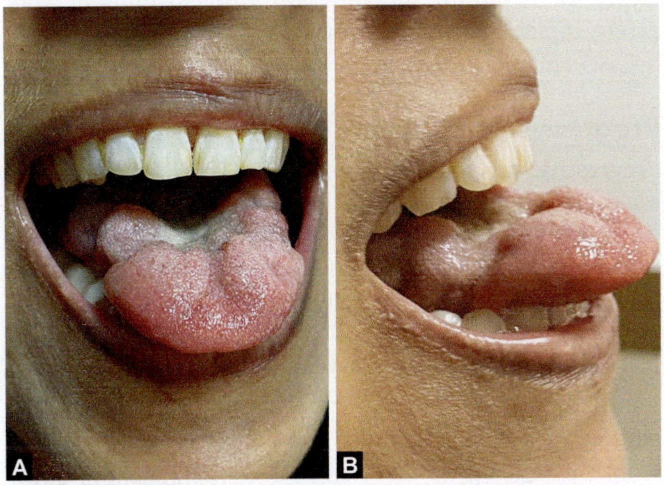

FIGS. 2A AND B: Atrophied tongue of a patient with amyotrophic lateral sclerosis (ALS). (A) As seen from the front; (B) As seen from the side.

It may manifest as nighttime awakenings, coughing and choking during meals or even fatal laryngospasm, and aspiration with the attendant complications, including death.

Respiratory Involvement

As the disease progresses and respiratory muscles are involved, patients often complain of dyspnea on exertion and/or rest, orthopnea, early morning headaches, and sleep disturbances. When observed in later stages, they may use accessory breathing muscles and show paradoxical abdominal movements, symptoms of carbon dioxide retention (such as bounding pulse, chemosis, papilledema, and cyanosis), and weak sniffing and coughing. The patient's voice may be frequently interrupted by sighs and can become weaker and softer at the end of long sentences, indicating poor breath support during speaking.

Other Features

Patients may complain of pain secondary to immobilization-induced joint pericapsulitis. Sleep can be disturbed and may lead to fatigue. ALS patients often have coexisting depression. They can have severe weight loss disproportionate to their caloric intake, which may represent a cachexia-like state.

Atypical Features

Atypical clinical features are less commonly found in patients with ALS. Aside from frontotemporal cognitive impairment, they should trigger a search for other possible diagnoses.

Cognition

Only 14% of ALS patients have frank frontotemporal dementia (FTD), compared to approximately 40% who have some form of cognitive impairment. Up to 30% of people may experience the beginning of FTD before developing ALS. The GGGGCC hexanucleotide repeat intronic expansion in the *C9orf72* gene has been linked to the inheritance of ALS and FTD as a single characteristic. In C9orf72-ALS and C9orf72-FTD/ALS, the whole clinical spectrum of ALS (which includes aberrant muscle tone and tendon reflexes, fasciculations, muscular cramps, and gait abnormalities) may be present.[7]

Bladder and Bowel Manifestations

In most cases, Onufrowicz's motor neurons that control the pelvic floor and sphincter muscles are unaffected by ALS. While frank urge incontinence and bowel dysfunction are uncommon, mild urinary urgency and retention may occur.

Sensory System Manifestations

The sensory system is typically spared, except in bulbospinal muscular atrophy (Kennedy's disease). Patients may experience nonspecific sensory symptoms in the distal extremities, which are not supported by objective examination. Visual and hearing impairment does not occur in ALS.

Extrapyramidal Manifestations

Extrapyramidal symptoms are generally absent in ALS. On occasion, patients with ALS may have features of retropulsion or postural reflex dysfunction, likely secondary to spasticity or mixed neurodegenerative disease, such as synucleinopathy.

Amyotrophic Lateral Sclerosis-plus Syndromes

Amyotrophic lateral sclerosis-plus syndrome comprises a diagnosis of ALS along with clinical features extending beyond the motor neuron pool and neuromuscular systems on neurological examination. Patients with this syndrome are more likely to have fALS and generally mutations in SOD1 or TDP-43. The valosin-containing protein (VCP)-associated ALS may show features of inclusion body myopathy (IBM) and Paget's disease. The additional features in ALS syndromes are combined into abnormalities of one of the four systems:

1. *Ocular motility abnormalities*: Gaze abnormalities, horizontal, upgaze, downgaze impersistence, and/or head movements
2. *Cerebellar features*: Ataxia and/or limb dysmetria
3. *Extrapyramidal features*: Resting tremor, masked face, startled appearance, bradykinesia, rigidity, dystonia, retropulsion, apraxia of eye closure, and/or gait apraxia
4. *Autonomic dysfunction*: Excessive sweating, special sensory, and/or loss of taste and smell[8]

Clinical Subtypes

Progressive Bulbar Palsy

Bulbar palsy may initially appear in 19–28% of ALS patients. It is most frequently observed in postmenopausal women, and its prognosis could be poorer. Dysarthria is typically the first symptom, followed by dysphagia, which progresses locally before affecting the cervical, thoracic, and lumbosacral segments, respectively. In rare cases, the disease may remain localized to just the bulbar region (true progressive bulbar palsy).[9]

Primary Lateral Sclerosis

Primary lateral sclerosis is a pure UMN disease that affects only 2–4% of all ALS patients and does not progress to involve the LMN. The disease begins between 50 and 55 years of age, and it advances extremely slowly. Clinically, pure PLS, which has a slower rate of progression than ALS and a higher degree of preserved function, can be identified after 4 years of only showing pure UMN symptoms. Very rarely, it may present as a paraneoplastic manifestation of breast cancer.[10]

Progressive Muscular Atrophy

Progressive muscular atrophy is a pure LMN condition with a generally good prognosis. Prior to being designated as PMA, the disease must by definition be pure LMN syndrome for an extended period, and it requires reevaluation to look for the emergence of UMN signs.

Familial Amyotrophic Lateral Sclerosis

Familial ALS, which can be autosomal dominant, autosomal recessive, or X-linked dominant, is seen in 5–10% of ALS patients globally. In 60–80% of fALS cases, a large-effect mutation (possibly pathogenic) can be found. *C9orf72* (~38%), *SOD1* (~20%), *FUS* (~4%), and *TDP-43* (4–5%) mutations are most often found. If there have been ALS cases in the same family for several generations, fALS should be suspected. These typically present at a younger age, affect men and women equally, have shorter disease durations, and favor the lower limbs. The Caucasian population is more likely than the Asian population to have the *C9orfF72* gene mutation, which typically causes FTD-ALS. More than 30 genes have recently been linked to fALS.[11]

Mills Hemiplegic Variant

This rare variant manifests with both UMN and LMN signs on one side of the body.

Flail Arm and Flail Leg Variant

Flail arm syndrome, which affects around 10% of ALS patients, is characterized by painless asymmetric proximal and distal limb wasting with positive Babinski's sign, whereas "flail leg variation," which affects about 6% of ALS patients, is characterized by pseudopolyneuritic syndrome in the lower limbs. Patients of both these variants survive longer than typical ALS patients.[12]

Western Pacific Amyotrophic Lateral Sclerosis

Guam, an island in the Western Pacific, is home to this particular variant of the disease. It is a combination of ALS, parkinsonism, and dementia in variable proportions. Nearly 5% of patients present with predominant ALS whereas 38% have a combination of parkinsonism and dementia. The cause of Guamanian ALS remains unknown. Environmental elements such as cycad seeds, aluminum, and silicon have all been investigated in relation to the etiology of this disease. Beta methylamino-L-alanine, which is found in cycad seeds, has neurotoxic properties.[13]

DIAGNOSIS

Clinical Evaluation

The diagnosis of ALS is based on a detailed history and thorough clinical examination, with ancillary testing used to support the clinical suspicion and rule out alternate diagnoses. The World Federation of Neurology provides a set of clinical, electrodiagnostic, and pathological criteria for the diagnosis of ALS called the El Escorial classification.[14] This criterion divides candidates into definite, probable, possible, and suspected ALS based on the pattern of LMN and UMN involvement in four anatomical regions: bulbar, cervical, thoracic, and lumbosacral regions.[14] A definite ALS diagnosis requires disease involvement in three anatomic parts and therefore is possible only after a length of time and significant disease progression. In order to recognize early cases of ALS, the Awaji criteria were proposed, which include fasciculations as an electrodiagnostic marker for active denervation.[15] The recent Gold Coast criteria permit the diagnosis of ALS even if only one region is affected.[16]

Electrodiagnosis

The clinical examination is supported by electrodiagnosis, which also aids in determining the nature of LMN disease (neurogenic vs. myogenic) in weak muscles and detects sensory involvement that should be typically absent in ALS.

Nerve Conduction Studies

In ALS, motor and sensory nerve conduction studies (NCSs) are often normal. One might see a decrease in compound motor action potentials (CMAPs) and borderline slow motor nerve conduction in later stages with large-size motor neuron loss and muscle atrophy. Sensory NCS may be abnormal in the weak and paralyzed limb from local pressure palsy. Neurophysiological index [CMAP amplitude/distal motor latency × F (frequency%)] is recorded in abductor digiti minimi by stimulating the ulnar nerve at the wrist. It may help in differentiating rapid from slow progressors in ALS.[17]

Electromyography

Electromyography (EMG) is done in at least three of four anatomical segments (i.e., face, upper limbs, trunk, and lower limbs), especially in the weak muscles. At least two muscles (one proximal and one distal) with separate root and nerve innervations must exhibit active denervation in the form of fibrillation, positive sharp waves, and/or fasciculations against a backdrop of chronic denervation in order to meet the diagnostic criteria. ALS patients also show a progressive linear decline in motor unit number estimation (MUNE). The number of functioning motor units within a muscle, as represented by motor unit index (MUNIX), can detect disease progression in presymptomatic muscles in ALS.[17] The compound muscle action potential scan tool (MScanFit) is another technique for motor unit estimation. However, these are not indicated in the diagnostic process but are important to monitor LMN loss as biomarkers to evaluate disease progression.[17]

Repeated Nerve Stimulation

Repeated nerve stimulation (RNS) studies are generally normal in patients with ALS. But some patients can show a drop in RNS, which portends recent reinnervation with immature terminal nerve branches.

Transcranial Magnetic Stimulation (TMS-EMG)

Slowing of the central motor conduction time is seen in ALS, which is a reflection of central motor track integrity and is the difference between the latency of the response elicited by cranial versus cervical or cranial versus lumbosacral stimulation. Resting motor threshold (RMT) is a reflection of cortical motor neuron excitability. It is found to be reduced early in the course of the disease, i.e., cortical hyperexcitability is seen early in ALS patients. This is followed by a progressive increase of RMT and eventual inexcitability.[17] Short-interval intracortical inhibition (SICI) is a technique to quantify inhibitory cortical motor circuits by a method called threshold tracking. It has been suggested that it can be used to permit early diagnosis, discriminate ALS from mimicking disorders, and detect changes by drugs reducing cortical excitability.[17]

Neuroimaging

To rule out alternative reasons for the patient's symptoms, imaging of the brain and spine is performed. For UMN signs, it is crucial to search for intrinsic/extrinsic compressive and noncompressive lesions, and for LMN symptoms, to image the roots.

Neuromuscular Ultrasound

Ultrasound can detect fasciculations better than EMG in the tongue and is less painful.

Magnetic Resonance Imaging

Patients with ALS may exhibit substantial corticospinal tract (CST) hyperintensity. Gray and white matter have been measured using voxel-based morphometry to identify brain shrinkage in ALS patients associated with cognitive impairment.[18] Thinning of the primary motor cortex is a sensitive diagnostic marker in brain imaging. **Figure 3** shows the atrophy of the frontal and temporal lobes in a patient with ALS.

Functional Neuroimaging

The combination of proton magnetic resonance spectroscopy (^{1}H-MRS) with transcranial magnetic stimulation (TMS) or diffusion tensor magnetic resonance imaging (MRI) has shown the potential to improve sensitivity in the detection of UMN degeneration in ALS patients. Positron emission tomography with 2-deoxy-2-(fluorine-18)-fluoro-D-glucose integrated with computed tomography (^{18}F-FDG PET/CT) can serve as a potentially important biomarker in ALS patients as it can differentiate them from controls with an accuracy of 93%.[18]

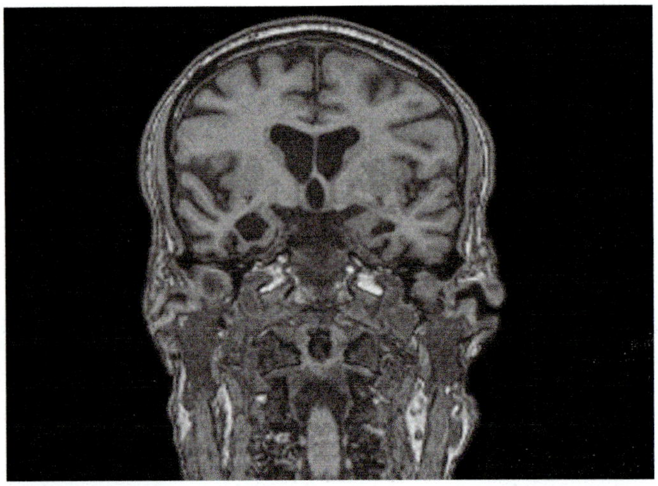

FIG. 3: MRI (coronal section) showing frontal and temporal lobe atrophy in a patient with ALS.

(ALS: amyotrophic lateral sclerosis; MRI: magnetic resonance imaging)

Laboratory Tests

To rule out conditions other than ALS that may mimic ALS, laboratory tests are conducted as enumerated in **Box 1**.

Genetic Testing

Genetic linkage studies are shown to identify pathological variants in 50–60% of ALS patients having a strong family history versus 10–20% of patients with sALS.[19] These studies can identify mutations in *SOD1*, *TARDBP*, *FUS*, *C9orf72*, and other pathogenic genes, and it may be helpful to identify underlying mechanisms to give targeted therapy in clinical trials.[19] Generally, genetic testing has been reserved for ALS patients with a positive family history. However, ALS-associated pathological variants have been identified in isolated cases as well. Moreover, there are no clinical differences in patients with fALS and sALS. Hence, early genetic testing is imperative in *all patients of ALS*, because drug development and gene therapy can also benefit those sporadic cases with clinically actionable

BOX 1 **Laboratory investigations in ALS patients.**

Essential investigations:

- Complete blood count and ESR
- Full biochemical profile including calcium
- CPK (>1,000 IU/L is unusual in ALS)
- Serum protein electrophoresis

Additional investigations in selected cases:

- Vitamin B12 level
- ANA by immunofluorescence, C-ANCA, P-ANCA
- Paraneoplastic antibody screen
- Serum leukocyte hexosaminidase levels
- Anti-AChR, anti-MuSK antibodies
- Anti-VGKC antibody
- HIV serology
- Lyme serology

Cerebrospinal fluid analysis (CSF)

Nerve and/or muscle biopsy:

- To look for ALS mimics

CECT chest and abdomen or whole-body PET:

- To look for occult malignancy

(AchR: acetylcholine receptor; ALS: amyotrophic lateral sclerosis; ANA: antinuclear antibody; C-ANCA: central antinuclear cytoplasmic antibody; CECT: contrast-enhanced computed tomography; CPK: creatine phosphokinase; ESR: erythrocyte sedimentation rate; HIV: human immunodeficiency virus; MuSK: muscle-specific kinase; P-ANCA: peripheral antinuclear cytoplasmic antibody; PET: positron emission tomography; VGKC: voltage-gated potassium channels) variants. Genetic testing and appropriate genetic counseling should be offered early to all ALS patients so that they can gain maximum benefit from available drugs and genetic therapies.[20]

DIFFERENTIAL DIAGNOSIS

The differential diagnosis of ALS along with corresponding investigations is given in **Table 4**.

TABLE 4: Differential diagnosis of ALS and appropriate investigations.

Disorders of muscle	Inclusion body myositis	EMG, CPK, and muscle biopsy
	Polymyositis	EMG, CPK, muscle biopsy, and autoimmune screen
	Dermatomyositis	EMG, CPK, and skin and muscle biopsy
	Distal myopathies	Family history, muscle biopsy
	Myotonic dystrophy	Systemic features, genetic testing of repeat nucleotides
	Oculopharyngeal muscular dystrophy	EMG, CPK, muscle biopsy, and genetic repeat nucleotide testing
Disorders of the neuromuscular junction	Myasthenia gravis	AChR and MuSK antibodies, RNS, and SFEMG
	Lambert–Eaton myasthenic syndrome	RNS, anti-VGCC antibodies
Disorders of a motor nerve and nerve root	Multifocal motor neuropathy	NCS, EMG, and GM1 antibodies
	Chronic inflammatory demyelinating neuropathy	NCS, EMG, CSF analysis—albuminocytological dissociation
	Motor neuropathy associated with POEMS syndrome	Skeletal survey, serum protein electrophoresis
	Cramp-fasciculation syndrome	NCS, EMG
	Neuromyotonia	Anti-VGKC antibodies
	Paraneoplastic syndrome	Serum tumor markers, imaging including whole-body PET, and bone marrow biopsy
	Heavy metal poisoning	Urine or blood screens, hair, and/or nail clippings
	Mononeuritis multiplex	NCS, EMG, vasculitis screen, serology, and nerve and muscle biopsy
	Radiculoplexopathy	NCS, EMG (changes only along the root distribution), MRI
Disorders of motor neurons	Spinal muscular atrophy	*SMN* gene deletion assay
	X-linked spinobulbar muscular atrophy (Kennedy's disease)	Increased CAG repeats in DNA from blood
	Poliomyelitis or post-polio syndrome	History, NCS, and EMG
	Monomelic spinal muscular atrophy (Hirayama disease)	EMG, MRI of cervical spine in flexion and extension
	Hexosaminidase A deficiency (late-onset Tay–Sachs disease)	Serum leukocyte Hex A activity and Hex A gene mutation analysis
CNS and spinal lesions	Syringomyelia or syringobulbia	MRI
	Tabes dorsalis	Syphilis serology
	Adrenomyeloneuropathy	Increased plasma levels of very-long-chain fatty acids
	Lyme disease	Lyme serology
	Hereditary spastic paraparesis	Family history, genetic testing
	Vacuolar myelopathy	HIV testing
	Tropical spastic paraparesis	Antibodies against HTLV1 may be detected in serum and CSF, MRI
	Spinocerebellar ataxia type 3 (Machado–Joseph disease)	Genetic testing
	Adult polyglucosan disease	NCS, EMG, and biopsy
	Subacute combined degeneration	Vitamin B12 concentration
Endocrine	Thyrotoxicosis	TFT
	Hyperparathyroidism	Serum calcium, parathyroid hormone levels

(AChR: acetylcholine receptor; ALS: amyotrophic lateral sclerosis; CAG: cytosine, adenine, guanine; CNS: central nervous system; CPK: creatine phosphokinase; CSF: cerebrospinal fluid; DNA: deoxyribonucleic acid; EMG: electromyography; GM1: ganglioside monosialic 1; HIV: human immunodeficiency virus; HTLV1: human T-lymphotropic virus type 1; MRI: magnetic resonance imaging; MuSK: muscle-specific kinase; NCS: nerve conduction study; POEMS: polyneuropathy, organomegaly, endocrinopathy, monoclonal gammopathy, and skin changes; RNS: repetitive nerve stimulation; SFEMG: single fiber electromyography; SMN: spinal motor neuron; TFT: thyroid function tests; VGCC: voltage-gated calcium channel; VGKC: voltage-gated potassium channel)

MANAGEMENT

Canadian best practice recommendations state that sending ALS patients to a multidisciplinary team early improves outcomes including survival, enhanced quality of life, increased use of adaptive equipment, and fewer hospital admissions.[21] Dedicated neurologists, rehabilitation specialists, pulmonary doctors, and gastroenterologists are frequently part of it. They address medical management as well as a broad range of issues including respiration and end-of-life care, nutrition and swallowing, cognition and psychosocial issues, communication, mobility, and activities of daily living. The ALS multidisciplinary clinic can be supplemented by telemedicine and telehealth monitoring with the clinic staff available for remote consultation between patient visits.[21]

Breaking the News

The news that a person or their family member has ALS can be devastating. It must be done with empathy, being careful not to take away hope and giving enough time for questions. It is important to find the right kind of words and use understandable terminology while checking for emotional responses and any distress to the family. It is best to disclose the diagnosis and its implication over more than one meeting and guide the patient to authentic resources where they can learn at their own pace. The neurologist can also direct these patients to local support groups. The SPIKES (Setting up, Perception, Invitation, Knowledge, Emotions with Empathy, and Strategy/Summary) protocol can be used as a template by healthcare professionals to break the bad news.[22]

Neurologists and caregivers should decide the timing of giving a diagnosis of ALS. An early diagnosis can give the patient the opportunity to enroll in a clinical trial and hence receive treatment that can potentially prolong their life. However, incorrectly diagnosing a patient with a terminal disease like ALS before being certain can cause a great deal of emotional distress. A lot of forethought should be given, and this decision should be carefully balanced.

Medical Therapy

There is no cure for ALS despite the disease being a focus of research for many decades. To date, only a few medications have somewhat increased survival rates.

- *Riluzole*: It is a glutamate antagonist and is dosed at 50 mg twice daily as a pill or in liquid form. It has demonstrated a 3-month increase in survival that continues into the illness's terminal clinical stage.[23]
- *Edaravone*: It is a free radical scavenger that is given intravenously at a dose of 60 mg per day for 2 weeks each month. After 6 months of treatment, there is a slight but significant reduction of functional decline according to the ALS functional rating scale—revised (ALSFRS-R), and a recent study revealed that the advantages are still there after 1 year.[24]
- *Sodium phenylbutyrate-taurursodiol*: Sodium phenylbutyrate is a histone deacetylase inhibitor that reduces endoplasmic reticulum stress by upregulating shock proteins. Taurursodiol reduces mitochondrial apoptosis by preventing the translocation of Bcl-2 Associated X-protein (BAX) into the mitochondrial membrane. Results of CENTAUR trial, a phase 2 randomized placebo-controlled clinical trial, showed that a co-formulated, fixed dose of sodium phenylbutyrate (3 g) and taurursodiol (1 g), when used as a therapy, can slow the rate of deterioration in ALSFRS-R score.[25] Sodium phenylbutyrate/taurursodiol was approved by FDA in September 2022.
- Nuedexta is a combination drug (dextromethorphan HBr 20 mg and quinidine sulfate 10 mg) indicated for pseudobulbar affect in ALS patients. It was Food and Drug Administration (FDA)-approved in 2011 and can reduce inappropriate crying and/or laughing episodes that happen unprovoked in ALS patients and often do not match how the patient is feeling.
- *High-dose methylcobalamin*: Japanese early stage trial of high-dose methylcobalamin for ALS (JETALS) done recently showed that the use of ultrahigh-dose methylcobalamin, i.e., 50 mg intramuscular injections, twice weekly for 16 weeks resulted in a 43% reduction in clinical deterioration as evaluated with the ALSFRS-R total score throughout the 16-week treatment period in patients with early stage ALS.[26]

Cellular and Gene Therapies

Cellular and gene therapies focus on delivering genetic material to cells that can modify gene expression by introducing functional copies of dysfunctional genes, delivering growth factors, or silencing the harmful expression of mutant genes. This is an active area of research, using results from genetic testing studies to design clinical trials for gene therapy. Antisense oligonucleotides (ASOs) are 8–50-base sequences of synthetic oligonucleotides that have shown success in clinical trials of spinal muscular atrophy (SMA) patients by inducing alternative splicing. These now serve as important proof-of-concept for ALS patients. A recent ASO intrathecal therapy in SOD1-associated fALS was found to be safe but failed to reach primary end-point efficacy.[27] In other pilot studies, ASOs in TDP-43[28] and FUS-linked fALS[29] were found to be feasible and safe. The ongoing research is focused both on understanding the disease mechanisms and on safe gene therapy platforms in fALS. ASO (Tofersen) was approved by SOD1-ALS by FDA based on biomarker changes in April 2023.

Noninvasive Brain Stimulation

The use of noninvasive brain stimulation (NIBS) in ALS treatment has the potential to be explored, as the biological effects of NIBS are being discovered. Proper standardization of technique and outcome measurement is required to fully evaluate the effect of NIBS in ALS patients.[30]

Symptom Management

It is necessary to manage the various symptoms in ALS patients in order to provide them with a better quality of life.

- *Pain*: It occurs late in the course of the disease but needs to be managed because it can significantly affect the quality of life of the patient. There are many different treatment options, and it is crucial to provide regular physical therapy to lessen the impact of immobilization as the disease advances.
- *Dysphagia*: To plan interventions and stop early deterioration, it is important to assess the swallowing function at the early stages of the disease. Despite the poor prognosis of ALS, effective management of dysphagia with diet and the use of postural compensation techniques delay the need for percutaneous endoscopic gastrostomy (PEG).
- *Nutrition management*: Significant dysphagia occurs in ALS patients as the disease progresses and involves bulbar muscles, which can cause them to become malnourished. Early preparation is necessary for identifying those who are at risk and for using PEG (or other alternative feeding techniques). This helps in maintaining body weight and improving the overall quality of life of the patient. The algorithm for PEG insertion in patients of ALS is given in **Flowchart 1**.[21]
- *Respiratory insufficiency management*: It is crucial to correctly diagnose and treat respiratory insufficiency in ALS. As soon as the signs of respiratory problems appear, an early discussion regarding all available treatment options, including noninvasive ventilation, invasive ventilation, and terminal palliative care, should take place. To facilitate advanced planning, patients and caregivers should be adequately informed about the management of respiration.
  - *Noninvasive ventilation*: Bilevel positive airway pressure or noninvasive intermittent positive pressure ventilation (NIPPVs) are recommended for noninvasive ventilation because both have been found to increase patient survival and quality of life.[31]
  - *Invasive ventilation*: When noninvasive breathing becomes inadequate (i.e., with progressive respiratory muscle involvement) or ineffective due to the course of the disease, invasive ventilation is an option. It should be considered on a case-by-case basis with prior counseling and the patient's living will. Although this method can prolong life, patients and caregivers must be thoroughly informed of

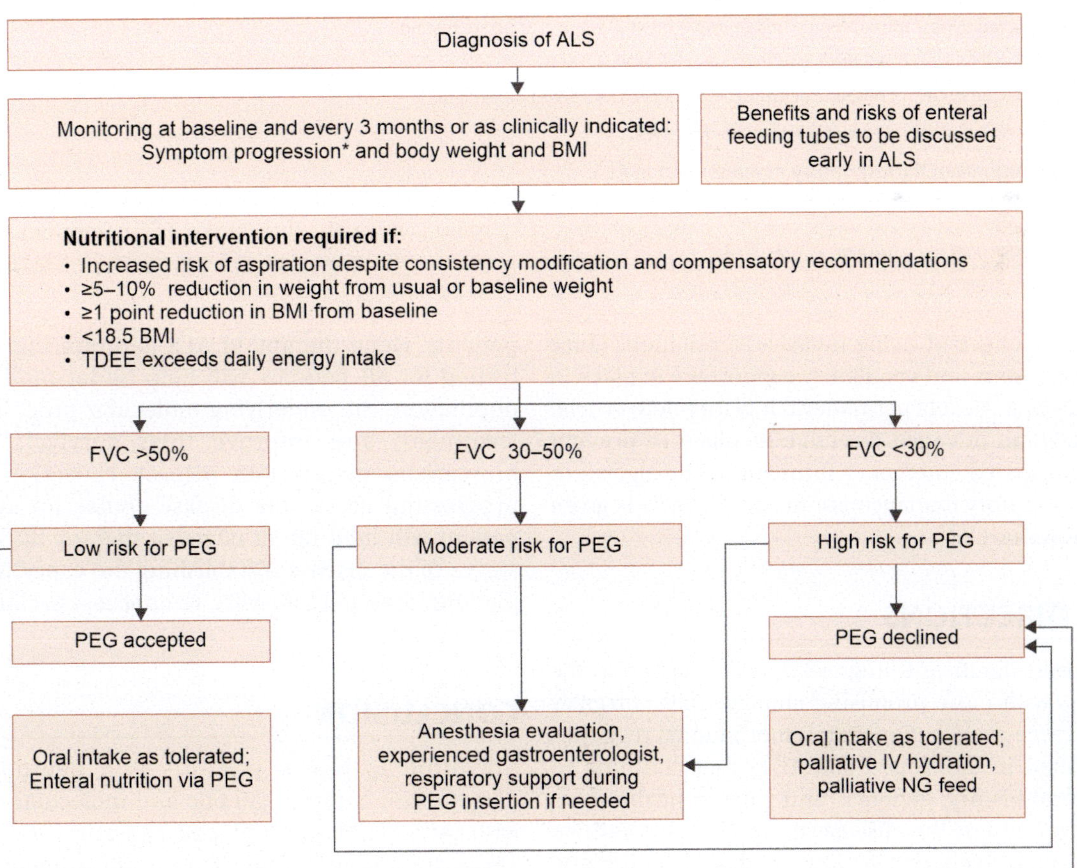

* Bulbar questions in amyotrophic lateral sclerosis functional rating scale-revised.

FLOWCHART 1: Algorithm for PEG insertion in patients with ALS.
(ALS: amyotrophic lateral sclerosis; BMI: body mass index; FVC: forced vital capacity; IV: intravenous fluid; NG: nasogastric tube; PEG: percutaneous enteral gastrostomy; TDEE: total daily energy expenditure)

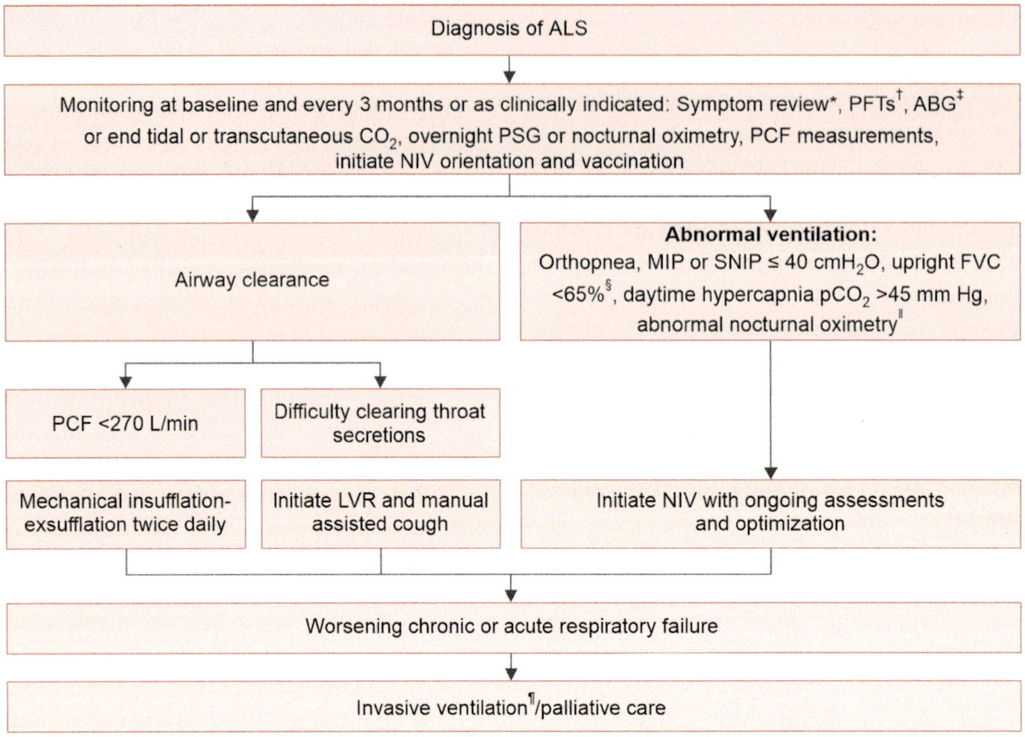

*Dyspnea, orthopnea, or morning headaches.

†Sitting FVC, supine FVC, or MIP and SNIP.

‡Perform when suspected hypercapnia or when bulbar impairment precludes accurate testing.

§FVC sitting or supine < 80% with respiratory insufficiency symptoms or signs.

‖Partial pressure of oxygen is <4% of baseline or symptomatic sleep disordered breathing.

¶If aligned with the patient's goals of care and advanced directives.

FLOWCHART 2: Algorithm for respiratory management in ALS.

(ABG: arterial blood gas; ALS: amyotrophic lateral sclerosis; FVC: forced vital capacity; H_2O: water; Hg: mercury; LVR: lung volume recruitment; MIP: maximal inspiratory pressure; NIV: noninvasive ventilation; PCF: peak cough flow; pCO_2: partial pressure of carbon dioxide; PFT: pulmonary function test; PSG: polysomnography; SNIP: sniff nasal inspiratory pressure)

the challenges of using invasive ventilation. Once tracheostomy and ventilatory support are in place in late ALS, it is likely permanent. It is therefore crucial to have an advance directive in place to prevent unanticipated emergency intubation. The algorithm for respiratory management in ALS patients is given in **Flowchart 2**.[21]

FUTURE DIRECTIONS

There has been significant progress in ALS research in the last 10 years with more promising clinical trials currently underway. Large-scale national and international registries are established in developed countries that continue to inform natural history, genetics, and gaps in health care. The heterogeneity of the disease makes it important to establish similar registries in low- and middle-income countries like India. Multidisciplinary care has shown improved survival rates, and it is important to identify and establish centers across India. The advent of telemedicine and telerehabilitation has improved access for some patients. Gene therapy in ALS is promising, and genetic testing for all patients will help understand our patient population, the underlying molecular processes, develop treatment, and improve their survival. Developing biomarkers involved in disease causation as well as progression across the disease course for an individual patient will help target effective therapy during different stages of the disease. Establishing the capacity to conduct platform trials in India will give us access to clinical trials for our patients.

CONCLUSION

Amyotrophic lateral sclerosis is a neurodegenerative disease with complex genetic and molecular mechanisms with varied etiology for disease causation and progression. There are currently four FDA-approved medications with modest effects in ALS. As the disease mechanisms in ALS are revealed, the future is promising with personalized treatment with drugs that target the underlying mechanisms in an individual.

REFERENCES

1. Longinetti E, Fang F. Epidemiology of amyotrophic lateral sclerosis: an update of recent literature. Curr Opin Neurol. 2019;32(5):771-6.
2. India State-Level Disease Burden Initiative Neurological Disorders Collaborators. The burden of neurological disorders across the states of India: the Global Burden of Disease Study 1990–2019. Lancet Glob Health. 2021;9(8):e1129-44.
3. Al-Chalabi A, Calvo A, Chio A, Colville S, Ellis CM, Hardiman O, et al. Analysis of amyotrophic lateral sclerosis as a multistep process: a population-based modelling study. Lancet Neurol. 2014;13(11):1108-13.
4. Bonafede R, Mariotti R. ALS pathogenesis and therapeutic approaches: the role of mesenchymal stem cells and extracellular vesicles. Front Cell Neurosci. 2017;11:80.
5. Hardiman O, Al-Chalabi A, Chio A, Corr EM, Logroscino G, Robberecht W, et al. Amyotrophic lateral sclerosis. Nat Rev Dis Primers. 2017;3:17071.
6. Opie-Martin S, Iacoangeli A, Topp SD, Abel O, Mayl K, Mehta PR, et al. The SOD1-mediated ALS phenotype shows a decoupling between age of symptom onset and disease duration. Nat Commun. 2022;13(1):6901.
7. Gossye H, Engelborghs S, Van Broeckhoven C, van der Zee J. C9orf72 Frontotemporal Dementia and/or Amyotrophic Lateral Sclerosis. In: Adam MP, Everman DB, Mirzaa GM, Pagon RA, Wallace SE, Bean LJH, et al. (Eds). GeneReviews®. Seattle: University of Washington; 2020
8. McCluskey L, Vandriel S, Elman L, Van Deerlin VM, Powers J, Boller A, et al. ALS-plus syndrome: nonpyramidal features in a large ALS cohort. J Neurol Sci. 2014;345(1-2):118-24.
9. Yunusova Y, Plowman EK, Green JR, Barnett C, Bede P. Clinical measures of bulbar dysfunction in ALS. Front Neurol. 2019;10:106.
10. Corcia P, Honnorat J, Guennoc AM, de Toffol B, Autret A. [Primary lateral sclerosis with breast cancer, a potential paraneoplastic neurological syndrome]. Rev Neurol (Paris). 2000;156(11):1020-2.
11. Chen S, Sayana P, Zhang X, Le W. Genetics of amyotrophic lateral sclerosis: an update. Mol Neurodegener. 2013;8(1):28.
12. Wijesekera LC, Mathers S, Talman P, Galtrey C, Parkinson MH, Ganesalingam J, et al. Natural history and clinical features of the flail arm and flail leg ALS variants. Neurology. 2009;72(12):1087-94.
13. Spencer PS, Fry RC, Palmer VS, Kisby GE. Western Pacific ALS-PDC: a prototypical neurodegenerative disorder linked to DNA damage and aberrant proteogenesis? Front Neurol. 2012;3:180.
14. Brooks BR, Miller RG, Swash M, World Federation of Neurology Research Group on Motor Neuron Diseases. El Escorial revisited: revised criteria for the diagnosis of amyotrophic lateral sclerosis. Amyotroph Lateral Scler Other Motor Neuron Disord. 2000;1(5):293-9.
15. Costa J, Swash M, de Carvalho M. Awaji criteria for the diagnosis of amyotrophic lateral sclerosis: a systematic review. Arch Neurol. 2012;69(11):1410-6.
16. Turner MR, UK MND Clinical Studies Group. Diagnosing ALS: the Gold Coast criteria and the role of EMG. Pract Neurol. 2022;22(3):176-8.
17. de Carvalho M. Electrodiagnosis of amyotrophic lateral sclerosis: a review of existing guidelines. J Clin Neurophysiol. 2020;37(4):294-8.
18. Chiò A, Pagani M, Agosta F, Calvo A, Cistaro A, Filippi M. Neuroimaging in amyotrophic lateral sclerosis: insights into structural and functional changes. Lancet Neurol. 2014;13(12):1228-40.
19. Smukowski SN, Maioli H, Latimer CS, Bird TD, Jayadev S, Valdmanis PN. Progress in amyotrophic lateral sclerosis gene discovery: reflecting on classic approaches and leveraging emerging technologies. Neurol Genet. 2022;8(3):e669.
20. Salmon K, Kiernan MC, Kim SH, Andersen PM, Chio A, van den Berg LH, et al. The importance of offering early genetic testing in everyone with amyotrophic lateral sclerosis. Brain. 2022;145(4):1207-10.
21. Shoesmith C, Abrahao A, Benstead T, Chum M, Dupre N, Izenberg A, et al. Canadian best practice recommendations for the management of amyotrophic lateral sclerosis. CMAJ. 2020;192(46):E1453-68.
22. Rosenzweig MQ. Breaking bad news: a guide for effective and empathetic communication. Nurse Pract. 2012;37(2):1-4.
23. Fang T, Al Khleifat A, Meurgey J-H, Jones A, Leigh PN, Bensimon G, et al. Stage at which riluzole treatment prolongs survival in patients with amyotrophic lateral sclerosis: a retrospective analysis of data from a dose-ranging study. Lancet Neurol. 2018;17(5):416-22.
24. Shefner J, Heiman-Patterson T, Pioro EP, Wiedau-Pazos M, Liu S, Zhang J, et al. Long-term edaravone efficacy in amyotrophic lateral sclerosis: post-hoc analyses of Study 19 (MCI186-19). Muscle Nerve. 2020;61(2):218-21.
25. Paganoni S, Macklin EA, Hendrix S, Berry JD, Elliott MA, Maiser S, et al. Trial of sodium phenylbutyrate–taurursodiol for amyotrophic lateral sclerosis. N Engl J Med. 2020;383(10):919-30.
26. Oki R, Izumi Y, Fujita K, Miyamoto R, Nodera H, Sato Y, et al.; Japan Early Stage Trial of Ultrahigh-Dose Methylcobalamin for ALS (JETALS) Collaborators. Efficacy and safety of ultrahigh-dose methylcobalamin in early stage amyotrophic lateral sclerosis: a randomized clinical trial. JAMA Neurol. 2022;79(6):575-83.
27. Miller T, Cudkowicz M, Shaw PJ, Andersen PM, Atassi N, Bucelli RC, et al. Phase 1–2 trial of antisense oligonucleotide tofersen for SOD1 ALS. N Engl J Med. 2020;383(2):109-19.
28. Brown A-L, Wilkins OG, Keuss MJ, Hill SE, Zanovello M, Lee WC, et al. TDP-43 loss and ALS-risk SNPs drive mis-splicing and depletion of UNC13A. Nature. 2022;603(7899):131-7.
29. Korobeynikov VA, Lyashchenko AK, Blanco-Redondo B, Jafar-Nejad P, Shneider NA. Antisense oligonucleotide silencing of FUS expression as a therapeutic approach in amyotrophic lateral sclerosis. Nat Med. 2022;28(1):104-16.
30. Edmond EC, Stagg CJ, Turner MR. Therapeutic noninvasive brain stimulation in amyotrophic lateral sclerosis: rationale, methods, and experience. J Neurol Neurosurg Psychiatry. 2019;90(10):1131-8.
31. Kim J, Bireley JD, Hayat G, Kafaie J. Effects of noninvasive ventilation in amyotrophic lateral sclerosis: the complication of bulbar impairment. Clin Transl Neurosci. 2020;4(1):8.

81

CHAPTER

Inherited Neuropathies

Shivani Sharma, Madhu Nagappa

INTRODUCTION

The inherited neuropathies are clinically and genetically heterogeneous groups of diseases affecting the peripheral nerves. These disorders may predominantly affect the peripheral nerves or may cause complex inherited neuropathy syndromes wherein neuropathy coexists with other phenotypes such as spasticity, ataxia, and global developmental delay among others. When peripheral nerves are the predominant or sole target, the following entities are recognized:

- *Diffuse neuropathies*: Hereditary motor and sensory neuropathy (HMSN) which involves both motor and sensory nerves, distal hereditary motor neuropathy (dHMN) which affects only motor nerves, and hereditary sensory and autonomic neuropathy (HSAN) which affects sensory and autonomic nerve fibers
- *Focal neuropathies*: Hereditary neuropathy with liability to pressure palsies (HNPP) and hereditary neuralgic amyotrophy (HNA). These disorders are either familial [autosomal dominant (AD), autosomal recessive (AR), or X-linked (XL)] or sporadic.[1]

HEREDITARY MOTOR AND SENSORY NEUROPATHY

Hereditary motor and sensory neuropathies constitute the most common inherited neuropathies and are also referred to as Charcot–Marie–Tooth diseases (CMTs). These are a heterogeneous group of disorders that have in common slowly progressive motor and sensory dysfunction leading to distal symmetrical weakness of the limbs, hypo/areflexia, and skeletal deformities, which are more pronounced in lower limbs as compared to upper limbs. They can be broadly categorized on the basis of electrophysiological studies:

- *Myelinopathies*: With predominant involvement of peripheral myelin wherein nerve conduction velocities are reduced
- *Axonopathies*: With predominant involvement of peripheral nerve axons wherein amplitudes of compound muscle action potentials are reduced with normal or slightly reduced nerve conduction velocities

Besides this, there are several other ways by which the CMTs can be classified.[2] Based on the age at onset, they may be neonatal/"congenital," early infantile (<2 years), childhood (2–10 years), juvenile (10–20 years), adult (20–50 years), and late adult onset (>50 years). Broadly, those with age at onset less than 10 years of age are classified as having an "early onset" CMT. In general, early onset CMT has rapid progression, greater disability, and worse prognosis as compared to late-onset CMT. Based on the patterns of inheritance, they are classified as AD, AR, and XL disorders. The AD pattern of inheritance is the most common. One of the early classifications of HMSN, which took into account the key clinical features, inheritance pattern, and electrophysiological and pathological characteristics, is as follows:

- HMSN IA, B
- HMSN II
- HMSN III (Dejerine–Sottas disease)
- HMSN IV (Refsum disease)
- HMSN V (+ paraplegia)
- HMSN VI (+ optic atrophy)
- HMSN VII (+ retinitis pigmentosa)

While HMSN is generally used interchangeably with CMT, this is most appropriate for HMSN I and II only, and there exists some degree of lack of concurrence among the nosological terms provided in the subsequent classifications. For example, recessively inherited demyelinating CMTs have been designated as CMT4, while in the earlier classification HMSN IV referred to Refsum disease. HMSN I or CMT1 and HMSN II or CMT2 refer to demyelinating and axonal neuropathies, respectively, that are autosomal dominantly inherited. In addition, the entity of CMTX is an XL disorder.

Likewise, HMSN III or the Dejerine–Sottas disease, which referred to a severe phenotype with onset in infancy or childhood and severe generalized neurologic deficit, has now been shown to be caused by mutations in several different genes, and this term is no longer used. Thus, with technological advances, it was considered appropriate to classify the CMTs based on genetic abnormality, and an alphabet was assigned to each subtype. But the number of genetic causes has now exceeded 26 letters; thus, there is no longer scope for a unique individual alphabet match. Further, a significant overlap was recognized not only in the inheritance patterns but also in the clinical-electrophysiological phenotypes of CMTs caused by any given genetic mutation. For example, mutations in *MPZ* were initially identified as a cause for the dominant demyelinating CMT1B, but were later found to be associated with dominant axonal the subtype (CMT2I/J) as well. Mutations in *TRPV4* were linked to CMT2C, and subsequently to dHMN. Even the pattern of inheritance varies; *GDAP1* mutations were initially linked to recessive demyelinating CMT4A, but were subsequently identified in dominant axonal CMT2K.

Hence, a revised classification has been proposed that incorporates the mode of inheritance (AD, AR, or XL), the phenotype (CMT, dHMN), electrophysiology (demyelinating: "de," axonal: "ax," intermediate: "in"), and causal gene. Thus, CMT1A would be redesignated as AD-CMTde-*PMP22dup*, CMT2A2 as AD-CMTax-*MFN2*, and CMTX as XL-CMTin-*GJB1*.[3]

The pathophysiology of HMSN has been elucidated to some extent. Schwann cells and axons are the key players in the efficient and rapid propagation of action potential along the nerve. They exhibit close anatomical and physiological interaction and regulate nerve function. Axons determine the survival, proliferation, and differentiation of Schwann cells. Schwann cells in turn play an important role in regulating ion channels, and the maintenance, survival, and regeneration of axons. Any disruption of this close-knit unit results in neuropathy. Abnormalities in several molecular and cellular mechanisms that control myelin formation and stability, membrane trafficking, and intracellular proteostasis, among others, lead to alteration in the structure and function of Schwann cells **(Table 1)**. Because of the close functional interaction, demyelinating neuropathies lead to functional axonopathies and clinically manifest secondary axonal degeneration. Thus, common secondary phenomena in CMTs include axonal loss, secondary Schwann cell proliferation, and acceleration of pathology due to immune-mediated mechanisms.[4]

Clinical Manifestations

Age at onset ranges from infancy to elderly, but the majority have onset within the first two decades of life. Since the clinical progression of CMT neuropathy is usually slow, the exact age at onset is often difficult to estimate.

TABLE 1: Molecular and cellular mechanisms implicated in various hereditary motor and sensory neuropathies (HMSNs).

Pathophysiological mechanisms	Genes
Myelin assembly	
Interaction of Schwann cells with extracellular matrix, regulating cell spreading, cell migration, and apoptosis	*PMP22, PMP2*
Myelin compaction	*MPZ*
Formation of gap junctions	*GJB1*
Cytoskeletal structure	
Actin polymerization	*INF2*
Membrane-protein interactions, stabilize myelin sheath	*PRX*
Intermediate filaments	*NEFL*
Cell signaling	*FGD4*
Axonal transport	*DYNC1H1*
Endosomal sorting and cell signaling	
Schwann cell associated	*LITAF, MTMR2, MTMR13, SBF1, SBF2, SH3TC2, NDRG1, FIG4, RAB7A, TFG, DNM2, SIMPLE*
Axons associated	*RAB7, DNM2, GNB4, WNK1, IKBKAP, NTRK1, NGF-β*
Synaptic transmission	*DCTN1, SLC5A7*
Membrane trafficking	*ARHGEF10, DNM2, LITAF, MTMR2, MTMR13, RAB7, SH3TC2, TFG*
Endoplasmic reticulum and Golgi	*ATL1, BSCL2, DGAT2, FAM134B, REEP1, TFG*
Proteasome and protein aggregation	
Microtubules	*HSPB1, HSPB8, CCT5, TUBB3*
Cell adhesion	*LRSAM1, PRNP, CADM3*
Ubiquitin ligase	*TRIM2, DCAF8*
Protein degradation	*DNAJB2, RNF170, PLEKHG5*
Mitochondria	
Mitochondrial dynamics, structure and function of respiratory chain	*MFN2, GDAP1, MT-ATP6, PDK3, DHTKD1, HK1, AIFM1, SURF1, SLC25A46*
Others	
Cell fusion–fission apparatus	*DNM2*
Calcium homeostasis	*TRPV4*
Glucose metabolism	*HK1*
Sphingolipid biosynthesis	*SPTLC1, SPTLC2*
Transcription	*EGR2, HINT1, PRPS1, AARS, GARS, HARS, KARS, MARS, NARS1, YARS, CTDP1, HINT1, SETX, IGHMBP2, MED25*
Chaperones	*HSPB1, HSPB3, HSPB8*
Motor proteins and axonal transport	*DCTN1, KIF21A, HSPB1, NEFL, BICD2, DYNC1H1, KIF1A, KIF5A, MYH14*

The common clinical features are the presence of distal symmetrical weakness, wasting, hypo/areflexia, and deformities which are more pronounced in lower limbs as compared to upper limbs. Deformities in the form of pes cavus and hammer toes can occur. Patients classically manifest with steppage gait and distal lower limb amyotrophy, giving an appearance of "jambes de coq" or an inverted champagne bottle **(Fig. 1A)**. Involvement of distal upper limbs occurs later in the course of the disease and results in "main en griffe" or claw hands **(Fig. 1B)**. Sensory symptoms and signs are relatively less prominent. About 20–30% of patients complain of pain, which is often musculoskeletal and rarely neuropathic. Other characteristic features such as abnormal gait and imbalance occur because of proprioceptive loss and skeletal deformities, namely pes cavus and hammertoes. Scoliosis may be present. Life expectancy is usually not affected. Severity is varied, spanning a spectrum from mildly symptomatic forms to severe disability. Demyelinating CMTs are characterized by reduced nerve conduction velocity. However, the clinical manifestations are the result of the reduced amplitude of compound muscle action potential, which is a reflection of axonal loss. Slowed velocities can be demonstrated even before the clinical manifestations and hence, they do not correlate with the severity.

A fraction of subjects develops neuropathy in the neonatal period or during infancy. This early onset CMT traditionally includes congenital hypomyelinating neuropathy and Dejerine–Sottas disease. Affected individuals typically manifest with foot deformities, delayed motor milestones, difficulty in walking, and impaired sensation. Severe phenotypes manifest with neonatal hypotonia, difficulty in feeding, and respiratory compromise. Most of these occur sporadically due to *de novo* dominant mutations or recessive alleles inherited from heterozygous carrier parents. Electrophysiological studies show features of demyelinating neuropathy in the majority, with marked slowing of conduction velocities. The most commonly implicated genes are *MPZ*, *PMP22*, and *EGR2*. Early and severe scoliosis is suggestive of, but not an exclusive feature of, *SH3TC2* mutations. The following sections describe the clinical, electrophysiological, and histological features of the most common demyelinating (*PMP22*, *MPZ*, *GJB1*) and axonal (*MFN2*) CMTs.[5]

PMP22-associated Neuropathies

Charcot-Marie-Tooth disease type 1A caused by duplication of *PMP22* is the most prevalent inherited neuropathy. It manifests commonly in late childhood or adolescence. The genetic abnormality has complete penetrance though the age at onset is varied. The clinical presentation is that of peroneal muscular atrophy, pes cavus, mild-to-moderate distal sensory loss, and uniform slowing of nerve conduction velocities. Calf hypertrophy instead of atrophy may be found. Intra- and interfamilial phenotypic variability concerning age at onset, motor deficit, sensory loss, and motor conduction velocities even between monozygotic twins is recognized, despite the common genetic change. It has been hypothesized that modifier genes such as single nucleotide polymorphism in *SH3TC2*, inflammation, or other factors may influence disability in CMT1A. Concomitant illnesses such as hypothyroidism, diabetes, obesity, and toxin exposure have been found to cause increased impairment in patients with CMT1A. Histological studies of the nerve show hypertrophic neuropathy with segmental demyelination and remyelination, and loss of large-diameter fibers and onion bulbs.

On the other hand, mutations in *PMP22* are uncommon and account for only 1–5% of all CMTs. These include single base substitutions (missense, nonsense, silent), deletions, and insertions in the coding region of *PMP22*. In addition, reciprocal translocation, splice-site mutations, and single base substitutions have also been reported in the noncoding exon 1A and three prime untranslated region (3′-UTR). The majority of these mutations are located in the four transmembrane domains of *PMP22*; nearly all

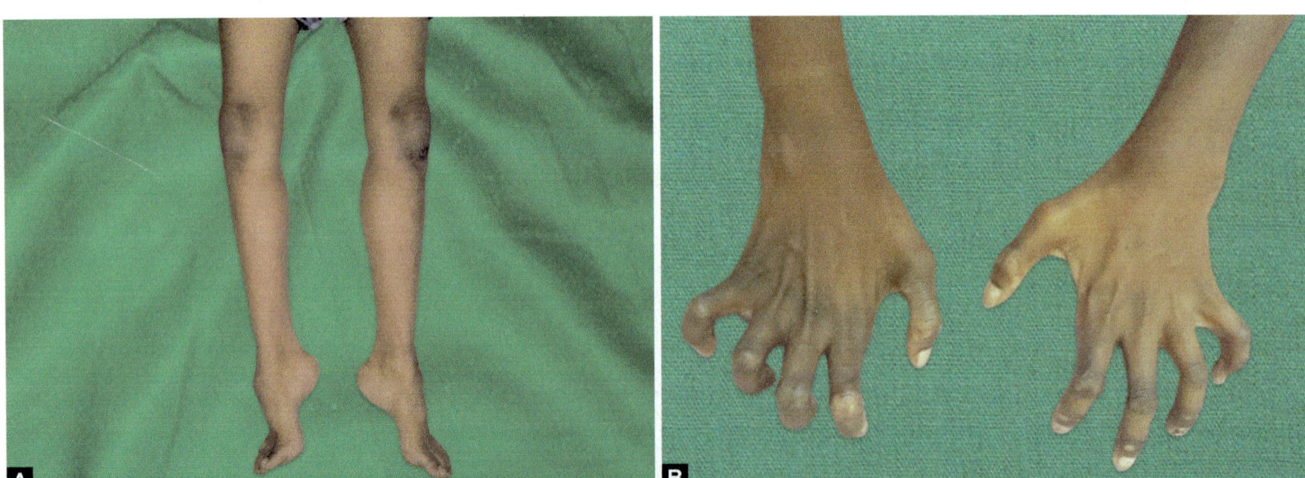

FIGS. 1A AND B: Patient with hereditary motor and sensory neuropathy with (A) pes cavus and (B) clawing of fingers.

are autosomal dominantly inherited, though uncommon mutations with AR and hemizygous states are also reported. Mutations in *PMP22* may be associated with the more severe phenotypes, Dejerine-Sottas syndrome type 1A, and congenital hypomyelinating neuropathy type 1A. Affected patients have slower conduction velocities and cranial nerve involvement such as ptosis, pale optic discs, facial weakness, and deafness. Other clinical features include nystagmus, lip or chin myokymia, and Ehlers-Danlos syndrome.[6]

MPZ-associated Neuropathy

Charcot-Marie-Tooth disease type 1B is caused by mutations in *MPZ* and is the second most common form of the AD hereditary demyelinating neuropathy. More than 200 different disease-causing mutations have been identified in *MPZ*. Clinical features include impaired hearing, scoliosis, optic atrophy, hip dysplasia, and delay in achieving the walking milestone. Very slow motor conduction velocities (<15 m/s) are observed among those with infantile onset. Intermediate slow (36–45 m/s) and normal (>45 m/s) motor conduction velocities are noted in patients with adult onset. Infantile onset correlates with a worse disability, slower conduction velocities, and increasing severity with age as compared to childhood or adult onset. Half of the subjects with infantile onset require aids or wheelchairs for ambulation.

Thus, mutations in *MPZ* that cause infantile-onset neuropathy disrupt the normal development of myelin such that it is not formed, and this is reflected as extremely slow nerve conduction velocities and symptom onset during the period of motor development. In childhood onset, myelin sheaths are more fully formed, but are abnormal, as evidenced by motor nerve conduction velocities that are in the range of 20–25 m/s. On the other hand, adult onset is characterized by normal myelin sheaths, degeneration of myelinated axons with normal or near normal nerve conduction velocities, and clinical appearance of an axonal neuropathy, even though *MPZ* is only expressed by myelinating Schwann cells. Specific mutations in *MPZ* are linked to specific phenotypes. For instance, mutations that introduce a cysteine into the extracellular loop (Tyr82Cys, Arg98Cys, Ser111Cys, and Ser123Cys) disrupt the disulfide bridge that is essential for maintaining the 3D structure of *MPZ*. This activates an intracellular process called the unfolded protein response, prevents myelination, and results in infantile-onset disease.[6]

GJB1-associated Neuropathy

X-linked CMT is usually caused by mutations in *GJB1*. It is the second most frequent form of CMT after CMT1A. Electrophysiologically, a mixed demyelinating and axonal pattern is seen with velocities often being in the "intermediate" range. The neuropathy manifests at a younger age and is more severe in males, while females are either asymptomatic or oligosymptomatic. Thus, males have higher functional disability scores. Clinical features include weakness, amyotrophy, impaired proprioception, and pes cavus. Other features include tremors and sensorineural hearing loss. Atrophy may be asymmetrical.

Central nervous system involvement is a recognized feature of *GJB1* mutations. Diffuse hyperintensity of cerebral white matter, which is prominent posteriorly, and involvement of splenium of the corpus callosum have been reported. Respiratory distress, pseudobulbar syndrome, transient and reversible weakness of limbs, dysarthria, aphasia, cranial nerve palsies, and white matter lesions in the brain have been reported. Multiaxial neurological involvement with cerebellar dysfunction, pyramidal signs, and sensorimotor polyneuropathy has been described.

The majority of the mutations in *GJB1* are located in the extracellular loop domains. The clinical severity and age at onset may be influenced by the nature and site of mutations. For example, Cys64Tyr and Val170Phe mutations are associated with a relatively severe phenotype, while Lys260Glu and His100Gln cause only moderate disability. Deletion of the entire coding sequence of *GJB1* has been reported to cause the early onset and severe phenotype in some but not in all cases. Nonfunctional mutations manifest in the first decade of life.[6]

MFN2-associated Neuropathy

The onset of *MFN2*-associated neuropathy ranges from the first to the sixth decade of life. Both the central and peripheral nervous systems can be affected in patients with *MFN2* variations. Patients present with the typical CMT phenotype with wasting and weakness of intrinsic muscles of the foot and ankle dorsiflexors (footdrop), deformities (pes cavus), and later involving leg muscles. The previously described HMSN VI (neuropathy and optic atrophy) is now recognized to be caused by *MFN2* mutations. Patients with optic atrophy manifest with severe visual impairment that develops subacutely, or sometimes acutely and mimics "optic neuritis." The ophthalmological evaluation shows central scotoma, defective color vision, pale optic discs, and normal intraocular tension. Optic atrophy may precede or follow the symptoms of neuropathy. A few patients have pyramidal signs in the form of brisk stretch reflexes and extensor plantar responses, a phenotype that was previously labeled as HMSN V. However, pyramidal signs are seen only when neuropathy is mild or moderate and they disappear when the severity of the disease increases. Acute onset mimicking an inflammatory polyradiculoneuropathy and psychomotor "regression" and subsequent significant recovery have been uncommonly described. Prominent sensory symptoms at the onset of disease in the form of burning or impaired sensations have also been reported rarely.

Other neurological features in patients with *MFN2*-associated neuropathy include motor developmental delay, mental retardation, ataxia, sensorineural hearing loss, hoarseness, diaphragmatic weakness, tremor, stroke, involuntary movements, scoliosis, contractures, asymmetrical neuropathy, and sleep disorders. Autonomic features such as erectile dysfunction, vasomotor dysfunction, increased sweating, and gastrointestinal dysmotility have also been described. Other uncommon features included low-set ears, high forehead, fetal pads, cryptorchidism, single transverse palmar crease, lipomatosis, lipodystrophy, hip dysplasia, and reduced vital capacity. *MFN2* variations can also cause mitochondrial depletion syndromes and result in fatal syndromes characterized by myopathy, hepatocerebropathy, and encephalomyopathy.

Most of the variations are located in the GTPase domain of the *MFN2*. Patients harboring the same variation have been shown to have disabilities ranging from mild to severe. Besides, there is nonuniformity in the penetrance and expressivity of different neurological features.[6]

Additional Features

In addition to the classical phenotype of distal wasting, weakness, and deformities, several additional features have been reported. Pupillary abnormalities have been reported in patients with copy number variations in *PMP22* and mutations in *MPZ* and *GJB1*. They include tonic pupils, miosis, mydriasis, anisocoria, and impaired pupillary reaction. Besides, pain and paresthesias, which are considered to be a feature of acquired neuropathies, have been described in patients with *PMP22, MPZ,* and other neuropathies. Patients with specific mutations in *MPZ*, namely Thr124Met and Gly123Ala, present with late-onset phenotype with pupillary abnormalities, shooting pains, and painful paresthesias, sometimes with rapid progression. Even autoimmune disorders such as systemic lupus erythematosus and autoimmune thyroiditis have been reported in association with *PMP22* duplication. Focal segmental glomerulosclerosis is seen in patients with mutations in *INF2*. The prevalence of restless leg syndrome (RLS) is significantly increased in patients with hereditary neuropathies as compared to the general population. Axonal loss, irrespective of the CMT subtype, increases axonal excitability in primary sensory units of leg muscles, leading to creeping sensations and RLS. Other features include deafness, vocal cord palsy, impaired cognition, dysphagia, respiratory insufficiency, tremor, dysphagia, dysarthria, fasciculations, cold-induced cramps, scoliosis, hip dysplasia, and hand deformities among others **(Table 2)**. Acute worsening resembling inflammatory polyradiculoneuropathies has also been reported.[5]

TABLE 2: Unusual neurological and systemic features in various hereditary motor and sensory neuropathies (HMSNs).

Clinical feature	Genes
Early proximal weakness	*MTMR2, MTM2, TFG*
Upper limb involvement	*GARS, REEP1, BSCL2, HSPB8*
Scoliosis	*MFN2, TRPV4, GARS, GDAP1, HSPB8, LMNA, PMP22, MPZ, PRX, EGR2, MTM2, MTM13, SH3TC2, NDRG1, ERG2, PRX, HK1, FDG4, FIG4, SLC12A6, GARS, NEFL, GNB4, LMNA, HINT1*
Optic atrophy	*MFN2, GDAP1, AIFM1, PRPS1, SLC25A46, INAD, SLC12A6, PDXK*
Glaucoma	*SBF2*
Cataract	*CTDP1, CMT2M, DNM2, PAHX, ABHD12*
Abnormal pupils	*MPZ, EGR2, PMP22, GJB1*
Restricted eye movements	*TUBB3*
Ptosis	*EGR2, DNM2, SLC12A6*
Macular degeneration	*FBLN5*
Deafness	*PMP22, NEFL, SH3TC2, NDRG1, GJB1, AIFM1, PRPS1, GJB3, INF2, PTRH2, MPZ, MFN2, TRPV4, EGR2, KARS, FDG4*
Vocal cord involvement	*PMP22, EGR2, MFN2, TRPV4, c, DCTN1, GARS, TRIM2*
Bulbar involvement	*PMP22, GJB1, HSPB1, GBF1, SPTLC3*
Hemifacial spasm	*MPZ*
Trigeminal neuralgia	*MPZ*
Diaphragm/respiratory involvement	*PMP22, TRPV4, MPZ, EGR2, GDAP1, MTM2, IGHMBP2, GARS, TRIM2, MTMR2, SLC12A6*
Upper motor neuron	*GDAP1, MFN2, KIF5A, SETX, GARS, BSCL2, NEFL, KARS*
Cognitive impairment/intellectual disability	*PMP22, HSPB1, DYNC1H1, INF2, KARS, FIG4, SLC12A6, AIFM1, SLC12A6, GAN, CTDP1, MCM3AP, MTMR13, EMILIN1, DYNC1H1, MCM3AP*
Seizures	*AARS, KARS, FIG4, SLC12A6*

Continued

Continued

Clinical feature	Genes
White matter involvement	*MFN2, GJB1, SLC12A6, INF2*
Ataxia	*PMP22, SH3TC2, SGJB1, NEFL, IFRD1, PNKP, MME, KARS, FIG4, NEFL (episodic ataxia)*
Tremor	*FBLN5, PDK3, MFN2, NEFL, SORD, KARS, SLC12A6*
Extrapyramidal signs	*AARS, KARS*
Transient encephalopathy/episodic weakness	*GJB1*
Microcephaly	*AARS, KARS, MTMR13*
Neuromyotonia	*HINT1*
Unilateral brachial plexopathy	*DRP2*
Cramps	*GARS, MPZ, PNKP, LRSAM1, HINT1, MME*
Fasciculation	*EGR2, HSPB1, HINT1, SORD*
Pain, paresthesias, dysesthesias	*PMP22, MPZ, MME, PNKP, GDAP1, LRSAM1, GNB4*
Contractures	*EGR2, NEFL, GARS, TRIM2, MME*
Arthrogryposis	*MFN2, TRPV4*
Carpal tunnel syndrome	*FBLN5*
Renal involvement	*INF2*
Hyperelastic skin, joint hypermobility	*FBLN5, EMILIN1*
Hyperkeratosis	*NEFL*
Neutropenia	*DNM2*

Electrophysiology

Nerve conduction studies (NCS) are essential to confirm the clinical diagnosis and further categorize patients broadly into demyelinating and axonal phenotypes. The key parameters that are measured are distal latencies, amplitudes, and velocities of motor and sensory nerves. Slowing of conduction velocities is an indirect measure of myelin function. Reduction in amplitudes of evoked motor responses and sensory potentials reflects the degree of axonal loss and this correlates with clinical disability irrespective of whether the patient has the primary axonal or demyelinating type of HMSN.

The median nerve conduction velocity of 38 m/s is the commonly used cutoff for differentiating demyelinating from axonal types. In addition, an intermediate form is recognized where the nerve conduction velocity ranging from 30 to 40 m/s, 25 to 45 m/s, and 35 to 45 m/s have been reported by different authors. In severely affected early onset demyelinating CMT, namely Dejerine–Sottas syndrome or congenital hypomyelinating neuropathy, there is profound slowing with median motor conduction velocity being <15 m/s. Based on nerve conduction velocities, CMTs have further been categorized into: (1) very slow (<15 m/s), (2) slow (15–35 m/s), (3) intermediate (35–45 m/s), and (4) normal (>45 m/s). This classification is useful for selecting genetic testing for patients with inherited neuropathies. Often patients present late in the course of their disease, and the compound muscle action potentials are not recordable. In this situation, it is challenging to distinguish primary axonal from demyelinating forms of CMT. Here, studies of proximal nerves, namely musculocutaneous, and radial nerves may be helpful.[5]

Slowing is usually uniform and diffuse in inherited neuropathies, unlike acquired etiologies, where the changes are nonhomogeneous and asymmetrical. However, in *GJB1*-associated neuropathy, motor conduction is nonuniform and heterogeneous within a single nerve and between multiple nerves, with the conduction velocity being more significantly reduced in the median as compared to the ulnar nerve. This internerve heterogeneity is prominent in females and is hypothesized to be due to the phenomenon of lyonization. On the other hand, demyelination is more pronounced and uniform in affected males as reflected by severely reduced conduction velocities. Likewise, temporal dispersion and conduction blocks are usually absent in inherited neuropathies, but exceptionally, temporal dispersion can occur in *GJB1* mutations.[1]

Imaging of Peripheral Nerves

With technological advances in imaging, it is now possible to visualize the morphological appearance of the nerves throughout their anatomical course, including the proximal plexuses and roots, which are not easily accessible for electrophysiological testing. Thus, magnetic resonance imaging (MRI) and high-resolution ultrasound (HRUS) complement the clinical evaluation and the data regarding the functional status of nerves provided by electrophysiology. HRUS, being available at the point of care, less time-consuming, and inexpensive, may be more advantageous as compared to MRI, but is operator dependent.

In inherited neuropathies, MRI and HRUS show markedly and diffusely enlarged nerves throughout their lengths, from the roots to the distal extremities. This has been consistently demonstrated in CMT1A caused by *PMP22* duplication. The nerve enlargement correlates with clinical disability and electrophysiological parameters. However, in other CMTs, this enlargement of nerves is not as consistent or as remarkable as in CMT1A. In patients with inexcitable electrophysiology, the presence of markedly enlarged nerves may guide the clinician to perform genetic testing for demyelinating HMSN, particularly to look for copy number variations in *PMP22*.[1]

Genetics

At the molecular genetic level, CMTs are very heterogeneous with mutations in more than 100 genes recognized so far, and the number is increasing. All possible modes of inheritance are recognized. The most frequently mutated gene is *PMP22*, and the most common genetic defect is duplication, leading to CMT1A. This copy number variation can be detected by a simple test such as multiplex ligation-dependent probe amplification (MLPA), which is quick, inexpensive, and reliable.

Sanger sequencing of the individual genes is the "gold standard" in molecular genetic diagnosis. However, given the large number of genes implicated in CMT and the lack of specific phenotypic distinguishing features, it is cumbersome and extremely time-consuming to sequentially analyze each gene. In this situation, the newer high-throughput genetic sequencing techniques, or next-generation sequencing (NGS), are gaining ground. They include whole genome sequencing (WGS), whole exome sequencing (WES), clinical exome sequencing (CES), and targeted gene panels that analyze only a limited number of genes. These are efficient concerning the cost, yield, and time taken to perform the test. They are useful if copy number variations in common genes (*PMP22*) are excluded. But the caveat is that they lead to the identification of a large number of variants of uncertain significance, whose causal relationship with the disease is often unclear.[5]

Next-generation sequencing by an unbiased analysis of several genes has also facilitated the identification of the simultaneous occurrence of variants in multiple genes in a given individual with CMT. These individuals may harbor multiple genetic variants in different combinations: (1) variations in multiple genes implicated in CMT, or (2) a combination of variations in genes implicated in CMT as well as genes implicated in other neurodegenerative disorders. *PMP22* triplication causes a more severe phenotype as compared to *PMP22* duplication, because of the increased dosage. Mutations in *PMP22* have been reported to occur simultaneously with other related genes such as *LITAF, SMN2, DCTN1, GJB1*, and *ABCD1*. Increased genetic "burden" arising from the simultaneous occurrence of multiple genetic variations may contribute to phenotypic variability, since these variants in different genes may cause mild phenotypes in isolation, but when present together may have an additive effect on the severity of symptoms by causing pathology at different sites. The non-CMT-related variants may act as "genetic modifiers" and impact the clinical phenotype.[7]

Histopathological Features

Though nerve biopsy is redundant in the era of genomics, morphological and ultrastructural changes in nerves including the axons, myelin, and nodes of Ranvier often aid in narrowing down the panel of genes for molecular analysis. These changes also help in understanding the functions of the mutated genes, and to some extent the pathways leading to disease, particularly when novel genetic variations of uncertain significance are identified. Nerve biopsy may also help in suspecting a genetic etiology in sporadic cases.

Findings on histological examination can be classified as nonspecific and specific. Nonspecific changes may be seen in any inherited neuropathy and include axonal loss, demyelination/remyelination, and features suggestive of inflammation. A varying degree of axon loss is a nonspecific feature of any chronic polyneuropathy. It involves both myelinated and unmyelinated axons, and is usually homogeneous between fascicles. Some of the specific histopathological findings include onion bulbs in *PMP22* duplication, uncompacted myelin and myelin outfoldings in *MPZ* mutation, abnormal paranodal loops in *PRX* mutations, giant axons in *NEFL* mutations, and abnormal mitochondria in *MFN2* and *GDAP1* mutations.[8]

Treatment of Hereditary Motor and Sensory Neuropathy

Targeted or disease-specific treatment is at present limited, though there are several pharmacotherapies in the pipeline **(Box 1)**. What can be practically offered is active physiotherapy and judicious use of orthotics that improve or maintain muscle strength and function, improve joint flexibility, range of movement and balance, and alleviate fatigue, pain, stiffness, and deformities. Orthosis, splinting, corrective surgeries, and tendon transfers may be advised on a case-to-case basis. Put together, these therapies improve the quality of life.

Apart from this, one also has to anticipate complications and treat them. Respiratory compromise is rare, and it can arise from severe neuropathy, diaphragmatic palsy, or spinal deformity. Some patients experience worsening neuropathy during pregnancy. Abnormal fetal lie and postpartum hemorrhage may necessitate appropriate intervention during delivery. Most importantly, drugs with neurotoxic

BOX 1	**Potential therapies for HMSNs.**

Agents that target PMP22 overexpression:

- Ascorbic acid, onapristone, geldanamycin, and rapamycin
- *PXT3003*: Baclofen + naltrexone + D-sorbitol

Curcumin: ↓ endoplasmic reticulum stress, MPZ neuropathy

Others:

- Agents that target axonal regeneration, regulators of gene expression, chaperones, calcium homeostasis, potassium channel blockers
- *Supplements*: Essential fatty acids, phospholipids, vitamin E, creatine- and bovine-derived ganglioside mixture

(HMSNs: hereditary motor and sensory neuropathies; MPZ: myelin protein zero)

effects such as chemotherapeutic agents should be avoided in these patients.[1]

DISTAL HEREDITARY MOTOR NEUROPATHIES

Distal hereditary motor neuropathies are a group of clinically and genetically heterogeneous inherited disorders characterized by lower motor neuron type of weakness of the distal extremities. The patients experience length-dependent weakness of lower limbs, but upper limb onset also occurs. The onset of symptoms is usually within the first 2 decades of life. The phenotype is characterized by insidious onset, slowly progressive weakness, wasting of distal limbs, and hypo-/areflexia. A clinician needs to distinguish distal weakness arising from intrinsic hand muscles from that of forearm flexors at the bedside, as the latter would indicate a distal myopathy. The recurrent laryngeal nerve may be involved; other cranial nerves are not affected. The clinical examination may also reveal minor sensory deficits as well as the presence of upper motor neuron involvement, and "overlap" with CMTs, amyotrophic lateral sclerosis (ALS), and hereditary spastic paraplegias (HSP) is now a recognized feature. Electroneuromyography (ENMG) shows evidence of motor axonopathy in the form of reduced amplitudes of evoked motor responses and chronic denervation.

Inheritance may be AD, AR, or XL. When the disease occurs "sporadically," particularly at a later age at onset, adequate efforts must be taken to reasonably exclude the acquired causes. Mutations in genes involved in protein misfolding, axonal transport, ribonucleic acid (RNA) metabolism, and cation-channel function have been implicated in the pathogenesis of dHMN **(Table 3)**. Genetic overlap with CMT2 is described. For example, mutations in *HSPB1* and *HSPB8* cause AD dHMN; in the presence of clinical and electrophysiological evidence of sensory involvement, the same phenotype would be reclassified as CMT2F and CMT2L, respectively. Some of the genes that have overlapping phenotypes with dHMN and CMT2, ALS, and HSP are summarized in **Table 4**.[9]

TABLE 3: Genes implicated in distal hereditary motor neuropathies (dHMNs).

Inheritance pattern/phenotype	Genes mutated
Autosomal dominant:	
• Lower limb onset	*HSPB1, HSPB8, BSCL2, TRPV4, GARS, DYNC1H1*
• Upper limb onset	*BSCL2, GARS*
• Vocal cord palsy	*TRPV4, DCTN1*
• Pyramidal signs	*HSPB1, BSCL2, SETX, DCTN1*
Autosomal recessive	*IGHMBP2, HSPB1*
X-linked	*ATP7A*

TABLE 4: Genes that have overlapping phenotypes with dHMN.

Overlapping clinical phenotype	Genes mutated
CMT2	*HSPB1, HSPB8, BSCL2, GARS, TRPV4*
Juvenile ALS	*SETX*
HSP	*BSCL2, HSPB1*

(ALS: amyotrophic lateral sclerosis; CMT: Charcot–Marie–Tooth disease; dHMN: distal hereditary motor neuropathy; HSP: hereditary spastic paraplegia)

HEREDITARY SENSORY AND AUTONOMIC NEUROPATHY

Hereditary sensory and autonomic neuropathies are a heterogeneous group of disorders that arise from the dysfunction of small myelinated and unmyelinated nerve fibers due to mutations in genes involved in the development and survival of neurons, including those involved in nociception. Several subtypes are recognized based on the clinical phenotype and genetic abnormality **(Table 5)**.

Hereditary sensory and autonomic neuropathy I is autosomal dominantly inherited and has onset in adolescence or adulthood, while the rest are AR disorders that manifest in the neonatal or infantile period. Sensory and autonomic dysfunctions occur early in the disease course. The affected individuals manifest with symmetrical impairment of pain and temperature sensation to varying extents. Severe and dramatic manifestations such as acral ulcerations, osteomyelitis, and autoamputation of digits are seen (HSAN II). Lancinating pain may be present. Other features that may be present in some subtypes of HSAN include impaired joint position sensation, reduced or absent corneal and gag reflexes, impaired taste sensations, and hypo-/areflexia. Weakness and atrophy occur in some forms (HSAN I, VI). Features of dysautonomia such as abnormal tearing and sweating, as well as cardiovascular and gastrointestinal dysfunctions are differentially present in various subtypes. Cognitive functions may be affected to varying extents. Again, overlap with CMT is recognized,

TABLE 5: Summary of key clinical features and genes implicated in hereditary sensory and autonomic neuropathy (HSAN).

HSAN	Inheritance	Genes mutated	Clinical features
HSAN I	Autosomal dominant	*SPTLC1* *SPLTC2* *ATL1* *RAB7* *DNMT1*	• Onset between second and fifth decades • Profound loss of pain and temperature sensation • Touch and pressure sensations lost to a lesser extent • Hypohidrosis in the distribution of sensory deficits • Acral ulcers, infected calluses, foot deformities • Intermittent lancinating pain • *Muscle stretch reflexes*: Absent • Moderate weakness • *Cognition*: Mild intellectual disability • *Others*: Dementia, hearing loss • Severe phenotypes are rare
HSAN II/ congenital insensitivity to pain	Autosomal recessive	*WNK1* *FAM134B* *KIF1A*	• Onset in infancy or early childhood • Developmental delay due to hypotonia • Severe feeding problems and frequent apnea in neonatal period • Profound sensory loss to all modalities (pain, temperature, and joint position sense) • Gastroesophageal reflux and vomiting • Erythematous blotching, episodic hyperhidrosis • Unintentional self-injury, painless fractures, acral ulcers, Charcot joints • Reduced taste sensation • Sensorineural hearing loss • *Corneal and gag reflexes*: Diminished • *Muscle stretch reflexes*: Sluggish • Scoliosis • *Cognition*: Mild intellectual disability or normal intelligence
HSAN III	Autosomal recessive	*IKBKAP*	• Onset at birth • Delayed developmental milestones, intellectual disability, delayed puberty, short-statured, scoliosis • Temperature sense more profoundly affected than pain • *Cutaneous and bone pain*: Diminished but not absent • Diminished corneal reflex • Optic neuropathy with predominant loss of papillomacular fibers • Reduced taste sensation, especially for sweet • Dysphagia, gastroesophageal reflux • *Autonomic crisis*: Vomiting, agitation, tachycardia, hypertension, blotchy erythema, and diaphoresis • Abnormal ventilatory drive in response to hypoxia and hypercapnia • Orthostatic hypotension without compensatory tachycardia, hypertension, tachycardia, chronic kidney disease • *Muscle stretch reflexes*: Decreased or absent • *Gait*: Ataxic • Hypersensitivity to sympathomimetics and parasympathomimetics
HSAN IV or congenital insensitivity to pain with anhidrosis	Autosomal recessive	*NTRK1 or TRKA*	• *Age at onset*: Birth • Profound insensitivity to pain, markedly reduced temperature sense • Self-mutilation, lip biting, corneal scarring, autoamputation of digits, poor healing • Charcot joints, osteomyelitis • Anhidrosis of trunk and upper extremities, episodic fevers and extreme hyperpyrexia • Thick, calloused skin, lichenification of palms, dystrophic nails, hypotrichosis of scalp • *Emotional tearing*: Normal • *Muscle stretch reflexes*: Sluggish/normal • *Cognition*: Intellectual disability, severe learning and behavioral problems, impulsivity, hyperactivity, and reckless behaviors

Continued

Continued

HSAN	Inheritance	Genes mutated	Clinical features
HSAN V	Autosomal recessive	*NGF*	• Similar to HSAN IV, except lack of anhidrosis and intellectual disability • Acral ulcers, painless fractures, and other trophic injuries • Loss of pain sensation, other sensations normal • *Corneal reflex*: Absent • Hypohidrosis to varying extent • *Muscle stretch reflexes*: Normal
HSAN VI	Autosomal recessive	*DST*	• Motionless open-mouthed facies • Impaired pain • Acral ulcerations, painless fractures, osteomyelitis, joint deformities • Hypo/hyperhidrosis sweating, heat intolerance, pupillary abnormalities, chronic diarrhea, sexual dysfunction • Weakness of intrinsic foot muscles, distal contractures • Syringomyelia • Sensorineural hearing loss • Severe psychomotor retardation • *Abnormal behavior*: Obsessive compulsive disorder, anxiety • Type 2 diabetes mellitus • Lethal in infancy, compound heterozygous mutations result in milder phenotypes
HSAN VII	Autosomal dominant	*SCN11A*	• Onset at birth • Reduced pain sensation • Recurrent bone fractures, joint dislocations, recurrent infections • Excessive sweating, itching • *Gastrointestinal dysmotility*: Failure to thrive, painful constipation, and diarrhea • Mild weakness
HSAN VIII	Autosomal recessive	*PRDM12*	• Onset at birth • Congenital insensitivity to pain • Acral ulcers, hypohidrosis, reduced tearing • *Corneal reflex*: Absent • Cutaneous and bone infection

e.g., mutations in *RAB7* cause CMT2B with severe sensory loss and weakness, a phenotype that has considerable overlap with HSAN I. NCS findings range from normal to severe abnormalities. Treatment is directed at managing the symptoms arising from sensory and autonomic dysfunctions as they carry significant morbidity and mortality.[10]

HEREDITARY NEUROPATHY WITH LIABILITY TO PRESSURE PALSIES

This is an AD disorder, with a prevalence of about 16 per 100,000. As the name suggests, the patients experience recurrent focal neuropathies, especially at the sites where the nerves are prone to entrapment or compression or trauma. These include the median nerve at the wrist, ulnar nerve at the elbow, and common peroneal nerve at the knee. In this context, even though carpal tunnel syndrome (CTS) is the most common entrapment neuropathy, and maybe a clinical manifestation or first manifestation of HNPP, HNPP is only a rare cause of CTS. The spectrum of manifestation ranges from an asymptomatic state to acute recurrent painless, focal, or mononeuropathy. Recovery occurs over days to weeks. An antecedent trauma or prolonged pressure over the vulnerable site may be obtained. A fulminant course, triggered by gastrointestinal or respiratory tract infection, may lead to the initial diagnosis of acute inflammatory demyelinating polyneuropathy (AIDP), especially if multiple nerves are involved. About one-third manifest with progressive polyneuropathy, reminiscent of the classical CMT. The onset is usually in adolescence, but uncommonly, younger children may be affected with motor developmental delay, hypotonia, or toe-walking.

Examination shows deficits in the distribution of the affected nerve, sluggish muscle stretch reflexes, and mild pes cavus. NCS shows features of a demyelinating neuropathy, which is generalized and beyond the clinically affected nerves. This is seen even in asymptomatic subjects. Characteristically, conduction blocks are seen across entrapment sites. The diagnosis is confirmed by demonstrating the deletion of a large segment of the *PMP22* gene. Rarely, single base-pair deletion/insertion, as well as point mutations in the *PMP22* gene, have been described. Nerve biopsy is redundant in the era of genetics, but when performed as a part of the workup when vasculitis or other causes of mononeuropathy or mononeuritis multiplex are suspected at the bedside. The histological hallmark of HNPP is the presence of tomaculae. These are sausage-shaped structures that are formed by the massively redundant and overfolded myelin sheath layers. In addition, segmental demyelination and remyelination are noted. The pathobiology is unclear, but is related to dosage effect; deletion of *PMP22* leads to reduced messenger RNA (mRNA) levels in contrast to CMT1A. Other mutations in HNPP also lead to the creation of a null allele or dominantly negatively interfere with the function of the PMP22 protein.

In the absence of a specific pharmacotherapy, the treatment consists of educating the patient to avoid trauma or compression at the sites that are prone to nerve entrapment. Excessive force/impact and/or repetitive movements, as well as prolonged awkward static joint positions are to be avoided. Splints, pads, and braces can also be used to stabilize the joints and avoid pressure/stretch to the nerves.[11]

HEREDITARY NEURALGIC AMYOTROPHY

Hereditary neuralgic amyotrophy is a rare AD disorder. It is typically characterized by acute onset of unilateral pain, followed by weakness and thereafter wasting of the upper limbs. The pain is aching, burning, or stabbing in nature and is usually located in the shoulder, arm, or neck. Weakness commonly occurs in the distribution of the long thoracic and suprascapular nerves, while the axillary, musculocutaneous, radial, and anterior interosseous nerves can also be affected. Impaired sensations, paresthesias, and vasomotor changes also occur in the affected limb. Bilateral involvement may occur, but even then, the weakness is asymmetrical. Sometimes, there is the involvement of regions outside the brachial plexus such as the lumbosacral plexus, phrenic nerve, recurrent laryngeal nerve, and facial nerve. Criteria for diagnosing HNA have been proposed **(Table 6)**.

TABLE 6: Diagnostic criteria for hereditary neuralgic amyotrophy.

Feature	Inclusion criteria	Compatible criteria
Age at onset	Second or third decade of life (median age = 28 years)	Earlier or later age at onset
Clinical manifestations	• Acute, uni-, or bilateral brachial plexopathy • Severe pain preceding the weakness by days to a few weeks • Predominantly motor deficits • *Number of episodes*: 1–20 • *Precipitating factors*: o Infections o Immunization o Surgery o Parturition o Strenuous exercise of affected limb o Cold exposure	• Attack recurrence (75%) • Sensory symptoms (70%) • Lumbar plexus (33%) and/or phrenic nerve (14%) involved • Cranial nerve involved • Dysmorphic features • Abortive attacks (pain not followed by weakness) • Weakness preceding onset of pain • Long intervals between attacks (up to years) • No pain during an attack (5%)
Family history	Autosomal dominant inheritance	Sporadic cases
Clinical examination	Patchy or multifocal distribution of abnormalities	• More prominent motor loss than sensory loss • Sensory abnormalities (80%) • Autonomic symptoms (15%) • Mononeuropathy • Absent or diminished tendon reflexes in affected limbs • Muscle weakness and atrophy
Course and severity	• Relapsing–remitting course • *Incomplete recovery*: Residual neurological deficit, especially after repeated attacks in the same limb	• Complete recovery between attacks • Chronic undulating course without complete symptom-free intervals
Electrophysiological findings	Signs of denervation/reinnervation in clinically weak muscles	• Reduced amplitude of compound muscle action potentials in muscles innervated by affected nerves • Reduced amplitudes of sensory nerve action potentials in affected nerves
Molecular genetics	• Identification of pathogenic variant or duplication in *SEPT9* • Linkage to the *SEPT9* locus on chromosome 17q25	Absence of linkage to the *SEPT9* locus on chromosome 17q25

Similar to the idiopathic neuralgic amyotrophy (INA) (nonhereditary form), the episodes of HNA are triggered by strenuous work involving the upper limbs, psychological stress, childbirth, infections, and immunizations. The age at onset ranges from infancy to adulthood and is most common in the second-to-third decade of life. Rarely, the onset may be at birth with Erb's or Klumpke-like paralysis. In contrast, INA is rare in the first decade of life. Besides, the presence of positive family history, more severe pain, and recurrent episodes distinguish HNA from INA. Because of the recurrent episodes, the prognosis for complete recovery is not as good as INA. A chronic undulating phenotype of HNA, with a protracted fluctuating course and lack of a clear asymptomatic period (remission) may also occur. Apart from this, individuals with HNA may have dysmorphic features such as hypotelorism, short palpebral fissures, epicanthal folds, long nasal bridge, small mouth, bifid uvula, cleft palate, pronounced neck folds, cutis verticis gyrata, partial syndactyly, and short stature.

Mutations in the septin 9 (*SEPT9*) gene, which has a role in cytoskeletal structure and cell division, have been implicated in HNA. Nevertheless, about 45% do not have mutations in *SEPT9*. Steroids may be administered during the acute phase to reduce pain and hasten recovery.[11]

OTHER INHERITED NEUROPATHIES

Apart from the classical inherited neuropathies, wherein the phenotype manifests either with predominant involvement of peripheral nerves, or a complex disorder wherein neuropathy is a part of a multiaxial disorder, there are other genetically determined syndromes, where neuropathy constitutes one of the key clinical manifestations. These are summarized in **Table 7**. Diagnosis is based on the clinical phenotype and confirmed by the relevant biochemical and genetic studies.

CONCLUSION

Inherited neuropathies constitute a heterogeneous group of genetically determined neuropathies with varying, but frequently overlapping, phenotypes and genetic abnormalities. Several systemic and neurological features unrelated to neuropathy may also coexist. It is important to make an accurate diagnosis by judicious use of electrophysiological and genetic testing to end the diagnostic odyssey and provide the appropriate genetic counseling, prognostication, and treatment.

TABLE 7: Other inherited neuropathies.

Category	Examples
Inherited ataxias	
Autosomal dominant	Spinocerebellar ataxia
Autosomal recessive	Friedrich's ataxia, vitamin E deficiency, ARSACS, AOA1
Hereditary spastic paraplegias	*BSCL2, REEP1, Atlastin, KIF1A*
Porphyrias	AIP, variegate porphyria, hereditary coproporphyria
Disorders of lipid metabolism	
Lipoprotein deficiencies	Tangier disease, abetalipoproteinemia, cerebrotendinous xanthomatosis
Leukodystrophies	Metachromatic leukodystrophy, Krabbe disease, adrenoleukodystrophy
Peroxisomal disorders	Refsum disease, Fabry's disease
Sphingomyelin lipidosis and gangliosidosis	
Mitochondrial disorders	MNGIE, NARP, SANDO
Defective DNA repair/maintenance disorders	Xeroderma pigmentosum, Cockayne's syndrome, ataxia telangiectasia
Others	Neuroacanthocytosis, neurofibromatosis types 1 and 2, myotonic dystrophy, familial amyloid polyneuropathy

(AIP: acute intermittent porphyria; AOA: ataxia with oculomotor apraxia; ARSACS: autosomal recessive spastic ataxia of Charlevoix–Saguenay; DNA: deoxyribonucleic acid; MNGIE: mitochondrial neurogastrointestinal encephalopathy; NARP: neuropathy, ataxia, retinitis pigmentosa syndrome; SANDO: sensory ataxic neuropathy, dysarthria, and ophthalmoparesis)

REFERENCES

1. Carroll AS, Burns J, Nicholson G, Kiernan MC, Vucic S. Inherited neuropathies. Semin Neurol. 2019;39(5):620-39.
2. Vallat JM, Mathis S, Funalot B. The various Charcot–Marie–Tooth diseases. Curr Opin Neurol. 2013;26(5):473-80.
3. Magy L, Mathis S, Le Masson G, Goizet C, Tazir M, Vallat JM. Updating the classification of inherited neuropathies: results of an international survey. Neurology. 2018;90(10):e870-6.
4. Jerath NU, Shy ME. Hereditary motor and sensory neuropathies: understanding molecular pathogenesis could lead to future treatment strategies. Biochim Biophys Acta. 2015;1852(4):667-78.
5. Klein CJ, Duan X, Shy ME. Inherited neuropathies: clinical overview and update. Muscle Nerve. 2013;48(4):604-22.
6. Fridman V, Reilly MM. Inherited neuropathies. Semin Neurol. 2015;35(4):407-23.
7. Bis-Brewer DM, Fazal S, Züchner S. Genetic modifiers and non-Mendelian aspects of CMT. Brain Res. 2020;1726:146459.
8. Weis J, Claeys KG, Roos A, Azzedine H, Katona I, Schröder JM, et al. Toward a functional pathology of hereditary neuropathies. Acta Neuropathol. 2017;133(4):493-515.
9. Frasquet M, Sevilla T. Hereditary motor neuropathies. Curr Opin Neurol. 2022;35(5):562-70.
10. Schwartzlow C, Kazamel M. Hereditary sensory and autonomic neuropathies: adding more to the classification. Curr Neurol Neurosci Rep. 2019;19(8):52.
11. Chance PF. Inherited focal, episodic neuropathies: hereditary neuropathy with liability to pressure palsies and hereditary neuralgic amyotrophy. Neuromolecular Med. 2006;8(1-2):159-74.

82

CHAPTER

Acquired Neuropathies

Vinod Puri, Neera Chaudhry, Divyani Garg

INTRODUCTION

Peripheral neuropathies are disorders affecting the peripheral nervous system, arising from a diverse etiological array. Various systems have been used to classify peripheral neuropathies, including categorization based on electrophysiology (axonal or demyelinating), onset and temporal profile (acute, subacute, and chronic), topography (polyneuropathy, mononeuropathy, and mononeuropathy multiplex), fiber involvement (large fiber, small fiber, mixed or sensory, motor, and mixed), presence of autonomic dysfunction, presence of facial nerve involvement, and etiology (inherited and acquired).[1] Acquired peripheral neuropathies form the largest etiological group encountered in clinical practice.[2] These disorders may be associated with systemic disorders such as diabetes or infections such as human immunodeficiency virus (HIV). Recognition of the underlying etiology is crucial to guide evaluation, and treatment of the causative factor frequently leads to the reversal or stabilization of peripheral neuropathy.[3] It is also vital to recognize treatable neuropathies in the early part of the temporal profile of the disease, before the occurrence of axonal damage, which is largely considered to be associated with prolonged recovery and residual sequelae.

The approach to peripheral neuropathy, particularly acquired peripheral neuropathies, hinges on meticulous history and clinical examination, which provide information regarding the pattern of involvement, associated autonomic dysfunction, distribution, and type of nerve fiber involvement, as well as the temporal course of the disease. Medical history is vital for discerning etiology and may provide essential clues toward the same. The presence of positive sensory phenomena, such as painful paresthesia, tingling, pins-and-needles sensation, etc., favors an acquired etiology, compared to inherited neuropathies, in which "numbness" or lack of sensation is usually described. "Burning feet" may be present in either inherited or acquired neuropathies. Asymmetric presentation, particularly at onset, is another feature that favors an acquired cause. The presence of prolonged fever and weight loss may point toward infectious etiology. History of drug use, including the previous history of chemotherapy, may point toward drug-related or paraneoplastic considerations. Similarly, the systemic examination is another crucial tool to ascertain etiology. Skin changes may be seen in nutritional deficiencies (e.g., knuckle hyperpigmentation in vitamin B12 deficiency).[4] Nail changes may be seen in toxin-related neuropathies (e.g., Mees' lines in thallium or arsenic toxicity). Hair loss may be another feature (thallium toxicity). Lymphadenopathy or liver/spleen enlargement may indicate lymphoproliferative or infective disorders. Hence, a thorough clinical history and examination anchor the diagnostic algorithm in acquired peripheral neuropathies.

Nerve conduction studies are used to characterize peripheral neuropathies as predominantly axonal or predominantly demyelinating, as well as the distribution of nerve involvement. Further evaluation is dictated by etiological possibilities and may include specialized tests, such as toxin or heavy metal screening, vasculitis panel, antiganglioside antibody panel, or infective work-up.[5] Occasionally, a nerve biopsy may be necessary.[6] Treatment includes symptom-based therapy and directed therapy, targeted at the reversal of etiology. In this chapter, we review the etiology, evaluation, and treatment of peripheral neuropathies of acquired origin.

EPIDEMIOLOGY

Compared to other chronic neurological disorders, epidemiological data is limited for peripheral neuropathy. Among neuropathies, mononeuropathies are more common than polyneuropathies. The most common mononeuropathy is carpal tunnel syndrome (estimated prevalence

5,000/100,000 population), followed by diabetic neuropathy (200–600/100,000 population), idiopathic (200/100,000 population), and toxic (100/100,000 population).[7]

Studies from India indicate a wide prevalence range, from 5 to 2,400 per 10,000 population.[8] Higher rates have been reported from Parsi communities and urban slums. In a study of 225 patients with peripheral neuropathy from Kolkata, the most common neuropathies included Guillain-Barré syndrome (GBS), diabetic neuropathy, hereditary sensory motor neuropathy, chronic inflammatory demyelinating polyneuropathy (CIDP), leprosy, and alcohol-related neuropathy.[9]

CLASSIFICATION

Acquired peripheral neuropathies are broadly categorized[10] into the following categories, based on the underlying etiology **(Table 1)**:
- Metabolic/nutritional
- Toxin/drug
- Immune-mediated
- Infectious

TABLE 1: Classification of acquired peripheral neuropathies.

Category	Types
Metabolic/nutritional	• Diabetes mellitus • Renal failure • Hepatic failure • B12 deficiency • Thiamine deficiency • Pyridoxine deficiency/excess • Vitamin E deficiency • Copper deficiency
Toxins	• Arsenic • Thallium • Lead
Drugs	• Chemotherapy agents • Antibiotics/antimycobacterial agents • Amiodarone
Immune-mediated	• Guillain–Barré syndrome • Chronic inflammatory demyelinating polyneuropathy • Multifocal motor neuropathy • Paraproteinemic neuropathy • Vasculitis • Sarcoidosis
Infectious	• Leprosy • HIV • Hepatitis C • Cytomegalovirus • Lyme disease • Varicella zoster • Diphtheria

Neuropathies due to Metabolic/Nutritional Disorders

These are symmetrical neuropathies, with sensory and motor involvement, and are usually axonal. Sensory complaints are frequently prominent.

Diabetes Mellitus

Peripheral neuropathy is common in both type 1 diabetes mellitus (T1DM) and type 2 diabetes mellitus (T2DM). It is a serious complication, associated with increased mortality and the risk of lower-limb amputations. Moreover, it leads to debilitating neuropathic pain. The prevalence ranges from 10 to 40% among diabetics, and nearly 50% of diabetics will eventually develop peripheral neuropathy.[11] It poses a major economic healthcare burden and accounts for nearly 50–75% of diabetic limb amputations.[12]

A diabetic foot ulcer is a serious complication, which may eventually lead to gangrene, Charcot's foot, and loss of limb.

Diabetic neuropathy has a wide heterogeneity of clinical presentations.[13] Various classifications have been proposed, broadly dividing the pattern into generalized and focal patterns **(Table 2)**.

Uremic Neuropathy

The incidence of uremic neuropathy has declined with the advent of earlier and more advanced dialysis and renal transplantation techniques.[14] The incidence reportedly

TABLE 2: Classification of neuropathy patterns in diabetes mellitus.

Generalized:	*Distal symmetrical polyneuropathy:* • Sensorimotor • Predominantly large fiber • Predominantly small fiber • Pure small fiber *Acute painful distal neuropathy:* • Hyperglycemic neuropathy *Autonomic neuropathy:* • Cardiovascular • Urogenital • Gastrointestinal • Sudomotor *Hypoglycemic neuropathy*
	Pupillary involvement
Focal/multifocal:	• Entrapment neuropathy • Cranial neuropathy • Limb mononeuropathy • Mononeuropathy multiplex • Thoracolumbar radiculoneuropathy • Lumbosacral radiculoplexoneuropathy • Cervical radiculoplexopathy

Source: Adapted from Sloan, et al (2021).[13]

ranges from 10 to 80%.[15] Usually, the presence of peripheral neuropathy indicates advanced renal disease. Patients with diabetes who have chronic kidney disease represent an especially vulnerable group for the development of peripheral neuropathy.

The pathogenesis is multifactorial and is believed to be a combination of the effects of uremic toxins and thiamine deficiency. The "middle" toxins, that is, uremic toxins with molecular mass in the middle range of 300–2000 Daltons, are not effectively removed by dialysis, and these may cause nerve injury. Other contributory factors include hyperparathyroidism and chronic hyperkalemia.

Peripheral nerves may be affected in the following manner in uremia:

- *Polyneuropathy*: Sensory complaints such as tingling paresthesias are prominent. The neuropathy is lower-limb predominant till the advanced stage when it involves the upper limb. Loss of vibration sense is an early feature.
- Entrapment neuropathy (e.g., carpal tunnel syndrome)
- *Restless legs syndrome (RLS)*: RLS has a definite association with renal dysfunction. It affects up to 25% of patients on dialysis.[16] RLS is characterized by an unpleasant sensation involving the lower limbs, during a period of rest or sleep, associated with an urge to move the legs, which leads to complete or partial relief of symptoms. RLS may disappear with the onset of frank neuropathy.
- Autonomic neuropathy

Vitamin B12 Deficiency

Vitamin B12 deficiency may be a result of low intake (in a strict vegan diet), problems with binding to intrinsic factor (pernicious anemia, atrophic gastritis, and prolonged antacids), or absorption (ileal resection or ileocecal diseases such as Crohn's disease or tuberculosis). A deficiency of vitamin B12 is associated mainly with myelopathy, with or without peripheral neuropathy (subacute combined degeneration) and optic neuropathy.[17] Peripheral neuropathy is usually large fiber and sensory dominant although mild motor weakness can occur.

Certain clinical clues are indicators of vitamin B12 deficiency.[18] These include:

- Development of sudden onset neuropathy
- Presence of associated myelopathy
- Onset in the upper limbs
- Concomitant upper and lower limb involvement
- Macrocytic anemia

Thiamine Deficiency

The deficiency of thiamine (vitamin B1) produces beriberi. Vitamin B1 catalyzes multiple enzymatic reactions, such as transketolase reaction and branched-chain amino acid metabolism.[19] Thiamine deficiency may occur in the context of severe malnutrition, alcoholism, and gastrectomy. Beriberi is characterized by the development of cardiovascular involvement and neuropathy. Neuropathy is distal axonal sensorimotor and is associated with neuropathic pain. It may progress to motor weakness and involvement of the cranial nerves, including tongue, facial, and laryngeal weakness. GBS-like presentations may also occur.[20]

Pyridoxine-related Neuropathy

Both an excess and deficiency of pyridoxine (vitamin B6) are implicated in the development of peripheral neuropathy.[21] Evidence of neuropathy related to pyridoxine deficiency largely stems from patients treated for tuberculosis with isoniazid (INH). However, the pathogenic role of associated other nutritional deficiencies has been posited in the development of neuropathy in these patients.[21] Pyridoxine excess (>50 mg/day), particularly megadoses (>2 g/day), has been reported to be associated with various forms of peripheral neuropathy:

- Sensory neuronopathy (most frequent)
- Sensory and autonomic neuropathy
- Sensory and motor axonal neuropathy
- Sensory and motor demyelinating neuropathy

Toxin and Drug-induced Neuropathy

Many toxins and drugs may lead to peripheral neuropathy **(Table 3)**. Toxins include alcohol, heavy metals, industrial agents, insecticides, and other chemicals. Native Indian medications may contain heavy metals, including lead, mercury, arsenic and silver, which may also trigger peripheral neuropathy on prolonged exposure.[22]

Some drugs and toxins are described in further detail below.

Toxin-induced Neuropathy

Alcohol-related Neuropathy

Alcohol-related neuropathy usually presents as a length-dependent, axonal neuropathy. It may involve small and/or large fibers, and autonomic dysfunction may be prominent. The course is usually progressive, with onset in the lower limbs.

The incidence of neuropathy is known to increase with the duration and severity of alcohol exposure.[23,24] Sensory features predominate, with burning and painful paresthesia. Motor features, including weakness, may also occur but are usually not prominent. Deep tendon reflexes are frequently attenuated or absent.

Nerve conduction studies show an axonal pattern. Electromyography may show reduced recruitment with features of active denervation (positive sharp waves/fibrillations).

Pathogenesis involves nutritional deficiency, including thiamine, although thiamine deficiency-related neuropathy has been reported to be a distinct clinical entity by some authors.[20] However, it is difficult to separate the role of

TABLE 3: Toxins and drugs causing peripheral neuropathy.

Toxins causing peripheral neuropathy clinical features	
Alcohol	**Sensory prominent axonal neuropathy**
Heavy metals:	
• Lead	• Motor prominent (wrist drop), encephalopathy
• Arsenic	• Sensory prominent, painful, length-dependent neuropathy/GBS mimic
• Thallium	• Painful sensory neuropathy/GBS mimic
• Mercury	• Ganglionopathy, encephalopathy
• Gold	• Axonal/demyelinating sensorimotor
Industrial agents:	
• n-Hexane	• Sensorimotor, length-dependent, coasting seen
• Carbon disulfide	• Sensorimotor, length-dependent
• Acrylamide	• Sensorimotor, length-dependent, ataxia, dermatitis
• Allyl chloride	• Sensorimotor, length-dependent
Organophosphates	Delayed onset, motor > sensory
Drugs causing peripheral neuropathy:	
Antiarrhythmic agents:	
• Amiodarone	• Sensorimotor, axonal/demyelinating
• Procainamide	• Sensorimotor, demyelinating
Antihypertensives:	
• Hydralazine	• Sensory prominent, axonal
Antibiotics:	
• Isoniazid	• Sensory prominent, axonal
• Ethambutol	• Sensory prominent, axonal, retrobulbar neuritis
• Dapsone	• Motor prominent, axonal
• Chloramphenicol	• Sensory prominent, axonal
• Metronidazole	• Sensory prominent, axonal
Chemotherapy agents: • Vinca alkaloids • Taxanes • Platinum-based agents • Epothilones • Bortezomib	All are sensorimotor, sensory prominent, axonal
Antiretrovirals: • Stavudine • Didanosine • Zalcitabine	All are sensory prominent, painful, axonal
Antiseizure medication:	
Phenytoin	Sensory and motor, axonal

alcohol per se versus the effects of malnutrition in these patients, in the pathogenesis of neuropathy.

Metal-related Neuropathy

Several heavy metals or metalloids may lead to metal-related neuropathy. Metals are usually not toxic in their elemental form. However, they may be toxic as their organic or inorganic compounds. Several industries use heavy metals, which may lead to occupational exposure.[25] In metal-related toxic neuropathy, clinching clues may include accompanying systemic/hematologic/dermatological features.

The diagnosis of metal-related neuropathy is made by demonstrating toxic levels of the concerned metal in the blood or urine (in the acute phase) or the hair and nails (in the chronic phase). Treatment necessitates chelation therapy with diverse heavy metal chelators, including ethylenediaminetetraacetic acid (EDTA), British anti-Lewisite (BAL), and D-penicillamine.

- *Arsenic*: Ground water exposure with high arsenic levels may lead to chronic exposure. Arsenic toxicity may also occur in the context of homicide or suicide. Gastrointestinal symptoms including vomiting and diarrhea are prominent. Acute neuropathy due to arsenic may lead to severe quadriparesis, mimicking GBS.[26] Paresthesias are usually prominent. Skin changes include hyperkeratosis of the palms and soles. Nails may show Mees' lines. Nerve conduction studies show axonal changes.
- *Lead:* Lead neuropathy is a predominantly motor axonal neuropathy, with a predilection to involve the radial nerve, leading to wrist drop. Associated symptoms include abdominal pain and anemia.

  Encephalopathy may also develop in severe cases.
- *Thallium*: Thallium is a component of many insecticides and rodenticides. Thallium poisoning leads to the development of painful sensorimotor neuropathy, in association with gastrointestinal symptoms. It competes with potassium intracellularly, interfering with intracellular energy generation.[27] Alopecia develops after 2–3 weeks. Thallium uniquely affects small fibers predominantly, as compared to other toxins. Sensory loss occurs in a stocking-and-glove pattern. Autonomic dysfunction may also be associated. Involvement of the respiratory muscles and quadriparesis may mimic GBS.[28] Nerve conduction studies reveal sensory > motor pattern of axonal loss.

Other Toxins

- *Organophosphates*: Neuropathy related to organophosphate poisoning is a delayed complication and is referred to as organophosphate-induced delayed polyneuropathy (OPIDP).[29] It occurs due to intoxication with some organophosphate esters. It sets in 1–4 weeks following exposure and is characterized by axonal degeneration. It is a sensorimotor peripheral neuropathy, which usually involves the lower limbs, but may also involve the upper limbs, leading to foot or wrist drops. Pure motor neuropathy has also been described.[30] Central axonal degeneration may account for spastic ataxia that may be associated with some patients. The neuropathy tends to worsen over the first few days of onset, and then slowly improves. It is believed to be a consequence of inhibition of neuropathy target esterase (NTE).[31]

- *Organic solvents*: Organic solvents are used in a wide range of industries, including paints, printing, coating industries (paints/varnishes), pesticides, etc. Several organic solvents are associated with the development of peripheral neuropathy. These include n-Hexane,[32,33] carbon disulfide, styrene,[34] and trichloroethane.[35] Occupational exposure to these compounds has been associated with sensorimotor neuropathy.

Drug-induced Neuropathy

Several drugs can damage the peripheral nerves, leading to neuropathy which is frequently irreversible. The typical pattern of involvement is in the glove-and-stocking distribution. Sensory features predominate, and motor involvement is less common.

The pathophysiological mechanisms may involve metabolic dysregulation, damage to organelles such as mitochondria and endoplasmic reticulum, covalent modification, inflammation, channelopathy, and disruption of axonal transport.[36] Dorsal root ganglions may also be affected.

Cardiovascular Agents

Amiodarone is a class-III antiarrhythmic agent. Although peripheral neuropathy with amiodarone use is infrequent,[37] it is influenced by the dose and the duration of exposure to the drug, with doses above 200 mg having a higher risk of neuropathy. The typical pattern of neuropathy is a length-dependent neuropathy, and demyelinating features may be evident on nerve conduction study. Perhexiline, an older antianginal agent, is associated with demyelinating neuropathy.

Chemotherapy Agents

The vinca alkaloids are chemotherapy agents associated with the development of peripheral neuropathy, particularly vincristine, and to a lesser extent, vinblastine and vinorelbine. The neuropathy may be severe in one-third of cases and is an ascending sensory neuropathy.[38] The platinum-based agents, including cisplatin and oxaliplatin, affect the dorsal root ganglia, leading to sensory neuronopathy, with predominant ataxia. The risk of development of neuropathy increases with increased dose. "Coasting" may be seen, which is a phenomenon characterized by the worsening of symptoms months after cessation of chemotherapy. Oxaliplatin may lead to cold-induced neuropathy.

Bortezomib, used in the treatment of multiple myeloma, leads to the involvement of unmyelinated C fibers, and hence, the neuropathy is characterized by severe burning and neuropathic pain. Thalidomide may also lead to predominantly sensory neuropathy in a length-dependent fashion, along with some motor dysfunction.

Ixabepilone is an epothilone used in the treatment of breast and prostate cancer and may induce sensory neuropathy.

Arsenic trioxide, used in the treatment of acute promyelocytic leukemia, is well known to lead to a mild and reversible sensorimotor neuropathy.

Taxanes (paclitaxel and docetaxel) are also implicated in the development of neuropathy.

Antibiotics

Among the antimycobacterial agents, INH and ethambutol are associated with peripheral neuropathy. The risk is dose-dependent and increases with high-dose INH therapy (>10 mg/kg/day). INH neurotoxicity is related to pyridoxine deficiency, as INH causes increased excretion of pyridoxine. Supplementation with pyridoxine prevents the development of neuropathy.

Linezolid can also lead to irreversible peripheral neuropathy, as well as optic neuropathy, which is used for the treatment of drug-resistant tuberculosis and *Staphylococcus aureus* infection.[39,40] Metronidazole can lead to sensory and motor peripheral neuropathy, as well as optic neuropathy and autonomic neuropathy, especially when used in doses >42 g total and >4 weeks.[41]

Several antiretroviral agents, particularly nucleoside reverse transcriptase inhibitors (NRTIs), may also lead to the development of peripheral neuropathy, including stavudine, lamivudine, didanosine, and zalcitabine.[42] The neuropathy may be painful and is predominantly sensory. The pathogenesis involves mitochondrial cytotoxicity due to the inhibition of mitochondrial DNA polymerase.

Withdrawal of the incriminating antibiotic agent may lead to varying degrees of recovery, which may occur over months.

Immune-mediated Neuropathy

These are a heterogeneous group of disorders due to immunological processes affecting the peripheral nerves or their blood supply. Since the initial descriptions of GBS, the spectrum of immune-mediated neuropathies continued to broaden, and now includes an array of disorders (**Box 1**).[43,44] These disorders share the pathogenetic mechanism of autoimmunity, either to proteins at the Node of Ranvier or myelin, or blood vessels supplying peripheral nerves.

Guillain–Barré Syndrome

Guillain–Barré syndrome is an acute-onset polyradiculoneuropathy. GBS may be associated with a preceding event in 60–70% of patients, such as infections (*Campylobacter jejuni, Cytomegalovirus*, Epstein-Barr virus, *Mycoplasma pneumoniae*, and *Haemophilus influenzae*), vaccination, or surgery, in the antecedent 1–4 weeks.[45] It has several variants:

- Acute inflammatory demyelinating polyradiculoneuropathy (AIDP)
- Acute motor and sensory axonal neuropathy (AMSAN)
- Acute motor axonal neuropathy (AMAN)

BOX 1 Immune-mediated neuropathies.[44]

- *Guillain–Barré syndrome (GBS) and its variants:*
  - AMAN
  - AMSAN
  - AIDP
  - MFS
  - Autonomic
  - Sensory neuronopathy/ganglionopathy
- *Chronic inflammatory demyelinating neuropathy (CIDP):*
  - CIPD (typical)
  - CIDP variants:
    - Distal acquired demyelinating sensory
    - Motor
    - Sensory
    - Lewis–Sumner syndrome
- Chronic immune sensory polyradiculopathy
- Autoimmune nodopathies
- Multifocal motor neuropathy (MMN)
- Paraproteinemic neuropathy
- *Vasculitis-related neuropathy:*
  - *Large and medium vessel*: Giant cell arteritis
  - *Medium and small vessel*: Polyarteritis nodosa
  - *ANCA-associated small vessel*: Granulomatosis with polyangiitis (Wegener's granulomatosis), eosinophilic granulomatosis with polyangiitis (Churg–Strauss syndrome), microscopic polyangiitis
  - *Small vessel vasculitis with immune complex*: Cryoglobulinemia
  - Vasculitis associated with systemic connective tissue disease
  - Isolated vasculitis of the peripheral nerves
- Sarcoidosis
- Behçet's disease
- Diabetic/nondiabetic radiculoplexopathy
- Brachial neuritis

(AMAN: acute motor axonal neuropathy; AMSAN: acute motor and sensory axonal neuropathy; ANCA: antineutrophil cytoplasmic antibody; AIDP: acute inflammatory demyelinating polyradiculoneuropathy; MFS: Miller–Fisher syndrome)

- Miller–Fisher syndrome (MFS)
- Acute pharyngeal-cervical-brachial variant (APCB variant)
- Autonomic neuropathy

Acute Inflammatory Demyelinating Polyradiculoneuropathy

AIDP is reported to be the most common GBS variant in Western countries. The typical pattern is of ascending weakness, although respiratory or upper limb involvement may begin concurrently or even before lower limb involvement. Back and limb pain is frequently reported. Paresthesias may be out of proportion to sensory findings, which are usually not prominent. The weakness progresses over 4 weeks to reach a nadir, and then begins to improve after 1–2 weeks. Respiratory and autonomic involvement may occur. Ventilation may be necessary in 25–30% of patients.[46] Mortality is 5%.

Acute Motor and Sensory Axonal Neuropathy

In comparison to AIDP, AMSAN is an axonal variant affecting motor and sensory nerve fibers.

It tends to worsen more rapidly, and recovery is slower and less complete.

Acute Motor Axonal Neuropathy

AMAN is the most frequent axonal variant of GBS and has been reported to be the most common variant in Asia and Central/South America. It is a pure motor variant that worsens more rapidly compared to AIDP. Although absent or attenuated reflexes are usual, some patients may have normal to even brisk reflexes. Antibodies to GM1 or GD1a may be present in 80% of patients. Two patterns of AMAN have been reported in electrophysiology which determines prognosis: axonal without conduction block and axonal with conduction block. In the former condition, axonal degeneration leads to Wallerian degeneration and is associated with prolonged and, some time, incomplete recovery. In the latter condition, the conduction block occurs due to transient nodopathy and is associated with rapid recovery.

Miller–Fisher Syndrome

MFS is characterized by the triad of ataxia, areflexia, and ophthalmoplegia. It is associated with anti-GQ1b antibodies.

Chronic Inflammatory Demyelinating Neuropathy

Chronic inflammatory demyelinating polyneuropathy is a chronic, progressive, or recurrent, symmetrical sensorimotor neuropathy. The diagnostic criteria for CIDP have recently been revised by the European Academy of Neurology/ Peripheral Nerve Society guidelines.[47] These consist of two levels of diagnostic certainty: CIDP and possible CIDP. The earlier term, "atypical CIDP," has now been replaced by CIDP "variants."

Typical chronic inflammatory demyelinating polyradiculoneuropathy (CIPD) is characterized by progressive or relapsing motor and sensory weakness of upper and lower limbs (proximal and distal), and sensory complaints in at least two limbs. The disease evolves over at least 8 weeks, and deep tendon reflexes are reduced or absent.

The CIDP variants consist of the following entities:

- Distal acquired demyelinating symmetric (DADS) neuropathy
- Multifocal CIDP or Lewis–Sumner syndrome
- Focal CIDP
- Motor CIDP
- Sensory CIDP

Multifocal Motor Neuropathy

Multifocal motor neuropathy (MMN) is a rare, pure motor neuropathy, characterized by asymmetrical weakness and conduction blocks on nerve conduction studies. Typically, onset is in the upper limbs in the distal muscles. Sensory loss, if present, is usually mild and confined to the lower limbs. Reflexes are attenuated in the affected extremity, and normal in the unaffected limbs. It is a differential diagnosis for Hirayama disease or amyotrophic lateral sclerosis.

The diagnosis of MMN requires objective evidence of weakness, in the absence of sensory loss, with the presence of a conduction block in two or more nerves in nonentrapment sites.[48]

Chronic Immune Sensory Polyradiculopathy

Patients with features of sensory CIPD but with normal nerve conduction studies may have chronic immune sensory polyradiculopathy (CISP). CISP affects sensory nerves proximal to the dorsal root ganglia.[49] On examination, these patients have marked large fiber sensory loss and gait ataxia. Somatosensory evoked potentials are abnormal. Magnetic resonance imaging (MRI) may show nerve root enhancement. CSF may show elevated protein levels. Immunotherapy results in good improvement.[50]

Nodopathies–Paranodopathies

Some patients with CIDP may harbor antibodies to nodal and paranodal proteins, including contactin-1 (CNTN1), neurofascin (155, 140, and 186), and contactin-associated protein 1 (Caspr-1). Patients with anti-CNTN1 antibodies have motor predominant form and respond poorly to IVIg therapy. These may have acute or subacute presentations. Patients with antibodies to Caspr-1 may also have acute to subacute onset, pain, cranial nerve involvement, and ataxia, and show poor response to IVIg therapy. Patients with antibodies to neurofascin share acute to subacute onset, younger age, presence of tremors, and respond poorly to IVIg therapy.[51] These patients usually respond to rituximab therapy.[52]

Paraproteinemic Neuropathy

Paraproteinemia or monoclonal gammopathy refers to clonal B cell expansion. Although most patients have monoclonal gammopathy of uncertain significance (MGUS) which is benign, approximately 1% per year may advance to develop multiple myeloma or other hematological neoplasms. Nearly one-third of patients with monoclonal gammopathy develop neuropathy **(Table 4)**.

IgG and IgA Gammopathy

IgG and IgA gammopathies may be associated with chronic demyelinating or axonal neuropathies.

TABLE 4: Peripheral neuropathy in paraproteinemias.[53]

Paraproteinemia	Neuropathy features
Monoclonal gammopathy: • MGUS: IgM ○ IgG/IgA • Multiple myeloma • Waldenstrom macroglobulinemia	• Large fiber, sensory ataxia, and demyelinating pattern • Uncommon, axonal • IgG > IgA, length dependent, sensorimotor or motor, axonal • IgM, large fiber, sensory prominent, axonal > demyelinating
POEMS syndrome	IgG or A, CIPD-like, demyelinating
Light chain amyloidosis	Lambda light chain, sensorimotor axonal, autonomic involvement

(MGUS: monoclonal gammopathy of uncertain significance; POEMS: polyneuropathy, organomegaly, endocrinopathy, M-protein, and skin changes)

POEMS Syndrome

POEMS is a rare syndrome. The acronym "POEMS" indicates polyneuropathy, organomegaly, endocrinopathy, M-protein, and skin changes. Up to 75% of patients develop osteosclerotic myeloma. The M-protein is composed of IgG or IgA lambda light chains. The clinical syndrome resembles typical CIPD, although axonal loss may be greater and slowing of conduction velocities more uniform on nerve conduction studies compared to typical CIDP. The disease is characterized by elevated vascular endothelial growth factor (VEGF) levels in the serum and cerebrospinal fluid (CSF).

IgM MGUS

IgM MGUS may occur in MGUS, Waldenstrom macroglobulinemia, and IgM-secreting lymphomas. Neuropathies tend to occur most commonly with IgM gammopathies, with nearly 50% of these patients having the presence of neuropathy. The most common neuropathy is DADS, characterized by chronic, symmetrical, distal onset, and sensory predominant demyelinating neuropathy. Nearly 70% of patients demonstrate anti-MAG antibodies.

Compared to typical CIPD, these patients rarely show conduction blocks or temporal dispersion in nerve conduction studies.

Vasculitis-related Neuropathy

Vasculitis-related neuropathies arise due to inflammation of the vasa nervorum of the peripheral nerves, leading to thrombosis and eventually, ischemic injury. It may be classified as small-, medium-, and large-vessel vasculitis **(Box 1)**. A common pattern is mononeuritis multiplex, which may be present in 35–65% of patients with vasculitis.[54] Distal sensorimotor pattern may also occur. Onset is usually acute or subacute. The neuropathy is painful. Systemic features (fever, weight loss, and joint pains) may be present in patients with systemic vasculitis. Extensive investigations are necessary to look for biomarkers of inflammation, including erythrocyte sedimentation rate, C-reactive protein, and vasculitis markers. A nerve biopsy is indicated if these investigations are noncontributory. Pathological features include intramural inflammation in the vessel wall. The neuropathy is predominantly axonal.

Infectious Neuropathy

Several infections may lead to neuropathies. The foremost of these are leprosy and HIV infection.

Leprosy

Leprosy, caused by *Mycobacterium leprae*, involves the skin and the peripheral nervous system. It tends to affect temperature sensation first, and large fibers and tendon reflexes tend to remain spared till the later disease stage. Patients may develop painless burn wounds **(Fig. 1)** due to loss of temperature sensation.

It is believed that *M. leprae* requires cooler temperatures for growth. Hence, sites of predilection include skin, superficial peripheral nerves, testes, and anterior one-third of the eye. The Ridley–Jopling classification is used to categorize the clinical features of leprosy. This consists of: Indeterminate (I), Tuberculoid (TT), Borderline tuberculoid (BT), Borderline (BB), Borderline lepromatous (BL), and Lepromatous (LL).

In lepromatous neuropathy, negative sensory symptoms predominate. The occurrence of positive sensory symptoms is a marker of possible lepra reactions. The most important clinical clue is nerve thickening with beading and tenderness. Superficially located easily palpable nerves include supraorbital and supratrochlear nerves, greater auricular nerve, ulnar, superficial radial, peroneal, and posterior tibial nerves.

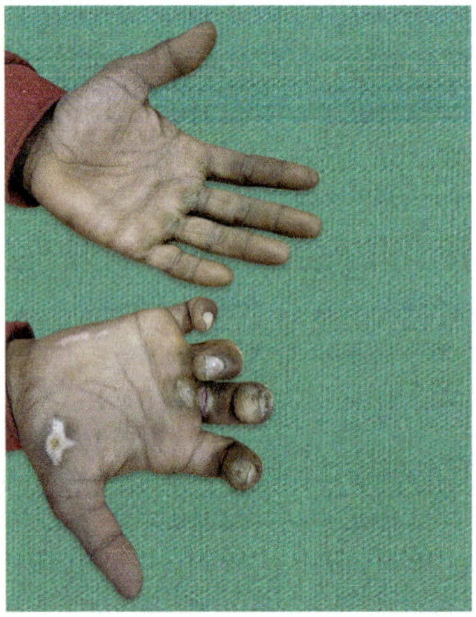

FIG. 1: Painless burns and ulnar clawing of the right hand in a patient with leprous neuritis.

Based on the pattern of nerve involvement, the following patterns are described:
- Mononeuropathy multiplex
- Small fiber, painful neuropathy
- Ganglionopathy
- Cranial neuropathy

Lepra reactions: These are immune-mediated syndromes that may occur after initiation of treatment for leprosy. They include:
- *Type I or reversal reaction*: These tend to occur in borderline leprosies and shift the pattern toward tuberculoid leprosy.
- *Type II reaction or erythema nodosum leprosum*: These are seen with lepromatous leprosy, and manifest as skin nodules, nerve pain, and inflammation in other body regions, such as lymph nodes, testes, etc.

Human Immunodeficiency Virus

The HIV infection can lead to several patterns of neuropathy. These include:
- Distal symmetrical sensorimotor neuropathy
- Mononeuropathy multiplex
- AIDP-like acute neuropathy
- CIPD-like chronic neuropathy
- Cranial neuropathy
- Lumbosacral radiculoplexopathy

Other Infectious Agents

Hepatitis C-related polyarteritis nodosa may present with a mononeuropathy multiplex-like presentation. This may be accompanied by systemic features, including fever, weight loss, and arthritis.

Varicella-zoster virus may present with dermatomal rash and focal neuropathy (herpes zoster), in immunocompromised individuals, such as those with diabetes, HIV, cancer, and aging.

Cytomegalovirus usually presents with a severely painful radiculoplexopathy, usually in association with HIV infection when the CD4 count is below 50 cells/μL. Diphtheria may lead to a rapidly progressive, descending quadriparesis with the bulbar onset and respiratory involvement. The GBS-like acute presentation may also be a manifestation of rabies, West Nile virus, and enterovirus infection.

EVALUATION

History

History is vital to neurological diagnosis. It is crucial to develop an accurate picture of the temporal profile of the illness, including onset and progression. Symptoms that are temporally correlated with exposure to a drug and improve

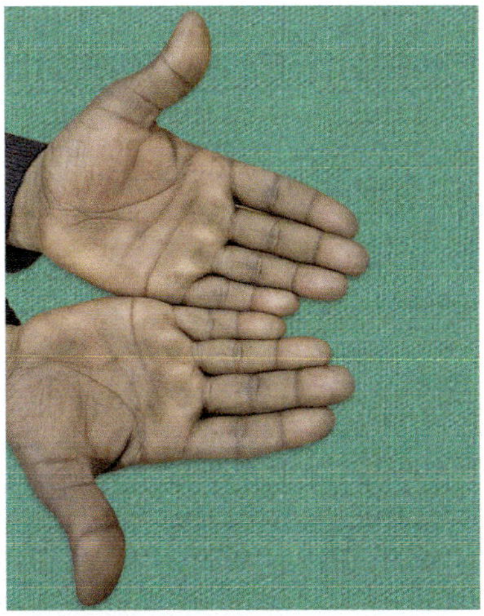

FIG. 2: Palmar hyperpigmentation seen in a patient with severe vitamin B12 deficiency.

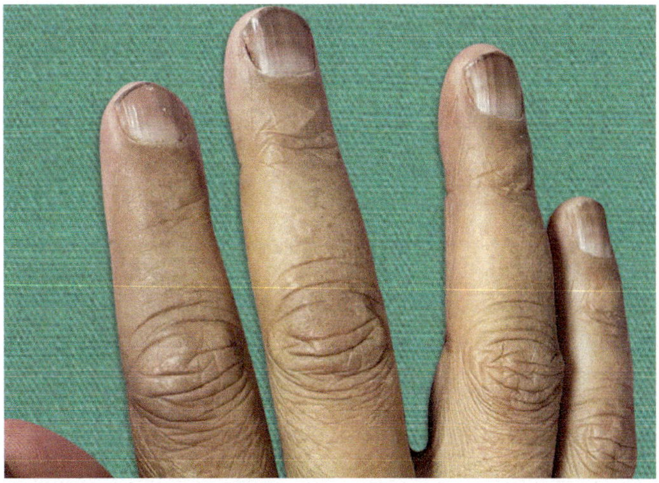

FIG. 3: Mees' lines seen in patients with arsenic/thallium toxicity.

after withdrawal incriminate the drug as the primary etiology. Similarly, the topographic pattern of neuropathic involvement is useful, i.e., whether the neuropathy has a length-dependent pattern or conforms to the pattern of mononeuropathy multiplex. Length-dependent patterns are common with toxin or drug-mediated or nutritional neuropathies. Mononeuropathy multiplex may be seen in diabetes, leprosy, HIV, or hepatitis C virus (HCV)-related neuropathy.

It is also important to decipher the pattern of fibers involved, i.e., large fiber or small fiber or mixed. Prominent autonomic dysfunction may be seen in certain acquired neuropathies, such as GBS and alcohol-induced neuropathy.

Apart from patient demographics, including age and gender, occupation is important to record. Heavy metal exposure may occur in battery manufacturing units, etc. Any exposure to drugs or chemotherapeutic agents must be explored. Dietary history, with predominant vegetarian fare, may predispose toward vitamin B12 deficiency. History of substance use, especially alcohol, must also be obtained. Presence of systemic complaints such as fever and weight loss points toward chronic infections such as HIV. Joint pains, arthritis, rash, and Raynaud's phenomenon indicate connective tissue disorders.

Examination

The examination is key in the evaluation of acquired peripheral neuropathies. Not only does examination confirm the pattern of neuropathic involvement, but it may also reveal vital clues indicating the etiology.

Diabetic neuropathy may be associated with diabetes-related dermopathy. Knuckle, palmar, and mucosal hyperpigmentation may be a feature of deficiency of vitamin B12 **(Fig. 2)**.

Lead toxicity can lead to Burton's line, a bluish line on the gums, which is formed due to the reaction between lead and sulfur compounds generated by oral bacteria. Mees' lines, also named Aldrich or Reynold's lines, are horizontal white bands that are seen on fingernails, and are associated with periods of stress **(Fig. 3)**. These are associated with arsenic and thallium poisoning. Hyperpigmentation of the skin (called "melanosis") and palmar and plantar hyperkeratosis are seen with arsenic poisoning, which may be due to chronic, low-level exposure. If exposure to arsenic continues, hypopigmented spots are formed, called the "raindrop" pattern.

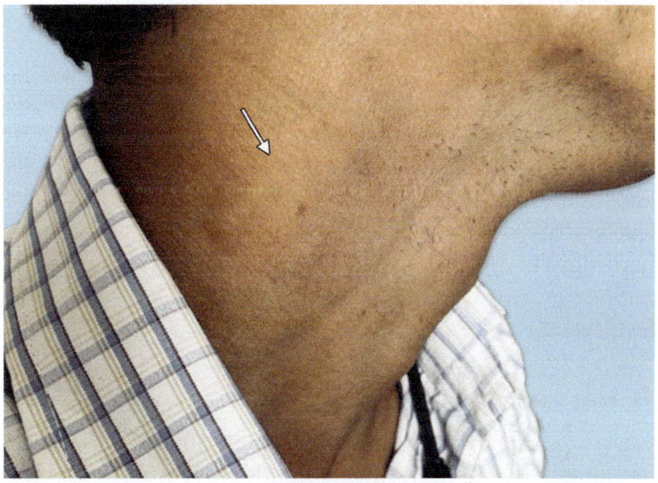

FIG. 4: Thickening of the greater auricular nerve (arrow) seen in leprosy, seen traversing parallel to the external jugular vein.

The presence of peripheral nerve thickening is seen in leprosy **(Fig. 4)**.

INVESTIGATIONS

Further evaluation is dictated by the patient's clinical presentation. Routine blood tests including complete blood count, liver function test, renal function test, thyroid function, vitamin B12 level, and blood sugar are widely available and must be performed for all patients with suspected neuropathy. A peripheral blood smear may show basophilic stippling in lead poisoning. Blood levels may be used in toxic neuropathies in the acute state in arsenic, thallium, and lead poisoning. Serum acetylcholinesterase (AChE) levels are low in acute organophosphate poisoning. Urinary 2,5-hexanedione levels are elevated in n-Hexane intoxication. Thiamine deficiency is indicated by reduced red blood cell transketolase level, although this is not required for diagnosis. Serum B12 (low), methylmalonic acid (high), and homocysteine (high) indicate vitamin B12 deficiency. A peripheral blood smear may show hypersegmented neutrophils. Low serum α-tocopherol level indicates vitamin E deficiency. Serum/urine electrophoresis for M band, evidence of end-organ damage in the form of hypercalcemia, anemia, and renal dysfunction indicates paraproteinemia.

Serological Tests

Serology is used for the diagnosis of HIV and hepatitis C. Serological tests for immune-mediated neuropathies include anti-ganglioside antibodies. Serum angiotensin-converting enzyme (ACE) levels may be elevated in sarcoidosis. Vasculitis markers are used in the diagnosis of vasculitis-related neuropathy, including complement levels, antinuclear antigen (ANA), c-ANCA, perinuclear anti-neutrophilic cytoplasmic antibodies (p-ANCA), anti-SSA/B antibodies, extractable nuclear antigen (ENA), cryoglobulin level, etc.

Nerve Conduction Studies

Nerve conduction studies of upper and lower limbs must be done. Routine motor nerve conduction studies include median, ulnar, peroneal, and tibial nerves and corresponding F waves. Routine sensory nerve conduction studies include median, ulnar, and sural nerves. Additional testing may include sympathetic skin response. Nerve conduction studies reveal a pattern of involvement, i.e., length-dependent pattern, mononeuritis pattern, entrapment neuropathy, etc. Nerve conduction studies may be normal in small-fiber sensory neuropathy and dorsal ganglionopathy.

The diagnosis of certain demyelinating neuropathies such as GBS, CIDP, MMN, and CISP is made based on electrophysiological criteria.[47,48,55,56]

Cerebrospinal Fluid

Cerebrospinal fluid assessment is sometimes used to demonstrate albuminocytological dissociation in immune-mediated neuropathies, including GBS, CIDP, and radiculoplexopathies. CSF may show increased cellularity in cytomegalovirus (CMV), HIV and Lyme disease, and other infective causes of radiculoneuropathy. CSF CMV PCR (polymerase chain reaction) is used for the diagnosis of CMV radiculoneuropathy.

Neuroimaging

Magnetic resonance imaging may show spinal nerve root enlargement and thickening in CIPD, and enhancement of nerve roots on contrast imaging in infective and inflammatory etiologies such as CMV, Lyme's, sarcoidosis, etc.

Nerve Biopsy

A nerve biopsy is indicated for suspected vasculitis-related neuropathy and may also support the diagnosis of CIDP.[6] Semithin sections allow a detailed overview of the nerve. Teased nerve fiber preparation allows the nerve to be assessed longitudinally, including the nodes of Ranvier. Ultrathin sections can be analyzed using electron microscopy for inclusions, myelin structure, and other details.

Skin Biopsy

A skin biopsy or slit skin smears may be useful in the diagnosis of leprosy. A skin biopsy may also be used to diagnose small-fiber neuropathy using intraepidermal nerve fiber density, which quantifies small fibers.

Others

Autonomic function tests may be used to demonstrate dysautonomia.

Toxicology screening may be used if heavy metal intoxication is suspected. In the acute phase, blood and urine samples may show elevated levels of toxins. In the chronic phase, hair and nail samples are useful.

Bone marrow biopsy is needed in patients with suspected paraproteinemia to quantify plasma cells. A skeletal survey is also done to look for bony involvement. Plasma VEGF level of >200 pg/mL supports POEMS syndrome. In suspected light chain amyloidosis, serum/urine immunofixation and immunoglobulin light-chain assay will show increased light chains, and subcutaneous fat pad biopsy or bone marrow biopsy may show the presence of amyloid deposits.

TREATMENT

All patients with acquired peripheral neuropathy should undergo therapy directed at the underlying etiology and symptomatic therapy.

Metabolic/Nutritional Neuropathies

In patients with diabetic neuropathy, stringent control of blood sugar can reverse symptoms and slow progression.

In vitamin-deficient neuropathies, supplementation of the deficient vitamin often leads to improvement of neuropathy. Vitamin B12 is administered as cyanocobalamin given as 1,000 μg parenterally once per week till the deficiency is corrected. Subsequently, it is administered at the same dose once a month (cyanocobalamin) or once in 2 months (hydroxocobalamin). Simultaneously, issues with oral absorption must also be explored. Acute thiamine deficiency requires intravenous thiamine. It is administered at a dose of 200 mg thrice daily till improvement or plateauing of symptoms.[19] Oral thiamine is then supplemented at a dose of 10 mg per day till complete recovery. In patients with alcoholic neuropathy, abstinence halts progression. Supplementation with thiamine, riboflavin, and B complex vitamins is needed as these patients are usually chronically malnourished.

Pyridoxine toxicity necessitates immediate cessation of pyridoxine supplementation and supportive treatment.

Drugs/Toxins

For heavy metal intoxication, chelation therapy is required. The antidote for thallium toxicity is Prussian blue, and it chelates thallium in the intestine. Other measures include forced diuresis, B complex and potassium supplementation, and hemodialysis.[57] In lead poisoning, chelation with disodium calcium edetate and dimercaprol, especially in cases with encephalopathy, is necessary. This is because the use of EDTA along may worsen features of encephalopathy. Disodium calcium edetate has a high affinity for lead, which is exchanged with calcium. Lead edetate is excreted renally. Other agents such as succimer and antioxidants like N-acetyl cysteine (NAC) are associated with a reduction in lead levels and may be used.[58] In arsenic toxicity, dimercaptosuccinic acid (DMSA) is the treatment of choice.

Immune-mediated Neuropathies

Among patients with GBS, treatment options include intravenous immunoglobulins (IVIg) and plasma exchange (PLEX). IVIg is administered at a dose of 2 g/kg, over 2–5 days. A second dose of IVIg in patients with poor prognosis did not provide any evidence of benefit in a randomized controlled trial.[59] PLEX is conducted as 5 cycles, with a total volume of exchange of 40–50 mL/kg per session. Supportive management in the form of nutrition, prevention of bedsore and deep vein thrombosis, and bladder and bowel care is essential.

In CIPD, the first line of treatment comprises steroids, IVIg, and PLEX. In case of nonresponse to one of these modalities, the others may be used.

Steroids may either be initiated as pulse intravenous methylprednisolone or high-dose oral steroids. Patients usually respond to steroids within 8–12 weeks. Steroid-sparing agents are added as the treatment is prolonged, and include azathioprine, methotrexate, and mycophenolate mofetil.

The IVIg is initiated at 2 g/kg over 5 days and maintained as monthly infusions of 1 g/kg.

In refractory cases, options include rituximab, tacrolimus, cyclophosphamide, and cyclosporine.

Even alemtuzumab and autologous hematopoietic stem cell transplantation are used.

For MMN, the first line of treatment comprises IVIg. Maintenance doses may be planned according to the individual's requirement. Steroids and PLEX are not useful in the treatment and may worsen weakness. In IVIg refractory cases, cyclophosphamide and rituximab therapies have been tried although the latter did not demonstrate a change in IVIg dose, frequency, or motor strength in an open-label trial.

Treatment of POEMS syndrome requires treatment of the underlying malignancy.

Treatment of IgA/IgG MGUS is managed along the lines of CIDP.

In patients with vasculitic neuropathy, steroids are the mainstay of treatment.[54] If the neuropathy is severe, pulse intravenous methylprednisolone may be initiated, followed by oral steroids. Another option is intravenous pulse cyclophosphamide (0.5–0.75 mg/m^2 monthly) along with mesna. Steroid-sparing agents include methotrexate, azathioprine, and mycophenolate. Rituximab is considered the first-line treatment for ANCA-associated vasculitis. For patients not responding to steroids or cyclophosphamide, IVIg may be considered.

Infections

Treatment of leprosy is based on the World Health Organization (WHO) leprosy classification **(Table 5)**.[60] In patients with neuritic involvement, steroids are shown to improve outcomes.[61] Steroids are given for 3–6 months or even longer. For type 2 lepra reaction, steroids are given for at least 3 months as per WHO recommendations. Thalidomide has also been used for this purpose.[62] Cyclosporine is also used in this condition.[63] Due to their toxicity, these agents may be considered in patients who do not respond adequately to steroids.

Symptom-based Therapy

Multiple options exist for symptom alleviation, including tricyclic antidepressants, gabapentinoids, serotonin-norepinephrine uptake inhibitors (SNRIs), etc. **(Table 6)**.[64]

TABLE 5: Multidrug treatment of leprosy (WHO guidelines).

Multibacillary leprosy (12 months)*	Paucibacillary leprosy (6 months)**
Dapsone: 100 mg once daily	*Dapsone*: 100 mg daily
Rifampicin: 600 mg once a month	*Rifampicin*: 600 mg once per month
Clofazimine: 300 mg once a month and 50 mg daily	–

*Paucibacillary leprosy: 1–5 skin lesions, absence of bacilli in slit skin smear.

**Multibacillary leprosy: >5 skin lesions, pure neuritis, presence of bacilli in slit skin smear.

TABLE 6: Symptomatic therapy for neuropathic pain.[64]

Drug class	Drugs	Dose range (minimum–maximum permissible)
Gabapentinoids	Gabapentin	200–3,600 mg
	Pregabalin	150–600 mg
Serotonin–norepinephrine reuptake inhibitors	Duloxetine	30–60 mg
	Venlafaxine	37.5–225 mg
Tricyclic antidepressants	Nortriptyline	10–150 mg
	Amitriptyline	10–150 mg
Tropical agents	5% lidocaine	Local application for 12 hours
	8% capsaicin	Local application for 1 hour
Opioids	Tramadol	50–400 mg

Patients with negative sensory symptoms must be advised about foot care, especially patients with diabetic neuropathy, as small ulcers or wounds can become infected and heal slowly, leading to complications such as cellulitis, sepsis, gangrene, and nonhealing ulcers.

CONCLUSION

Acquired peripheral neuropathies may arise from a wide spectrum of disorders, which include metabolic/nutritional, drugs/toxins, and immune-mediated and infectious causes. History and examination are the cornerstones of diagnosis. Systemic examination, especially dermatological, must be meticulously performed to glean underlying etiology. Most of the acquired neuropathies are eminently treatable, and many are reversible. Early diagnosis and treatment are crucial to ensure a good prognosis before the irreversible axonal loss is established. Treatment is twofold and comprises symptom-based therapy and specific therapy directed at the underlying etiology.

REFERENCES

1. Siao P, Kaku M. A Clinician's approach to peripheral neuropathy. Semin Neurol. 2019;39(5):519530.
2. Lozeron P, Trocello JM, Kubis N. Acquired neuropathies. J Neurol. 2013;260(9):2433-40.
3. Katona I, Weis J. Diseases of the peripheral nerves. Handb Clin Neurol. 2017;145:453-74.
4. Neau JP, Godeneche G, Mathis S, Guillet G. Neurodermatology. Handb Clin Neurol. 2014;121:15611594.
5. Levine TD, Saperstein DS. Laboratory evaluation of peripheral neuropathy. Neurol Clin. 2013;31(2):363-76.
6. Sommer C, Carroll AS, Koike H, Katsuno M, Ort N, Sobue G, et al. Nerve biopsy in acquired neuropathies. J Peripher Nerv Syst. 2021;26(Suppl 2):S21-S41.
7. Hanewinckel R, Ikram MA, Van Doorn PA. Peripheral neuropathies. Handb Clin Neurol. 2016;138:263-82
8. Trivedi S, Pandit A, Ganguly G, Das SK. Epidemiology of peripheral neuropathy: An indian perspective. Ann Indian Acad Neurol. 2017;20(3):173-84.
9. Ghosh B, Sengupta S, Bhattacharjee R, Pal S, Saha SP, Ganguly G, et al. Spectrum of peripheral neuropathy in eastern India. J Indian Med Assoc. 2006;104(4):168, 170-3.
10. Chalk CH. Acquired peripheral neuropathy. Neurol Clin. 1997;15(3):501-28.
11. Feldman EL, Callaghan BC, Pop-Busui R, Zochodne DW, Wright DE, Bennett DL, et al. Diabetic neuropathy. Nat Rev Dis Primers. 2019;5(1):41.
12. Vinik AI, Nevoret ML, Casellini C, Parson H. Diabetic neuropathy. Endocrinol Metab Clin North Am. 2013;42(4):747-87.
13. Sloan G, Selvarajah D, Tesfaye S. Pathogenesis, diagnosis and clinical management of diabetic sensorimotor peripheral neuropathy. Nat Rev Endocrinol. 2021;17(7):400-20.
14. Said G. Uremic neuropathy. Handb Clin Neurol. 2013;115:607-12.
15. Baluarte JH. Neurological complications of renal disease. Semin Pediatr Neurol. 2017;24(1):25-32.
16. Novak M, Winkelman JW, Unruh M. Restless legs syndrome in patients with chronic kidney disease. Semin Nephrol. 2015;35(4):347-58.
17. Staff NP, Windebank AJ. Peripheral neuropathy due to vitamin deficiency, toxins, and medications. Continuum (Minneap Minn). 2014;20(5 Peripheral Nervous System Disorders):1293-306.
18. Kumar N. Neurologic aspects of cobalamin (B12) deficiency. Handb Clin Neurol. 2014;120:915-26.
19. Wiley KD, Gupta M. (2022). Vitamin B1 Thiamine Deficiency. [online] Available from http://www.ncbi.nlm.nih.gov/books/NBK537204/. [Last accessed February, 2023].
20. Koike H, Iijima M, Sugiura M, Mori K, Hattori N, Ito H, et al. Alcoholic neuropathy is clinicopathologically distinct from thiamine-deficiency neuropathy. Ann Neurol. 2003;54(1):19-29.
21. Ghavanini AA, Kimpinski K. Revisiting the evidence for neuropathy caused by pyridoxine deficiency and excess. J Clin Neuromuscul Dis. 2014;16(1):25-31.
22. Saper RB, Kales SN, Paquin J, Burns MJ, Eisenberg DM, Davis RB, et al. Heavy metal content of ayurvedic herbal medicine products. JAMA. 2004;292(23):2868-73.
23. Vittadini G, Buonocore M, Colli G, Terzi M, Fonte R, Biscaldi G. Alcoholic polyneuropathy: a clinical and epidemiological study. Alcohol Alcohol. 2001;36(5):393-400.
24. Agelink MW, Malessa R, Weisser U, Lemmer W, Zeit T, Majewski T, et al. Alcoholism, peripheral neuropathy (PNP) and cardiovascular autonomic neuropathy (CAN). J Neurol Sci. 1998;161(2):135-42.
25. Koszewicz M, Markowska K, Waliszewska-Prosol M, Poreba R, Gac P, Szymanska-Chabowska A, et al. The impact of chronic co-exposure to different heavy metals on small fibers of peripheral nerves. A study of metal industry workers. J Occup Med Toxicol. 2021;16(1):12.
26. Vahidnia A, van der Voet GB, de Wolff FA. Arsenic neurotoxicity--a review. Hum Exp Toxicol. 2007;26(10):823-32.
27. Little AA, Albers JW. Clinical description of toxic neuropathies. Handb Clin Neurol. 2015;131:253296.
28. Liu H, Liao G. Long-term misdiagnosis and neurologic outcomes of thallium poisoning: A case report and literature review. Brain Behav. 2021;11(3):e02032.
29. Lotti M, Moretto A. Organophosphate-induced delayed polyneuropathy. Toxicol Rev. 2005;24(1):37-49.
30. Shukla A, Anand D, Urkude R. Organophosphate induced delayed pure motor neuropathy. J Neurol Neurosurg Psychiatry. 2017;88(5):e1-e1.
31. Kobayashi S, Okubo R, Ugawa Y. Delayed polyneuropathy induced by organophosphate poisoning. Intern Med. 2017;56(14):1903-5.

32. Chang CM, Yu CW, Fong KY, Leung SY, Tsin TW, Yu YL, et al. N-hexane neuropathy in offset printers. J Neurol Neurosurg Psychiatry. 1993;56(5):538-42.
33. Herskowitz A, Ishii N, Schaumburg H. N-hexane neuropathy. A syndrome occurring as a result of industrial exposure. N Engl J Med. 1971;285(2):82-5.
34. Gobba F, Cavalleri F, Bontadi D, Torri P, Dainese R. Peripheral neuropathy in styrene-exposed workers. Scand J Work Environ Health. 1995;21(6):517-20.
35. House RA, Liss GM, Wills MC. Peripheral sensory neuropathy associated with 1,1,1trichloroethane. Arch Environ Health. 1994;49(3):196-9.
36. Jones MR, Urits I, Wolf J, Corrigan D, Colburn L, Peterson E, et al. Drug-induced peripheral neuropathy: A narrative review. Curr Clin Pharmacol. 2020;15(1):38-48.
37. Manji H. Drug-induced neuropathies. Handb Clin Neurol. 2013;115:729-42.
38. Seretny M, Currie GL, Sena ES, Ramnarine S, Grant R, MacLeod MR, et al. Incidence, prevalence, and predictors of chemotherapy-induced peripheral neuropathy: A systematic review and meta-analysis. Pain. 2014;155(12):2461-70.
39. Legout L, Senneville E, Gomel JJ, Yazdanpanah Y, Mouton Y. Linezolid-induced neuropathy. Clin Infect Dis. 2004;38(5):767-8.
40. Rho JP, Sia IG, Crum BA, Dekutoski MB, Trousdale RT. Linezolid-associated peripheral neuropathy. Mayo Clin Proc. 2004;79(7): 927-30.
41. Goolsby TA, Jakeman B, Gaynes RP. Clinical relevance of metronidazole and peripheral neuropathy: a systematic review of the literature. Int J Antimicrob Agents. 2018;51(3):319-25.
42. Margolis AM, Heverling H, Pham PA, Stolbach A. A review of the toxicity of HIV medications. J Med Toxicol. 2014;10(1):26-39.
43. Kieseier BC, Mathey EK, Sommer C, Hartung HP. Immune-mediated neuropathies. Nat Rev Dis Primers. 2018;4(1):31.
44. Allen JA, Parry GJ. Acquired immunologic neuropathies. Semin Neurol. 2015;35(4):398-406.
45. Hadden RD, Karch H, Hartung HP, Zielasek J, Weissbrich B, Schubert J, et al. Preceding infections, immune factors, and outcome in Guillain-Barré syndrome. Neurology. 2001;56(6):758-65.
46. Malek E, Salameh J. Guillain-Barre Syndrome. Semin Neurol. 2019;39(5):589-95.
47. Van den Bergh PYK, van Doorn PA, Hadden RDM, Avau B, Vankrunkelsven P, Allen JA, et al. European Academy of Neurology/ Peripheral Nerve Society guideline on diagnosis and treatment of chronic inflammatory demyelinating polyradiculoneuropathy: Report of a joint Task Force—Second revision. J Peripher Nerv Syst. 2021;26(3):242-68.
48. Olney RK, Lewis RA, Putnam TD, Campellone JV, American Association of Electrodiagnostic Medicine. Consensus criteria for the diagnosis of multifocal motor neuropathy. Muscle Nerve. 2003;27(1):117-21.
49. Khadilkar S, Patel B, Mansukhani KA, Jaggi S. Two cases of chronic immune sensorimotor polyradiculopathy: Expanding the spectrum of chronic immune polyradiculopathies. Muscle Nerve. 2017;55(1):135-7.
50. Shelly S, Shouman K, Paul P, Engelstad J, Amrami KK, Spinner RJ, et al. Expanding the spectrum of chronic immune sensory polyradiculopathy: CISP-Plus. Neurology. 2021;96(16):e2078-89.
51. Martín-Aguilar L, Lleixà C, Pascual-Goñi E, Caballero-Ávila M, Martínez-Martínez L, Díaz-Manera J, et al. Clinical and laboratory features in anti-NF155 autoimmune nodopathy. Neurol Neuroimmunol Neuroinflamm. 2022;9(1):e1098.
52. Fehmi J, Vale T, Keddie S, Rinaldi S. Nodal and paranodal antibody-associated neuropathies. Pract Neurol. 2021:practneurol-2021-002960.
53. Chaudhry HM, Mauermann ML, Rajkumar SV. Monoclonal gammopathy-associated peripheral neuropathy: Diagnosis and management. Mayo Clin Proc. 2017;92(5):838-50.
54. Blaes F. Diagnosis and therapeutic options for peripheral vasculitic neuropathy. Ther Adv Musculoskelet Dis. 2015;7(2):45-55.
55. Leonhard SE, Mandarakas MR, Gondim FAA, Bateman K, Ferreira MLB, Cornblath DR, et al. Diagnosis and management of Guillain–Barré syndrome in ten steps. Nat Rev Neurol. 2019;15(11):671-83.
56. Ong S, Cassidy A. Chronic immune sensory polyradiculopathy (CISP). Pract Neurol. 2022;22(1):57-9.
57. Misra UK, Kalita J, Yadav RK, Ranjan P. Thallium poisoning: emphasis on early diagnosis and response to haemodialysis. Postgrad Med J. 2003;79(928):103-5.
58. Wani AL, Ara A, Usmani JA. Lead toxicity: a review. Interdiscip Toxicol. 2015;8(2):55-64.
59. Walgaard C, Jacobs BC, Lingsma HF, Steyerberg PEW, van den Berg B, Doets AY, et al. Second intravenous immunoglobulin dose in patients with Guillain-Barré syndrome with poor prognosis (SID-GBS): a double-blind, randomised, placebo-controlled trial. Lancet Neurol. 2021;20(4):275-83.
60. World Health Organization. (2023). Leprosy. [online] Available from https://www.who.int/news-room/fact-sheets/detail/leprosy. [Last accessed February, 2023].
61. Rao PN, Suneetha S. Pure neuritic leprosy: Current status and relevance. Indian J Dermatol Venereol Leprol. 2016;82(3):252-61.
62. Upputuri B, Pallapati MS, Tarwater P, Srikantam A. Thalidomide in the treatment of erythema nodosum leprosum (ENL) in an outpatient setting: A five-year retrospective analysis from a leprosy referral centre in India. PLOS Negl Trop Dis. 2020;14(10):e0008678.
63. Lambert SM, Alembo DT, Nigusse SD, Yamuah LK, Walker SL, Lockwood DNJ. A randomized controlled double-blind trial of ciclosporin versus prednisolone in the management of leprosy patients with new Type 1 reaction, in Ethiopia. PLoS Negl Trop Dis. 2016;10(4):e0004502.
64. Bates D, Schultheis BC, Hanes MC, Jolly SM, Chakravarthy KV, Deer TR, et al. A comprehensive algorithm for management of neuropathic pain. Pain Med. 2019;20(Suppl 1):S2-S12.

83

CHAPTER

Diseases of the Autonomic Nervous System

Ajith Sivadasan, Aditya Vijayakrishnan Nair

INTRODUCTION

The autonomic nervous system (ANS) controls the body's vital functions and maintains homeostasis. Functions include regulation of heart rate, blood pressure, sleep, rate of respiration, bladder, and bowel functions. The system functions autonomously without a person's conscious effort.

Autonomic dysfunction is highly prevalent and remains underdiagnosed. Clinical presentations are varied and often nonspecific. A high index of suspicion is needed for an early diagnosis. Delayed diagnosis can potentially lead to increased morbidity and even mortality, especially in the setting of cardiovascular autonomic dysfunction. Objective confirmation of autonomic dysfunction is desirable. Simple bedside tests often complement a good clinical examination. The advent of newer autonomic function tests which are noninvasive, simple, reproducible, and quantitative has revolutionized the care of patients with autonomic dysfunction.

FUNCTIONAL ANATOMY OF THE AUTONOMIC NERVOUS SYSTEM

The ANS was divided by Langley into three parts—(1) the sympathetic, (2) parasympathetic, and (3) enteral (intestinal) nervous systems. The sympathetic nervous system can be further subclassified as noradrenergic, adrenergic, and cholinergic.[1-3] The main neurotransmitter in the parasympathetic nervous system is acetylcholine (ACh).

The processing centers in the central nervous system integrate afferent stimuli from the body and external environment.[4] The centers include the hypothalamus (paraventricular, dorsomedial nucleus), nucleus of solitary tract, reticular formation, amygdala, hippocampus, and the olfactory cortex. The bulbopontine level regulates respiration and circulation, pontomesencephalic level controls pain modulation, and the forebrain is involved in goal-related autonomic and endocrine responses for maintenance of homeostasis and adaptation. The autonomic outflow is subsequently modified to enable the functions of the organs systems according to the needs of the body.

Sympathetic Nervous System

The preganglionic neurons leave the intermediolateral horn of spinal cord between T1 and L2 (thoracolumbar pathway). The postganglionic cell bodies are located adjacent to the spine and include the superior cervical, celiac, superior mesenteric, inferior mesenteric, and aortorenal ganglia. The postganglionic nerve fibers from the ganglia reach the effector organs. The main effector organs include the smooth muscles of the blood vessels, viscera, pupils, and lungs. The other effector organs include the heart, sweat, salivary, and digestive glands.

Parasympathetic Nervous System

The preganglionic cell bodies are located in brainstem (cranial nerves III, VII, IX, and X) and sacral portion of spinal cord (craniosacral pathway). The postganglionic cell bodies are located close to the effector organs. These include the ciliary, sphenopalatine, submandibular, otic, and pelvic ganglia as well as the ganglion cells located in the wall of the heart and gastrointestinal (GI) tract. The effector organs include blood vessels of head, neck and thoracoabdominal viscera, lacrimal and salivary glands, smooth muscles of the glands, and viscera and pupillary muscle.

The responses to activation of the sympathetic and parasympathetic nervous system are often reciprocal and have been depicted in **Table 1**. The main neurotransmitters are ACh and norepinephrine (NE). ACh (nicotinic) is the preganglionic neurotransmitter for both the sympathetic and parasympathetic divisions. ACh (muscarinic) is also the postganglionic neurotransmitter in the parasympathetic nervous system. NE is the neurotransmitter for postganglionic sympathetic neurons except the eccrine glands which are innervated by cholinergic neurons.

Autonomic Immune Axis

The ANS has an important role in regulation of immune function and inflammation.[5,6] Splenic innervation by the vagus and sympathetic splanchnic nerves helps in downregulating inflammation. However, the sympathetic nervous system could also accentuate local inflammation and be activated in the setting of chronic inflammation.

Baroreflex Pathway and Abnormalities

The baroreflex pathway is responsible for moment-to-moment control of blood pressure in response to external stimuli, orthostasis, and stress.[2] Separate pathways from the relay station in the nucleus of tractus solitarius (NTS) control the sympathetic vasomotor [rostral ventrolateral medulla (RVLM)] and cardiovagal outputs (nucleus ambiguus). Afferent discharges are relayed from the carotid sinus and aortic arch by the glossopharyngeal and vagus nerves, respectively. The activation of premotor sympathetic neurons in the RVLM leads to increased sympathetic noradrenergic output and α1-mediated vasoconstriction, increased peripheral vascular resistance and elevations in blood pressure. The cardiovagal output is mediated by the nucleus ambiguus neurons innervating the heart which results in bradycardia. Sympathetic noradrenergic innervation to the heart is mediated by β1-receptors. The nucleus tractus solitarius acts as the relay station coordinating reciprocal changes in heart rate and blood pressure for maintenance of homeostasis. A schematic representation of the baroreflex pathway has been provided in **Flowchart 1**.

Orthostatic hypotension (OH) results from abnormalities in the baroreflex efferent pathway involving the RVLM, intermediolateral column in the spinal cord, preganglionic neurons, sympathetic ganglia, or postganglionic noradrenergic neurons. Baroreflex afferent failure manifests with labile blood pressures, hypertensive crisis, tachycardia or bradycardia, and unpredictable responses to antihypertensives and vasoconstrictor drugs. Baroreflex afferent failure could occur following surgery to the neck, radiation or be a manifestation of autonomic neuropathies such as Guillain–Barré syndrome (GBS) or familial dysautonomia.[7,8]

TABLE 1: Functions of the sympathetic and parasympathetic nervous system.

	Sympathetic nervous system	Parasympathetic nervous system
Blood pressure	Increased	Decreased (mildly)
Heart rate	Increased	Decreased
Lung	Bronchodilation	Bronchoconstriction
Bladder	Increased sphincter tone	Decreased sphincter tone (voiding)
Bowel	Decreased motility	Increased motility
Pupils	Dilation	Constriction
Sweat glands	Sweating	–
Sexual functions	Ejaculation	Erection

Thermoregulatory Pathways

The thermoreceptor afferents from the sympathetic innervation of the skin enter the dorsal horn of the spinal cord and relay in the parabrachial nucleus.[2,9] The neurons in the parabrachial nucleus acts as a relay station that conveys the peripheral inputs to the median preoptic area in the hypothalamus. The heat-sensitive neurons are located in the medial preoptic area and cold-sensitive neurons in the dorsomedial nucleus of the hypothalamus. Sympathetic responses to cold are mediated by the dorsomedial nucleus to the nucleus raphe pallidus and subsequent skin vasoconstriction via α1 receptors and thermogenesis via β2 receptors in the adipose tissue. The heat responses are mediated via the medial preoptic nucleus to rostral medulla and subsequently the intermediolateral column of the spinal cord. Sympathetic cholinergic innervation occurs to the sweat glands via M3 receptors and skin vasodilation also occurs.

CLINICAL FEATURES OF AUTONOMIC DYSFUNCTION

Clinical manifestations of autonomic dysfunction can occur due to loss of function or overactivity of the ANS. Symptoms can be episodic, situational, or persistent.

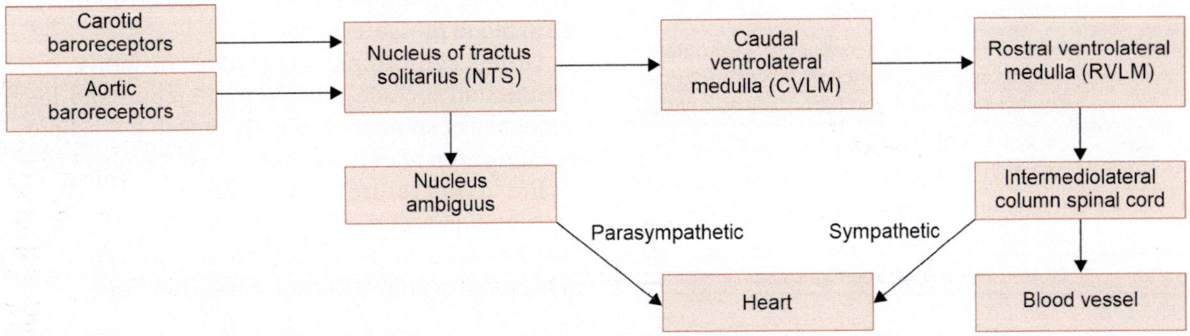

FLOWCHART 1: Schematic representation of the baroreflex pathway.

The details regarding temporal profile of disease—onset, progression, antecedent illness, comorbidities and concomitant disorders, lifestyle changes, and medication history are paramount to establishing a definite diagnosis. The symptoms include multiple organ systems including the cardiovascular, GI, genitourinary, secretomotor, and the thermoregulatory system.[2,3,10] The symptoms may be generalized or restricted to specific domains **(Table 2)**. Comprehensive self-reported questionnaires such as the Autonomic Symptom Profile (169 point) or Composite Autonomic Symptom Score (COMPASS-84 point) have been used traditionally for assessing the extent of involvement.[11,12] A COMPASS 31 score with 31 questions in 6 domains has been found to be refined, simplified, and suitable for widespread use in clinical practice in disorders of the ANS.[13]

Sympathetic Dysfunction

Sympathetic noradrenergic hyperactivity results in palpitations, tachycardia, hypertension, mydriasis, and piloerection. Sympathetic noradrenergic hypofunction/failure results in OH, ptosis, lack of piloerection, and ejaculatory failure.

Sympathetic adrenergic hyperactivity causes palpitations, facial pallor, impaired GI motility, and mydriasis. Sympathetic adrenergic failure causes generalized fatigue and orthostatic intolerance.

Sympathetic cholinergic hyperactivity results in generalized or focal hyperhidrosis. Sympathetic cholinergic failure causes hypohidrosis or anhidrosis with impaired thermoregulation and abnormal responses to fever and hot temperatures. A drug history to exclude concomitant use of anticholinergics, carbonic anhydrase inhibitors, or serotonin reuptake inhibitors is mandatory to exclude secondary causes of cholinergic dysfunction.

TABLE 2: System specific manifestations of autonomic dysfunction.

System	Manifestations
Cardiovascular	Orthostatic hypotension (OH), labile hypertension, arrhythmias, supine hypertension, and syncope
Gastrointestinal	Gastroparesis, dysphagia, early satiety, bloating, constipation, and diarrhea
Genitourinary	Retention, urgency, incontinence, incomplete voiding, erectile dysfunction, loss of nocturnal penile tumescence, and retrograde ejaculation
Secretomotor	Lack of sweating, excess sweating, gustatory sweating, dryness of mouth, and eyes
Skin	Hypothermia, hyperpyrexia, loss of hair, and nail discoloration
Pupillomotor	Blurred vision, impaired night vision

Parasympathetic Dysfunction

Parasympathetic hyperactivity results in hypersalivation, vomiting, diarrhea, urinary urgency, and bradycardia. Parasympathetic failure causes dry mouth, tachycardia, mydriasis, bladder retention, erectile dysfunction, and constipation.

ORTHOSTATIC INTOLERANCE

Orthostatic intolerance is commonly reported in disorders of the ANS. This need not always be attributable to OH and other causes such as postural orthostatic tachycardia syndrome (POTS) and reflex syncope also need to be considered. OH is diagnosed when there is sustained drop in blood pressure (systolic ≥ 20 mm Hg, diastolic ≥ 10 mm Hg) within 3 minutes of standing. Delayed OH is defined as a sustained drop in blood pressure after 3 minutes of upright posture. Long-term follow-up of patients with delayed OH has revealed a progression to OH with increased mortality and development of neurodegenerative disorders like multiple system atrophy (MSA).[14] The symptoms of orthostatic intolerance are diverse and include light headedness, generalized tiredness, blurred vision, diaphoresis, vertigo, nausea, and palpitations. It is important to note that the elderly population can present with "reversible" cognitive dysfunction because of cerebral hypoperfusion.[15] Syncope occurs when there is significant drop in blood pressure impairing cerebral perfusion. The relationship of orthostatic symptoms to meals (pooling in splanchnic circulation), standing on early morning awakening (intravascular volume depletion), warming (vasodilatation), or exercise (muscle arteriolar dilatation) should be elicited. Drugs aggravating OH include diuretics, antihypertensives, alpha blockers, levodopa, tricyclic antidepressants, and vasodilators. OH precipitated by drugs could also be the first sign to suggest the presence of or unmask an underlying autonomic disorder. Non-neurogenic causes of OH include cardiac pump failure, reduced intravascular volume due to dehydration or blood loss, and metabolic causes like hypocortisolemia. Other indicators of impaired baroreflex function include supine hypertension, postprandial hypotension, fixed heart rate irrespective of changes in posture, and elevated nocturnal blood pressures. POTS is diagnosed by the increase in heart rate (>30 beats/min, tachycardia >120 beats/min) without a fall in blood pressure on standing.

Other symptoms suggestive of early autonomic dysfunction include erectile dysfunction and decrease in frequency of spontaneous early morning erections. Lack of sweating even after heavy exercise, hot bath, or on exposure to hot temperatures may indicate sudomotor failure. Constipation and diarrhea indicate visceral GI dysfunction. Diarrhea occurs due to GI dysmotility with contribution due to bacterial overgrowth contributed by stasis.

CLINICAL AUTONOMIC DISORDERS

The disorders can be broadly categorized as central (involving brain and spinal cord) or peripheral autonomic disorders (autonomic neuropathies). The classification is as described in the **Table 3**.

Synucleinopathies

Autonomic dysfunction in synucleinopathies is secondary to neurodegeneration and dysfunction associated with abnormal aggregates of α-synuclein proteins in the cytoplasm of nuclei and glia.[16,17] There is emerging evidence of cell-to-cell spread of α-synuclein in a "prion-like" manner.[18] The pattern and location of abnormal aggregates lead to distinct phenotypes involving the central or peripheral nervous system. The disorders are characterized by autonomic dysfunction in addition to motor, cognitive, and behavioral deficits. Prominent autonomic dysfunction is seen in MSA, pure autonomic failure (PAF), and dementia with Lewy body (DLB).

Multiple system atrophy is a progressive disorder which includes autonomic dysfunction with parkinsonism (MSA-P) or cerebellar involvement (MSA-C). The neuropathological hallmark is oligodendroglial cytoplasmic inclusions. In addition, there is neuronal loss and gliosis in the brainstem, cerebellum, striatum, and intermediolateral columns of the spinal cord. There is usually symptomatic OH within 1 year of onset of parkinsonism. Evidence of a generalized and severe autonomic dysfunction is present. OH could coexist with supine hypertension. Diagnostic criteria for OH in MSA warrant a fall by at least 30/15 mm Hg.[16,17] Genitourinary autonomic abnormalities with erectile dysfunction, urinary incontinence, and increased postvoid residual volumes are common and early manifestations. Rapid eye movement (REM) sleep behavioral disorder (RBD) and nocturnal stridor could be present. A central pattern of autonomic dysfunction with global anhidrosis on the thermoregulatory sweat test (TST) and relatively preserved sweat volumes on the quantitative sudomotor axon reflex tests (QSART) is a discriminating feature from PAF.[16]

Pure autonomic failure is characterized by symptoms of OH, defective sweating, impotence, and bladder dysfunction.[16,19] The pathology is at the level of postganglionic efferent peripheral sympathetic nerves. The disorder usually affects middle-aged women and though the symptoms are disabling, life span does not shorten. There could be antibodies to ganglionic ACh receptor in some cases of PAF which implies that the etiology could be immune mediated in some cases. The progression is slow, and patients may tolerate substantial drops in blood pressure with relatively minor symptoms (light headedness and coat-hanger distribution pain) due to compensations in cerebral autoregulation.[16] Supine hypertension could be seen in nearly 50% and could lead to secondary end organ (cardiac and renal dysfunction). From a therapeutic perspective, supine hypertension often interferes with optimal management of OH. This is attributed to receptor denervation hypersensitivity and baroreflex dysfunction.[16] A postganglionic pattern of sweating dysfunction with abnormal QSART volumes corresponding to

TABLE 3: Classification of clinical autonomic disorders based on site of neuraxis involved.

Autonomic disorders with brain involvement	
Multisystem degeneration	• Multiple system atrophy • Diffuse Lewy body disease • Parkinson's disease (advanced)
Focal CNS disorders	• Insular cortex involvement (stroke) • Limbic encephalitis • Diencephalic syndromes • Posterior fossa tumors
Autonomic disorders with spinal cord involvement	• Traumatic myelopathy • Syringomyelia • Tetanus • Stiff person syndrome • Neuromyelitis optica and multiple sclerosis
Autonomic disorders with peripheral nervous system involvement	Autonomic neuropathies (described in **Table 4**)

(CNS: central nervous system)

TABLE 4: Classification of neuropathies with prominent autonomic involvement.

Systemic disease	Diabetes mellitus, chronic kidney disease, and amyloidosis
Autoimmune causes	Autoimmune autonomic ganglionopathy (AAG), Sjögren's syndrome, Guillain–Barré syndrome, and Lambert–Eaton syndrome
Hereditary	HSAN, Fabry disease, Tangier disease, familial amyloid neuropathy, and mitochondrial neurogastrointestinal encephalomyopathy (MNGIE)
Infectious	HIV, botulism, and diphtheria
Toxin/drug induced	Alcohol, pyridoxine, vincristine, and cisplatin
Localized forms	Horner's syndrome, Adie pupil, gustatory sweating, palmar/axillary hyperhidrosis, reflex sympathetic dystrophy, and Chagas disease
Phenotypes possibly associated with ganglionic AChR antibody (low titers and positivity)	AAG, POTS, chronic idiopathic anhidrosis, chronic intestinal pseudo-obstruction, and PAF

(AChR: acetylcholine receptor; HSAN: hereditary sensory and autonomic neuropathy; HIV: human immunodeficiency virus; PAF: pure autonomic failure; POTS: postural orthostatic tachycardia syndrome)

areas of areas of anhidrosis on the TST is characteristic. In addition to abnormal QSART, the autonomic dysfunction in PAF (postganglionic) can be differentiated from MSA (preganglionic) by low supine NE levels with minimal response to standing, and an impaired cardiac sympathetic innervation on metaiodobenzylguanidine (MIBG).[20] A subset of patients with PAF can have a phenotype conversion to MSA (typically within 3 years of diagnosis) and DLB (can occur up to 8 years).[21]

The severity of autonomic dysfunction in DLB and advanced Parkinson disease is often less severe.[16] Both peripheral and central patterns of autonomic dysfunction are seen. Treatment with dopaminergic drugs potentially aggravates OH.

Autonomic Hyperactivity Syndromes

Involvement of the neuraxis at multiple levels could cause autonomic hyperactivity. Sympathetic hyperactivity could be secondary to increased activation of the excitatory pathways and/or interruption of the descending inhibitory pathways.[22] Early recognition of autonomic hyperactivity is important to avoid complications including hypertensive crisis, intracerebral hemorrhage, seizures, encephalopathy, cardiac arrhythmias, stress cardiomyopathy, acute pulmonary edema, and renal failure. Parasympathetic dysfunction could lead to heart blocks and asystole. Overwhelming sepsis, hypovolemia, pulmonary embolism, and intoxication could mimic or coexist in the setting of autonomic hyperactivity. Malignant hyperthermia, neurolept malignant syndrome, serotonin syndrome, and acute porphyria are important differentials.

Autonomic Dysreflexia

Autonomic dysreflexia is a potentially life-threatening neurological emergency affecting patients with spinal cord injury above T6 level (major splanchnic outflow). This results from widespread reflex activity of the sympathetic nervous system below the level of injury which is isolated from the normal regulatory vasomotor centers in the brainstem.[22] There is hypertension due to widespread sympathetic mediated vasoconstriction of the splanchnic bed. Reflex bradycardia might occur. Other clinical features include pounding headache, flushing of skin with profuse sweating above the spinal level, blurred vision, and shortness of breath with anxiety. Potential complications include intracranial hemorrhage, seizures, encephalopathy, and cardiac arrhythmias as mentioned above. Common precipitating factors include bladder distension, constipation, fecal impaction, tight clothing, catheter obstruction, catheter insertion, or a urinary tract infection. Treatment consists of head end elevation, lowering the legs, loosening tight clothing, and judicious use of antihypertensives. The precipitating cause needs to be identified and properly addressed.

Paroxysmal Sympathetic Hyperactivity

Paroxysmal sympathetic hyperactivity (PSH) is classically described in the setting of young patients with severe traumatic brain injuries involving the deep structures.[22-24] The phenomenon is often seen in the acute and subacute phase in patients with hypoxic-ischemic encephalopathy (HIE), autoimmune encephalitis, cerebral fat embolism, and other cerebral catastrophes including subarachnoid hemorrhage and malignant infarction. Increased catecholamine surges have been documented during the paroxysms. Disconnections within the central inhibitory areas (insula and cingulate) and lower sympathetic activating areas (hypothalamus to brainstem) are documented. Maladaptive plasticity changes with the spinal cord and reflex responses to external triggers may perpetuate the PSH interfering with long-term rehabilitation. Clinical features include fever, tachycardia, tachypnoea, diaphoresis, hypertension, pupillary dilatation, rigidity, and dystonic posturing. Differentiation from seizures is often difficult. Paroxysms could last up to 30 minutes if left untreated. Medications proven to be useful include benzodiazepines, morphine, labetalol, propranolol, dexmedetomidine, propofol, and clonidine.

Autonomic Dysfunction after Cerebrovascular Accident

It is frequently encountered. During acute stroke, there could be elevated blood pressure and cardiac arrhythmias. These can occur in the absence of primary cardiac involvement. Involvement of the right insular cortex, cingulate cortex, inferior parietal lobule, and brainstem has shown to be associated with autonomic dysfunction. There could be increased morbidity and mortality secondary to the same. ANS modulation is emerging as a new therapeutic target for stroke management.

Ictal bradycardia and rarely asystole can occur with temporal lobe epilepsy. Diencephalic involvement can be seen with autoimmune encephalitis, cerebral malaria, rabies, alcohol intoxication, and deep venous cerebral venous thrombosis. Baroreflex failure can occur in GBS, familial dysautonomia, and porphyria.[2,8]

Guillain–Barré Syndrome

Autonomic dysfunction is frequently encountered in both the axonal and demyelinating variants of GBS. A variant with isolated pan dysautonomia has also been well described. The dysfunction correlates with the clinical severity and most patients tend to have severe neuropathic pain. Fluctuations in blood pressure, heart rate, paralytic ileus, and urinary retention are well recognized features. Temporary pacing may be warranted in cases with severe autonomic dysfunction and risk of bradyarrhythmia. Severe GBS presentations mimicking brain death with full recovery are well documented in literature. In particular, paralytic ileus is a difficult condition with an overlap secondary to infections, metabolic disturbances, and drugs. The ileus may be refractory and necessitates the use of nasogastric, rectal tubes, and therapeutic colonoscopies for decompression.[22]

Diabetic Autonomic Neuropathy

Diabetic autonomic neuropathy is often under recognized and has significant impact on morbidity, mortality, and quality of life.[25] Factors in the pathogenesis include altered metabolism, vascular insufficiency, oxidative stress, loss of growth factor trophism, and autoimmune destruction of nerves. Involvement can be generalized or restricted to individual organ systems. Subclinical autonomic dysfunction has been described to occur within 1–2 years of diagnosis in both type 1 and type 2 diabetes mellitus. Cardiovascular autonomic neuropathy (CAN) can result in life-threatening complications including arrhythmias, silent myocardial ischemia, and sudden cardiac death.[26] Longitudinal studies have revealed a mortality risk two- to threefold higher in patients with CAN compared to those with only diabetes mellitus. Rapid correction of blood sugars could result in "treatment induced neuropathy in diabetes" (insulin neuritis) with severe small fiber and autonomic dysfunction.

Autoimmune Autonomic Disorders

Autoimmune Autonomic Ganglionopathy

Autoimmune autonomic ganglionopathy (AAG) is an immune-mediated form of generalized, severe autonomic failure.[27,28] Onset could be acute, or some cases may present with chronic illness resembling degenerative forms of autonomic failure like PAF. OH with severe GI dysmotility is often the prominent symptom. A viral prodrome is noted in 60%. About 50% of patients with AAG have antibodies against the neuronal nicotinic ACh receptor found in autonomic ganglia (ganglionic AChR). Motor strength, deep tendon reflexes and nerve conduction studies are usually normal. The clinical presentation and severity correlate with the antibody titers. Focal and restricted patterns such as postural orthostatic tachycardia, and intestinal pseudo-obstruction are reported with lower antibody titers.[6,29] The specificity of low antibody titers has been recently debated. Immunotherapy has been shown to have therapeutic benefit in these patients. AAG can also occur as part of a paraneoplastic syndrome.

Other autoimmune causes of autonomic dysfunction include paraneoplastic autoimmune syndromes (anti-Hu, anti-CRMP5, and PCA-2), Sjögren syndrome, Eaton-Lambert myasthenic syndrome, and autoimmune encephalitis related to antibodies to N-methyl-D-aspartate (NMDA) receptor, voltage-gated potassium channel (VGKC, with peripheral nerve hyperexcitability syndromes), and dipeptidyl-peptidase-like protein 6 (DPPX). Chronic idiopathic anhidrosis (not associated with ganglionic AChR autoantibodies) could be responsive to immunotherapies.[6]

Postural Orthostatic Tachycardia Syndrome

Postural orthostatic tachycardia syndrome is the most common and most under-recognized cause of orthostatic intolerance.[30] A symptomatic and sustained increase in heart rate (>30 beats/min, and >40 beats/min in individuals 12–19 years of age) is seen without OH.[31] The standing heart rate reaches values above 120 beats/min. Symptoms reported include orthostatic light headedness, presyncope, vision blurring, cognitive changes, generalized tiredness, palpitations, tremors, cold extremities, and exercise intolerance. There is a significant overlap with functional autonomic disorders such as migraine, irritable bowel syndrome, fibromyalgia, inappropriate sinus tachycardia, and chronic fatigue syndrome. Coexistent severe orthostatic headache should warrant evaluation for a cerebrospinal fluid (CSF) leak, which could be seen in patients with POTS and collagen dysfunction. Antecedent viral illness and concomitant autoimmune markers (mainly thyroid antibodies) have been reported in nearly 50% and 33%, respectively.[31] Autonomic neuropathies with lower limb involvement and impaired sympathetic vasomotor tone can manifest as POTS (neuropathic POTS). Primary and secondary hyperadrenergic (due to drugs) can cause POTS with elevated plasma NE levels. Volume dysregulation with low plasma volumes, reduced renin, aldosterone, and angiotensin-converting enzyme 2 (ACE-2) activity could predispose to POTS. Hypermobile joints (Ehler-Danlos syndrome), physical deconditioning, and mast-cell activation syndrome (MCAS) have been associated with POTS.[31] Physical counter-maneuvers, volume replacement, graded exercise program, compression stockings, and drugs (propranolol and ivabradine) can help in symptomatic relief.

Amyloidosis

Clinical features include skin changes (ecchymosis), macroglossia, organomegaly, renal (proteinuria, renal failure) and cardiac involvement (restrictive cardiomyopathy, cardiac failure). Significant small fiber and autonomic dysfunction should always warrant a comprehensive evaluation for amyloidosis.[32,33] AL amyloidosis which is associated with plasma cell dyscrasias is the most common acquired form. Kappa and lambda type immunoglobulin light chains accumulate and deposit as amyloid. An increase in serum free light chains might be the earliest change warranting dedicated evaluation and follow-up for AL amyloidosis.[32] Immunofixation electrophoresis and pathological evaluation of abdominal fat aspirate, rectal mucosa, or minor salivary gland help in establishing the diagnosis. Melphalan, dexamethasone, lenalidomide, bortezomib, cyclophosphamide, and stem cell transplantation offer valuable treatment options.

Mutations in TTR gene lead to the most common form of inherited amyloidosis and are associated with significant dysautonomia.[32,34] Phenotypes can be heterogenous and a high index of suspicion is often needed for establishing an early diagnosis. The prognosis of hereditary amyloid neuropathies has improved with orthotopic liver transplantation, RNA-targeted interventions (patisiran and inotersen), and mutant transthyretin stabilizers (tafamidis and diflunisal). AA amyloid is rarely associated with neurological involvement. Serum amyloid P scan, abdominal fat pad, or rectal biopsy could help in establishing the diagnosis.

Porphyria

Nearly 10–40% of patients with porphyria develop neuropathy. Porphyric neuropathies are often misdiagnosed early in the disease. Moreover, administration of provocative drugs leads to further complications and prolonged hospital stay.[35] Abdominal pain in porphyria reflects a visceral autonomic neuropathy with gastric hypomotility, constipation, and pseudo-obstruction. Somatic involvement is characterized by a motor axonal polyneuropathy mimicking a GBS-like illness. Other causes of a visceral autonomic neuropathy include mitochondrial disorders and amyloid polyneuropathies. The classification of neuropathies with prominent autonomic involvement is as given in **Table 4**.

AUTONOMIC FUNCTION TESTS

The recent advent of noninvasive, quantitative, and reproducible tests has significantly influenced the evaluation of autonomic disorders.[36,37] The objectives of autonomic function testing include: (1) to establish the presence of clinical/subclinical autonomic dysfunction, (2) quantify the severity and distribution of dysfunction, (3) localize the dysfunction as central, peripheral, or mixed, (4) prove clues regarding the underlying etiology by observations of the patterns of dysfunction (length vs. nonlength dependent, adrenergic vs. cardiovagal, and central vs. peripheral), (5) guide pharmacological treatment strategies and need for interventions such as cardiac pacing, and (6) prognosis, serial follow-up, and a research tool to study the natural history and efficacy of therapeutic strategies.

It is useful in identifying restricted forms of autonomic dysfunction and the cause of orthostatic intolerance (POTS, OH, and syncope). The severity is calculated using a composite autonomic severity score (CASS).[37] Beat-to-beat monitoring devices (Finapres) continuously track blood pressure (using finger cuffs) and heart rate changes and compute the systolic and diastolic blood pressures, cardiac output, peripheral resistance, and baroreflex sensitivity. Brachial artery blood pressure is reconstructed from finger arterial pressure. A description of the autonomic function tests (adrenergic and cardiovagal) has been provided in **Table 5**. The pictorial representation of abnormalities in the autonomic function tests has been shown in **Figures 1 and 2**.

TABLE 5: Autonomic function tests (cardiovagal and adrenergic).

Cardiovagal (parasympathetic cholinergic)	Comments
HR response to deep breathing (rate of 6 breaths/min, regular, continuous)	E:I ratio 1.2 (age-dependent)
30:15 ratio: RR interval at 30th second/15th second while standing	Ratio <1.04 considered abnormal
HR response to Valsalva: Maximum HR during the Valsalva/minimum HR within 30 seconds of the peak heart rate	Ratio <1.21 considered abnormal
Adrenergic (sympathetic noradrenergic)	
Head-up tilt test: • Tilt to 60–70° • Continue test for 20–45 minutes when delayed OH is suspected	• HR increases by 5–20 bpm • BP fall >20/10 mm Hg suggestive of OH • *Other abnormalities*: POTS and syncope
BP response to Valsalva (abnormal in neurogenic orthostatic hypotension)	• Maximal drop of blood pressure during phase 2 • Recovery during late phase 2 • Phase 4 overshoot • Pressure recovery time (PRT)
Cold pressor test: Immersion of the uncuffed hand into cold water (4°C) for 60–180 seconds	• Increase in BP systolic (15–20 mm Hg), diastolic (10–15 mm Hg), HR increase of around 10 bpm • Peak response at 60–90 seconds
Isometric hand grip: Hand-held dynamometer at one-third of maximal contraction strength for 3–5 minutes in uncuffed arm	Diastolic BP rise <15 mm Hg is considered abnormal

(BP: blood pressure; HR: heart rate; POTS: postural orthostatic tachycardia syndrome; OH: orthostatic hypotension)

Orthostatic Hypotension: Neurogenic versus Non-neurogenic Causes

Non-neurogenic OH occurs in the setting of relatively elder patients with physical deconditioning, volume depletion, anemia, systemic illness, drug-induced OH, and hypocortisolemia. A heart rate increase of >0.5 beats/min for every 1 mm fall in systolic blood pressure usually indicates non-neurogenic OH.[38] Reduced heart rate responses, absent phase 4 overshoot during Valsalva, and reduced/attenuated NE response during standing are features consistent with neurogenic OH.[38]

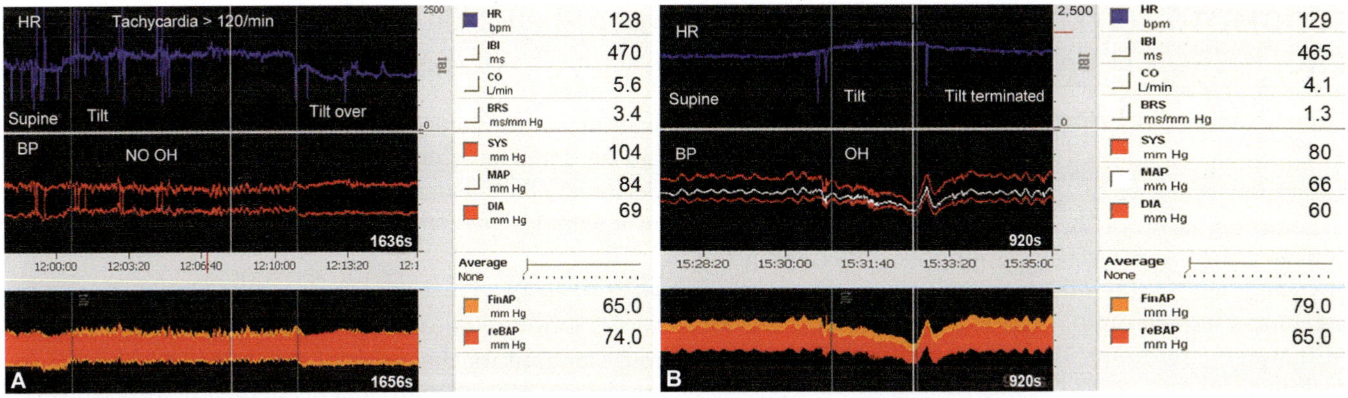

FIGS. 1A AND B: Autonomic function tests using beat to beat monitoring shows (A) disproportionate sustained increase in heart rate (HR) without any fall in blood pressure (BP) during tilt consistent with postural orthostatic tachycardia syndrome (POTS). (B) Fall in BP with reflex increase in HR during the tilt phase consistent with OH.

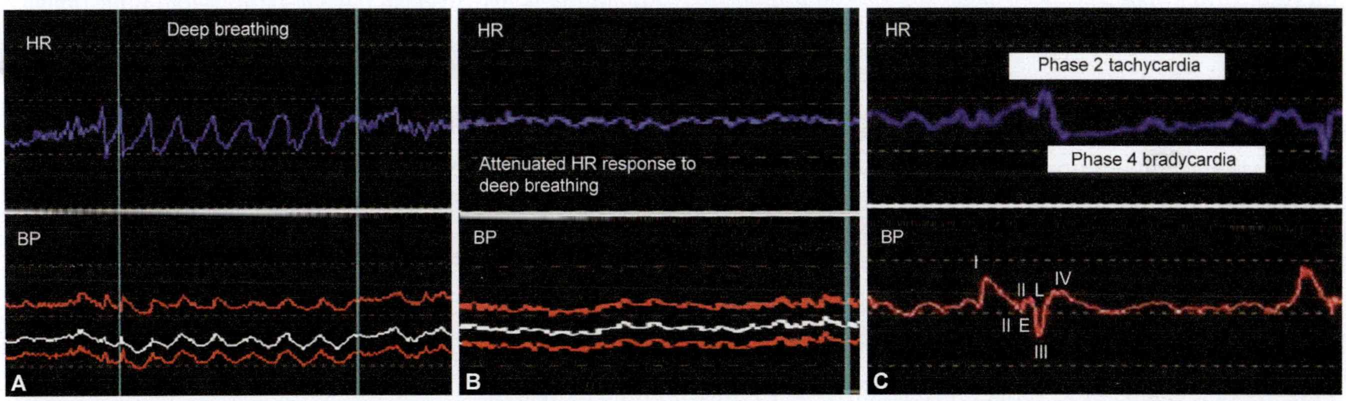

FIGS. 2A TO C: Autonomic function tests using beat to beat monitoring shows (A) normal heart rate (HR) responses to deep breathing, (B) attenuated HR responses to deep breathing suggestive of cardiovagal dysfunction, and (C) normal blood pressure (BP) and HR responses during the different stages of the Valsalva maneuver.

CARDIOVASCULAR AUTONOMIC REFLEX TESTS

In addition to the tests mentioned for cardiovagal and adrenergic testing, the cardiovascular autonomic reflex tests include heart rate variability (HRV) analysis, electrocardiogram-Holter analysis (including arrhythmias and QT interval), continuous ambulatory blood pressure monitors (for nondippers), baroreflex sensitivity, catecholamine assays, and cardiac scintigraphy. Features of CAN include loss of circadian rhythm of blood pressure changes (nondippers), resting tachycardia, OH, impaired HRV, blunted cardiac output response to exercise, intraoperative cardiovascular lability, cardiomyopathy, and arrhythmias.[39] Power spectral analysis of HRV could indicate attenuation of signals in the high-frequency spectrum (0.25 Hz) indicating abnormal cardiovagal (parasympathetic) function, altered "sympathovagal" balance, and the risk of arrhythmias. These are useful biomarkers being evaluated especially in the context of clinical trials and role of autonomic neuromodulation.

Catecholamine Levels

Norepinephrine levels are reduced in peripheral autonomic disorders. The test should be interpreted with caution as some disorders could have overlap and both central and peripheral autonomic dysfunction. The test should be deferred in patient already taking NE precursors or reuptake inhibitors. Peripheral disorders with reduced plasma NE levels include PAF, DLB, amyloid, and autoimmune autonomic neuropathies.[38] Plasma NE level is an important biomarker to decide optimal treatment in patients with refractory OH.[38] Patients with low baseline levels associated with peripheral autonomic disorders show a robust response to droxidopa. Central autonomic disorders such as MSA with higher baseline serum NE levels respond better to atomoxetine.[16,38]

SUDOMOTOR (SYMPATHETIC CHOLINERGIC) FUNCTION

Quantitative Sudomotor Axon Reflex Test

Quantitative sudomotor axon reflex test evaluates the functional integrity of the postganglionic sympathetic sudomotor axon. ACh iontophoresed into the skin activates the axon terminal. Impulses travel along the postganglionic sudomotor axon, initially antidromically, reaching a branch point, then orthodromically to release ACh at nerve terminal. The released ACh activates muscarinic receptors on sweat glands. The sweat response is recorded from the forearm, proximal leg, distal leg, and foot and compared with normatives. It is important to note that the patient is not on medicines such as anticholinergics and carbonic anhydrase inhibitors which interfere with sweat production. QSART has an important role in differentiating peripheral from central autonomic disorders.

Thermoregulatory Skin Test

The core body temperature is increased by warming to 38°C. The resultant sweat production is recognized by the change in color of an indicator powder (starch-iodine) applied to the body. The sweat pattern and distribution are recorded by digital photography. Patterns of intact sweating and anhidrosis can be recognized. The test evaluates the integrity of the central, preganglionic, postganglionic pathways, and eccrine sweat glands. A pictorial representation of TST has been depicted in **Figure 3**.

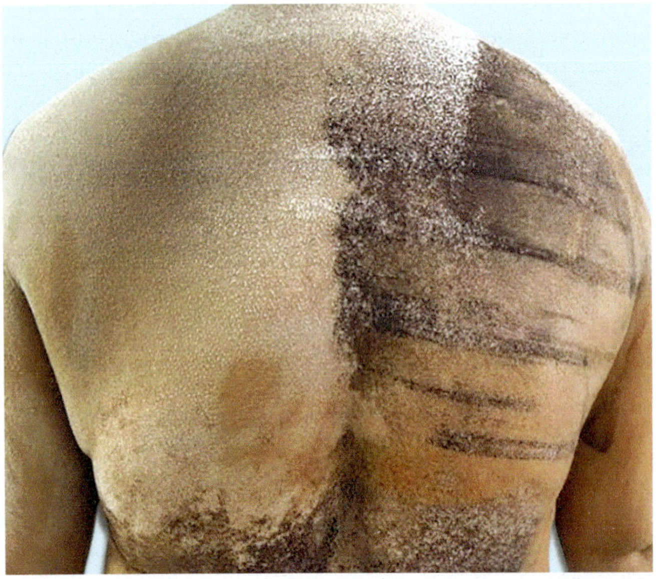

FIG. 3: A representative picture of the thermoregulatory skin test (TST) in a patient demonstrating anhidrosis on one side of the trunk.

Sympathetic Skin Response

Sympathetic skin response (SSR) tests sudomotor function by activation of sympathetic sudomotor fibers. Electrical, acoustic, or inspiratory gasp stimuli can be used. Recording can be obtained from the hands and feet with reference electrode at the dorsum. Presence/absence of SSR is noted and an amplitude difference of >50% can be considered abnormal.

Skin Biopsy

Punch biopsies have been traditionally considered the gold standard for diagnosis of small fiber neuropathy by assessment of intraepidermal nerve fiber density (IENFD). In addition, assessment of pilomotor nerve fibers and sweat glands can also be done.[40] Sympathetic adrenergic innervation of arrector pili muscles can be visualized using immunochemical stains, such as tyrosine hydroxylase or dopamine β-hydroxylase. Sweat gland nerve fiber density can help assess sympathetic cholinergic innervation with the use of immunostaining to vasoactive intestinal polypeptide. Amyloid deposits and synuclein aggregates can also be detected in skin biopsy specimens expanding the indications for skin biopsy in assessment in autonomic disorders.[40] A checklist of the investigations which can be considered in the evaluation of a patient with autonomic dysfunction has been provided in **Box 1**.[2]

BOX 1 **Check list of investigations for evaluation of autonomic dysfunction.**

List of investigations:

- Routine blood tests including complete blood counts, blood sugars, HbA1c, thyroid functions, creatinine, liver function tests, serum protein electrophoresis (immunofixation and serum free light chains as indicated), and serum cortisol
- Quantitative autonomic function tests for cardiovagal, adrenergic, and sudomotor dysfunction
- Nerve conduction studies
- Serological tests for Sjögren's syndrome, HIV screening, and antibodies to ganglionic AChR
- Biochemical tests for catecholamines (supine and standing), metanephrines (pheochromocytoma), 5-hydroxy indoleacetic acid (carcinoid), plasma histamine, and tryptase levels (mast cell activation syndrome)
- Subcutaneous fat pad aspiration, rectal, or minor salivary gland biopsy
- Genetic testing for TTR amyloid, Fabry's disease (including α-galactosidase)
- Schirmer test and Rose Bengal test (lacrimal function), pupillary response to pharmacological tests
- Gastrointestinal motility studies
- Post void urine and urodynamic studies
- Cardiac PET and scintigraphy (to look for denervation)
- Scratch test (cutaneous flare response)

(AChR: acetylcholine receptor; HbA1c: glycated hemoglobin; HIV: human immunodeficiency virus; PET: positron emission tomography; TTR: transthyretin)

MANAGEMENT

Treatment

The main cornerstone of treatment includes (1) identification and treatment of the etiology, (2) removal of the precipitating/offending agent, and (3) specific treatment for autonomic dysfunction. Patient should be well educated about the potential stressors which include heavy exercise, physical deconditioning, heavy meals, hot weather, and offending drugs such as diuretics, alpha blockers, and dopamine agonists.

Nonpharmacological Management of OH

Lifestyle Modification

Exercises in recumbent or seated position (stationary bicycle or rowing machine) are often recommended.[38,41,42] Frequent, small meals with low glycemic index are preferable to reduce postprandial hypotension. Alcohol and heavy carbohydrate intake deferred till bedtime can theoretically help counteract supine hypertension. Adequate salt and fluid intake (at least 2.5 L/day) should be encouraged. Bolus water drinking can provide short periods of symptomatic relief. Avoid abrupt changes in position and sitting for a short while before standing can help reduce the symptoms of OH. Valsalva-like maneuvers need to be avoided.

Physical counter maneuvers include leg crossing, standing on tip toes, stooping, and squatting.[43] Elastic compression stockings (waist-high) and abdominal binders can help reduce the OH.[44] Sleeping with the head end elevated 30–45° can help decrease the nocturnal supine hypertension.[42] The resultant reduction in natriuresis and overnight volume depletion helps improve the orthostatic tolerance the next day morning.

Pharmacological Strategies in OH

Adequate caution should be exercised to ensure care of offending drugs, precipitating factors, and optimal use of nonpharmacological strategies before prescribing drugs for treatment of OH.

- Fludrocortisone (0.1–0.2 mg/day) is a synthetic mineralocorticoid which increases intravascular volume by enhancing renal sodium and water reabsorption. Side effects of fludrocortisone include pedal edema, supine hypertension, and hypokalemia. Contraindications include heart failure and renal failure. Long-term use is discouraged because of risk of hypertension and related organ damage.[45,46]
- Midodrine (2.5–10 mg thrice daily) is a selective α1 agonist which constricts arteriolar and venous vasculature [Food and Drug Administration (FDA) approved in 1996]. Midodrine is relatively short-acting with the duration of action lasting 1–3 hours. It has been shown to increase standing systolic blood pressure and increase standing and walking time.[38,47] It should not be taken after midafternoon to avoid nocturnal supine hypertension. Piloerection, scalp itching, and urinary retention have been described as potential side effects.[38,48]
- Droxidopa (100–600 mg up to three times/day) is a NE precursor which is used to treat symptomatic OH (FDA approved in 2014). Indications include OH in DLB, familial amyloidosis, and dopamine β-hydroxylase deficiency.[49] The effect lasts for 3.5 hours, and careful dose titration needs to be done.[38,49] Therapeutic responses are better in patients with low baseline serum NE levels (<220 pg/mL).[38,50] Carbidopa blocks the conversion of droxidopa to the active metabolite NE limiting use in patients with concurrent parkinsonism.[51] Side effects include hypertension, headache, and nausea. Concomitant use with other sympathomimetic drugs including midodrine is discouraged.
- Atomoxetine (10–18 mg, two times a day) is a short-acting NE reuptake inhibitor which is particularly useful in patients with OH associated with central autonomic disorders such as MSA.[38,52] In contrast to droxidopa, the responses are better in patients with higher baseline serum NE levels.[38,53] Side effects include anorexia, supine hypertension, and insomnia.
- Pyridostigmine (60–180 mg/day) improves ganglionic transmission in the sympathetic baroreflex pathway (which is activated mainly during standing). Hence, the drug improves OH and peripheral resistance without causing supine hypertension.[38,54] Combination of pyridostigmine (60 mg/day) and midodrine (5 mg/day) is more effective than pyridostigmine alone. Similarly, a synergistic effect with atomoxetine has been reported.[38]
- Erythropoietin can be used in chronic OH and acts by increasing the hematocrit. A dose of 25–75 IU/thrice weekly followed by maintenance of 25 IU/kg thrice weekly can be used particularly in the setting with associated anemia of chronic disease.[38]

Concurrent supine hypertension is seen in a significant proportion (up to 50%) of patients with neurogenic OH.[38,55] Untreated high supine hypertension can potentially cause hypertensive end organ damage. Treatment strategies include head end elevation at bedtime, high carbohydrate meal at bedtime, and short-acting antihypertensives such as captopril and losartan.[56] Beta-blockers and ivabradine can help in alleviating the hyperadrenergic symptoms in POTS. Postprandial OH can be reduced with frequent small low carbohydrate meals. Acarbose, midodrine with meals, and octreotide are useful in treatment of postprandial OH.

Gastroparesis can be addressed by lowering fat content of feeds and judicious use of prokinetics such as metoclopramide, domperidone, and erythromycin. Constipation may require high-fiber diet, stool softeners, and laxatives. Bladder involvement may necessitate timed voiding schedules, anticholinergics (for overactive bladder), and intermittent self-catheterization (for impaired detrusor activity). Erectile dysfunction might need phosphodiesterase 5 inhibitors (sildenafil and tadalafil). Caution should be exercised in ischemic heart disease and concomitant nitrate therapy. Hyperhidrosis is treated with anticholinergics (trihexyphenidyl and glycopyrrolate) and intradermal botulinum toxin. Focal hyperhidrosis can also be treated with topical antiperspirants, tap water iontophoresis, and sympathotomy.

REFERENCES

1. Low PA, Benarroch EE. Clinical Autonomic Disorders, 3rd edition. Philadelphia: Lippincott Williams & Wilkins; 2009.
2. Benarroch EE. Physiology and pathophysiology of the autonomic nervous system. Continuum (Minneap Minn). 2020;26(1):12-24.
3. Mathias C. Autonomic diseases: clinical features and laboratory evaluation. J Neurol Neurosurg Psychiatry. 2003;74(Suppl 3):iii31-iii41.
4. Cersosimo MG, Benarroch EE. Central control of autonomic function and involvement in neurodegenerative disorders. Handb Clin Neurol. 2013;117:45-57.
5. Bellocchi C, Carandina A, Montinaro B, Targetti E, Furlan L, Rodrigues GD, et al. The interplay between autonomic nervous system and inflammation across systemic autoimmune diseases. Int J Mol Sci. 2022;23(5):2449.
6. Vernino S. Autoimmune autonomic disorders. Continuum (Minneap Minn). 2020;26(1):44-57.
7. Timmers HJ, Karemaker JM, Lenders JW, Wieling W. Baroreflex failure following radiation therapy for nasopharyngeal carcinoma. Clin Auton Res. 1999;9(6):317-24.
8. Lamotte G, Coon EA, Suarez MD, Sandroni P, Benarroch EE, Cutsforth–Gregory JK, et al. Natural history of afferent baroreflex failure in adults. Neurology. 2021;97(2):e136-e144.
9. Benarroch EE. Thermoregulation: Recent concepts and remaining questions. Neurology. 2007;69(12):1293-7.
10. Cheshire WP Jr. Autonomic history, examination, and laboratory evaluation. Continuum (Minneap Minn). 2020;26(1):25-43.
11. Low PA. Composite autonomic scoring scale for laboratory quantification of generalized autonomic failure. Mayo Clin Proc. 1993;68(8):748-52.
12. Suarez GA, Opfer-Gehrking TL, Offord KP, Atkinson EJ, O'Brien PC, Low PA, et al. The Autonomic symptom profile: A new instrument to assess autonomic symptoms. Neurology. 1999;52(3):523-8.
13. Sletten DM, Suarez GA, Low PA, Mandrekar J, Singera W. COMPASS 31: a refined and abbreviated Composite Autonomic Symptom Score. Mayo Clin Proc. 2012;87(12):1196-201.
14. Pilleri M, Facchini Gibbons CH, Freeman R. Clinical implications of delayed orthostatic hypotension: a 10-year follow-up study. Neurology. 2015;85(16):1362-7.
15. Pilleri M, Facchini S, Gasparoli E, Biundo R, Bernardi L, Marchetti M, et al. Cognitive and MRI correlates of orthostatic hypotension in Parkinson's disease. J Neurol. 2013;260(1):253-9.
16. Coon EA, Singer W. Synucleinopathies. Continuum (Minneap Minn). 2020;26(1):72-92.
17. Consensus statement on the definition of orthostatic hypotension, pure autonomic failure, and multiple system atrophy. Neurology. 1996;46(5):1470.
18. Woerman AL, Stöhr J, Aoyagi A, Rampersaud R, Krejciova Z, Watts JC, et al. Propagation of prions causing synucleinopathies in cultured cells. Proc Natl Acad Sci U S A. 2015;112(35):E4949-58.
19. Kaufmann H, Norcliffe-Kaufmann L, Palma JA, Biaggioni I, Low PA, Singer W, et al. Natural history of pure autonomic failure: A United States prospective cohort. Ann Neurol. 2017;81(2):287-97.
20. Yoshida M, Fukumoto Y, Kuroda Y, Ohkoshi N. Sympathetic denervation of myocardium demonstrated by 123I-MIBG scintigraphy in pure progressive autonomic failure. Eur Neurol. 1997;38(4):291-6.
21. Singer W, Berini SE, Sandroni P, Fealey RD, Coon EA, Suarez MD, et al. Pure autonomic failure: predictors of conversion to clinical CNS involvement. Neurology. 2017;88(12):1129-36.
22. Rabinstein AA. Autonomic hyperactivity. Continuum (Minneap Minn). 2020;26(1):138-53.
23. Meyfroidt G, Baguley IJ, Menon DK. Paroxysmal sympathetic hyperactivity: the storm after acute brain injury. Lancet Neurol. 2017;16(9):721-9.
24. Scott RA, Rabinstein AA. Paroxysmal sympathetic hyperactivity. Semin Neurol. 2020;40(5):485-91.
25. Verrotti A, Prezioso G, Scattoni R, Chiarelli F. Autonomic neuropathy in diabetes mellitus. Front Endocrinol (Lausanne). 2014;5:205.
26. Vinik AI, Ziegler D. Diabetic cardiovascular autonomic neuropathy. Circulation. 2007;115(3):387-97.
27. Vernino S, Low PA, Fealey RD, Stewart JD, Farrugia G, Lennon VA, et al. Autoantibodies to ganglionic acetylcholine receptors in autoimmune autonomic neuropathies. N Engl J Med. 2000;343(12):847-55.
28. Golden EP, Vernino S. Autoimmune autonomic neuropathies and ganglionopathies: epidemiology, pathophysiology, and therapeutic advances. Clin Auton Res. 2019;29(3):277-88.
29. Sandroni P, Low PA. Other autonomic neuropathies associated with ganglionic antibody. Auton Neurosci. 2009;146(1-2):13-7.
30. Benarroch EE. Postural tachycardia syndrome: A heterogeneous and multifactorial disorder. Mayo Clin Proc. 2012;87(12):1214-25.
31. Cutsforth-Gregory JK. Postural tachycardia syndrome and neurally mediated syncope. Continuum (Minneap Minn). 2020;26(1):93-115.
32. Freeman R. Autonomic peripheral neuropathy. Continuum (Minneap Minn). 2020;26(1):58-71.
33. Kaur D, Tiwana H, Stino A, Sandroni P. Autonomic neuropathies. Muscle Nerve. 2021;63(1):10-21.
34. Plante-Bordeneuve V. Transthyretin familial amyloid polyneuropathy: an update. J Neurol. 2018;265(4):976-83.
35. Kazamel M, Desnick RJ, Quigley JG. Porphyric neuropathy: Pathophysiology, diagnosis, and updated management. Curr Neurol Neurosci Rep. 2020;20(12):56.
36. Low PA, Tomalia VA, Park KJ. Autonomic function tests: some clinical applications. J Clin Neurol. 2013;9(1):1-8.
37. Novak P. Quantitative autonomic testing. J Vis Exp. 2011;53:2502.
38. Palma JA, Kaufmann H. Management of orthostatic hypotension. Continuum (Minneap Minn). 2020;26(1):154-77.
39. Spallone V, Ziegler D, Freeman R, Bernardi L, Frontoni S, Pop-Busui R, et al. Cardiovascular autonomic neuropathy in diabetes: clinical impact, assessment, diagnosis, and management. Diabetes Metab Res Rev. 2011;27(7):639-53.
40. Gibbons CH, Wang N, Kim JY, Campagnolo M, Freeman R. Skin biopsy in evaluation of autonomic disorders. Continuum (Minneap Minn). 2020;26(1):200-12.
41. Cheshire WP Jr. Clinical classification of orthostatic hypotensions. Clin Auton Res. 2017;27(3):133-5.
42. Gibbons CH, Schmidt P, Biaggioni I, Frazier-Mills C, Freeman R, Isaacson S, et al. The recommendations of a consensus panel for the screening, diagnosis, and treatment of neurogenic orthostatic hypotension and associated supine hypertension. J Neurol. 2017;264(8):1567-82.

43. Krediet CT, van Lieshout JJ, Bogert LW, Immink RV, Kim YS, Wieling W. Leg crossing improves orthostatic tolerance in healthy subjects: a placebo-controlled crossover study. Am J Physiol Heart Circ Physiol. 2006;291(14):H1768-72.
44. Smit AA, Wieling W, Fujimura J, Denq JC, Opfer-Gehrking TL, Akarriou M, et al. Use of lower abdominal compression to combat orthostatic hypotension in patients with autonomic dysfunction. Clin Auton Res. 2004;14(3):167-75.
45. Chobanian AV, Volicer L, Tifft CP, Gavras H, Liang CS, Faxon D. Mineralocorticoid-induced hypertension in patients with orthostatic hypotension. N Engl J Med. 1979;301(2):68-73.
46. Grijalva CG, Biaggioni I, Griffin MR, Shibao CA. Fludrocortisone is associated with a higher risk of all-cause hospitalizations compared with midodrine in patients with orthostatic hypotension. J Am Heart Assoc. 2017;6:pii:e006848.
47. Wright RA, Kaufmann HC, Perera R, Opfer-Gehrking TL, McElligott MA, Sheng KN, et al. A double-blind, dose-response study of midodrine in neurogenic orthostatic hypotension. Neurology. 1998;51(1):120-4.
48. Smith W, Wan H, Much D, Robinson AG, Martin P. Clinical benefit of midodrine hydrochloride in symptomatic orthostatic hypotension: a phase 4, double-blind, placebo-controlled, randomized, tilt-table study. Clin Auton Res. 2016;26(4):269-77.
49. Kaufmann H, Norcliffe-Kaufmann L, Palma JA. Droxidopa in neurogenic orthostatic hypotension. Expert Rev Cardiovasc Ther. 2015;13(8):875-91.
50. Palma JA, Norcliffe-Kaufmann L, Martinez J, Kaufmann H. Supine plasma NE predicts the pressor response to droxidopa in neurogenic orthostatic hypotension. Neurology. 2018;91(16):e1539-44.
51. Claassen D, Lew M. Initiating droxidopa for neurogenic orthostatic hypotension in a patient with Parkinson disease. Clin Auton Res. 2017;27(suppl 1):13-14.
52. Ramirez CE, Okamoto LE, Arnold AC, Gamboa A, Diedrich A, Choi L, et al. Efficacy of atomoxetine versus midodrine for the treatment of orthostatic hypotension in autonomic failure. Hypertension. 2014;64(6):1235-40.
53. Shibao C, Martinez J, Palma JA, Kaufmann H, Biaggioni I. Norepinephrine levels predicts the improvement in orthostatic symptoms after atomoxetine in patients with neurogenic orthostatic hypotension (P5.320). Neurology. 2017;88.
54. Singer W, Sandroni P, Opfer-Gehrking TL, Suarez GA, Klein CM, Hines S, et al. Pyridostigmine treatment trial in neurogenic orthostatic hypotension. Arch Neurol. 2006;63(4):513-8.
55. Arnold AC, Biaggioni I. Management approaches to hypertension in autonomic failure. Curr Opin Nephrol Hypertens. 2012;21:481-5.
56. Di Stefano C, Maule S. Treatment of supine hypertension in autonomic failure: A case series. Clin Auton Res. 2018;28(2):245-6.

84
CHAPTER

Myasthenia Gravis and Lambert–Eaton Myasthenic Syndrome

Seena Vengalil, Saraswati Nashi, Deepak Menon, Samim MM, Atchayaram Nalini

INTRODUCTION

Myasthenia gravis (MG) is an antibody-mediated postsynaptic disorder of the neuromuscular junction (NMJ). Fatigable muscle weakness, worsening with activity, is the hallmark of the disease. Diurnal variation, with worsening towards evening, is seen. The spectrum of muscle involvement may vary from purely ocular involvement to severe weakness of bulbar, limb, or respiratory muscles. The age of onset is variable; however, peaks occur in young women and older men.[1] MG is an antibody-mediated disease caused by antibodies directed against the acetylcholine receptor (AChR), muscle-specific kinase (MuSK), low-density lipoprotein receptor-related protein 4 (LRP4), agrin, or antistriational antibodies like those against titin, ryanodine receptor, etc. Though, predominantly an antibody-mediated disease, T cells and their cytokines also play a role in pathogenesis. In this chapter, we review the epidemiology, clinical manifestations, pathology, pathophysiology, diagnosis, and management of MG.

EPIDEMIOLOGY

The incidence rate of MG is around 5.3 per million person-years (range 1.7–21.3)[2] and the prevalence rate is around 150–200 per million.[3] Incidence is higher in African American women. The Asian population has an earlier age of onset and juvenile MG is more common in Asians.[4] The peak age of onset of MG is between 20–39 years in women and 50–70 years in men.[5] Early-onset MG (EOMG) (<50 years) affects women more commonly with a female:male ratio of 3:1. At 50 years of age, the ratio is equal and after 50 years, men have a higher incidence with a male:female ratio of 3:2. A study from India showed a median age of onset to be 48 years (males 53 years and in females 34 years).[6]

Genetic factors and environmental risk factors play a role in the induction of MG. There are numerous HLA associations with MG and its subtypes. EOMG is associated with HLA-B8 and HLA-DRw3.[5] Sex hormones may play a role in MG pathogenesis as evidenced by a female preponderance in EOMG and the increased risk of thymic hyperplasia in young women. Estrogen induces epigenetic changes in the autoimmune regulator (*AIRE*) gene leading to reduced expression of AIRE, thus increasing the susceptibility of females to autoimmune diseases.[7] Various infectious agents such as Epstein–Barr virus, West-Nile virus, Zika virus as well as immune-checkpoint inhibitors in cancer immunotherapy have been implicated in the pathogenesis of MG.[8]

PATHOPHYSIOLOGY OF MYASTHENIA GRAVIS

Effective transmission of impulse across a NMJ requires the release of acetylcholine (ACh) from presynaptic terminals and its binding to the AChR on the postsynaptic membrane. An action potential opens up calcium channels in the presynaptic membrane, leading to efflux of ACh from the synaptic vesicles. The binding of ACh to its receptor AChR on the postsynaptic membrane leads to activation of voltage-dependent sodium channels, thereby triggering a muscle fiber action potential and subsequent muscle contraction. The amount of ACh released is usually higher than the amount needed for the generation of an action potential, thus accounting for the safety factor of transmission.

Antibodies involved in MG can be classified into (1) transmembrane or extracellular and (2) intracellular. Antibodies against extracellular proteins such as AChR, anti-MuSK, anti-LRP4, or anti-agrin directly or indirectly affect the function of AChR at the postsynaptic membrane, leading to impaired neuromuscular transmission. Antibodies against intracellular proteins such as titin, Ryanodine receptor (RyR), and cortactin are not directly pathogenic but may be markers of disease severity, presence of thymoma, etc.[1]

Anti-acetylcholine receptor (found in 80% of patients with MG) activates complement, leading to the formation of membrane attack complex (MAC), thus leading to the destruction of postsynaptic membrane. Some antibodies also bind to ACh binding site, thereby blocking ACh from binding to receptors and thus reducing signaling. AChR antibodies also cause cross-linking of AChR leading to accelerated internalization and destruction of AChR.

The LRP4 and agrin cause phosphorylation of MuSK and the activated MUSK along with rapsyn causes AChR clustering in the postsynaptic membrane. Anti-MuSK, anti-LRP4, and anti-agrin antibodies cause reduced AChR clustering. Anti-MuSK antibodies are found in 1–10% of patients with MG and anti-LRP4 in 7–33% of double seronegative cases of MG.

Antibodies against intracellular proteins such as titin and ryanodine receptor are not directly pathogenic and are usually associated with thymoma, late-onset MG (LOMG), and severe MG **(Fig. 1)**.

Loss of Immune Tolerance and Role of Thymus in Myasthenia Gravis

The thymus plays a key role in the pathogenesis of MG as evidenced by (1) frequent occurrence of thymic follicular hyperplasia or thymoma in MG, (2) correlation between the degree of follicular hyperplasia and levels of AChR antibodies, and (3) the beneficial effect of thymectomy. AChR and proteins like titin are expressed by thymic epithelial cells and myoid cells. Autoreactive T cells normally undergo negative selection in the thymus by clonal deletion or conversion to regulatory T cells (Tregs). Autoimmune regulator also causes expression of peripheral proteins by thymic epithelial cells and T cells which recognize these proteins and then undergo negative selection, thus causing tolerance over autoimmunity.[3] There is defective AIRE expression as well as impaired T cell selection in patients with MG and thymic hyperplasia. Defective T cell subsets also cause activation of B cells in germinal centers, leading to the production of autoreactive B cells and plasma cells.

Myasthenia gravis patients have anti-AchR Th1 CD4+ T cells in the blood which are capable of inducing B cells to produce AChR antibodies. Anti-AChR Th2 cells and cytokines produced by them such as interleukin-6 (IL-6) and IL-10 also contribute to the pathogenesis of MG. Tregs which are CD4+ T cells with a CD25 maker are very important in maintaining self-tolerance. Tregs are functionally impaired in MG and their levels improve post-thymectomy.[9]

Classification and Clinical Features of Myasthenia Gravis

Myasthenia gravis is classified into (1) EOMG—onset <50 years of age, more in females, and associated with thymic hyperplasia; (2) LOMG >50 years of age, more in males; (3) thymomatous MG 10–15%; (4) ocular MG—symptoms remain restricted to extraocular muscles; and (5) antibody positive (AChR or MuSK positive) or double seronegative (no detectable antibodies to AChR or MuSK) **(Table 1)**.[10]

The cardinal clinical feature of MG is fatigability, fluctuating muscle weakness worsening with repeated activities, and improving with rest. Infection, heat, and stress may aggravate the weakness. Diurnal fluctuations may be seen, with improvement noticed on waking up in the morning. Weakness may affect the ocular, bulbar, limb, or respiratory muscles.

Ocular muscle involvement is the most common initial symptom of MG, occurring in 85% of the patients. Up to 50–80% of them progress to generalize MG, the majority progressing within 2 years of onset of the disease.

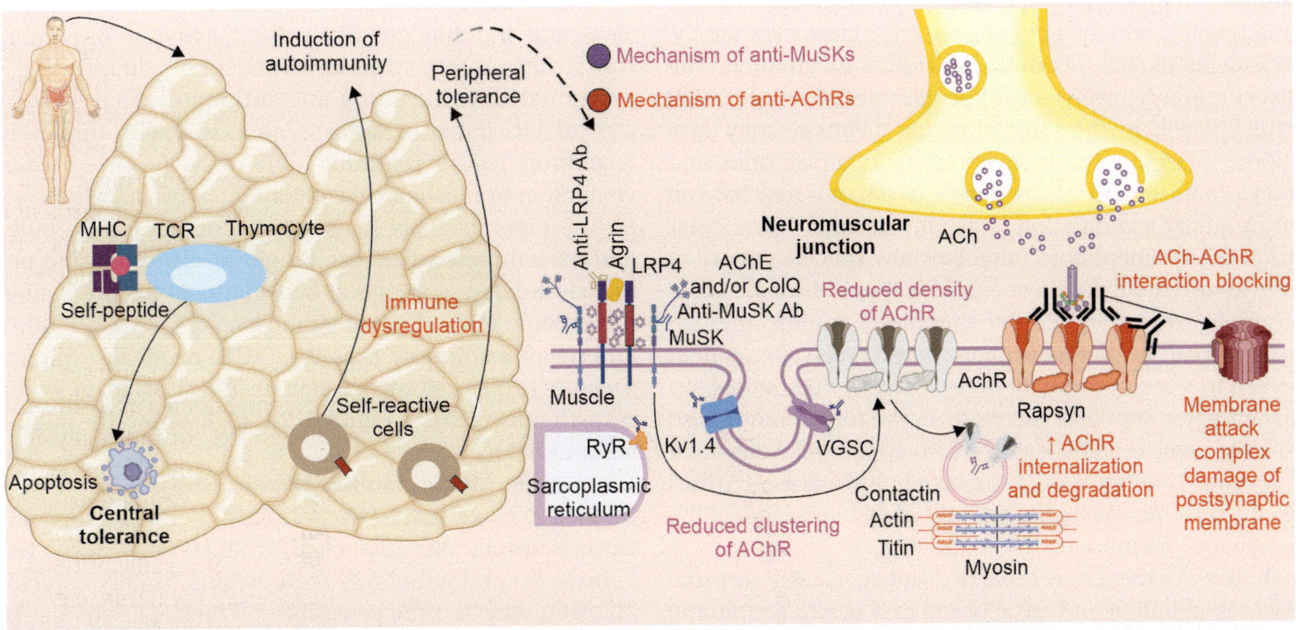

FIG. 1: The pathophysiology of myasthenia gravis (MG).

(AChR: acetylcholine receptor; ColQ: collagen Q; LRP4: low-density lipoprotein receptor-related protein 4; MHC: major histocompatibility complex; MuSK: muscle-specific kinase; RyR: ryanodine receptor; TCR: T cell receptor; VGSC: voltage-gated sodium channel)

TABLE 1: The clinical features of different types of myasthenia gravis (MG).

	EOMG	LOMG	Thymomatous	Anti-MuSK	Ocular	Double seronegative
Frequency	20%	45%	10–15%	6%	15%	4%
Age at onset	<50 years	>50 years	Any age (40–60 years)	Young females	Any age	Any age
Predominant weakness	Generalized	Generalized	Generalized	Facial and bulbar	Ocular	Generalized
Sex ratio (male:female)	1:3	5:1	1:1	1:3	1:2	-
Antibodies	AChRAb	AChR and antistriational	AChR and antistriational	Anti-MuSK	AChR	Anti-LRP4 and anti-agrin
Thymic pathology	Thymic hyperplasia	Atrophy	Thymoma A-5% AB, B1–3 95%	Normal	–	–
Thymectomy	Indicated	–	Indicated	–	–	–
Response to immunotherapy	Good +++	+++	+	+	+++	+

(AChR: acetylcholine receptor; EOMG: early-onset myasthenia gravis; LOMG: late-onset myasthenia gravis; MuSK: muscle-specific kinase)

Extraocular muscle fibers have a higher rate of synaptic firing than other muscles, thus making them more prone to fatigue. The tonic muscle fibers for sustained gaze have fewer AChR receptors, hence receptor loss occurs early.[11] Ptosis occurs due to the involvement of levator palpebrae superioris (LPS) and can be unilateral or bilateral; if bilateral, it is asymmetric. Prolonged upgaze can be used to elicit eyelid fatigue. Other clinical signs are (1) enhancement of ptosis of the contralateral eye when the more ptotic eyelid is lifted and (2) Cogan's lid twitch sign—when the patient is asked to look up after a sustained downgaze for 20–30 seconds, there is an upward shooting of upper eyelid followed by downward movement and few twitches may occur before settling. Orbicularis oculi are also weak and result in peek sign—opening of eyes resulting in sclera being visible when the patient is asked to close eyes tightly. Extraocular muscle involvement results in diplopia. The most commonly involved extraocular muscle is the medial rectus followed by the superior rectus.[12] Patients may have hypometric large saccades, hypermetric small saccades, and intersaccadic fatigue.[13] Gaze paretic nystagmus may be seen and pupillary examination is usually normal. Extraocular muscle involvement does not follow any specific pattern of nerve involvement and hence differentiates MG from other causes of gaze paresis or ophthalmoplegia. Improvement in ptosis and extraocular movements may be seen after patient is asked to sleep or rest with eyes closed for 30 minutes. An ice pack when kept over the ptotic eyelid for 2 minutes also results in improvement of ptosis, with upper eyelid elevation of >2 mm. Cooling reduces acetylcholinesterase (AChE) activity, thus increasing the amount of ACh available at the postsynaptic membrane.

Bulbar weakness may result in dysphagia and dysarthria. Nasal regurgitation and nasal twang may occur. Dysphonia may occur due to laryngeal involvement. Iced drink test may show improvement in nasal twang and bulbar symptoms.[14] Bulbar involvement can occur in 80% of MuSK-MG patients and may cause rapid deterioration and myasthenic crisis. Atrophy of muscles is another significant feature of MuSK-MG, especially those of facial muscles and tongue causing a triple furrowed appearance of the tongue.[15,16] Atrophy of limb girdle and paraspinal muscles may also occur. Voice fatigue may be tested by making the patient count 50–100. Axial muscle weakness, especially those of neck extensors, may result in a head drop. Jaw muscles may be weak causing difficulty in chewing solid food. Severe jaw weakness may cause the jaw to drop, necessitating the support of fingers to lift the jaw. The face may be expressionless and when asked to smile, there may be a myasthenic snarl due to failure of contraction of the upper corner of the mouth.[17]

Limb muscle fatigue manifests as proximal muscle weakness and difficulty in overhead activities or climbing stairs. Respiratory muscle involvement, manifesting as exertional breathlessness and orthopnea, may occur in 40% of MG patients. Myasthenic crisis, with impending respiratory failure, requiring noninvasive positive pressure ventilation or mechanical ventilation, may occur in 10–15% of MG patients. This is usually accompanied by bulbar and neck muscle weakness. Single breath count and neck muscle weakness are good bedside tools for predicting a myasthenic crisis. Forced vital capacity (FVC) <20 mL/kg and mean inspiratory pressure (MIP) or mean expiratory pressure (MEP) <40 cm of water are indicators of impending myasthenic crisis.[18] **Figures 2A to E** show the clinical features of MG.

Juvenile MG is another distinct subset occurring in 11–24% of cases that have their onset before adolescence. Onset is usually after 10 years of age and is rare before 1 year. Female preponderance is seen, begins usually as ocular MG, and may become generalized. Transient neonatal MG occurs in 10–15% of neonates born to mothers with MG due to the transplacental transfer of antibodies. They have a

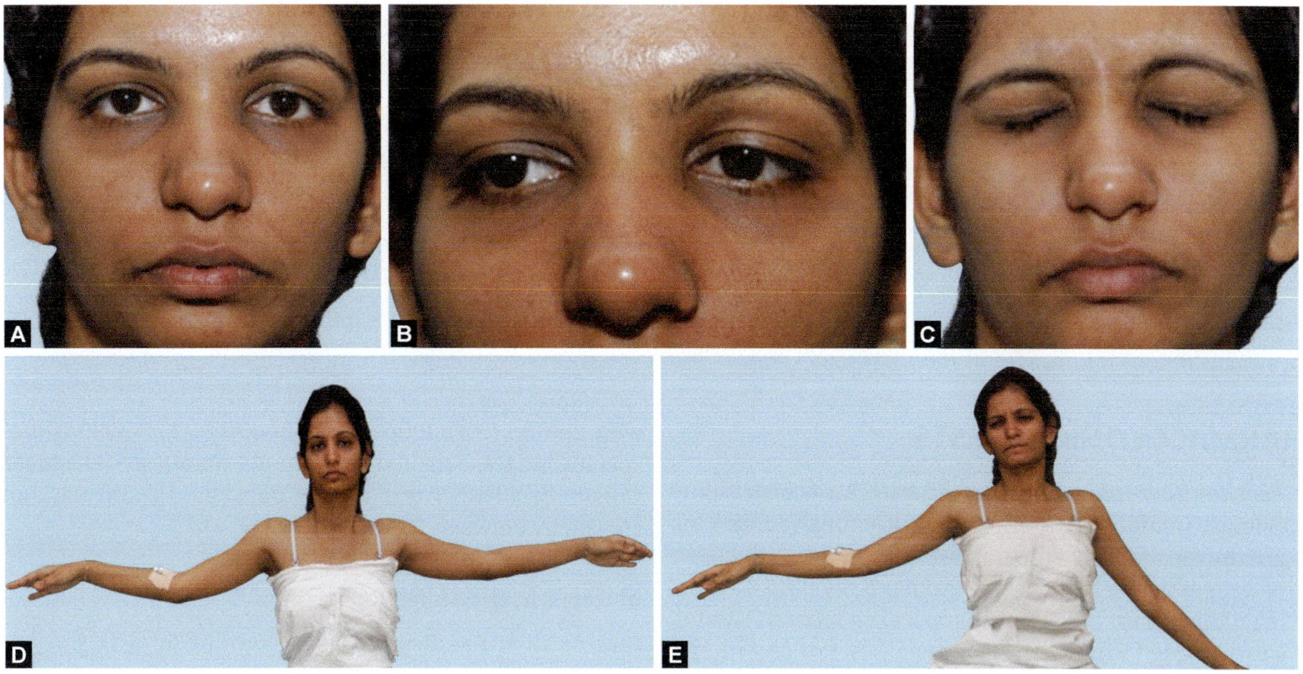

FIGS. 2A TO E: (A and B) A 20-year old with AChR antibody positive myasthenia gravis with fatigable ptosis, (C) weakness of orbicularis oculi, (D and E) shows fatigable limb weakness.

weak cry, poor feeding, breathing difficulties, and hypotonia and arthrogryposis. Weakness lasts a few days to weeks and responds to AChE inhibitors. The severity of weakness does not correlate with antibody titers nor with the severity of weakness in the mother.[18]

The Myasthenia Gravis Foundation of America (MGFA) classification of MG[19] into clinical classes based on severity is as follows:

- *Class I MG is characterized by the following*: Any ocular muscle weakness (may have weakness of eye closure, all other muscle strength is normal)
- *Class II MG is characterized by the following*: Mild weakness affecting muscles other than ocular muscles, may also have ocular muscle weakness of any severity.
    - *Class IIa MG is characterized by the following*: Predominantly affecting limb, axial muscles, or both, may also have lesser involvement of oropharyngeal muscles.
    - *Class IIb MG is characterized by the following*: Predominantly affecting oropharyngeal, respiratory muscles, or both, may also have lesser or equal involvement of limb, axial muscles, or both.
- *Class III MG is characterized by the following*: Moderate weakness affecting muscles other than ocular muscles, may also have ocular muscle weakness of any severity.
    - *Class IIIa MG is characterized by the following*: Predominantly affecting limb, axial muscles, or both, may also have lesser involvement of oropharyngeal muscles.
    - *Class IIIb MG is characterized by the following*: Predominantly affecting oropharyngeal, respiratory muscles, or both, may also have lesser or equal involvement of limb, axial muscles, or both.
- *Class IV MG is characterized by the following*: Severe weakness affecting muscles other than ocular muscles, may also have ocular muscle weakness of any severity.
    - *Class IVa MG is characterized by the following*: Predominantly affecting limb, axial muscles, or both, may also have lesser involvement of oropharyngeal muscles.
    - *Class IVb MG is characterized by the following*: Predominantly affecting oropharyngeal, respiratory muscles, or both, may also have lesser or equal involvement of limb, axial muscles, or both.
- *Class V MG is characterized by the following*: Intubation with or without mechanical ventilation, except when employed during routine postoperative management, and the use of a feeding tube without intubation places the patient in class IVb.

DIAGNOSIS OF MYASTHENIA GRAVIS

Common bedside tests are the icepack test, sustained upgaze test, and the rest test (sleep test). However, a combination of pharmacological tests, electrophysiological, and serological tests is used to ascertain the diagnosis.

Ice pack test: An ice pack is placed on the eyelid for 2 minutes. An improvement of ≥ 2 mm in the vertical palpebral aperture is considered positive. The test is sensitive, however, lacks specificity.[20] A combination of ice test and single-fiber electromyography (SFEMG) is more accurate for the diagnosis of MG **(Figs. 3A and B)**.

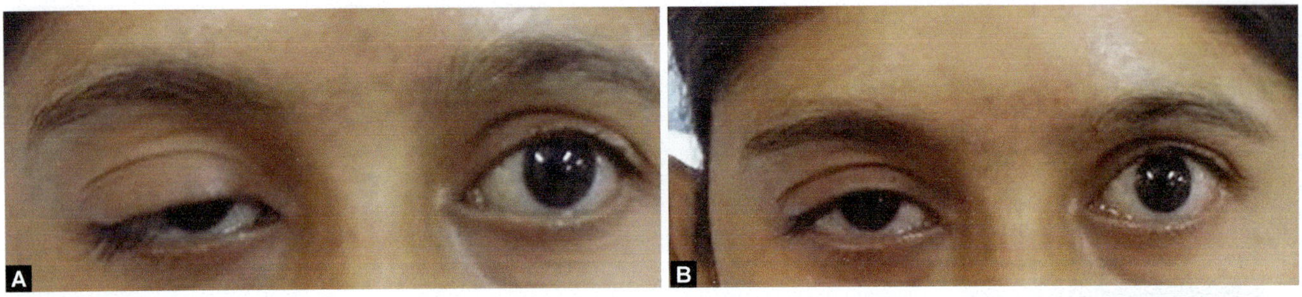

FIGS. 3A AND B: Ice pack test, (A) the left-sided image shows ptosis of right eye preice pack test; and (B) the right image shows improvement in ptosis following ice pack application for 2 minutes.

PHARMACOLOGICAL TESTS

- *Tensilon (edrophonium chloride test)*: An acetylcholinesterase inhibitor administered intravenously to look for unequivocal improvement in symptoms. An initial dose of 2 mg is given, followed by another 8 mg if no adverse reactions occur. It has a rapid onset (30 seconds) and is short-acting (5 minutes). However, it is not commonly used as there is a risk of hypotension, bronchospasm, and arrhythmias. The sensitivity is 70–95%.[9] However, false positivity may be seen in other lower motor neuron disorders and brainstem tumors.[17]
- *Neostigmine test*: It is another acetylcholine esterase inhibitor that can be used to assess improvement. Peak action is seen around 30 minutes after intramuscular injection and the effect lasts several hours. The usual dose in adults is 1.5 mg. The sensitivity is about 83% and specificity 97%.[21]

Electrophysiological Tests

Repetitive nerve stimulation (RNS): A supramaximal stimulation of the nerve at a low frequency of 2-3 Hz is used. A 10% decrement in compound muscle action potential (CMAP) between the first and fourth/fifth evoked potential is a positive response. Decrement is absent in normal individuals.

If decrement is absent, the test may be done postexercise when postactivation exhaustion causes decrement. It has a sensitivity of 75% in generalized MG and 50% in ocular MG.[22] Decrement may also be seen in Lambert-Eaton myasthenic syndrome (LEMS), motor neuron disease, and myopathies. Technical factors such as appropriate immobilization of muscle, choice of muscle (recommended to test in weak muscles), and withholding acetylcholine esterase inhibitors at least 12 hours before testing will increase the yield of RNS.[17]

In general, proximal muscles such as the trapezius, deltoid, and facial muscles such as nasalis have a good yield. Deltoid had the highest yield among all muscles in select studies while trapezius was better in others.[23] The highest diagnostic yield of the RNS test in an Indian study was with deltoid and nasalis (78.8% each), followed by trapezius (65.5%) and the highest mean patient discomfort score was with deltoid (2.4), followed by nasalis (1.3).[24] RNS is more specific but less sensitive than the ice pack test.[20] Diagnostic sensitivity of RNS test ranges between 14 and 94% and specificity between 73 and 100% **(Fig. 4)**.[21]

Serological Tests

Anti-AchR antibodies are highly specific for MG. Enzyme-linked immunosorbent assay (ELISA) testing kits are commonly used to detect these antibodies but the gold standard is radioimmunoprecipitation (RIPA).[25] However, there may be false positive values especially in LEMS (5%), motor neuron disease (3–5%), and polymyositis (<1%).[26] The sensitivity of this test is approximately 85% for generalized MG and 50% for ocular MG. In seronegative generalized MG, low-affinity anti-AChR antibodies binding to clustered AChRs are found in 66% of patients. Cell-based assays are used to detect clustered AChR antibodies because conventional testing with RIPA assay does not detect clustered AChR.[18]

Anti-AChR antibody response is heterogeneous, three types are described—(1) binding, (2) blocking, and (3) modulating antibodies. Approximately 4% of patients with negative AChR binding antibodies have an elevated AChR modulating antibody assay, and 1% of patients with negative AChR binding antibodies have elevated AChR blocking antibodies.[17,21]

In about 40% of cases who are seronegative for anti-AchR antibodies, anti-MuSK has been identified. The specificity of anti-MuSK antibodies is very high (94–100%).[21] Neither AChR nor anti-MuSK antibodies are present in the sera of about 10% of MG patients. These cases are called double-seronegative MG. Patients with thymoma are known to be positive for anti-titin and antistriational antibodies. These antibodies are also commonly found in patients with LOMG. Anti-titin antibodies are present in about 49–95% of thymoma-associated myasthenia gravis (TAMG), antiryanodine receptor antibodies in 70–80% while antiKv1.4 is found in around 40–70% of TAMG patients. Several other antigenic targets have been reported in MG; these include the proteins agrin, rapsyn, cortactin, AChE, collagen Q (ColQ), and collagen XIII. The pathogenicity, specificity for MG, and diagnostic or prognostic value are not fully characterized **(Tables 2 and 3)**.[27,28]

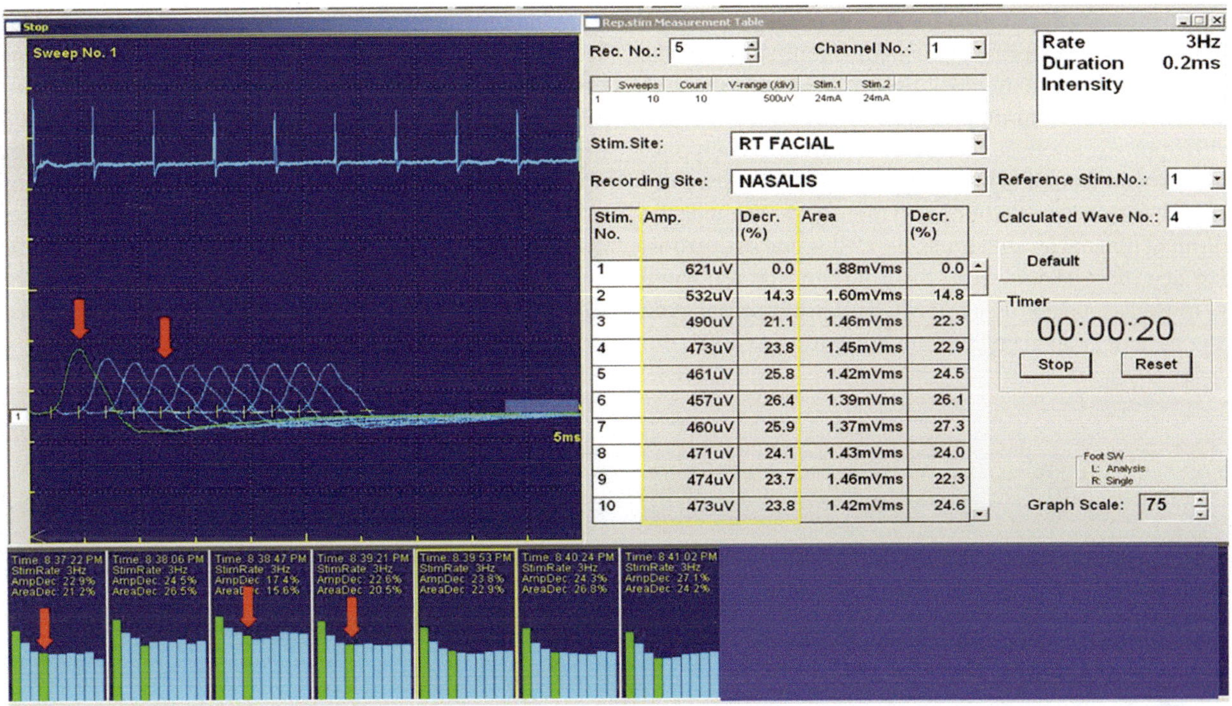

FIG. 4: Decremental pattern of repetitive nerve stimulation (RNS) at 3 Hz seen in nasalis muscle; significant decrement is seen; arrows indicate the decrement between the first and fourth compound muscle action potential (CMAP).

TABLE 2: Autoantibodies in myasthenia gravis.

Antibody	Anti-AchR	Anti-MuSK	Anti-LRP4
Frequency	80%	7–10% (40% of AchRAb negative cases)	2–27% of double seronegative
Subclass	IgG1, IgG3	IgG4	IgG1/IgG2
Pathogenesis	• Binding, blocking or modulating • Complement-mediated damage	• Bind to Ig-like domain • Cell-mediated cytotoxicity	Disrupt activation of MuSK, and reduce AchR clustering[28]

(AChRAb: acetylcholine receptor antibodies; IgG: Immunoglobulin G; MuSK: muscle-specific kinase; TAMG: thymoma-associated myasthenia gravis)

Single Fiber Electromyography

The activation of a normal motor unit, results in nearly simultaneous excitation of all the muscle fibers supplied by the corresponding motor axon. SFEMG measures the time interval between two or more adjacent muscle fibers action potentials (MFAPs) (inner potential interval—IPI) of the same motor unit, and the variation between IPIs is called the "jitter".[29] This is mathematically expressed as mean consecutive difference (MCD) which is the mean of the differences in consecutive IPI recorded between a pair of MFAPs. In neuromuscular disorders, especially in MG, due to the failure of neuromuscular transmission, there is an increase in jitter between adjacent MFAPs of the same motor unit, which can be measured by an appropriate EMG needle. At times, due to impairment of NM transmission, the threshold for depolarization fails to be reached and a muscle

TABLE 3: Autoantibodies in myasthenia gravis (MG): Sensitivity and specificity of various modalities in diagnosing MG.[21]

Test	Sensitivity (%)	Specificity (%)
Neostigmine test: All cases of MG	83	97
Neostigmine test: Ocular MG	93	–
Neostigmine test: Generalized MG	98	–
Ice pack test: All cases of MG	28–96	31–100
Ice pack test: Ocular MG	85	33
Ice pack test: Generalized MG	90	–
Ice pack test and SFEMG	79	64
Ice pack test and RNS	24	92
Anti-AChR Ab: All cases of MG	50–97	95–100
Anti-AChR Ab: Ocular MG	38–75	–
Anti-AChR Ab: Generalized MG	73–94	–
Anti-AChR Ab: Clustered	13–66	100
Anti-MuSK-Ab	27–70*	93–100
Anti-LRP4 Ab	3	–
RNS: All cases of MG	15–92	73–100
RNS: Ocular MG	14–67	91
RNS: Generalized MG	32–94	–
SFEMG: All cases of MG	64–100	22–97
SFEMG: Ocular MG	73–100	22–100
SFEMG: Generalized MG	85–99	91–100

*In those who are seronegative for anti-AChR antibody.

(Ab: antibody; AChR: acetylcholine receptor; MG: myasthenia gravis; MuSK: muscle-specific kinase; RNS: repetitive nerve stimulation; SFEMG: single-fiber electromyography)

fiber may fail to get depolarized, referred to as "blocking". SFEMG studies are performed most commonly in frontalis, orbicularis oculi, or extensor digitorum communis. A minimum of 15–20 separate pairs are recorded from 2 or 3 sites with approximately 50 firings recorded from each pair. The study is abnormal if (1) >10% of the total pairs (two out of twenty) show increased jitter or (2) mean jitter exceeds the upper limit of normal for that muscle.[29,30] It is one of the most sensitive test (95–99%) for NMJ disorders in that a normal SFEMG in weak muscle rules out MG and is abnormal even when the patient is on acetylcholine inhibitors (AChEI). But its specificity is low and can be abnormal in anterior horn cell diseases, myopathies, or in patients who have received botulinum toxin injections and are technically demanding. SFEMG is currently performed with facial concentric EMG needles unlike the single fiber EMG needles of the previous era and the muscles can be studied either by voluntary or stimulated activation. Standard reference values are available for concentric needle SFEMG for both voluntary and axonal stimulation for various muscles.[30] **Figures 5A to D** show a sample of an abnormal SFEMG report performed from the right frontalis muscles.

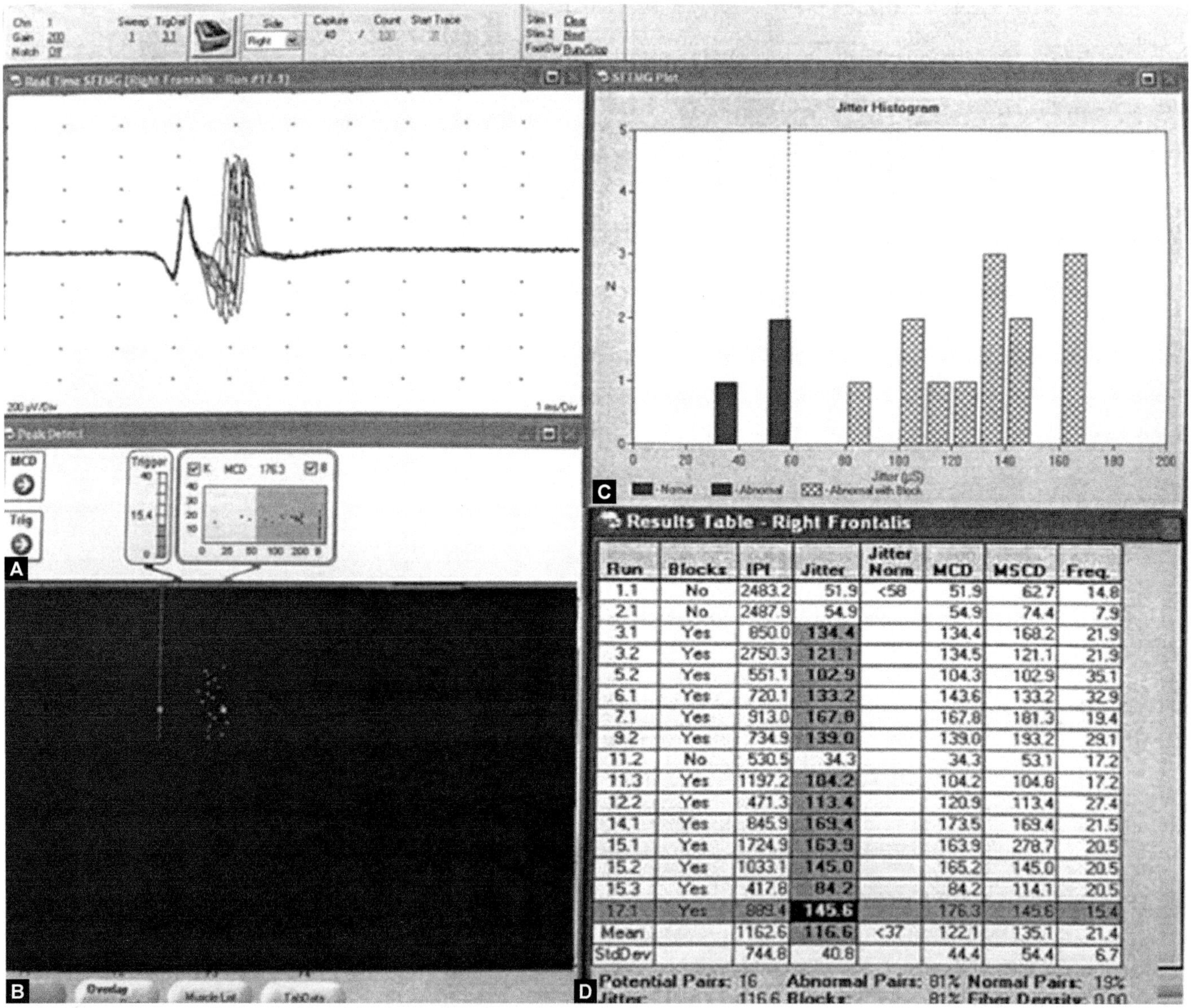

Run	Blocks	IPI	Jitter	Jitter Norm	MCD	MSCD	Freq.
1.1	No	2483.2	51.9	<58	51.9	62.7	14.8
2.1	No	2487.9	54.9		54.9	74.4	7.9
3.1	Yes	850.0	134.4		134.4	168.2	21.9
3.2	Yes	2750.3	121.1		134.5	121.1	21.9
5.2	Yes	551.1	102.9		104.3	102.9	35.1
6.1	Yes	720.1	133.2		143.6	133.2	32.9
7.1	Yes	913.0	167.8		167.8	181.3	19.4
9.2	Yes	734.9	139.0		139.0	193.2	29.1
11.2	No	530.5	34.3		34.3	53.1	17.2
11.3	Yes	1197.2	104.2		104.2	104.8	17.2
12.2	Yes	471.3	113.4		120.9	113.4	27.4
14.1	Yes	845.9	169.4		173.5	169.4	21.5
15.1	Yes	1724.9	163.9		163.9	278.7	20.5
15.2	Yes	1033.1	145.0		165.2	145.0	20.5
15.3	Yes	417.8	84.2		84.2	114.1	20.5
17.1	Yes	889.4	145.6		176.3	145.6	15.4
Mean		1162.6	116.6	<37	122.1	135.1	21.4
StdDev		744.8	40.8		44.4	54.4	6.7

FIGS. 5A TO D: Single-fiber electromyography (SFEMG) performed from right frontalis muscle in a patient suspected of having ocular myasthenia gravis (MG) using a facial concentric needle EMG with a sensitivity of 200 microvolt and 1 ms per division, low-frequency filter at 500 Hz, high-frequency filter at 1 kHz. (A) Superimposed tracing from a pair showing increased jitter. (B) A vertical sequential plot of the consecutive IPI between the two pairs in A showing increased jitter. (C) The jitter histogram of the 16 pairs of muscle fiber action potentials recorded. The vertical line represents the threshold. Note that the mean consecutive difference (MCD) from all except two pairs were above the normal MCD for frontalis muscle. (D) Table summarizing the various parameters from the 16 pairs of muscle fiber action potentials recorded from the right frontalis. Note that jitter (MCD) values were significantly increased in almost all the pairs (highlighted) with blocking seen in several pairs. The mean MCD was also increased. Pairs with MCD above 150 µs should not be ideally used for calculating mean MCD.

Thymic hyperplasia/thymoma screening—a computed tomography (CT) chest is mandatory in all patients to screen for thymic hyperplasia/thymoma. Magnetic resonance imaging (MRI)/positron emission tomography (PET)-CT may be needed in select cases;[31] however, existing literature suggests that it may be difficult to distinguish between thymic hyperplasia and normal thymus on these imaging modalities **(Fig. 6)**. About 10–15% patients have thymoma. MuSK MG is rarely associated with thymic pathologies.[10] Thymomas are further classified histopathologically into subtypes A, AB, B1, B2, and B3. This classification is used to guide further management.[32]

Besides these tests, newer modalities such as ocular vestibular-evoked myogenic potentials, otoacoustic emissions, and disease-specific circulating miRNAs in serum for autoimmune myasthenia are being investigated as diagnostic markers.[21]

TREATMENT OF MYASTHENIA GRAVIS

Myasthenia gravis is the prototype example of an autoimmune disease, one that is initiated by CD4+ T cells, driven by B cells and mediated by autoantibodies and complement cascade. Immunomodulation therapies, both conventional and novel agents, act by suppressing the various steps of this complex immunological interplay, and this remains the cornerstone of MG treatment.[33-35]

Symptomatic Treatment

The discovery of AChEI and their benefit in MG is a major landmark in the history of pharmacology and neurology. In minimally symptomatic patients, they alone may be sufficient as treatment. AChEIs are quaternary ammonium compounds that prolong the action of ACh in NMJ by reversibly inhibiting the AChE enzyme.[36] Pyridostigmine and neostigmine are the most commonly used AChEIs and are available in oral, sustained-release preparations, syrup, and for parenteral dosing. The side effects include increased sweating, hypersalivation, excess bronchial secretions, and increased gut motility resulting in abdominal cramps and diarrhea due to the action of muscarinic receptors and less frequently muscle cramps and fasciculations due to nicotinic receptor action. Either dose reduction or use of glycopyrrolate and loperamide can be used to deal with troublesome side effects. Caution must be exercised when administering AChEI to MuSK MG since paradoxical worsening has been observed probably due to postsynaptic AChR declustering. Beta-agonists such as ephedrine at 45–200 mg/day and salbutamol such as 4–12 mg/day and even higher have been effective in the treatment of congenital MG.[37-40] Their role in autoimmune MG due to their permissive role in NMJ transmission is being explored.

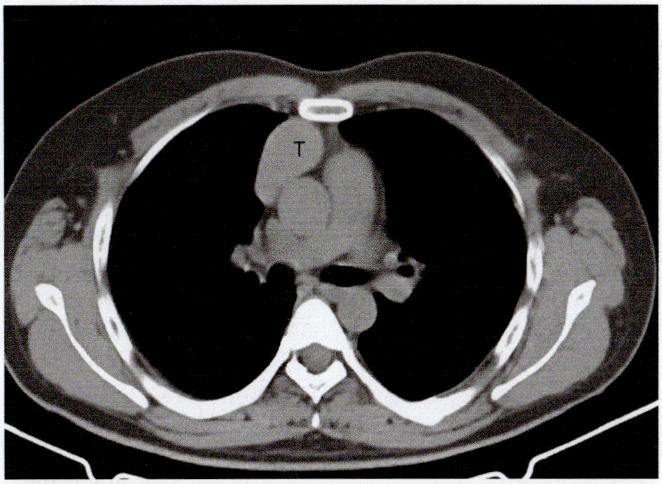

FIG. 6: Anterior mediastinal mass suggestive of thymoma (T) in a patient with myasthenia gravis.

Conventional IST Agents

The introduction of corticosteroids was the game changer in the management of MG and despite many advances, continues to be the first-line treatment, mainly because of the rapidity of action and low cost. About a third of the patients can worsen with high-dose initiation especially elderly and those with bulbar symptoms and thymoma.[41-43] Initiation at low doses and gradual weekly dose up-titration according to the patient' symptoms is preferred in most situations.[44] If the response remains poor despite adequate dosage and time, or an attempt at corticosteroid taper fails alternate immunosuppressants and steroid-sparing agents may be initiated. The obvious disadvantage is the side effect profile and patients must be educated about the need for monitoring.

Azathioprine (AZA) along with mycophenolate mofetil (MMF) is two of the most preferred steroid-sparing immunosuppressants. AZA is a purine analog, and its active metabolites bring about lymphocyte suppression by inhibiting DNA and RNA synthesis. Although monotherapy with AZA was shown to be efficacious and better tolerated than corticosteroids in some studies, the long gap of 6 months for initial treatment response rarely makes them an ideal agent as monotherapy.[45,46] But when combined with corticosteroids, AZA leads to earlier tapering and lower maintenance dose of steroids with fewer treatment failure and longer remissions.[47] It also has the advantage of being safe during pregnancy.[48,49] Slow dose up-titration seldom cause idiosyncratic reactions and routine screening for thiopurine methyltransferase (TPMT) and inosine triphosphate pyrophosphatase (ITPase) enzymes may not be warranted. Patients have to be educated about the potential for hematological, gastrointestinal side effects, increased risks of infections, and the need for weekly and subsequent monthly and 3-monthly blood monitoring.[50,51] There is minimally increased long-term risk of lymphoma (OR 1.2) at higher cumulative doses.[52]

Mycophenolate mofetil acts by inhibiting purine synthesis in T and B cells by inhibiting the inositol monophosphate dehydrogenase enzyme.[53] Although the only phase III study employing MMF at 2 g/day failed to show clinical benefit or steroid-sparing effect in MG, real-world data and expert opinions recommend MMF as a first- or second-line immunosuppressant in MG.[36,54,55] An early taper of steroids and suboptimal duration of MMF treatment might have been the reasons for negative trial results as it takes at least 12 months for the maximum benefit of MMF. Hematological and gastroenterological side effects demand monitoring as in AZA but most studies show MMF to be well tolerated with minimal side effects. But unlike AZA, MMF is teratogenic and not recommended during pregnancy.[36]

Cyclosporine (CsA) and tacrolimus (FK506) are calcineurin inhibitors that block cytokine gene transcription and hence inhibit T cell proliferation. Primarily used to prevent transplant rejection, both agents are beneficial in MG and are the preferred IST in many centers across China and Japan.[56] Other than steroids, CsA is one IST that has an equally rapid onset of action; as early as 2 weeks. The main limiting factor of these agents is the side effect profile including nephrotoxicity, hypertension, paresthesia, gum sensitivity, altered taste, hirsutism, headache, muscle cramps, and diarrhea which can be seen in up to 20% of patients. FK506 has a better side effect profile but the evidence favoring its efficacy in MG is less robust.[57] Both agents require monitoring of renal and liver functions, blood glucose levels, and the dose adjustments would require trough level monitoring. These agents have their role in refractory MG in patients who fail the first- and second-line agents or those who are dependent on therapeutic plasma exchange (PLEX) and intravenous immunoglobulin (IVIG) maintenance.

Cyclophosphamide (CyC) is the prototypical alkylating agent that was broadly employed in oncology and several autoimmune disorders and has been found to improve muscle strength, with steroid-sparing action in MG.[58] The effect is, however, not sustained and starts to wane after 1 year.[59] This along with their side effect profile, reserves their use in refractory MG when alternate second-line agents are not an option.

Methotrexate (MTX) besides being a folate anti-metabolite has several anti-inflammatory functions that lead to a reduction of T cell proliferation. The relative ease of administration and the inexpensiveness makes MTX an attractive IST in refractory MG but randomized controlled trials (RCTs) failed to show any steroid-sparing effect or reduction in MG scores.[60] It was well tolerated in trials with nonspecific pain being the most common side effect. Frequent monitoring of liver function tests is required and there is an increased risk of infections.

Therapeutic plasma exchange or IVIG is routinely employed for acute worsening of MG, for patients with severe MG refractory to first-line agents or before thymectomy. They also have a role in the maintenance treatment of MG as 3 or 4 weekly maintenance regimens, though because of various financial and logistic reasons, are not popularly used for this purpose in our country. Systematic reviews and meta-analyses have found both agents to have comparable efficacy and tolerability with one not being superior to the other.[61-63] Each procedure has its advantages. IVIG may offer some safety advantages such as easier administration, lesser vasovagal reactions, cardiac events, lesser systemic infections, and shorter hospital stay while PLEX in some studies have noted faster recovery and early extubation.[64,65] But overall, the choice between the IVIG and PLEX is largely decided by patient preferences, financial and institutional preferences. Subcutaneous intravenous immunoglobulin (SCIG) preparations are also available in many countries and offer effective maintenance treatment.[66,67] Having a slower absorption rate, lower peak levels, and longer steady-state levels negates several of the infusion-related adverse reactions related to IVIG infusion and patients benefitting from IVIG can be transitioned to equivalent doses of SCIG.[68] SCIG also allows greater patient autonomy since the infusion system can be assembled and self-administered by patients or their caregivers. SCIG is not yet marketed in India.

Thymectomy in nonthymomatous AChR positive generalized MG, was conclusively demonstrated to be beneficial, leading to a reduction in MG severity, IST dosage, hospitalizations, and relapses.[69] The benefit takes up to 1 year to manifest but continues to persist during subsequent years. Less invasive transcervical and videoscopy or robotic-assisted techniques result in lesser morbidity, but trans-sternal thymectomy offers maximal resection and a hence better chance at complete remission.[41,70,71] Thymectomy is recommended in AChR negative generalized MG but not in anti-MuSK, LRP4 or agrin-related MG, ocular MG, or in patients >65 years. Stabilizing of patient's condition is mandatory before thymectomy is contemplated and it has no role during acute crisis. Patients with thymoma should undergo thymectomy more from an oncological perspective but benefits in terms of MG will take longer to manifest. The benefit is less clear in ocular MG and is not usually performed unless refractory, and is not recommended in MuSK-positive MG.

Table 4 summarizes the mechanism of action, time to onset of action, and dosage of conventional IST.

Novel Immunomodulatory Agents

With advances in the understanding of immunopathology, drug development, and translational research, the focus of treatment in MG is shifting from the conventional broad-spectrum IST to target-specific biologicals which offer better efficacy, lesser side effects, and offer patient-specific personalized treatment. Recent years have seen several novel agents of great promise that act at various levels of MG immunopathogenesis. But their current role such as when to initiate, duration of treatment, and long-term safety is still evolving.[34]

Table 5 summarized the newer biological agents recently approved and under evaluation in MG.

TABLE 4: Mechanism of action, time to onset of action and dosage of conventional IST.

Agent	Mechanism of action	Minimum time to onset of clinical benefit	Dose
Corticosteroids	Inhibition of T cells and monocyte-macrophage activation	2–12 weeks	Initiation at 10/20 mg daily and weekly uptitration to 50/60 mg daily
Azathioprine	Purine analog inhibiting DNA and RNA replication	12 months	Initiation at 50 mg daily and increased weekly to 2–3 mg/kg/day
Mycophenolate mofetil	Inhibition of inositol monophosphate dehydrogenase	6–12 months	1–2 g/day in divided doses
Cyclosporine	Inhibits calcineurin	2–12 months	Initiation at 3 mg/kg/day and increased to 6 mg/kg/day, titration based on clinical efficacy, therapeutic drug monitoring (400-600 ng/mL) and/or serum creatinine levels
Tacrolimus	Macrolide antibiotic that inhibits calcineurin	2–12 months	3 mg/kg/day with further titration based on clinical efficacy or therapeutic drug monitoring (7–8 ng/mL)
Methotrexate	Folic acid antimetabolite	3–6 months	Initiation at 10 mg/week single dose, increased weekly up to 20–25 mg/week
Cyclophosphamide	Alkylating agent preventing DNA replication	3–4 months	Pulse of 1–1.5 mg/m^2 given over 5 days repeated monthly for 6 months
IVIG	Multiple mechanisms, predominantly FcRn saturation	10–15 days	2 g/kg divided over 2–5 days
SCIG	Same as IVIG but with lower peak and trough immunoglobulin levels and steadier state	2 weeks	Weekly dose is calculated by multiplying the maintenance dose of IVIG in grams by 1.37 divided by the interval between IVIG doses
PLEX	Removal of pathogenic antibodies by "apheresis"	2–4 days	30–40 mL/kg of plasma exchanged per day for 5 days

(IVIG: intravenous immunoglobulin; PLEX: therapeutic plasma exchange; SCIG: subcutaneous immunoglobulin)

Complement Inhibitors

Binding of Ig G1 and G3 antibodies to the postsynaptic AChR receptors results in complement cascade and cleavage of C5 complement that in turn triggers the formation of MACs leading to postsynaptic damage.[72-74] Eculizumab is a humanized monoclonal antibody against C5 complement and in 2017, following the results of the REGAIN trial, was the first complement inhibitor approved by the United States Food and Drug Administration (USFDA) for clinical use in refractory AChR positive generalized MG. However, the cost remains prohibitive even high-income countries and continues to be beyond the grasp of low and middle-income countries until biosimilars are available. Ravulizumab and zilucoplan are other C5 complement inhibitors being explored in MG and the latter have received orphan drug status for the treatment of severe AChR positive generalized MG. While these are very well tolerated the major concern with this class of agents is the increased risk of *Neisseria meningitidis* infection and is mandatory to have the patient vaccinated at least 2 weeks before the first dose.

FcRn Inhibitors

The neonatal Fc receptor (FcRn) is a beta 2 microglobulin that selectively rescues IgG from lysosomal degradation by binding to the Fc receptor. Hence FcRn maintains circulating IgG levels and prolongs its half-life.[75] Efgartigimod, rozanolixizumab, nipocalimab, and batoclimab are FcRn inhibitors undergoing clinical trials in MG. By blocking FcRn, they bring about a rapid drop in levels of IgG akin to a "chemical plasma exchange" and this has shown to parallel clinical improvement. Efgartigimod in December 2021 received FDA approval for use in AChR positive generalized MG.

B Cell Inhibitors

Rituximab is the prototype example of a B cell inhibitor and is a chimeric monoclonal antibody against CD20 transmembrane protein expressed by the B cell subpopulation, bringing about their depletion through complement and antibody-mediated mechanisms.[76] Due to its efficacy, relative ease of maintenance and comparatively favorable side effect profile RTX has become a popular choice for autoimmune disorders. It has been tried in MG since 2008 and two meta-analyses, done in 2014 and 2021 showed RTX to be safe and effective in MG; with improvement in clinical scores, steroid-sparing effect and adverse events ranging from 4 to 19% but most being mild. The efficacy is far more in MuSK-positive MG than AChR MG.[77,78] However the data was from case series and case reports and the only RCT which looked into RTX in AChR MG showed that while safe, RTX had neither clinical benefit nor steroid-sparing effect

TABLE 5: Summary of the newer biological agents recently approved and under evaluation in myasthenia gravis (MG).

Agent (pharmaceutical company)	Mechanism of action	Dose	Adverse effects	Current status
Eculizumab (Alexion)	C5 complement inhibitor	900 mg IV qwk × 4, then 1,200 mg IV q2wk	Risk of *Neisseria meningitidis*	*Approved* for AChR positive GMG in 2017
Efgartigimod (Argenx)	FcRn inhibitor	10 mg/kg qwk IV	Mild; headache, reduced monocyte count, rhinorrhea, myalgia, pruritus, injection site pain, herpes zoster reactivation	*Approved* for AChR positive GMG by FDA in December 2021
Zilucoplan (UCB)	C5 and C5b complement inhibitor	0.3 mg/kg QD SC	Mild; injection site reactions, headache	Orphan drug status for moderate to severe AChR positive MG; ongoing phase III trial
Ravulizumab (Alexion)	C5 complement inhibitor with extended half-life	Weight based (<60 kg–2,400 mg, 60–100 kg–2,700 mg, >100 kg–3,000 mg) IV; second dose 15 days after first dose, then q8wk maintenance	Risk of *Neisseria meningitidis*	Ongoing phase III trial
Rozanolixizumab (UCB)	High-affinity FcRn blocker	7 mg/kg qwk SC	Mild-to-moderate headache	Positive phase III trial results
Nipocalimab (Johnson & Johnson)	High-affinity FcRn blocker	60 mg/kg IV q2wk	Well-tolerated	Ongoing phase III trial
Batoclimab (Immunovant)	FcRn blocker	340 mg or 680 mg SC qwk × 4, then 340 mg every 2 weeks	Influenza-like illness	Ongoing phase II trial
Rituximab (Genentech, Roche)	Anti-CD20 antibody	Induction with 375 mg/m^2 IV qwk × 4 or 1 g q2wk × 1 and repeat in 6 m	Infusion reactions, minor risk of infections	MuSK MG and as a second line agent for refractory AChR MG
Inebilizumab (Viela Bio)	Anti-CD19 antibody	300 mg IV q2k × 1, then 300 mg IV in 6 m	Fever, urinary infection	Ongoing phase II trial
Mezagitamab (Takeda)	Anti-CD 38 antibody	600 mg SC qwk	Fever, headache, postural hypotension	Ongoing phase II trial
CAR and CAAR T cell therapy	Chimeric auto-antibody receptor-expressing T cells directed against autoreactive B cells	–	Serious cytokine release syndrome	Ongoing phase I trial
Hematopoietic stem cell therapy	Eradication of all autoreactive T and B cells	–	Toxicity related to conditioning regime	Ongoing phase 1 trial

(AChR: acetylcholine receptor; C5: complement 5; FcRn: neonatal Fc receptor; GMG: generalized myasthenia gravis; FDA: Food and Drugs Administration; q: every; Wk: week, D: day; IV: intravenous; SC: subcutaneous; CAR: chimeric antigen receptor; CAAR: chimeric autoantigen receptor)

compared to placebo.[79] Despite lacking class I evidence, the current consensus opinion and expert recommendation are that RTX is a treatment option for MuSK MG and treatment-refractory AChR positive generalized MG.[30,41] This may change as studies exploring early initiation of RTX and low-dose protocols show promise.

Several other B cell inhibitors such as inebilizumab (anti-CD19), iscalimab (anti-CD40), and mezagitamab (anti-CD38) are being evaluated in MG.[80,81]

Chimeric Antigen Receptor T Cell Therapy

Chimeric antigen receptor (CAR) T cell therapy is based on the principle of adoptive T cell transfer in which the patient's T cells are primed for destroying the tumor cells and are reinfused after ex vivo expansion. These modified T cells express target-specific CARs thus equipping them with high selectivity.[82,83] CAR T cell therapy is revolutionizing the treatment of hemato-oncological conditions and currently phase 1 and 2 studies in MG (Descartes-8) are underway with early promising results.[84,85]

Hematopoietic Stem Cell Transplantation

The perpetuation of autoimmunity in MG is by long-lived plasma cells, which survive in bone marrow niches and are not targeted by current immunosuppressants.[86] Hematopoietic stem cell therapy (HSCT) theoretically reboots the immune system by eradicating all T and B cells and offers a potential cure for several refractory autoimmune disorders. Though a phase I study of HSCT in MG had to be terminated due to recruitment failure a phase 2 trial is currently recruiting patients with various refractory autoimmune neurological disorders including MG.[87]

TREATMENT IN SPECIAL SITUATIONS

- *Children*: The treatment of pediatric and juvenile MG is essentially similar to that in adults, but the differential diagnosis is broader and conditions such as congenital myasthenic syndromes, congenital myopathies, and muscular dystrophies can sometimes be mistaken for autoimmune MG. First-line IST would be steroid and is initiated when symptomatic treatment fails and second-line treatment is initiated when steroids fail or when the disease recurs with steroid taper.[88] There is no data to recommend one agent over the other. The evidence favoring thymectomy is less robust but is recommended in the presence of thymoma and seropositive generalized MG even in the absence of thymoma although it is generally deferred in very young children due to immunological development.[88]
- *Pregnancy*: While there are differences in data depending on centers, in general, pregnancy, especially the first trimester and postpartum period and discontinuation of treatment just before or during pregnancy are risk factors associated with worsening of MG.[89] A stable period of 6 months to 1 year is advisable before conception. In most series, there was no increase in cesarean rates though there is a small but increased risk of neonatal MG due to transplacental migration of antibodies.[49,90] Complication rates are low but include prolonged labor due to patient fatigue and fetal distress. Steroids and AZA are drugs of choice in pregnancy and patients in crisis may require IVIG or PLEX.[49,90]
- *Elderly*: Elderly constitutes a unique population due to the comorbidities and medications that can raise difficulties; delay diagnosis and overlap with symptoms that pose difficulties in management.[91,92] The most common phenotype is generalized MG with oculobulbar onset, but the response to treatment and prognosis is not necessarily poor. Care must be taken to screen the drug list to exclude medications that can worsen MG.

LAMBERT–EATON MYASTHENIC SYNDROME

Introduction

Lambert–Eaton myasthenic syndrome is a disorder of NMJ resulting from the loss of function of presynaptic P/Q type voltage-gated calcium channels (VGCC). Circulating antibodies bind to these VGCCs and impair neurotransmission.[93] Etiologically, it can be due to the presence of underlying cancer (cancer-associated LEMS—CA-LEMS) or autoimmune disorders(nontumor LEMS—NT-LEMS).[94] Cancers usually are small cell lung carcinomas (SCLC) and the prognosis depends on the stage of these cancers. Clinically, they present with fatigable limb weakness with autonomic symptoms and sluggish reflexes.

Epidemiology

The prevalence rate was estimated to be around 2.6 per million in the US Veterans Affairs Population study.[95] CA-LEMS constitutes around 60% of cases of LEMS. Usual cancers are SCLC; however, other lung and nonlung carcinomas are implicated too. The median age at onset of CA-LEMS is around 60 years. Males constitute 59–70% of these cases. CA-LEMS is more frequently seen in men reflecting smoking habits while NT-LEMS has no sex preponderance.[94] The age of onset in NT-LEMS shows a double peak with one peak at around 35 years and another at around 60 years and a range between 7 and 80 years.[94]

Pathophysiology

Lambert–Eaton myasthenic syndrome is caused by Anti-VGCC antibodies which reduce the quantal release of ACh into the NMJ by impairing calcium influx into the presynaptic terminal.[96,97] Direct downregulation of VGCC and also decrease in a number of active zones are known.[98] These autoantibodies also impair neurotransmission at the parasympathetic and sympathetic neurons causing autonomic dysfunction.

Voltage-gated calcium channel is expressed on the surface of cells of SCLC in patients with CA-LEMS. They induce autoantibodies that cross-react with VGCC present on presynaptic terminals thereby impairing neurotransmission.[98]

Genetic susceptibility has also been described in NT-LEMS which shows a strong association with HLA-DR3-B8. In about 15% of cases where anti-VGCC antibodies are absent, other potential antibody targets are synaptotagmin-1, M1 type presynaptic muscarinic AChR.[99]

Clinical Presentation

Clinically, patients present with fatigable proximal limb weakness, usually beginning in the lower limbs. Symptoms are known to spread caudally to cranial, involving ocular and bulbar muscles later in the course of illness.[100] This is contrary to MG where the weakness usually spreads in the craniocaudal direction. Proximal muscles are usually involved first followed by the distal. Dysphagia, dysarthria, dyspnea, ptosis, and double vision may be seen and are described in varying frequencies in different studies.[101]

In a study comparing 101 patients with MG and 38 with LEMS, it was observed that in MG, initial weakness involved extraocular muscles in 59%, bulbar muscles in 29%, and limb muscles in 12% of the patients. However, in LEMS no patient had an ocular weakness, 5% had bulbar weakness, and 95% had weakness of the limbs as the first symptom. At the peak of illness, weakness in MG was purely ocular in 25%, oculobulbar in 5%, exclusively involving limbs in 2%, and present in both oculobulbar muscles and limbs in 68%. However, none of the LEMS patients had weakness restricted to extraocular or bulbar muscles at the peak of illness. The legs were affected in all LEMS patients, whereas in 12 patients with generalized MG, weakness was restricted to the arms.[100] However, others report ocular symptoms in 0–80% and bulbar in 5–80% of patients, probably explained by different times of assessment.[94] There is a variable latency to diagnosis ranging from months to years.

Autonomic symptoms include dry mouth (the most frequent), dry eyes, male impotence, constipation, orthostatic dysfunction, blurred vision, and hypohidrosis. Autonomic dysfunction is found in 80–96% of patients with LEMS.[94] Areflexia/hyporeflexia is noted in about 40%;[94] however, reflexes may be well elicited immediately following a brief exercise which is characteristic of the disease and known as postexercise facilitation.[102] Hence, the reflexes should be tested after a period of rest.

The symptoms in CA-LEMS show a rapid downhill course when compared to NT-LEMS and the survival is determined by the stage of the associated tumor.[103] In contrast, patients with NT-LEMS have a near-normal survival.[98] Cerebellar ataxia may be a feature of CA-LEMS.[104,105]

Investigations

Antibodies to VGCC are detected in nearly 85% of all cases of LEMS, detected by RIPA.[106] Electrophysiological studies are helpful in diagnosis.[107] The usual abnormalities are (1) reduced resting CMAP, (2) decrements in CMAP after low-frequency RNS, and (3) increments in CMAP amplitude of over 100% above resting values seen after maximal voluntary contraction of 10 seconds especially in the distal muscles such as abductor digit minimi, anconeus, and abductor pollicis brevis rather than in proximal muscles such as trapezius.[108] In normal individuals, the physiological increment is usually <40% of the initial CMAP **(Fig. 7)**.[109] An interesting feature in LEMS is the decremental pattern with low-rate RNS becomes progressively greater with repeated trains of stimuli, whereas in MG, the decrement becomes less pronounced and hence we see a U-shaped curve in MG.[110] This is in contrast to the clinical pattern of weakness which is predominantly proximal. A partial explanation for this discrepancy could be the technical difficulties inherent while stimulating the proximal muscles of both upper and lower limbs.[111] Oh et al. reported that 60% facilitation postexercise had 97% sensitivity and 99% specificity for diagnosing LEMS and suggested it as an alternative to the gold standard of 100% increment.[112] High-frequency RNS (20–50 Hz) is often cumbersome and painful for patients.[113] Apart from RNS, SFEMG may be used.

Cancer screening is recommended in all patients to screen for both lung and nonlung carcinomas. It should continue every 3–6 months for at least 2 years after symptom onset, preferably with fluorodeoxyglucose (FDG)-PET CT.[107]

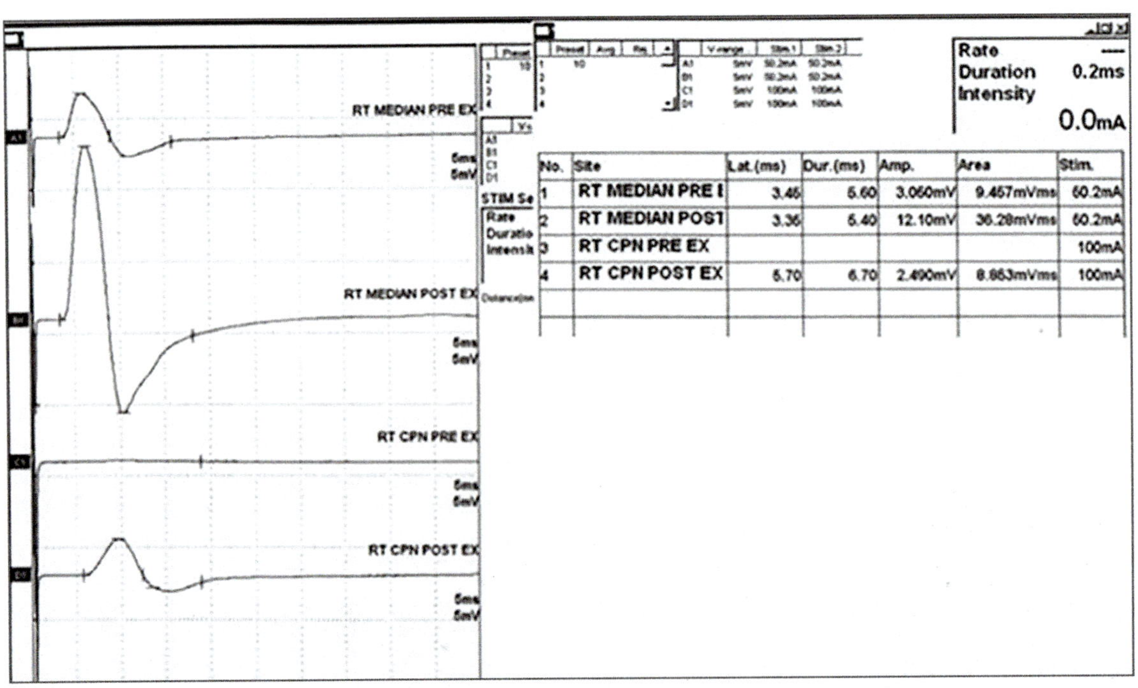

FIG. 7: Increment in compound muscle action potential (CMAP) seen post 10 seconds maximal voluntary contraction compared to baseline in median (top two graphs) and peroneal nerves (bottom two graphs).

The association with tumors after 5 years into the illness is only anecdotal.[101] Tumors in LEMS have been detected many years before too many years after the diagnosis of LEMS. A DELTA-P (Dutch English LEMS Tumor Association Prediction) score has been developed to determine the risk of SCLC based on six independent risk factors, including, (1) age at onset, (2) smoking habits, (3) weight loss, (4) bulbar involvement, (5) erectile dysfunction, and (6) Karnofsky Performance Status. The score ranges from 0 to 6, with a higher score indicating higher risk.[94] The probability for SCLC varies from 0 to 2.6% with a DELTA-P score of 0–1, up to 83.9–100% with a score of 3–6.[94]

Differential Diagnosis

Lambert–Eaton myasthenic syndrome may be confused with MG, amyotrophic lateral sclerosis, and inflammatory myositis. However, appropriate clinical and electrophysiological examination gives clues to the diagnosis.[102]

Treatment

Symptomatic treatment: The use of 3,4 diaminopyridine (DAP) resulted in significant improvement in clinical symptoms, muscle strength score or myometric limb measurement compared to placebo in four RCTs.[114,115] There was an improvement in the resting CMAP too.[115] 3,4-DAP broadens the presynaptic action potential allowing more time for calcium channels to remain open. It is known to block voltage-gated potassium channels and also has a partial agonist action on the calcium channels (CaV1 subtype, L type).[97,114] Calcium channel agonists too have been tried in experimental studies in the past.[116] Pyridostigmine has been used but has shown conflicting results with some studies reporting benefits while others reported no additional benefit. Guanidine has been used in the past but is best avoided due to significant adverse effects.

Symptomatic treatment with 3,4-DAP is advised at a usual dose of 10–20 mg/dose. Improvement may be seen at 3–8 hours of intake of 3,4-DAP. The maximum dosage is 80 mg/day. It has a good safety profile and tolerability. However, there are dose-limiting adverse effects in the form of paresthesias, gastrointestinal symptoms and seizures, and supraventricular tachycardias in cases of intoxication.[107] Amifampridine phosphate (the salt form of 3,4-DAP) has been shown to have superior stability (it can be stored at room temperature) compared with the base.[107]

The mainstay of treatment in CA-LEMS is the treatment of the underlying tumor.[117] In acute severe cases, plasmapheresis and IVIG may be tried. Long-term immunosuppressants are required in patients without adequate symptomatic improvement and commonly used agents are prednisolone, AZA. Rituximab has been tried in a few cases with moderate benefit. In a study on the long-term outcome of NT-LEMS, favorable outcomes were noted, however, the muscle strength scores improved after a median duration of use of immunosuppressants for 6 years.[118] Modest benefits of prednisone and AZA are recognized.[119] A study on 73 patients with LEMS (42% with lung cancer) demonstrated that high-dose prednisolone often achieved only mild to moderate improvement in symptoms, which was not sustained when the dose was reduced.

CONCLUSION

The diagnosis and management of NMJ disorders including MG and LEMS are challenging. MG is more common than LEMS and presents usually with typical fatigable weakness of oculobulbar and limb muscles. The typical clinical triad of LEMS consists of proximal muscle weakness, autonomic symptoms, and areflexia. Accurate clinical, electrophysiological, and serological tests give a clue to the diagnosis. There is a wide array of newer drugs available for the treatment of MG. Appropriate treatment including the treatment of underlying malignancy in CA-LEMS is a must.

REFERENCES

1. Gilhus NE, Tzartos S, Evoli A, Palace J, Burns TM, Verschuuren JJGM. Myasthenia gravis. Nat Rev Dis Primer. 2019;5(1):30.
2. Carr AS, Cardwell CR, McCarron PO, McConville J. A systematic review of population based epidemiological studies in Myasthenia Gravis. BMC Neurol. 2010;10(1):46.
3. Dresser L, Wlodarski R, Rezania K, Soliven B. Myasthenia gravis: Epidemiology, pathophysiology and clinical manifestations. J Clin Med. 2021;10(11):2235.
4. Bubuioc AM, Kudebayeva A, Turuspekova S, Lisnic V, Leone MA. The epidemiology of myasthenia gravis. J Med Life. 2021;14(1):7-16.
5. Keesey JC. Clinical evaluation and management of myasthenia gravis. Muscle Nerve. 2004;29(4):484-505.
6. Singhal B, Bhatia N, Umesh T, Menon S. Myasthenia gravis: A study from India. Neurol India. 2008;56(3):352.
7. Dragin N, Bismuth J, Cizeron-Clairac G, Biferi MG, Berthault C, Serraf A, et al. Estrogen-mediated downregulation of AIRE influences sexual dimorphism in autoimmune diseases. J Clin Invest. 2016;126(4):1525-37.
8. Benfaremo D, Manfredi L, Luchetti MM, Gabrielli A. Musculoskeletal and rheumatic diseases induced by immune checkpoint inhibitors: A review of the literature. Curr Drug Saf. 2018;13(3):150-64.
9. Jayam Trouth A, Dabi A, Solieman N, Kurukumbi M, Kalyanam J. Myasthenia gravis: A review. Autoimmune Dis. 2012;2012:1-10.
10. Melzer N, Ruck T, Fuhr P, Gold R, Hohlfeld R, Marx A, et al. Clinical features, pathogenesis, and treatment of myasthenia gravis: A supplement to the Guidelines of the German Neurological Society. J Neurol. 2016;263(8):1473-94.
11. Sommer N, Melms A, Weller M, Dichgans J. Ocular myasthenia gravis: A critical review of clinical and pathophysiological aspects. Doc Ophthalmol. 1993;84(4):309-33.

12. Nair A, Patil-Chhablani P, Venkatramani D, Gandhi R. Ocular myasthenia gravis: A review. Indian J Ophthalmol. 2014;62(10): 985-91.
13. Yee RD. Rapid eye movements in myasthenia gravis: II. Electro-oculographic Analysis. Arch Ophthalmol. 1976;94(9):1465-72.
14. Turner C. A review of myasthenia gravis: Pathogenesis, clinical features and treatment. Curr Anaesth Crit Care. 2007;18(1):15-23.
15. Rodolico C, Bonanno C, Toscano A, Vita G. MuSK-Associated myasthenia gravis: Clinical features and management. Front Neurol. 2020;11:660.
16. Matta APC, Ferreira ACAF, Kirmse A, Damm AC, Farinhas JGDIB, Barbosa MD, et al. Anti-musk positive myasthenia gravis and three semiological cardinal signs. Neurol Int. 2017;8(4):6361.
17. Juel VC, Massey JM. Myasthenia gravis. Orphanet J Rare Dis. 2007;2(1):44.
18. Hehir MK, Silvestri NJ. Generalized myasthenia gravis. Neurol Clin. 2018;36(2):253-60.
19. Jaretzki A, Barohn RJ, Ernstoff RM, Kaminski HJ, Keesey JC, Penn AS, et al. Myasthenia gravis: Recommendations for clinical research standards. Task Force of the Medical Scientific Advisory Board of the Myasthenia Gravis Foundation of America. Neurology. 2000;55:16-23.
20. Lo YL, Najjar RP, Teo KY, Tow SL, Loo JL, Milea D. A reappraisal of diagnostic tests for myasthenia gravis in a large Asian cohort. J Neurol Sci. 2017;376:153-8.
21. Yoganathan K, Stevenson A, Tahir A, Sadler R, Radunovic A, Malek N. Bedside and laboratory diagnostic testing in myasthenia. J Neurol. 2022;269(6):3372-84.
22. Oh SJ, Kim DE, Kuruoglu R, Bradley RJ, Dwyer D. Diagnostic sensitivity of the laboratory tests in myasthenia gravis. Muscle Nerve. 1992;15(6):720-4.
23. Amandusson Å, Elf K, Grindlund ME, Punga AR. Diagnostic utility of repetitive nerve stimulation in a large cohort of patients with myasthenia gravis. J Clin Neurophysiol. 2017;34(5):400-7.
24. Misra UK, Kalita J, Srivastava A. A study of diagnostic yield, technical ease and patient discomfort of low rate repetitive nerve stimulation test in patients with myasthenia gravis. Electromyogr Clin Neurophysiol. 2006;46(6):337-41.
25. Oger J, Frykman H. An update on laboratory diagnosis in myasthenia gravis. Clin Chim Acta Int J Clin Chem. 2015;449:43-8.
26. Koneczny I, Herbst R. Myasthenia gravis: Pathogenic effects of autoantibodies on neuromuscular architecture. Cells. 2019;8(7):671.
27. Lazaridis K, Tzartos SJ. Autoantibody specificities in myasthenia gravis; implications for improved diagnostics and therapeutics. Front Immunol. 2020;11:212.
28. Fichtner ML, Jiang R, Bourke A, Nowak RJ, O'Connor KC. Autoimmune pathology in myasthenia gravis disease subtypes is governed by divergent mechanisms of immunopathology. Front Immunol. 2020;11:776.
29. Sanders DB, Stålberg EV. AAEM minimonograph #25: Single-fiber electromyography. Muscle Nerve. 1996;19(9):1069-83.
30. Sanders DB, Arimura K, Cui L, Ertaş M, Farrugia ME, Gilchrist J, et al. Guidelines for single fiber EMG. Clin Neurophysiol. 2019;130(8):1417-39.
31. Sussman J, Farrugia ME, Maddison P, Hill M, Leite MI, Hilton-Jones D. Myasthenia gravis: Association of British Neurologists' management guidelines. Pract Neurol. 2015;15(3):199-206.
32. den Bakker MA, Roden AC, Marx A, Marino M. Histologic classification of thymoma: A practical guide for routine cases. J Thorac Oncol. 2014;9(9):S125-30.
33. Menon D, Barnett C, Bril V. Novel treatments in myasthenia gravis. Front Neurol. 2020;11:538.
34. Menon D, Urra Pincheira A, Bril V. Emerging drugs for the treatment of myasthenia gravis. Expert Opin Emerg Drugs. 2021;26(3):259-70.
35. Menon D, Bril V. Pharmacotherapy of Generalized myasthenia gravis with special emphasis on newer biologicals. Drugs. 2022;82(8):865-87.
36. Sanders DB, Wolfe GI, Benatar M, Evoli A, Gilhus NE, Illa I, et al. International consensus guidance for management of myasthenia gravis: Executive summary. Neurology. 2016;87(4):419-25.
37. Bestue-Cardiel M, Sáenz de Cabezón-Alvarez A, Capablo-Liesa JL, López-Pisón J, Peña-Segura JL, Martin-Martinez J, et al. Congenital endplate acetylcholinesterase deficiency responsive to ephedrine. Neurology. 2005;65(1):144-6.
38. Lashley D, Palace J, Jayawant S, Robb S, Beeson D. Ephedrine treatment in congenital myasthenic syndrome due to mutations in DOK7(LOE Classification). Neurology. 2010;74(19):1517-23.
39. Sadeh M, Shen XM, Engel AG. Beneficial effect of albuterol in congential myasthenic syndrome with epsilon subuint mutations. Muscle Nerve. 2011;44(2):289-91.
40. Liewluck T, Selcen D, Engel AG. Beneficial effects of albuterol in congenital endplate acetylcholinesterase deficiency and DOK-7 myasthenia. Muscle Nerve. 2011;44(5):789-94.
41. Narayanaswami P, Sanders DB, Wolfe G, Benatar M, Cea G, Evoli A, et al. International Consensus Guidance for Management of Myasthenia Gravis. Neurology. 2021;96(3):114-22.
42. Sugimoto T, Ochi K, Ishikawa R, Tazuma T, Hayashi M, Mine N, et al. Initial deterioration and intravenous methylprednisolone therapy in patients with myasthenia gravis. J Neurol Sci. 2020;412: 116740.
43. Bae JS, Go SM, Kim BJ. Clinical predictors of steroid-induced exacerbation in myasthenia gravis. J Clin Neurosci Off J Neurosurg Soc Australas. 2006;13(10):1006-10.
44. Seybold ME, Drachman DB. Gradually increasing doses of prednisone in myasthenia gravis. Reducing the hazards of treatment. N Engl J Med. 1974;290(2):81-4.
45. Mantegazza R, Antozzi C, Peluchetti D, Sghirlanzoni A, Cornelio F. Azathioprine as a single drug or in combination with steroids in the treatment of myasthenia gravis. J Neurol. 1988;235(8):449-53.
46. Witte AS, Cornblath DR, Parry GJ, Lisak RP, Schatz NJ. Azathioprine in the treatment of myasthenia gravis. Ann Neurol. 1984;15(6): 602-5.
47. Palace J, Newsom-Davis J, Lecky B. A randomized double-blind trial of prednisolone alone or with azathioprine in myasthenia gravis. Myasthenia Gravis Study Group. Neurology. 1998;50(6):1778-83.
48. Skorpen CG, Hoeltzenbein M, Tincani A, Fischer-Betz R, Elefant E, Chambers C, et al. The EULAR points to consider for use of antirheumatic drugs before pregnancy, and during pregnancy and lactation. Ann Rheum Dis. 2016;75(5):795-810.
49. Alharbi M, Menon D, Barnett C, Katzberg H, Sermer M, Bril V. Myasthenia gravis and pregnancy: Toronto Specialty Center Experience. Can J Neurol Sci J Can Sci Neurol. 2021;48(6):767-71.
50. Fonseca V, Havard CW. Long-term treatment of myasthenia gravis with azathioprine. Postgrad Med J. 1990;66(772):102-5.
51. Hohlfeld R, Michels M, Heininger K, Besinger U, Toyka KV. Azathioprine toxicity during long-term immunosuppression of generalized myasthenia gravis. Neurology. 1988;38(2):258-61.
52. Pedersen EG, Pottegård A, Hallas J, Friis S, Hansen K, Jensen PEH, et al. Use of azathioprine for non-thymoma myasthenia and risk of cancer: a nationwide case-control study in Denmark. Eur J Neurol. 2013;20(6):942-8.
53. Allison AC, Eugui EM. Mycophenolate mofetil and its mechanisms of action. Immunopharmacology. 2000;47(2-3):85-118.
54. Hehir MK, Burns TM, Alpers J, Conaway MR, Sawa M, Sanders DB. Mycophenolate mofetil in AChR-antibody-positive myasthenia gravis: outcomes in 102 patients. Muscle Nerve. 2010;41(5):593-8.
55. Li ZY. China guidelines for the diagnosis and treatment of myasthenia gravis. Neuroimmunol Neuroinflammation. 2016;3: 1-9.

56. Lavrnic D, Vujic A, Rakocevic-Stojanovic V, Stevic Z, Basta I, Pavlovic S, et al. Cyclosporine in the treatment of myasthenia gravis. Acta Neurol Scand. 2005;111(4):247-52.
57. Zhou L, Liu W, Li W, Li H, Zhang X, Shang H, et al. Tacrolimus in the treatment of myasthenia gravis in patients with an inadequate response to glucocorticoid therapy: randomized, double-blind, placebo-controlled study conducted in China. Ther Adv Neurol Disord. 2017;10(9):315-25.
58. De Feo LG, Schottlender J, Martelli NA, Molfino NA. Use of intravenous pulsed cyclophosphamide in severe, generalized myasthenia gravis. Muscle Nerve. 2002;26(1):31-6.
59. Nagappa M, Netravathi M, Taly AB, Sinha S, Bindu PS, Mahadevan A. Long-term efficacy and limitations of cyclophosphamide in myasthenia gravis. J Clin Neurosci. 2014;21(11):1909-14.
60. Pasnoor M, He J, Herbelin L, Burns TM, Nations S, Bril V, et al. A randomized controlled trial of methotrexate for patients with generalized myasthenia gravis. Neurology. 2016;87(1):57-64.
61. Barth D, Nabavi Nouri M, Ng E, Nwe P, Bril V. Comparison of IVIG and PLEX in patients with myasthenia gravis. Neurology. 2011;76(23):2017-23.
62. Gajdos P, Chevret S, Toyka KV. Intravenous immunoglobulin for myasthenia gravis. Cochrane Database Syst Rev. 2012;2012(12):CD002277.
63. Ipe TS, Davis AR, Raval JS. Therapeutic plasma exchange in myasthenia gravis: A Systematic literature review and meta-analysis of comparative evidence. Front Neurol. 2021;12:1355.
64. Alipour-Faz A, Shojaei M, Peyvandi H, Ramzi D, Oroei M, Ghadiri F, et al. A comparison between IVIG and plasma exchange as preparations before thymectomy in myasthenia gravis patients. Acta Neurol Belg. 2017;117(1):245-9.
65. Jensen P, Bril V. A comparison of the effectiveness of intravenous immunoglobulin and plasma exchange as preoperative therapy of myasthenia gravis. J Clin Neuromuscul Dis. 2008;9(3):352-5.
66. Adiao KJB, Espiritu AI, Roque VLA, Reyes JPBT. Efficacy and tolerability of subcutaneously administered immunoglobulin in myasthenia gravis: A systematic review. J Clin Neurosci Off J Neurosurg Soc Australas. 2020;72:316-21.
67. Alcantara M, Sarpong E, Barnett C, Katzberg H, Bril V. Chronic immunoglobulin maintenance therapy in myasthenia gravis. Eur J Neurol. 2021;28(2):639-46.
68. Menon D, Sarpong E, Bril V. Practical aspects of transitioning from intravenous to subcutaneous immunoglobulin therapy in neuromuscular disorders. Can J Neurol Sci. 2021;49(2):161-7.
69. Wolfe GI, Kaminski HJ, Aban IB, Minisman G, Kuo HC, Marx A, et al. Randomized Trial of Thymectomy in Myasthenia Gravis. N Engl J Med. 2016;375(6):511-22.
70. Bril V, Kojic J, Ilse WK, Cooper JD. Long-term clinical outcome after transcervical thymectomy for myasthenia gravis. Ann Thorac Surg. 1998;65(6):1520-2.
71. Instituto Nacional de Ciencias Medicas y Nutricion Salvador Zubiran. (2019). Transsternal Versus Transcervical Thymectomy for the Management of Myasthenia Gravis: A Randomized Controlled Trial With a Mean Follow-up of 10 Years. [online] Available from https://clinicaltrials.gov/ct2/show/NCT03825185 [Last accessed February, 2023].
72. Howard JF. Myasthenia gravis: The role of complement at the neuromuscular junction. Ann N Y Acad Sci. 2018;1412(1):113-28.
73. Huda R, Tüzün E, Christadoss P. Targeting complement system to treat myasthenia gravis. Rev Neurosci. 2014;25(4):575-83.
74. Christadoss P, Tüzün E, Li J, Saini SS, Yang H. Classical complement pathway in experimental autoimmune myasthenia gravis pathogenesis. Ann N Y Acad Sci. 2008;1132:210-9.
75. Pyzik M, Sand KMK, Hubbard JJ, Andersen JT, Sandlie I, Blumberg RS. The neonatal fc receptor (FcRn): A misnomer? Front Immunol. 2019;10:1540.
76. Pescovitz MD. Rituximab, an anti-cd20 monoclonal antibody: history and mechanism of action. Am J Transplant. 2006;6(5 Pt 1):859-66.
77. Iorio R, Damato V, Alboini PE, Evoli A. Efficacy and safety of rituximab for myasthenia gravis: a systematic review and meta-analysis. J Neurol. 2015;262(5):1115-9.
78. Zhao C, Pu M, Chen D, Shi J, Li Z, Guo J, et al. Effectiveness and safety of rituximab for refractory myasthenia gravis: A systematic review and single-arm meta-analysis. Front Neurol. 2021;12:736190.
79. Nowak RJ, Coffey CS, Goldstein JM, Dimachkie MM, Benatar M, Kissel JT, et al. Phase 2 trial of rituximab in acetylcholine receptor antibody-positive generalized myasthenia gravis: The BeatMG Study. Neurology. 2022;98(4):e376-89.
80. Novartis Pharmaceuticals. (2021). Safety, Tolerability, Pharmacokinetics and Efficacy of CFZ533 in Moderate to Severe Myasthenia Gravis. [online] Available from https://clinicaltrials.gov/ct2/show/NCT02565576 [Last accessed February, 2023].
81. Novartis Pharmaceuticals. (2017). Myasthenia gravis. [online] Available from https://www.novctrd.com/ctrdweb/trialresult/trialresults/pdf?trialResultId=17276 [Last accessed February, 2023].
82. June CH, Sadelain M. Chimeric Antigen Receptor Therapy. N Engl J Med. 2018;379(1):64-73.
83. Feins S, Kong W, Williams EF, Milone MC, Fraietta JA. An introduction to chimeric antigen receptor (CAR) T-cell immunotherapy for human cancer. Am J Hematol. 2019;94(S1):S3-9.
84. Cartesian Therapeutics. (2023). Autologous T-Cells Expressing A Chimeric Antigen Receptor Directed To B-Cell Maturation Antigen (BCMA) In Patients With Generalized Myasthenia Gravis (MG). [online] Available from https://clinicaltrials.gov/ct2/show/NCT04146051 [Last accessed February, 2023].
85. Wexier W. (2021). CAR T-cell Therapy Descartes-08 Eased Myasthenia Gravis Symptoms. [online] Available from https://myastheniagravisnews.com/news-posts/2021/09/09/car-t-cell-therapy-descartes-08-myasthenia-gravis-symptoms/ [Last accessed February, 2023].
86. Chang HD, Tokoyoda K, Hoyer B, Alexander T, Khodadadi L, Mei H, et al. Pathogenic memory plasma cells in autoimmunity. Curr Opin Immunol. 2019;61:86-91.
87. Fred Hutchinson Cancer Research Center. (2021). High-Dose Immunosuppressive Therapy Using Carmustine, Etoposide, Cytarabine, and Melphalan (BEAM) + Thymoglobulin Followed by Syngeneic or Autologous Hematopoietic Cell Transplantation for Patients With Autoimmune Neurologic Diseases. [online] Available from https://clinicaltrials.gov/ct2/show/study/NCT00716066 [Last accessed February, 2023].
88. O'Connell K, Ramdas S, Palace J. Management of juvenile myasthenia gravis. Front Neurol. 2020;11:743.
89. Bansal R, Goyal MK, Modi M. Management of myasthenia gravis during pregnancy. Indian J Pharmacol. 2018;50(6):302-8.
90. Chaudhry SA, Vignarajah B, Koren G. Myasthenia gravis during pregnancy. Can Fam Physician. 2012;58(12):1346-9.
91. Vijayan J, Menon D, Barnett C, Katzberg H, Lovblom LE, Bril V. Clinical profile and impact of comorbidities in patients with very-late-onset myasthenia gravis. Muscle Nerve. 2021;64(4):462-6.
92. Zivković SA, Clemens PR, Lacomis D. Characteristics of late-onset myasthenia gravis. J Neurol. 2012;259(10):2167-71.
93. Schoser B, Eymard B, Datt J, Mantegazza R. Lambert–Eaton myasthenic syndrome (LEMS): a rare autoimmune presynaptic disorder often associated with cancer. J Neurol. 2017;264(9):1854-63.
94. Titulaer MJ, Lang B, Verschuuren JJ. Lambert–Eaton myasthenic syndrome: from clinical characteristics to therapeutic strategies. Lancet Neurol. 2011;10(12):1098-107.

95. Abenroth DC, Smith AG, Greenlee JE, Austin SD, Clardy SL. Lambert-Eaton myasthenic syndrome: Epidemiology and therapeutic response in the national veterans affairs population: Epidemiology of LEMS. Muscle Nerve. 2017;56(3):421-6.
96. Takamori M. Lambert–Eaton myasthenic syndrome: Search for alternative autoimmune targets and possible compensatory mechanisms based on presynaptic calcium homeostasis. J Neuroimmunol. 2008;201-202:145-52.
97. Meriney SD, Tarr TB, Ojala KS, Wu M, Li Y, Lacomis D, et al. Lambert-Eaton myasthenic syndrome: mouse passive-transfer model illuminates disease pathology and facilitates testing therapeutic leads: The LEMS mouse passive-transfer model. Ann N Y Acad Sci. 2018;1412(1):73-81.
98. Gilhus NE. Lambert-Eaton myasthenic syndrome; pathogenesis, diagnosis, and therapy. Autoimmune Dis. 2011;2011:1-5.
99. Ginebaugh SP, Badawi Y, Tarr TB, Meriney SD. Neuromuscular active zone structure and function in healthy and Lambert-Eaton myasthenic syndrome states. Biomolecules. 2022;12(6):740.
100. Wirtz PW. Difference in distribution of muscle weakness between myasthenia gravis and the Lambert-Eaton myasthenic syndrome. J Neurol Neurosurg Psychiatry. 2002;73(6):766-8.
101. Pellkofer HL, Armbruster L, Linke R, Schumm F, Voltz R. Managing non-paraneoplastic Lambert–Eaton myasthenic syndrome: Clinical characteristics in 25 German patients. J Neuroimmunol [Internet]. 2009;217(1–2):90-4.
102. Hülsbrink R, Hashemolhosseini S. Lambert–Eaton myasthenic syndrome—diagnosis, pathogenesis and therapy. Clin Neurophysiol. 2014;125(12):2328-36.
103. Wirtz PW, Wintzen AR, Verschuuren JJ. Lambert–Eaton myasthenic syndrome has a more progressive course in patients with lung cancer. Muscle Nerve. 2005;32(2):226-9.
104. Romics L, McNamara B, Cronin PA, O'Brien ME, Relihan N, Redmond HP. Unusual paraneoplastic syndromes of breast carcinoma: a combination of cerebellar degeneration and Lambert–Eaton myasthenic syndrome. Ir J Med Sci. 2011;180(2):569-71.
105. Titulaer MJ, Wirtz PW, Kuks JBM, Schelhaas HJ, van der Kooi AJ, Faber CG, et al. The Lambert–Eaton myasthenic syndrome 1988–2008: A clinical picture in 97 patients. J Neuroimmunol. 2008;201-202:153-8.
106. Giannoccaro MP, Avoni P, Liguori R. Presynaptic paraneoplastic disorders of the neuromuscular junction: An update. Brain Sci. 2021;11(8):1035.
107. Kesner VG, Oh SJ, Dimachkie MM, Barohn RJ. Lambert-Eaton myasthenic syndrome. Neurol Clin. 2018;36(2):379-94.
108. Oh SJ. Distinguishing features of the repetitive nerve stimulation test between Lambert–Eaton myasthenic syndrome and myasthenia gravis, 50-year reappraisal. J Clin Neuromuscul Dis. 2017;19(2):66-75.
109. Ivanovski T, Miralles F. Lambert-Eaton Myasthenic syndrome: early diagnosis is key. Degener Neurol Neuromuscul Dis [Internet]. 2019;9:27-37.
110. Sanders DB, Cao L, Massey JM, Juel VC, Hobson-Webb L, Guptill JT. Is the decremental pattern in Lambert–Eaton syndrome different from that in myasthenia gravis? Clin Neurophysiol. 2014;125(6):1274-7.
111. Maddison P, Newsom-Davis J, Mills KR. Distribution of electrophysiological abnormality in Lambert-Eaton myasthenic syndrome. J Neurol Neurosurg Psychiatry. 1998;65(2):213-7.
112. Oh SJ, Kurokawa K, Claussen GC, Ryan HF. Electrophysiological diagnostic criteria of Lambert-Eaton myasthenic syndrome. Muscle Nerve. 2005;32(4):515-20.
113. Chiou-Tan FY, Gilchrist JM. Repetitive nerve stimulation and single-fiber electromyography in the evaluation of patients with suspected myasthenia gravis or Lambert-Eaton myasthenic syndrome: Review of recent literature: Electrodiagnosis in MG and LEMS. Muscle Nerve. 2015;52(3):455-62.
114. Ojala KS, Ginebaugh SP, Wu M, Miller EW, Ortiz G, Covarrubias M, et al. A high-affinity, partial antagonist effect of 3,4-diaminopyridine mediates action potential broadening and enhancement of transmitter release at NMJs. J Biol Chem. 2021;296:100302.
115. Keogh M, Sedehizadeh S, Maddison P. Treatment for Lambert-Eaton myasthenic syndrome. Cochrane Database Syst Rev. 2011;2011(2):CD003279.
116. Tarr TB, Lacomis D, Reddel SW, Liang M, Valdomir G, Frasso M, et al. Complete reversal of Lambert-Eaton myasthenic syndrome synaptic impairment by the combined use of a K+ channel blocker and a Ca2+ channel agonist: Reversal of LEMS synaptic impairment. J Physiol. 2014;592(16):3687-96.
117. Tarr TB, Wipf P, Meriney SD. Synaptic pathophysiology and treatment of Lambert-Eaton myasthenic syndrome. Mol Neurobiol. 2015;52(1):456-63.
118. Maddison P. Long term outcome in Lambert-Eaton myasthenic syndrome without lung cancer. J Neurol Neurosurg Psychiatry. 2001;70(2):212-7.
119. Maddison P. Treatment in Lambert-Eaton myasthenic syndrome: Treatment in Lambert-Eaton myasthenic syndrome. Ann N Y Acad Sci. 2012;1275(1):78-84.

85

CHAPTER

Hereditary Myopathies

Satish V Khadilkar, Rakhil S Yadav, Bhagyadhan Patel

INTRODUCTION

Inherited myopathies comprise many groups, each containing a large number of genetically mediated diseases. These are broadly grouped into muscular dystrophies, congenital myopathies (CMs), metabolic myopathies, myotonic disorders, etc. Muscular dystrophies are the primary diseases of the muscles resulting from cytoskeletal protein abnormalities or enzymopathies, resulting in muscle degeneration and regeneration and clinically leading to progressive muscle weakness.[1-3] CMs, as a group, present very early in life and are a result of the maldevelopment of the myofibers. Metabolic myopathies are diseases of energy production for the muscles and present with exercise intolerance or progressive muscle weakness. Myotonias are characterized by the inability of the muscle to relax after a sustained contraction. The dystrophic types are associated with muscle weakness and extramuscular manifestation.[4,5]

In addition to this basic categorization, within each category, individual diseases have some peculiarities of their own and these clinical and laboratory aspects help the differential diagnosis. The number of diseases that need to be covered in this chapter is very large and hence a tabulated approach has been adopted and comments on pathophysiology and therapeutic advances have been grouped in this manuscript.

PATHOPHYSIOLOGY OF INHERITED MYOPATHIES

Various mechanisms are involved in the pathophysiological cascades of inherited myopathies. A common theme in muscular dystrophies is cytoskeletal protein abnormalities. The cytoskeleton stretches from the subsarcolemmal proteins, such as the dystrophin, to the sarcolemmal proteins such as the sarcoglycans and the dystroglycans, and their connections to the laminin and the collagen tissues. The cytoskeleton holds the structures together and protein abnormalities lead to the weakening of this structure and the resultant events namely, cytoskeletal disruption, membrane instability, mechanical stress, altered membrane permeability, and abnormal calcium homeostasis leading to cell disintegration. Enzymopathies can also result in muscular dystrophies. CMs result from the defective formation of the muscle, e.g., nemaline rods, central nucleation, fiber type preponderance, and disproportion.

COMMON INHERITED MYOPATHIES

Duchenne Muscular Dystrophy/Becker Muscular Dystrophy

Duchenne muscular dystrophy/Becker muscular dystrophy (DMD/BMD) is common X-linked muscular dystrophy. The incidence is about 1 in 3,500 live male births. It is commonly seen in boys and occasionally in girls when there is only one X chromosome or when an unaffected paternal X chromosome becomes inactive and the mutant maternal X chromosome expresses abnormal protein.[6-9]

The dystrophin gene is located on the short arm of the X chromosome at Xp21 and it is one of the largest genes. It consists of 79 exons and codes for a 14kb mRNA. It is expressed in the skeletal, cardiac, and smooth muscles of the body and also in the brain. The rate of spontaneous mutations is high. Deletion or duplication of gene segments is seen in two-thirds of patients. Deletions are commonly seen at two *hot spots*, between exons 43 and 52 and between exons 2 and 21. Duplication is less common and point mutations are uncommon. Up to 90% of cases of DMD and BMD follow the reading frame rule proposed by Koenig. Out-of-frame deletions lead to DMD while in-frame deletions lead to BMD. Dystrophin is a cytoskeletal subsarcolemmal protein. Its absence leads to cytoskeletal disruption, membrane instability, increased susceptibility to mechanical stress, altered membrane permeability, and abnormal calcium homeostasis.

Most patients are present between 3 and 5 years of age with complaints of delayed motor milestones or abnormal gait. Affected boys have clumsiness of gait, difficulty in running, climbing, and getting up from the ground and frequent falls. Some walk on their toes. Uncommon presentations are language delay or global developmental delay. Important signs are Gower's maneuver, calf hypertrophy, and tendo-Achilles contracture.

Apparent improvement is seen between 2 and 6 years of age due to a normal growth spurt. After 6 years of age, weakness of paraspinal, gluteal, and quadriceps muscles causes lumbar lordosis a protuberant abdomen, waddling gait, and buckling of the knee with frequent falls, respectively. Later in life, when patients become wheelchair-bound, contracture in many muscles hampers comfort and progressive kyphoscoliosis causes respiratory dysfunctions.

Examination shows hypertrophy of calves, deltoid, brachioradialis, infraspinatus, glutei, temporalis, and tongue. Except for calves and deltoids, all muscles reduce in size. Ocular, facial, bulbar, and hand muscles are usually spared. Gower's sign is seen as the child gets up from the ground **(Figs. 1A to E)**. The Valley sign is best seen on the posterior shoulder girdle while the arm is abducted to 90° (or best possible abduction if 90° abduction is not possible) and the hand facing upward **(Fig. 1F)**.

It is visible because of simultaneous hypertrophy of the deltoid superolaterally, infraspinatus inferomedially, and wasting of the posterior axillary fold. Deep tendon reflexes are depressed in weak muscles. Ankle reflexes are present till late in the disease.[6,9]

Other system involvement: Overt cardiac symptoms begin after 10 years of age, one-third of patients are symptomatic by 14 years and it is present in all patients over 18 years of age. Cardiac hypocontractility is more common than conduction defects. Restrictive lung disease is common. Vital capacity begins to diminish around 10 years of age, reducing at the rate of 10%/year approximately. As the vital capacity goes below 1 liter, the complication rates increase. Average intelligence and attention deficit disorders are seen.

Becker muscular dystrophy is a milder clinical form with onset at a later age. Patients usually walk well. Cardiac involvement is less frequent. Carrier females are asymptomatic or have muscle pain or cramps with subclinical cardiac involvement.

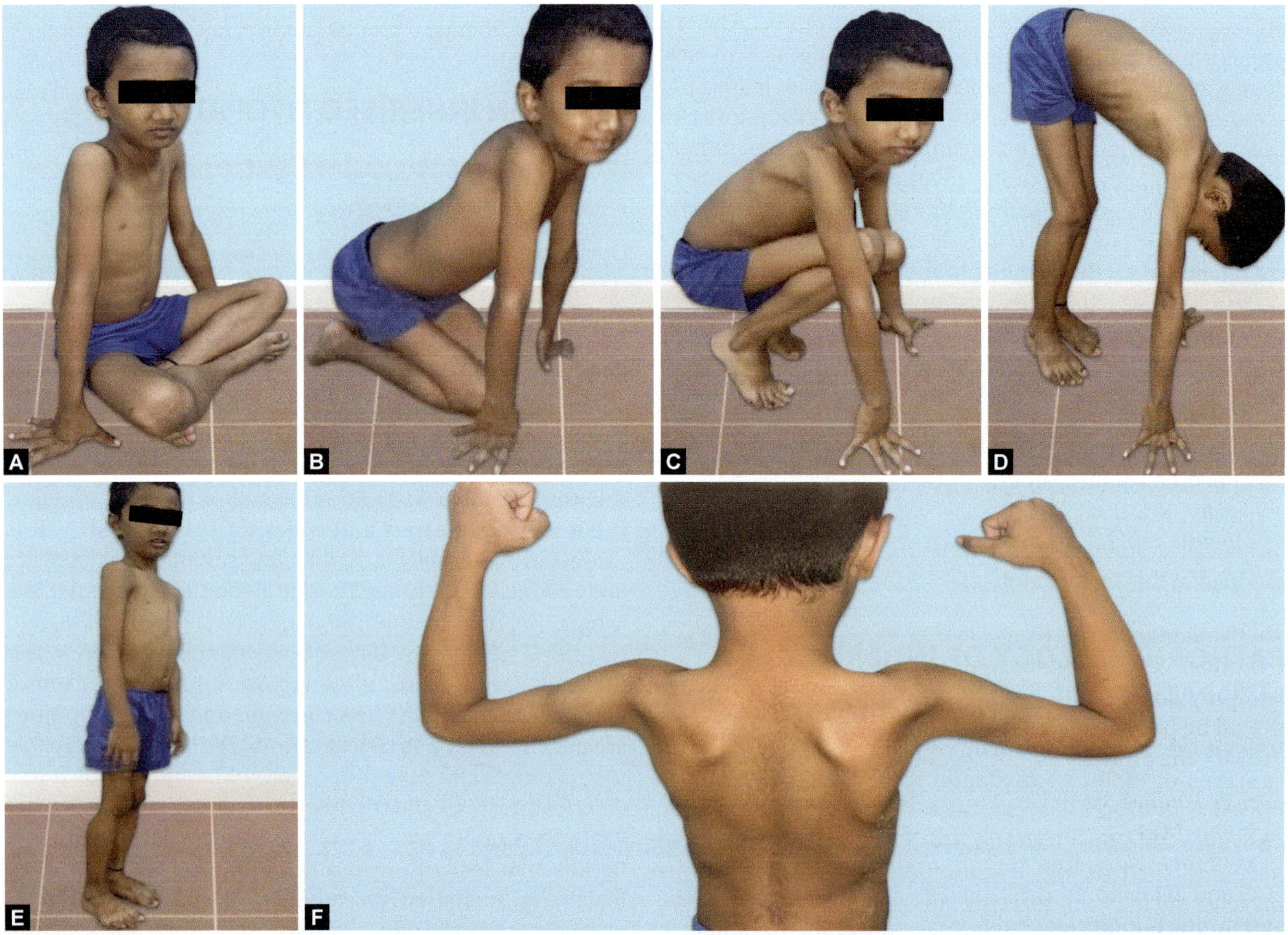

FIGS. 1A TO F: (A to E) Gower's sign; (F) Valley sign.

Other phenotypes associated with dystrophinopathies: (1) Exercise intolerance; (2) myalgia; (3) exertional myoglobinuria; (4) isolated cardiomyopathy; and (5) asymptomatic hyperCKemia. In general, familial cases with DMD seem to follow similar clinical courses but on occasions, striking intrafamilial phenotypic variability has been seen. Intrafamilial variation with the same in-frame mutation is reported. Approximately 30% of patients have no family history of the disease and these represent spontaneous mutations.

Creatine kinase (CK) level is markedly elevated but decreased in later stages as muscle wasting occurs.

Multiplex polymerase chain reaction (PCR) techniques study 19–32 exons covering the hot spots. They can detect common deletions. Multiplex ligation-dependent probe amplification (MLPA) is a more sensitive technique for detecting deletions. MLPA test studies all 79 exons and can detect duplications as well, increasing the yield by about 10%. If MLPA testing is negative, the *DMD* gene can be tested for point mutations. Direct sequence analysis of the *DMD* gene is not widely available and exorbitantly expensive. Previously unidentified deep intronic mutations have recently been identified by a targeted high-density oligonucleotide microarray technique. Carrier detection requires the MLPA test, as it studies the dosing effect.

Electromyography (EMG) shows myopathic patterns. Muscle magnetic resonance imaging (MRI) can reflect the order, extent, and degree of skeletal muscle involvement. The order of affection is gluteus maximus, adductor magnus, quadriceps femoris, rectus femoris, and biceps muscle of the thigh. Semimembranosus, semitendinosus, sartorius, and gracilis are selectively affected and in decreasing order.

Muscle biopsy: Indication of biopsy in recent years is limited to situations where the clinical phenotype is atypical or the genetic test is negative. Light microscopy shows degenerating necrotic muscle fibers with the invasion of macrophages and clusters of regenerating muscle fibers with basophilic cytoplasm. Increased variability of muscle fiber size is common; fibers are initially larger than normal and become smaller later on. Histochemistry with ATPase shows type-1 fiber predominance. In advanced stages, significant replacement of fibers by fat and endomysial connective tissue is seen. Immunostaining confirms the absence of dystrophin. Three antibodies (Dys 1, 2, and 3) are available against dystrophin. They cover the carboxy terminus, central region, and amino terminus. As each antibody covers only a portion of the protein, all three should be preferably used. In dystrophin deficiency as seen in BMD, the protein staining is irregular and fragmented.

Carrier females: CK levels are raised in half of the known carriers. MLPA can detect the carrier status. Cardiac surveillance should be started after 10 years of age with ECG and 2D Echo. If rhythm disturbance is present, Holter monitoring is indicated. Pulmonary function tests should be done annually before the loss of ambulation and frequently after the loss of ambulation.

Management

Drug Therapy:

- *Corticosteroid therapy*: Alteration of regulation of genes in muscle fibers, slowing of the rate of skeletal muscle breakdown, reducing cytotoxic T-cells, lowering cytosolic calcium concentrations, and increasing myogenic repair have been proposed as the likely mechanisms of corticosteroid. The optimum dose of prednisolone/prednisone is 0.75 mg/kg/day. Other dosing regimens are 1.25 mg/kg and 2.5 mg/kg alternate day doses; 10 days ON and 10 days OFF; 10 days ON and 20 days OFF; followed by 5 mg/kg/dose twice weekly; or 10 mg/kg/weekends. Deflazacort 0.9 mg/kg/day is another option. In India, where the prevalence of tuberculosis is high, corticosteroid treatment may flare up underlying tuberculosis.
- Vamorolone, a first-in-class dissociative steroidal anti-inflammatory drug, that preserves anti-inflammatory efficacy and decreases steroid-associated safety concerns, has been used in DMD.
- AdipoRon, a small AdipoR agonist, shows beneficial effects on the Mdx mouse model and better alternative for glucocorticoid.
- *Givinostat [ITF2357]*: A histone deacetylase inhibitor with potential anti-inflammatory, antiangiogenic, and anti-neoplastic activities. It is in phase-II DMD clinical trials.
- *Isosorbide dinitrate with ibuprofen*: Altered synthesis of nitric oxide (NO) due to a reduction of NO synthase (nNOS) activity is also present in DMD. Isosorbide dinitrate, a NO donor, restores NO and ibuprofen, a nonsteroidal anti-inflammatory drug induces a beneficial effect.
- Nuclear factor kappa B (NF-κB) is central in causing muscle damage and preventing muscle regeneration. Edasalonexent, which is NF-κB inhibitor, is under phase-1 trial.
- *Myostatin inhibitors*: Talditercept alpha, a weekly, subcutaneous human IgG1 (Fc)–adnectin fusion that binds myostatin, is currently being evaluated in an ongoing phase-3 clinical trial.
- Idebenone (phase-3 trial), pamrevlumab (phase-2 trial), and CAP-1002 contain allogeneic cardiosphere-derived cells (CDCs) (phase-2 trial)

Gene Therapy

The *DMD* gene is very large and, hence, it is difficult to have a viral vector to carry the entire gene. Critical fragments of the gene can be carried by adeno-associated viral vectors. Such microdystrophin and minidystrophin genes have been injected in mice and dystrophin has been successfully expressed.

- *Antisense oligonucleotide exon skipping*: This technique can be used to redirect splicing which induces exon skipping and thus helps the production of the functioning dystrophin. However, the antisense oligonucleotide is to be tailored to the deletion, which is a limitation.

Providing sustained therapy is another unanswered issue. Golodirsen (exon 53 skipping), eteplirsen (exon 51 skipping), and casimersen (exon 45 skipping) are antisense oligonucleotides used in treatment.

- *Read-through stop-codon strategies*: Gentamicin and PTC-124 have been studied. Gentamicin has not been successful in clinical trials. PTC-124 (Ataluren, now Translarna™) is one of the identified agents, it is an oral nonaminoglycoside drug that has read-through activity with no antibiotic properties. Ataluren was granted conditional marketing authorization in the European Union under the trade name Translarna™ for the treatment of nmDMD in ambulatory patients aged 5 years and older.
- *Utrophin modulation: SMT C1100 [2-arylbenzoxazole {5-(ethyl sulfonyl)-2-(naphthalen-2-yl) benzo(d) oxazole}]*: Utrophin upregulator; recently, phase 1b has been completed but the results are not yet published

Stem Cell Therapy

Myoblast transfer and bone marrow-derived stem cell transfer have been used in research settings. Mesenchymal stem cell sources presently appear most promising.

Genome editing using CRISPR technology may permanently cure the disease once its efficacy, safety, and delivery issues have been resolved. This technology is used in DMD to bypass mutations.[10-22]

Limb Girdle Muscular Dystrophies

Limb girdle muscular dystrophy (LGMD) is a group of genetic disorders characterized by slowly progressive pelvic and shoulder girdle weakness.[3,23] Apart from symmetrical proximal limb girdle weakness, a few subtypes have distinctive features such as ethnic preponderance, joint contractures, distal weakness, scapular winging, cardiac involvement, etc. Genetic testing should be performed to confirm the diagnosis of LGMD. Ancillary testing such as EMG and muscle biopsy is used to differentiate LGMD from anterior horn cell diseases and inflammatory myopathies.[2,4,5,24,25] Broad genetic testing is now increasingly used to diagnose genetic muscle disease. At present, more than 100 genes can present with the LGMD phenotype.[26] The salient features of common LGMDs are described below in **Table 1**[1,27-30] and the uncommon ones in **Table 2**.

Autosomal dominant LGMDs (D1-4) and many recessive LGMDs are seen from time to time and some have been described only in a few families. The details of these have been summarized in **Table 2.**[1,4,25,31-33] Among these, keloids give a clue to the Bethlem myopathy **(Fig. 4A)** and excessive laxity of the distal joints and contractures of the proximal joints point to the Ullrich myopathy **(Fig. 4B)**.

European Neuromuscular Center (ENMC) has laid down criteria for new inclusions in the LGMD group and these are as follows:[1,34,35] Genetically inherited conditions in two unrelated family members, proximal muscle weakness, the patient must have achieved independent walking at or before 2 years, and the presence of dystrophic features (elevated CK levels, degenerative features on MRI skeletal muscles, muscle biopsy showing fatty degeneration with muscle necrosis). According to new criteria, ten conditions no longer fulfill the diagnostic criteria for LGMD **(Table 3)**.

Investigation for the group of LGMDs comprises serum CK estimation, electrophysiological testing, muscle MRI imaging, and genetic testing. Over the last few years, MRI

TABLE 1: Salient features of commonly occurring LGMDs.[1,27-30]

Disease	Gene (protein)	Pathophysiology	Key features
LGMD R1	*CAPN3* (Calpain 3)	An important role in sarcomere and regulates calcium outflow in sarcoplasmic reticulum	Onset in the second decade, prominent scapular winging **(Fig. 2A)**, severe hip adductor weakness, toe walking, ankle contractures, abdominal hernia (truncal weakness), marked serum CK elevation
LGMD R2	*DYSF* (Dysferlin)	An important role in muscle membrane repair, homeostasis, and signal transduction	Onset in the second decade, 4 presentations: 1. Early calf involvement (Miyoshi) 2. Proximal limb girdle weakness (LGMD 2B) 3. Proximodistal form (most common) 4. Distal myopathy with anterior tibial weakness (DMAT) Biceps lump **(Fig. 2B)** and diamond on quadriceps **(Fig. 3A)**, wasting of calves **(Fig. 3B)** episodes of calf pains and swelling, marked serum CK elevation
LGMD R3–R6	*SGC* (Sarcoglycan)	Tetrameric structure stabilizing linkage of dystrophin and dystroglycan	Onset usually in the first decade, DMD mimics, calf hypertrophy, proximal muscle weakness, hip abduction sign, ankle contractures, toe walking, scapular winging, marked serum CK elevation
LGMD R12	*ANO5* (Anoctamin)	Calcium-activated channel involved in phospholipid scrambling and membrane fusion and repair	Adult-onset, severe affection in males, prominent calf involvement (Miyoshi-like), striking asymmetry, hip girdle and quadriceps weakness, very gradual progression, myalgias and exercise intolerance, marked serum CK elevation

(CK: creatine kinase; DMD: Duchenne muscular dystrophy; LGMD: limb girdle muscular dystrophy)

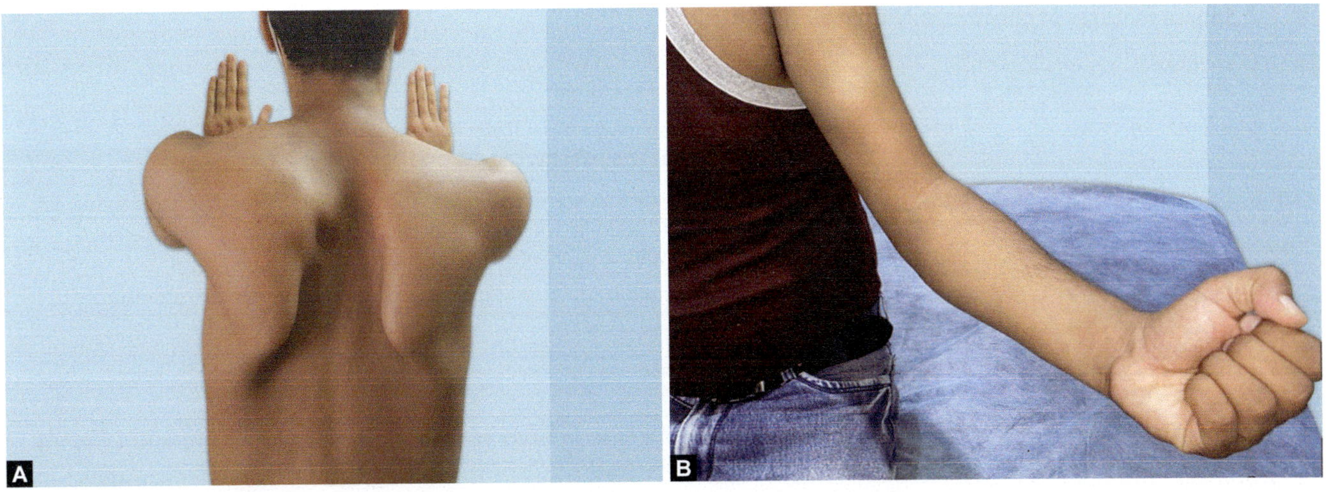

FIGS. 2A AND B: (A) Scapular winging in calpainopathy and (B) biceps lump in dysferlinopathy.

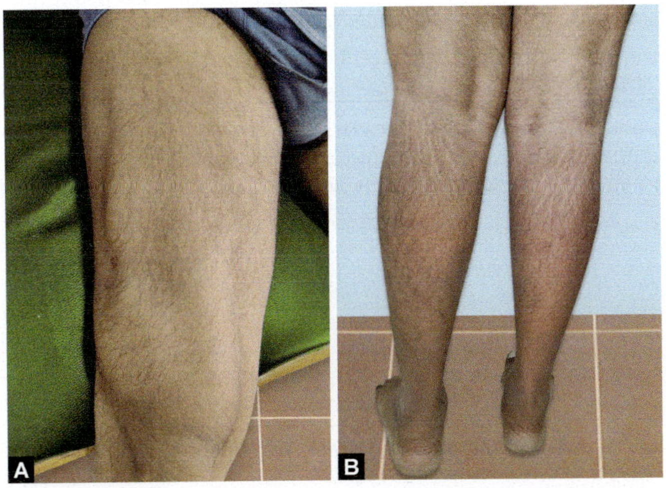

FIGS. 3A AND B: (A) Diamond on quadriceps and (B) wasted calves in dysferlinopathy.

has been gainfully employed in the studies of LGMD and patterns have emerged. These have been listed in **Table 4**.

Management of LGMDs

Supportive management consists of physical, occupational, and speech therapy along with orthotic devices to decrease morbidity and increase muscle strength,[5,35] assessment of cardiac and pulmonary involvement and its management, correction of spinal and joint deformities, maintaining adequate nutrition and body weight, and genetic counseling to prevent transmission from one generation to another.

Future therapies such as viral vector gene therapy have been found effective in animal models of LGMD namely calpain, dysferlin, and sarcoglycan, and invention of gene editing through CRISPR/Cas9 (clustered regularly interspaced short palindromic repeats/CRISPR associated-9) 53 and other technologies may allow for perinatal correction of disease.

Myotonic Disorders

This group of diseases presents with myotonia and weakness in different proportions. Myotonia is a clinical phenomenon, of inability to relax after sustained muscle contractions, and is elicited by the bedside by asking the patient to release the grip after 15 seconds of full contraction (grip myotonia) and by percussion of the muscles (percussion myotonia). Myotonic disorders are primarily divided into dystrophic and nondystrophic, depending upon the presence or absence of dystrophic changes in the affected muscles.

Myotonic Dystrophy Type 1

Myotonic dystrophy (DM) is an autosomal dominant disorder characterized by a triad of myotonia, progressive weakness, and early onset cataracts. The facies tend to be characteristic, exhibiting frontal baldness, ptosis, facial weakness, long thin face, and myopathic mouth **(Fig. 6)**.

Myotonic dystrophy is a multisystem disorder involving muscles, ocular lens, heart, endocrine organs, gastrointestinal tract, and central nervous system. There are two types: myotonic dystrophy type 1 (DM1) and myotonic dystrophy type 2 (DM2). DM1 is caused by the expansion of CTG repeats in the myotonic dystrophy protein kinase (DMPK) gene and DM2 is caused by CCTG expansion in the zinc finger protein 9 (*ZFN9*) gene. Due to the difference in the number of CTG alleles in normal individuals of different ethnicities, the prevalence of DM1 varies in different ethnic populations.[36] As DM is an autosomal dominant disorder and clinical manifestations of DM can be protean, clinical examination of apparently normal family members is of utmost importance. Based on the number of CTG repeats, age at onset, and severity of weakness, DM1 can be classified into the following subtypes:

- *Congenital DM1*: Most severe form; CTG repeats >1,000; onset at birth **(Table 5)**[37-42]
- *Classical DM1*: Most common form; CTG repeats 150–1,000; onset in adolescence or adulthood

TABLE 2: Salient features of uncommonly occurring LGMDs.[1,4,25,31-33]

Disease (previous nomenclature)	Inheritance	Gene (protein)	Key features
LGMD D1 (LGMD 1D)	AD	*DNAJB6* (HSP40)	Adulthood-onset lower limb weakness; cardiac involvement is unusual and few patients can develop bulbar weakness
LGMD D2 (LGMD1F)	AD	*TNPO3* (Transportin)	Onset can occur from infancy to adulthood; shoulder girdle weakness and scapular winging can occur; distal weakness in late cases and respiratory impairment can occur early
LGMD D3 (LGMD 1G)	AD	*HNRNPDL*	Onset in adulthood; limitation of finger flexion is characteristic
LGMD D4 (LGMD 1I)	AD	*CAPN3* (Calpain 3)	
LGMD D5 (Bethlem myopathy)	AD	*COL6A1* (Collagen 6 subunits A1)	Childhood to adolescent onset; early joint contractures; keloids
LGMD R7 (LGMD 2G)	AR	*TCAP* (Telethonin)	Early onset in first or second decade, prominent TA weakness, scapular winging, calf hypertrophy, and cardiomyopathy
LGMD R8 (LGMD 2H)	AR	*TRIM 32*	Described only in Hutterite population in North America; onset in second or third decade; slow progression; contractures occur frequently
LGMD R9 (LGMD 2I)	AR	*FKRP* (Fukutin-related protein)	Early diaphragmatic weakness, calf and other muscles hypertrophy, respiratory failure, and cardiomyopathy are common
LGMD R10 (LGMD 2J)	AR	*TTN* (Titin)	Second or third decade onset; early tibialis anterior; slow progression; and absence of cardiomyopathy
LGMD R11 (LGMD 2K)	AR	*POMT1* (O-mannosyltransferase 1)	Early onset in infancy and first decade; proximal weakness; calf hypertrophy; cognitive abnormalities; epilepsy; contractures; microcephaly and eye abnormalities can occur
LGMD R13 (LGMD 2M)	AR	*FCMD* (Fukutin)	
LGMD R14 (LGMD 2N)	AR	*POMT2* (O-mannosyltransferase 2)	
LGMD R 15 (LGMD 2O)	AR	*POMGnT1*	
LGMD R 16 (LGMD 2P)	AR	*DAG1* (Dystroglycan 1)	
LGMD R17 (LGMD 2Q)	AR	*PLEC1* (Plectin)	Childhood onset; proximal weakness; microcephaly and cognitive impairment
LGMD R18 (LGMD 2S)	AR	*TRAPPC11*	Childhood onset; prominent scapular winging; chorea, ataxia, and cognitive decline can occur
LGMD R19 (LGMD 2T)	AR	*GMPPB* (GDP mannose phosphorylase B)	Variable age of onset; calf hypertrophy; CNS involvement such as hypotonia, intellectual disabilities, and seizures in childhood
LGMD R20 (LGMD 2U)	AR	*CRPPA*	Childhood-onset; relatively rapid progression; muscle hypertrophy and *CM* can occur
LGMD R21 (LGMD 2Z)	AR	*POGLUT1*	Third-decade onset; proximal weakness; scapular winging; respiratory involvement
LGMD R22 (Bethlem myopathy)	AD	*COL6A1/2/3* (Collagen 6 subunits A1/2/3)	Childhood to adolescent-onset; early joint contractures; keloids
LGMD R23 (MDC1A)	AR	*LAMA2* (laminin 2)	Childhood-onset; multiple contractures; mental retardation; seizure; dysmorphic features
LGMD R24	AR	*POMGNT2*	

(AD: autosomal dominant; AR: autosomal recessive; CNS: central nervous system; LGMD: limb girdle muscular dystrophy)

- *Mild DM1*: Mild form; CTG repeats 50–150; onset after 40 years of age

Investigations

Investigations consist of CK estimation, thyroid profile and sugar monitoring, slit-lamp examination for cataracts, EMG study to show myopathic potentials, myotonic discharges and mild peripheral neuropathy, ECG to detect cardiac arrhythmias, polysomnography, and the gene diagnosis. Genetic diagnosis is the gold standard for DM1. Confirmation of CTG repeats can be done by southern blot and triplet primed PCR.

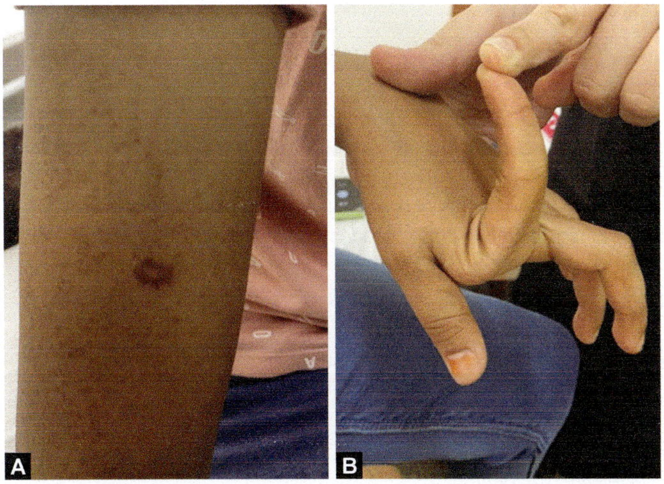

FIGS. 4A AND B: (A) Keloids in Bethlem myopathy and (B) hyperlaxity in Ullrich myopathy.

TABLE 3: Exclusions as per the new ENMC criteria.

Old name	Gene	New nomenclature	Reason for exclusion
LGMD 1A	*MYOT*	Myofibrillar myopathy	Distal
LGMD 1B	*LMNA*	EDMD	High risk of cardiac arrhythmias and EDMD phenotype
LGMD 1C	*CAV3*	Rippling muscle disease	The main clinical features are rippling muscle disease and myalgias
LGMD 1E	*DES*	Myofibrillar myopathy	Distal weakness and cardiomyopathy
LGMD 1H	?	Not confirmed	False linkage
LGMD 2R	*DES*	Myofibrillar myopathy	Distal weakness
LGMD 2V	*GAA*	Pompe's disease	Known disease entity and histological features

(EDMD: Emery–Dreifuss muscular dystrophy; ENMC: European Neuromuscular Center)

Myotonic Dystrophy Type 2

Myotonic dystrophy type 2 is caused by CCTG expansion in the *ZFN9* gene. Although systemic features of DM2 are similar to DM1, the following features occur in DM2 which help to differentiate it from DM1.[43,44] These are—the later age of onset, prominent muscle pain, stiffness and proximal weakness, milder wasting, facial and bulbar weakness, presence of calf hypertrophy, and lesser impairment of cognitive functions.

Management of DM1 and DM2

Mexiletine (150-200 mg three times per day) is most efficacious to reduce myotonia. Other drugs that can be helpful are phenytoin, carbamazepine, amitriptyline, and

TABLE 4: Distinct MRI features of different LGMDs.[1,34]

LGMD type	MRI features
Calpainopathy	Predominant involvement of posterior thigh, adductor magnus, and medial gastrocnemius; vastus lateralis and sartorius relative sparing
Dysferlinopathy	Early involvement of medial gastrocnemius, hamstrings, and paraspinals
Sarcoglycanopathy	Early involvement of hip adductor, hamstrings, and glutei; relative sparing of calf muscles and vasti
LGMD R9 (FKRP)	Early involvement of gluteus maximus, iliopsoas, and hip adductors
Anoctaminopathy	Medial gastrocnemius, soleus, hamstrings, and hip adductors asymmetrical affected; anterior thigh and iliopsoas spared
Bethlem myopathy	Sandwich sign—peripheral fatty infiltration of vastus lateralis with central sparing **(Fig. 5)**; central atrophy of rectus femoris

(LGMD: limb girdle muscular dystrophy; MRI: magnetic resonance imaging)

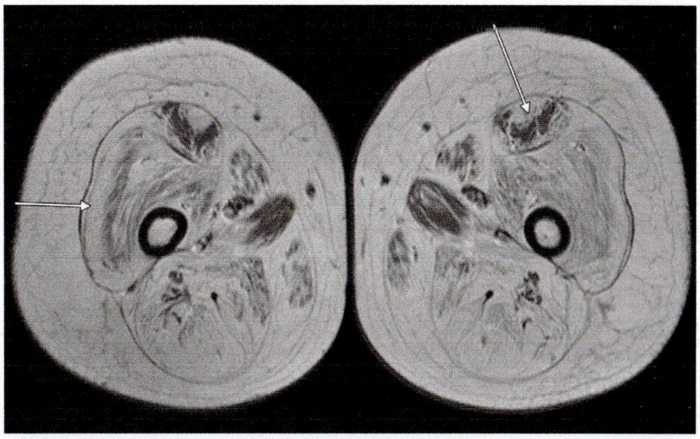

FIG. 5: Sandwich sign in Bethlem myopathy.

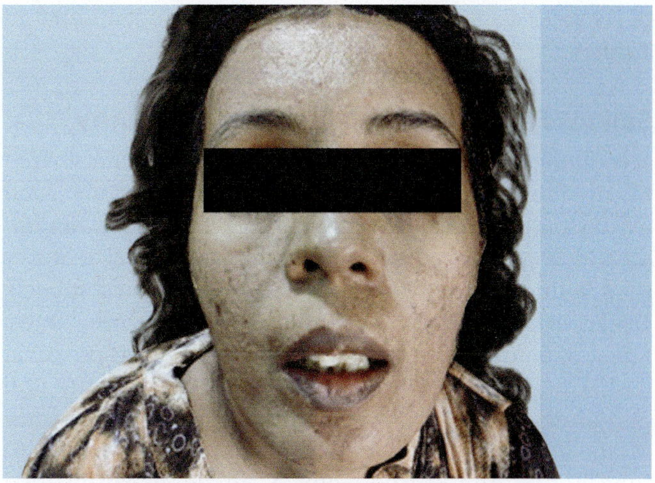

FIG. 6: Characteristic facies in myotonic dystrophy.

TABLE 5: Salient features of DM1.[37-42]

Musculoskeletal	• Myotonia, i.e., delayed after sustained voluntary contraction can be elicited on action (finger grip, eye closure, and jaw opening) and percussion (thenar eminence, wrist extensors, and tongue) • Myotonia improves with exercise (warmup phenomenon) and worsens with rest and cold • *Myopathic features* ***(Fig. 6)***: Ptosis, wasting and weakness of temporalis, masseter, facial muscles, and sternocleidomastoid (hatchet face and swan neck appearance); early involvement of bulbar muscles and neck flexors; weakness and wasting of the forearm with relative sparing of the arm (shank of an animal appearance); prominent involvement of ankle dorsiflexors; respiratory weakness can lead to breathlessness and excessive daytime sleepiness • *Fatigue*: Fatigue is the most impactful symptom due to muscle weakness, excess daytime sleepiness and respiratory insufficiency
Heart	Cardiac conduction abnormalities such as PR prolongation, AV block, atrial tachycardia, and ventricular dysfunction
Eyes	Premature cataracts (Christmas tree appearance)
Central nervous system	Behavior changes; cognitive dysfunction; psychomotor slowing
Endocrine	Testicular atrophy; balding; erectile dysfunction; insulin resistance
Gastrointestinal and liver	Gallbladder stones; constipation; elevated liver enzymes
Malignancy	Higher risk of thyroid and ovary cancer; choroidal melanoma

(AV: atrioventricular; DM1: myotonic dystrophy type 1)

acetazolamide.[36,45,46] Moderate-intensity aerobic exercise can be helpful with fatigue and weakness. Regular cardiac monitoring to detect arrhythmias and intervention like pacemaker or defibrillator insertion in severe conduction defects is recommended. Modafinil and overnight bilevel positive airway pressure (BiPAP) support to reduce features of sleep apnea. Standard surgical therapy is needed for cataracts. Regular screening for diabetes, thyroid dysfunction, and testosterone deficiency should be done.

Distal Myopathies

These myopathies preferentially affect distal or semidistal muscles of extremities, mostly affecting either anterior or posterior compartments of legs. At least 20 different genetic disorders have been described in patients with apparently similar phenotypes.[47] A small subgroup has the characteristic deposition of myofibrillar degradation products and is known as myofibrillar myopathies (MFMs). Salient features of classical distal myopathies and MFM are mentioned in **Table 6.**[1,47,48-53]

Salient Features of Myofibrillary Myopathy

Myofibrillary myopathy refers to a small group characterized by myofibrillar degeneration of Z-disk proteins such as desmin, alpha-B crystallin, myotilin, ZASP, filamin C, and Bag3. Most MFMs have similar clinical features that include late adulthood onset progressive muscle weakness predominantly in distal muscles of lower limbs. Some patients can have prominent weakness in proximal and scapuloperoneal distribution. Cardiomyopathy and peripheral neuropathy are common associated features. Mode of transmission is usually autosomal dominant inheritance and infrequently X-linked or autosomal recessive. Despite having similar clinical features, MFM can be classified pathologically into desminopathy, alpha-B crystallinopathy, myotilinopathy, Zaspopathy, filaminopathy, and Bag3opathy.

Congenital Muscular Dystrophies

Congenital muscular dystrophy (CMD) is a group of rare muscular dystrophies with clinical and genetic heterogeneity and onset within the first 2 years of life. New gene discovery is a continuous ongoing process resulting in expansion of its clinical and molecular spectrum. The final diagnosis achieved in around 60% of patients using comprehensive gene panels indicates that new genes or unusual mutations of currently known genes are likely to be the cause. CMDs are commonly autosomal recessive, but few cases are autosomal dominant due to spontaneous mutations, direct inheritance, or mosaicism. Progressive skeletal muscle weakness and hypotonia are cardinal manifestations. Details of common subtypes are described in **Table 7**. Regular evaluation for pulmonary, cardiac, and swallowing functions is important aspect of supportive care.[54]

Facioscapulohumeral Muscular Dystrophies

Facioscapulohumeral muscular dystrophy (FSHD) is an autosomal dominant and third common muscular dystrophy, with variable age of presentation and rate of progression. Patients present with facial weakness resulting in an inability to whistle or drink from a straw and often their eyes remain open when they sleep. There is severe winging and riding of scapulae **(Fig. 8A)** and wasting and weakness of the pectoral muscles. The arms are wasted while the forearms maintain bulk, the Popeye arms.[55-59] Patients often exhibit Beevor's sign **(Fig. 8B)**, lordosis and visceroptosis.

TABLE 6: Salient features of classical distal myopathies.[1,47-53]

Name and pathogenesis	Salient features	CK level, muscle biopsy, and MRI features
GNE myopathy: GNE (GNE) encodes for an epimerase-kinase enzyme involved in sialic acid biosynthesis, important in the sialylation of glycoproteins and glycolipids	Usually third-decade onset; early and prominent ankle dorsiflexor weakness **(Fig. 7A)**; proximal weakness as the disease progresses but quadriceps remain spared; FDI atrophy can occur **(Fig. 7B)**; uncommonly asymmetrical	Modestly elevated; RV; prominent involvement of anterior leg; milder involvement of calves; sparing VM
Dysferlinopathy: DYSF (dysferlin)—dysferlin is a ubiquitous transmembrane protein most probably acts in calcium-mediated sarcolemmal fusion events and resealing	Onset in later teens and adults; calf swelling and pain; calf weakness and atrophy; inability to stand tiptoe and hop; proximal weakness as the disease progresses; DMAT variant with onset in ankle dorsiflexors	Moderate to severely elevated CK; myopathy + inflammatory infiltrate; prominent calf and posterior thigh involvement
Anoctaminopathy: ANO5 (anoctamin 5), a cytoplasmic calcium-activated chloride channel, with a possible role in membrane fusion and repair	Onset in second or third decade; male preponderance; calf pain and transient swelling; calf weakness and atrophy; asymmetry is common; proximal weakness later on	Similar to dysferlinopathy
Zaspopathy LDB3 (ZASP): LDB3 encodes the LIM domain-binding 3 protein, also called Z-band alternatively spliced PDZ motif-containing protein (ZASP) that interacts with other Z-disk proteins	Onset in >40–50 years; foot drop at onset; wrist and finger extensor weakness; cardiomyopathy	Normal to mildly elevated; RV and myopathy; anterior leg and hamstrings affected
Laing myopathy: MYH7 (beta myosin heavy chain)	Childhood-onset; foot drop and toe extensor weakness; neck flexor, finger and wrist extensor weakness; neck and axial weakness later on	Moderately elevated; RV absent; anterior leg and thigh affected; calf spared
Udd myopathy: TTN (titin) interacts with key proteins, including calpain-3 that binds the C-terminal portion of titin	Onset >35–40 years; ankle dorsiflexors weakness at onset; hamstring weakness; upper limbs sparing	Modestly elevated; RV and myopathic changes; anterior > posterior leg involved
Welander myopathy: TIA1 encodes an RNA-binding protein and is a key molecule in stress granules, regulators of RNA translation, and metabolism	Onset >50 years; wrist flexors and small muscles of hands weakness at onset; later on, ankle dorsiflexor and toe weakness	

(CK: creatine kinase; DMAT: distal myopathy with anterior tibial; MRI: magnetic resonance imaging)

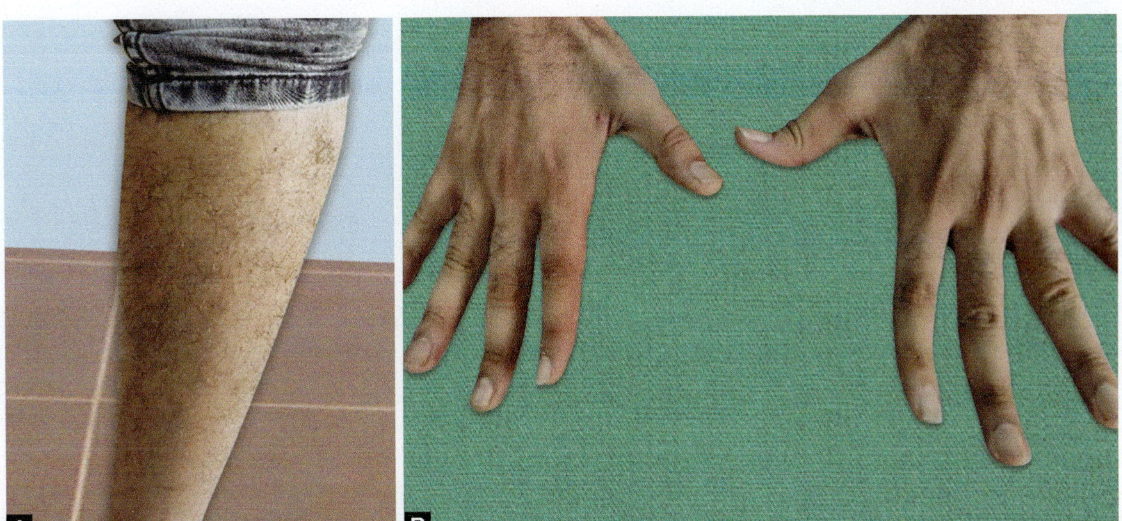

FIGS. 7A AND B: (A) Wasting of the anterior leg muscles in GNE myopathy and (B) FDI wasting in GNE myopathy.

There is a variable degree of lower limb weakness, which manifests in proximal as well as distal muscles. FSHD1 is a monogenic disorder resulting from a contraction in the number of D4Z4 repeats on one copy of 4q in the presence of a distal A polymorphism, while FSHD2 is a digenic disease requiring at least one permissive A polymorphism on 4q and a mutation in a methylating gene (e.g., *SMCHD1*) on chromosome 18. Both FSHD1 and -2 link up to a common downstream pathway that causes depression of the *DUX4* gene and results in disease manifestation by toxic gain of function. A normal person has more than 10 units of D4Z4 repeats. In FSHD, it becomes <10. Less the number of repeats more severe the manifestation. FSHD1 and -2 have similar presentations. It is variable between families and also among the same family. The most common initial symptom is overhead abduction of the upper limbs. Asymmetry and absence of contracture around weak muscles differentiate it from other muscular dystrophies.[60]

Oculopharyngeal Muscular Dystrophy

Oculopharyngeal muscular dystrophy (OPMD) is a rare late-onset muscle weakness, caused by the abnormal expansion of GCG repeats in exon 1 of the poly (A) binding protein, nuclear 1 (*PABPN1*) gene on chromosome 14. It can be autosomal recessive or dominant **(Fig. 9)**. EMG studies show myopathic changes with or without peripheral neuropathy.[61,62]

Emery–Dreifuss Muscular Dystrophy

Emery–Dreifuss muscular dystrophy (EDMD) is characterized by early onset joint contractures, proximal weakness, and cardiac involvement. Joint contractures involve elbow flexors (inability to extend elbow), ankle plantar flexors (early toe walking), and spine (rigid spine) **(Fig. 10)**.[63]

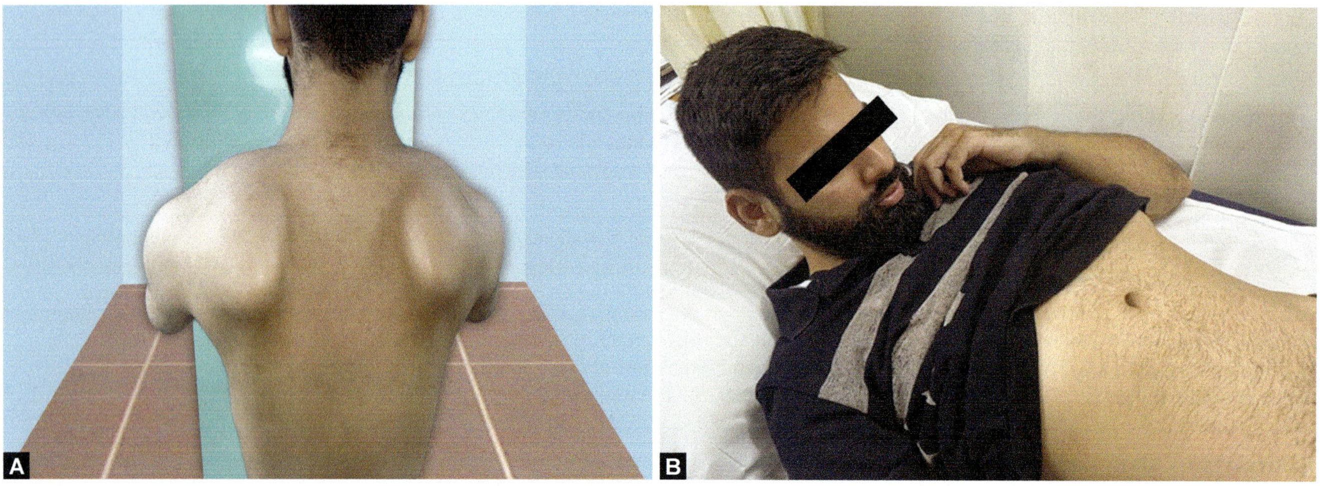

FIGS. 8A AND B: (A) Winging and riding of the scapulae in FSHD; (B) Beevor's sign in FSHD.
(FSHD: facioscapulohumeral muscular dystrophy)

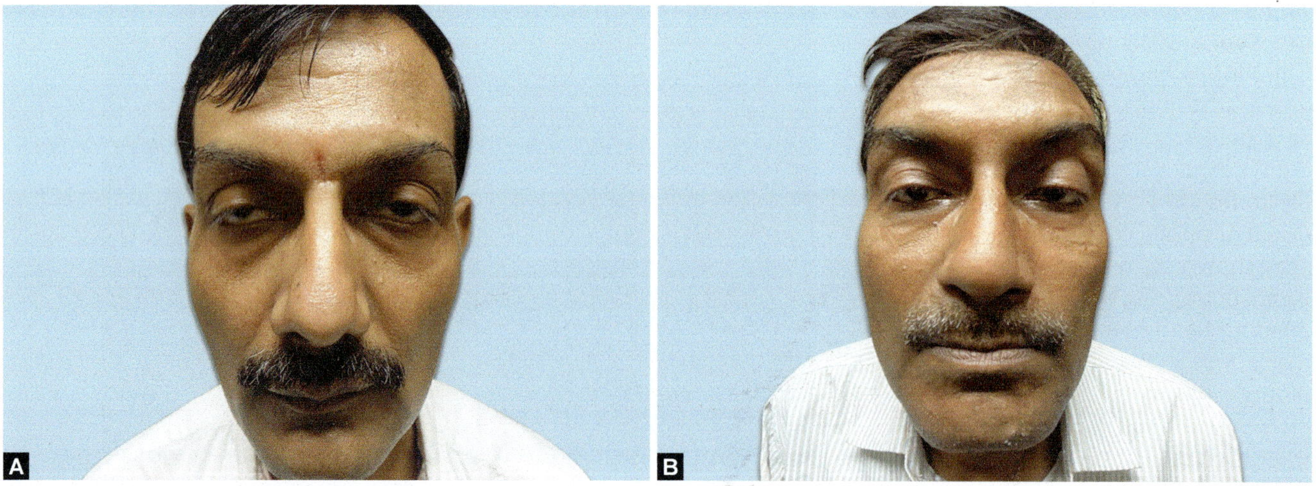

FIGS. 9A AND B: Brothers with bilateral ptosis in OPMD.
(OPMD: oculopharyngeal muscular dystrophy)

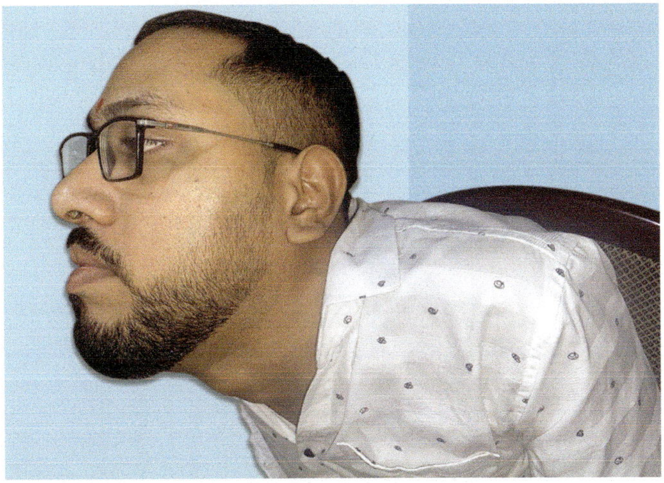

FIG. 10: Neck contracture in EDMD.
(EDMD: Emery–Dreifuss muscular dystrophy)

Progressive muscle weakness involves biceps, triceps, and ankle dorsiflexors with preservation of deltoid (humeroperoneal distribution).[64,65] Cardiac involvement is in the form of cardiac arrhythmias, conduction defects, and dilated cardiomyopathy. Immunohistochemistry shows changes in emerin, FHL1, and lamin A/C.[64,66]

Table 7 summarizes the distinctive clinical and investigative features and the current and potential therapies.

Congenital Myopathies

Congenital myopathy is similar to CMD, a heterogeneous group of muscle disorders present in the neonatal age group. It is classified as per their histopathological findings. This spectrum of disorders is constantly evolving due to the identification of new genes and their various clinical and histological expressions.[67] There are five main types. Clinical presentations usually range from mild forms presenting as hypotonia and weakness to severe forms presenting as reduced fetal movements and congenital arthrogryposis. Symptoms are usually static or slowly progressive in mild form while rapidly progressive and lead to death in severe form. Floppy babies with a frog-like posture, dysmorphic face, ophthalmoparesis, sucking and respiratory problems, chest deformities, congenital hip dysplasia, bone and joint deformities, loss of muscle mass, and delayed motor milestones are some of the common features. CK levels are normal or mildly elevated. EMG can be normal, myopathic, or can show a mixed myopathic and neurogenic pattern. The diagnostic approach comprises a detailed clinical evaluation including family history, muscle MRI, and muscle biopsy. Muscle MRI is a noninvasive diagnostic tool that helps in identifying specific patterns of muscle involvement. These patterns are correlated more with specific gene defects rather than specific histological findings. Next-generation sequencing (NGS) can detect abnormal genes. However, nonspecific clinical presentations, overlapping skeletal muscle biopsy findings, and genetic heterogeneity form hurdles in interpreting the results. The management goal is to preserve basic functions, prevent complications, and provide a good quality of life. Regular evaluation for pulmonary/cardiac/swallowing functions, spine deformities, muscle contractures, and bone mineral density is important for the maintenance of function. N-acetylcysteine corrects oxidative metabolism-related abnormalities. Dantrolene, 5-aminoimidazole-4-carboximide ribonucleoside, and 1,4-benzothiazepine derivatives JTV519 and S107 modulate calcium release from the sarcoplasmic reticulum in central core disease due to mutations in RYR1. AAV8-based gene therapy is under trial for XLMTM-associated myopathy. **Table 8** summarizes the pathophysiology and clinical features of the main CMs and **Table 9**[67-71] describes the genetic aspects and muscle MRI findings.

Metabolic Myopathies

Metabolic myopathies are genetic disorders that impair energy metabolism. Disorders of mitochondrial functions (mitochondrial myopathies), lipid metabolism, and glycogen storage commonly result in muscle diseases (metabolic myopathies). Muscle weakness, exercise intolerance, and rhabdomyolysis in varying severity are cardinal features of metabolic myopathy. Usually, most metabolic myopathies have muscle involvements alone, except for glutaric aciduria type II and mitochondrial myopathies which result in multiorgan dysfunctions.[72,73]

Mitochondrial Myopathies

Mitochondrial myopathies present with fatigue and muscle weakness that are exercise-induced or fixed. The absence of muscle stiffness, and muscle cramps, and the presence of extraskeletal involvement help to differentiate them from metabolic myopathies. The clinical features of mitochondrial myopathies are highly variable concerning the age at onset, the spectrum of organ dysfunctions, and severity. However, salient features of major clinical phenotypes have been described in **Table 10**.[74,75]

Salient investigational findings in mitochondrial myopathies are elevated CK, lactic acid, alanine and growth/differentiation factor (GDF-15) in serum, elevated urine organic acids (tricarboxylic acid intermediates, 3-methylglutaconic aciduria), normal EMG, red-ragged fibers, and cytochrome oxidase negative fibers on muscle histopathology. Genetic testing should be done to confirm the diagnosis, explain the prognosis, and change the therapy.

Management

Even though precise definitive treatment for mitochondrial myopathy is lacking, the following molecules are commonly prescribed—coenzyme Q (ubiquinol), riboflavin, thiamine, levocarnitine, and levoarginine.

TABLE 7: Salient clinical, investigative, and therapeutic details of various inherited myopathies.

Hereditary myopathy	Pathology/ pathophysiology	CK	Muscle MRI	Other evaluations	Clinical features	Treatment trial
DMD/BMD	• Deletion > duplication > point mutation • DMD: Out-of-frame deletion • BMD: In-frame deletion • *Mechanism of muscle damage*: Cytoskeletal disruption, membrane instability, mechanical stress, alter membrane permeability, abnormal calcium homeostasis	Markedly elevated	Selective involvement of gluteus maximus, adductor magnus, quadriceps femoris, rectus femoris and biceps muscle of the thigh, semimembranosus, semitendinosus, sartorius and gracilis	• *Muscle histopathology*: Degenerating and regenerating muscle fibers with variability in fiber size • *Genetic testing*: Multiplex PCR, MLPA, direct sequence analysis, targeted high-density oligonucleotide microarray technique	• *Important signs*: Gower's maneuver, calf hypertrophy, tendo-Achilles contracture, Valley sign and sparing of facial, bulbar and hand muscles. Lumbar lordosis with protuberant abdomen, waddling gait, and buckling of the knee with frequent falls • *Other system involvements*: Cardiac hypocontractility, restrictive lung disease, attention deficit	*Drug therapy*: 1. Corticosteroid 2. Vamorolone 3. AdipoRon 4. Givinostat [ITF2357] 5. Edasalonexent 6. Talditercept alpha 7. Idebenone 8. Pamrevlumab 9. CAP-1002 *Gene therapy*: 1. Antisense oligonucleotide exon skipping 2. Read through stop codon strategy 3. PTC 124 4. Utrophin modulation: SMT C1100 5. Stem cell therapy 6. Genome editing using CRISPR technology
CMD: 1. LAMA2/merosin	Merosin is one of a large family of glycosylated proteins found in the basement membrane and attaches to the dystroglycan complex	5×	Involvement of muscle periphery in the anterior thigh with sparing of gracilis and sartorius	• *Brain MRI*: White matter changes with sparing of the internal capsule, corpus callosum, and other dense fiber tracts. Subcortical cyst • *Muscle or skin biopsy*: Absence of laminin α2 staining in complete laminin α2 deficiency. Partial deficiency can be seen in both primary LAMA2-RD and αDG-RD	• *Complete deficiency*: Present at birth, significant hypotonia and weakness of the extremities, sparing face and extraocular muscles and arthrogryposis. • *Partial deficiency*: Milder and more variable phenotypes. Seizure (30%)	*Three main purposes of treatment*: Basement membrane treatment, modulating cellular events caused by laminin-α-2 loss, and genetic correction by exon skipping or CRISPR/Cas9
2. Alpha dystroglycan-related dystrophies (αDG-RD)	18 identified genes, the spectrum is broad	2–5×		*Muscle biopsy*: Dystrophic changes. Western-blot analysis for glycosylated α-dystroglycan differentiate primary and secondary α-dystroglycan deficiency	Fukuyama CMD patients have less weakness, CNS and ocular involvement and significant cardiac and respiratory involvement as compared to muscle–eye–brain disease (MEB) and walker Warburg disease (WWD). WWD has a more severe eye and CNS changes than MEB	*Treatment strategies*: Use of small molecules, gene therapy, and cell therapy

Continued

Continued

Hereditary myopathy	Pathology/ pathophysiology	CK	Muscle MRI	Other evaluations	Clinical features	Treatment trial
3. *Collagenopathy*: Severe Ullrich CMD (UCMD) to milder Bethlem myopathy (BM)	Being an important component of the muscle extracellular matrix, collagen 6 interacts with the basement membrane of all muscle fibers	Normal–5×	Peripheral involvement with central sparing of vastus lateralis and hamstrings	• *Rectus femoris ultrasound*: Fatty infiltration of central fascia known as "central shadow sign" • *Muscle biopsy*: From minimal myopathic changes or features of fiber type disproportion to severe dystrophic features • *Collagen 6 immunoreactivity*: Absent from the sarcolemma/ basement membrane specifically in dominantly acting mutations, while overall absent in patients with recessive null mutations	• Distal joint hypermobility and proximal joint contracture with characteristic skin lesions are diagnostic clues • Cognition and cardiac system are not affected	Cyclosporin A and Omigapil were tried as an anti-apoptotic agent. Oligonucleotide-based allele-specific silencing demonstrates restoration of collagen 6 fibrils in 2 studies
4. SEPN1-related myopathy	It protects human cells against oxidative stress	1–3×	Selective involvement of sartorius, semimembranosus and adductor muscles with sparing of the gracilis is specific finding	*Muscle biopsy*: Small focal areas of mitochondrial depletion and sarcomere disorganization (mini cores) on oxidative stains in muscle fibers, together with type-1 fiber predominance and variable atrophy, protein aggregates, and/or endomysial fibrosis	Poor head control in the 1st month of life is the most common presenting sign. In later infancy and childhood, prominent muscle weakness is noticed in the axial group, especially neck flexors. Limb strength is preserved till the fourth decade of life. Other features are relative atrophy of the inner thigh muscles, mild hyperlaxity of hands and wrists, mild facial weakness, typical nasal voice, mild ophthalmoparesis, hirsutism, signs of insulin resistance, spinal stiffness, and thoracic lordoscoliosis with lateral translation. Progressive restrictive respiratory failure	
5. Recessive RYR1-related myopathy (RYR1-RM)	It encodes for sarcoplasmic reticulum calcium release channel	Mildly elevated		*Muscle biopsy*: Extreme fiber atrophy, frequent central nucleation, fiber type uniformity, irregular oxidative enzyme stains including core-like areas	Significant congenital onset hypotonia, early onset severely progressive scoliosis, feeding and swallowing difficulties, and pulmonary insufficiency. Ophthalmoplegia/paresis may be absent	
6. LMNA-related CMD (LMNA-CMD)	Missense, deletions (in-frame) and duplications in exon 4 c.745 C>T of lamin A/C gene	Mild-to-moderate elevation	Selective involvement of vastus lateralis and gastrocnemius medialis and sparing of cranial, psoas and forearm muscles	*Muscle biopsy*: Variable, even in a given section and in-between different muscles. The immuno-histochemical examination is normal even in severe disease	Weakness presents in early life and usually follows an axial-scapuloperoneal pattern. Dropped head syndrome; pronounced lumbar hyperlordosis; and arm, hand, and peroneal region weakness with preservation of hip flexors. Contracture in the spine and lower limbs with preservation of the upper limbs joint differentiates it from EMD and COL6-RD. Pulmonary and cardiac involvements are common. Cognition remains unaffected	

Continued

Continued

Hereditary myopathy	Pathology/ pathophysiology	CK	Muscle MRI	Other evaluations	Clinical features	Treatment trial
7. Choline kinase B-related CMD	It is involved in phosphatidylcholine biosynthesis and leads to mitochondrial dysfunction	Mildly elevated		• *Muscle biopsy*: Giant mitochondria with abnormal structure on electron microscopy • *MRI brain*: Normal despite significant CNS involvement	Proximal weakness and muscle wasting present in early life. Congenital heart defects and dilated cardiomyopathy (40%). CNS involvement (100%). Skin manifestation (80%)	
FSHD	Expression of DUX4 in muscle tissue results in apoptosis, oxidative stress, and interference with myogenic differentiation	<10×		• *Muscle biopsy*: Nonspecific myopathic changes. In a few patients, characteristic perivascular inflammatory infiltrate, typically CD4 or CD8 cells are seen • *Genetic testing*: D4Z4 contraction using Southern blot shows contraction between 10 and 38 kb. If the Southern blot is negative then determination of the presence of at least one A allele and very low methylation (less than 20%) confirms a diagnosis of FSHD2	• *Face*: Brow furrow decrease; inability to tightly close the eyes; flattened, transverse smile; and an inability to tense the platysma when asking the patient to growl • *Shoulder*: Round shape because of selective preservation of deltoid muscles, Poly-hill appearance due to selective involvement of lower part of trapezius muscle • *Upper limb*: Popeye arm appearance due to wasting of biceps and triceps with preservation of distal forearm muscles. Later in the disease, selective involvement of the finger and wrist extensors • *Chest wall*: Pectoral muscles wasting, decreased normal clavicular angle, posterior and lateral winging of scapula on shoulder abduction or forward flexion, pectus excavatum • *Abdomen*: Protuberant, Beevor sign due to sparing of upper abdominal muscles in the initial stage, specific for FSHD • *Back and spine*: Camptocormia or lumbar lordosis may happen due to involvement of abdominal and paraspinal muscles • *Lower limb*: Tibialis anterior weakness, hip girdle muscles involved later in disease course • *Other systems*: Restrictive respiratory patterns, dilated ventricles, reduced cardiac function, asymptomatic supraventricular arrhythmias, incomplete right bundle branch block, retinal vasculopathy, asymptomatic high-frequency hearing loss, cognitive changes, mental retardation, and seizures	• Regular screening for pulmonary function, heart, eyes, and hearing • Scapular fixation in patients with preserved upper limb strength • Regular physiotherapy • Pain management *There are 2 approaches to genetic therapies*: 1. Targeting DUX4 at the DNA, RNA, and protein levels by oligonucleotide, CRISPR technology 2. Inhibiting the effects of DUX4-mediated toxicity

Continued

Continued

Hereditary myopathy	Pathology/ pathophysiology	CK	Muscle MRI	Other evaluations	Clinical features	Treatment trial
OPMD	Expanded PABPN1 has the following effects: • Toxic intranuclear aggregates cause endoplasmic reticulum stress and mitochondrial dysfunction • Inactivation of native wild-type protein and mRNA quality control will disturb • Sequestration of molecular chaperons, RNA-binding proteins, and RNA by intranuclear aggregates which cause abnormal transcription and translation in muscles The end result of the above effects is muscle wasting and fibrosis	Correlates with disease stage, low in mild and advanced cases, high in severe cases	Fatty replacement of muscle fibers commonly involving—adductor magnus, soleus, and tongue muscles	• *Muscle biopsy*: Shows the following changes: (1) Fiber size varies, (2) small rounded or angular fibers, (3) rimmed vacuoles in small fibers, (4) occasionally necrotic and regenerative myofibers, (5) mitochondrial abnormalities—COX-negative fibers and ragged-red fibers, (6) PABPN1-positive insoluble intranuclear aggregates (100% sensitive and 96% specific) • *Genetic study*: Abnormal expansion of (GCN)n repeats in the *PABPN1* gene, located on chromosome 14	Ptosis (100%), Dysphagia (62–100%), proximal weakness (20–81%)	*Symptomatic treatment*: • *Dysphagia*: Injection botulism toxin in cricopharyngeal muscle • *Ptosis with good levator function*: Levator advancement or resection • *Ptosis with poor levator function*: Frontalis suspension *Therapeutic strategies*: • Knockdown of mutant PABPN1 and/or augmentation of wild-type PABPN1 using adeno-associated virus (AAV) vectors • Boosting muscle growth using myostatin inhibitor • Reduction and dispersal of intranuclear aggregates using cystamine, doxycycline, trehalose, guanabenz, and intrabodies • Autologous myoblast transplantation combined with cricopharyngeal myotomy • Mitochondrial restoration
EMD	*X-linked*: Emerin, FHL1	Normal to mild elevation	Diffuse muscle involvement	*EMG*: Neuropathy + myopathy	Contracture > weakness	
	AD/AR: Lamin A/C				Weakness > contracture, high risk of cardiomyopathy	

(AD: autosomal dominant; AR: autosomal recessive; BMD: Becker muscular dystrophy; CMD: congenital muscular dystrophy; CNS: central nervous system; DMD: Duchenne muscular dystrophy; EMG: electromyography; FSHD: facioscapulohumeral muscular dystrophy; MRI: magnetic resonance imaging)

TABLE 8: Pathophysiology and clinical features of major congenital myopathies.

Name and pathology/pathophysiology	Clinical features
• *Nemaline myopathy*: Small rod-like inclusion, made up of alpha-actinin, actin, and other Z-band filaments in muscle fibers • *Cap myopathy*: Subsarcolemmal cap-like (triangular) inclusions • *Zebra body myopathy*: Elongated filamentous structures with thin, dark bands alternating with wider dark ones	• *Severe*: Hyposthenia, hypotonia, poor sucking, weak swallowing, arthrogryposis, and dilated cardiomyopathy • *Milder*: Characteristic faces (elongated face, high-arched palate, and tented upper lip), delayed motor milestones, dysarthria, dysphagia, high-arched feet, muscle contracture, and respiratory involvement
Core myopathy: Presence of a rounded structure known as a "core", where oxidative activities are either absent or reduced in contrast to normal activities in the surrounding areas *Two types*: Central core and multi-mini core myopathy	*Central core myopathy*: • *Severe*: Fetal akinesia, congenital arthrogryposis • *Milder*: Delayed motor milestones, ophthalmoparesis, eyelid ptosis, proximal and axial muscles weakness and hypotonia, minimum or no respiratory involvement *Multi-mini core myopathy*: • Axial, proximal, and eye muscle weakness • Scoliosis or stiffness of the spine, arthrogryposis, and torticollis • Respiratory involvement • Severe neonatal manifestations
Centronuclear myopathy: The nucleus is exactly in the center of the myocytes, vesicular appearance, and larger than normal	Polyhydramnios, reduced fetal movements, hypotonia, arthrogryposis, dysphagia, ophthalmoparesis, eyelid ptosis, malformations such as pyloric stenosis, inguinal hernias, and cryptorchidism. Cardiac functions are preserved. Repeated miscarriages of male fetuses on the mother's side of the family are an important clue
Congenital fiber type disproportion: The type-1 fibers are significantly and consistently smaller than the type-2 fibers	Facial and proximal muscle weakness, mild-to-severe respiratory involvement, significant dysphagia, and contractures
Myosin storage myopathy	*Three common patterns*: (1) Early-onset distal myopathy with cores, (2) late-onset distal myopathy without cores and with the variable association of cardiomyopathy and/or fiber-type disproportion, and (3) limb-girdle involvement with myofibrillar damage

TABLE 9: Gene defects and muscle MRI findings in major congenital myopathies.[67-71]

Gene defects in congenital myopathies	Muscle MRI

RYR1	• Thigh > leg, anterior > posterior thigh compartment
	• *Involved muscles*:
	  ○ *Pelvis*: Gluteus maximus
	  ○ *Thigh*: Adductor magnus, vastus lateralis, sartorius > adductor longus, rectus femoris, and gracilis
	  ○ *Leg*: Soleus > gastrocnemius lateralis > gastrocnemius medialis. Peroneus group > tibialis anterior group

SEPN1	*Involved muscles*: • *Thigh*: Sartorius, adductor, and biceps femoris • *Leg*: Gastrocnemius, toe extensors, and peroneal • *Relatively spared muscles*: Gracilis, rectus femoris, vastus, semimembranosus, semitendinosus, tibialis anterior, and soleus
NEB	• Selective involvement of the anterior leg compartment muscles, especially the tibialis anterior • *Other involved muscles*: Rectus femoris, vastus lateralis and gracilis
ACTA1	• Widespread involvement in thigh and leg muscles • Sartorius, soleus > gracilis, gastrocnemius • *Diagnostic clue*: Tibialis posterior muscle involvement
MYH7	• Leg > thigh • *Earliest and most commonly affected muscle*: Tibialis anterior • *Other involved muscles*: Peroneal, soleus, tibialis posterior, and vastus • *Spared muscles*: Gastrocnemius lateralis, rectus femoris, adductor longus, sartorius, and gracilis

Continued

Continued

Gene defects in congenital myopathies	Muscle MRI
TMP2	Selective involvement of leg and posterior thigh muscles
DNM2	• *Important clue*: Early involvement of the plantar flexors • *Involved muscles*: ○ *Thigh*: Adductor longus, semimembranosus, biceps femoris, rectus femoris, and vastus intermedius ○ *Leg*: Soleus, gastrocnemius medialis, and tibialis anterior • *Spared muscles*: Vastus lateralis, vastus medialis, sartorius, gracilis, and semitendinosus
BIN1	Sparing of thigh muscles and soleus differentiates it from DNM2 mutation
MTM1	• *Involved muscles*: Anterior thigh compartment muscles, adductor magnus, and soleus • *Spared muscles*: Adductor longus, sartorius, gracilis, and gastrocnemius medialis

(MRI: magnetic resonance imaging)

TABLE 10: Salient clinical features and pathogenesis of major clinical phenotypes of mitochondrial myopathies.[72,74-77]

Disease	Pathogenesis	Salient features
Kearns–Sayre syndrome (KSS)	Mitochondrial DNA (mtDNA) deletion; usually sporadic; rarely maternal	Triad of onset before age of 20: extraocular muscle weakness and retinitis pigmentosa + one of the following: • Ataxia • Cerebrospinal fluid protein level >100 mg/dL • Cardiac conduction blocks
Chronic progressive external ophthalmoplegia (CPEO) and CPEO-plus	mtDNA point mutation; maternal inheritance	Adult-onset progressive ophthalmoplegia, sometimes associated with skeletal myopathy in CPEO-plus **(Fig. 11)**
Mitochondrial encephalomyopathy, lactic acidosis, and stroke-like episodes (MELAS)	mtDNA point mutation; m.A3243G most common mutation	Onset from infancy to adulthood, stroke-like episodes in the parieto-occipital region, epilepsy, short stature, cognitive decline, myopathy, sensorineural hearing loss (SNHL), vomiting spells, gastroparesis, atypical migraine
Myoclonic epilepsy with red-ragged fibers (MERRF)	Mutations in mtDNA tRNALys m.A8344G	Progressive myoclonic jerks, epilepsy, ataxia, cervical lipomas, short stature, dementia, SNHL, cardiomyopathy, myopathy, and optic atrophy
mtDNA deletion and depletion syndromes	mtDNA deletion/ nuclear DNA mutation affecting mtDNA replicase function	Epileptic encephalopathy, global development delay, progressive external ophthalmoplegia (PEO), and myopathy
POLG spectrum disorders	Mutation in *POLG* gene	• *Myocerebrohepatopathy*: Onset at infancy, lactic acidosis, liver failure, variable muscle, and brain involvement • *Alpers–Huttenlocher syndrome (AHS)*: Epileptic encephalopathy, vision loss, and extreme valproate sensitivity • Autosomal dominant and recessive PEO

Lipid Myopathies

Lipid myopathies are genetic disorders involving the metabolism of fats that cause exercise or fasting-induced muscle weakness and myalgias. Some patients can have static weakness, fasting hypoglycemia, and rhabdomyolysis. Pathophysiology primarily consists of β-oxidation and carnitine metabolism, which are responsible for shuttling the free fatty acids into the mitochondrial matrix. Such defects lead to abnormal accumulation of lipids in the cytoplasm.[76]

The three common subtypes of lipid myopathies are—carnitine palmitoyltransferase (CPT) type II, very long-chain acyl CoA (VLCA) deficiency, and multiple acyl-Co-A dehydrogenase (MADD) deficiency.

Investigations

Creatine kinase, acylcarnitine, and lactate levels are normal at rest while elevated during exacerbations. Urine organic acids (dicarboxylic acid) may be elevated. Skin biopsy can study for acylcarnitine levels in fibroblasts, muscle biopsy

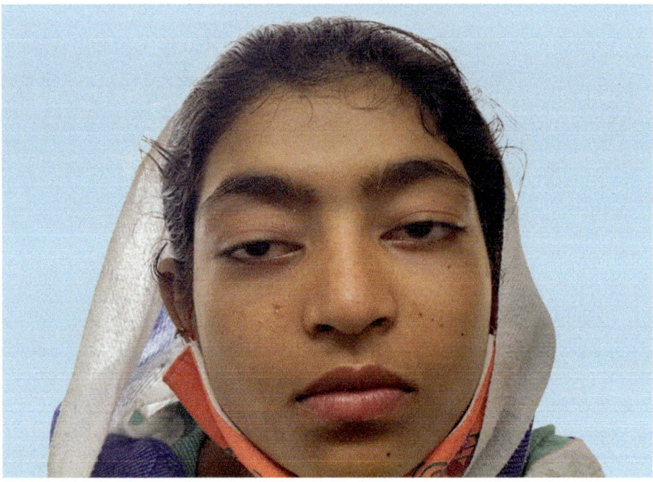

FIG. 11: Ptosis in mitochondrial myopathy.

TABLE 11: Salient features of types of glycogen storage diseases.[78-80]

GSD subtype	Pathophysiology	Salient features
McArdle's disease (GDS5)	Myophosphorylase deficiency leads to impaired phosphorylation of glycogen; PYGM mutation	Childhood-onset; muscle weakness and cramping with exertion and rhabdomyolysis; second wind phenomenon
Pompe's disease (GSD2)	Acid maltase deficiency; mutation in *GAA* gene Alpha-glucosidase deficiency leads to accumulation of glycogen	Infants present with floppy babies; respiratory failure and cardiomyopathy; adults present with fixed muscle weakness and respiratory distress but no rhabdomyolysis
Cori's disease (GSD3)	Mutation in *AGL* gene; deficiency in glycogen debrancher enzyme	Infants present with fasting hypoglycemia; failure to thrive and hepatomegaly but no rhabdomyolysis

with Sudan black or Oil red O shows lipid deposition, and the genetic testing is used for definitive diagnosis.

Management

Management consists of preventing exacerbations by avoiding fasting, high-carbohydrate intake, increasing fluids during exercise, and levocarnitine supplementation. Treatment of rhabdomyolysis during exacerbations is important and involves multidisciplinary management.

Glycogen Storage Disease Myopathy

Clinical manifestations of glycogen storage diseases (GSDs) vary from fasting hypoglycemia and liver involvement in childhood to exercise intolerance and rhabdomyolysis in adulthood. Some patients may exhibit the second wind phenomenon (improvement in exercise tolerance after 10 minutes of exercise) and out of wind phenomenon (glucose intake before exercise can exacerbate symptoms). GSDs result from deficiencies in the enzymes that build glycogen, as well as those that interfere with the degradation of glycogen and subsequent mobilization of glucose. Salient features of common subtypes of GSD are mentioned in **Table 11**.

Management

Dietary therapy is the mainstay of treatment for GSDs. A frequent high simple carbohydrate diet is helpful, especially for McArdle's disease. High protein with complex carbohydrates is recommended. Patients should avoid strenuous exercise and fasting and perform moderate aerobic exercises to improve endurance. Enzyme replacement therapy is indicated for symptomatic patients with Pompe's disease.

INDIAN PERSPECTIVE

While the spectrum of inherited myopathies seen in India is broadly similar to that described from other parts of the world, some points need a mention.

The lack of awareness of these conditions in the population and to an extent, amongst the medical practitioners, limited availability of modern investigations such as muscle biopsy with histochemistry and immunocytochemistry and new-generation sequencing and funding limitations result in a large fraction of inherited myopathies undefined and hence not effectively prevented from passing on to the successive generations.[81]

Duchenne muscular dystrophy, as expected, is the most common dystrophy of childhood and the genetic spectrum seems similar. However, it is not uncommon to see more than one affected child in a family, related to lack of awareness, the short gap between children, delay in the diagnosis, and the desire to have a normal male child.

Limb girdle dystrophies are the most common dystrophies of adulthood and adolescence and within this large group, the available literature suggests that calpainopathy, dysferlinopathy, sarcoglycanopathies, and collagen 6 diseases are more often documented in hospital-based data. GNE myopathy is also common and has been amply documented. Founder mutations are known in calpainopathy in the Agarwal community and GNE myopathy among people originating from Rajasthan. Myotonic dystrophy is not as common as in the western populations, and this probably relates to the average triplet repeat size in the Indian population. Pompe disease has been documented in its infantile and late forms and is important to diagnose as it is treatable. Information on other metabolic and mitochondrial diseases, CMs, and CMDs is slowly evolving and the available hospital-based data is limited.[82-84]

CONCLUSION

As we have seen, inherited myopathies comprise a wide variety of muscle disorders. Their clinical features are protean and a single gene can present with multiple phenotypes and vice versa. Some diseases have tell-tale clinical features and others are nonspecific. Thorough history taking, detailed clinical examination, and appropriate use of modern investigations often lead to an accurate diagnosis. While the majority of diseases are not modifiable, prevention is feasible in many, using genetic information and counseling, and the course of some others can be changed, e.g., Pompe disease. The field is expanding and newer therapies are likely to develop in the coming years.

ACKNOWLEDGMENT

Authors wish to thank Dr Darshan Pandya for his help in the preparation of the manuscript.

REFERENCES

1. Khadilkar SV, Patel BA, Lalkaka JA. Making sense of the clinical spectrum of limb girdle muscular dystrophies. Pract Neurol. 2018;18(3):201-10.
2. Khadilkar SV, Faldu H, Patil S, Singh R. Limb-girdle muscular dystrophies in India: a review. Ann Indian Acad Neurol. 2017;20(2):87-95.
3. Khadilkar SV, Yadav RS, Patel BA. (2018). Limb–Girdle Muscular Dystrophies. Neuromuscular Disorders [Internet]. [online] Available from http://link.springer.com/10.1007/978-981-10-5361-0_12. [Last accessed April, 2023].
4. Angelini C, Giaretta L, Marozzo R. An update on diagnostic options and considerations in limb-girdle dystrophies. Expert Rev Neurother. 2018;18(9):693-703.
5. Bushby K. Diagnosis and management of the limb girdle muscular dystrophies. Pract Neurol. 2009;9(6):314-23.
6. Venugopal V, Pavlakis S. (2022). Duchenne Muscular Dystrophy. [online] Available from https://www.ncbi.nlm.nih.gov/books/NBK482346/. [Last accessed April, 2023].
7. Arora H. Duchenne muscular dystrophy: Still an incurable disease. Neurol India. 2019;67(3):717.
8. van Ruiten HJA, Straub V, Bushby K, Guglieri M. Improving recognition of Duchenne muscular dystrophy: a retrospective case note review. Arch Dis Child. 2014;99(12):1074-7.
9. Goyal M, Gupta A, Agarwal K, Kapoor S, Kumar S. Duchenne Muscular Dystrophy: Genetic and Clinical Profile in the Population of Rajasthan, India. Ann Indian Acad Neurol. 2021;24(6):873.
10. Buyse GM, Goemans N, van den Hauwe M, Thijs D, de Groot IJM, Schara U, et al. Idebenone as a novel, therapeutic approach for Duchenne muscular dystrophy: Results from a 12 month, double-blind, randomized placebo-controlled trial. Neuromuscul Disord. 2011;21(6):396-405.
11. Voit T. Safety and efficacy of drisapersen for the treatment of Duchenne muscular dystrophy (DEMAND II): an exploratory, randomised, placebo-controlled phase 2 study. Lancet Neurol. 2014;13:987-96.
12. Birnkrant D. Diagnosis and management of Duchenne muscular dystrophy, part 3: primary care, emergency management, psychosocial care, and transitions of care across the lifespan. Lancet Neurol. 2018;17:445-55.
13. Fujikura Y, Kimura K, Yamanouchi K, Sugihara H, Hatakeyama M, Zhuang H, et al. A medium-chain triglyceride containing ketogenic diet exacerbates cardiomyopathy in a CRISPR/Cas9 gene-edited rat model with Duchenne muscular dystrophy. Sci Rep. 2022;12(1):11580.
14. Birnkrant D. Diagnosis and management of Duchenne muscular dystrophy, part 1: diagnosis, and neuromuscular, rehabilitation, endocrine, and gastrointestinal and nutritional management. Lancet Neurol. 2018;17:251-67.
15. Birnkrant DJ, Bushby K, Bann CM, Alman BA, Apkon SD, Blackwell A, et al. Diagnosis and management of Duchenne muscular dystrophy, part 2: respiratory, cardiac, bone health, and orthopaedic management. Lancet Neurol. 2018;17(4):347-61.
16. Ferizovic N, Summers J, de Zárate IBO, Werner C, Jiang J, Landfeldt E, et al. Prognostic indicators of disease progression in Duchenne muscular dystrophy: A literature review and evidence synthesis. PLoS One. 2022;17(3):e0265879.
17. Landfeldt E, Thompson R, Sejersen T, McMillan HJ, Kirschner J, Lochmüller H. Life expectancy at birth in Duchenne muscular dystrophy: a systematic review and meta-analysis. Eur J Epidemiol. 2020;35(7):643-53.
18. Kim S, Zhu Y, Romitti PA, Fox DJ, Sheehan DW, Valdez R, et al. Associations between timing of corticosteroid treatment initiation and clinical outcomes in Duchenne muscular dystrophy. Neuromuscul Disord. 2017;27(8):730-7.
19. Houde S, Filiatrault M, Fournier A, Dubé J, D'Arcy S, Bérubé D, et al. Deflazacort Use in Duchenne Muscular Dystrophy: An 8-Year Follow-Up. Pediatr Neurol. 2008;38(3):200-6.
20. Bello L, D'Angelo G, Villa M, Fusto A, Vianello S, Merlo B, et al. Genetic modifiers of respiratory function in Duchenne muscular dystrophy. Ann Clin Transl Neurol. 2020;7(5):786-98.
21. Angelini C, Pegoraro E, Turella E, Intino MT, Pini A, Costa C. Deflazacort in Duchenne dystrophy: Study of long-term effect. Muscle Nerve. 1994;17(4):386-91.
22. Charleston J. Eteplirsen treatment for Duchenne muscular dystrophy. Neurology. 2018;90:e2146-54.
23. Pegoraro E, Hoffman EP. (1993) Limb-Girdle Muscular Dystrophy Overview. GeneReviews® [Internet]. [online] Available from http://www.ncbi.nlm.nih.gov/pubmed/20301582. [Last accessed April, 2023].
24. Liewluck T, Milone M. Untangling the complexity of limb-girdle muscular dystrophies. Muscle Nerve. 2018;58(2):167-77.
25. Thompson R, Straub V. Limb-girdle muscular dystrophies - international collaborations for translational research. Nat Rev Neurol. 2016;12(5):294-309.
26. Bushby KMD. Diagnostic criteria for the limb-girdle muscular dystrophies: Report of the ENMC consortium on limb-girdle dystrophies. Neuromuscul Disord. 1995;5(1):71-4.
27. Magri F, Nigro V, Angelini C, Mongini T, Mora M, Moroni I, et al. The Italian limb girdle muscular dystrophy registry: Relative frequency, clinical features, and differential diagnosis. Muscle Nerve. 2017;55(1):55-68.
28. Guglieri M, Bushby K. How to go about diagnosing and managing the limb-girdle muscular dystrophies. Neurol India. 2008;56(3): 271-80.
29. Iyadurai SJP, Kissel JT. The limb-girdle muscular dystrophies and the dystrophinopathies. Continuum (Minneap Minn). 2016;22(6):1954-77.
30. Wicklund MP. The limb-girdle muscular dystrophies. Continuum (Minneap Minn). 2019;25(6):1599-618.
31. Straub V, Bertoli M. Where do we stand in trial readiness for autosomal recessive limb girdle muscular dystrophies? Neuromuscul Disord. 2016;26(2):111-25.

32. Straub V, Murphy A, Udd B. 229th ENMC international workshop: Limb girdle muscular dystrophies - Nomenclature and reformed classification Naarden, the Netherlands, 17-19 March 2017. Neuromuscul Disord. 2018;28(8):702-10.
33. Angelini C. LGMD. Identification, description and classification. Acta Myologica. 2020;39(4):207.
34. Wang L, Zhang VW, Li S, Li H, Sun Y, Li J, et al. The clinical spectrum and genetic variability of limb-girdle muscular dystrophy in a cohort of Chinese patients. Orphanet J Rare Dis. 2018;13(1):1-14.
35. Dam L ten, van der Kooi AJ, van Wattingen M, de Haan RJ, de Visser M. Reliability and accuracy of skeletal muscle imaging in limb-girdle muscular dystrophies. Neurology. 2012;79(16):1716-23.
36. Meola G. Clinical aspects, molecular pathomechanisms and management of myotonic dystrophies. Acta Myologica. 2013;32(3):154-65.
37. Thornton CA. Myotonic dystrophy. Neurol Clin. 2014;32(3):705-19.
38. Thornton C. The myotonic dystrophies. Semin Neurol. 1999;19(1):25-33.
39. Ricker K. Myotonic dystrophy and proximal myotonic myopathy. J Neurol. 1999;246(5):334-8.
40. Udd B, Krahe R. The myotonic dystrophies: molecular, clinical, and therapeutic challenges. Lancet Neurol. 2012;11(10):891-905.
41. Pennock E, Mahadevan MS. Therapeutics development in myotonic dystrophy type. Muscle Nerve. 2011;44(2):160-9.
42. Magana JJ, Cisneros B. Perspectives on gene therapy in myotonic dystrophy type 1. J Neurosci Res. 2011;89(3):275-85.
43. Meola G, Moxley RT. Myotonic dystrophy type 2 and related myotonic disorders. J Neurol. 2004;251(10):1173-82.
44. Meola G, Cardani R. Myotonic dystrophy type 2 and modifier genes: an update on clinical and pathomolecular aspects. Neurol Sci. 2017;38(4):535-46.
45. Turner C, Hilton-Jones D. Myotonic dystrophy: Diagnosis, management and new therapies. Curr Opin Neurol. 2014;27(5):599-606.
46. LoRusso S, Weiner B, Arnold WD. Myotonic Dystrophies: Targeting Therapies for Multisystem Disease. Neurotherapeutics. 2018;15(4):872-84.
47. Dimachkie MM, Barohn RJ. Distal myopathies. Neurol Clin. 2014;32(3):817-42.
48. Narayanaswami P, Weiss M, Selcen D, David W, Raynor E, Carter G, et al. Evidence-based guideline summary: Diagnosis and treatment of limb-girdle and distal dystrophies: Report of the Guideline Development Subcommittee of the American Academy of Neurology and the Practice Issues Review Panel of the American Association of Neuromuscular & Electrodiagnostic Medicine. Neurology. 2014;83(16):1453-63.
49. Felice KJ. Distal Myopathies. Neurol Clin. 2020;38(3):637-59.
50. Shaibani A. Distal Myopathies: Case Studies. Neurol Clin. 2016;34(3):547-64.
51. Milone M, Liewluck T. The unfolding spectrum of inherited distal myopathies. Muscle Nerve. 2019;59(3):283-94.
52. Palmio J, Udd B. Myofibrillar and distal myopathies. Rev Neurol (Paris). 2016;172(10):587-93.
53. Savarese M, Sarparanta J, Vihola A, Jonson PH, Johari M, Rusanen S, et al. Panorama of the distal myopathies. Acta Myologica. 2020;39(4):245-65.
54. Khadilkar SV, Yadav RS, Patel BA. (2018). Congenital Muscular Dystrophies. Neuromuscular Disorders. [online] Available from http://link.springer.com/10.1007/978-981-10-5361-0_14. [Last accessed April, 2023].
55. Statland JM, Tawil R. Facioscapulohumeral Muscular Dystrophy. Continuum (Minneap Minn). 2016;22(6):1916-31.
56. Tawil R, van der Maarel SM. Facioscapulohumeral muscular dystrophy. Muscle Nerve. 2006;34(1):1-15.
57. Statland JM, Tawil R. Risk of functional impairment in facioscapulohumeral muscular dystrophy. Muscle Nerve. 2014;49(4):520-7.
58. Pradhan S. Poly-hill sign in facioscapulohumeral dystrophy. Muscle Nerve. 2002;25(5):754-5.
59. Lutz KL, Holte L, Kliethermes SA, Stephan C, Mathews KD. Clinical and genetic features of hearing loss in facioscapulohumeral muscular dystrophy. Neurology. 2013;81(16):1374-7.
60. Van der Kooi EL, Vogels OJM, van Asseldonk RJGP, Lindeman E, Hendriks JCM, Wohlgemuth M, et al. Strength training and albuterol in facioscapulohumeral muscular dystrophy. Neurology. 2004;63(4):702-8.
61. Yamashita S. Recent Progress in Oculopharyngeal Muscular Dystrophy. J Clin Med. 2021;10(7):1375.
62. Brais B, Rouleau GA, Bouchard JP, Fardeau M, Tomé FMS. Oculopharyngeal muscular dystrophy. Semin Neurol. 1999;19(1):59-66.
63. Kubo S, Tsukahara T, Arahata K. Emery-Dreifuss muscular dystrophy. Nippon Rinsho. Japan J Clin Med. 1997;55(12):3186-9.
64. Bonne G, Mercuri E, Muchir A, Urtizberea A, Bécane HM, Recan D, et al. Clinical and molecular genetic spectrum of autosomal dominant Emery-Dreifuss muscular dystrophy due to mutations of the Lamin A/C gene. Ann Neurol. 2000;48(2):170-80.
65. Zacharias AS, Wagener ME, Warren ST, Hopkins LC. Emery-Dreifuss muscular dystrophy. Semin Neurol. 1999;19(1):67-79.
66. Helbling-Leclerc A, Bonne G, Schwartz K. Emery-Dreifuss muscular dystrophy. Eur J Hum Genet. 2002;10(3):157-61.
67. Claeys KG. Congenital myopathies: an update. Dev Med Child Neurol. 2020;62(3):297-302.
68. Sharma MC, Jain D, Sarkar C, Goebel HH. Congenital myopathies - A comprehensive update of recent advancements. Acta Neurol Scand. 2009;119(5):281-92.
69. Wallgren-Pettersson C, Sainio K, Salmi T. Electromyography in congenital nemaline myopathy. Muscle Nerve. 1989;12(7):587-93.
70. Pelin K. (2021). Genetics of the congenital myopathies. [online] Available from https://onlinelibrary.wiley.com/doi/10.1002/9780470015902.a0029175. [Last accessed April, 2023].
71. Cassandrini D, Trovato R, Rubegni A, Lenzi S, Fiorillo C, Baldacci J, et al. Congenital myopathies: clinical phenotypes and new diagnostic tools. Ital J Pediatr. 2017;43(1):101.
72. Berardo A, DiMauro S, Hirano M. Diagnostic algorithm for metabolic myopathies. Curr Neurol Neurosci Rep. 2010;10(2):118-26.
73. Volpi L, Ricci G, Orsucci D, Alessi R, Bertolucci F, Piazza S, et al. Metabolic myopathies: Functional evaluation by different exercise testing approaches. Musculoskelet Surg. 2011;95(2):59-67.
74. Sharp LJ, Haller RG. Metabolic and mitochondrial myopathies. Neurol Clin. 2014;32(3):777-99.
75. Cohen BH. Mitochondrial and Metabolic Myopathies. Continuum (Minneap Minn). 2019;25(6):1732-66.
76. Khadilkar S, Desai M. Editorial Commentary: Lipid Storage Myopathies. Ann Indian Acad Neurol. 2022;25(1):5-6.
77. van Adel BA, Tarnopolsky MA. Metabolic myopathies: Update 2009. J Clin Neuromuscul Dis. 2009;10(3):97-121.
78. Tsujino S, Nonaka I, DiMauro S. Glycogen storage myopathies. Neurol Clin. 2000;18(1):125-50.
79. DiMauro S, Bresolin N, Hays AP. Disorders of glycogen metabolism of muscle. CRC Crit Rev Clin Neurobiol. 1984;1(2):83-116.
80. Amato AA. Acid maltase deficiency and related myopathies. Neurol Clin. 2000;18(1):151-65.
81. Savarese M, di Fruscio G, Torella A, Fiorillo C, Magri F, Fanin M, et al. The genetic basis of undiagnosed muscular dystrophies and myopathies. Neurology. 2016;87(1):71-6.
82. Chakravorty S, Nallamilli BRR, Khadilkar SV, Singla MB, Bhutada A, Dastur R, et al. Clinical and Genomic Evaluation of 207 Genetic Myopathies in the Indian Subcontinent. Front Neurol. 2020;11:1305.
83. Benarroch L, Bonne G, Rivier F, Hamroun D. The 2020 version of the gene table of neuromuscular disorders (nuclear genome). Neuromuscul Disord. 2019;29(12):980-1018.
84. Attri S, Gahlawat S. Challenges and Advances in Molecular Diagnosis of Myopathies and Dystrophies in Perspective of Their Use in Developing Countries: Past, Present, and Future. Neurol India. 2021;69(4):797.

86

CHAPTER

Acquired Myopathies

Atchayaram Nalini, Deepak Menon, Seena Vengalil, Saraswati Nashi

INTRODUCTION

Acquired myopathies are a heterogenous group of disorders of variable etiology, diverse clinical manifestations, and prognosis. In-depth knowledge of clinical profile is needed for timely diagnosis and treatment. In this review, we discuss about common acquired myopathies, predominantly inflammatory myopathies, and also on endocrine, drug-induced, toxic, infective, and critical illness myopathy (CIM).

ENDOCRINE MYOPATHY

Early recognition of endocrine myopathies is vital given their potential reversibility and also in preventing multisystemic and life-threatening manifestations. The usual presentation is as a painful proximal myopathy and hence is often confused with inflammatory myopathies. Moreover, systemic clinical features may not often be readily apparent especially in early stages and a high index of suspicion is needed.

Osteomalacia is the adulthood manifestation of vitamin D deficiency and should be suspected in any form of painful proximal myopathy and waddling gait along with brisk tendon reflexes. Patients have associated fatigue and lethargy and can develop kyphoscoliosis and progressive later in the disease course.[1] The underlying pathology is a low serum calcium due to vitamin D deficiency with compensatory hyperparathyroidism mobilizing bone calcium stores, but at the expense of serum phosphorous and bone mineralization. This is reflected in the biochemical picture which reveals elevated alkaline phosphatase, which is a good screening parameter, low-normal serum calcium, low phosphorous, low 25 hydroxy vitamin D, "losers zones" in skeletal survey, and high serum parathormone although the latter is not mandatory for a diagnosis. Patients usually have a rapid clinical improvement with vitamin D replacement. An exploration into the etiology of vitamin D deficiency such as a history suggesting malabsorption should also be made.

Unlike in osteomalacia, where it is one of the most common manifestation, myopathy is rare in hypoparathyroidism and when present is mild.[2] The predominant symptoms are features axonal hyperexcitability such as tetany and carpopedal spasms although there are very reports of isolated proximal myopathies.[3,4] The most common etiology is iatrogenic following thyroidectomy. Biochemically, patients will have low calcium, high phosphate, with low parathormone levels.

Primary hyperparathyroidism manifests due to a hyperfunctioning parathyroid adenoma and less frequently a carcinoma. Myopathy though infrequent is characteristically proximal with associated myalgia and preserved deep tendon reflexes (DTRs).[5] There will be other associated features of hypercalcemia which can sometimes be dismissed as "nonspecific" symptoms such as fatigue, lethargy, mild irritability, abdominal pain, constipation and cramps, headache, and polydipsia. The classical teaching of proximal muscle and tongue wasting with brisk reflexes resembling amyotrophic lateral sclerosis (ALS) has not been reported in subsequent case series.[5,6] In classical hyperparathyroidism, both serum calcium and parathormone are high but the clinical features does not correlate with the level of calcium.[7] Patients rapidly improve with parathyroidectomy.

Secondary hyperparathyroidism may be encountered more frequently and can present with similar clinical features with lower limb tending to be involved predominantly.[8] It is usually seen in chronic kidney disease, with vitamin D deficiency leading to compensatory increased parathormone levels. Uremia and carnitine deficiency are proposed to be contributory causes. Patients generally improve with vitamin D replacement.

Chronic proximal myopathy with myalgia can be seen in as many as 60% of patients with thyrotoxicosis with associated fatigue, cramps, and sensory neuropathy in a minority. The weakness predominantly affects iliopsoas and quadriceps but weakness is seldom profound.[9] Patients respond to beta blockers and hormonal correction but too

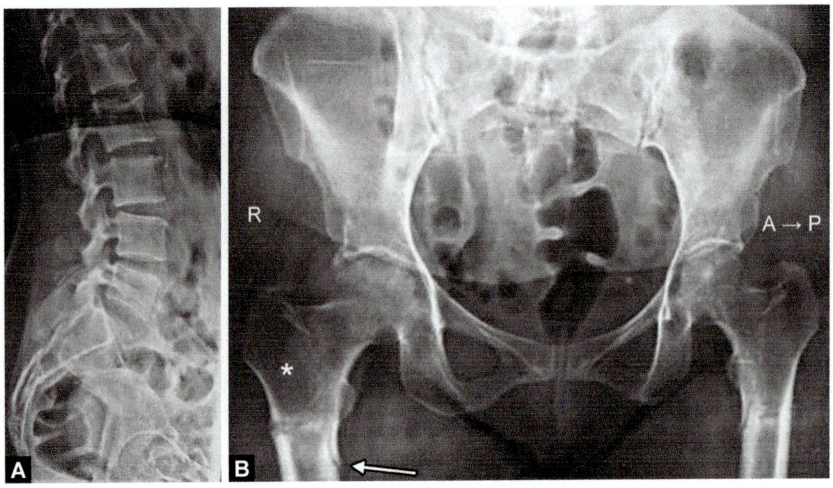

FIGS. 1A AND B: Skeletal survey showing decreased bone density (*), pathological fracture in vertebra and subtrochanteric fracture (arrow) suggestive of osteomalacia-related myopathy.

rapid a correction is also associated with myopathy.[10,11] Thyroid toxic periodic paralysis is another entity to be borne in mind when patients with thyrotoxicosis present with severe weakness.

In hypothyroid myopathy patients report muscle stiffness, aches, and pains along with proximal weakness and can be only symptoms of hypothyroidism. The classical clinical features such as myoedema which is a local nonpainful visible and palpable firm muscle swelling at the site of percussion or muscle flick, muscle enlargement, and delayed relaxation of ankle and other systemic signs of hypothyroidism are clues to diagnosis.[12] Rarely, rhabdomyolysis and respiratory involvement have also been described. Unlike other causes of endocrine, creatine kinase (CK) can be elevated several folds in hypothyroid myopathy and falls with successful treatment.

Proximal myopathy is seen in around 60% of patients with Cushing's disease and the clues to endogenous glucocorticoid excess are given by the classical clinical features.[13] Despite hormonal correction, clinical improvement may not be complete with age and associated hyperglycemia being determining factors. Muscle symptoms are part of Addison's disease, but the associated constitutional symptoms predominate and a presentation with isolated myopathy is unusual. Besides the gamut of systemic symptoms, unusual flexion contractures of abdomen, pelvic girdle, and limb muscles have been described in both primary and secondary hypoaldosteronism.[14,15] Plasma cortisol, adrenocorticotropic hormone (ACTH) levels, and ACTH suppression tests aid in diagnosis of these disorders.

Both growth hormone (GH) excess as in acromegaly and GH deficiency in hypopituitarism can have neuromuscular manifestations such as muscle weakness, decreased endurance, and muscle fatigue and is seen in up to 50% of patients. Other clinical symptoms and signs are usually prominent and should raise the clinician' suspicion.

Case 1 (Figs. 1A and B)

A 52-year-old lady with pain in pelvic girdle and difficulty in rising from the floor 2 years. Examination showed painful restriction of hip joints, mild hip weakness, and exaggerated DTR. Alkaline phosphatase was 200 U/L, serum calcium 8.9 mg/dL, serum phosphorous 1.8 mg/dL (2.5–4.5), serum parathormone 144.2 pg/mL (15–65), and vitamin D <15 ng/mL.

Case 2 (Figs. 2A to D)

A 10-year-old girl was referred to us as a case of spinal muscular atrophy (SMA). She had weakness of all four limbs.

Case 3 (Figs. 3A to E)

A 24-year-old man presented with exertional myalgia, cramps and weakness, progressive generalized muscle hypertrophy of 6 months, and a muscular build (A to E). With a suspicion of rhabdomyosarcoma, he had undergone gastrocnemius muscle biopsy elsewhere and was normal. His CK was 2,442 U/L, TSH > 100 mIU/L, free T4 < 1 μg/L, free T3 < 40 ng/dL suggestive of severe hypothyroidism. He recovered completely with eltroxin replacement.

DRUG-INDUCED/TOXIC MYOPATHIES

Dalakas defines drug-induced myopathies as a subacute rarely acute syndrome of muscle weakness, pain, and fatigue with elevated CK or myoglobinuria in a patient who did not have a preexisting muscle disorder.[16] The termination of exposure generally leads to improvement but at times weakness can be progressive or irreversible. The mere temporal sequence of exposure and symptom is not sufficient to conclude a toxic myopathy which is a diagnosis

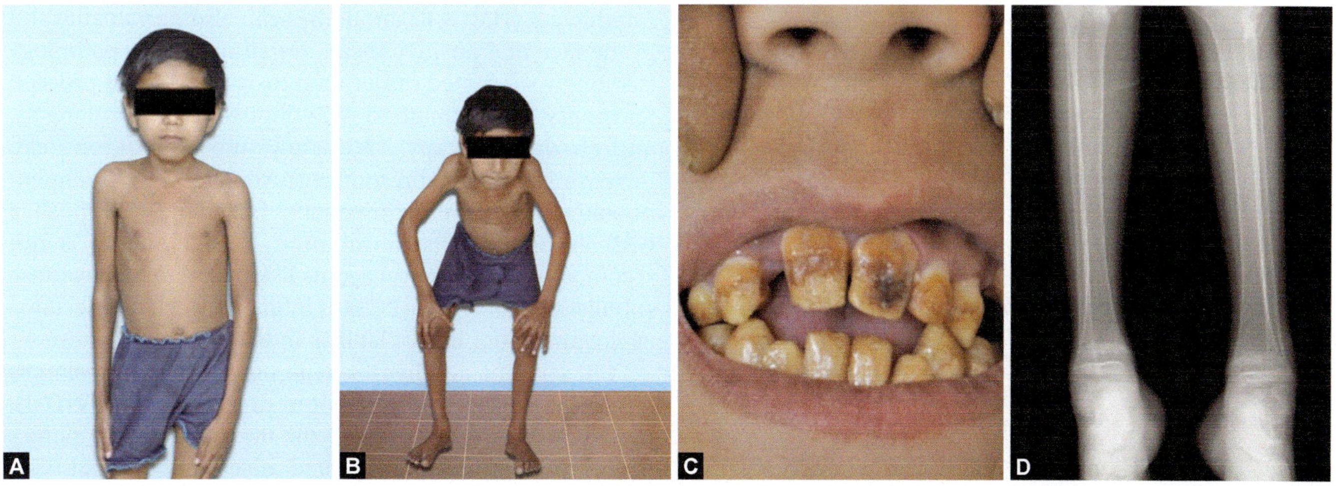

FIGS. 2A TO D: Case 2 distal renal tubular acidosis—10-year-old girl with lean body habitus (A), severe pain and difficulty to sit down and get up from floor (B), discolored teeth (C), X-ray both legs showing osteopenia, mild splaying and irregularity of distal metaphysis of bilateral tibia.

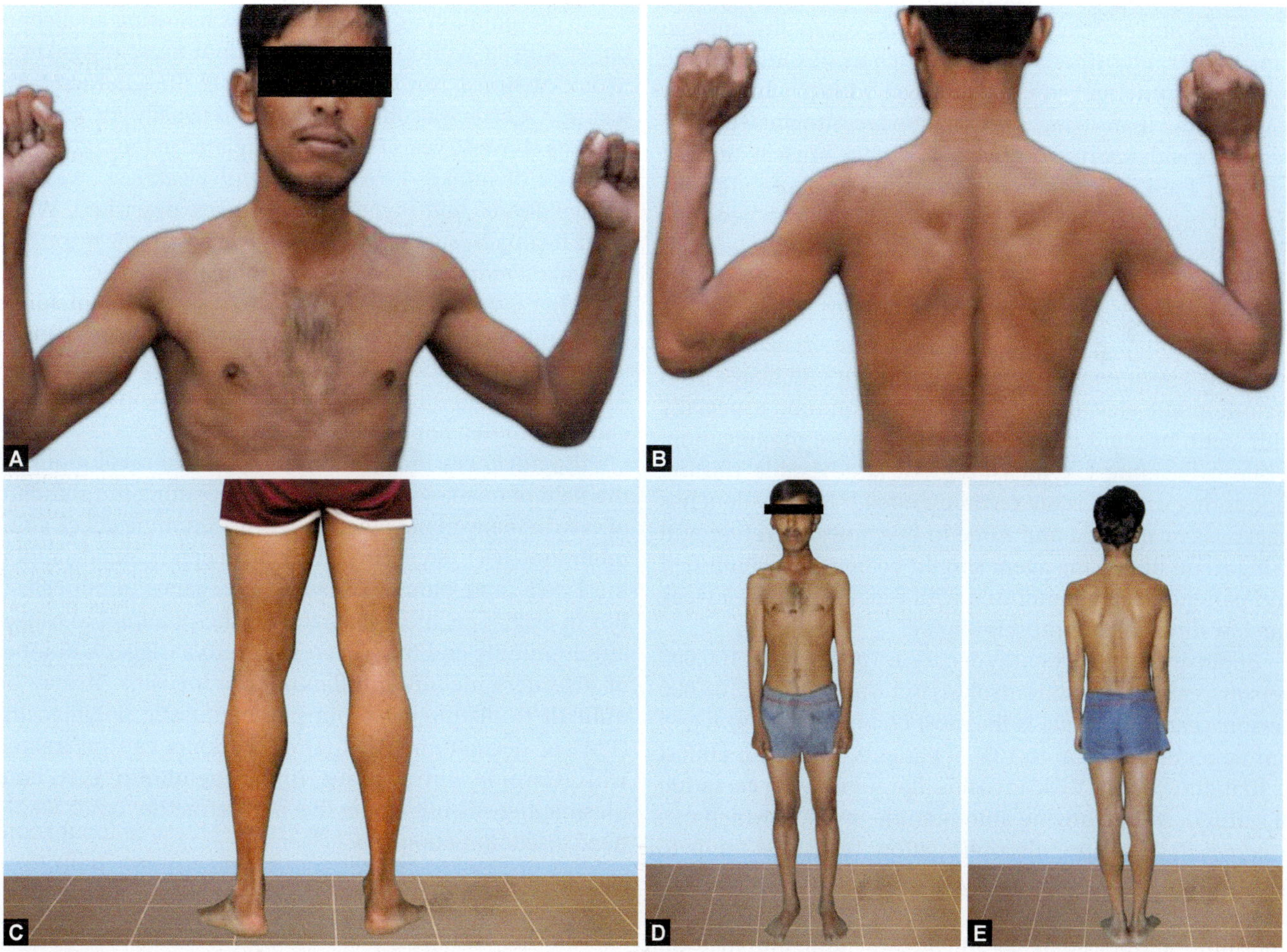

FIGS. 3A TO E: Case 3 with hypothyroid myopathy. (A to C) Muscle hypertrophy of deltoid, biceps, triceps, rhomboids, latissimus dorsi and calf muscles. (D and E) After treatment with thyroxine, symptoms subsided and muscle bulk is normal.

TABLE 1: Common drugs causing myopathy, the type, and histological pattern.[16,19]

Drugs	Histological pattern
Statins, fibrates, penicillamine, and interferons	Necrotizing and inflammatory myopathy—MHC I upregulation, T cell and macrophage invasion, and necrosis
Steroid	Type II fiber atrophy
Zidovudine	Mitochondrial myopathy
Chloroquine, hydroxychloroquine, and amiodarone	Lysosomal storage myopathy, presence of autophagic vacuoles
Colchicine	Antimicrotubular myopathy, lysosomal accumulation, and autophagic vacuoles
Alcohol	Necrotizing myopathy in acute setting, type II atrophy in chronic cases

of exclusion, and a muscle biopsy is often part of diagnostic armamentarium **(Table 1)**.

Steroid use results in type II muscle fiber atrophy and with normal CK and electromyogram (EMG), "myopathy" may be a misnomer. Fluorinated steroids such as dexamethasone are more prone and are usually seen with prednisone at doses greater than 30 mg. Presentation is as proximal muscle weakness with sparing of bulbar and neck muscle, normal reflexes. Pain is prominently absent. An acute steroid-induced myopathy has also been described which develops within days of initiation.[17] Discontinuation usually leads to gradual improvement.

Asymptomatic or mildly symptomatic hyperkalemia in patients on at-risk medications who are on agents such as statins are often a cause for concern for clinicians. Mild asymptomatic elevation of CK is not uncommon especially with statin use and do not warrant any dose modification. While a baseline CK measurement is advisable routine monitoring with CK is not recommended.[18] If the patient has weakness or myalgia and three to five times elevation and rising trend of CK, the agent should be better discontinued and patient closely monitored with repeat CK after 1 week and low threshold for muscle biopsy.

Statin-induced myopathy occurs in 5 patients per 100,000 person-years, and rhabdomyolysis in 1.6 patients per 100,000 person-years.[19] Myalgia is the most common symptom and can be reported by up to 10% of patients, but can manifest as rhabdomyolysis, toxic myositis that remits with cessation of statin or to necrotizing autoimmune myositis which can progress despite drug discontinuation. Weakness tends to be proximal and symmetric, and patients can report pain, fatigue, and cramps. Some reports suggest higher risk for lipophilic statins such as simvastatin and atorvastatin compared to hydrophilic agents such as rosuvastatin and pravastatin.[19] It usually manifests in the initial few months but cases as late as 20 years have been described but in such scenarios alternate causes such as hypothyroidism have to be excluded. Testing for 3-hydroxy-3-methylglutaryl-coenzyme A reductase (HMGCR) antibodies can also be valuable and in the face of a positive result, an autoimmune pathology is strongly suspected rather than toxic and should proceed for biopsy.[20] Combination with fibrates, azole antifungals, antiretroviral therapy, verapamil, and amiodarone can increase the risk of statin-induced myopathy.[16] The treatment in statin-induced toxic myopathy is generally supportive with immediate discontinuation. Rechallenging is not recommended and novel agents like proprotein convertase subtilisin-kexin type 9 (PCSK9) inhibitors such as injectable evolocumab may be available in India, in the near future.

Chloroquine and hydroxychloroquine are antimalarials that received much attention during the COVID-19 pandemic and are also used for their anti-inflammatory properties in rheumatological diseases. Myopathy is precipitated at high-dose chronic use and the CK level can be normal. Histologically and even clinically, it can resemble Pompe's disease with acid phosphatase positive vacuoles and respiratory involvement. Macular involvement and peripheral neuropathy have also been associated.

Alcohol can cause both acute and chronic myopathy. Acute presentation as rhabdomyolysis following an alcohol binge with or without painful proximal muscle weakness which at times can be asymmetric is the characteristic feature.[21] Chronic alcoholic myopathy is usually encountered patients above 40 years of age and is related to the cumulative quantity of intake. Proximal painful weakness, wasting, fasciculations, and myotonia have been described. While acute myopathy subsides in days to weeks, chronic myopathy may take 2 months–1 year to remit after abstinence.

Other less common causes of toxic myopathy included organophosphorus poisoning, epsilon aminocaproic acid used as antifibrinolytic agent, and D-penicillamine. Although commonly cited, zidovudine myopathy is not common Indian population.[22]

The advances in immunotherapy have revolutionized the field of oncology and is rapidly becoming the standard of care in many malignancies. In brief, immune check point inhibitors (ICI), target certain T cell receptors and disinhibit the T cells, and stimulate their action against tumor cells.[23] But in exchange, these agents have the potential to trigger autoimmunity and have been shown to a trigger a number of disorders including inflammatory myositis. It may be difficult to distinguish from paraneoplastic polymyositis (PM) or dermatomyositis (DM). Patients can be treated with steroids, intravenous immunoglobulin IVIG and plasmapheresis but aggressive and refractory cases would need discontinuation of ICI.[24]

INFECTIVE MYOPATHIES

A wide variety of agents can lead to myositis including viral, bacterial, parasitic, and rarely fungal with the course ranging from acute, subacute to chronic. Viral infections are the most common cause for an infective myositis and is often an under recognized entity. Viral agents including human immunodeficiency virus (HIV) to severe acute respiratory syndrome coronavirus 2 (SARS-CoV2) have been implicated in myositis with influenza and enteroviruses being the more common ones.[25] It is more common in children, often triggered by an exercise, and can closely resemble inflammatory myositis and even more confusing in the presence of a viral exanthem. The presence of a preceding upper respiratory or gastrointestinal "flu" could be pointers. The involvement of muscles can be focal and asymmetric, tending to involve calves more frequently, and occasionally be severe enough to cause rhabdomyolysis. HIV myositis on the other hand tends to be proximal and symmetrical and can be seen at any stage of illness. It can pose a diagnostic challenge since other causes such as drug-induced, autoimmune inflammatory, and opportunistic infection-related myositis can present in a similar fashion. A muscle magnetic resonance imaging (MRI) followed by biopsy is often required to settle the diagnosis. Treatment is generally supportive although IVIG has been occasionally tried in severe HIV-associated myopathy.

Pyomyositis refers to the localized bacterial infection and abscess formation in the muscle due to a hematogenous (primary) or extension from a contiguous structure or foreign body (secondary). Signs of local inflammation will be extravagant, with imaging or biopsy showing evidence of abscess. The most common organism implicated is *Staphylococcus aureus* (90%), followed by *Streptococcus pyogenes*, *Salmonella*, *Escherichia coli*, and pneumococci.[25] A diffuse or multiple involvement of muscles due to bacterial infection without local abscess formation is referred to as bacterial myositis. *S. aureus* and group A streptococci are incriminated in most cases. Clostridial myositis is another life-threatening bacterial myositis notorious to cause gas formation with crepitations and cutaneous blebs.

Among parasitic infections of muscle, trichinella, taenia, and toxoplasma are the most common in India. In majority of cases, patients remain asymptomatic, with the larvae reaching the muscle through gut and remain encapsulated with eventual calcification. Rarely, systemic symptoms of acute infection may be followed by myalgia, weakness, and muscle hypertrophy. Fungal myositis are rare and disseminated candidiasis, cryptococcosis, histoplasmosis, and microsporidium may be seen in severely immunocompromised individuals.

CRITICAL ILLNESS MYOPATHY

Critical illness myopathy is suspected in difficult to wean-ventilated patients who have been in intensive care unit (ICU) with multiorgan dysfunction and failures, with flaccid limbs, proximal more than distal weakness, diminished reflexes, and normal sensations **(Box 1)**.[26] Vascular, metabolic, electrical, and mitochondrial dysfunction have all been cited as contributory causes. Pathologically CIM can be divided into thick filament myopathy, acute myopathy with scattered or diffuse necrosis, diffuse cachectic myopathy, and rarely rhabdomyolysis.[27] Other treatable causes for a flaccid weakness such as Guillain–Barré syndrome (GBS) may become difficult to exclude and features such a cranial nerve involvement, diffuse areflexia and cerebrospinal fluid (CSF) albuminocytological dissociation are not seen in CIM. In the absence of any effective treatment, preventive strategies such as limiting use of neuromuscular blocking and steroids, control of hyperglycemia, and early mobilization should be initiated whenever possible in patients in ICU.

BOX 1 Diagnostic criteria for critical illness myopathy.[26]

- Background of critical illness
- Limb weakness or difficulty weaning patient from ventilator after non-neuromuscular causes have been excluded
- CMAP amplitudes <80% of the lower limit of normal in two or more nerves without conduction block
- SNAPs >80% of the lower limit of normal
- Needle EMG showing with short duration, low-amplitude motor unit potentials with early or normal full recruitment, with or without fibrillation potentials in conscious and collaborative patients; or increased CMAP duration or reduced muscle membrane excitability on direct muscle stimulation in noncollaborative patients
- Absence of a decremental response on RNS
- Muscle histopathological findings of primary myopathy

(CMAP: compound muscle action potential; EMG: electromyogram; RNS: repetitive nerve stimulation; SNAP: sensory nerve action potential)

INFLAMMATORY MYOPATHIES

Introduction

Idiopathic inflammatory myopathies/myositis (IIM) are a heterogenous group of treatable myopathies with diverse clinical manifestations with variable treatment response and prognosis.[28] Muscle weakness and myalgia are common but extramuscular manifestations such as skin rashes, arthralgia, and interstitial lung disease (ILD) also occur. The major advancement in the diagnosis and management of IIM was the discovery of myositis-specific antibodies (MSAs), specific for myositis, mutually exclusive, each with distinct disease phenotypes, organ involvement, prognosis, and thus facilitating a more personalized approach to diagnosis and management.[29] MSAs are present in nearly 50–60% of patients with IIM. 20% of IIM patients may have antibodies which are found in other autoimmune conditions such as systemic lupus erythematosus (SLE), Sjogren's syndrome, or systemic sclerosis and these antibodies are called myositis-associated antibodies (MAA).[29] Common MAAs are anti-Ro-52, anti-KU, anti-Pm-Scl, and anti-U1RNP. Nearly 20–30% of IIM patients lack antibodies and are classified as seronegative.

Though PM dominated as a major subtype of IIM historically, the discovery of MSAs has made its presence disputed. The major sub-types of IIM based on distinct clinical, histopathological features, and presence of MSAs are DM (juvenile and adult onset), antisynthetase syndrome (ASS), immune mediated necrotizing myopathy (IMNM), overlap myositis (OM), inclusion body myositis (IBM), and PM.

Various criteria have been used in the classification of IIM, the predominant ones being Bohan and Peter criteria, Dalakas criteria, and Tanimato criteria. The 2017 European League Against Rheumatism/American College of Rheumatology (EULAR/ACR) criteria were developed to circumvent the flaws of previous classification systems and provide a properly validated, weighted system for different variables which may help in better discrimination of IIM form mimickers.[30] **Table 2** gives EULAR/ACR criteria. However, with more widespread testing of MSAs and use of muscle MRIs, the current criteria may soon require revision.

Epidemiology

The incidence of IIM is 1.16–19/million/year and prevalence varies from 2.4 to 33.8 per 100,000.[31] DM, IMNM, and PM are more common in women while IBM is more common in men.[31-33] Peak age of incidence is around 50–59 years.[31,32] Infectious agents such as HIV, hepatitis B and C, and human T cell leukemia virus type 1 (HTLV1) are proposed to act as triggers for PM, DM, and IBM.[28] Extensive physical exertion, UV, radiation and smoking may be other risk factors. The major genetic risk factor for IIM localizes to human leukocyte antigen (HLA) alleles and alleles of the 8.1 ancestral haplotype are strongly associated with PM and DM.[33] Mortality varies between 10 and 30%[34,35] and is highest in the first year after diagnosis.[36] The main prognostic factors are cardiac and respiratory involvement.[36]

Pathogenesis

Complex interplay of genetic and environmental risk factors with native and adaptive immune responses plays a key role in the pathogenesis. Each subtype of IIM has unique histopathological features and transcriptome analysis has revealed unique gene expression profiles that may help in identifying IIM subtypes with >90% accuracy.[37]

Dermatomyositis is mediated by adaptive immune response with humoral B cell-mediated response, T-cell infiltration and complement deposition leading to vessel damage, ischemia, and perifascicular atrophy. Endomysial capillaries in these regions are reduced and have endothelial cell loss with membrane attack complex (MAC) deposition.[38] Intermediate-sized perimysial blood vessels are destroyed by innate immune response of plasmacytoid dendritic cells which are sources of interferons. Type 1 interferon-inducible genes are upregulated in muscles and myofibers/capillaries stain for interferon alpha/beta inducible protein MxA.[39] Immune mediated vascular damage causes ischemia and muscle fiber atrophy in watershed areas, distant from avascular regions of perimysium.

TABLE 2: EULAR/ACR classification criteria for adult and juvenile idiopathic inflammatory myopathies.

Variable	Score point without muscle biopsy	Score point with muscle biopsy
Age of onset ≥18 years and <40 years	1.3	1.5
Age of onset >40 years	2.1	2.2
Objective, symmetrical weakness, and progressive of proximal upper limbs	0.7	0.7
Objective, symmetrical weakness, and progressive of proximal lower limbs	0.8	0.5
Neck flexors weaker than neck extensors	1.9	1.6
Proximal limb weakness more than distal in lower limbs	0.9	1.2
Heliotrope rash	3.1	3.2
Gottron's papules	2.1	2.7
Gottron's sign	3.3	3.7
Dysphagia or esophageal dysmotility	0.7	0.6
Presence of anti-Jo-1 autoantibody	3.9	3.8
Elevated levels of creatine kinase (CK), lactate dehydrogenase (LDH), aspartate aminotransferase (AST), or alanine aminotransferase (ALT)	1.3	1.4
Muscle biopsy shows endomysial infiltration of mononuclear cells surrounding but not invading myofibers		1.7
Muscle biopsy shows perimysial/perivascular infiltration of mononuclear cells		1.2
Muscle biopsy shows perifascicular atrophy		1.9
Muscle biopsy shows rimmed vacuoles		3.1

Note: Definite IIM, at least 90% probability, >7.5 score without biopsy and >8.7 with biopsy, probable IIM (>55% probability)— 5.5–7.5 without biopsy and 6.7–8.7 with biopsy, possible IIM (50–55% probability) —5.3–5.5 without biopsy and 6.5–6.7 with biopsy, Non-IIM, <5.3 without biopsy and 6.5 with biopsy.

Immune response with antibodies against one of the aminoacyl transfer RNA (tRNA) synthetases as well as CD4 cells with reactivity against tRNA synthetase leads to the damage of endothelial cells, muscle, and lung tissue in ASS. Antibodies against signal recognition particle (SRP) and HMGCR are implicated in the pathogenesis of IMNM. HLA class II DRB1*11:01 allele is strongly associated with anti-HMGCR antibodies[40] and exposure to statins may further aggravate the risk of IMNM in these individuals by reducing tolerance. Antibody-mediated complement activation is proposed to cause muscle damage in IMNM, however, complement inhibitors did not cause significant improvement in IMNM patients.

Inclusion body myositis is characterized by muscle inflammation and degeneration. Inflammation is mediated by antibodies against cyclic nucleotidase NT5C1A protein as well as by CD4 and CD8+ T cells. These cells are resistant to apoptosis and hence IBM has poor response to treatment. p62 and TDP43 proteins are accumulated in muscle, thus signifying muscle degeneration too in IBM. Myositis of PM is dependent on predominant cytotoxic immune response. PM is a rare entity now and most of the studies of PM involved patients who have now been reclassified as DM, ASS, IMNM, etc. Hence, further studies are needed for understanding pathogenesis of PM.

Clinical Features

Dermatomyositis

Dermatomyositis patients present with acute or insidious onset proximal muscle weakness accompanied by a skin rash. Patients usually present with difficulty in rising from floor, climbing stairs, or lifting weights. It is usually painless. Breathlessness due to ILD or respiratory muscle weakness, congestive cardiac failure, or arrythmias due to myocarditis, dysphagia due to pharyngeal or esophageal involvement, and gastrointestinal hemorrhage due to vasculopathy may occur.[41]

The characteristic skin rashes of DM include (1) heliotrope rash—violaceous erythema of upper eyelids with edema. This may be overlooked in dark-skinned individuals. (2) Malar erythema, (3) erythema involving lower anterior neck and upper part of chest—V sign, (4) erythema over posterior neck, upper back, and shoulders extending to lateral part of arms—shawl sign, (5) Gottron's papules—erythematous/violaceous papules or plaques over extensor aspects of metacarpophalangeal/interphalangeal joints, (6) Gottron's sign—erythematous macules and patches over elbows and knees, (7) inverse Gottron's papules—on palmar aspect of hands, (8) Holster sign—erythema over lateral aspect of hips and upper thighs, (9) vasculopathic lesions such as ulceration, telangiectasias, and livedo reticularis, (10) panniculitis, alopecia, and poikiloderma. Nailfold capillary examination may show dilated and tortuous blood vessels and avascular areas.[42]

Figure 4 shows cutaneous manifestations in an adult case of DM.

Amyopathic DM has cutaneous manifestations without muscle weakness while DM sine dermatitis (adermatopathic DM) presents with isolated myositis. Juvenile dermatomyositis (JDM) occurs in children <18 years of age and has multisystem involvement and calcinosis cutis. **Figure 5** shows cutaneous manifestations in a case of JDM. CK is elevated 10–20-fold in patients with DM.

The antibodies associated with DM include—(1) anti-Mi2 (nucleosome remodeling deacetylase complex), 10–20% of cases, presents with classical clinical features and rash; (2) anti-TIF1γ (transcription intermediary factor 1γ), 8–40% of cases, has increased risk of malignancy, poikiloderma, and ovoid palatal patch;[43] (3) anti-NXP2 (nuclear matrix protein), 3–30% of cases, increased risk of malignancy, intestinal vasculopathy, dysphagia, calcinosis, and distal weakness; (4) anti-MDA5 (melanoma differentiation-associated gene; (5), nearly 10% of cases, characterized by amyopathic DM, ILD, arthritis, cutaneous ulcers, alopecia, and calcinosis; (6) anti-SAE (small ubiquitin-like modifier activating enzyme),

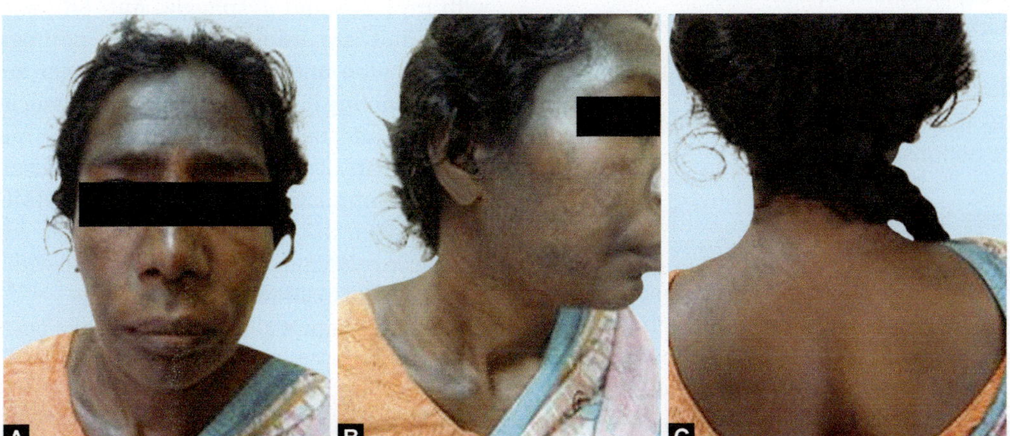

FIGS. 4A TO C: Hyperpigmentation involving face, neck, upper chest, and back in a 42-year-old lady with anti-Mi2 positivity.

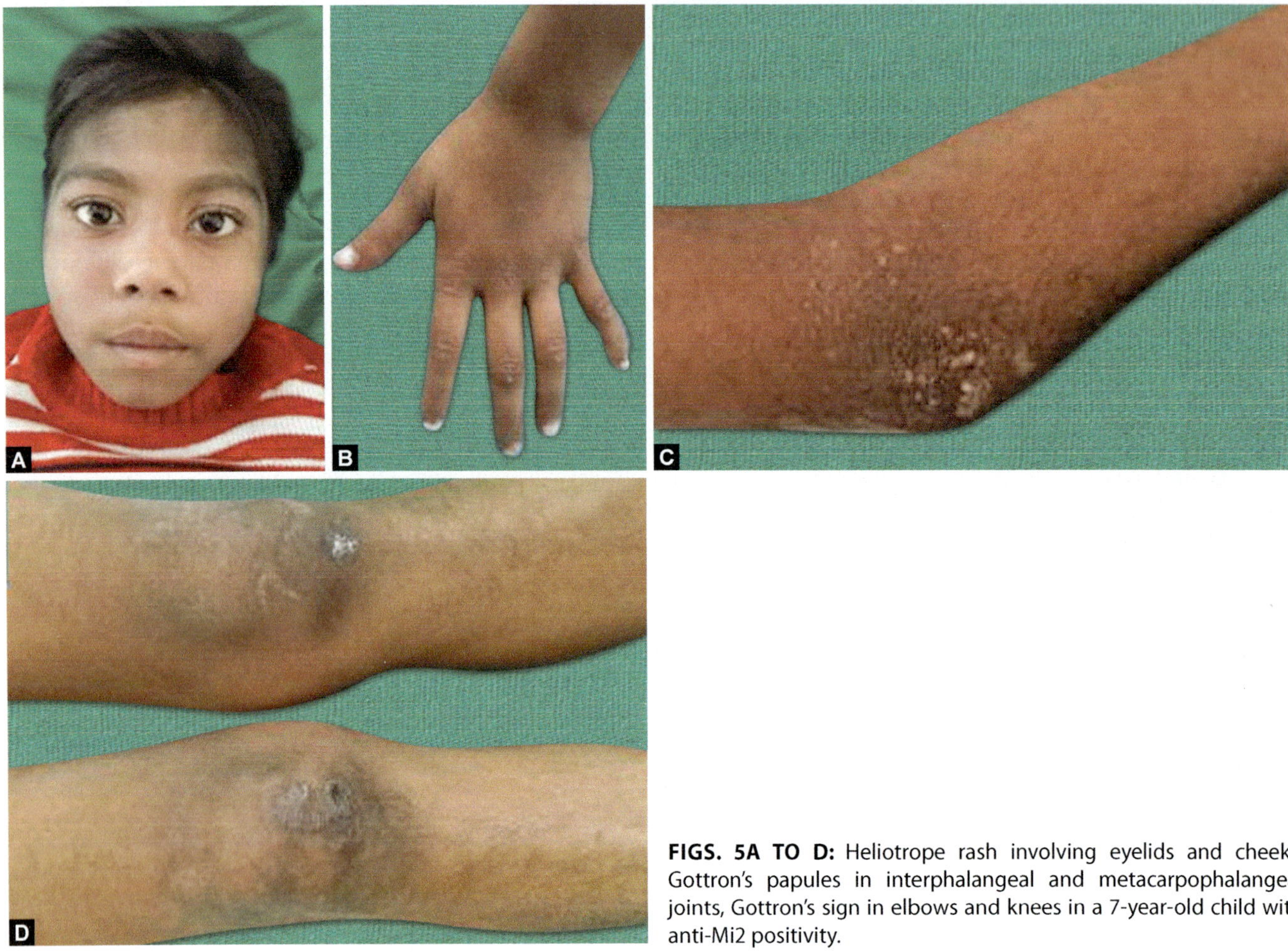

FIGS. 5A TO D: Heliotrope rash involving eyelids and cheeks, Gottron's papules in interphalangeal and metacarpophalangeal joints, Gottron's sign in elbows and knees in a 7-year-old child with anti-Mi2 positivity.

5–10% of cases, skin changes may precede myositis, "angel wing" rash on back.[44]

Dermatomyositis patients have nearly fivefold increased risk of malignancy,[45] most common malignancies associated being cancer of lung, breast, ovary, colon, cervix, pancreas, esophagus, and lymphoma. Risk of malignancy is highest in those with antibodies against NXP2 or TIF1γ.

Interstitial lung disease is common in ASS and in those with anti-MDA5 antibodies. Rapidly progressive ILD with consolidation in lower lung zones can affect those with anti-MDA5 antibodies and has a poorer prognosis.[46]

Table 3 gives the list of antibodies associated with IIM and clinical associations.

Antisynthetase Syndrome

Antisynthetase syndrome is a constellation of ILD, arthritis, fever, and Raynaud's phenomenon with antibodies against aminoacyl tRNA synthetases. Eight autoantibodies have been described in ASS and patients with antibodies against PL-7 or PL-12 have higher risk of ILD than those with anti-JO1 antibodies, Mechanic's hands (thickened, cracked skin on dorsal and ventral aspect of hands) and Hiker's feet (hyperkeratosis of toes and plantar aspect of feet) may occur in ASS.[41,47]

Figure 6 shows mechanics hands and hikers' feet in a case of ASS.

Immune-mediated Necrotizing Myopathy

Immune mediated necrotizing myopathy develops as a subacute, rapidly progressive limb weakness without skin rash. Weakness is more severe and may be associated with myalgias and dysphagia. Anti-SRP and anti-HMGCR antibodies are implicated in the pathogenesis. IMNM patients with anti-SRP may be younger and may have a more disabling illness. IMNM may be associated with statin exposure and risk of developing disease may persist even after 10 years of statin initiation or may occur many months after discontinuation. Patients with anti-HMGCR antibodies have higher risk of malignancy, lesser risk of ILD, and cardiac involvement compared to those with anti-SRP.[48] CK is elevated 20 to 50-fold.

Figure 7 shows clinical features in a case with anti-SRP positivity.

Overlap Myositis

Overlap myositis indicates myositis with other connective tissue diseases such as SLE, systemic sclerosis, or Sjögren's

TABLE 3: Antibodies implicated in IIM and clinical associations.

Antibody	Frequency (%)	Clinical manifestations
Myositis specific antibodies (MSA)		
Anti-Mi2 (nucleosome remodeling deacetylase complex)	5–20	Classical DM
Anti-NXP2 (nuclear matrix protein)	3–30	DM, malignancy, calcinosis, myalgia, dysphagia, intestinal vasculopathy, and distal weakness
Anti- MDA5 (melanoma differentiation-associated gene 5)	13–30	Amyopathic DM, arthritis, ILD, and calcinosis
Anti-TIF1γ (transcription intermediary factor 1γ)	10–20	DM, malignancy, ovoid palatal patch, and poikiloderma
Anti-SAE (small ubiquitin-like modifier activating enzyme)	5–10	Skin disease preceding myositis, "angel-wing" rash on back, and dysphagia
Anti-SRP (signal recognition particle)	5–15	IMNM, ILD, cardiac involvement
Anti-HMGCR (3-hydroxy-3-methylglutaryl CoA reductase)	6–10	IMNM, statin association
Anti-Jo-1 (histidyl tRNA synthetase)	15–30	ASS, ILD (nonspecific interstitial pneumonia), and nonerosive arthritis
Anti- PL-7 (threonyl tRNA synthetase)	5–10	ASS, more severe ILD
Anti-PL-12 (alanyl tRNA synthetase)	<5	ASS, ILD
Anti-OJ (isoleucyl tRNA synthetase)	<2	ASS
Anti-EJ (glycyl tRNA synthetase)	<2	ASS
Anti-KS (asparaginyl tRNA synthetase)	<2	ASS, especially ILD and arthritis
Anti-Ha/YRS (tyrosyl tRNA synthetase)	<1	ASS
Anti-Zo (phenylalanyl tRNA synthetase)	<1	ASS
Anti-FHL-1 (four and a half LIM-domains 1)	5–10	IIM with severe muscle involvement
Myositis-associated antibodies (MAA)		
Anti-Pm-Scl (human exosome protein complex)	8–10	PM, DM, and scleroderma overlap
Anti-U1RNP (U1 small nuclear RNP)	10	Mixed connective tissue disease
Anti-Ku (Regulatory subunit of DNA-dependent protein kinase)	<2	Overlap with scleroderma and ILD
Anti-Ro (TRIM21, ring-shaped protein binding Y RNAs)	10–40	Severe disease
Anti-RuvBL1 and anti-RuvBL2 (nuclear proteins RuvBL1/2)	3	Overlap with scleroderma
Anti-cN-1A (cytosolic 5′-nucleotidase 1a)	5–20	IBM, SLE, and Sjogren's syndrome

(ASS: antisynthetase syndrome; DM: dermatomyositis; IBM: inclusion body myositis; IIM: idiopathic inflammatory myopathy; ILD: interstitial lung disease; IMNM: immune-mediated necrotizing myopathy; PM: polymyositis; SLE: systemic lupus erythematosus)

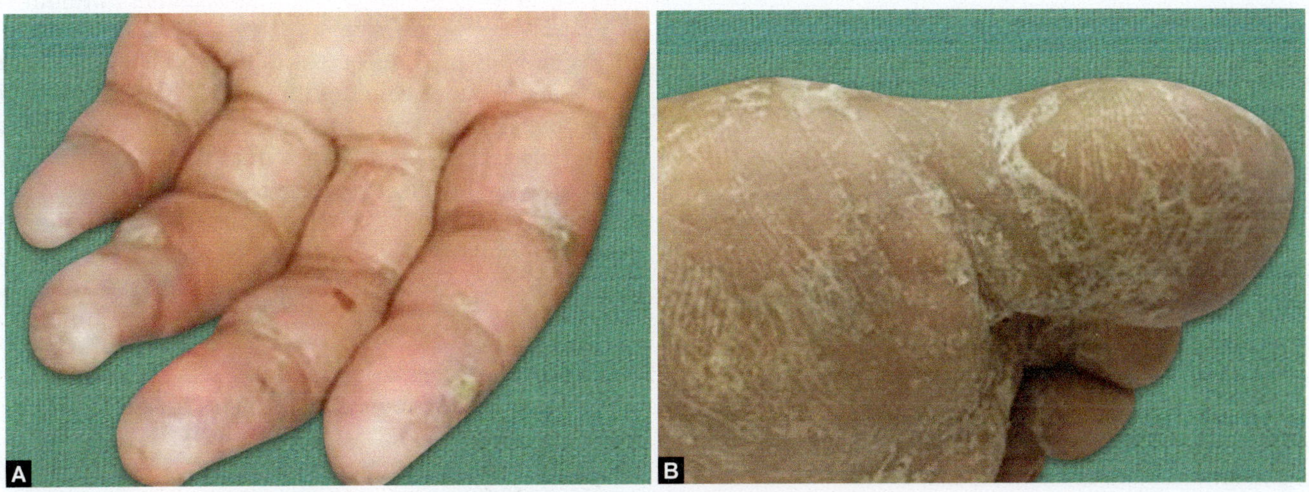

FIGS. 6A AND B: Mechanics hands and Hikers feet in a patient with antisynthetase syndrome.

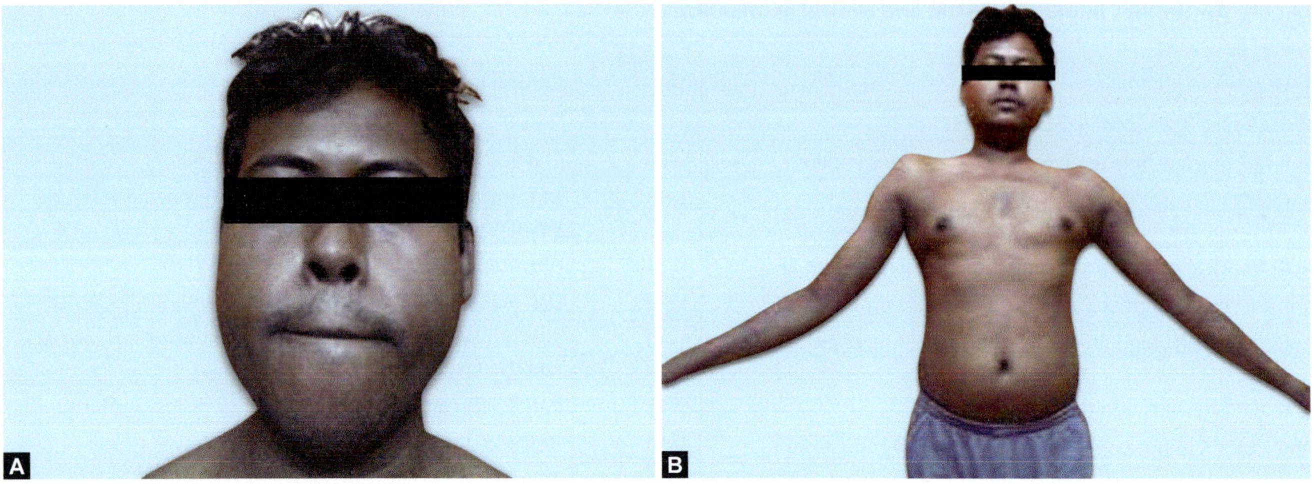

FIGS. 7A AND B: Hyperpigmentation of face, bifacial weakness, proximal muscle wasting, and upper limb weakness in a 34-year-old man with antisignal recognition particle positivity.

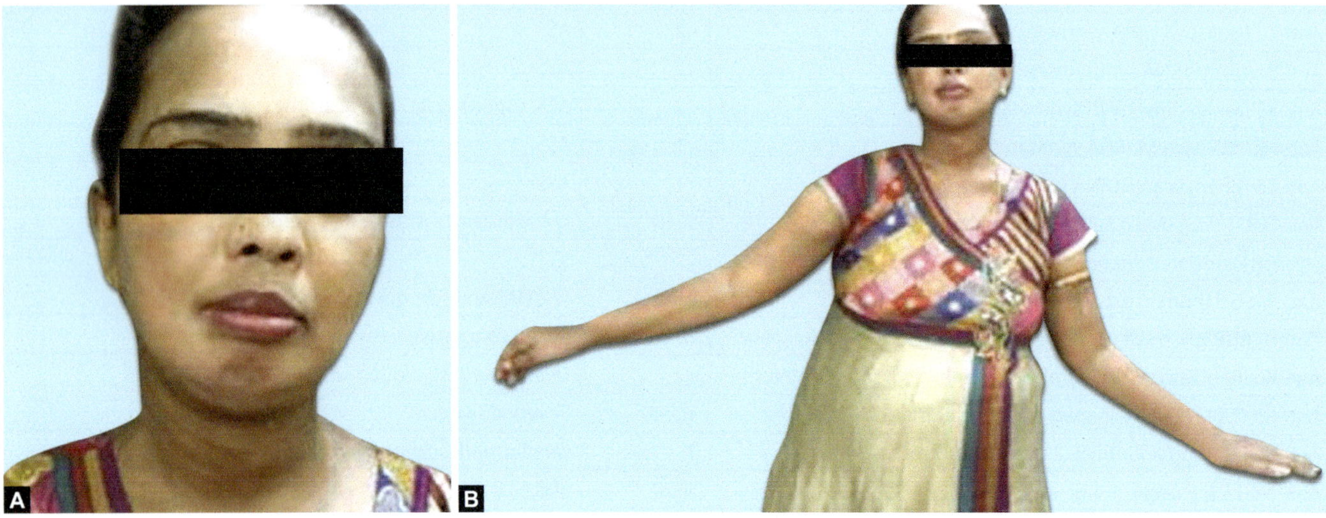

FIGS. 8A AND B: Malar rash and severe proximal weakness in a 35-year-old lady with anti-OJ positivity.

syndrome. Antibodies found in these patients include anti-Pm Scl, anti-U1 RNP, anti-RuvBL1, anti-RuvBL2, anti-Ku, anti-Ro/SS-A, and anti-La/SS-B. Patients with scleroderma and myositis are termed scleromyositis. Head drop, distal weakness, and extramuscular manifestations may occur.

Figure 8 shows a patient with OM due to anti-OJ positivity.

Polymyositis

Polymyositis is a diagnosis of exclusion and presents with muscle and extramuscular involvement similar to DM. It is more common in women above 20 years of age and may present with subacute or chronic progressive proximal limb and neck flexor weakness. Dysphagia may occur in one-third of patients. ILD and myocarditis may occur.

Inclusion Body Myositis

Inclusion body myositis occurs in patients above 40 years of age and is more common in men. It has an insidious onset and slow progression, involving both proximal and distal muscles. Forearm flexors, quadriceps, and anterior tibial muscles are affected leading to early falls. Dysphagia is common. Cytosolic 5'nucleotidase 1A is the antibody associated with IBM.

Indian Experience

There are several case reports and case series from India.[49-52] In an unpublished cohort of 104 patients from our institute, there were 30 cases of DM, 22 cases of IMNM, 43 cases of OM, and 9 cases of ASS. Age at onset in adult patients ranged

TABLE 4: The pattern of antibody positivity.

MSA		MAA	
Mi2b	27	PM-Scl 100 and PM-Scl 75	14
SRP	20	Ro-52 alone	18
PL-7 PL-12	7	Sm-RNP	3
OJ	2	Ro-52 with Sm-RNP	2
NXP-2	2	Ku	2
MDA5	1	Ku + Ro	1
HMGCR	2	ANA (more than 1:80) homogenous/ nucleolar/cytoplasm	3
		PM-Scl 100 and PM-Scl 75	14
		Ro-52 alone	18

(ANA: antinuclear antibody; HMGCR: 3-hydroxy-3-methylglutaryl CoA reductase; MAA: myositis-associated antibodies; MDA5: melanoma differentiation-associated gene 5; MSA: myositis-specific antibodies; PM: polymyositis; SRP: signal recognition particle)

from 6–67 years (mean 37.7 ± 15.5) and age at evaluation ranged from 7 to 67.5 years (mean 39.3 ± 15.8). There were nine cases of JDM, age of onset 10.4 ± 4 years and age at evaluation 11 ± 4.1 years.

Hyperpigmentation and proximal limb weakness were most common presenting features. Dysphagia was more common in ASS and IMNM while respiratory involvement was more common in ASS and DM. ILD was seen in three cases each of OM and IMNM and two cases of DM with anti-Mi2 positive status. Paraneoplastic profile was positive in three cases of DM (anti-Yo in 2, anti-titin-1), and OM each (anti-SOX-1, Anti-titin-1, and anti-CV2/CRMP5-1) **(Table 4)**.

LABORATORY INVESTIGATIONS

The diagnostic repertoire of inflammatory myositis has expanded hugely with exciting developments in the pipeline. The current laboratory investigation are listed in **Table 5**.

Creatine kinase may be elevated 10–50 times the normal limits in DM, the values are usually much higher in necrotizing myositis and OM. However, the values may be normal.[53] Also, note that the decrease in CK alone is not a sign of improvement.[54] In some cases with normal CK, serum aldolase may be elevated.

Histopathology

The pathological features of DM include:

- Perifascicular atrophy (specificity > 90%, sensitivity 25–50%, detected by routine histochemistry)
- Perimysial inflammation
- Perifascicular expression of MHC class I, binding of complement to capillaries, and the surface of sarcolemma (less sensitive and specific)
- Perifascicular human myxovirus resistance protein 1[55] and retinoic acid-inducible gene 1 expression (sensitivity—71% and 50% respectively, detected by immunohistochemistry)
- Cellular infiltrates of dendritic cells, B cells, CD4 T cells, and macrophages
- Microtubular inclusions in intramuscular capillaries (electron microscopy) and capillary drop-out.[39,54,56]
- Vacuolated/punched out fibers in anti-TIF1γ antibody disease; microinfarctions in anti-NXP2 antibody disease **(Figs. 9A to D)**.

TABLE 5: Recommended investigations.

Muscle enzymes	Creatine kinase, AST, ALT, LDH, rarely aldolase
Autoantibodies	Serum myositis-specific and myositis-associated autoantibodies
Muscle biopsy	H&E, MGT, NADH-TR, SDH, ATPase, and immunostaining for expression of MHC class I and MHC class II, CD4, and CD8
Muscle special stains	Immunohistochemistry, electron microscopy if available
Electrophysiology	NCS and EMG
Imaging of muscle	MRI of muscle
Pulmonary function test	FVC and DLCO
Lung imaging	High-resolution CT thorax
Cardiac evaluation	Electrocardiogram and echocardiogram
	Video fluoroscopy for dysphagia
Screening for malignancy	Whole body PET-MRI/malignancy work-up like mammography, colonoscopy, chest, and abdomen scans
	Bone density scan in patients on steroids

(ALT: alanine transaminase; AST: aspartate transaminase; ATPase: adenosine triphosphatase stain; CT: computed tomography; DLCO: diffusing capacity of lung for carbon monoxide; EMG: electromyography; H&E: hematoxylin & eosin stain; LDH: lactate dehydrogenase; MHC: major histocompatibility complex; MGT: modified Gomori trichrome stain; MRI: magnetic resonance imaging; NADH-TR: nicotinamide adenine dinucleotide dehydrogenase-tetrazolium reductase stain; NCS: nerve conduction study; SDH: succinate dehydrogenase stain)

Polymyositis

Histopathologically, invasion of muscle fibers with endomysial cytotoxic CD8+ T cells and upregulation of MHC class I, macrophages surrounding, and invading non-necrotic muscle fibers is a characteristic feature seen but this histological feature is not just unique for PM, but even more common in IBM.[57]

Necrotizing Myopathy

Pathologically, there are scattered necrotic fibers with focal upregulation of MHC class I; binding of complement to sarcolemma and surface of capillaries and MAC deposition on non-necrotic fibers. Histopathology findings in necrotizing myopathy (NM) do not show primary inflammatory lesions as well as there are no tubuloreticular

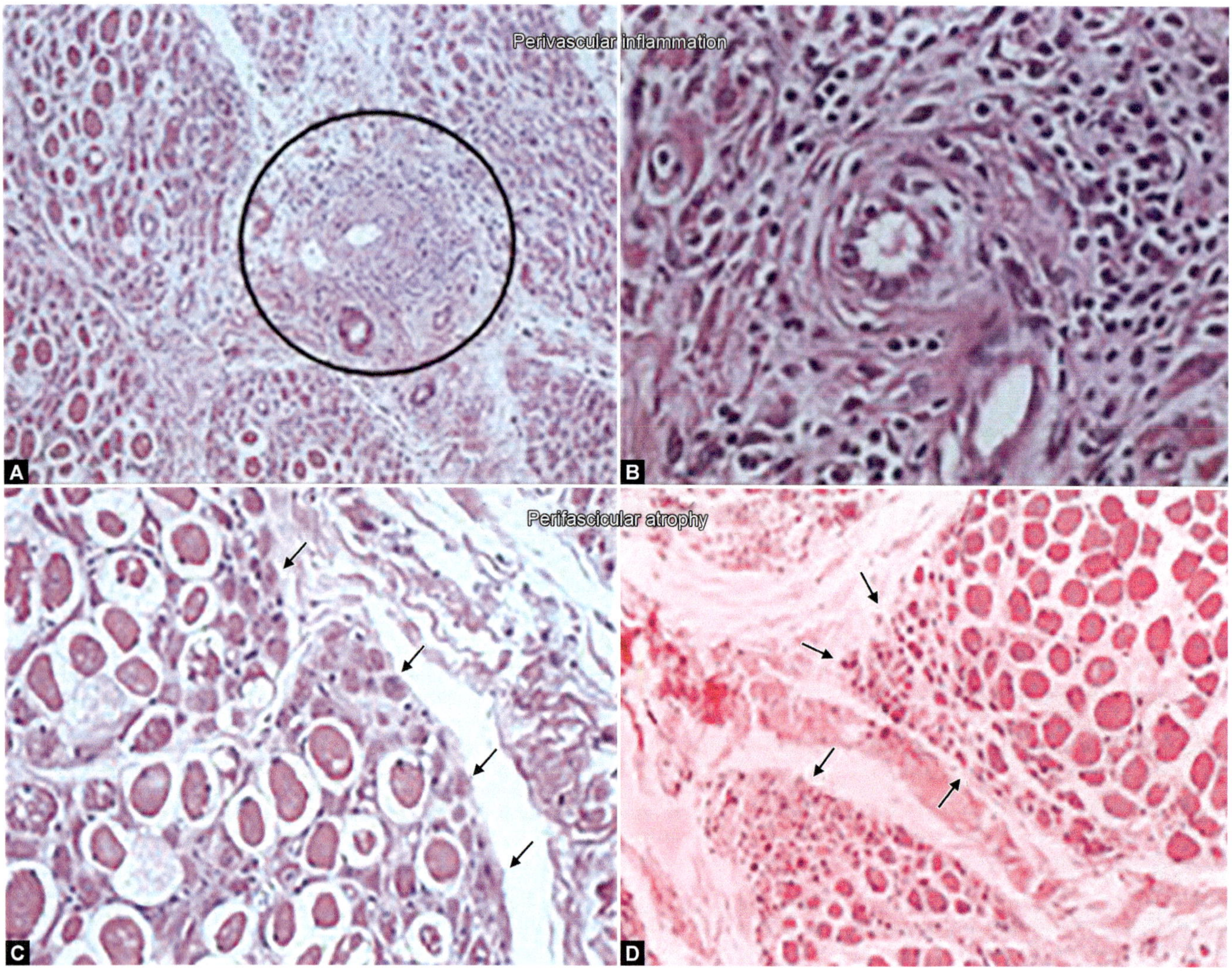

FIGS. 9A TO D: Muscle biopsy in a case of dermatomyositis showing perifascicular inflammation and atrophy.

inclusions found in the endothelial cells.[58] However, some cases with anti-SRP or anti-HMGCR antibodies may have lymphocytic infiltrates.[48]

Overlap Myositis

Perifascicular necrosis and perifascicular binding of MHC class 1 and class 2 antibodies and complement binding to sarcolemma are the histological findings in OM. Compared to DM, the amount of necrosis is more in ASS biopsies. Nuclear actin aggregation is another feature on electron microscopy which is specific for this group.

Inclusion Body Myositis

Histologically, IBM is characterized by endomysial inflammation, invasion of non-necrotic muscle fibers by mononuclear cells especially CD8 T cells, up regulation of MHC class 1; amyloid deposition and presence of protein accumulation, tubulofilament inclusions in electron microscopy; and signs of mitochondrial damage in the form of excessive cytochrome oxidase c negative fibers and paracrystalline inclusions.[59]

Imaging Findings in Inflammatory Muscle Diseases

The inflammation is usually symmetrical and involves the proximal muscle groups in PM and DM, but the muscle involvement can be patchy and asymmetric. Short tau inversion recovery (STIR) can be used to differentiate between involved and uninvolved muscles. STIR and fat-saturated gadolinium-enhanced T1-weighted images often show high signal intensity (HSI) in the active phase. In other times, inflammation may extend only along individual muscles and muscle groups along the myofascial distribution. In chronic phase, fatty atrophy of the musculature is seen on T1-weighted images.

In DM, the subcutaneous adipose tissue, fasciae, and the muscle show HSI on STIR MRI sequences. The HSI is situated more peripherally and in a honeycomb pattern in muscles in DM. JDM generally takes a more severe clinical course, which is shown by the extent and intensity of cutaneous, subcutaneous, and muscular signal abnormalities on MRI. In IMNM, MRI shows more widespread muscle edema, atrophy, and fatty replacement as compared to DM, PM, and IBM.

Magnetic resonance imaging in IBM shows focally increased signal is seen on STIR and fat-saturated gadolinium-enhanced T1-weighted images, more in the anterior thigh compartment.[60] Overall, MRI of muscles can be used to assess disease activity, and choose appropriate biopsy sites in myositis **(Figs. 10A to C)**.

Positron emission tomography (PET) MRI is another important diagnostic modality which helps detecting associated systemic malignancy in early stages. Breast and ovarian cancers are common in women, whereas lung and prostate cancers predominate in men. Other malignancies include lymphoma, colon, pancreatic, and bladder cancer.[41] While in the Asian population, nasopharyngeal carcinoma is reported to be the most common followed by gastric and hepatobiliary tract cancers **(Fig. 11)**.[61]

High-resolution Computed Tomography of the Chest

Organizing pneumonia pattern is common, especially in anti-SAE and anti-MDA5 antibody subgroups. Organizing pneumonia and nonspecific interstitial pneumonia patterns were almost equally frequent in patients with aminoacyl tRNA synthetase antibodies. Nonspecific interstitial pneumonia pattern was associated with a mild clinical course. Rapidly progressive ILD in DM is commonly associated with lower lung zone consolidation.[46] Usual interstitial pneumonia pattern is rare. Acute lung injury and diffuse alveolar damage may be seen in acute presentations.[62-64]

Cardiac Manifestations

Cardiomyopathy, arrhythmias, myocarditis, pericarditis, and cardiac failure are known complications and screening for these is essential.[65]

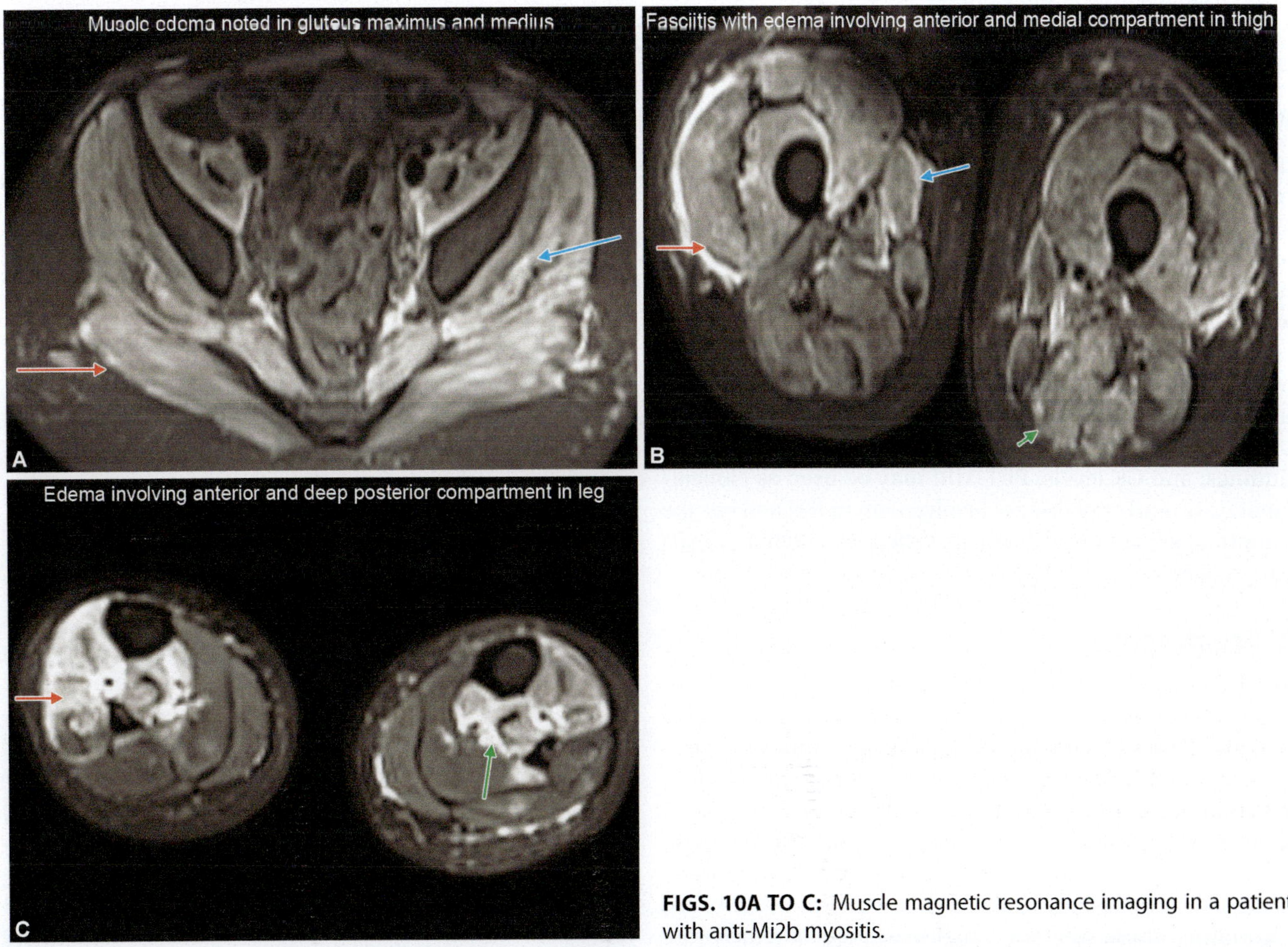

FIGS. 10A TO C: Muscle magnetic resonance imaging in a patient with anti-Mi2b myositis.

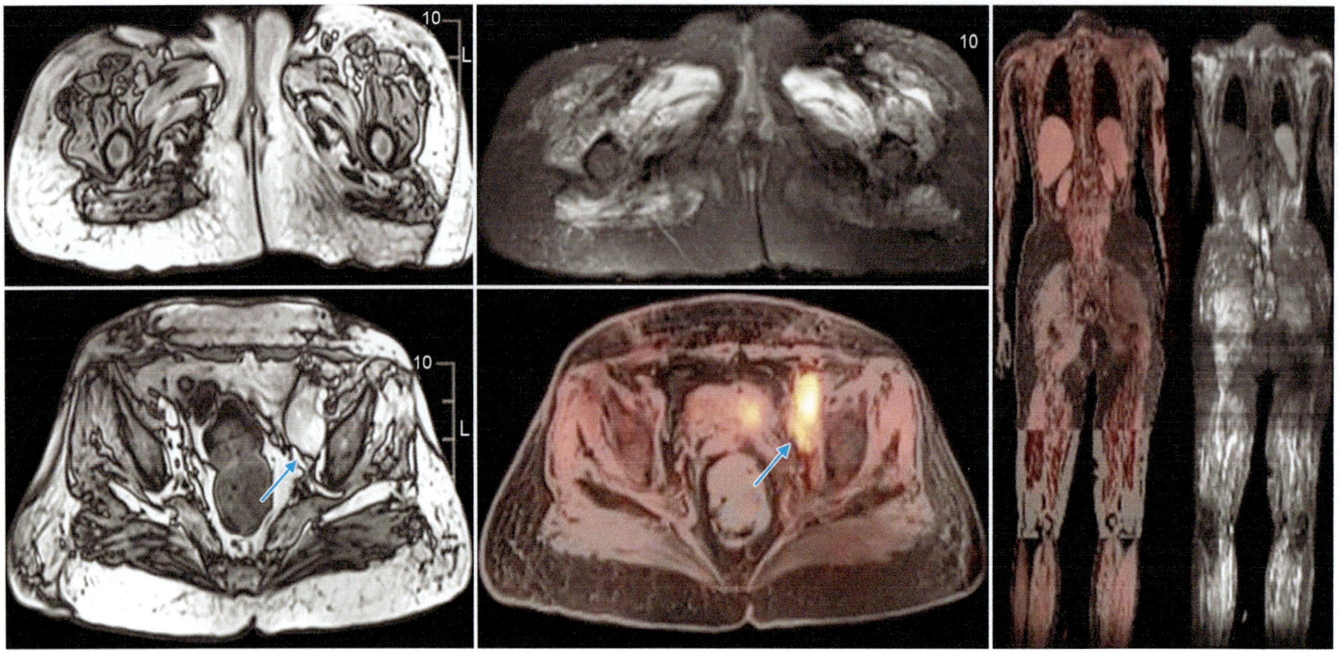

FIG. 11: PET-MRI in a patient with IIM. A 40-year-old female, operated for Ca cervix 7 years back, 5-month history of progressive painful proximal weakness of UL and LL and neck flexor weakness and dysphagia. No rash. CK was 3,000. Anti-SRP strong positive, Ro52 strong positive. PET MR showed diffuse myoedema and hypermetabolic, necrotic left inguinal lymph nodes (blue arrow).

(CK: creatine kinase; MRI: magnetic resonance imaging; PET: positron emission tomography; SRP: signal recognition particle)

Our Experience

In unpublished data from our center, muscle MRI revealed more severe muscle edema in anti-Mi2b group compared to anti-SRP myositis. Fasciitis was present in all patients with anti-Mi2b myositis. It was observed that peroneal group was specifically affected in anti-Mi2b group but spared in anti-SRP group, however, we are awaiting results on a larger cohort. In another unpublished study on PET-MRI in 30 cases of IIM from our center, PET reflected the severity of muscle inflammation, showing good association with severity of muscle weakness, Mi2B positivity, histopathological findings, and CK levels. PET-MRI may be used as clinical/laboratory marker of disease involvement in IIM and has the important advantage of detecting systemic malignancy in its early stages.

Treatment

The treatment of inflammatory myopathies is individual-centric, based both on clinical and investigation profile of the patients. Several factors play a key role including the age of patient, rapidity of onset, the severity of illness, coexistence of other immune/nonimmune-mediated diseases such as infections, diabetes, respiratory/bulbar involvement, antibody profile, and so on. Often, the decision at bedside is guided by these factors rather than strict protocol-based algorithms. These subgroups of diseases are extremely rare and so it is difficult to organize a randomized-controlled trial (RCT) to recommend a particular class of treatment.

The inflammatory myopathies respond well to immunomodulation. However, the response may not be adequate in some patients especially when the treatment is delayed as the muscle tissue gets fibrosed or undergoes fatty changes. Some patients may worsen even on treatment. Steroids constitute the initial therapeutic intervention unless a situation like infections demand otherwise.

The usual immunomodulation to start with are glucocorticoids except in the case of IBM.[66] This is accepted universally and given at a dose of 0.5–1 mg/kg/day; however, the authors rarely use beyond 60 mg/day in view of significant adverse effects. For acute and severe cases, intravenous glucocorticoids are initiated at a dose of around 1,000 mg IV daily for 3–5 days and later switched over to oral medication. The duration of treatment is guided by the clinical response and generally lasts up to 12 weeks followed by a slow taper initially by 10 mg every 1 or 2 weeks followed by 5 mg every week. Patients may require long-term maintenance treatment and hence have to be monitored for adverse effects such as diabetes, hypertension, osteoporosis, cataracts, weight gain, mood swings, and infections.[54] They can be given calcium supplements as prophylaxis for osteoporosis. The patients with DM have to be explained regarding skin manifestations including use of sunscreens, avoiding UV exposure, and topical glucocorticoids.

In two RCTs on refractory IIM, IVIG caused improvement in manual muscle testing (MMT) scores compared to placebo.[67-69] However, in the trial by Miyasaka et al., patients on placebo too noted similar improvement, however, the time to major improvement was shorter in patients on IVIG. IVIG can be given at 2 g/kg over 5 days every month. Subcutaneous immune globulin has also been tried to sustain remission. Several retrospective case series on IVIG have shown benefit for both muscular and extramuscular manifestations such as lung involvement, skin, and respiratory manifestations. It is particularly useful in patients where glucocorticoids are contraindicated as in the case of concomitant infections. Both dosage and time interval between successive pulses of IVIG have to be individualized as per response. It is generally well tolerated; however, there are adverse effects.

Steroid-sparing immunomodulation is necessary in most cases. First-line agents include azathioprine, mycophenolate, and methotrexate which are commonly used. Second-line agents are cyclosporin and tacrolimus, but are not routinely used due to their side-effect profile. Other commonly used immunosuppressants include cyclophosphamide, IVIG, and rituximab (RTX). Experimental treatments such as abatacept, leflunomide, baricitinib, tocilizumab, anakinra, sifalimumab, and Janus kinase (JAK) inhibitors (tofacitinib and ruxolitinib) are rarely used. There are reports of tumor necrosis factor alpha (TNFα) inhibitors worsening and/or inducing myositis, hence they are best avoided. Though not supported by RCTs, plasmapheresis has been used in few case series with some therapeutic benefit.[70]

The detailed description of the mechanism of action and adverse events of these immunosuppressants has been discussed in another chapter on Myasthenia Gravis by the same authors. Few relevant points have been discussed in this chapter. Azathioprine, given at a usual dose of 2–3 mg/kg/day, is prescribed only in patients with normal thiopurine methyltransferase activity. However, the authors prefer other drugs in view of the delay in onset of action with azathioprine. There was no significant difference between azathioprine and methotrexate in terms of efficacy and adverse effects in a recent study on 102 antisynthetase antibody positive patients.[71] Another study comparing azathioprine with mycophenolate in myositis associated ILD reported similar efficacy but reduced risk of adverse reactions with mycophenolate.[72] Methotrexate (10–25 mg every week) should be avoided in patients with ILD. Cyclophosphamide in a dose of 1 g/m^2 in monthly pulses may be used in patients with severe disease, ILD, and in systemic sclerosis.[73,74]

Rituximab, a commonly used drug, is a chimeric monoclonal antibody against the CD20 antigen expressed on B lymphocytes. Shockingly, the first placebo-phase trial of RTX in refractory myositis did not show a significant difference between the two treatment groups, but its study design was faulty and hence the results are not accurate. The largest RCT on RTX, i.e., RTX in myositis (RIM) showed significant improvement in 83% of the 195 individuals refractory to steroids and one another immunosuppressant.[75] Another study found a significant clinical improvement in patients with antisynthetase antibody (ARS-ab) subtype.[76] In a review of 458 patients with myositis treated with RTX, 78.3% responded well especially those with positive myositis-specific autoantibodies.[77]

Some patients develop secondary complications such as rhabdomyolysis and myocarditis. Special attention is a must to these factors. We have to look for symptoms of heart failure, arrhythmias, look for electrocardiogram (ECG) changes, Echocardiogram (Echo), troponin I levels, and NT-pro BNP levels (N-terminal pro-brain natriuretic peptide) as markers of heart failure and manage accordingly. Cardiac MRI in these cases shows myocardial edema, early gadolinium enhancement, late gadolinium enhancement in ventricular septal, basal and mid-cavity segments, subendocardium, and intramural myocardium.[78]

Extramuscular manifestations require multispecialty care; referrals to dermatology, pulmonology, rheumatology, and oncology in case of manifestations are mandated. Gastrointestinal bleeding is known in children with JDM due to vasculopathy. All patients should benefit from a structured rehabilitation program and physiotherapy.[54]

Management of Inclusion Body Myositis

Even though IBM has been extensively studied, currently no effective treatment plan is available. There was no significant improvement with usual immunosuppressants such as steroids and methotrexate in several clinical trials. However, alemtuzumab provided transient improvement in a study. In another study, downmodulation of inflammatory markers was seen, without any change in the degenerative molecules.[57] Three placebo-controlled clinical trials assessed effects of IVIG in IBM given for 3–6 months. The results are contradictory, mostly with no significant impact on muscle strength and most studies have only a short follow-up period.[69] Drugs targeting degenerative pathways such as arimoclomol, rapamycin, bimagrumab, follistatin, and oxandrolone have been tried without much benefit and some are in trial phase.[59]

Nearly two-thirds of the patients suffer from impaired swallowing due to functional stenosis of the upper esophageal sphincter, which is detected by video fluoroscopy or real-time MRI.[79] Certain local treatments include cricopharyngeal myotomy, pharyngoesophageal balloon dilatation, and botulinum toxin to temporarily inactivate the muscle by injecting into the upper esophageal sphincter. Cricopharyngeal myotomy is an effective technique, but it is irreversible; hence patients may later present with reflux or other swallowing difficulties.[41] Percutaneous feeding tube can be advised.

Trials targeting muscle-inhibiting transforming growth factor beta (TGF-β) molecules or muscle growth factors are being done. Resistance exercises with occupational and rehabilitation therapies are known to improve ambulation and balance and also avoid disuse atrophy and prevent joint contractures which are seen particularly in certain subgroups like anti-NXP2 myositis.[20]

CONCLUSION

Acquired myopathies comprise a heterogeneous group of muscle diseases. A high index of suspicion will help us identify endocrine or drug-induced myopathies as they may mimic other chronic degenerative myopathies.

Inflammatory myopathies are a group of rare muscle diseases with diverse clinical manifestations including a range of extramuscular manifestations. The diagnosis is usually made by a combination of clinical manifestations, laboratory tests, myositis-specific and myositis-associated antibodies, and muscle biopsy. Additional investigations to look for ILD, malignancies, dysphagia assessment, and other rheumatologic manifestations are needed. The mainstay of treatment of IIM includes steroids and other immunosuppressants which are tailored individually based on the clinical profile of the patient. Patients have to be carefully monitored for the side effects of these immunosuppressive drugs and also other systemic involvement. Newer drugs are added to the armamentarium including biologics. Early diagnosis and a comprehensive treatment, however, remain crucial to the management. With the discovery of new antibodies, it is expected that treatment can be further individualized and more targeted.

REFERENCES

1. Russell JA. Osteomalacic myopathy. Muscle Nerve. 1994;17(6): 578-80.
2. Bhadada SK, Bhansali A, Upreti V, Subbiah S, Khandelwal N. Spectrum of neurological manifestations of idiopathic hypoparathyroidism and pseudohypoparathyroidism. Neurol India. 2011;59(4):586.
3. Nora DB, Fricke D, Becker J, Gomes I. Hypocalcemic myopathy without tetany due to idiopathic hypoparathyroidism: case report. Arq Neuro-Psiquiatr. 2004;62:154-7.
4. Policepatil SM, Caplan RH, Dolan M. Hypocalcemic Myopathy Secondary to Hypoparathyroidism. WMJ. 2012;111(4):173-5.
5. Frame B, Heinze EG, Block MA, Manson GA. Myopathy in primary hyperparathyroidism. Ann Intern Med. 1968;68(5):1022-7.
6. Turken SA, Cafferty M, Silverberg SJ, De La Cruz L, Cimino C, Lange DJ, et al. Neuromuscular involvement in mild, asymptomatic primary hyperparathyroidism. Am J Med. 1989;87(5):553-7.
7. Zhu CY, Sturgeon C, Yeh MW. Diagnosis and management of primary hyperparathyroidism. JAMA. 2020;323(12):1186-7.
8. Mallette LE, Patten BM, Engel WK. Neuromuscular disease in secondary hyperparathyroidism. Ann Intern Med. 1975;82(4):474-83.
9. Duyff RF, den Bosch JV, Laman DM, van Loon BJP, Linssen WHJP. Neuromuscular findings in thyroid dysfunction: a prospective clinical and electrodiagnostic study. J Neurol Neurosurg Psychiatry. 2000;68(6):750-5.
10. Olson BR, Klein I, Benner R, Burdett R, Trzepacz P, Levey GS. Hyperthyroid myopathy and the response to treatment. Thyroid. 1991;1(2):137-41.
11. Li Q, Liu Y, Zhang Q, Tian H, Li J, Li S. Myopathy in hyperthyroidism as a consequence of rapid reduction of thyroid hormone: A case report. Medicine. 2017;96(30):e7591.
12. Vignesh G, Balachandran K, Kamalanathan S, Hamide A. Myoedema. A clinical pointer to hypothyroid myopathy. Indian J Endocrinol Metab. 2013;17(2):352.
13. Vogel F, Braun LT, Rubinstein G, Zopp S, Künzel H, Strasding F, et al. Persisting muscle dysfunction in cushing's syndrome despite biochemical remission. J Clin Endocrinol Metabol. 2020;105(12):e4490-8.
14. Ebinger G, Six R, Bruyland M, Somers G. Flexion contractures: A forgotten symptom in Addison's disease and hypopituitarism. Lancet. 1986;328(8511):858.
15. Nishlkawa T. Flexion contractures possibly reflect the existence of hypocortisolism. Intern Med. 2003;42(8):629-31.
16. Dalakas MC. Toxic and drug-induced myopathies. J Neurol Neurosurg Psychiatry. 2009;80(8):832-8.
17. Haran M, Schattner A, Kozak N, Mate A, Berrebi A, Shvidel L. Acute steroid myopathy: a highly overlooked entity. QJM. 2018;111(5):307-11.
18. Wiklund O, Pirazzi C, Romeo S. Monitoring of lipids, enzymes, and creatine kinase in patients on lipid-lowering drug therapy. Curr Cardiol Rep. 2013;15(9):397.
19. Valiyil R, Christopher-Stine L. Drug-related myopathies of which the clinician should be aware. Curr Rheumatol Rep. 2010;12(3):213-20.
20. Selva-O'Callaghan A, Alvarado-Cardenas M, Pinal-Fernández I, Trallero-Araguás E, Milisenda JC, Martínez MÁ, et al. Statin-induced myalgia and myositis: an update on pathogenesis and clinical recommendations. Expert Rev Clin Immunol. 2018;14(3):215-24.
21. Simon L, Jolley SE, Molina PE. Alcoholic myopathy: Pathophysiologic mechanisms and clinical implications. Alcohol Res. 2017;38(2):207-17.
22. Sagar A, Mohanty AP, Bahal A. Zidovudine-induced myopathy: A study in Indian patients. J Neurosci Rural Pract. 2010;1(2):63-6.
23. Robert C. A decade of immune-checkpoint inhibitors in cancer therapy. Nat Commun. 2020;11(1):3801.
24. Solimando AG, Crudele L, Leone P, Argentiero A, Guarascio M, Silvestris N, et al. Immune checkpoint inhibitor-related myositis: from biology to bedside. Int J Mol Sci. 2020;21(9):3054.
25. Narayanappa G, Nandeesh BN. Infective myositis. Brain Pathol. 202127;31(3):e12950.
26. Latronico N, Bolton CF. Critical illness polyneuropathy and myopathy: a major cause of muscle weakness and paralysis. Lancet Neurol. 2011;10(10):931-41.
27. Zhou C, Wu L, Ni F, Ji W, Wu J, Zhang H. Critical illness polyneuropathy and myopathy: a systematic review. Neural Regen Res. 2014;9(1):101-10.
28. Lundberg IE, Fujimoto M, Vencovsky J, Aggarwal R, Holmqvist M, Christopher–Stine L, et al. Idiopathic inflammatory myopathies. Nat Rev Dis Primers. 2021;7(1):86.
29. Betteridge Z, McHugh N. Myositis-specific autoantibodies: an important tool to support diagnosis of myositis. J Intern Med. 2016;280(1):8-23.
30. Leclair V, Lundberg IE. New myositis classification criteria—What we have learned since Bohan and Peter. Curr Rheumatol Rep. 2018;20(4):18.
31. Svensson J, Arkema EV, Lundberg IE, Holmqvist M. Incidence and prevalence of idiopathic inflammatory myopathies in Sweden: a nationwide population-based study. Rheumatology. 2017;56(5):802-10.
32. Furst DE, Amato AA, Iorga ŞR, Gajria K, Fernandes AW. Epidemiology of adult idiopathic inflammatory myopathies in a U.S. managed care plan: Epidemiology of idiopathic inflammatory myopathies. Muscle Nerve. 2012;45(5):676-83.
33. Rothwell S, Cooper RG, Lundberg IE, Miller FW, Gregersen PK, Bowes J, et al. Dense genotyping of immune-related loci in idiopathic inflammatory myopathies confirms HLA alleles as the strongest genetic risk factor and suggests different genetic

background for major clinical subgroups. Ann Rheum Dis. 2016;75(8):1558-66.

34. Bronner IM, van der Meulen MFG, de Visser M, Kalmijn S, van Venrooij WJ, Voskuyl AE, et al. Long-term outcome in polymyositis and dermatomyositis. Ann Rheum Dis. 2006;65(11):1456-61.
35. Dobloug GC, Svensson J, Lundberg IE, Holmqvist M. Mortality in idiopathic inflammatory myopathy: results from a Swedish nationwide population-based cohort study. Ann Rheum Dis. 2018;77(1):40-7.
36. Dankó K, Ponyi A, Constantin T, Borgulya G, Szegedi G. Long-term survival of patients with idiopathic inflammatory myopathies according to clinical features: a longitudinal study of 162 cases. Medicine. 2004;83(1):35-42.
37. Pinal-Fernandez I, Casal-Dominguez M, Derfoul A, Pak K, Miller FW, Milisenda JC, et al. Machine learning algorithms reveal unique gene expression profiles in muscle biopsies from patients with different types of myositis. Ann Rheum Dis. 2020;79(9):1234-42.
38. Pestronk A, Schmidt RE, Choksi R. Vascular pathology in dermatomyositis and anatomic relations to myopathology. Muscle Nerve. 2010;42(1):53-61.
39. Greenberg SA, Pinkus JL, Pinkus GS, Burleson T, Sanoudou D, Tawil R, et al. Interferon-α/β-mediated innate immune mechanisms in dermatomyositis. Ann Neurol. 2005;57(5):664-78.
40. Mammen AL, Gaudet D, Brisson D, Christopher-Stine L, Lloyd TE, Leffell MS, et al. Increased frequency of DRB1*11:01 in anti-HMG-CoA reductase-associated autoimmune myopathy. Arthritis Care Res(Hoboken). 2012;64(8):1233-7.
41. Malik A, Hayat G, Kalia JS, Guzman MA. Idiopathic inflammatory myopathies: clinical approach and management. Front Neurol. 2016;7:64.
42. Fiorentino D, Marvi U, Chung L. Clinical presentation and evaluation of dermatomyositis. Indian J Dermatol. 2012;57(5):375.
43. Bernet LL, Lewis MA, Rieger KE, Casciola-Rosen L, Fiorentino DF. Ovoid palatal patch in dermatomyositis: A novel finding associated with anti-TIF1γ (p155) antibodies. JAMA Dermatol. 2016;152(9):1049.
44. Inoue S, Okiyama N, Shobo M, Motegi S, Hirano H, Nakagawa Y, et al. Diffuse erythema with 'angel wings' sign in Japanese patients with anti-small ubiquitin-like modifier activating enzyme antibody-associated dermatomyositis. Br J Dermatol. 2018;179(6):1414-5.
45. Olazagasti JM, Baez PJ, Wetter DA, Ernste FC. Cancer risk in dermatomyositis: a meta-analysis of cohort studies. Am J Clin Dermatol. 2015;16(2):89-98.
46. Zuo Y, Ye L, Liu M, Li S, Liu W, Chen F, et al. Clinical significance of radiological patterns of HRCT and their association with macrophage activation in dermatomyositis. Rheumatology. 2020;59(10):2829-37.
47. Cox JT, Gullotti DM, Mecoli CA, Lahouti AH, Albayda J, Paik J, et al. "Hiker's feet": a novel cutaneous finding in the inflammatory myopathies. Clin Rheumatol. 2017;36(7):1683-6.
48. McGrath ER, Doughty CT, Amato AA. Autoimmune myopathies: updates on evaluation and treatment. Neurotherapeutics. 2018;15(4):976-94.
49. Malaviya A. Idiopathic inflammatory myopathies: Contributions from India. Indian J Rheumatol. 2020;15(6):209.
50. Prasad ML, Sarkar C, Roy S, Bagchi U, Singh RR, Singh YN, et al. Idiopathic inflammatory myopathy: clinicopathological observations in the Indian population. Rheumatology. 1992;31(12):835-9.
51. Khadilkar S, Patil S, Amin S. Study of idiopathic inflammatory myopathies with special reference to borderland between idiopathic inflammatory myopathies and muscular dystrophies. Neurol India. 2008;56(3):356.
52. Challa S, Hui M, Jakati S, Uppin M, Rajasekhar L, Kannan M, et al. Juvenile idiopathic inflammatory myopathies: A clinicopathological study with emphasis on muscle histology. Indian J Pathol Microbiol. 2019;62(1):61.
53. Kuruvilla A, Sarma P, Radhakrishnan V, Ramesha K. Clinical, electrophysiologic, and histopathologic profile, and outcome in idiopathic inflammatory myositis: An analysis of 68 cases. Ann Indian Acad Neurol. 2010;13(4):250.
54. Schmidt J. Current classification and management of inflammatory myopathies. JND. 2018;5(2):109-29.
55. Tanboon J, Inoue M, Saito Y, Tachimori H, Hayashi S, Noguchi S, et al. Dermatomyositis: Muscle pathology according to antibody subtypes. Neurology. 2022;98(7):e739-49.
56. Uruha A, Nishikawa A, Tsuburaya RS, Hamanaka K, Kuwana M, Watanabe Y, et al. Sarcoplasmic MxA expression: A valuable marker of dermatomyositis. Neurology. 2017;88(5):493-500.
57. Selva-O'Callaghan A, Pinal-Fernandez I, Trallero-Araguás E, Milisenda JC, Grau-Junyent JM, Mammen AL. Classification and management of adult inflammatory myopathies. Lancet Neurol. 2018;17(9):816-28.
58. Allenbach Y, Benveniste O, Goebel HH, Stenzel W. Integrated classification of inflammatory myopathies. Neuropathol Appl Neurobiol. 2017;43(1):62-81.
59. Naddaf E, Barohn RJ, Dimachkie MM. Inclusion body myositis: update on pathogenesis and treatment. Neurotherapeutics. 2018;15(4):995-1005.
60. Ukichi T, Yoshida K, Matsushima S, Kawakami G, Noda K, Furuya K, et al. MRI of skeletal muscles in patients with idiopathic inflammatory myopathies: characteristic findings and diagnostic performance in dermatomyositis. RMD Open. 2019;5(1):e000850.
61. Ungprasert P, Leeaphorn N, Hosiriluck N, Chaiwatcharayut W, Ammannagari N, Raddatz DA. Clinical features of inflammatory myopathies and their association with malignancy: A systematic review in asian population. ISRN Rheumatol. 2013;2013:1-7.
62. Karadimitrakis S, Plastiras SC, Zormpala A, Chatzikonstantinou K, Boki KA, Tzelepis GE, et al. Chest CT findings in patients with inflammatory myopathy and Jo1 antibodies. Euro J Radiol. 2008;66(1):27-30.
63. Laporte A, Mariampillai K, Allenbach Y, Pasi N, Donciu V, Toledano D, et al. Idiopathic inflammatory myopathies: CT characteristics of interstitial lung disease and their association(s) with myositis-specific autoantibodies. Eur Radiol. 2022;32(5):3480-9.
64. Lega JC, Reynaud Q, Belot A, Fabien N, Durieu I, Cottin V. Idiopathic inflammatory myopathies and the lung. Eur Respir Rev. 2015;24(136):216-38.
65. Amato AA, Greenberg SA. Inflammatory myopathies: Continuum (Minneap Minn). 2013;19:1615-33.
66. Carstens PO, Schmidt J. Diagnosis, pathogenesis, and treatment of myositis: Recent advances. Clin Exp Immunol. 2014;175(3):349-58.
67. Dalakas MC, Illa I, Dambrosia JM, Soueidan SA, Stein DP, Otero C, et al. A Controlled Trial of High-dose Intravenous Immune Globulin Infusions as Treatment for Dermatomyositis. N Engl J Med [Internet]. 1993;329(27):1993-2000.
68. Miyasaka N, Hara M, Koike T, Saito E, Yamada M, Tanaka Y, et al. Effects of intravenous immunoglobulin therapy in Japanese patients with polymyositis and dermatomyositis resistant to corticosteroids: a randomized double-blind placebo-controlled trial. Mod Rheumatol. 2012;22(3):382-93.
69. Anh-Tu Hoa S, Hudson M. Critical review of the role of intravenous immunoglobulins in idiopathic inflammatory myopathies. Semin Arthritis Rheum. 2017;46(4):488-508.
70. Cozzi F, Marson P, Pigatto E, Tison T, Polito P, Galozzi P, et al. Plasma-exchange as a "rescue therapy" for dermato/polymyositis in acute phase. Experience in three young patients. Transf Apheresis Sci. 2015;53(3):368-72.
71. Casal-Dominguez M, Pinal-Fernandez I, Huapaya J, Albayda J, Paik JJ, Johnson C, et al. Efficacy and adverse effects of methotrexate compared with azathioprine in the antisynthetase syndrome. Clin Exp Rheumatol. 2019;37(5):858-61.

72. Huapaya JA, Silhan L, Pinal-Fernandez I, Casal-Dominguez M, Johnson C, Albayda J, et al. Long-term treatment with azathioprine and mycophenolate mofetil for myositis-related interstitial lung disease. Chest. 2019;156(5):896-906.
73. Ge Y, Peng Q, Zhang S, Zhou H, Lu X, Wang G. Cyclophosphamide treatment for idiopathic inflammatory myopathies and related interstitial lung disease: a systematic review. Clin Rheumatol. 2015;34(1):99-105.
74. Bae S, Charles-Schoeman C. Oral cyclophosphamide in treatment of patients with refractory idiopathic inflammatory myopathies: a retrospective observational study. Clin Rheumatol [Internet]. 2018 Aug [cited 2022 Aug 3];37(8):2113-23. Available from: http://link.springer.com/10.1007/s10067-018-4174-3
75. Oddis CV, Reed AM, Aggarwal R, Rider LG, Ascherman DP, Levesque MC, et al. Rituximab in the treatment of refractory adult and juvenile dermatomyositis and adult polymyositis: A randomized, placebo-phase trial. Arthritis Rheum. 2013;65(2):314-24.
76. Leclair V, Galindo-Feria AS, Dastmalchi M, Holmqvist M, Lundberg IE. Efficacy and safety of rituximab in anti-synthetase antibody positive and negative subjects with idiopathic inflammatory myopathy: a registry-based study. Rheumatology. 2019;58(7):1214-20.
77. Fasano S, Gordon P, Hajji R, Loyo E, Isenberg DA. Rituximab in the treatment of inflammatory myopathies: A review. Rheumatology. 2017;56(1):26-36.
78. Liu Y, Fang L, Chen W, Zhu Y, Lin X, Wang Y, et al. Identification of characteristics of overt myocarditis in adult patients with idiopathic inflammatory myopathies. Cardiovasc Diagn Ther. 2020;10(3):405-20.
79. Olthoff A, Carstens PO, Zhang S, von Fintel E, Friede T, Lotz J, et al. Evaluation of dysphagia by novel real-time MRI. Neurology. 2016;87(20):2132-8.

87

CHAPTER

Channelopathies of the Peripheral Nerves and Muscles

Salman Bhai, Natalia Gonzalez Caldito

INTRODUCTION

Ion channel dysfunction or channelopathies are a group of heterogeneous disorders characterized by episodic or fluctuating symptoms. These ion channels are expressed throughout the body, therefore affecting different organ systems, and causing a wide range of disorders. In the nervous system, ion channels are involved in action potentials and synaptic transmission, which are key in neuronal signaling.[1,2] Although channelopathies can have both central and peripheral nervous system manifestations,[3] this chapter is focused on the disorders affecting the peripheral nerves and muscles.

Most of the channelopathies are inherited, but they can be acquired as well such as autoimmune or toxin induced.

EPIDEMIOLOGY

Neuromuscular channelopathies are rare disorders, and although there has been a significant advancement in the understanding of the physiopathology and presentation, their prevalence is still incompletely characterized. According to the current knowledge, some disorders have been better evaluated than others, but the estimated prevalence in inherited channelopathies ranges between 1/100,000 and 1/1,000,000 and it differs significantly across disorders.[4,5] Toxin-induced and autoimmune channelopathies also have significant variations in prevalence.

Nondystrophic myotonias are usually inherited in an autosomal dominant manner except a recessive form of myotonia congenita. As expected, the autosomal dominant form of myotonia congenita (Becker disease) is more common than the recessive form (Thomsen disease), with a prevalence of 1:25,000 and 1:400,000, respectively.[6] Men tend to be more affected than women. The estimated prevalence of paramyotonia congenita is 1:250,000, and the prevalence of periodic paralysis varies across subtypes.[7] It ranges from 1:200,000 in hyperkalemic periodic paralysis to 1:1,000,000 in hypokalemic periodic paralysis and Andersen–Tawil syndrome.[8] The prevalence of ryanodinopathies such as malignant hyperthermia is difficult to accurately estimate as patients only present after receiving depolarizing muscle relaxants (succinylcholine) and volatile anesthetic agents (halothane). However, its incidence during anesthesia is between 1:10,000 and 1:250,000. All ethnic groups are affected, and the highest incidence is in young patients, half of them presenting below the age of 15 years.[9] Ultimately, the estimated prevalence of congenital myasthenic syndromes is 2.5–12/1,000,000.[10]

Channelopathies affecting the peripheral nerves tend to be inherited in an autosomal dominant fashion but there has not been an accurate estimate of its worldwide prevalence. Erythromelalgia and paroxysmal pain disorder usually start in childhood, whereas the prevalence of small fiber neuropathy rises with increasing age. There is intrafamilial variability in age of onset and severity.[11]

Autoimmune channelopathies include well-known disorders such as myasthenia and Lambert–Eaton myasthenic syndrome. These are discussed elsewhere in this textbook and will not be discussed here. Regarding other autoimmune channelopathies, due to their novelty and ongoing research, an accurate prevalence is not yet established. There have been around 200 cases reported of Isaac's syndrome (acquired neuromyotonia) but its prevalence is likely higher.[12]

Toxin-induced channelopathies differ greatly depending on the geographic location. Ciguatera toxin approaches 10% in the Caribbean but outside of this area, the cases are sparse and result from fish transportation. On the other hand, the intoxication of tetrodotoxin is mainly seen in the Pacific Ocean (Japan) and Baja California coastal region with an incidence of 30–50 cases per year. Botulism occurs more frequently, although it depends on the subtype. Infant botulism, the most common form, has an incidence of 2/100,000 live births a year with a median of 4 months of age. Foodborne botulism incidence is 1/10,000,000, but adult intestinal colonization is rarer and every year there are single-digit cases reported.[13]

PATHOPHYSIOLOGY

Ion channels are transmembrane proteins, and they are crucial in action potential generation and synaptic transmission. They have ion selectivity, and their proper functioning determines electrical differences between the two sides of the membrane, which is key in action potential generation.[14]

Signaling in skeletal muscle occurs when an action potential reaches the axon of a motoneuron and travels, terminating in the neuromuscular junction. Briefly, this leads to calcium influx in the presynaptic membrane and the release of acetylcholine at the neuromuscular junction. Acetylcholine binds to receptors in the motor endplate of the muscle fiber and this initiates a skeletal muscle action potential. In the sarcolemma, voltage-gated sodium channels are activated and there is depolarization with a rapid influx of sodium. As the membrane potential becomes less negative, these channels start to inactivate. In addition, as this occurs, there is the activation of voltage-gated potassium channels with potassium efflux that contributes to repolarization and recovering of the resting action potential. With repeated stimulation, there is a rundown of potassium in the cell, and chloride channels contribute to recovering and stabilization of the resting membrane potential.[14]

Depending on the type of channel dysfunction, symptoms vary. Interestingly, the malfunction of a channel does not always explain all the symptoms described in that disorder, indicating that the pathophysiology may be more complex. For example, with chloride channel malfunctioning, there is delayed recovery in the resting membrane potential, leading to myotonia (delayed relaxation of the muscle). However, this model does not explain the "warm up" phenomenon (improvement with exercise).

Other ion channelopathies result in an excitable sarcolemma, which leads to different clinical manifestations. For example, malfunctioning of the sodium channels can cause defects in the inactivation of these channels and sometimes the improvement of activation. This can result in enhanced hyperexcitability with sodium influx (paramyotonia congenita), but it can also result in sustained depolarization of the resting potential causing the fibers to be inexcitable (seen in hyperkalemic periodic paralysis or tetrodotoxin poisoning). In hypokalemic periodic paralysis, there is a loss of function of the skeletal muscle L-type calcium or voltage-gated sodium channel, which leads to an inexcitable sarcolemma causing episodic paralysis.[8,15] On the other hand, with potassium channelopathies as these channels are involved in the recovery of the resting action potential, a lack of function can result in hyperexcitability (acquired neuromyotonia or Isaac's syndrome).

Calcium channels are also important in the contraction-relaxation coupling in muscle function. Ryanodinopathies are sarcoplasmic reticulum calcium channelopathies in which calcium channels are hypersensitive, thus releasing excessive calcium, resulting in generalized rigidity and increased metabolism. **Figure 1** shows the structure of different ion channels and conditions associated with them.

In addition to the skeletal muscle, channelopathies can affect other structures of the peripheral nervous system (nociceptors or neuromuscular junction). Ion channels have a key role in detecting and transmitting stimuli by nociceptors. Transient receptor potential (TRP) family of ion channels as well as sodium channels is an example, and malfunctioning of these channels can lead to episodic pain due to a gain of function (erythromelalgia) or absence of pain (congenital insensitivity pain). Malfunctioning of the acetylcholine receptors (such as in myasthenia gravis due to antibody blockage) can lead to decreased synaptic transmission and result in fatigable weakness.

CLINICAL PRESENTATIONS

Skeletal Muscle Inherited Channelopathies

Most of them are autosomal dominant inherited disorders and although they usually have high penetrance, there can be significant differences phenotypically between and within families. They are known for their fluctuating symptoms or paroxysmal attacks, which are precipitated by physiologic stresses (intense exercise, fever, or lack of sleep) and environmental factors (temperature changes). They are broadly classified as nondystrophic myotonias and periodic paralysis, although both are inherited disorders **(Table 1)**.[1,2]

Nondystrophic Myotonias

Nondystrophic myotonias are divided by the mutation type, such as those affecting the chloride (*CLCN1* gene) and sodium (*SCN4A* gene) channels. Myotonia is defined as a delay in the relaxation of the skeletal muscles upon contraction, which can be elicited upon voluntary action or with percussion over the muscle. It usually worsens with cold temperatures, pregnancy, emotional stress, fatigue, and dietary potassium. Patients typically present with muscle stiffness in the absence of muscle weakness or atrophy. Stiffness can be painful, but this is more common in sodium channelopathies. Fatigue has a big impact on patients' lives as well.

Chloride channelopathies are also called myotonia congenita. Becker disease, the recessive form, is more severe and has an earlier onset. Patients with Thomsen disease, autosomal dominant form, usually have normal strength whereas those with Becker disease can have a transient weakness that improves with exercise. Myotonia begins

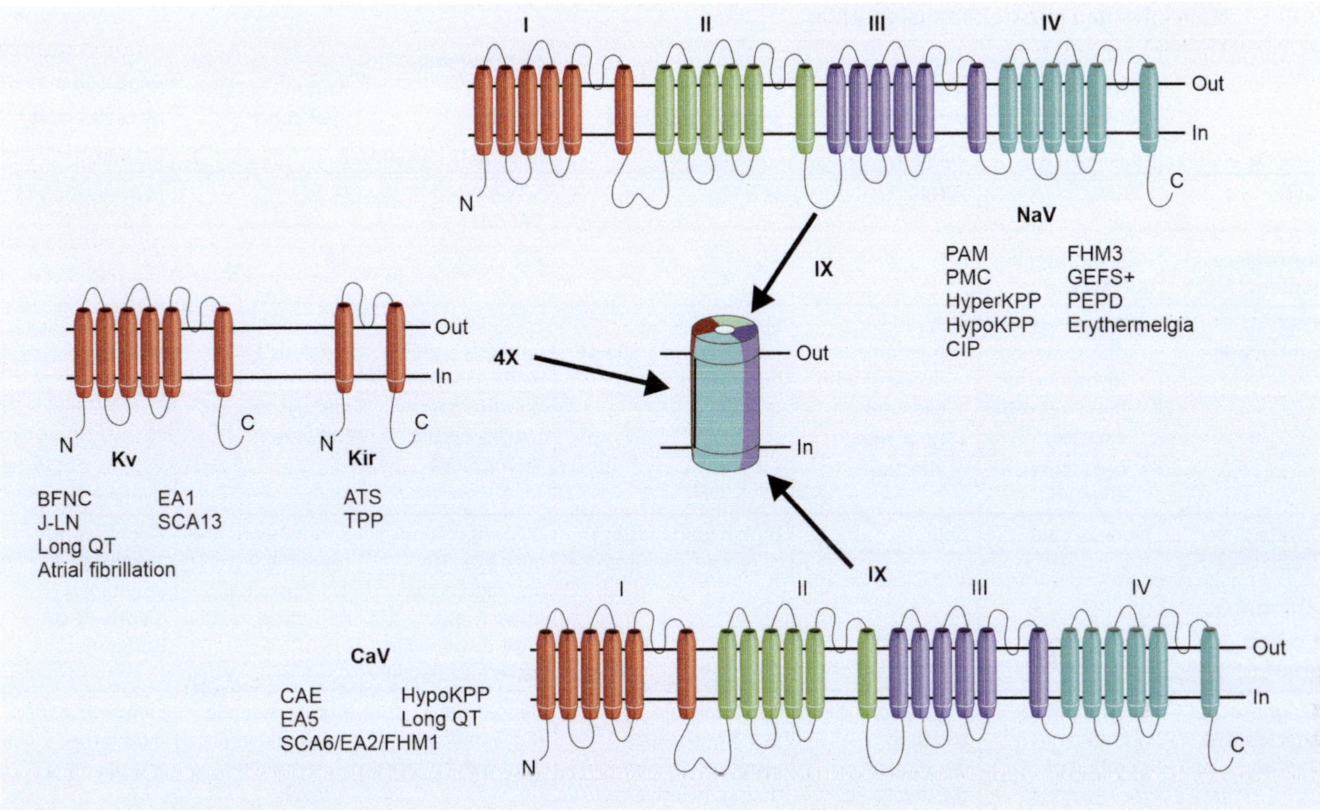

FIG. 1: Schematic diagram showing the structure of different ion channels and conditions associated with them.

(ATS: Andersen–Tawil syndrome; BFNC: benign familial neonatal convulsions; CAE: childhood absence epilepsy; CaV: voltage-gated calcium channel; CIP: congenital insensitivity to pain; EA1: episodic ataxia type 1; EA2: episodic ataxia type 2; EA5: episodic ataxia type 5; FHM1: familial hemiplegic migraine type 1; FHM3: familial hemiplegic migraine type 3; GEFS+: genetic epilepsy with febrile seizures plus; HyperKPP: hyperkalemic periodic paralysis; HypoKPP: hypokalemic periodic paralysis; J-LN: Jervell and Lange–Nielsen syndrome; Kir: inward-rectifier potassium channel; Kv: voltage-gated potassium channel; NaV: voltage-gated sodium channel; PAM: potassium-aggravated myotonia; PEPD: paroxysmal extreme pain disorder; PMC: paramyotonia congenita; SCA6: spinocerebellar ataxia type 6; SCA13: spinocerebellar ataxia type 13; TPP: thyrotoxic periodic paralysis)

in the first or second decade of life, and patients have a muscular build. It affects the legs more commonly, and it can cause falls, although more commonly, patients describe difficulties releasing grip after handshaking and slowing with quick movements. It improves with exercise, and patients usually experience the "warm up" phenomenon. On the other hand, they are the most symptomatic with rapid movements after a phase of inactivity (active myotonia). Anesthetic complications are known in myotonia congenita, and it usually presents with generalized spams that complicate intubation and mask ventilation. This could be the presenting symptom in some cases.[16]

Sodium channelopathies are a group of disorders that include paramyotonia congenita and sodium channel myotonias. Paramyotonia congenita (also known as Eulenburg disease) is autosomal dominant and is characterized by painful, prolonged, and cold-induced myotonia. Contrary to myotonia congenita, patients experience paradoxical myotonia as their symptoms worsen with exercise. Myotonia is also more pronounced in the face, clinically presenting as facial stiffness and eye closure myotonia. Patients can experience weakness after exercise that can last from hours to days. Sodium channel myotonias typically have myotonia as the only symptom. In some cases, myotonia can improve with acetazolamide (acetazolamide-responsive myotonia), fluctuate (myotonia fluctuans), or be permanent (myotonia permanens). They are triggered by potassium and contrary to paramyotonia congenita, they are not sensitive to temperature changes. The warm up phenomenon can also be seen.[16]

Primary Periodic Paralysis

Primary periodic paralysis is associated with mutations in the sodium channel gene *SCN4A*, calcium channel gene *CACNA1S*, or potassium channel gene *KCNJ2*. Patients experience episodes of attacks of flaccid muscle weakness, which are triggered by changes in potassium levels. They are triggered by the ingestion of carbohydrate-rich foods or resting after exercise. These attacks typically start before the second decade of life.

Hyperkalemic periodic paralysis is caused by mutations in the sodium channel SCN4A. Their attacks last minutes to hours with a frequency of around 16 per month and are triggered by high potassium foods, fasting, or resting after

TABLE 1: Main inherited muscle channelopathies.

	Myotonia congenita	Paramyotonia congenita	Hyperkalemic periodic paralysis	Hypokalemic periodic paralysis	Andersen–Tawil syndrome	Malignant hyperthermia
Channelopathy	Chloride	Sodium	Sodium	Sodium or calcium	K	Calcium
Gene	*CLCN1*	*SCN4A*	*SCN4A*	*SCNA4A* or *CACNA1S*	*KCNJ2*	*RYR1* and *SCN4A*
Inheritance pattern	AD (Thomsen) or AR (Becker)	AD	AD	AD	AR	AD
Clinical presentation	• "Warm up" phenomenon. Myotonia that improves with exercise • Legs more affected	• Paradoxical myotonia (worsens with exercise) • Face more affected	Episodic flaccid paralysis and areflexia lasting minutes to hours	Episodic flaccid paralysis and areflexia lasting hours to days. Usually occurs during sleep	Episodic flaccid paralysis, EKG abnormalities, and dysmorphic features	Muscle rigidity, rhabdomyolysis, hyperthermia
Triggers	None or cold	Cold	High K foods, fasting, or resting after exercise	Alcohol, resting after exercise, and factors that lower K (e.g., high-carbohydrate foods and insulin)	Spontaneous and the same factors as hypokalemic periodic paralysis	Depolarizing anesthetic agents (e.g., halothane or isoflurane)
Diagnostic characteristics	Low amplitude and short duration of the myotonic discharges on EMG	High amplitude and long duration of the myotonic discharges on EMG	Hyperkalemia ($K > 5$ mmol/L or increases >1.5 mmol/L) during the attacks	Hypokalemia ($K < 3$ mmol/L) during the attacks	• Hypokalemia, hyperkalemia, or normal K levels • Long QT or QU interval on EKG	Elevated CK during the attacks
Acute treatment	NA	NA	Mild exercise and K-lowering agents	Mild exercise and K supplementation	K supplementation	Dantrolene
Chronic treatment	Mexiletine, lamotrigine	Mexiletine, lamotrigine	Acetazolamide	Acetazolamide and K-rich diet	K-rich diet	NA

(AD: autosomal dominant; AR: autosomal recessive; CK: creatine kinase; EKG: electrocardiogram; EMG: electromyography; K: potassium; NA: not applicable)

exercise. Patients are areflexic during the attack and have normal strength outside of episodes. However, there can be a mild fixed limb-girdle weakness. Myotonia or paramyotonia can also be a clinical symptom.

Hypokalemic periodic paralysis can be caused by mutations in the calcium channel gene *CACNA1S* or the sodium channel gene *SCN4A*. Attacks start in the second decade of life with the highest frequency between 15 and 35 years, decreasing afterward. Attacks can be mild-to-complete paralysis. They can last hours to days, and the frequency is usually less than 10 per month. They usually occur during sleep, and the triggers include alcohol, resting after exercise, and factors that lower potassium (such as high-carbohydrate foods and insulin). Patients can have fixed limb-girdle weakness. Stiffness or heaviness can be a vague prodrome and with mild exercise, the attack can be aborted.

Andersen-Tawil syndrome is caused by a mutation in the potassium channel *KCNJ2* gene. The clinical triad is episodic flaccid muscle paralysis, electrocardiogram abnormalities (ventricular arrhythmias and prolonged QT interval), and dysmorphic features (short stature, low-set ears, ocular hypertelorism, broad nasal root, small mandible, fifth digit clinodactyly, and second and third toe syndactyly). Attacks can occur spontaneously or triggered by the same factors as hypokalemic periodic paralysis.[17]

Other Inherited Muscle Channelopathies

Other inherited muscle channelopathies and related syndromes are comprised of a heterogeneous group of disorders.

Thyrotoxic periodic paralysis is the most common periodic paralysis and although the mechanism is not clearly understood, it is thought to require a mutation of the potassium channel KCNJ18, which is regulated by the thyroid hormone. It requires both an inherited predisposition to paralysis attacks and thyrotoxicosis and hyperkalemia.

Malignant hyperthermia and central core disease are both ryanodinopathies caused by a mutation of the ryanodine receptor gene (*RYR1*), with the protein located in the calcium channel. In some cases, with malignant hyperthermia, there have been mutations of the sodium channel gene *SCN4A* as well. In malignant hyperthermia, depolarizing agents cause massive calcium release, which then leads to skeletal muscle rigidity, accelerated metabolism, rapid rise in body temperature, and tachycardia. In central core disease, there is a risk of malignant hyperthermia as well, but patients can also develop a progressive myopathy (proximal weakness) and hypotonia.

Severe neonatal episodic laryngospasm is caused by mutations of the sodium channel gene *SCN4A*. Patients present with face or limb myotonia and episodes of life-threatening laryngeal spasms. In the most severe scenario, cases can lead to sudden infant death.

Congenital myasthenic syndromes are most often caused by postsynaptic genetic defects of the neuromuscular junction, but they can also be caused by presynaptic or synaptic defects. Mutations can cause slow and fast congenital myasthenic syndromes. Further discussion is reserved for the dedicated section within this textbook.

Peripheral Nerve Inherited Channelopathies

Nociceptors are the sensory neurons involved in detecting high-threshold stimuli that can potentially cause tissue injury, including pain and temperature. Channelopathies affecting those neurons lead to sensory abnormalities such as increased or absence of pain sensation. This results in pain or insensitivity syndromes, depending on if there is a channel gain or loss of function. Interestingly, nociceptors overlap with channels involved in the function of autonomic neurons, therefore autonomic dysfunction can be also observed.[18]

Most of these diseases are due to mutations in the sodium channel gene *SCN9A* [voltage-gated sodium channel (NaV1.7)]. A gain of function of this channel causes primary erythromelalgia. It consists of episodes of burning pain, warmth, and redness. They are precipitated by prolonged standing, exercise, heat, or alcohol, although a trigger is not always identified. Pain is relieved with cooling and in some instances, patients can experience secondary injuries due to severe cold exposure or prolonged water immersion. The distal extremities are most involved, but they can also affect the acral parts such as the nose or ears.[19]

Other disorders with a gain of function mutations of the same channel are paroxysmal extreme pain disorder and small fiber neuropathy. Paroxysmal extreme pain disorder is also known as familial rectal pain. It presents with episodic ocular, mandibular, and rectal pains. It is occasionally associated with autonomic dysfunction. It can be triggered by eating or defecation.

Inactivation of the sodium channel NaV1.7 due to loss of function mutations of the *SCN9A* gene causes congenital insensitivity to pain. Patients present with a complete lack of pain with other somatosensory modalities being spared. The first symptoms noted are a lack of response to injuries or immunizations. In the first year, patients accumulate bruises and cuts. Other evidence can be seen with the eruption of the teeth, which then can lead to injuries to the lips and gums. Due to the lack of pain, patients unknowingly engage in harmful behavior and tend to accumulate fractures and other bodily injuries. In addition, some families can be accused of physical child abuse due to injuries.[11,18] Similarly, hereditary sensory and autonomic neuropathy type IID is another disorder caused by a loss of function mutation of *SCN9A*. In addition to the absence of pain and temperature, patients have autonomic dysfunction.[18]

Sodium channel, voltage-gated, type XI (NaV1.9) is another sodium channel present in nociceptors. Mutations in this channel (gene *SCN11A*) can also lead to congenital insensitivity to pain (loss of function mutation) and familial episodic pain syndrome (gain of function mutation). Interestingly, the latter can also be caused by mutations involving a completely different channel, ankyrin-type TRP (TRPA) channel (*TRPA1* gene). Patients usually present with episodic pain on the chest and arms radiating to the abdomen and legs (type I, *TRPA1* mutation) or distally, hands and feet (type II, *SCN11A* mutation). These attacks are triggered by hunger, fatigue, and cold.[18]

Transient receptor potential vanilloid 4 (TRPV4) is an encoded calcium-permeable cation channel that is activated by heat, mechanical stimuli, and endogenous and synthetic agonists. Mutations in this channel can be divided into inherited neuropathies and skeletal dysplasias, although there can be an overlap between both groups.[20] The underlying mechanisms explaining this wide range of manifestations are not completely understood but it can partially be explained by the multiple activities in which TRPV4 is involved, such as chondrocyte homeostasis and differentiation and maturation of neuron cells. TRPV4 may have other functions as well.[20] TRPV4-mediated neuropathies have a wide spectrum of manifestations. Hereditary sensory motor neuropathy type II C (Charcot–Marie–Tooth type 2C) is a progressive sensorimotor neuropathy, and patients have distinct features such as bilateral sensorineural hearing loss, vocal cord paralysis, and bladder urgency or incontinence. Another disease is congenital distal spinal motor neuropathy, which is a lower motor neuron syndrome affecting the lower body. Patients have clubfoot as well as knee and hip contractures but no sensory deficits. Scapuloperoneal spinal muscular atrophy is also a TRPV4-mediated neuropathy in which there is a congenital reduction of the peroneus and shoulder muscles (scapular winging) with progressive weakness and sensory deficits. Patients also have vocal cord paresis.[20]

There are mutations in the potassium channel (genes *KCNQ1* and *KCNQ2*) that result in peripheral nerve hyperexcitability. They are a heterogenous group of disorders that present with myokymia, muscle cramps, stiffness, and fasciculations.[21]

Acquired Nerve and Skeletal Muscle Channelopathies

Most acquired muscle channelopathies are toxin or autoimmune induced **(Table 2)**. Ciguatera toxin is perhaps the most common toxin-induced channelopathy (sodium channel activation). Gastrointestinal symptoms such as nausea, diarrhea, and abdominal pain are the first to emerge. These can last up to 7 days and, as they improve, sensory symptoms (paresthesia, cold allodynia, pruritus) and myalgias develop. Cold allodynia is pathognomonic. Ataxia and tremors can be present as well as arrhythmias.

Another neurotoxin found in other fish (mostly pufferfish) is tetrodotoxin. It is mostly produced by the *Vibrio* species. It blocks fast-type sodium channels, depressing action potential generation. Symptoms are dose dependent, with onset as early as a few hours. Systemic symptoms are vomiting, diarrhea, bradycardia, blisters, and petechiae. Neurological symptoms are dysesthesias and paresthesia progressing to weakness (and in the most severe cases, flaccid quadriparesis).

Botulism, caused by the botulinum toxin produced by *Clostridium botulinum*, leads to inhibition of acetylcholine release. It can present as infantile, foodborne, wound, adult intestinal, and iatrogenic botulism.[13] Infantile botulism is the most common and usually caused by the ingestion of honey. It presents as dilated pupils, constipation, weak cry/suck, hypotonia, ptosis, and weakness including respiratory muscles. Food or adult intestinal botulism has a similar presentation with gastrointestinal symptoms that precede neurological deficits (fixed mydriasis, blurry vision, rapid progressive descending paralysis including the cranial nerves). Wound and iatrogenic botulisms are also similar but without gastrointestinal symptoms.

Black widow spider venom has α-latrotoxin, which inserts into the presynaptic neuronal membrane, becoming a channel and allowing calcium influx (leading to acetylcholine release). This inhibits other neurotransmission reuptake causing generalized pain and rigidity due to sustained muscle contraction, cramps, and autonomic disturbances.

Autoimmune channelopathies are a group of disorders caused by antibodies to specific ion channels on neurons, nerves, or muscles.[12] They can be idiopathic, but commonly are seen in the setting of a paraneoplastic process. Antibodies against the voltage-gated potassium channel complex proteins, leucine-rich glioma-inactivated 1 (LGI1) and Caspr2, have central and peripheral clinical manifestations.[22] LGI1 is primarily linked to limbic encephalitis and faciobrachial dystonic seizures, while Caspr2 has more peripheral manifestations. Isaac's syndrome or acquired neuromyotonia is a peripheral hyperexcitability syndrome that has an insidious onset of generalized muscle stiffness, myokymia, and muscle hypertrophy. Burning pain in the setting of small fiber neuropathy is another clinical feature that can be observed.[22] In addition, there is Morvan's syndrome, which is a combination of neuromyotonia with autonomic and central nervous system (CNS) dysfunction,

TABLE 2: Main acquired peripheral nerve and muscle channelopathies.

	Ciguatera fish poisoning	Tetrodotoxin poisoning	Botulism	Latrotoxin	Isaac's syndrome (acquired neuromyotonia)
Etiology	Ciguatoxin-contaminated fish in tropical and subtropical areas (e.g., bass and snapper)	Tetrodotoxin in contaminated pufferfish	Botulinum toxin	α-latrotoxin from the black widow spider	Autoimmune or paraneoplastic due to LGI1 and Caspr2 antibodies
Channelopathy	Sodium	Sodium	Neuromuscular junction	Calcium	Potassium
Clinical presentation	GI symptoms • Cold allodynia, paresthesia, and myalgias	GI symptoms • Paresthesia, perioral numbness that later progress to generalized weakness (respiratory failure)	GI symptoms • Progressive descending weakness (respiratory failure). • CN involvement and miosis	• Generalized pain and rigidity due to sustained muscle contraction • Autonomic disturbances	• Muscle stiffness, cramps, and fasciculations • Myokymia or neuromyotonia on EMG • It can present concomitantly with Morvan's syndrome*
Treatment	Supportive care	Supportive care	Botulism antitoxin and supportive care	Supportive care	• Immunosuppressive therapy (e.g., high-dose steroids and plasmapheresis) • If malignancy, treating underlying cancer

**Morvan's syndrome*: Peripheral nerve hyperexcitability, autonomic dysfunction (e.g., hyperhidrosis), sleep disturbances (e.g., insomnia and REM sleep disorders), and encephalopathy.

(CN: cranial nerve; EMG: electromyography; GI: gastrointestinal; LGI1: leucine-rich glioma-inactivated 1; REM: rapid eye movement)

including insomnia.[23] Neuromyotonia and Morvan's syndrome have been associated with thymoma, but malignancy association is not very common.[23]

In addition, other autoimmune channelopathies affect the neuromuscular junction and the autonomic system. The former is myasthenia gravis and Lambert-Eaton myasthenic syndrome, and the latter is autoimmune autonomic ganglionopathy. Those are covered elsewhere.[12,24]

DIAGNOSIS AND INVESTIGATIONS

Muscle Inherited Myopathies

Physical Examination

The neurologic exam is of immense diagnostic value, as patients can have distinct features on the exam. The patient's appearance can be characteristic of patients with myotonia congenita, especially Becker disease, which can have a strong muscular build or muscular hypertrophy of muscles.[16] In addition, observing gait and the speed of grip release can provide important information.

Myotonia is a relevant finding on the exam, and there are bedside tests that can be completed to evaluate for it. Action myotonia can be tested by active muscle contraction such as with repeated handgrip or blinking. Reported stiffness (myotonia) can improve with repeated action due to the warm up phenomenon (myotonia congenita) or worsen with activity (paramyotonia). Myotonia can also be tested by percussion of the muscles with a reflex hammer (to observe if there is the presence of a catch or slowing in the relaxation phase). It is performed over the thenar eminence, forearm extensor, trapezius, quadriceps, calf, or tongue muscles. Furthermore, transient hemiparesis (tested in the biceps) can be seen with Becker disease, which resolves upon repetitive action. Also, there can be a lid lag when quickly looking downward after upgaze (eyelid myotonia), which is seen in sodium channelopathies.[16] Some patients with nondystrophic myotonias can complain of weakness, although it is reported more often than detected on the exam. If weakness is present, it is usually mild (4/5 strength on the Medical Research Council scale).

Patients with primary periodic paralysis have areflexia and flaccid paralysis during the attacks, usually sparing the facial and respiratory muscles. In between attacks, the examination is usually normal. Overall, there is not a characteristic phenotype except in Andersen-Tawil syndrome. They have short stature, low-set ears, ocular hypertelorism, broad nasal root, small mandible, fifth digit clinodactyly, and second-and-third toe syndactyly.

Diagnostic Testing

Electrodiagnostic Testing

When a physical examination reveals myotonia, electrodiagnostic testing should be completed to confirm electrical myotonia and to guide genetic testing. Needle electromyography (EMG) is used to detect myotonic discharges. Myotonic potentials are repetitive 20–80 Hz discharges with an amplitude and frequency that wax and wane. Depending on the channelopathy, there are differences between the myotonic discharges. In chloride channelopathies, there is a loss of function that leads to resting membrane potential instability resulting in a self-maintained activity. Because of this, the myotonic discharges tend to have a low amplitude (<0.4 mV) and short duration (<1 second) with the "dive bomber" sound (smoothly increasing in frequency). On the other hand, in sodium channelopathies, there is a decrease in sodium channel inactivation leading to a tonic depolarization, and the myotonic discharges tend to have a higher amplitude (>0.4 mV) and longer duration (>2 seconds) with a "slowly deceleration motorcycle" sound. In addition, the first inner discharge interval is usually longer than 30 milliseconds in chloride channelopathies versus shorter than 30 milliseconds in sodium channelopathies.[25]

Once a diagnosis of muscle channelopathy is suspected, short and long exercise tests (SETs and LETs, respectively) can be performed to further distinguish between the various syndromes. The sensitivity of the SET is 53–100% in myotonia congenita, 83–100% in paramyotonia congenita, and 60% in sodium channel myotonia.[25] The test can be repeated with cooling of the limb (20–25°C) and it leads to improved sensitivity. In primary periodic paralysis, LET is a valuable test to reach the diagnosis as paralysis attacks usually occur with resting after exercise.

Between attacks, needle EMG can show positive sharp waves and myotonia in hyperkalemic periodic paralysis but not in hypokalemic periodic paralysis.[4,26]

Laboratory Testing

During an attack, in hypokalemic periodic paralysis, potassium levels can be significantly low (<3 mmol/L). In hyperkalemic periodic paralysis, they can be elevated (>5 mmol/L or increases >1.5 mmol/L), but around 50% of patients will have normal potassium levels. In Andersen-Tawil syndrome, potassium levels can be elevated, normal, or low. Thyroid function tests should also be obtained as thyrotoxic hypokalemic periodic paralysis can resemble hypokalemic periodic paralysis.

Transient elevations in creatine kinase can be seen in hypokalemic periodic paralysis, but otherwise the levels are normal between attacks.[7]

Genetic Testing

After confirmation of myotonia or when periodic paralysis is suspected, genetic testing is recommended to further characterize the disease and the pathogenic variant. Over 100 pathogenic variants of *CLCN1* and *SCN4A* gene mutations have been identified. Most of the chloride and sodium channelopathies are due to missense mutations but deletions, duplications, insertions, and frameshift mutations have also been identified throughout the entire coding sequence. With the development of new genetic testing techniques such as next generation sequencing, the diagnostic yield has improved significantly.[27,28]

Additional Testing

Andersen–Tawil syndrome can have heart conduction abnormalities, and an electrocardiogram should be part of the diagnostic evaluation. Typical findings are long-QT or QU interval at rest and with normokalemia. Patients are at risk for arrhythmias, which are usually ventricular. However, sudden cardiac death is rare.[7]

Testing for malignant hyperthermia can be complex, and only high-risk patients should be tested. The first is to screen for personal and family anesthetic history. However, it is not uncommon that patients at risk for malignant hyperthermia have had one-to-two exposures to triggering agents without events (up to 50% of the cases).[29] Fevers and muscle cramping with heat and exercise can be indicators as well. The most sensitive test is the contracture test. While it is sensitive, it has a 20% false-positive rate. The test evaluates *in vitro* response of the patient's muscle to RYR1 agonists such as halothane and caffeine. The disadvantage is that the muscle tissue must be fresh so the geographical location of the patient is a limiting factor. A combination of clinical, electrophysiologic, *in vitro* assays, and genetic testing should help guide clinical diagnosis and management.

Peripheral Nerve Inherited and Acquired Channelopathies

When the clinical presentation is highly suspicious for a neuropathic genetic disorder, genetic testing is obtained. Despite advances in diagnostics, the etiology of small fiber neuropathy is most often idiopathic.[18]

In small fiber neuropathy, a skin biopsy may reveal a reduction of intraepidermal nerve fiber density, though this is a nonspecific finding. Similar findings are seen in erythromelalgia as it can also show a decreased epidermal and perivascular nerve density. Another test that can be performed is thermography, which reveals an increased temperature of the affected areas in primary erythromelalgia. Another supportive study when evaluating small fiber neuropathy is quantitative sensory testing, which shows an increased thermal threshold.[19]

Nerve conduction studies are completed to evaluate for concurrent large fiber neuropathies. They should be normal in isolated small fiber neuropathies; however, the combination of large and small fiber involvement is disease specific. For example, in hereditary sensory and autonomic neuropathies, there can be a reduction in sensory compound action potentials, whereas in congenital insensitivity to pain, a mild reduction in the sensory and motor conduction velocities can be found.[18]

Peripheral hyperexcitability syndromes can have characteristic findings on exam. Myokymia can be observed, which consists of continuous, rippling, undulating movement of the muscle. EMG can be particularly useful, revealing neuromyotonic and myokymic discharges. Neuromyotonic discharges are specific but less frequently seen. They appear as motor units firing at high frequencies ranging from 150 to 250 Hz (continuously or in bursts with decrementing amplitudes and frequency), and they produce a "pinging sound" and a funnel or tornado shape in a 100-millisecond division. Myokymic discharges are defined as one or a few motor unit action potential discharges that fire repetitively sounding like "soldiers marching" in irregular steps. The intraburst spike frequency is about 30–40 Hz while the repeating discharge interval varies between 1 and 5 Hz. Their occurrence can be intensified by increasing axonal excitability (e.g., with hyperventilation-induced hypocapnia). Genetic or antibody testing can be performed to further evaluate the findings.[30]

Isaac's syndrome or acquired neuromyotonia has similar electrodiagnostic findings as the inherited peripheral nerve hyperexcitability disorders described above. LGI1 and Caspr2 antibodies are surface-cell antibodies and they can be identified in serum and cerebrospinal fluid.[31] This syndrome can present as a paraneoplastic process in the setting of cancer, therefore an evaluation to rule out malignancy should be completed.[12]

Differential Diagnosis

A detailed history and physical examination are crucial in attaining the correct diagnosis. This can provide valuable information to help guide further diagnostic evaluation. For example, understanding whether the patient's symptoms improve or worsen with exercise can help differentiate myotonia from paramyotonia. Also, the presence of myotonia narrows the differential diagnosis to a limited number of diseases. Importantly, with greater accessibility to genetic testing, variants of unknown significance are commonly found. These are best resolved with deep clinical and electrophysiologic phenotyping to correlate with the mutation.

Myotonic dystrophy (DM) is perhaps the best-known myotonic disorder. It is an autosomal dominant inherited disorder with systemic manifestations. Usually, it presents with myotonia, muscular dystrophy, cardiac conduction defects, posterior cataracts, and endocrine disorders. It can be divided into two subtypes with distinct clinical features:[32] Myotonic dystrophy type 1 (DM1, Steinert disease) is characterized by cranial muscle weakness/wasting providing a characteristic appearance and leading to ptosis, dysphagia, dysarthria, and in some cases, eye movement abnormalities. Patients also have a distal weakness (foot drop or impaired hand dexterity), and reflexes are decreased. Progression is slow but later in the disease, patients can experience respiratory muscle weakness, cardiovascular abnormalities, (such as arrhythmias), and cancer, which can shorten life expectancy. In addition, patients develop cataracts early in life and frontal bolding. Among the endocrine abnormalities, type 2 diabetes mellitus is more common than in the general population. Cognitive decline can be observed as well. Myotonic dystrophy type 2 [DM2, proximal myotonic myopathy (PROMM)] is adult-onset DM (primarily limited to Europe descent), which is similar to DM1 with the difference of being late-onset and affecting primarily the proximal muscles instead of the distal ones. In addition, it has a more benign course with rare-to-exceptional face and respiratory muscle weakness and no cognitive impairment. Tremors and pain can be present.

Another myotonic disorder is Schwartz–Jampel syndrome (chondrodystrophic myotonia), which is an inherited disorder characterized by short stature, chondrodysplasia, ocular and facial abnormalities, and joint contractures. There are no warm up phenomena, and EMG reveals persistent myotonia resembling complex repetitive discharges and neuromyotonia.

Pompe disease (late-onset glycogen storage type II) is another disorder that can have myotonia on EMG without clinical myotonia. It is due to acid maltase deficiency resulting in glycogen accumulation in tissues, mostly in the skeletal muscle. Patients can present with respiratory muscle weakness but also with cardiomyopathy.[33]

Although less frequent, certain medications can lead to electrical myotonia without clinical myotonia. Among them, there are colchicine, chloroquine, and statins.[33]

In addition to these disorders, other disorders that clinically appear similar to myotonia and need to be considered are other disorders presenting with cramps after exercise, such as glycogen storage disorders like McArdle disease or rippling muscle disease as well as hypothyroid myopathy.[34] Muscle stiffness in some cases can be mistaken for myotonia. Interestingly, fibromyalgia and chronic fatigue syndrome have turned out to be misdiagnoses for myotonia congenita.[34]

MANAGEMENT

Management depends on the underlying etiology. The treatment of acquired channelopathies varies greatly, and it is beyond the scope of this chapter. The treatment of inherited muscle channelopathies is mostly symptomatic and preventive. There are different therapeutic options for myotonia. Mexiletine is usually the first-line therapy with the most evidence. It is an antiarrhythmic medication that enhances the fast inactivation of sodium channels. Lamotrigine also inhibits sodium channels, and it has shown to be effective in treating myotonia.[16] It has even been suggested as the first-line therapy.[35] Additional sodium channel blockers with less evidence are ranolazine, flecainide, phenytoin, and carbamazepine among others.[16] There are other medications with a different mechanism of action used in treating myotonia. Acetazolamide is one of them. It is the treatment of choice in the named acetazolamide-responsive myotonia.[8] Interestingly, it can worsen paramyotonia congenita in some patients.[16]

The treatment in primary periodic paralysis can be divided into abortive and preventive therapies. In abortive therapy, mild exercise at the beginning of symptom onset can abort the attack. In hypokalemic periodic paralysis or Andersen–Tawil syndrome, potassium supplementation can also be effective in terminating the attack. In hyperkalemic periodic paralysis, oral carbohydrates can be efficacious as well as beta agonist inhalers and intravenous calcium gluconate (if hyperkalemia is severe).[8] For preventive therapy, the treatment also differs between the subtypes of periodic paralysis. Patients with hypokalemic periodic paralysis and Andersen–Tawil syndrome should keep a specific diet (low salt and carbohydrates and no alcohol), and even take daily potassium supplementation. Acetazolamide has been also recommended and in some cases potassium-sparing diuretics such as triamterene. Hyperkalemic periodic paralysis patients should also have specific dietary changes with avoiding potassium-rich foods. Acetazolamide can be used as well. The mechanism of this medication is not well understood in periodic paralysis.[8] The treatment for malignant hyperthermia is mainly supportive care in addition to dantrolene, which blocks the release of calcium from the sarcoplasmic reticulum of muscle cells, thus decreasing muscle contraction.[29]

The treatment of inherited nerve channelopathies is also focused on symptomatic management. In primary erythromelalgia, prevention of the attacks is the cornerstone. Avoiding intense exercise, heat, and prolonged standing, which are common triggers, can help in decreasing the flare frequency. Alcohol and spicy foods can lead to an episode as well but in some cases, the trigger is not known. As the underlying physiopathology is the gain of function of sodium channels, medications targeting those such as mexiletine and other antiepileptic drugs such as carbamazepine are used.[36] A promising drug under development for treating primary erythromelalgia is vixotrigine, which is a voltage- and use-dependent sodium channel blocker (NaV1.7).[37] For acute therapy, safe cooling with a vent or cool water immersion can provide significant relief. In addition, local anesthetics can also be effective.[36]

The prevention of the attacks in paroxysmal extreme pain disorder is also obtained with carbamazepine, which reduces the frequency of the attacks. They are triggered by mechanical pressure, so avoiding it can also help in preventing them. Neuropathic pain in small fiber neuropathy can be treated as other painful neuropathies.

CONCLUSION

As this chapter describes, channelopathies are a diverse group of disorders with different etiologies and unique findings on examination. Overall, they are rare disorders, and it is possible that trainees and more seasoned neurologists have never encountered some of these. Although inherited channelopathies are more common than acquired etiologies, it is equally important to be able to recognize the acquired ones. Despite the rarity of these diagnoses, an open mind and systematic approach can prompt the astute clinician toward these diagnoses to embark on targeted workup and management.

REFERENCES

1. Genevieve B, Shevell M. Channelopathies: a review. Pediatr Neurol. 2008;38:73-85.
2. Kim JB. Channelopathies. Korean J Pediatr. 2014;57:1-18.
3. Ryan DP, Ptáček LJ. Episodic neurological channelopathies. Neuron. 2010;68:282-92.
4. Statland JM, Fontaine B, Hanna MG, Johnson NE, Kissel JT, Sansone VA, et al. Review of the diagnosis and treatment of periodic paralysis. Muscle Nerve. 2018;57:522-30.
5. Horga A, Raja Rayan DL, Matthews E, Sud R, Fialho D, Durran SC, et al. Prevalence study of genetically defined skeletal muscle channelopathies in England. Neurology. 2013;80:1472-5.
6. Lehmann-Horn F, Jurkat-Rott K, Rüdel R. Diagnostics and therapy of muscle channelopathies: guidelines of the Ulm Muscle Center. Acta Myol. 2008;27:98-113.
7. Statland JM, Barohn RJ. Muscle channelopathies: the nondystrophic myotonias and periodic paralyses. Contin Lifelong Learn Neurol. 2013;19:1598-614.
8. Phillips L, Trivedi JR. Skeletal muscle channelopathies. Neuro-therapeutics. 2018;15:954-65.
9. Rosenberg H, Pollock N, Schiemann A, Bulger T, Stowell K. Malignant hyperthermia: a review. Orphanet J Rare Dis. 2015;10:93.
10. Finsterer J. Congenital myasthenic syndromes. Orphanet J Rare Dis. 2019;14:57.
11. Hisama FM, Dib-Hajj SD, Waxman SG. SCN9A Neuropathic Pain Syndromes. In: Adam MP, Everman DB, Mirzaa GM, Pagon RA, Wallace SE, Bean LJH, et al (Eds). GeneReviews® [Internet]. Seattle (WA): University of Washington; 2006 [updated 2020]. pp. 1993-2023.
12. Huang K, Luo YB, Yang H. Autoimmune channelopathies at neuromuscular junction. Front Neurol. 2019;10:516.
13. Janecek J, Kushlaf H. Toxin-induced channelopathies, neuromuscular junction disorders, and myopathy. Neurol Clin. 2020;38:765-80.
14. Grider MH, Jessu R, Kabir R. Physiology, Action Potential. In: StatPearls. Treasure Island (FL): StatPearls Publishing; 2022.
15. Phuyal P, Nagalli S. Hypokalemic Periodic Paralysis. In: StatPearls. Treasure Island (FL): StatPearls Publishing; 2022.
16. Stunnenberg BC, LoRusso S, Arnold WD, Barohn RJ, Cannon SC, Fontaine B, et al. Guidelines on clinical presentation and management of nondystrophic myotonias. Muscle Nerve. 2020;62:430-44.
17. Veerapandiyan A, Statland JM, Tawil R. Andersen–Tawil Syndrome. In: Adam MP, Everman DB, Mirzaa GM, Pagon RA, Wallace SE (Eds). GeneReviews®. Seattle (WA): University of Washington; 1993.
18. Bennett DLH, Woods CG. Painful and painless channelopathies. Lancet Neurol. 2014;13:587-99.
19. Mann N, King T, Murphy R. Review of primary and secondary erythromelalgia. Clin Exp Dermatol. 2019;44:477-82.
20. Nilius B, Voets T. The puzzle of TRPV4 channelopathies. EMBO Rep. 2013;14:152-63.
21. Spillane J, Kullmann DM, Hanna MG. Genetic neurological channelopathies: molecular genetics and clinical phenotypes. J Neurol Neurosurg Psychiatry. 2016;87:37-48.
22. van Sonderen A, Ariño H, Petit-Pedrol M, Leypoldt F, Körtvélyessy P, Wandinger KP, et al. The clinical spectrum of Caspr2 antibody-associated disease. Neurology. 2016;87:521-8.
23. Irani SR, Alexander S, Waters P, Kleopa KA, Pettingill P, Zuliani L, et al. Antibodies to Kv1 potassium channel-complex proteins leucine-rich, glioma inactivated 1 protein and contactin-associated protein-2 in limbic encephalitis, Morvan's syndrome, and acquired neuromyotonia. Brain. 2010;133:2734-48.
24. Golden EP, Vernino S. Autoimmune autonomic neuropathies and ganglionopathies: epidemiology, pathophysiology, and therapeutic advances. Clin Auton Res. 2019;29:277-88.
25. Drost G, Stunnenberg BC, Trip J, Borm G, McGill KC, Ginjaar IH, et al. Myotonic discharges discriminate chloride from sodium muscle channelopathies. Neuromuscul Disord. 2015;25(1):73-80.
26. Hehir MK, Logigian EL. Electrodiagnosis of myotonic disorders. Phys Med Rehabil Clin N Am. 2013;24:209-20.
27. Trip J, Drost G, Verbove DJ, van der Kooi AJ, Kuks JB, Notermans NC, et al. In tandem analysis of CLCN1 and SCN4A greatly enhances mutation detection in families with nondystrophic myotonia. Eur J Hum Genet. 2008;16(8):921-9.
28. Ferradini V, Cassone M, Nuovo S, Bagni I, D'Apice MR, Botta A, et al. Targeted next generation sequencing in patients with myotonia congenita. Clin Chim Acta. 2017;470:1-7.
29. Ellinas H, Albrecht MA. Malignant hyperthermia update. Anesthesiol Clin. 2020;38:165-81.
30. Katirji B. Peripheral nerve hyperexcitability. Handb Clin Neurol. 2019;161:281-90.
31. Dalmau J, Rosenfeld MR. Paraneoplastic syndromes of the CNS. Lancet Neurol. 2008;7:327-40.
32. Meola G, Cardani R. Myotonic dystrophies: an update on clinical aspects, genetic, pathology, and molecular pathomechanisms. Biochim Biophys Acta. 2015;1852:594-606.
33. Miller TM. Differential diagnosis of myotonic disorders. Muscle Nerve. 2008;37:293-9.
34. Graves TD, Hanna MG. Neurological channelopathies. Postgrad Med J. 2005;81:20-32.
35. Andersen G, Hedermann G, Witting N, Duno M, Andersen H, Vissing J. The antimyotonic effect of lamotrigine in nondystrophic myotonias: a double-blind randomized study. Brain J Neurol. 2017;140:2295-305.
36. Tham SW, Giles M. Current pain management strategies for patients with erythromelalgia: a critical review. J Pain Res. 2018;11:1689-98.
37. Biogen. (2018). An exploratory, randomized, double-blind, crossover study to compare the efficacy and safety of BIIB074 versus placebo in the treatment of primary inherited erythromelalgia. [online] Available from https://clinicaltrials.gov/ct2/show/NCT02917187.

Part 4H: Ataxias

88 CHAPTER

Ataxias

Divyani Garg, Achal Kumar Srivastava

INTRODUCTION

Coordinated movement of the limbs and eyes is reliant on a complicated network that connects the basal ganglia, cerebellar structures, and the cortex. Disruption in this complex machinery leads to incoordination of gait, limbs, and abnormalities of eye movements. Motor coordination also depends on sensory and proprioceptive inputs via the afferent system. Disturbance of this afferent circuitry leads to sensory ataxia. Clinical features of cerebellar dysfunction may be anatomically correlated to the cerebellar structure. Gait and truncal ataxia correlate with midline/vermis dysfunction, and limb incoordination correlate with dysfunction of the ipsilateral cerebellar hemisphere. Gaze abnormalities correlate with flocculonodular lobe malfunction. Cerebellar dysfunction may also arise due to problems with cerebellar connections, that is, cerebellar peduncles or brainstem. The presence of long tract signs, internuclear ophthalmoplegia, and cranial nerve dysfunction indicates brainstem origin. The presence of cerebellar dysarthria and nystagmus indicates cerebellar pathology. Other less common features of cerebellar dysfunction include cerebellar cognitive affective syndrome, cerebellar mutism, and cerebellar "fits". Details of these clinical correlates may be found in several standard textbooks.

Sensory ataxia may arise due to dysfunction of the sensory peripheral nerve fibers, dorsal root ganglia and posterior column, resulting from disruption of proprioceptive input. Clinically, this manifests as ataxia which worsens with the removal of visual input, as in the dark or on closing eyes. The associated loss of other large fiber sensations and sensory symptoms (tingling and numbness) may be apparent. Deep tendon reflexes are usually attenuated or absent. Pseudoathetosis may be seen in the limbs. These features aid in distinguishing the two broad categories of cerebellar and sensory ataxia.

Pragmatically, cerebellar ataxia is categorized based on etiology as inherited, acquired, or sporadic ataxia. Acquired cerebellar dysfunction is crucial to recognize, as it usually represents treatable or reversible causes, such as infectious, immune-mediated, toxin/drug-induced, or paraneoplastic. Otherwise, the larger group of inherited ataxias is degenerative and irreversible. As is the paradigm in neurological disorders, history and clinical examination are imperative to localize where in the neuraxis the lesion lies, and also to uncover etiology. Further evaluation is dictated by the clinical picture that subsequently emerges. In general, structural imaging may reveal a host of acquired disorders, including neoplasms, demyelination, infections, vascular pathology, and the like. Occasionally, inherited or degenerative ataxias may also have signature radiological findings, such as multiple system atrophy (MSA), Joubert syndrome, and autosomal recessive spastic ataxia of Charlevoix–Saguenay (ARSACS). In the Indian context, it is important to recognize the occurrence of spinocerebellar ataxia (SCA) type 12 in the "Vaniya" ethnic group. This ethnic correlation was first recognized in India, and its clinical phenotype and genotype have expanded since, with multiple descriptions from India. The presence of tremors is the hallmark clinical feature of this SCA type.

In this chapter, we describe the clinical spectrum, clinical features, biochemical and radiological findings, as well as paradigms for evaluation and treatment in ataxia, specifically focusing on cerebellar disorders.

EPIDEMIOLOGY

Among the SCAs, SCA3 is the most common subtype, followed by SCA2 and SCA6.[1] The overall prevalence of ataxia in children has been reported to be 26/100,00. Among the SCAs, polyglutamine repeat disorders are most common, including SCA 1, 2, 3, 6, 7, 17, and dentatorubral-pallidoluysian atrophy (DRPLA).[2] Ataxic cerebral palsy contributes to the overall prevalence of ataxias in children.[3] For dominant ataxias, it is 2.7/100,000 and for recessive ataxias, it is 3.3/100,000.[4] Friedreich's ataxia (FA) is the most common autosomal recessive ataxia, followed by ataxia telangiectasia (AT) and ataxia with oculomotor apraxia (AOA). In a large epidemiological Korean study that included 820 patients with cerebellar ataxia, 16.6% were familial and the remaining 83.4% were nonfamilial. Sporadic cerebellar ataxias were the most common, occurring in 62.9% of patients, followed by genetic (20.7%), secondary (5.2%) and 11.1% were undetermined. In this series, the most common genetic ataxia was SCA, with SCA3 being the most common subtype.[5] In India, SCA2 and SCA12 have been reported to be the most common dominant ataxias from India, followed by SCA1,[6] albeit with better quality of life compared to SCA1 and SCA2.[7] Analysis of molecular data from a central laboratory from India revealed SCA12 to be the most common subtype.[8]

PATHOLOGY AND PATHOPHYSIOLOGY

The cerebellum comprises a midline portion, the vermis, and two lateral portions, the cerebellar hemispheres. It consists of three major segments—(1) the anterior lobe, (2) the posterior lobe, and (3) the flocculonodular lobe. The superficial cortex lines the deep white matter. There are three pairs of deep nuclei—(1) the dentate, (2) emboliform and globose (together called the nucleus interpositus), and (3) fastigial nuclei. The superficial cortex comprises three layers—(1) an outer molecular layer, (2) the middle Purkinje layer, and (3) the deepest granule cell layer. The Purkinje cells form the efferent outflow of the cerebellum. Phylogenetically, the cerebellum consists of three units—(1) the archicerebellum (flocculonodular lobe), (2) the paleocerebellum (vermis, pyramid, uvula, and paraflocculus), and (3) the neocerebellum (midportion of the vermis and cerebellar hemispheres). The fastigial nucleus controls muscles in stance and gait. Lesions of the fastigial nucleus lead to problems with the maintenance of stance and gait. The nucleus interpositus enables stability by aiding segmental reflexes and halts unwanted movement. Problems with nucleus interpositus lead to abnormal rapid alternating movement, loss of check response, limb incoordination, and truncal titubation. The dentate nucleus controls fine dexterity. The three cerebellar peduncles connect the cerebellum to the brainstem—(1) the superior cerebellar peduncle (brachium conjunctivum) connects it to the midbrain, (2) the middle cerebellar peduncle (brachium pontis) connects to the pons, and (3) the inferior cerebellar peduncle (restiform body) connects to the medulla. Of these, the middle cerebellar peduncle carries only afferent fibers.

ACQUIRED CEREBELLAR ATAXIA

Acquired cerebellar ataxias form the largest etiological group among cerebellar ataxias. Broadly, these may be categorized as:

- Metabolic/nutritional
- Toxin/drug-mediated
- Immune-mediated
- Infectious
- Neoplastic
- Vascular

Metabolic/Nutritional Cerebellar Ataxia

These disorders arise from a host of metabolic factors, including vitamin deficiencies. Broadly, they tend to be symmetrical disorders and may have other systems of the neuraxis involved, in addition to cerebellar dysfunction. These are detailed below. Ataxia with vitamin E deficiency (AVED) is an inherited disorder, and is highlighted in the section on "Inherited Ataxias". Acquired vitamin E deficiency is described below.

Vitamin B1 Deficiency

The deficiency of vitamin B1 (thiamine) leads to two distinct syndromes—(1) Wernicke's encephalopathy and (2) Korsakoff psychosis. Wernicke's encephalopathy is characterized by the triad of ataxia, ophthalmoplegia, and encephalopathy.[9] Thiamine deficiency often occurs in individuals with chronic alcohol dependence syndrome. However, it may occur also in malnutrition, prolonged fasting or excessive vomiting. The regions affected include the dorsomedial thalamus, mammillary bodies, periaqueductal gray matter, walls of the third ventricle, and tectal plate. These areas may also demonstrate increased T2-weighted/fluid-attenuated inversion recovery (T2/FLAIR) signal change. Atrophy of the mammillary bodies and dorsomedial thalamus is associated with an amnestic syndrome. Involvement of the superior cerebellar vermis accounts for ataxia and abducens nucleus and midbrain/pons involvement accounts for ophthalmoplegia. Wernicke's encephalopathy is reversible with prompt treatment. However, untreated Wernicke's encephalopathy may progress to become irreversible, with the development of confabulations and gait impairment. This latter condition is referred to as Korsakoff's psychosis and develops in nearly 80% of patients with Wernicke's encephalopathy.

Vitamin B12 Deficiency

Deficiency of vitamin B12 leads to involvement of the posterior and lateral columns of the spinal cord, termed "subacute combined degeneration".[10] This is usually seen in a strictly vegetarian or vegan diet. The ataxia due to vitamin B12 deficiency is therefore, sensory or afferent ataxia. There may be associated optic nerve involvement and peripheral neuropathy in a nonlength-dependent pattern. Magnetic resonance imaging (MRI) of the spinal cord shows a hyperintense signal in the posterior column, referred to as the "inverted V" sign.

Vitamin E Deficiency

Acquired vitamin E deficiency may arise as a result of malabsorption due to surgery, celiac disease, etc. Clinically, it manifests with ataxia, peripheral neuropathy, myopathy, and retinitis pigmentosa.

Toxin-/Drug-related Ataxia

A large number of drugs can lead to ataxia, of which antiseizure medications are most commonly incriminated **(Table 1)**.[11] Antiseizure medications that may cause ataxia include phenytoin, carbamazepine, gabapentin, and phenobarbitone. Chemotherapy agents include cytarabine, fluorouracil, and platinum-based compounds (cisplatin, oxaliplatin, and paclitaxel). Psychiatric drugs that cause ataxia include lithium. Several antibiotics can cause ataxia including metronidazole.

Toxins that can lead to ataxias include toluene or benzene derivatives, heavy metals, and drugs of abuse (cocaine, heroin, and phencyclidine). The most important of these is alcohol.

TABLE 1: Drugs/toxins that may induce ataxia.[11]

Class	Agent	Mechanism/ Comments
Drugs		
Antiseizure medications	• Phenytoin • Carbamazepine • Phenobarbitone • Gabapentin • Vigabatrin	• Damage to Purkinje cells • Patients with cerebellar atrophy are more susceptible • Although it may cause transient initial ataxia, it is useful for the treatment of ataxia
Chemotherapy agents	• 5-Fluorouracil • Cytosine arabinoside • Cisplatin, oxaliplatin, paclitaxel • Methotrexate • Capecitabine • Epothilone D	• Pancerebellar syndrome • Cumulative doses >24 g predispose • Sensory ataxia • More likely with intrathecal doses • Encephalopathy
Antibiotics	• Metronidazole • Mefloquine	Cerebellar nuclei show edema
Other agents	• Lithium • Amiodarone, Procainamide • Ciclosporin, calcineurin inhibitors • Bismuth • Bromide	5–7% develop the cerebellar syndrome
Toxins		
Stimulant drugs	• Alcohol • Cocaine • Heroin • Phencyclidine • Kava	Disruption of GABAergic pathways
Heavy metals	• Mercury • Lead • Manganese • Aluminum • Thallium	Celphos poisoning was reported from Varanasi, India
Toxins	• Toluene/benzene • Carbon monoxide • Organophosphate	

Immune-mediated Ataxias

Immune-mediated cerebellar ataxia encompasses disorders such as acute disseminated encephalomyelitis (ADEM) and multiple sclerosis (MS), as well as autoimmune cerebellar ataxias which specifically target the cerebellum, including paraneoplastic cerebellar degeneration (PCD).[12] A new entity called primary autoimmune cerebellar ataxia (PACA) has been proposed, with the establishment of diagnostic criteria.[13]

Paraneoplastic Cerebellar Degeneration

Paraneoplastic cerebellar degeneration is the most frequent among paraneoplastic neurological disorders.[14] PCD is defined by the onset of acute or subacute symmetrical ataxia in a patient with cancer diagnosed within 5 years of ataxia onset. PCD may also be defined by the presence of ataxia in combination with an onconeural antibody. Onconeural antibodies associated with ataxia include anti-Yo, anti-Ri, anti-Ma2, anti-CV2/CRMP5, anti-VGCC, anti-Tr, and anti-VGCC antibodies and are associated with specific malignancies.

The following **Table 2** summarizes the known associations with specific antibodies in immune-mediated cerebellar ataxias.

Non-paraneoplastic Autoimmune Cerebellar Ataxia

Certain autoantibodies may also be associated with the development of acute to subacute onset of ataxia, in the absence of underlying malignancy. These include anti-glutamic acid decarboxylase (GAD) 65, anti-CASPR2, anti-mGluR1, and anti-Homer-3. In patients with anti-CASPR2 antibodies, gait ataxia is prominent, and nystagmus and dysarthria are uncommon. Patients may also develop

TABLE 2: Antibodies and associations in immune-mediated cerebellar ataxia.

Antibody	Condition/Association
Antigliadin, transglutaminase-2 and 6	Celiac disease/gluten ataxia
Anti-Yo	Breast, and ovarian cancer
Anti-Hu	Small cell lung cancer
Anti-CV2	Thymoma, small cell lung cancer
Anti-Ma2	Testicular cancer, lung cancer
Anti-Ri	Breast cancer
Anti-Tr	Hodgkin's lymphoma
Anti-VGCC	Lambert–Eaton syndrome
Anti-DPPX	Limbic encephalitis, diarrhea, ataxia
Anti-LGI1	Limbic encephalitis, ataxia
Anti-CASPR2	Limbic encephalitis, peripheral nerve hyperexcitability syndrome, ataxia
Anti-mGluR1	Ataxia
Anti-GAD65	Ataxia, stiff person syndrome
Others: Anti-Zic4, anti-glycine R, anti-PCA-2, anti-Homer-3, etc.	

transient attacks of cerebellar ataxia resembling episodic ataxia (EA) syndromes. Cerebellar atrophy does not develop usually. In patients with antibodies to GAD65, ataxia is symmetrical and progressive and afflicts women in the sixth decade. Cerebellar atrophy may develop. Insulin-dependent diabetes mellitus may also develop. The prognosis remains guarded despite immunotherapy. Intravenous immunoglobulin (IVIG) therapy is preferred.

Opsoclonus-myoclonus-ataxia Syndrome

This rare disorder usually has an onset in the second year of life. The combination of opsoclonus, myoclonus, and ataxia, called opsoclonus-myoclonus-ataxia syndrome (OMAS), may also be associated with cognitive issues and sleep abnormalities. In children with OMAS, nearly 50% will have associated neuroblastoma.[15] Nearly 40% of adult patients with OMAS may harbor an underlying malignancy and may be associated with paraneoplastic antibodies, such as anti-Ri, anti-Ma2, anti-CRMP5, etc. One-third of these cases have a parainfectious origin. Infectious agents associated with OMAS include human immunodeficiency virus (HIV), West Nile virus, Epstein–Barr virus (EBV), *Salmonella*, *Streptococcus*, scrub typhus, etc. Paraneoplastic OMAS may be differentiated from nonparaneoplastic OMAS by older age at onset. Opsoclonus is characterized by rapid, chaotic, and multidirectional saccades without any intersaccadic interval. OMAS may result in long-term cognitive issues. Early and aggressive immunotherapy may improve outcomes.

Hashimoto's Thyroiditis

Also known as steroid-responsive encephalopathy associated with autoimmune thyroiditis (SREAT), elevated antithyroid (antithyroid peroxidase or less commonly, antithyroglobulin) antibodies occur in combination with altered mental status, memory issues, myoclonus, seizures, tremors, ataxia, and sleep abnormalities.[16] Neuroimaging may be normal, but may show dural enhancement.

Gluten Ataxia

Gluten sensitivity, which manifests as celiac disease, is characterized by gastrointestinal complaints and gluten sensitivity. IgG and IgA antibodies to gliadin and tissue transglutaminase (TG2 and TG6) are used for diagnosis. These antibodies cross react with cerebellar cells.[17]

Gluten ataxia is clinically characterized by a combination of ataxia, brisk reflexes, and peripheral neuropathy. Other manifestations include chorea and myoclonus. MRI may show cerebellar atrophy. The presence of enteropathy is not required for the diagnosis. The majority of the patients with gluten ataxia do not have clinical or histological features of enteropathy. Treatment required a gluten-free diet, which prevents further progression and may stabilize ataxia.

Infectious Ataxias

Acute cerebellitis is an infectious or parainfectious process, more commonly occurring among children. Pathogens incriminated include varicella-zoster virus (VZV), EBV, mycoplasma, mumps virus, and entero- and parvoviruses. In adults, usually EBV and VZV are implicated. Patients usually develop profound truncal ataxia, and features of raised intracranial pressure may also develop. Usually brainstem signs are absent, and their presence should raise concerns for alternative etiology. MRI may show an increase signal in the cerebellum and/or leptomeningeal enhancement. Usually, the process is self-limited with good recovery in children. Residual sequelae may persist in adults.

Coronavirus disease 2019 (COVID-19) is also associated with the development of post-infective ataxia syndrome, which may occur as OMAS.[18]

Chronic infections such as HIV[19] and syphilis[20] have also been described to lead to ataxia.

Neoplasms

Ataxia may be a result of primary cerebellar tumors, or secondaries. In children, the common neoplasms include pilocytic astrocytoma and medulloblastoma. In adults, metastases are more common. Features of raised intracranial pressure are common among patients with posterior fossa tumors.

Vascular

Stroke, either ischemic or hemorrhagic, involving the cerebellar blood supply may present as acute onset ataxia.[21] Usually, this is unilateral and brainstem signs may be associated. Features of raised intracranial pressure may also develop.

Superficial siderosis is a syndrome characterized by subpial hemosiderin deposition due to subarachnoid hemorrhage occurring at a slow rate.[21] Iron from blood is neurotoxic, and initially, apoferritin binds free iron in the subarachnoid space to form ferritin and hemosiderin, preventing injury. However, with continued bleeding, these neuroprotective mechanisms are overpowered. The most common clinical features include ataxia, due to involvement of the cerebellum, and the eighth nerve, leading to sensorineural hearing loss. This is because the posterior fossa structures receive the earliest irrigation of blood-stained CSF.

Hemosiderin deposition is represented by cortical T2 hypointensity, which is best seen on iron-sensitive sequences such as GRE. Clinically, superficial siderosis leads to hearing impairment and cerebellar ataxia. The most common source of chronic low-grade bleeding is a dural tear, which may occur due to trauma or disk disease. Other sources include intracranial tumors, vascular malformation, surgery, etc. Management required correction of the source of bleeding. Iron chelating agent deferiprone has been used without success, and is not recommended for management.

INHERITED ATAXIAS

Inherited ataxias are a large group of disorders. Based on the mode of inheritance, inherited ataxias are classified as autosomal dominant (including EAs), autosomal recessive, X-linked, and mitochondrial disorders.

Autosomal Dominant Cerebellar Ataxia

Spinocerebellar Ataxia

Autosomal dominant cerebellar ataxias (ADCA) are also and more popularly known as spinocerebellar ataxias. SCAs are a heterogeneous group, characterized by cerebellar and brainstem involvement. Based on Anita Harding's classification, three types were defined. ADCA type I (ADCA I) consists of ataxia in combination with other neurological features, such as peripheral neuropathy, e.g., SCA1, 2 and 3; ADCA II consists of ataxia associated with pigmentary retinopathy. SCA7 is the only SCA that belongs to this category. ADCA III consists of pure ataxia syndromes, e.g., SCA6.

Based on genetics and molecular mechanisms, SCAs may be classified as ataxias due to repeat expansion and nonrepeat mutations.[22] These are summarized in **Table 3**. Repeat expansion mutations are characterized by the phenomenon of anticipation, that is, disease onset at an earlier age group than the previous generation. Clinical anticipation refers to the worsening of the disease in subsequent generations, which occurs due to the lengthening of the repeats. SCAs up to type 48 have been described.[23]

TABLE 3: Genotype and phenotype of some spinocerebellar ataxias (SCAs).

SCA	Genetic mutation	Phenotype
Repeat mutations		
SCA1	*ATXN1*	Ataxia, pyramidal involvement, neuropathy, and bulbar symptoms
SCA2	*ATXN2*	Slow saccades, ataxia, and neuropathy
SCA3	*ATXN3*	Ophthalmoplegia, ataxia, pyramidal signs, peripheral neuropathy, amyotrophy, and fasciculations
SCA6	*CACNA1A*	Pure ataxia and downbeat nystagmus
SCA7	*ATXN7*	Ataxia, retinopathy, and pyramidal signs
SCA8	*ATXN8*	Ataxia, pyramidal signs, neuropathy, and cognitive issues
SCA10	*ATXN10*	Ataxia, seizures
SCA12	*PPP2R2B*	Ataxia, tremors
SCA17	*TBP*	Ataxia, pyramidal and extrapyramidal involvement, dementia, and psychiatric issues
SCA31	*BEAN1*	Pure ataxia
SCA36	*NOP56*	Ataxia, hearing issues, and amyotrophy
SCA37	*DAB1*	Ataxia, vertical gaze issues
Nonrepeat mutations		
SCA5	*SPTBN2*	Pure ataxia
SCA13	*KCNC3*	Ataxia, cognitive issues
SCA14	*PRKCG*	Ataxia, myoclonus
SCA15/16	*ITPR1*	Pure ataxia
SCA19/22	*KCND3*	• SCA22: Pure ataxia • SCA19: Ataxia, dementia, and myoclonus
SCA28	*AFGL3L2*	Ataxia, pyramidal signs, ophthalmoplegia

However, some autosomal recessive and X-linked disorders are also called SCA, SCA(R), and SCA(X), respectively.

Spinocerebellar ataxias have wide clinical heterogeneity. The predominant manifestation is cerebellar ataxia, although vestibular and sensory ataxias are also contributors. Nonataxia features include motor features such as spasticity and amyotrophy, extrapyramidal features such as parkinsonism, dystonia, chorea and myoclonus, peripheral neuropathy, seizures, and oculomotor abnormalities. The latter include saccadic slowing or under- or overshooting, broken pursuits, and retinal degeneration as seen in SCA7. Cognitive dysfunction, sleep disorders, and neurobehavioral issues such as mood problems have also been reported among SCA patients.

Other Ataxias of Autosomal Dominant Inheritance

Autosomal dominant cerebellar ataxia, deafness and narcolepsy (ADCA-DN): This occurs because of mutations in DNMT1 protein, and is characterized by cerebellar ataxia, sensorineural hearing loss, and sleep abnormalities, typically narcolepsy and cataplexy.[24]

Hypomyelination with atrophy of the basal ganglia and cerebellum (H-ABC): This occurs because of mutations in the *TUBB4A* gene.[25] This disorder presents in infancy or childhood, with developmental delay, ataxia, and extrapyramidal features. MRI shows features of hypomyelination, cerebellar atrophy, and putaminal dysgenesis, with atrophy of the caudate head, with preserved globus pallidus and thalamus.

CAPOS syndrome: This is a childhood disorder that occurs due to mutations in the *ATP1A3* gene.[26] CAPOS is an acronym for cerebellar ataxia, areflexia, pes cavus, optic atrophy, and sensorineural hearing loss.

Episodic Ataxias

Episodic ataxias are dominantly inherited disorders, characterized by episodes of usually profound ataxia, which vary in duration from minutes to days.[27]

Episodic ataxia 1: EA1 occurs due to mutations in the *KCNA1* gene. It usually presents in adolescence, but may present up to the second decade. Ataxia usually lasts from seconds to minutes. Attacks may be precipitated by abrupt postural change, stress/emotion, vestibular stimulation, and exercise.[27] Myokymia is observed in the hand muscle and the face.

Episodic ataxias 2: EA2 is the most frequent of the EAs, and is associated with mutations in the *CACNA1* gene, which it shares with familial hemiplegic migraine 1 (FHM1). The age at onset is in infancy or childhood. The duration of attacks is from hours to days, and attacks are usually severe. Precipitants include physical exertion, emotional stress or excitement, and fatigue. Patients have interictal ataxia and may develop cerebellar atrophy.

In total, eight subtypes have been described which are summarized in **Table 4**.

TABLE 4: Episodic ataxias (EA).

Episodic ataxia	Gene/s affected	Clinical features
EA1	*KCNA1*, chr. 12p13	• Attacks last seconds-minutes • Ataxia, vertigo, tremor, seizures • Interictal myokymia
EA2	*CACNA1A*, chr. 19p13	• Attacks last hours • Ataxia, vertigo, diplopia, tonic upgaze, seizure, confusion • Interictal ataxia/nystagmus
EA3	Chr. 1q42	• Attacks last minutes to hours • Vertigo, dysarthria, diplopia, and headache • Interictal myokymia
EA4	Unknown	• Attacks last minutes • Vertigo, diplopia
EA5	*CACNB4*, chr. 2q	• Attacks last hours • Vertigo, dysarthria
EA6	*SLC1A3*, chr. 5p13	• Attacks last hours to days • Vertigo, seizures • Interictal ataxia, nystagmus
EA7	Unknown, chr. 19q13	• Attacks last hours to days • Vertigo, dysarthria
EA8	*UBR4*, chr. 1p36	• Attacks last from minutes to up to 24 hours • Vertigo • Interictal nystagmus, ataxia, myokymia

Autosomal Recessive Cerebellar Ataxia

These are a large and heterogeneous group of disorders with onset in childhood or adolescence. The most common autosomal recessive cerebellar ataxia is FA worldwide.

The classification of these disorders is challenging due to the large number of genes involved. Clinically, it may be pragmatic to approach them based on the presence of associated sensorimotor abnormalities **(Table 5)**.

The Society for Research on the Cerebellum and Ataxias Task Force classified autosomal recessive cerebellar ataxia broadly into three groups:

1. *Primary AR cerebellar ataxias*: These constitute around 15 disorders.
2. *Rare ataxias*: These are reported in small numbers of families.
3. *Complex ataxias*: Such as metabolic ataxias. Ataxia is a part of a multisystem syndrome.

Another pragmatic classification is based on age at onset:

- *Congenital*: Joubert syndrome and Cayman ataxia
- *Infancy*: AT and ARSACS
- *Childhood or adolescence*: FA, AOA1, AOA2, polymerase gamma (POLG)-related ataxia, and AVED
- *Adulthood*: Autosomal recessive cerebellar ataxia type 1 (ARCA1), ARCA3, and spastic paraplegia 7 (SPG7)

Some of these disorders are detailed below. The associated genetic defects are enumerated in **Table 6.**

Joubert Syndrome

Joubert syndrome is a rare neurodevelopmental disorder that is defined by the presence of the "molar tooth sign" on neuroimaging. Molar tooth sign develops resultant to aplasia or hypoplasia of the cerebellar vermis, combined with a deepened interpeduncular fossa and lengthened superior cerebellar peduncle. It is a multisystemic disorder, with involvement of the ophthalmic, hepatic, renal, and skeletal systems. It is a part of disorders called ciliopathies, associated with primary ciliary abnormalities.[28]

Friedreich's Ataxia

Friedreich's ataxia is the most common inherited ataxia.[29] It is caused usually by GAA expansion in the first intron of the frataxin (*FXN*) gene on chromosome 9q21.11. The

TABLE 5: Approach to autosomal recessive cerebellar ataxias based on features of neuropathy.

Features of neuropathy	Disorder	MRI findings
Sensory axonal	• Friedreich's ataxia • Ataxia with vitamin E deficiency • Abetalipoproteinemia • Infantile onset spinocerebellar ataxia (SCA)	• Cervical cord atrophy • Cerebellar atrophy • Cerebellar atrophy • Cerebellar, brainstem and cortical atrophy
Sensory and motor axonal	• Ataxia telangiectasia • Ataxia telangiectasia-like • Ataxia with oculomotor apraxia 1 • Ataxia with oculomotor apraxia 2 • Autosomal recessive spastic ataxia of Charlevoix–Saguenay • Cerebrotendinous xanthomatosis	• Vermian atrophy • Cerebellar atrophy • Cerebellar atrophy • Cerebellar atrophy
Sensory and motor demyelinating	• Refsum disease • Marinesco–Sjögren syndrome	• Cerebellar atrophy • Cerebellar atrophy, small anterior pituitary

TABLE 6: Genetic abnormalities in autosomal recessive cerebellar ataxia.

Ataxia syndrome	Molecular defect
Ataxia telangiectasia	*ATM* gene on chromosome 11q22
Ataxia telangiectasia-like disease	*MRE11* on chromosome 11q21, *RNF168*
Ataxia with oculomotor apraxia 1	*APTX* on chromosome 9
Ataxia with oculomotor apraxia 2	*SETX* on chromosome 9
Ataxia with vitamin E deficiency	*TTPA* on chromosome 8
Abetalipoproteinemia	*MTP* on chromosome 4
Autosomal recessive spastic ataxia of Charlevoix–Saguenay (ARSACS)	*SACS* on chromosome 13q11
Coenzyme Q10 deficiency	*COQ2* on chromosome 4q21.23
Friedreich's ataxia	*FXN* on chromosome 9q13
Mitochondrial recessive ataxia syndrome (MIRAS)	*POLG* on chromosome 15q22.26
Refsum disease	*PHYH, PEX7*

usual age of onset is in the second decade (around 15 years of age). However, late-onset FA (age at onset >25 years) and very late-onset FA (age at onset >40 years) have been reported. These differ from typical FA in slower progression, greater spasticity, and less frequent diabetes and cardiac involvement.

Neurological manifestations include ataxia, which is a combination of afferent, cerebellar, and vestibular components. Sensory involvement occurs due to neuronopathy and posterior column involvement. Deep tendon reflexes are usually absent but may be normal. The plantar response is usually extensor. Square wave jerks are pathognomonic, but other abnormalities include saccadic dysmetria. Optic atrophy is present in 20% of patients. Patients may also develop hearing loss. Non-neurological manifestations include skeletal muscle deformities (scoliosis and pes cavus), diabetes mellitus, and cardiomyopathy (hypertrophic/dilated).

Ataxia Telangiectasia

Ataxia telangiectasia is a rare DNA repair disorder.[30] It occurs due to mutations in the ataxia telangiectasia-mutated (*ATM*) gene. Due to defective DNA repair, these patients have an enhanced risk of malignancy and immune deficiency disorder. AT may occur as the classic form or variant AT. The classic form is characterized by the total absence of ATM kinase activity. The usual age of onset is in early childhood.

Neurological features include ataxia, dystonia, chorea, tremor, and ocular abnormalities.[31] The latter typically comprises oculomotor apraxia, saccadic slowing, and nystagmus. Telangiectasias appear on the skin, conjunctiva, or pharynx, usually by 10 years of age. Central nervous system tumors and lymphoproliferative disorders occur at increased rates. Patients may also have a history of recurrent respiratory tract infections, leading eventually to bronchiectasis. MRI usually shows prominent cerebellar atrophy. Patients with variant AT demonstrate reduced levels of ATM kinase activity, and have increased lifespan and milder disease severity.

Ataxia telangiectasia-like disorders, characterized by milder disease and slower progression, are rare disorders. Mutations in *MRE11* and *RNF168* genes may lead to AT-like disorders.

Ataxia with Oculomotor Apraxia

Ataxia with oculomotor apraxia type 1is childhood-onset ataxia due to mutations in the aprataxin (*APTX*) gene.[32] Oculomotor apraxia is a hallmark finding. As the disease progresses, extraocular movement restriction may develop. Axonal motor neuropathy is also associated with distal atrophy. Chorea and dystonia may also develop. AOA2 is caused by mutations in the senataxin (*SETX*) gene.[33]

Autosomal Recessive Spastic Ataxia of Charlevoix–Saguenay

Autosomal recessive spastic ataxia of Charlevoix–Saguenay is early-onset, hereditary ataxia which occurs due to mutations in the sacsin gene.[34] Spasticity is a hallmark feature, with onset in infancy. The plantar response is extensor, and nystagmus and saccadic intrusions into pursuits may be present. Retinal examination may show the presence of myelinated retinal nerve fibers. Distal amyotrophy and skeletal deformities may develop in advanced cases.[35] Peripheral neuropathy is mainly axonal with some demyelinating features. MRI shows cerebellar atrophy, prominently affecting the vermis, along with spinal atrophy. Typical hypointense transverse "pontine stripes" on T2-weighted MRI are observed.

Cerebrotendinous Xanthomatosis

Cerebrotendinous xanthomatosis is a rare disorder of bile acid metabolism, which occurs due to mutations in the *CYP27A1* gene, leading to a deficiency of the mitochondrial sterol 27-hydroxylase enzyme.[36] Neurological features include cognitive and psychiatric impairment, pyramidal involvement, ataxia, and dystonia.[37] Presence of tendon xanthomas, while pathognomonic, is not essential, as tendon xanthomas may not be visible. Cataracts may develop. Chronic diarrhea and premature atherosclerosis may also develop.

Mitochondrial Ataxias

POLG-related Ataxia

Polymerase gamma-related neurological disorders comprise a large group of syndromes that occur due to mutations in the mitochondrial *POLG* gene.[38] Six major syndromes are associated.

1. Alpers–Huttenlocher syndrome
2. Myocerebrohepatopathy
3. Myoclonic epilepsy myopathy sensory ataxia
4. Ataxia neuropathy spectrum includes mitochondrial recessive ataxia syndrome (MIRAS), sensory ataxia neuropathy dysarthria and ophthalmoplegia (SANDO) syndrome.[39]
5. Progressive external ophthalmoplegia
6. Spinocerebellar ataxia with epilepsy[40]

X-linked Cerebellar Ataxias

These include fragile X-associated tremor ataxia syndrome (FXTAS) and X-linked adrenoleukodystrophy, and other rarer syndromes.[41,42] These are summarized in **Table 7**.

TABLE 7: Features of X-linked cerebellar ataxias.

Ataxia syndrome	Features	Gene affected
• Fragile X syndrome • Fragile X-associated tremor ataxia syndrome	• Cognitive impairment, elongated facies, cryptorchidism • Cognitive impairment, ataxia, tremor, peripheral neuropathy	*FMR1* • CGG triplet expansion • Significant reduction in the posterior vermis
X-linked adrenoleukodystrophy	White matter and dentate involvement, lead to pyramidal tract and cerebellar involvement	*ABCD1* • Elevated long chain fatty acids
X-linked Opitz syndrome	Midline malformations, developmental delay	*MID1* gene
Menkes syndrome	• Delayed milestones, intellectual disability, lax skin, kinky, steel-colored hair • Milder phenotype: occipital horn syndrome	*ATP7A* copper transporter gene
Rett syndrome	Developmental regression, midline hand wringing stereotypy, seizures, ataxia, hypotonia	*MECP2* gene at Xq28
Xq28 microduplication syndrome	Infantile hypotonia, intellectual decline, autism	*MECP2* duplication
Allan–Herndon–Dudley syndrome	Psychomotor retardation, intellectual disability, thyrotoxicosis, elongated facies	*MCT8* mutations

SPORADIC DEGENERATIVE ATAXIA

These mainly include MSA and idiopathic late-onset cerebellar ataxia (ILOCA)/sporadic adult-onset ataxia (SAOA).

Multiple System Atrophy

This is an adult-onset, neurodegenerative disorder characterized by a combination of parkinsonism, ataxia, and autonomic dysfunction.[43-46] The two subtypes, MSA-parkinsonism (MSA-P) and MSA-cerebellar (MSA-C) are distinguished clinically based on predominant motor manifestations of parkinsonism or cerebellar ataxia. Autonomic dysfunction is the hallmark, based on orthostatic fall in blood pressure or urinary dysfunction (fall in systolic BP by 20 mm Hg and/or diastolic BP by 10 mm Hg at 3 minutes of standing). Pathology typically shows the presence of glial cytoplasmic inclusions. In MSA-C, MRI may show the presence of typical findings such as the "hot cross bun" sign and middle cerebellar peduncle hyperintensities. Treatment is symptomatic.

Late-onset Cerebellar Ataxia/Sporadic Adult-onset Ataxia

This is a late-onset form of ataxia, arising from heterogeneous causes. Autonomic dysfunction may be present, but does not meet the criteria for MSA. Up to 25% of patients characterized initially as ILOCA may develop MSA over the subsequent 4–5 years.[47]

DIAGNOSIS

Diagnosis is based on clinical features, in combination with evaluation.

Diagnosis of acquired ataxias requires the presence of an incriminating agent (such as infection/drug, etc.) followed by the development of ataxia, and improvement or stabilization of features on removal or treatment of the underlying cause. Diagnosis of hereditary ataxias is based on the presence of a typical phenotype, family history, and molecular testing, along with relevant ancillary tests. MSA is diagnosed based on diagnostic criteria.

Further details of diagnostic tests are outlined in the section on investigations.

DIFFERENTIAL DIAGNOSIS

The differential diagnosis for cerebellar ataxia includes other ataxias such as afferent or vestibular ataxia. However, cerebellar and afferent ataxias may occur concomitantly in the same patient. Afferent ataxias may be distinguished from cerebellar ataxias by the presence in the form of features of sensory impairment, and worsening of the ataxia in the dark. Additionally, the presence of cerebellar dysarthria and nystagmus are seen only in cerebellar involvement. Features of incoordination worsen dramatically on the closing of eyes or removal of visual inputs in sensory or afferent ataxia.

INVESTIGATIONS

Blood Tests

Routine blood tests, including complete blood count, hepatic and renal function tests, and electrolytes should be done in all patients with ataxia. Additional tests include blood sugar level, thyroid function test, vitamin B12/methylmalonic acid/homocysteine level, serum copper, or vitamin E levels. In patients with suspected autoimmune ataxias, autoimmune antibodies may be evaluated. These include anti-GAD65, antigliadin or tissue transglutaminase antibodies, anti-thyroid peroxidase (anti-TPO), antinuclear antibody, anti-Ro and anti-La antibodies, as well as cerebellar antibodies. The latter include anti-Yo, anti-Hu, anti-Ri, anti-Tr, mGluR1, anti-VGKC/CASPR, anti-Ma1, and Zic4. In suspected infection, HIV, syphilis, Lyme, and human T-lymphotropic virus (HTLV) serology may be tested.

Cerebrospinal Fluid

Cerebrospinal fluid (CSF) testing may be useful in patients with suspected CNS infections, autoimmune etiology (elevated protein relative to cells), or neoplastic infiltration of the meninges (to look for atypical cells). CSF 14-3-3 is useful in the diagnosis of Creutzfeldt-Jakob disease.

Imaging

All patients with cerebellar ataxia should undergo neuroimaging to look for structural causes. MRI brain, with or without contrast, is the preferred test to assess the posterior fossa in detail. Due to bony artifacts, computed tomography (CT) is not sensitive to evaluation of the posterior fossa structures. However, in the right clinical context, hemorrhage may be ruled out in the acute setting by using a CT scan. Structural lesions which may be identified include demyelination or tumors. The use of contrast enables detection of leptomeningeal inflammation, and better characterization of tumors or demyelinating lesions.

In long-standing ataxia, the presence of cerebellar atrophy should be sought whether it is vermian, hemispheric or pancerebellar. The presence of cerebellar atrophy points to degenerative ataxias although this may not be present in the earlier stages of the disease.

However, specific MRI findings may be apparent in specific disease entities. Hot-cross bun sign: Atrophy of myelinated transverse pontine fibers gives rise to this appearance, which is usually associated with MSA-C, but may also be seen in SCAs. The presence of transverse pontine stripes, or linear pontine hypointensities, seen on T2-weighted imaging, is suggestive of ARSACS. "Molar tooth" sign: This refers to the appearance of elongation of the superior cerebellar peduncles, which in combination with the midbrain, appears like a molar tooth. SCAs in general, show brainstem, and cerebellar atrophy. Superficial siderosis shows the presence of hemosiderin deposition on leptomeninges.

Genetic Testing

There are above 100 hereditary ataxia syndromes. With the advent of next-generation sequencing, clinical exome sequencing or large multigene panel testing is considered to be an efficient way to achieve a molecular diagnosis. However, trinucleotide disorders are not covered by these tests. For nucleotide repeat disorders, specific assays are required. Smaller repeats may be captured by polymerase chain reaction (PCR)-based tests. Highly expanded repeats may not be detected by PCR, and require advanced tests such as Southern blotting or triplet repeat primed PCR.[48]

Single gene testing may be indicated in the presence of suggestive clinical features, family history, and certain ethnic groups, e.g., presence of a progressive visual loss in a patient with suspected SCA suggests SCA7. The workflow for molecular diagnosis is outlined in **Flowchart 1**.

Metabolic Testing

These tests include assessing enzymes or substrates, e.g., phytanic acid (Refsum disease), cholestanol (CTX), very long chain fatty acids (adrenoleukodystrophy), urine organic acids, plasma amino acids (aminoacidurias), and lysosomal enzymes (Niemann-Pick disease type C).

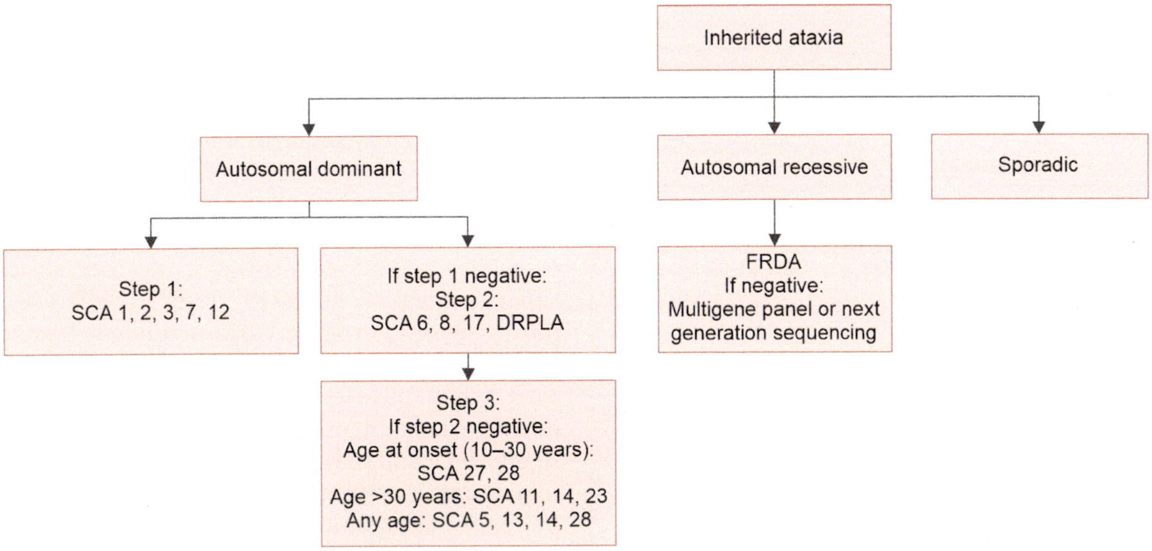

FLOWCHART 1: Molecular diagnostics workflow.

(DRPLA: dentatorubral-pallidoluysian atrophy; FRDA: Friedreich's ataxia; SCA: spinocerebellar ataxia)

Other Tests

Muscle biopsy, and elevated arterial lactate levels may be useful in suspected mitochondrial ataxias.

MANAGEMENT

Although treatment remains symptomatic in most degenerative ataxias, the focus of evaluation should be on those ataxias which are considered to be treatable.[49,50]

The treatable ataxia with disease-specific therapy is enlisted in **Table 8**.

Although mesenchymal stem cell therapy has been tried in neurodegenerative cerebellar ataxia and was found to be safe, efficacy remains unproven.[51]

SPECIAL FEATURES IN THE INDIAN CONTEXT

The first description of SCA2, which is the most common SCA in India, was provided by Wadia and Swami in 1971, who described the presence of slowing of saccades in patients with ADCA with cerebellar and pontine atrophy.[52] Presence of neuropathy was subsequently described, making this a distinct phenotype of SCA. He further characterized the extraocular movement abnormalities in SCA2 by describing that saccadic slowing was consequent to the reduced synaptic density of excitatory burst neurons in the caudal pons.

Spinocerebellar ataxia 12 was also described from India, in the specific ethnic community of Agarwals.[53] SCA2 and SCA12 overlaps have also been reported.[54] A lower pathogenic threshold for CAG repeats of 43 has been defined in SCA12.[55] Cognitive impairment in SCA12 has also been reported, in executive control and new learning ability.[56]

TABLE 8: Management of treatable ataxias.

Ataxia	Treatment	Comments
Acquired ataxia		
Gluten ataxia	Gluten-free diet	Improvement in ataxia with strict diet reported
Anti-GAD ataxia/ other autoimmune ataxia	Immunotherapy	Methylprednisolone, IVIG or plasma exchange
Steroid responsive encephalopathy with autoimmune thyroiditis	Immunotherapy	Steroids, IVIG, plasma exchange
Superficial siderosis	Removal of the underlying cause	
Opsoclonus myoclonus ataxia syndrome	Removal of underlying neoplasm, immunotherapy	MIBG scan may be needed in children
Paraneoplastic cerebellar degeneration	Removal of underlying neoplasm, immunotherapy	Steroids, IVIG, plasma exchange, rituximab, cyclophosphamide
Drug/toxin-related ataxia	Removal of offending drug/ toxin	
Inherited ataxia		
Ataxia with vitamin E deficiency	Vitamin E 800 mg per day	Given in divided doses
Abetalipoproteinemia	• Large dose of vitamin E and vitamin A • Vitamin E (100–300 mg/kg per day) • Vitamin A (100–400 IU/kg per day)	Low fat diet should be supplemented

Continued

Continued

Ataxia	Treatment	Comments
Cerebrotendinous xanthomatosis	Chenodeoxycholic acid (CDCA) 250 mg thrice daily	CDCA is shown to improve cognition
Ataxia with CoQ10 deficiency	Coenzyme Q supplementation	30 mg/kg in three divided doses
Refsum disease	Low phytanic acid diet	Plasma exchange for acute worsening
Episodic ataxia 2	Acetazolamide 4-aminopyridine	
Friedreich's ataxia	Idebenone	May improve cardiac hypertrophy
Niemann–Pick disease type C	Miglustat 200 mg thrice daily	
GLUT1 deficiency	Ketogenic diet	

(GAD: glutamic acid decarboxylase; GLUT1: glucose transporter type 1; IVIG: Intravenous immunoglobulin; MIBG: metaiodobenzylguanidine)

CONCLUSION

Ataxias are a heterogeneous group of disorders, arising from a plethora of etiologies, ranging from acquired to inherited causes. Possible anatomical localization includes cerebellar, afferent sensory pathways, or vestibular dysfunction. The temporal profile often gives a clue to possible etiologies. Throughout the evaluation of ataxia, every effort must be expended to uncover a treatable disorder. In acute and subacute ataxias, the usual causes include infectious or postinfectious, drug or toxin-mediated, and immune-mediated causes, such as gluten ataxia or PCD. In chronic ataxias, both inherited and sporadic nonhereditary causes must be kept in mind. Family history is of immense significance and may provide a paradigm for the mode of inheritance if present. Inherited ataxias, accordingly, may be autosomal dominant, autosomal recessive, X-linked, or mitochondrial disorders. Sporadic disorders include MSA and ILOCA. Treatment is focused on symptomatic and supportive therapy for all patients. Certain ataxias, considered remediable, require specific therapy.

REFERENCES

1. Scott SS de O, Pedroso JL, Barsottini OGP, França-Junior MC, Braga-Neto P. Natural history and epidemiology of the spinocerebellar ataxias: Insights from the first description to nowadays. J Neurol Sci. 2020;417:117082.
2. Klockgether T, Mariotti C, Paulson HL. Spinocerebellar ataxia. Nat Rev Dis Primers. 2019;5(1):24.
3. Musselman KE, Stoyanov CT, Marasigan R, Jenkins ME, Konczak J, Morton SM, et al. Prevalence of ataxia in children: A systematic review. Neurology. 2014;82(1):80-9.
4. Salman MS. Epidemiology of cerebellar diseases and therapeutic approaches. Cerebellum. 2018;17(1):4-11.
5. Kim JS, Kwon S, Ki CS, Youn J, Cho JW. The etiologies of chronic progressive cerebellar ataxia in a Korean population. J Clin Neurol. 2018;14(3):374-80.
6. Sinha KK, Worth PF, Jha DK, Sinha S, Stinton VJ, Davis MB, et al. Autosomal dominant cerebellar ataxia: SCA2 is the most frequent mutation in eastern India. J Neurol. Neurosurg Psychiatry. 2004;75(3):448-52.
7. Dabla S, Garg D, Aggarwal R, Kumar N, Faruq M, Rajan R, et al. Spinocerebellar ataxia 12 patients have better quality of life than spinocerebellar ataxia 1 and 2. Ann Indian Acad Neurol. 2022;25(4):647-53.
8. Bhanushali AA, Venkatesan R, Das BR. Spinocerebellar ataxias in India: Three-year Molecular Data from a Central Reference Laboratory. Neurol India. 2020;68(1):86.
9. Sinha S, Kataria A, Kolla BP, Thusius N, Loukianova LL. Wernicke encephalopathy-clinical pearls. Mayo Clin Proc. 2019;94(6): 1065-72.
10. Qudsiya Z, De Jesus O. Subacute Combined Degeneration of the Spinal Cord. StatPearls Publishing; 2022.
11. Manto M. Toxic agents causing cerebellar ataxias. In: Subramony SH, Dürr A (Eds). Handbook of Clinical Neurology, Vol 103. Philadelphia: Elsevier; 2012. pp. 201-13.
12. Mitoma H, Manto M, Hadjivassiliou M. Immune-mediated cerebellar ataxias: Clinical Diagnosis and treatment based on immunological and physiological mechanisms. J Mov Disord. 2021;14(1):10-28.
13. Hadjivassiliou M, Graus F, Honnorat J, Jarius S, Titulaer M, Manto M, et al. Diagnostic criteria for primary autoimmune cerebellar ataxia-guidelines from an International Task Force on Immune-Mediated Cerebellar Ataxias. Cerebellum. 2020;19(4):605-10.
14. Joubert B, Rostásy K, Honnorat J. Immune-mediated ataxias. Handb Clin Neurol. 2018;155:313-32.
15. Rossor T, Yeh EA, Khakoo Y, Angelini P, Hemingway C, Irani SR, et al. Diagnosis and management of opsoclonus-myoclonus-ataxia syndrome in children: An International Perspective. Neurol Neuroimmunol Neuroinflamm. 2022;9(3):e1153.
16. Laurent C, Capron J, Quillerou B, Thomas G, Alamowitch S, Fain O, et al. Steroid-responsive encephalopathy associated with autoimmune thyroiditis (SREAT): Characteristics, treatment and outcome in 251 cases from the literature. Autoimmun Rev. 2016;15(12):1129-33.
17. Hadjivassiliou M, Grünewald RA. Gluten ataxia: An underdiagnosed condition. Cerebellum. 2022;21(4):620-2.
18. Chan JL, Murphy KA, Sarna JR. Myoclonus and cerebellar ataxia associated with COVID-19: a case report and systematic review. J Neurol. 2021;268(10):3517-48.
19. Guedes BF, Vieira Filho MAA, Listik C, Carra RB, Pereira CB, da Silva ER, et al. HIV-associated opsoclonus-myoclonus-ataxia syndrome: early infection, immune reconstitution syndrome or secondary to other diseases? Case report and literature review. J Neurovirol. 2018;24(1):123-7.
20. Garg D, Vibha D, Pandit AK, Srivastava AK. Neurosyphilis presenting as pure cerebellar ataxia: An atypical manifestation. BMJ Case Rep. 2019;12(8):e231058.
21. Kumar N. Superficial Siderosis: A Clinical Review. Ann Neurol. 2021;89(6):1068-79.
22. Mundwiler A, Shakkottai VG. Autosomal-dominant cerebellar ataxias. Handb Clin Neurol. 2018;147:173-85.
23. De Michele G, Galatolo D, Barghigiani M, Iacovo DD, Trovato R, Tessa A, et al. Spinocerebellar ataxia type 48: last but not least. Neurol Sci. 2020;41(9):2423-32.

24. Winkelmann J, Lin L, Schormair B, Faraco J, Plazzi G, Melberg A, et al. Mutations in DNMT1 cause autosomal dominant cerebellar ataxia, deafness and narcolepsy. Hum Mol Genet. 2012;21(10):2205-10.
25. van der Knaap MS, Linnankivi T, Paetau A, Feigenbaum A, Wakusawa K, Haginoya K, et al. Hypomyelination with atrophy of the basal ganglia and cerebellum: follow-up and pathology. Neurology. 2007;69(2):166-71.
26. Salles PA, Mata IF, Brünger T, Lal D, Fernandez HH. ATP1A3-related disorders: An Ever-expanding clinical spectrum. Front Neurol. 2021;12:637890.
27. Jen JC, Wan J. Episodic ataxias. Handb Clin Neurol. 2018;155: 205-15.
28. Bachmann-Gagescu R, Dempsey JC, Bulgheroni S, Chen ML, D'Arrigo S, Glass IA, et al. Healthcare recommendations for Joubert syndrome. Am J Med Genet A. 2020;182(1):229-49.
29. Bürk K. Friedreich Ataxia: Current status and future prospects. Cerebellum Ataxias. 2017;4:4.
30. Tiet MY, Horvath R, Hensiek AE. Ataxia telangiectasia: what the neurologist needs to know. Pract Neurol. 2020;20(5):404-14.
31. Rothblum-Oviatt C, Wright J, Lefton-Greif MA, McGrath-Morrow SA, Crawford TO, Lederman HM. Ataxia telangiectasia: A review. Orphanet J Rare Dis. 2016;11(1):159.
32. Coutinho P, Barbot C, Coutinho P. Ataxia with Oculomotor Apraxia Type 1. I GeneReviews®. 2015.
33. Moreira MC, Koenig M. Ataxia with Oculomotor Apraxia Type 2. GeneReviews®. 2018.
34. Bouhlal Y, Amouri R, El Euch-Fayeche G, Hentati F. Autosomal recessive spastic ataxia of Charlevoix-Saguenay: an overview. Parkinsonism Relat Disord. 2011;17(6):418-22.
35. Agarwal A, Garg D, Kharat A, Qavi A. Autosomal recessive spastic ataxia of charlevoix-saguenay (ARSACS): Case report of a novel nonsense mutation in the *SACS* gene. Ann Indian Acad Neurol. 2020;23(3):395.
36. Nie S, Chen G, Cao X, Zhang Y. Cerebrotendinous xanthomatosis: A comprehensive review of pathogenesis, clinical manifestations, diagnosis, and management. Orphanet J Rare Dis. 2014;9:179.
37. Federico A, Gallus GN. Cerebrotendinous Xanthomatosis. GeneReviews®. 2022.
38. Rahman S, Copeland WC. POLG-related disorders and their neurological manifestations. Nat Rev Neurol. 2019;15(1):40-52.
39. Hanisch F, Kornhuber M, Alston CL, Taylor RW, Deschauer M, Zierz S. SANDO syndrome in a cohort of 107 patients with CPEO and mitochondrial DNA deletions. J Neurol Neurosurg Psychiatry. 2015;86(6):630-4.
40. Rahman S. Mitochondrial disease and epilepsy. Dev Med Child Neurol. 2012;54(5):397-406.
41. Zanni G, Bertini ES. X-linked disorders with cerebellar dysgenesis. Orphanet J Rare Dis. 2011;6:24.
42. Zanni G, Bertini E. X-linked ataxias. Handb Clin Neurol. 2018; 155:175-89.
43. Palma JA, Norcliffe-Kaufmann L, Kaufmann H. Diagnosis of multiple system atrophy. Auton Neurosci. 2018;211:15-25.
44. Fanciulli A, Wenning GK. Multiple-system atrophy. N Engl J Med. 2015;372(3):249-63.
45. Wenning GK, Stankovic I, Vignatelli L, Fanciulli A, Calandra-Buonaura G, Seppi K, et al. The Movement Disorder Society Criteria for the Diagnosis of Multiple System Atrophy. Mov Disord. 2022;37(6):1131-48.
46. Lamotte G, Kaufmann H. Movement disorder society criteria for the diagnosis of multiple system atrophy-what's new? Clin Auton Res. 2022;32(3):163-5.
47. Barbosa R, Lampreia T, Bugalho P. The aetiology of Idiopathic Late Onset Cerebellar Ataxia (ILOCA): Clinical and imaging clues for a definitive diagnosis. J Neurol Sci. 2016;365:156-7.
48. Wallace SE, Bird TD. Molecular genetic testing for hereditary ataxia. Neurol Clin Pract. 2018;8(1):27-32.
49. Agarwal A, Garg D, Faruq M, Rajan R, Goyal V, Srivastava AK. Treating Hereditary Ataxias—Where Can We Help? Ann Nat Acad Med Scie (India). 2019;55(04):182-8.
50. KP D, Kishore A. Treatable cerebellar ataxias. Clin Park Relat Disord. 2020;3:100053.
51. Bhartiya M, Kumar A, Singh RK, Radhakrishnan DM, Rajan R, Srivastava AK. Mesenchymal Stem cell therapy in the treatment of neurodegenerative cerebellar ataxias: A systematic review and meta-analysis. Cerebellum (London, England). 2022.
52. Wadia NH, Swami RK. A new form of heredo-familial spinocerebellar degeneration with slow eye movements (nine families). Brain. 1971;94(2):359-74.
53. Srivastava AK, Choudhry S, Gopinath MS, Roy S, Tripathi M, Brahmachari SK, et al. Molecular and clinical correlation in five Indian families with spinocerebellar ataxia 12. Ann Neurol. 2001; 50(6):796-800.
54. Faruq M, Shakya S, Garg A, Srivastava AK. Spinocerebellar ataxia 2 and 12 mutations in an Indian family with cerebellar ataxia and slow saccades. Mov Disord Clin Pract. 2014;1(3):267-70.
55. Srivastava AK, Takkar A, Garg A, Faruq M. Clinical behaviour of spinocerebellar ataxia type 12 and intermediate length abnormal CAG repeats in PPP2R2B. Brain. 2017;140(1):27-36.
56. Agarwal A, Kaur H, Agarwal A, Nehra A, Pandey S, Garg A, et al. Cognitive impairment in spinocerebellar ataxia type 12. Parkinsonism Relat Disord. 2021;85:52-6.

Part 4I: Miscellaneous

89 CHAPTER

Neurological Care in High Income and Low Middle Income Countries Including India

Senthil Amudhan, HV Srinivas

INTRODUCTION

Neurological care has two challenges—acute care and rehabilitation phase. Acute is exemplified by stroke and seizure disorder while rehabilitation is the main component of treatment, not only for the poststroke residual deficit but also for other relentlessly progressive neurodegenerative disorders—Parkinson's disease (PD), dementia, motor neuron disease, muscular dystrophy, and others. While there are several hospitals to take care of acute neurological conditions, several lacunae exist in the long-term care of chronic neurological disorders, which require a group of several specialists such as physiotherapists, psychiatrists, and speech therapists.

Globally, neurological disorders are the leading cause of disability, accounting for 276 million (11·6%) of global disability-adjusted life years (DALYs), and the second leading cause of death, accounting for 9 million deaths (16.5% of global deaths).[1] The recent atlas on resources for neurological disorders by the World Health Organization (WHO) and World Federation of Neurology drew attention to the low priority and dearth of resources available to tackle neurological disorders, particularly in low- and middle-income countries (LMICs) where around 70% of people with neurological disorders live and huge treatment gap persists with far-reaching consequences.[2] Neuroinfections—viral, bacterial, and parasitical—are an additional burden in LMICs, and some countries in Saharan Africa still have no neurologists.[2]

Even though neurological care is available at the level of primary healthcare centers (PHCs) in 94% of countries, it is not known for the quality of services and expertise available.[2] Though there are several organizations to create community awareness for common neurological disorders, societal attitude and the stigma attached to them still persist and prevent timely help-seeking. Among LMICS, India, accounting for 18% of the global population and 16% of global DALYs due to neurological disorders, has huge potential to impact global neurological care.[1] This chapter provides an overview of neurological care in high-income countries (HICs) and LMICs including India with emphasis on neurological disorders that have global, regional, and temporal relevance (epilepsy, stroke, dementia, and PD). Though this chapter focuses on specific neurological disorders, the findings and implications could be extended to a number of other neurological disorders that were not explicitly mentioned, particularly in terms of delivery of neurological care.

GLOBAL HEALTHCARE SYSTEMS AND NEUROLOGIC CARE

The health system's expenditure on neurological disorders is considerably low across the globe, and only 24% countries have stand-alone neurological health policies.[2] In most of the countries, neurological care is provided through the existing three-tiered primary, secondary, and tertiary care.[3] Primary care is the first point of contact within the healthcare system and offers basic preventive and curative healthcare by a nonspecialist with complex cases being referred to a higher level.[3] General practitioner (GP), nurse, other healthcare workers, nonmedical staff based in rural areas, and practitioners of traditional medicine (in some countries) are primarily involved in primary neurological care.[4] Secondary care is provided by district or regional hospitals for the management of severe cases and patients requiring access to diagnostic and technological expertise. The staff at secondary health centers includes neurologists, internists, residents, nurses, and trained technicians.[4] Tertiary care is often delivered by teaching hospitals, which offers the most advanced forms of neurological diagnosis, treatment, and rehabilitation through multidisciplinary approach.[3] In some countries, there are also other public or private facilities (polyclinics, multispecialty clinics) offering wide range of neurological services.

Healthcare Systems and Neurological Care in High-income Countries

Healthcare systems in HICs are relatively well organized and structured, with an efficient functioning, monitoring, and funding mechanism. Some countries such as the United Kingdom have national health systems where primary care practices are community-based and serve as gateways for referrals to more specialized care, while hospitals typically operate within set budgets and with salaried specialists.[5] The United States has a mix of publicly and privately financed insurance with high percentage of uninsured people. Majority of the hospitals in the United States are private. According to the WHO, quality of health services is not adequate even in HICs.[6] Even when neurological care is accessible, it is often regarded as delayed, inconvenient, and inefficient in many HICs.[7] Fragmented care, poor coordination across health and social sectors, limited accession to neurologist, and sustainability issues are some neurological care challenges reported in HICs.[8] Many rural areas in HICs face severe workforce shortage, resulting in limited access to healthcare services and inequities.[9] Timely access to care is another challenge in HICs where patients are left with long waiting times, especially for publicly funded or specialist care services.[10] Despite the availability of cutting-edge treatments and researches in HICs, the health system challenges and disparities in HICs have significant potential to adversely impact the provision of comprehensive, integrated, and quality care for neurological disorders, the majority of which are chronic in nature.

Healthcare Systems and Neurological Care in Low- and Middle-income Countries

Huge disparities exist for neurological services, needs, and resources between HICs and LMICs **(Table 1)**. Despite increasing awareness of neurological disorders there is

TABLE 1: Key findings on neurological care and resources in HICs and LMICs.

Domain	Parameter	HICs	LMICs	Inference
Dedicated policy for neurological health	Presence of policy	Present in 64% of the high-income countries and 33% of upper middle-income countries	Present in 28% of the low-income countries and 23% of lower middle-income countries	Overall deficit in dedicated or stand-alone neurological policies, in LMICs. This will have negative impact on the organization and quality of neurological service delivery, accessibility, and community care
Legislation for neurological disorders	Legislation for people with epilepsy	Present in 78% of the high-income countries and 42% of upper middle-income countries	Present in 17% of the low-income countries and 17% of lower middle-income countries	There is a deficit in legislation on epilepsy and dementia, particularly in LMICs. Without legislation, people with epilepsy and dementia are at an increasing risk of further stigmatization and loss of socioeconomic rights
	Legislation for people with dementia	Present in 60% of the high-income countries and 35% of upper middle-income countries	Present in 13% of the low-income countries and 7% of lower middle-income countries	
Financing for neurological disorders	Separate budget line for neurological disorders	Present in 14% of the high-income countries and 16% of upper middle-income countries	Present in 4% of the low-income countries and 12% of lower middle-income countries	Financing is not adequate in both HICs and LMICs. There is an ongoing lack of prioritization, earmarking, and planning of financial resources for the care of people with neurological disorders globally
Social welfare support for neurological disorders	Monetary support	Offered in 86% of the high-income countries and 69% of upper middle-income countries	Offered in 24% of the low-income countries and 42% of lower middle-income countries	In general, LMICs report a lower level of social welfare support services, which adversely affects access to treatment and care
	Nonmonetary support	Offered in 86% of the high-income countries and 44% of upper middle-income countries	Offered in 12% of the low-income countries and 27% of lower middle-income countries	
	Residential care	Offered in 83% of the high-income countries and 31% of upper middle-income countries	Offered in 8% of the low-income countries and 18% of lower middle-income countries	

Continued

Continued

Domain	Parameter	HICs	LMICs	Inference
Neurological workforce	The median number of neurological workforce* per 100,000 population	7.1 in high-income countries and 3.1 in upper middle-income countries	0.1 in low-income countries and 1.4 in lower middle-income countries	A specialist neurology workforce is not only essential for comprehensive neurological care but also important for the provision of training, support and supervision for nurses, other paramedical staff, and primary healthcare providers providing ancillary care. The overall shortage of a neurology workforce causes significant strain on care for the vulnerable population of patients with neurological conditions, which is especially felt in rural areas in low- and lower middle-income countries
	The median number of adult neurologists per 100,000 population	4.75 in high-income countries and 1.09 in upper middle-income countries	0.03 in low-income countries and 0.13 in lower middle-income countries	
	Neurologist in a rural area	Present in 45% of the high-income countries and 19% of upper middle-income countries	Present in 0% of the low-income countries and 17% of lower middle-income countries	
Neurological care by primary healthcare providers	Primary healthcare physicians offering neurological care	Present in 90% of the high-income countries and 100% of upper middle-income countries	Present in 88% of the low-income countries and 87% of lower middle-income countries	Primary healthcare physicians form a significant resource for neurological care in both HICs and LMICs where no specialist neurologists exist
Access to essential medications at the primary care level	At least one anticonvulsant (carbamazepine, phenobarbital, phenytoin, valproic acid)	Available in 79% of the high-income countries and 48% of upper middle-income countries	Available in 47% of the low-income countries and 42% of lower middle-income countries	In general, LMICs report an inadequate supply of essential medications at the primary care lower level, which adversely affects compliance and health outcomes in neurological care
	Antiparkinsonian medicine (levodopa + carbidopa)	Available in 77% of the high-income countries and 30% of upper middle-income countries	Available in 0% of the low-income countries and 19% of lower middle-income countries	
	Warfarin	Available in 73% of the high-income countries and 30% of upper middle-income countries	Available in 5% of the low-income countries and 13% of lower middle-income countries	
Neurological services quality	Guidelines for the care of neurological disorders	Available in 79% of the high-income countries and 68% of upper middle-income countries	Available in 23% of the low-income countries and 44% of lower middle-income countries	Overall deficit in guidelines for the care of neurological disorders, in LMICs. This will have a negative impact on the quality standards and performance metrics for those providing and commissioning health and social care services
Neurological information gathering system	No neurological disorder data compiled in the last 2 years	Not compiled in 17% of the high-income countries and 38% of upper middle-income countries	Available in 58% of the low-income countries and 59% of lower middle-income countries	Data reporting systems help to monitor trends in disease burden, identify high-priority healthcare issues, and develop plans for improvements in health services. There is a deficit of data reporting systems for neurological disorders in LMICs

*Neurological workforce (defined as the total number of adult neurologists, neurosurgeons, and child neurologists).

(HICs: high-income countries; LMICs: low- and middle-income countries)

Source: Adapted from World Health Organization, World Federation of Neurology. Atlas: Country Resources for Neurological Disorders, 2nd edition. Geneva: World Health Organization; 2017.

no matching financial resources or governmental policies in LMICs. Several systems (lack of adequate services and resources, inadequate drugs/medical supplies, lack of intersectoral action, high diagnostic and treatment cost, poor quality care), societal (lack of support system, inadequate disability benefits, stigma, discrimination), and individual (inability to pay, loss of wages, access to care, poor help-seeking) level barriers exist in LMICs. Unlike

HICs, where the government and insurance companies bear the majority of the cost of treatment, the patient and their family have to bear the majority of the cost in LMICs. The financial burden associated with neurological care is heavy and includes direct costs (investigation charges, outpatient treatment, cost of medications, inpatient care, and transport), indirect cost (loss of time, productivity, and wages), and intangible costs (psychosocial pain, stigma, and suffering). In LMICs, there are very few or no neurologists, and most of the patients with neurological disorders are seen by GPs/primary care physician who have limited knowledge of neurological disorders. Further, most of the neurological care in LMICs is concentrated in urban cities, making it inaccessible for rural population. There is also a severe shortage of trained nurses and paramedical staff, resulting in inadequate preventive, promotive, and rehabilitative neurological care services in LMICs. Inadequate supply of essential drugs for neurological care in primary care centers leading to poor compliance and high treatment cost is not uncommon in LMICs. Practitioners of indigenous medicine and faith healers are frequently preferred due to high cost and nonavailability of essential drugs.[4] Advanced treatment modalities such as deep brain stimulation, thrombolysis, intravenous immunoglobulin, plasmapheresis, and epilepsy surgery are largely confined to few selected centers and demand a huge cost, leading to poor access and affordability. Further, confinement of neurological care to hospitals, proliferation of vertical disease-specific programs, competing reproductive and child health priorities, and lack of adequate population level data on disease distribution, risk-factors, and help-seeking patterns are some of the challenges for providing integrated evidence-informed care for neurological disorders in LMICs.[11]

Healthcare Systems and Neurological Care in India

In India, a gross mismatch exists between the burden of neurological disorders and the availability of neurologists, other health professionals, and infrastructure.[12] In India, there are only about 2,500 neurologists to serve a huge population of 1.4 billion people, equating to one neurologist for 1 million people.[13] The prevalence of neurological disorders in rural areas was twice as common as in urban areas, emphasizing the need to attend to rural population too, which is often neglected.[14] Most of the neurologists are concentrated in a few metropolitan and larger cities with <3% of neurologists serving in some rural areas covering a population of 84.59 million.[15] Nearly 1 billion people live in areas where there is no practicing neurologist, and around 700 million people living in rural India have to travel a distance of 75–100 km for a tertiary consultation.[15] GPs from private sector form the major source of delivering primary neurological care in both rural and urban India. Like other LMICs, delivery of comprehensive neurological care in India becomes difficult with shortage of trained support staff, shortage of essential drugs, diagnostics and beds, high treatment cost, poor community support and rehabilitation services, health disparities, and limited research activities.

CARE FOR SPECIFIC NEUROLOGICAL DISORDERS

Though there are numerous neurological disorders with varying prevalence, incidence, morbidity, and mortality, this chapter focuses on four neurological disorders (epilepsy, stroke, dementia, and PD) that are associated with high burden, and have distinctive relevance for delivery of neurological care and practice.

Epilepsy

Epilepsy affects nearly 50 million people worldwide, with 80% of them living in LMICs.[16] It is associated with an increased risk of disability, psychiatric comorbidity, social isolation, reduced quality of life, huge healthcare costs, lost productivity, and premature death.[16] Epilepsy has negative impact on education, employment, marriage, and other social opportunities due to stigma, discrimination, and violations of human rights.[16] Nearly a quarter of epilepsy cases are preventable, and 70% of people with epilepsy (PWE) can live seizure-free lives with the help of low-cost and effective drugs.[16] Across the globe, variety of interventions ranging from population-based interventions (targeting risk factors, stigma, awareness, legislation), self-management, pharmacological interventions, surgical management, and alternative therapies (dietary therapies) exist for the prevention, management, and care for PWE.

Epilepsy Care in HICs

High-income countries have adequate resources, better care, and a lower burden of epilepsy than LMICs. Most of the HICs have guidelines for the care of PWE.[17] In the United Kingdom, GPs provide epilepsy care under the shared care model, where epilepsy is diagnosed and treated only under the supervision of a specialist with an annual review. However, a recent evaluation from the United Kingdom highlighted several shortcomings in the care of PWE, particularly the community-based care.[17] In the United States, epilepsy care is delivered through a 4-level comprehensive team model: level 1 (primary care physician/emergency room), level 2 (general neurologist), level 3 (specialized epilepsy center with interdisciplinary epilepsy care), and level 4 (specialized epilepsy center with comprehensive diagnostic and surgical treatment capabilities).[18] Access to antiepileptic drugs (AEDs) is still a challenge for those uninsured in the United states. For persons with drug-resistant epilepsy (DRE), HICs have better resources and facilities to provide access to expensive surgical intervention, dietary therapy, or investigational trials. In HICs, stroke being the leading potentially preventable cause attributing to 12% of epilepsies emphasizes the importance of coordination with stroke care.[16] The average cost per person with epilepsy in HICs, where minority of the world's epilepsy population lives, was estimated as $11,432, indicating a need to enhance epilepsy care delivery efficiency.[19]

Epilepsy Care in LMICs

The burden of epilepsy is high in LMICs (8.75 per 1,000 vs. 5.18 per 1,000 in HICs). However, LMICs continue to have substantial deficit in policies, programs, resources, services, and financial coverage for epilepsy care.[16] Despite the effectiveness and low cost of antiseizure medications, which can cost as low as US$ 5 per year, treatment gap in several LMICs ranged from 50 to >75%.[16] In LMICs, primary healthcare providers with limited training and limited access to AEDs manage most PWE. In most of the LMICs, nurses are often the primary providers of epilepsy care particularly in rural areas; diagnostic facilities and specialist care are not available outside urban centers.[16] Additionally, indigenous or traditional healers provide a more affordable epilepsy care to PWE in developing countries. The mortality associated with epilepsy is also significantly higher in LMICs, than in HICs, due to lack of access to or poor healthcare facilities for status epilepticus, drowning, head trauma, and burns.[16] Vital challenges and possible solutions to improve epilepsy care in LMIC are provided in **Table 2**.

Another key driver for epilepsy care in LMICs is the availability and affordability of AEDs. AEDs are available in the public sector in less than half of the time in LMICs.[16] Availability of AEDs was lower, and even when available either their costs were disproportionately high or they were marketed in substandard or falsified form in LMICs.[16] Suboptimal distribution of providers with neurological training, pharmacists and out-of-pocket payment for AEDs, misconceptions about epilepsy, and absence of community-based care model are other major barriers for epilepsy care in LMICs.[20] Treatments for people with DRE is limited, and the average annual cost per person with epilepsy was estimated to be $204, reflecting the lack of epilepsy care services.[19] Perinatal insults accounting for 11% of all epilepsies, neurocysticercosis, and cerebral malaria being other causes of epilepsy in LMICs indicate a need for larger public health response through integration with maternal and child health and communicable disease programs.

TABLE 2: Vital challenges and possible solutions to improve epilepsy care in LMICs.

Vital challenges	Possible solution
Access to primary care diagnosis and treatment	• Needs primary care providers, epilepsy educators, training of specialists, etc. • International working group to access the problem in more detail and develop an action plan
Access to antiseizure medicine	• Provision of subsidized or free first-line antiseizure medicines • Examine implementable policies to control the costs of antiseizure medicines
Limited implementation of epilepsy guidelines and standards of care	• Each country should highlight the referral cascade for the delivery of epilepsy care • Existing guidelines should be adapted to the local context, and efforts to ensure their dissemination are needed
Lack of epilepsy and healthcare data	• There is a need for standardized data collection through national health information systems • Use of standardized definitions, developed by the ILAE with support from the WHO

(ILAE: International League Against Epilepsy; LMICs: low- and middle-income countries; WHO: World Health Organization)

Source: World Health Organization, International League Against Epilepsy, International Bureau for Epilepsy. Epilepsy: A Public Health Imperative. Geneva: World Health Organization; 2019.

Epilepsy Care in India

Among the 50 million PWE worldwide, nearly 10–12 million PWE are expected to reside in India, contributing to nearly one-sixth of the global burden. The epidemiological study in India shows a prevalence rate of 5/1,000 and incidence rate of 50/100 thousand.[21] Though epilepsy is an eminently treatable condition, attitudes toward epilepsy were far more negative, and there is a large treatment gap (70–95%) in India for various reasons—lack of awareness, stigma attached to epilepsy, inadequate supply of drugs, poor compliance in view of the long duration of treatment.[22-24] Indian Epilepsy Association with its large number of branches all over the country has been in the forefront of creating awareness. In India, psychiatrists, medical graduates, physicians, pediatricians, and primary care health workers provide majority of epilepsy care. The rural population with epilepsy has higher mortality than the urban population due to limited access and availability of services.[25] In rural India, people often present to practitioners of indigenous medicine and traditional healers before consulting primary care providers, owing to cultural beliefs, easy accessibility, and affordability.[16] Nurses and other primary care providers receive little or no training in epilepsy care in India. Despite the fact that India's healthcare system is organized into levels, there is no formal referral mechanism for PWE. A recent multicountry assessment revealed that though India has specific clinical protocols and standards for epilepsy care, several deficiencies exist for access to diagnosis and treatment **(Table 3)**.[16] However, epilepsy surgery in India has seen remarkable advances in the last decade with 39+ centers undertaking epilepsy surgeries regularly with high-end technologies.[26] Despite this, only 2 out of 1,000 eligible

TABLE 3: Comprehensive epilepsy care in India compared with other countries—overview.

Domain	High-income countries			Upper middle-income countries				LMICs	Low-income countries		LMICs
	Chile	The United Kingdom	The United States of America	Kazakhstan	China	Russian Federation	South Africa	Kenya	Uganda	Tanzania	India
Available diagnostic technology											
Availability of basic* diagnostic technology in a rural area	✓	✓	✓	EEG and CT only	✓	EEG and CT only	–	–	–	–	–
Availability of basic* diagnostic technology in an urban area	✓	✓	✓	✓	✓	✓	✓	✓	✓	✓	✓
Availability of advanced* diagnostic technology in a rural area	–	✓	✓	–	–	–	–	–	–	–	–
Availability of advanced* diagnostic technology in an urban area	✓	✓	✓	–	✓	PET only	✓	–	–	–	PET only
Availability of antiseizure medicines											
Availability of essential[†] medicines in a rural area	✓	✓	✓	✓	✓	✓	✓	✓	✓	–	✓
Availability of essential[†] medicines in an urban area	✓	✓	✓	✓	✓	✓	✓	✓	✓	✓	✓
Availability of newer[†] medicines in a rural area	✓	✓	✓	✓	–	✓	–	–	–	–	–
Availability of newer[†] medicines in an urban area	✓	✓	✓	✓	✓	✓	✓	–	–	–	✓
Nonpharmacological epilepsy treatment											
Nonpharmacological epilepsy treatment in a rural area	–	✓	✓	–	–	–	–	–	–	–	–
Nonpharmacological epilepsy treatment in an urban area	✓	✓	✓	✓	✓	✓	✓	Surgery only	–	Surgery only	✓
Epilepsy training for healthcare providers											
Advanced training for epilepsy specialist physicians	✓	✓	✓	✓	✓	✓	✓	–	–	–	✓
Formal training for primary healthcare providers (physicians, nurses, others)	✓	✓	✓	✓	✓	✓	✓	✓	✓	✓	–
Formal training for nonmedically trained providers	–	–	–	–	–	–	–	✓	–	✓	✓

Continued

Continued

Domain	High-income countries			Upper middle-income countries				LMICs	Low-income countries		LMICs
	Chile	The United Kingdom	The United States of America	Kazakhstan	China	Russian Federation	South Africa	Kenya	Uganda	Tanzania	India
Treatment and care management of epilepsy											
Initial treatment by specialist	✓	✓	✓	✓	✓	✓	–	✓	–	✓	✓
Initial treatment by generalist primary care provider, the nurse	✓	✓	✓	✓	✓	✓	✓	✓	✓	✓	✓
Initial treatment by nonmedically trained provider	–	–	–	–	–	–	–	✓	–	✓	✓
Long-term treatment and care management by specialist	✓	✓	✓	✓	✓	✓	✓	✓	–	–	✓
Long-term treatment and care management by generalist primary care provider, the nurse	✓	✓	✓	✓	✓	✓	✓	✓	✓	✓	✓
Long-term treatment and care management by nonmedically trained provider	–	–	–	–	–	–	–	–	–	–	✓
Epilepsy advocacy and social support groups											
Professional neurology associations	✓	✓	✓	✓	✓	✓	✓	✓	✓	–	✓
Consumer organizations	✓	✓	✓	–	–	–	✓	–	✓	–	–

*Basic diagnostic technology included electroencephalography—sleep/awake, inpatient monitoring, magnetic resonance imaging, and computed tomography scans; advanced diagnostic technology included single-photon emission computed tomography, positron emission tomography, and magnetoencephalography.

†Essential medicines include phenobarbital, phenytoin, sodium valproate, and carbamazepine. Newer medicines include lamotrigine, levetiracetam, oxcarbazepine, and topiramate.

Nonpharmacological epilepsy treatment includes behavioral, dietary, vagus nerve stimulation, surgery and deep brain stimulation, and/or responsive neurostimulation.

(CT: computed tomography; EEG: electroencephalography; LMICs: low- and middle-income countries; PET: positron emission tomography)

Source: Adapted from World Health Organization, International League Against Epilepsy, International Bureau for Epilepsy. Epilepsy: A Public Health Imperative. Geneva: World Health Organization; 2019.

patients in India receive epilepsy surgery, resulting in a huge surgical treatment gap.[26]

Currently, the National Mental Health Program provides limited follow-up and referral care for PWE in India. A National Epilepsy Control Program is proposed to facilitate proper treatment of epilepsy at every level.[27] To reduce the treatment gap in India, various models of delivery of epilepsy care ranging from fixed satellite clinic model, camp approach (specialists or trained physicians engaging in rural camps), mobile clinic approach (single visit by neurologist), rural approach (integrating epilepsy care in primary healthcare), GPs approach (training GPs in epilepsy care), community health worker approach (for identification, referral, and follow-up), to community-based rehabilitation model have been demonstrated.[28] Though these models could be cost-effective and complementing, no large-scale replication and evaluation studies have been reported till date in India.

Stroke

Stroke is the world's second leading cause of death and the third leading cause of DALYs. The majority of the stroke burden were attributed to lower-income countries and LMICs, which accounted for 86.0% of global deaths and 89.0% of global DALYs due to stroke.[29,30] An ideal stroke service would encompass seamless interdisciplinary (medical, nursing, and allied healthcare) care from prevention to rehabilitation by integrating specialized services with other services (e.g., ambulance, emergency department, neurology, rehabilitation, care of older patients, and palliative care).[31] Globally, the rehabilitation needs of stroke far exceed the available resources and when available, their quality falls well short of evidence-based standards.

Stroke Care in HICs

As the timely delivery of stroke care becomes increasingly crucial to enhance patient outcomes, the organization of stroke services has gained more importance in HICs. Lack of public awareness, preference to contact primary care physician rather than emergency medical services, and inequitable access to modern imaging techniques in hospitals are significant barriers for reaching the hospital on time.[32,33] Some HICs have mobile stroke unit ambulances that include a specialized stroke team (advanced nurse practitioners, stroke specialists, with or without telemedicine support) as well as computed tomography (CT) scanning, a point-of-care laboratory, and the ability to provide thrombolysis to eligible patients to expedite diagnosis, triage, and treatment before they arrive at the hospital.[34] Acute telestroke has now become common in many regions while telerehabilitation is still less developed. The various stoke services to overcome these barriers in high-income health systems are summarized in **Table 4**.[31,35,36]

Stroke Care in LMICs

Low- and middle-income countries currently account for over 90% of stroke burden with an increasing trend.[30] Several barriers exist for stroke care in LMICs. The patient level barriers include inadequate awareness of stroke symptoms, sociocultural beliefs, poor and delayed help-seeking (inability to reach the stroke centers within the window period) while the system level barrier includes lack of advocacy materials on stroke, inadequate funding and medical transportation, ill-equipped emergency care services for acute stroke, very few stroke centers with facility for hyperacute investigations and treatment, treatment and

TABLE 4: Stroke care needs and the required service components in high-income health systems.[31]

Stroke care needs	Stroke service component	Expected outcome
Early recognition and timely help-seeking (prehospital)	Education campaign for the general public	Reduced time to diagnosis and treatment initiation
Early diagnosis and treatment before reaching the hospital (prehospital)	• Training campaigns for primary care and emergency medical care staff • Mobile stroke unit ambulances • Stroke unit • Acute telemedicine • Stroke centers (comprehensive or primary)	Improved prehospital diagnosis and management
Hospital care (intrahospital)	• Stroke unit • Acute telemedicine • Stroke centers (comprehensive or primary) • Telerehabilitation	• Prevent early complications • Promote early recovery
Transfer from hospital to the community (post hospital)	• Early supported discharge services • Stroke unit • Community rehabilitation services • Stroke centers (comprehensive or primary) • Telerehabilitation	Accelerated discharge to home from the hospital, increased rehabilitation in the home setting, continuing rehabilitation, and reintegration into regular living

Source: Adapted from Langhorne P, et al (2020).[31]

telesupport, shortage of dedicated workforce for stroke care, insufficient training of existing staff, low access to health insurance or to universal health coverage, rehabilitation not offered as standard stroke care, absence of community support systems, prevention strategies, and standard poststoke care protocol.[37] Acute stroke care in LMICs is usually provided by internists or family physicians with limited training and expertise.[37] Even though for acute management thrombolytic therapy is required, it is very expensive and the number of eligible patients to get this treatment is infinitesimally small.[38] In LMICs, <30% of patients with stroke were found to attend hospital within 3 hours of symptom onset, and the usual delay in attending the hospital ranged from 17 to 60 hours.[37] People, especially from rural region, often believe that the stroke is better managed by alternate medicine. There is huge scarcity of speech and language pathologists in LMICs. Funding is a major barrier for implementation of various stroke care models in LMICs.[37]

Stroke Care in India

Stroke is India's fourth major cause of death and fifth leading cause of disability with an annual incidence rate of 145 per 100 thousand population.[39] In India, stroke care is included in the National Program for Prevention and Control of Cancer, Diabetes, Cardiovascular Disease, and Stroke (NPCDCS), which provides national guidelines and specific strategies to provide cost-effective stroke management, prevention, and rehabilitation at all levels of healthcare.[40] Stroke Registry Program was initiated in 2012 by National Centre for Disease Informatics and Research to facilitate and support programs of surveillance of stroke. It has 62 institutions across India registered as on 2016.[41] In addition, an Indo-US Collaborative Stroke Registry was also established with five major teaching institutes from India and one major institute from the United States to generate high-quality stroke data.[42] Despite these initiatives, India faces several challenges similar to other LMICs in delivering organized care for stroke. Prehospital delays (~12 hours), increased door-to-needle time, lack of neuroimaging and thrombolysis facilities in the first hospital of arrival, high cost, and nonaffordability contribute to lower rates of thrombolysis (0.5%) in India.[43,44] Tenecteplase, which costs about half as much as alteplase, has now been approved by the Indian government for use in acute stroke during the first 3 hours of symptom onset.[40]

Stroke units in India were disproportionately less compared to its population size and are mostly concentrated in urban regions, particularly in private and tertiary care hospitals.[45] Stroke rehabilitation in India is not well established due to a paucity of professionals. Several stroke care models [multidisciplinary team (MDT) care, physician-led care, hub and spoke model, telestroke services, and task sharing] are being implemented in various regions across India to improve stroke care.[37] Recently, state-of-the-art Mobile Stroke Unit was established in Tezpur and Dibrugarh areas of Assam to bring the services of hospital to the patient's doorsteps in remote areas by providing acute stroke care management with CT scanner, provision of telemetry, and thrombolytic therapy.[46] Several technology-based initiatives such as SMART INDIA app to provide low-cost telestroke services to doctors in rural India, IMPETUS and CARE-DAT to improve the quality of life of disabled stroke patients, and StrokeSOS app to reduce prehospital delays among stroke patients have been launched to improve stroke care in India. Though India has integrated stroke into its national program and has a dedicated national stroke association and research network, several challenges exist for enhancing stroke chain of survival in India.[42] A national action plan for stroke grounded in public health approach will be crucial, to overcome several bottlenecks in providing optimal accessible, affordable, acceptable, and optimal stroke care in India.

Dementia

With increasing longevity, dementia emerges as one of the major causes of disability and dependency among older people, both in HICs and in LMICs. With no specific treatment available, relentlessly progressive disease, and crumbling social structure, it has become the responsibility of government/society to take care of people living with dementia (PwD). Globally, it is estimated that over two billion individuals would be over the age of 60 by 2050.[47] According to the latest WHO estimates, more than 55 million individuals globally have dementia, with approximately 10 million new cases diagnosed each year.[47] The prevalence is estimated to increase to 78 million by 2030 and to 139 million by 2050.[47] The physical, psychological, social, and economic impacts of dementia can be devastating not only for PwD but also for carers, families, and society as a whole. Care required for PwD includes primary healthcare, specialist care, and adequate postdiagnostic support care (memory groups, support groups, respite care etc.). Emphasizing the importance of dementia, the WHO has developed a Global Dementia Observatory, while the Alzheimer's Disease International and British United Provident Association (BUPA) have provided guidance for developing and implementing National Dementia Plans.[48]

Dementia Care in HICs

High-income countries account for majority (74%) of global dementia cost that is attributable equally by informal and social care costs.[47] Long-term institutional care is the major contributor of social care costs in HICs. Nongovernmental organizations (NGOs) often play a crucial role in delivering dementia care in many HICs.[47] HICs had a median of 2.2 (psycho)geriatricians per 100,000 people.[47] In HICs, GPs were the primary point of access to dementia care followed by neurologists, geriatricians, and psychiatrists as second point of access before reaching specialized dementia care (memory clinics).[49] However, dementia training for GPs is neither adequate nor incentivized.[50] In HICs, more than half of patients with dementia are still undiagnosed, and only 50–75% of dementia cases are correctly identified by GPs.[50] Only Denmark and United Kingdom have established targets to improve diagnosis rates.[50] In comparison with LMICs (52.9 ± 114.9 weeks), time taken from dementia symptom onset to the first contact with the healthcare system in HICs was relatively shorter (25.8 ± 52.3 weeks), and there was more collaboration between psychiatric and geriatric outpatient units in the dementia care pathway.[49] Though many HICs have introduced paid leave for carers, lack of norms for memory clinics, inconsistent availability of training, and support to caregivers remain a challenge for improved dementia care in HICs.[49,50]

Access to medications, hygiene products, assistive technologies, community-based services, and carer services are relatively higher in HICs. However, ethical challenges persist for the integration of palliative care and use of intelligent assistive technology for PwD. National dementia plans with risk reduction guidelines exist in many HICs and most of them tend to be stand-alone plans rather than integrated or subnational.[51] Some HICs have dementia-specific legislation or legal provisions to protect the rights of people with dementia.[51] Some of the newer initiatives include Dementia Networks (DemNet-D) in Germany to overcome the fragmentation of dementia care, dependency law in Spain to provide financial support for patients with dementia and their dependent family members, dementia-friendly communities in the USA, International Dementia Alliance (IDEAL) in Europe to guide the organization of dementia care, and the Japanese initiatives toward promoting a healthy aging society.[52]

Dementia Care in LMICs

About two-thirds of PwD live in LMICs.[53] In LMICs, majority of dementia care costs are attributable to informal care. Dementia is generally under-recognized, underdisclosed, undertreated, and undermanaged in LMICs.[54] In many LMICs, dementia is often viewed as a natural part of the aging, and even when identified, there are still issues related to stigma, lack of resources, and variations in how dementia is perceived and addressed in noncommunicable disease (NCD) policies and programs.[55] Primary healthcare providers (GPs and nurses) play a crucial role in diagnosis of dementia. Lack of awareness, stigma, and lack of effective brief screening questionnaires limit early dementia detection in LMICs.[55] Dementia-specific legislation, dedicated funding, fostering inclusive and dementia-friendly environments, availability of MDT, responsive referral pathways, continuity of health information, dementia-specific clinical guidelines, and standards as well as social and financial support to carers are relatively absent in many LMICs.[47] LMICs had a median of 0.02 (psycho)geriatricians per 100,000 people, and very few LMICs have dementia plans.[47] Strengthening Responses to Dementia in Developing Countries (STRiDE) and 10/66 Dementia Research Group are some key initiatives toward improved dementia care in LMICs. A mix of nonprofit, public, and commercial entities provides caregiver services and supports, with NGOs providing the majority of services in LMICs. Nonavailability of family caregivers as a result of social-economic transitions poses additional challenge to dementia care in LMICs.[56]

Dementia Care in India

In India, it is estimated that there are currently about 5.29 million people with dementia and this is expected to double by 2030 and triple by 2050.[57] Dementia care services in India are largely hospital-based, expensive, fragmented, and inequitable.[58] Only 1 out of every 10 patients with dementia receives any kind of diagnosis, treatment, or care in India.[58] The major causes attributed to this treatment gap include a lack of awareness among the general public and healthcare professionals, paucity of expert or trained human resource capacity for dementia care, and a lack of public health priority for dementia.[57] As a result, practically all dementia care is provided by the family at home, with little knowledge or financial assistance. Currently, India does not have a national dementia plan with allocated fund to prioritize dementia care. As general physicians are tasked with recognizing dementia in India, there are efforts underway to implement physician training modules for dementia care in India.[59] Diagnosis is further complicated by availability of screening and diagnostic tools that can be used only in predominantly English-speaking and formally educated people.[59] Hence, a culturally appropriate Indian Council of Medical Research-Neurocognitive Tool Box (ICMR-NCTB) has been developed in many Indian languages and for people who are illiterate/low literate to accommodate the linguistic diversity and educational heterogeneity in India.[60] Current support systems for caregivers are grossly inadequate, and caregivers rarely have access to dementia-related support.[57] Implementation of biomarker-based dementia diagnosis and dementia-friendly community approach to develop inclusive societies for PwD is very limited in India.[57,59]

Several healthcare delivery models for dementia in India include dementia India report model with seven core strategies,[57] cost-sharing models of care, integrated care model, task-shifted models of care, and collaborative community-based care (CCBC).[58] The Alzheimer's and Related Disorders Society of India (ARDSI), an NGO established in 1992, spearheaded the dementia movement in India and published the dementia India report in 2010.[57] The Tata Longitudinal Study on Aging (TLSA); Srinivaspura Aging, Neuro Senescence, and COGnition (SANSCOG) study; and Advancing Approaches for Dementia and Associated Research (AADAR) are some important ongoing prospective cohort programs for dementia in India.[61] India is part of STRiDE and for the first time in India, the

Longitudinal Aging Study in India-Diagnostic Assessment of Dementia (LASI-DAD) was established to provide population-representative data on cognition, dementia, and genetic risks to inform evidence-based dementia care.[62] In India, out-of-pocket expenditures account for the majority of healthcare spending. The recently launched Ayushman Bharat Scheme by Government of India with scope to cover the cost of hospitalization and establish health and wellness centers, which incorporate elderly care services and coverage for costs of essential drugs and diagnostics, are significant steps toward universal health coverage for dementia care.[59] In India, NPCDCS has implications toward dementia risk reduction, while the geriatric care at various levels of healthcare is strengthened through National Program for Health Care of the Elderly (NPHCE).[63] Though Mental Health Care Act of 2017 provides a legal framework and promotes inclusion for PwD, it is unlikely to have an impact unless dementia is recognized as a health priority.

Parkinson's Disease

Parkinson's disease is one of the most rapidly growing neurological disorders in terms of prevalence, disability, and fatalities due to aging. The burden of PD has more than doubled worldwide in the last decade. While there is no cure, PD requires an integrated multidisciplinary management approach besides pharmacotherapy for optimal health outcomes. A survey among members of the International Parkinson and Movement Disorders Society indicated significant disparities in PD care across the countries that varied by income level **(Table 5)**.[64]

PD Care in HICs

In many HICs, majority of the PD diagnosis was made by specialist PD neurologist or general neurologist.[65] Diagnostic delay and misdiagnosis of PD were common among GPs, and the time it takes to consult specialist after referral is considerable.[65] Waiting times to consult a geriatrician,

TABLE 5: Availability of PD treatment across countries by income group.

Domain	Parameter	HICs	LMICs	Inference
Professional care	Consultation of >200 PD patients per year per neurologist	Reported in 57.9% of neurologists in HICs	Reported in 11.4% of neurologists in LMICs	Delayed referral, delayed diagnosis, misdiagnosis, poor help-seeking and follow-up in LMICs
Availability of conventional drugs	Levodopa/Carbidopa	Available in 99.3% of HICs	Available in 99.0% of LMICs	Availability of levodopa in LMICs is comparable with HICs
	Others (MAO-B inhibitor, dopamine agonist, COMT inhibitor, amantadine)	Available in >96% of HICs	Availability ranged from 52.5% for COMT inhibitors to 80.8% for dopamine agonists in LMICs	LMICs report an inadequate supply of other classes of PD medications at the hospital level, which can have adverse health outcomes in PD
Frequency of use of conventional drugs	>75% of PD patients on levodopa/carbidopa	Reported in 80% of HICs	Reported in 68.4% of LMICs	The affordability and utility of levodopa for PD is limited in LMICs
	MAO-B inhibitors and COMT inhibitors	Used in 25–75% of PD patients in most HICs	Used in <25% of PD patients in most LMICs	Lower availability of MAO-B inhibitors and COMT inhibitors in LMICs due to their higher costs
Availability of device-aided therapies	Deep brain stimulation	Available in 94.5% of HICs	Available in 52.5% of LMICs	Device-aided therapies were less available in LMICs
	Apomorphine	Available in 76.0% of HICs	Available in 27.3% of LMICs	
	Levodopa, carbidopa, intestinal gel	Available in 95.2% of HICs	Available in 8.1% of LMICs	
Availability of nonpharmacological therapy	Physiotherapy, occupational therapy, and SALT	Physiotherapy is available in >90% of HICs while occupational therapy and SALT are available in around 80% of HICS	Physiotherapy is available in >90% of LMICs while occupational therapy and SALT available in around 50% of LMICs	Occupational therapy and SALT were less available in LMICs
Availability of CATs	Mucuna pruriens	Available in 30.1% of HICs	Available in 9.1% of LMICs	The use of CATs was limited in LMICs due to the high cost
	Ayurveda	Available in 0.0% of HICs	Available in 8.1% of LMICs	
	Cannabinoid	Available in 2.1% of HICs	Available in 0.0% of LMICs	

(CATs: complementary and alternative therapies; COMT: catechol-O-methyltransferase; HICs: high-income countries; LMICs: low- and middle-income countries; MAO-B: monoamine oxidase-B; PD: Parkinson's disease; SALT: speech and language therapy)

Source: Adapted from Goh ZHK, et al (2022).[64]

PD nurse specialist (PDNS), or therapist were usually large, reflecting the limited availability of allied healthcare professionals.[65] ParkinsonNet in Netherlands that includes "participatory medicine" and Düsseldorf Parkinson network in Germany are some of the notable patient-centered MDT approaches for PD. PD patients in rural areas often receive delayed diagnosis and poor care due to limited access and availability.[66] PD care close to home (homespital), remote monitoring, and telerehabilitation through digital technology often face challenges from existing insurance models and technology divide.[66] Palliative care for PD is limited and generally provided by clinicians without certification in palliative care, specialist (certification in neurology and palliative care), or through collaboration (neurologist with a palliative care physician/clinician).[67]

PD Care in LMICs

In most LMICs, care to PD patients is provided by GPs, and access to neurological care is very limited due to shortage of neurologists.[68] Patients, caregivers, healthcare professionals, and the general public all have significant knowledge gaps about PD, which has negative effects for help-seeking behavior, access to appropriate care, timely diagnosis, and medication adherence. Patients often seek treatment from traditional healers as well as complementary and alternative medicines, owing to cultural attributions and misconceptions.[68] The availability and access to device-assisted therapies, surgeries, and a MDT of well-trained healthcare professionals to support PwD are extremely constrained.[69,70] Despite several challenges, feasibility of telerehabilitation model for developing countries in PD care, training, and research has recently been demonstrated.[71]

PD Care in India

In India, there are around 80 PD cases per 100,000 population, and the number is expected to increase rapidly in the coming years as population ages.[72] India faces most challenges faced by other LMICs with regard to PD care. Neurologists, neurosurgeons, physiotherapists, and nurses trained in the field of movement disorders are very few.[73] Movement disorder clinics are very few with limited access to rural India where around 70% of total population live.[73,74] Given that most of the PD patients are diagnosed and treated by GPs and internists, misdiagnosis, delayed diagnosis, and referral are more likely.[74] Nearly 50% of PD patients attending movement disorder clinics were found to use complementary and alternative (ayurveda and homeopathy) medicines.[75] Adaptation and large-scale expansion of tele-neurorehabilitation services to provide PD care at various health system levels and across the country remain a significant challenge.[76] The PD and Movement Disorder Society of India registered in 2014 is active in uplifting the specialty in India by raising awareness, hosting workshops, and encouraging young students and neurologists to better understand and treat PD patients and undertake research in the field.[73] A need for improved psychoeducation, social support, and support services (respite) has emphasized for caregivers of PD patients in India.[77]

CONCLUSION

The burden, presentations, needs, services, and impact of neurological disorders vary considerably across the HICs and LMICs. LMICs are expected to see an increasing burden of stroke, dementia, and PD, owing to the sociodemographic transition, lifestyle changes, and aging. It is thus important to initiate a comprehensive, coordinated response at the global level to overcome the existing challenges and strengthen the existing health systems to provide improved preventive, promotive, curative, and rehabilitative services for neurological disorders in LMICs. In LMICs, an emphasis on neurology is urgently needed with support from national, global stakeholders, and funding agencies to improve neurological training, access to diagnostics and treatment, and support quality research locally. PHCs can now be connected to nearby high-technology centers, and patients can be better managed through telemedicines. Teleneurology appears to be a potentially powerful and promising strategy in shaping and redefining the future neurological care in both LMICS and HICs. Though India has made tremendous progress in neurological care when compared to other LMICs, more concentrated efforts and commitments are urgently required to deliver safe, efficient, high-quality, patient-centered, timely, and integrated neurologic care. Brain Health Initiative with establishment of Brain Health Clinics, a first-of-its-kind program in the country, launched by NIMHANS in association with NITI Aayog is a step toward developing successful models for improved care of neurological disorders in India.

REFERENCES

1. Feigin VL, Nichols E, Alam T, Bannick MS, Beghi E, Blake N, et al. Global, regional, and national burden of neurological disorders, 1990–2016: a systematic analysis for the Global Burden of Disease Study 2016. Lancet Neurol. 2019;18(5):459-80.
2. World Health Organization, World Federation of Neurology. Atlas: Country Resources for Neurological Disorders, 2nd edition. Geneva: World Health Organization; 2017.
3. World Health Organization. (2006). Neurological disorders: public health challenges. [online] Available from https://apps.who.int/iris/handle/10665/43605. [Last accessed December, 2022].
4. Singhal BS, Khadilkar SV. Chapter 114: Neurology in the developing world. In: Biller J, Ferro JM (Eds). Handbook of Clinical Neurology. Amsterdam: Elsevier; 2014. pp. 1773-82.

5. Schoen C, Osborn R, Squires D, Doty MM, Pierson R, Applebaum S. How health insurance design affects access to care and costs, by income, in eleven countries. Health Aff (Millwood). 2010;29(12):2323-34.
6. World Health Organization, Organization for Economic Cooperation and Development, International Bank for Reconstruction and Development. Delivering Quality Health Services: A Global Imperative for Universal Health Coverage. Geneva: World Health Organization; 2018.
7. Dorsey ER, Glidden AM, Holloway MR, Birbeck GL, Schwamm LH. Teleneurology and mobile technologies: the future of neurological care. Nat Rev Neurol. 2018;14(5):285-97.
8. The Neurological Alliance. (2018). The long term plan for the NHS: Getting it right for neurology patients. [online] Available from https://www.neural.org.uk/assets/pdfs/2018-08-long-term-plan-for-nhs.pdf [Last accessed April, 2023].
9. Parlier AB, Galvin SL, Thach S, Kruidenier D, Fagan EB. The road to rural primary care: a narrative review of factors that help develop, recruit, and retain rural primary care physicians. Acad Med. 2018;93(1):130-40.
10. Schoen C, Osborn R, Squires D, Doty M, Pierson R, Applebaum S. New 2011 survey of patients with complex care needs in eleven countries finds that care is often poorly coordinated. Health Aff (Millwood). 2011;30(12):2437-48.
11. Thakur KT, Albanese E, Giannakopoulos P, Jette N, Linde M, Prince MJ, et al. Neurological disorders. In: Patel V, Chisholm D, Dua T, Laxminarayan R, Medina-Mora ME (Eds). Mental, Neurological, and Substance Use Disorders: Disease Control Priorities, 3rd edition (volume 4). Washington (DC): The International Bank for Reconstruction and Development/The World Bank; 2016.
12. Gourie-Devi M. Organization of neurology services in India: unmet needs and the way forward. Neurol India. 2008;56(1):4-12.
13. Singh G, Khadilkar S, Jayalakshmi S. (2020). The future of neurology in India. A report of the 27th annual meeting of the Indian Academy of Neurology. [online] Available from https://worldneurologyonline.com/article/the-future-of-neurology-in-india/. [Last accessed December, 2022].
14. Gourie-Devi M, Gururaj G, Satishchandra P, Subbakrishna DK. Prevalence of neurological disorders in Bangalore, India: a community-based study with a comparison between urban and rural areas. Neuroepidemiology. 2004;23(6):261-8.
15. Ganapathy K. Distribution of neurologists and neurosurgeons in India and its relevance to the adoption of telemedicine. Neurol India. 2015;63(2):142.
16. World Health Organization, International League Against Epilepsy, International Bureau for Epilepsy. Epilepsy: A Public Health Imperative. Geneva: World Health Organization; 2019.
17. Minshall I, Buckels L, Cox P, Jamroze H, Jeyam T, Newman A, et al. UK general practice: continuing to fail in the care of people with epilepsy? Epilepsy Behav. 2021;124:108354.
18. Ostendorf AP, Ahrens SM, Lado FA, Arnold ST, Bai S, Bensalem Owen MK, et al. United States Epilepsy Center characteristics: a data analysis from the National Association of Epilepsy Centers. Neurology. 2022;98(5):e449-58.
19. Begley C, Wagner RG, Abraham A, Beghi E, Newton C, Kwon CS, et al. The global cost of epilepsy: a systematic review and extrapolation. Epilepsia. 2022;63(4):892-903.
20. Singh G, Sharma M, Krishnan A, Dua T, d'Aniello F, Manzoni S, et al. Models of community-based primary care for epilepsy in low- and middle-income countries. Neurology. 2020;94(4):165-75.
21. Sridharan R, Murthy BN. Prevalence and pattern of epilepsy in India. Epilepsia. 1999;40(5):631-6.
22. Mani KS, Rangan G, Srinivas HV, Kalyanasundaram S, Narendran S, Reddy AK. The Yelandur study: a community-based approach to epilepsy in rural South India—epidemiological aspects. Seizure. 1998;7(4):281-8.
23. Radhakrishnan K, Pandian JD, Santhoshkumar T, Thomas SV, Deetha TD, Sarma PS, et al. Prevalence, knowledge, attitude, and practice of epilepsy in Kerala, South India. Epilepsia. 2000;41(8): 1027-35.
24. Jain S, Satishchandra P. Chapter 293: Organization of health care in India. In: Engel J, Pedley TA, Aicardi J (Eds). Epilepsy: A Comprehensive Textbook. Philadelphia: Lippincott Williams and Wilkins; 2008. pp. 2885-8.
25. Amudhan S, Gururaj G, Satishchandra P. Epilepsy in India I: Epidemiology and public health. Ann Indian Acad Neurol. 2015;18(3):263.
26. Rathore C, Radhakrishnan K. Epidemiology of epilepsy surgery in India. Neurol India. 2017;65(Supplement):S52-9.
27. Tripathi M, Jain DC, Devi MG, Jain S, Saxena V, Chandra PS, et al. Need for a national epilepsy control program. Ann Indian Acad Neurol 2012;15(2):89-93.
28. Amudhan S, Gururaj G, Satishchandra P. Epilepsy in India II: Impact, burden, and need for a multisectoral public health response. Ann Indian Acad Neurol. 2015;18(4):369.
29. GBD 2019 Stroke Collaborators. Global, regional, and national burden of stroke and its risk factors, 1990–2019: a systematic analysis for the Global Burden of Disease Study 2019. Lancet Neurol. 2021;20(10):795-820.
30. Feigin VL, Brainin M, Norrving B, Martins S, Sacco RL, Hacke W, et al. World Stroke Organization (WSO): Global Stroke Fact Sheet 2022. Int J Stroke. 2022;17(1):18-29.
31. Langhorne P, Audebert HJ, Cadilhac DA, Kim J, Lindsay P. Stroke systems of care in high-income countries: what is optimal? Lancet. 2020;396(10260):1433-42.
32. Meretoja A, Keshtkaran M, Tatlisumak T, Donnan GA, Churilov L. Endovascular therapy for ischemic stroke: save a minute–save a week. Neurology. 2017;88(22):2123-7.
33. Coutts SB, Menon BK. Late thrombolysis for stroke works, but how do we do it? Lancet. 2019;394(10193):97-8.
34. Audebert H, Fassbender K, Shazam Hussain M, Ebinger M, Turc G, Uchino K, et al. The PRE-hospital stroke treatment organization. Int J Stroke. 2017;12(9):932-40.
35. McDermott M, Skolarus LE, Burke JF. A systematic review and meta-analysis of interventions to increase stroke thrombolysis. BMC Neurol. 2019;19(1):86.
36. Lachkhem Y, Rican S, Minvielle É. Understanding delays in acute stroke care: a systematic review of reviews. Eur J Public Health. 2018;28(3):426-33.
37. Pandian JD, Kalkonde Y, Sebastian IA, Felix C, Urimubenshi G, Bosch J. Stroke systems of care in low-income and middle-income countries: challenges and opportunities. Lancet. 2020;396(10260):1443-51.
38. Berkowitz AL, Mittal MK, McLane HC, Shen GC, Muralidharan R, Lyons JL, et al. Worldwide reported use of IV tissue plasminogen activator for acute ischemic stroke. Int J Stroke. 2014;9(3):349-55.
39. Das SK, Banerjee TK, Biswas A, Roy T, Raut DK, Mukherjee CS, et al. A prospective community-based study of stroke in Kolkata, India. Stroke. 2007;38(3):906-10.
40. National Health Mission. (2022). National Program for prevention and control of cancer, diabetes, cardiovascular diseases and stroke (NPCDCS). [online] Available from https://nhm.gov.in/index1.php?lang=1andlevel=2andsublinkid=1048andlid=604. [Last accessed December, 2022].
41. National Center for Disease Informatics and Research. National Stroke Registry Programme. [online] Available from https://stroke.ncdirindia.org/. [Last accessed December, 2022].
42. Srivastava MVP, Bhatia R, Vishnu VY, Goyal M. Essential workflow and performance measures for optimizing acute ischemic stroke treatment in India. Stroke. 2020;51(7):1969-77.
43. Ashraf VV, Maneesh M, Praveenkumar R, Saifudheen K, Girija AS. Factors delaying hospital arrival of patients with acute stroke. Ann Indian Acad Neurol. 2015;18(2):162-6.

44. Khurana D, Padma MV, Bhatia R, Kaul S, Pandian J, Sylaja PN, et al. Recommendations for the early management of acute ischemic stroke: a consensus statement for healthcare professionals from the Indian Stroke Association. J Stroke Med. 2018;1(2):79-113.
45. Pandian JD, Sudhan P. Stroke epidemiology and stroke care services in India. J Stroke. 2013;15(3):128-34.
46. Indian Council of Medical Research. (2020). ICMR's mobile stroke care unit for northeast region inaugurated. [online]. Available from https://main.icmr.nic.in/sites/default/files/photo-gallery-docs/ICMR_Press_Release_Mobile_Stroke_Care_Unit_NER.pdf. [Last accessed December, 2022].
47. World Health Organization. (2021). Global status report on the public health response to dementia. [online] Available from https://www.who.int/publications/i/item/9789240033245. [Last Accessed December, 2022].
48. Burns A, Robert P; IDEAL steering group. Dementia care: international perspectives. Curr Opin Psychiatry. 2019;32(4): 361-5.
49. Volpe U, Amin H, Ayinde OO, Burns A, Chan WC, David R, et al. Pathways to care for people with dementia: an international multicenter study. Int J Geriatr Psychiatry. 2020;35(2):163-73.
50. OECD Policy Brief. (2018). Renewing priority for dementia: where do we stand? [online] Available from https://www.oecd.org/health/health-systems/Renewing-priority-for-dementia-Where-do-we-stand-2018.pdf. [Last accessed December, 2022].
51. Alzheimer's Disease International, Bliss A, Lynch C, Dabas L, Barbarino P. (2020). From plan to impact III: maintaining dementia as a priority in unprecedented times. [online] Available from https://www.alzint.org/resource/from-plan-to-impact-iii/. [Last accessed December, 2022].
52. Lobo A, Lobo E, De-la-Cámara C. Dementia care in high-income countries. Curr Opin Psychiatry. 2019;32(5):465-70.
53. Patterson C, Alzheimer's Disease International. (2018). World Alzheimer report 2018: the state of the art of dementia research: new frontiers. [online] Available from https://www.alzint.org/resource/world-alzheimer-report-2018/. [Last accessed December, 2022].
54. Comas-Herrera A, Guerchet M, Karagiannidou M, Prince M, Knapp M. (2016). World Alzheimer report 2016: improving healthcare for people living with dementia: coverage, quality, and costs now and in the future. [online] Available from https://www.alz.co.uk/research/WorldAlzheimerReport2016.pdf. [Last accessed December, 2022].
55. Ferri CP, Jacob KS. Dementia in low-income and middle-income countries: different realities mandate tailored solutions. PLoS Med. 2017;14(3):e1002271.
56. Fam J, Mahendran R, Kua EH. Dementia care in low- and middle-income countries. Curr Opin Psychiatry. 2019;32(5):461-4.
57. Alzheimer's and Related Disorders Society of India. (2010). Dementia India report 2010: prevalence, impact, costs, and services for dementia. [online] Available from https://ardsi.org/pdf/annual%20report.pdf. [Last accessed December, 2022].
58. Nulkar A, Paralikar V, Juvekar S. Dementia in India—a call for action. J Glob Health Rep. 2019;3:e2019078.
59. Alladi S, Rajagopalan J. (2021). Early diagnosis of dementia: a complex problem requiring a multidimensional approach for India. In: Gauthier S, Rosa-Neto P, Morais JA, Webster C (Eds). World Alzheimer Report 2021: Journey Through the Diagnosis of Dementia. London: Alzheimer's Disease International; 2021. pp. 221-2.
60. Iyer GK, Paplikar A, Alladi S, Dutt A, Sharma M, Mekala S, et al. Standardizing dementia diagnosis across linguistic and educational diversity: study design of the Indian Council of Medical Research-neurocognitive toolbox (ICMR-NCTB). J Int Neuropsychol Soc. 2020;26(2):172-86.
61. Ravindranath V, Sundarakumar JS. Changing demography and the challenge of dementia in India. Nat Rev Neurol. 2021;17(12): 747-58.
62. Lee J, Khobragade PY, Banerjee J, Chien S, Angrisani M, Perianayagam A, et al. Design and methodology of the Longitudinal Aging Study in India-Diagnostic Assessment of Dementia (LASI-DAD). J Am Geriatr Soc. 2020;68(Suppl 3):S5-10.
63. Ministry of Health and Family Welfare. (2022). Efforts by the government to reduce dementia cases, address mental disorders, and curb the use of tobacco. [online] https://pib.gov.in/PressReleaseIframePage.aspx?PRID=1796437. [Last accessed December, 2022].
64. Goh ZHK, Cheong JLY, Marras C, Tanner CM, Kasten M, Korczyn AD, et al. Surveying global availability of Parkinson's disease treatment. J Parkinsons Dis. 2022;12(3):1023-34.
65. Schrag A, Khan K, Hotham S, Merritt R, Rascol O, Graham L. Experience of care for Parkinson's disease in European countries: a survey by the European Parkinson's Disease Association. Eur J Neurol. 2018;25(12):1410-e120.
66. Bloem BR, Henderson EJ, Dorsey ER, Okun MS, Okubadejo N, Chan P, et al. Integrated and patient-centered management of Parkinson's disease: a network model for reshaping chronic neurological care. Lancet Neurol. 2020;19(7):623-34.
67. Oliver D, Borasio GD, Veronese S, Voltz R, Lorenzl S, Hepgul N. Current collaboration between palliative care and neurology: a survey of clinicians in Europe. BMJ Support Palliat Care. 2020; bmjspcare-2020-002322.
68. Bhidayasiri R, Virameteekul S, Sukoandari B, Tran TN, Lim TT. Challenges of Parkinson's disease care in southeast Asia. In: Riederer P, Laux G, Nagatsu T, Le W, Riederer C (Eds). NeuroPsychopharmacotherapy. New York: Springer International Publishing; 2020. pp. 1-21.
69. Kaiyrzhanov R, Rizig M, Aitkulova A, Zharkinbekova N, Shashkin C, Kaishibayeva G, et al. Parkinson's disease in central Asian and Transcaucasian countries: a review of epidemiology, genetics, clinical characteristics, and access to care. Parkinsons Dis. 2019;2019:e2905739.
70. Bhidayasiri R, Phokaewvarangkul O, Sakdisornchai K, Boonpang K, Chaudhuri KR, Parsons J, et al. Establishing apomorphine treatment in Thailand: understanding the challenges and opportunities of Parkinson's disease management in developing countries. Expert Rev Neurother. 2020;20(6):523-37.
71. Leochico CFD, Espiritu AI, Ignacio SD, Mojica JAP. Challenges to the emergence of telerehabilitation in a developing country: a systematic review. Front Neurol. 2020;11:1007.
72. Dhiman V, Menon GR, Kaur S, Mishra A, John D, Rao Vishnu MV, et al. A systematic review and meta-analysis of prevalence of epilepsy, dementia, headache, and Parkinson disease in India. Neurol India. 2021;69(2):294.
73. Behari M. Movement disorders: the genesis and progression in India: neurological perspective. Neurol India. 2018;66(7):3.
74. Surathi P, Kamble N, Bhalsing KS, Yadav R, Pal PK. Prescribing pattern for Parkinson's disease in Indian community before referral to tertiary center. Can J Neurol Sci. 2017;44(6):705-10.
75. Pandit AK, Vibha D, Srivastava AK, Shukla G, Goyal V, Behari M. Complementary and alternative medicine in Indian Parkinson's disease patients. J Tradit Complement Med. 2015;6(4):377-82.
76. Khanna M, Gowda GS, Bagevadi VI, Gupta A, Kulkarni K, S Shyam RP, et al. Feasibility and utility of tele-neurorehabilitation service in India: experience from a quaternary center. J Neurosci Rural Pract. 2018;9(4):541-4.
77. Sanyal J, Das S, Ghosh E, Banerjee TK, Bhaskar LV, Rao VR. Burden among Parkinson's disease care givers for a community based study from India. J Neurol Sci. 2015;358(1):276-81.

90

CHAPTER

Tropical Ataxic Neuropathy and Konzo

Archana B Netto, AB Taly, Manju Netto

INTRODUCTION

Neurological syndromes from tropical countries, classified as "tropical myeloneuropathies," include a spectrum of the predominantly spastic syndrome of human T cell lymphotropic virus (HTLV)-associated myelopathy, tropical spastic paraparesis, Konzo, and lathyrism at one end, and the tropical ataxic neuropathies (TAN) at the other.[1] In between this spectrum is the tobacco/nutritional amblyopia, epidemic optic neuropathy and peripheral neuropathy of Cuba, prisoner of war neuropathy (that includes burning feet or happy feet, camp eyes, camp deafness, and camp giddiness),[2] and various other opticomyeloneuropathies (the syndrome of optic nerve spinal cord and peripheral nerve involvement) and polyneuropathies described from Tanzania, West Indies, Senegal,[3] etc., with minor variations.[4] The clinical constellation of bilateral optic atrophy, bilateral sensory neural deafness, predominant posterior column, and pyramidal tract myelopathy, with ataxic polyneuropathy, is termed as the TAN. Despite the fact that TAN is known for more than a century, effective treatment is still not discovered. In this chapter, we review the history, and current knowledge of epidemiology, clinical features, controversies in pathogenesis, and differential diagnoses, and identify areas where further research is needed.

BOX 1 **Historical milestones of TAN.[5-19]**

- 1897: Strachan described syndrome in West Indies—postmortem of 510 cases
- 1911: Scott published detailed account—implicated nutritional etiology (syndrome came to be known as Strachan–Scott syndrome)
- 1928: Wright described in Sierra Leone in children and puerperal ladies
- 1928: Bradley reported syndrome from Seychelles
- 1929: Sharples described syndrome from British Guiana
- 1930: Shelley from East Africa
- 1930: Moore invoked cassava
- 1934: Nicholls from Ceylon
- 1936: Clark invoked high cyanogens in cassava
- 1937: Egypt
- 1940: Pallister—Chinese POW in Malay
- 1945: Spillane and Scott, German POW in Middle East
- 1956: Cruickshank—syphilitic etiology
- 1958: Nigeria
- 1959: Money coined TAN. Thiamine and riboflavin deficiency TAN
- 1960: Senegal
- 1965: Wilson–thiocyanate levels in TAN
- 1973: Uganda, Ghana, Kenya, Rhodesia, and Malaysia
- 1975: Krishnaswamy from India
- 1999: Mathangi animal models for TAN from India

(POW: prisoners of war; TAN: tropical ataxic neuropathy)

HISTORY OF TROPICAL ATAXIC NEUROPATHY

The major milestones pertaining to TAN, from the time the disease was first described in 1897, are detailed in **Box 1**.[3-19]

EPIDEMIOLOGY

Figure 1 discusses cohorts of more than 3,000 participants aged above 10 years were followed up for 2 years in southwest Nigeria (Ososo) where the incidence was found to be 64 per 10,000 individuals (male:female = 1:3).[20] A door-to-door census from the same region, screening all participants aged above 10 years, placed the prevalence at 6% (male:female = 1:2). The highest prevalence of 24% was found in the ages 60–69 years. The prevalence progressively increased with each decade, with a decline after the age of 70 years[14] probably due to patients' death.

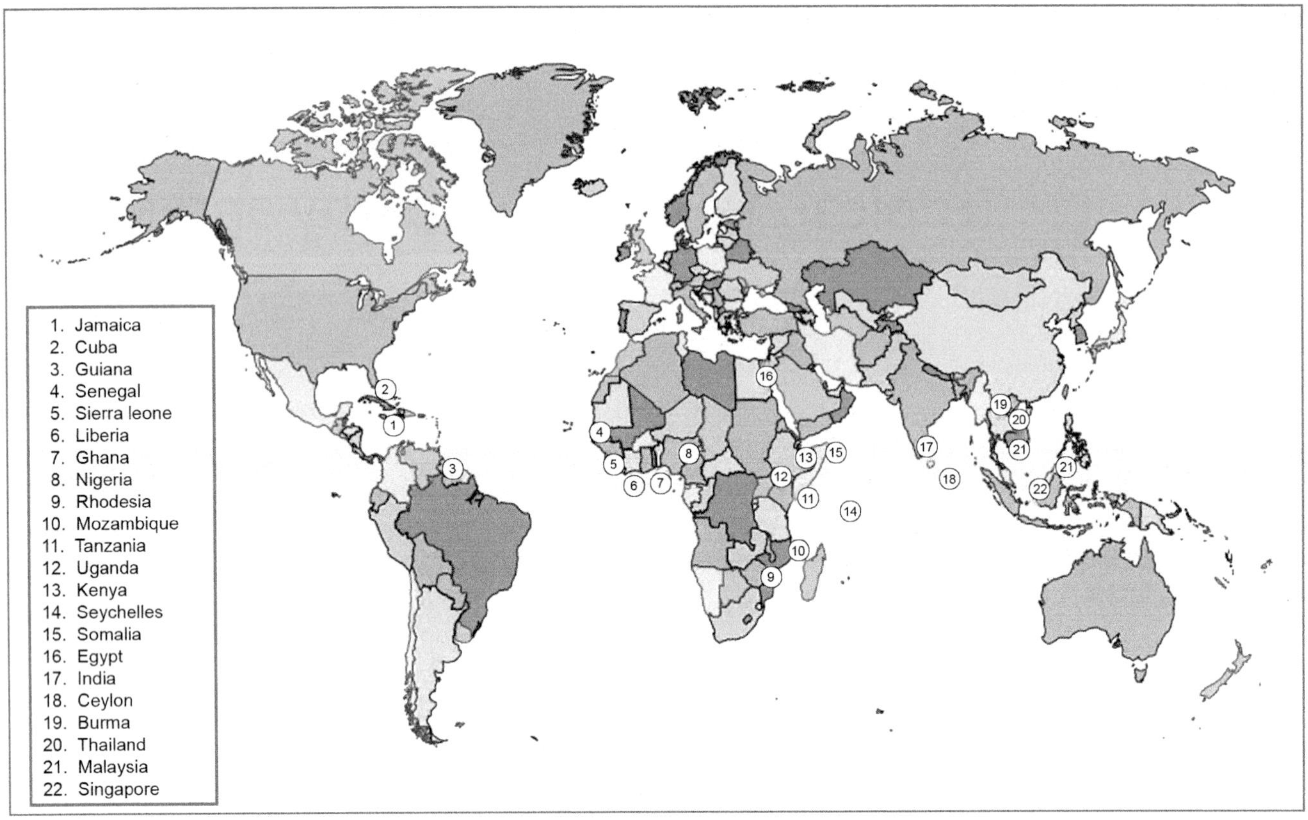
1. Jamaica
2. Cuba
3. Guiana
4. Senegal
5. Sierra leone
6. Liberia
7. Ghana
8. Nigeria
9. Rhodesia
10. Mozambique
11. Tanzania
12. Uganda
13. Kenya
14. Seychelles
15. Somalia
16. Egypt
17. India
18. Ceylon
19. Burma
20. Thailand
21. Malaysia
22. Singapore

FIG. 1: World map with affected countries. Countries which have reported tropical ataxic neuropathy, or nutritional ataxic neuropathy or prisoner of war neuropathy are numbered and the corresponding names of the states/countries given in the lower left corner.

Interestingly, the disease appears nonexistent in temperate countries barring a single report from Birmingham[8] of the "prisoners of war neuropathy" who were held captive in tropical countries **(Fig. 1)**.

INDIAN SCENARIO

Tropical ataxic neuropathy remains one of the least reported neurological disorders in India. The first published account was by Krishnaswamy and Kalamangalam in 1975.[21] The next report was from Kerala in 2008.[22] There are no large-scale epidemiological studies of TAN from India that compare Indian data with African data. The female preponderance in Indian literature conforms to African studies.[19] However, the highest prevalence was noted in the third decade, unlike the African population where TAN predominantly affects the elderly population.[22,14]

CLINICAL FEATURES

Careful scrutiny of the literature reveals the presence of two neurological syndromes under TAN. The first is a syndrome that affects adolescent children, with mucocutaneous manifestations of malnourishment and retrobulbar neuropathy, which improves with dietary modification and supplementation with autoclaved dried yeast.[14] Spinal ataxia was noted in half of the patients.[20] The second syndrome affects the middle-aged and elderly with varying combinations of sensory polyneuropathy, gait ataxia, optic atrophy, and sensory neural deafness. In contrast to the adolescent syndrome, mucocutaneous manifestations of malnutrition are less frequent (0–30%) and neurological symptoms do not respond to dietary modifications or vitamin supplementation.[14]

The authors' experience from a tertiary care institute, a referral center catering exclusively to patients with neurological disorders from all over the country over 6 years are mentioned here alongside other data to get a perspective of the Indian scenario.[4] 31 cases were evaluated (16 from Karnataka, 10 from Andhra Pradesh, 3 from Tamil Nadu, and 1 each from Kerala and West Bengal). Among these, Kerala is the only state where cassava is grown on a large scale as a staple diet. Seven were men and 24 were women aged between 13 and 68 years. The majority were in the age group of 15–25 (n = 13) followed by 26–35 (n = 10), and 36–45 (n = 5). Two patients were aged less than 15 years and one patient was 68 years old.

The most common presenting symptom was abnormal gait followed by sensory symptoms **(Table 1)**. 85% had exaggeration of gait difficulty in the dark suggestive of sensory ataxia and half of them had positive washbasin

TABLE 1: Symptomatology of tropical ataxic neuropathy.

	Osuntokun *n* = 84 (%)	Oluwole *n* = 66 (%)	Madhusudhan *n* = 40 (%)	Our cohort *n* = 31 (%)
Sensory symptoms	68 (81)		34 (85)	28 (90)
Visual	60 (71)	44 (72)	20 (50)	19 (61)
Abnormal gait	47 (56)	35 (57)	40 (100)	31 (100)
Weakness of lower limbs	30 (35)	–	10 (25)	17 (55)
Tinnitus	29 (34)		2 (5)	4 (13)
Deafness	23 (26)	30 (48)	32 (80)	24 (77)
Abdominal pain	4 (5)	–	–	1 (3)
Sphincter disturbance	3 (4)	–	–	3 (9)
Dysarthria	–	–	6 (15)	7 (23)
Dysphagia	–	–	2 (5)	3 (9)
Dyspnea	–	–	2 (5)	1 (3)
Dysphonia				2 (6)

Parentheses indicate the percentage of patients in each study.[11,13,20]

phenomenon. The various sensory symptoms included burning, tingling, pins and needles, worms/ants crawling sensation, tight band around legs, feeling of heat or cold, inability to feel the footwear/ground, feeling of walking on cotton/pebbles, numbness, etc. The Nigerian synonym for the disease originates from the Yoruba word "Ralerale", which means the reflex of rubbing the soles of the feet on the ground to remove phantom soilage. Sensory symptoms in the trunk have been in the form of girdle pains. The sensory symptoms mostly involved the legs. A third to half of the patients' reported symptoms in the upper limbs with clumsy hands and painful paresthesias. As noted in other reports, exacerbation of symptoms occurs in the rainy season.[10,12,14] Lower cranial symptoms in the form of dysarthria, dysphagia, and dysphonia occurred in a minority of patients. Dysphonia was manifested (especially common in women) as a high-pitched hypophonic voice with an inability to shout loudly. Dysphonia has not been reported previously. Night blindness was reported in 2 out of 84 patients by Osuntokun, which was attributed to coexistent vitamin A deficiency. The typical gait is wide-based and ataxic which becomes high steppage if associated with foot drop. The patient's eyes remain glued to the floor. Approximately, two-thirds of the patients reported worsening at night and a half gave a history of falls.[12] One-third of the patients reported the use of walking aids.[22]

Evidence of malnourishment included angular stomatitis, cheilitis, glossitis, hair loss, discoloration of hair, premature greying of hair, etc., **(Table 2)**. Cognitive impairment was noted in two patients, who developed psychosis with associated visual, auditory hallucinations, and paranoia in tandem with the neurological symptoms. One of these patients had a history of mental retardation from childhood and the other had developed neuro-psychiatric syndrome in the postpartum period. Visual

TABLE 2: Physical signs in tropical ataxic neuropathy.

	Osuntokun *n* = 84 (%)	Oluwole *n* = 66 (%)	Madhusudhan *n* = 40 (%)	Our cohort *n* = 31 (%)
Malnutrition signs	33	–	0	4 (13)
Cognitive impairment	7 (8)	1 (1.5)	–	2 (6)
Vision loss			20 (50)	25 (81)
Bilateral optic atrophy	50 (55)	32 (48.5)	8 (20)	18 (60)
Seventh nerve palsy	–	3 (4.5)	–	1 (3)
Sensory neural deafness	36 (43)	11 (16)	36 (90)	26 (84)
Palatal weakness	–	–	2 (5)	0
Wasting of tongue	–	–	2 (5)	0
Diaphragmatic palsy			3 (7.5)	–
Nystagmus				4 (13)
Motor wasting and weakness	27 (32)	22	30	10 (32)
Hypotonia	16 (19)	–	–	27 (87)
Spasticity	6 (7)		10 (25)	4 (13)
Loss of DTRs	–	–	18 (45)	27 (87)
Extensor plantar	10 (12)	2 (3)	10 (25)	6 (19)
Incoordination	56 (67)	2 (3)	–	8 (26)
Primitive reflexes		25 (38)		0
Sensory gait ataxia	57 (68)	48 (73)	36 (90)	29 (93)
Positive Romberg's	50 (60)	18 (27)	40 (100)	29 (93)
Sensory loss to pin	17 (20)	66 (100)	20 (50)	19 (61)
Sensory loss to cotton				17 (57)
Loss of joint position	54 (65)	19 (29)	36 (90)	29 (96)
Loss of vibration	68 (81)	39 (59)		26 (89)

Note: Parentheses indicate the percentage of patients in each study.[11,13,20]

acuity of 6/36 or more was categorized as visual impairment, evident in 32/36. Optic atrophy in the form of temporal pallor of the disk or white contracted disk was considered. Sensorineural hearing loss (present in 24 patients) was evaluated by bedside tuning fork tests. Audiometry was available for 20 patients, of which 19 had confirmed sensorineural deafness. Gaze-evoked nystagmus was seen in four patients. Apart from the sensory loss in glove and stocking distribution, hyperesthesia was seen in a minority of patients ($n = 2$). The sensory level was not seen in any of the patients. Even though incoordination of lower limbs elicited by the heel knee test was present, other cerebellar tests such as decomposition of movement, intention tremor, and rebound phenomenon adiadochokinesia were absent. Extrapyramidal syndrome of Parkinson's disease was found in a single patient with TAN is believed to be coincidental.[12] Lack of extrapyramidal involvement is intriguing, considering the fact that cyanide mainly affects the extrapyramidal system, as implicated in etiopathogenesis. Choreoathetoid movements of lower limbs have been reported in a few patients from the Indian series, however, whether this is extrapyramidal in origin or pseudoathetosis due to loss of proprioception needs clarification. The presence of primitive reflexes that were not age-related probably suggests diffuse cortical involvement and might reflect a degenerative etiology.[14] Two-thirds of the patients ($n = 21$) were dependent for mobility and activities of daily living at the time of admission. At discharge, 75% (22/37) felt their symptoms were status quo whereas eight patients reported mild-to-significant improvement.

LABORATORY FEATURES

Anemia is rare.[12,22] Hemoglobin, serum albumin, total protein, and albumin—globulin ratios, indices of protein nutrition, have been reported to be normal in TAN.[12] Serum cholesterol level, accepted as an index of calorie consumption,[23] has been found to be lower in patients compared to the control group.[12] The total serum level of vitamin B12 and its metabolism are normal in these patients.[13] Vitamin B nutrition parameters in the Nigerian TAN were compared with normal controls on the cassava diet and controls who were not on cassava. The serum riboflavin levels were significantly lower in the patients. Thiamine status, as assessed by transketolase activity of RBC hemolysate, was reported to be marginally deficient.[24] Microbiological assays of nicotinic acid, folate, pantothenic acid, and pyridoxine were normal.[24] The serum and urinary thiocyanate level, an indirect measure of cyanide load were significantly elevated,[12,22] and the sulfur-containing amino acids cysteine, which is thiol donor for the cyanide to form thiocyanate, were reduced. Cerebrospinal fluid (CSF) studies are reported to be normal in most[12,22] and elevation in protein does not exceed 60 mg/dL, with pleocytosis being mild (in 18 and 15% of patients, respectively). CSF Kahn test for syphilis is consistently negative.[25]

Electrophysiological studies have revealed slowing of motor conductions in the nerves of lower limbs without conduction blocks.[12,22,26] Sensory conductions reveal a complete absence of sural sensory nerve action potentials in all patients.[22] The reduced conduction velocities in the affected nerves suggest a demyelinating disorder. Pathologic or autopsy studies of TAN patients are sparse in the literature. The histopathology of sural nerve biopsy is consistent with predominantly axonal involvement affecting both unmyelinated and myelinated fibers. The latter were most affected without signs of regeneration, suggesting a sensory neuronopathy.[27] Anterior tibial nerve biopsy specimens have revealed perineural infiltration with lymphocytes and perineurial fibrosis in patients with polyneuropathy. The vasa nervora are usually normal.[12]

In the epidemic Cuban neuropathy, which presented as either retrobulbar neuropathy, sensory peripheral neuropathy, dorsolateral myeloneuropathy, or as mixed forms, the morphological findings in sural nerve biopsies revealed alterations ranging from mild-to-severe axonal damage in all the cases. In a minority of patients, axonal damage was accompanied by perineural fibrosis and vascular abnormalities. Axonal regeneration was noted in 23% and remyelination in 26%. Morphometric analysis revealed a predominant loss of myelinated fibers in 92% of the patients involving large-caliber fibers. Scarce mononuclear cells were observed in half of the cases. No virus-like elements were detected. The morphological features in this study indicate that, regardless of the clinical presentation, peripheral nerve lesions of the epidemic neuropathy in Cuba correspond to axonal neuropathy. These features are compatible with nutritional, toxic, or metabolic etiologies, but are incompatible with an inflammatory etiology.[28] Whether the biopsy findings of epidemic Cuban neuropathy can be extrapolated to TAN is controversial because cassava is not implicated in the etiopathogenesis of Cuban neuropathy.

Whereas these two studies described a predominant axonopathy or sensory neuronopathy in TAN,[27,28] other studies provide evidence of demyelinating neuropathy. Anterior tibial nerve biopsy in the Nigerian tropical ataxic neuropathy revealed sudanophilic granules in the perineurium and endoneurium suggestive of myelin breakdown. There was also a reduction in the number of myelin sheaths. Axonal changes were not found to be as striking or extensive as myelin alterations. The blood vessels were congested with a moderate proliferation of endothelial cells and occasional ones showing small areas of infiltration of lymphocytes plasma cells and mononuclear cells. The perineural connective tissue was thickened by dense fibrous tissue in some nerves and hyalinized collagen in others. Electron microscopy revealed abundant unmyelinated fibers compared to myelinated fibers.[29]

ETIOPATHOGENESIS

Tropical ataxic neuropathy has been associated with malnutrition, vitamin B deficiencies, chronic cyanide intoxication from excessive cassava consumption, tropical malabsorption, vegetarian diets, poor protein intake, viral, degenerative, and genetic factors.[30] No single factor has been implicated conclusively.

The interest in cyanide-containing cassava in etiopathogenesis was rekindled in the 1960s. Cassava is described as a food security crop because of its resistance to drought and poor soil. All cassava species contain cyanogenic glycosides in their leaves and roots. The two cyanogenic glycosides are linamarin and lotaustralin (in a ratio of 97:3).[31] During drought conditions, cassava plant produces more linamarin and bitter cassava has higher linamarin content than sweet species.[18] Various processing methods such as fermenting, sun drying, soaking, boiling, roasting, and grinding can reduce the cyanide content by up to 98%.[18] This is achieved by the release of the enzyme linamarinase in the cell wall, which catalyzes the hydrolysis of linamarin to hydrogen cyanide and acetone. The resulting hydrogen cyanide escapes into the atmosphere making the processed cassava edible and safe for consumption.[32] If the cassava is inadequately processed, then the cyanide reaches the body. Cyanides are highly toxic and inhibit the enzyme cytochrome c oxidase (aa3) in the mitochondria effectively causing histotoxic hypoxia. The body tries to avoid this by providing hydroxycobalamin, ferric ions from hemoglobin or thiols donated by sulfur-containing amino acids, etc. Hydroxycobalamin reacts with cyanide to form cyanocobalamin, which is excreted through urine and bile. Minor amounts get converted to formic acid and are excreted in the urine. However, the major pathway of the detoxification of cyanide is the reaction with cysteine to form an iminothiazolidine compound excreted in the saliva and urine. The thiocyanate level in the urine and saliva is considered to be an indirect measure of cyanide load in the body. Hence, effectively, detoxification is dependent on nutritional status, protein malnutrition, and sulfur-containing amino acids.[32] Experiments to identify the specific cause for neuropathy caused by cassava have been considered using Wistar strain albino rats as the experimental animal model.[17] Cassava fed rats were compared control animals, animals given cyanide, malnourished animals fed cyanide to identify the causative factors. This study revealed that, although the behavioral pattern in motor coordination of the cassava-fed animals was similar to the other groups studied, the neurochemical basis for the observed behavioral pattern was unique for cassava. Hence, the neurotoxicity of cassava could be attributed to nonmetabolized linamarin, more than its nutritional status and/or cyanide toxicity.[17] Demyelination due to cyanide, high thiocyanate levels in serum urine, and nerve specimens of patients, reduction of these levels following diet modification, the strong geospatial correlation between endemic areas for TAN, and cassava cultivation all favored cyanide in etiopathogenesis of TAN.[31]

Although cyanide hypothesis is rather appealing, it is challenged by various other studies that found high thiocyanate levels in Swedish smokers with no disease,[33] and in unaffected family members of the patients, and low prevalence in a community where cassava consumption was very high,[34] and case reports from noncassava consuming areas.[35] It is interesting that cassava was introduced to Africa from South America sometime after the 11th century AD, and curiously TAN is not common in South America.

The absence or diminution of sulfur-containing amino acids has also been implicated.[12] The hypothesis that deficient intake of sulfur-containing essential amino acids due to a cassava-dominated diet may compromise cyanide metabolism to thiocyanate by rhodanese[36,37] needs more research and therapeutic trials.

A novel unifying hypothesis that TAN might be caused by nitriles, compounds containing a cyano (R-CN) group, via neurotoxic action independent of cyanide,[38] in a manner akin to lathyrism, has been suggested recently. There is increasing evidence from limited human and several animal studies that nitriles show a wide variety of neurotoxic properties. Nitriles cause degeneration of vestibular hair cells (loss of balance), auditory hair cells (deafness), corneal clouding, retinal detachment and degeneration (vision loss), and degeneration of olfactory mucosa (anosmia). It also causes neurofilament accumulation with swelling of axons resulting in axonopathy, particularly targeting the larger neurons of dorsal root ganglia and spinal cord motor neurons. The neurotoxic properties of nitriles are determined by its concentration, type of compound structure, isomeric forms, metabolic bioactivation in the body, as well as gender and species differences in disease susceptibility.[38]

It has been suggested that certain trace metals such as copper may be of etiological significance because deficiency of copper is known to cause sheep "sway-back".[39]

The relationship of TAN to parasitic diseases, especially schistosomiasis, has intrigued several researchers in the past.[40]

There have been reports of a possible association between a TAN-like illness with HTLV-2 in four females with ataxic gait and prominent mental changes. Though serology showed HTLV-2 positivity in all, CSF showed HTLV-2 antibodies in only two of them.[41] Recent studies have reevaluated thiamine deficiency as the etiological mechanism. The thiamine nutritional status, as assessed by the transketolase activity and thymine pyrophosphate effect, was found to indicate significant thiamine deficiency in patients with TAN. The clinical manifestations of sensory polyneuropathy, optic atrophy, and gait ataxia are compatible with thiamine deficiency.[18] A dramatic and statistically significant improvement in the mean ataxia score of TAN patients as compared to controls occurred in the first week after receiving 100 mg of thiamine.[20]

There might be a complex relationship between the toxicant and the neurological disease, which may be relevant to other toxic or neurodegenerative diseases.

TREATMENT

Detoxification of cyanide is carried out by hydroxycobalamin (not cyanocobalamin) and the enzyme rhodanese, both of which are stored in the liver.[42] Sulfur-containing amino acids act as thiol donors, which combine with cyanide to form thiocyanate. In a controlled clinical trial, treatment with hydroxycobalamin had no effect.[43] A subsequent placebo-controlled, double-blind clinical trial with cysteine, hydroxycobalamin, and riboflavin for 48 weeks also did not find any benefit.[44] Hence, currently, no effective treatment is available.

Prognosis and Natural History

There is paucity of information regarding the natural history and age-specific mortality of the disease, even though follow-up studies suggest a higher mortality compared to community.[14] In Nigeria, where 84 patients were followed up for less than a decade, no deaths occurred among the patients, none were paraplegic, and two had signs of myelopathy; those who had optic atrophy and deafness at presentation developed definite polyneuropathy on follow-up, confirmed by electrophysiological tests. In most patients with deafness, myelopathy, and optic atrophy, the symptoms started within weeks of each other. In a few cases, there was a clear history that symptoms of myelopathy preceded visual impairment and nerve deafness. The spinal nerves are the last to be involved.[12] The longest follow-up study is of exprisoners of war from the Far East, who had developed nutritional neuropathy, optic atrophy sensorineural deafness, etc., and was studied after an interval of 23–36 years in Europe. Follow-up of 898 former prisoners of war neuropathy patients after a mean period of 32 years after release and treatment revealed a persistent neurological deficit in 5.5%. The residual deficits included peripheral neuropathy, optic atrophy, sensory neural deafness, and myelopathy.[3] In the Indian series, with a median follow-up period of 2 years, sensory ataxia was noted to have improved in 60%, however, the improvement was mild in half of the patients and moderate in the other half. The patients who had initially been chair-bound were able to walk unaided within 1 year. None showed improvement in visual and hearing deficits and there were no fatalities.[22] The ataxic neuropathy with nutritional mucocutaneous manifestations, especially in adolescents and young adults improved with diet and nutritional supplementation whereas the TAN in the elderly attributed to cassava did not show improvement in neurological symptoms.[14]

DIFFERENTIAL DIAGNOSIS

A combination of ataxia (sensory and cerebellar) along with pyramidal signs may be seen in high cervical cord lesion, craniovertebral junction (CVJ) anomalies, or vascular malformations of the area. A combination of deafness or optic atrophy may be seen in a small percentage of patients with syrinx and CVJ anomaly. In the presence of peripheral neuropathy, the syndrome becomes myeloneuropathy, and the possibility of a structural lesion gets excluded. The etiology of myeloneuropathies could be nutritional, toxic, paraneoplastic, autoimmune, metabolic, or infectious, as enumerated in **Box 2.**[4,45] A detailed history covering dietary habits including cassava consumption, malabsorption symptoms, systemic symptoms for autoimmune or infectious diseases, epidemiologic, genetic factors, recent illnesses, surgeries, toxin exposure, and drug intake needs to be obtained. A magnetic resonance imaging (MRI) of

BOX 2 **Differential diagnosis of tropical ataxic neuropathy.**[45]

- *Nutritional and toxic*:
  - Subacute combined degeneration of spinal cord
  - Copper deficiency myeloneuropathy
  - Thiamine deficiency
  - Folate deficiency
  - Vitamin E deficiency
  - Drugs and toxins (pyridoxine, cisplatin, NO, OP compound, and clioquinol)
- *Autoimmune and paraneoplastic*:
  - Paraneoplastic sensory neuronal disease
  - Sjögren's syndrome
  - Autoimmune hepatitis-associated sensory neuronopathy
  - Chronic ataxic neuropathy due to paraproteinemias
  - Multiple sclerosis
  - Sarcoidosis
- *Metabolic and heredodegenerative*:
  - Refsums
  - Frederick's ataxia
  - Ataxia with vitamin E deficiency
  - Cerebrotendinous xanthomatosis
  - Adrenomyeloneuropathy
  - Hereditary spastic paraparesis plus syndromes
  - Mitochondrial cytopathies
- *Structural spinal cord pathology*:
  - Craniovertebral junction anomaly
  - Arteriovenous malformation
- *Infections*:
  - HIV vacuolar myelopathy
  - HTLV-associated myelopathy
  - Tabes dorsalis
  - Hepatitis C

(HIV: human immunodeficiency virus; HTLV: human T cell lymphotropic virus; NO: nitrous oxide; OP: organophosphorus) the spine should be performed to detect any structural pathology. Laboratory evaluation should include nutritional indices, peripheral smear, various vitamin levels, homocysteine, methylmalonic acid, copper levels, autoantibodies, onconeural antibodies, paraproteins, and screening for various infections, genetic studies, liver biopsy, minor salivary glands, or nerve biopsies tailored to the patients' clinical picture.[4]

KONZO

Konzo is an acute upper motor neuron disease causing paralysis of the legs which is mostly irreversible and affects women of childbearing age and children. It is associated with the consumption of bitter cassava containing high cyanide, especially in those with protein depleted diets. The word Konzo means "tied legs". The word originated from Yaka tribe in Democratic Republic of Congo (DRC) to designate a fetish used by hunters to weaken legs and catch wild animals.[46] The literature suggests that Konzo was known from the Yaka indigenous population of the Bandundu province in Zaïre, presently known as the DRC, since the end of the 19th century. However, the disease was first reported in Congo in 1938 by Dr Trolli. The disease is also known as Mantakassa in certain regions of Africa.[46]

Epidemiology

Konzo occurs amongst very poor rural people in DRC, Mozambique, Tanzania, Cameroon, and Central African Republic and has recently been reported in Angola (Banea 2012) and Zambia. Accurate prevalence estimates (as high as 5% in certain rural areas) have been difficult because of unreliable demographic data and poor surveillance systems.[46]

Though the disease occurs as isolated cases the majority occurs as outbreaks of epidemics.[46] Konzo epidemics occur as a result of (1) war such as the recent civil war in DRC, where people were forced from their homes and had to eat poorly processed bitter cassava from the bush, (2) drought which stresses the cassava plant and causes it to produce much more cyanogen than normal, and (3) as a result of short cut processing methods.[47] Persistent Konzo also occurs in very deprived areas in Mozambique, DRC, and Tanzania.[47,48] Most epidemiological studies have shown a link between outbreaks of Konzo, agroecological collapse, and consumption of insufficiently processed bitter cassava (*Manihot esculenta Crantz*), a staple for millions of people in sub-Saharan Africa[46] (kashala).

Pathophysiology

The universal mechanism in animals to detoxify cyanide is its conversion catalyzed by the enzyme rhodanese, to produce thiocyanate, which is water soluble and removed in the urine. The reaction consumes essential S-containing amino acids methionine and cysteine (cysteine) which must be obtained from ingested protein. If there is a shortfall of protein in the diet, such as occurs in these very poor communities where many people have only one meal per day, then priority removal of essential S-containing amino acids to detoxify ingested poisonous cyanide may lead to protein malnutrition and stunting, as has been observed in DRC.[47] Furthermore, if there is a shortage of S-containing amino acids to detoxify ingested cyanide, then this would lead to an increase in the concentration of cyanide in the blood which could cause Konzo, perhaps via the formation of the neurotoxin cyanate.[47]

The general belief is that cyanide probably impairs mitochondria function, which successively leads to adenosine triphosphate (ATP) depletion and blockage of orthograde axonal transport, which, in turn, leads to total ATP depletion and subsequent cell death.[49]

While the exact biological mechanisms that cause this disease have largely remained elusive, host genetics, and environmental components such as the gut microbiome have been explored (bramble). It appears that children of high Konzo prevalent zones (HPZ) not only harbor enrichments of bacteria that have been demonstrated to hydrolyze linamarin, but also contain an overall higher abundance of genes that code for beta-D-glucosidase, which is the bacterial enzyme in gut which hydrolyzes linamarin. When assessing genes that could serve to detoxify cyanogenic compounds, it was found that the children from low Konzo prevalent zones (LPZ) on average have a higher abundance of both bacterial thiosulfate sulfurtransferase/rhodanese) and 3-mercaptopyruvate sulfurtransferase (MPST) as compared to the children from HPZ. This means bacterial abundance and functional genes could exacerbate the release of cyanide after ingesting cyanogenic glucosides in the children from HPZ, as well as a possible scenario of added bacterial protection/detoxification in LPZ. Though studies on gut microbiome indicate enrichments of bacteria capable of hydrolyzing linamarin as well as genes coding for beta-D-glucosidase in the children from HPZ, the development of Konzo is multifactorial in nature with numerous environmental variables and stressors.[50]

Clinical Features

Konzo occurred abruptly in less than 1 day in 90% of cases and over 2–7 days in the remainder. The acute symptoms are usually precipitated by physical exertion like prolonged walk. Apart from weakness patients complain of heaviness, trembling, stiffness, cramps, etc., the sensory symptoms if at all present are transient and disappear in a few days. These include paresthesia, numbness, muscle ache, and a sensation of electrical discharge in the back of the legs.[46] About half the patients have optic neuropathy with decreased visual acuity and alterations of the visual fields. A small number of Konzo patients have an ocular motor disturbance leading to pendular nystagmus and abnormal pursuit eye movements and saccades. The nystagmus starts at the onset of the disease and it may be unilateral or bilateral. Dysphagia if present is of pseudobulbar nature and transient in the initial phase. The severity of the neuro-ophthalmologic involvement is not parallel to the severity of the motor disturbance in Konzo.[49]

Examination

The main clinical picture of Konzo consists of an isolated symmetric spastic paraparesis with exaggerated deep tendon reflexes of the lower limbs and extensor plantar responses. The ankle clonus is frequently found, as well as pathological reflexes of the upper extremities in severely affected subjects, with a clearly noticeable palmomental reflex. Severely affected patients may have quadriparesis with truncal weakness, dysarthria and dysphagia of pseudobulbar nature clinical examination may reveal defects in visual fields, atrophy of the temporal part of the retinal nerve fiber layer linked with the temporal pallor of the optic disk.[49] The field defects are in the form of concentric constriction, centrocecal scotoma, and temporal constriction. Hearing and sensory function, as well as urinary, bowel, and sexual functions appear to be clinically normal.[46]

The World Health Organization (WHO) has adopted the following definition and epidemiological criteria for the disease:[46]

- Heavy reliance on cassava as a staple food
- Abrupt onset (<1 week) of leg weakness and
- A nonprogressive course of the disease in a formerly healthy person
- A symmetric spastic abnormality when walking and/or running
- Bilaterally exaggerated knee and/or ankle jerks without signs of disease of the spine in an endemic area.

Based on the ability to walk, the following WHO classification of severity has been proposed: mild form = subject is able to walk without support, moderate form = subject has to use one or two sticks, and severe form = subject is unable to walk. Neuropsychological findings suggest impaired neurocognition in children from Konzo-affected areas compared to those from nearby nonaffected areas, raising concerns that the overall human burden of the disease could be underestimated.[46]

Investigations

Central and peripheral nerve conduction studies have shown a prominent dysfunction of the pyramidal system with evidence of subclinical involvement of sensory pathways. About half of the Konzo patients also have abnormal visual evoked potentials, with both delayed latency and reduced amplitude.[49]

Nonepileptic electroencephalographic abnormalities are found while MRI from two subjects has remained unremarkable.[51,52] To date, the only observation that was done on an autopsied brain in the 1930's was not conclusive.[46] Levels of urine and plasma thiocyanate have been found to be significantly elevated in these patients,[46] however, diagnostic utility of this as a biomarker is questionable.

Differential Diagnosis

The closest differential for myelopathy of nutritional toxicity origin is lathyrism due to the consumption of *Lathyrus Sativus*/grass pea. The other differentials are tropical spastic paraparesis/HTLV-associated myelopathy, primary lateral sclerosis, etc. However, Konzo differs from all these tropical myelopathy syndromes in that the onset is acute and the disease is nonprogressive after the initial presentation. Other causes of noncompressive myelopathy. These include but are not limited to the subacute myelo-optic neuropathy (SMON) due to clioquinol (5-chloro-7-iodo-8-quinolinol; iodochlorhydroxyquin) intoxication, infections or liver failure, hereditary spastic paraplegia (HSP), or amyotrophic lateral sclerosis (ALS).[46,49]

Treatment

There is no effective treatment for Konzo. Prevention is the only way to eradicate the disease. This could be achieved by diversifying the diet in the region, developing plant breeding methods to reduce the cyanogen content in cassava, and better removal of toxins from cassava through more efficient processing methods.[53] Recently, a method called wetting for cassava flour has been shown to drastically reduce the cyanogen content and prevent outbreaks of Konzo.[47]

Prognosis

In a 14 years follow-up of Konzo patients, it was found that the neurological signs of spastic paraparesis remained constant. Functional improvement occurred, however, even in severely affected patients with contractures:[54] Previous studies have concluded that after initial weeks of improvement, the disability remained unchanged over the years and decades. A follow-up of Konzo patients in Tanzania 9–18 months after onset found that all patients still needed support to walk and the signs were unchanged 2 years later.[48] A quarter of the patients are left with permanently reduced visual acuity (Mwanza).[49]

CONCLUSION

"Whatever the agents responsible for these myeloneuropathies turn out to be the history of lathyrism warns us that the exact role of a suspected food stuff may long elude us."[10] Lathyrism is one of the oldest neurotoxic diseases known to mankind. Hippocrates (460–377 BC) is believed to have been aware of the toxic pea causing persistent paralysis of the legs. It remained a mystery for centuries until two groups of Indian scientists in 1964 identified beta-N-oxalylamino-L-alanine after primate feeding studies.[10] If cassava consumption is indeed responsible for cases of TAN, there are significant public health implications. It is the poorest populations of subsistence farmers who are most dependent on cassava for food and nutritional security, and would therefore be at the most risk for developing the neurological effects of TAN.[55] In areas with high consumption, proper processing of cassava may need to be emphasized, as improper processing yields higher toxic food products. For detoxification of cyanide, sulfur-containing amino acids are necessary and often lacking in tropical diets, which may be countered with measures to combat protein malnutrition.

Although TAN has been attributed to cyanide from cassava, it is clinically different from Konzo and has never been reported in areas where Konzo is encountered. It is, however, difficult to understand how presumably the same agent may result in several distinct clinical entities.

Cassava can be grown in relatively hostile environments and has high-calorie content.[55] As such, any food that may be promoted instead would have to adequately substitute these important qualities.

Tropical ataxic neuropathy being a serious and disabling health problem and multifactorial in etiopathogenesis provides unsurpassed opportunities for research and international cooperation to identify new avenues for treatment and unravel the pathogenesis of this mysterious toxic-metabolic neuropathy. It is rather astonishing how little literature has come from India where the disease is not at all uncommon!

REFERENCES

1. Bucher B, Poupard JA, Vernant, JC, Defreitas EC. Tropical Neuromyelopathies and Retroviruses: A review. Rev Infect Dis. 1990;12:5:890-9.
2. Gill GV, Bell DR. Persisting nutritional neuropathy among former war prisoners. J Neurol Neurosurg Psychiatry.1982;45:861-5.
3. Roman GC, Spencer PS, Schonberg BS. Tropical Myeloneuropathies: The hidden endemias. Neurology. 1985;35:1158-70.
4. Netto AB, Netto CM, Mahadevan A, Taly AB, Agadi J B. Tropical ataxic neuropathy—a century old enigma. Neurol India. 2016;64: 1151-9.
5. Strachan H. On a form of multiple neuritis prevalent in the West Indies. Practitioner. 1897;59:477-84.
6. Scott HH. An investigation into an acute break of 'central neuritis'. Ann Trop Med Parasitol. 1918;12:109-96.
7. Stannus HS. Deficiency diseases in Sierra Leone and pellagra. Trans R Trop Med Hyg. 1930;6:627-32.
8. Stannus HS. Some problems inn riboflavin and allied deficiencies. Br Med J. 1944;2:103-4.
9. Spillaine JD. Presidents address on Tropical Neurology. Proc Royal Soc Med.1969;62:403-10.
10. Money GL. Clinical aspects of tropical ataxic neuropathies related to malnutrition. West Afr Med J. 1959;8:3-17.
11. Montgomery RD, Cruickshank EK, Robertson WB, McMenemey WH. Clinical and pathological observations on Jamaican neuropathy: A report on 206 cases. Brain 1964;87:425-62.
12. Osuntokun BO. An ataxic neuropathy in Nigeria: A clinical biochemical and electrophysiological study. Brain. 1968;91:215-48.
13. Osuntokun BO. Cassava diet chronic cyanide intoxication and neuropathy in the Nigerian Africans. World Nutr Diet. 1981;36: 141-73.
14. Oluwole OSA, Onabolu AO, Link H, Rosling H. Persistence of tropical ataxic neuropathy in a Nigerian community. J NeurolNeurosurg Psychiatry. 2000;69:96-101.
15. Moore DGF. Partial loss of central acuity of vision for reading and distance in school-children and its possible association with food deficiency. W Afr Med J. 1930;3:46-51.
16. Makene WJ, Wilson J. Bichemical studies in Tanzanian patients with ataxic tropical neuropathy. J Neurol Neurosurg Psychiatry. 1972;35:31-3.
17. Mathangi DC, Namasivayam A. Neurochemical and behavioural correlates in cassava-induced neurotoxicity in rats. Neurotox Res. 2000;2:29-35.
18. Adamolekun B. Neurological disorders associated with cassava diet: A review of putative etiological mechanism. Metab Brain Dis. 2011;26:79-85.
19. Oluwole OSA, Onabolu AO, Catgreave IA, Rosling H, Persson A, Link H. Incidence of endemic ataxic polyneuropathy and its relation to exposure to cyanide in a Nigerian community. J Neurol Neurosurg Psychiatry. 2003;74:1417-22.
20. Monekosso GL, Annan WGT. Clinical epidemiological observations on an ataxic syndrome in Western Nigeria. Trop Geogr Med. 1964;16:316-23.
21. Krishnaswamy K, Kalamegham R. Tropical ataxic myelopathy. Trop Geogr Med. 1975;27:249-52.
22. Madhusudhan M, Menon MK, Ummer K, Radhakrishnan K. Clinical and etiological profile of topical ataxic neuropathy in Kerala, South India. Eur Neurol. 2008;60:21-6.
23. Edozien JC. A biochemical evaluation of the state of nutrition in Nigeria. W Afr Sci Ass. 1965;10:22-38.
24. Osuntokun BO, Aldetoyinbo A, Bademosi O. Vitamin B nutrition in the Nigeria topical ataxic neuropathy. J Neurol Neurosurg Psychiatry. 1985;48(2):154-6.
25. Cruickshank EK, Montgomery RD, Spillane JD. Obscure neurologic disorders in Jamaica. World Neurol. 1961;2:199-211.
26. Cragg BG, Thomas PK. Changes in nerve conduction in experimental allergic neuritis. J Neurol Neurosurg psychiatry. 1964;27: 106-15.
27. Dalakkas MC. Chronic idiopathic ataxic neuropathy. Ann Neurol. 1986;19(6):545-54.
28. Borrajero I, Perez JL, Dominiguez C, Chong A, Coro RM, Rodriguez H, et al. Epidemic neuropathy in Cuba: morphological charecterization of peripheral nerve lesions in sural nerve biopsies. J Neurolsci. 1994;127:68-76.
29. Williams AO, Osuntokun BO. Peripheral neuropathy in tropical (nutritional) ataxia in Nigeria light and electron microscopic study. Arch Neurol.1969;21:475-92.
30. Adamolekun B. Thiamine deficiency and the etiology of tropical ataxic neuropathy. Int Health. 2010;2:17-21.
31. Oluwole OSA, Oludiran A. Geospatial association of endemicity of ataxic polyneuropathy and highly cyanogenic cassava cultivars. Int J Health Geograp.2013;12:41.
32. Dhas PK, Chitra P, Jayakumar S, Mary AR. Study of the effects of hydrogen cyanide exposure in Cassava workers Indian J Occup Environ Med. 2011;15(3):133-6.

33. Tylleskar T, Banea M, Bikangi N Cooke RD, Poulter NH, Rosling H. Cassava cyanogens and Konzo, an upper motor neuron disease found in Africa. Lancet. 1992;339:208-11.
34. Oluwole OSA, Onabula AO, Cotgreave IA, Persson A, Link H. Low prevalence of ataxic polyneuropathy in a community with high exposure to cyanide from cassava foods. J Neurol. 2002;249: 1034-40.
35. Haddock DRW. Neurological disorders in Ghana. In: Spillane JD (ed). Tropical Neurology. London: Oxford University Press; 1973. pp. 207-22.
36. Cliff J, Lundquist P, Martenson J, Rosling H, Sorbo B. Association of high cyanide and low sulfur intake in cassava induced spastic paraparesis. Lancet 1985;326:1211-3.
37. Llorens J, Soler-Martín C, Saldaña-Ruíz S, Cutillas B, Ambrosio S, Vaello PB A new unifying hypothesis for lathyrism, konzo and tropical ataxic neuropathy: Nitriles are the causative agents. Food Chem Toxicol.2011;49:563-70.
38. Llorens J, Demêmes D, Sans A. The behavioral syndrome caused by 3,3'- iminodipropionitrile and related nitriles in the rat is associated with degeneration of the vestibular sensory hair cells. Toxicol Appl Pharmacol. 1993;123:199-210.
39. Lee HJ. The occurrence and correction of cobalt and copper deficiency affecting sheep in south Australia. Australian Veterin J. 1950;26:152-9.
40. Cowper SG. Schistosomiasis in Nigeria. Ann Trop Med Parasitol. 1963;57:307.
41. Sheremata WA, Harrington WJ, Bradshaw PA, Foung SK, Raffanti S P, Berger JR, et al Association of '(tropical) ataxic neuropathy' with HTLV-II. Virus Res. 1993;29:71-7.
42. Cipollone R, Ascenzi P, Tomao P, Imperi F, Visca PJ. Enzymatic detoxification of cyanide: clues from Pseudomonas aeruginosa Rhodanese. Mol Microbiol Biotechnol. 2008;15(2-3):199-211.
43. Osuntokun BO, Langman MJ, Wilson J, Aladetoyinbo A. Controlled trial of hydroxocobalamin and riboflavine in Nigerian ataxic neuropathy. J Neurol Neurosurg Psychiatry. 1970;33:5:663-6.
44. Osuntokun BO, Langman MJ, Wilson J, Adeuja AGO, Aladetoyinbo MA. Controlled trial of combinations of hydroxocobalamincystine and riboflavine-cystine, in Nigerian ataxic neuropathy. J Neurol Neurosurg Psychiatry. 1974;37(1):102-4.
45. Spinazi M, Angelini C, Patrini C. Subacute sensory ataxia and optic neuropathy with thiamine deficiency. Nat Rev Neurol. 2010;6: 288-93.
46. Kashala-Abotnes E, Okitundu D, Mumba D, Boivin MJ, Tylleskär T, Tshala-Katumbay D. Konzo: A distinct neurological disease associated with food (cassava) cyanogenic poisoning. Brain Res Bull. 2019;145:87-91.
47. Banea JP, Nahimana G, Mandombi C, Bradbury JH, Denton IC, Kuwa N. Control of konzo in DRC using the wetting method on cassava flour. Food Chem Toxicol. 2012;50(5):1517-23.
48. Howlett WP, Brubaker GR, Mlingi N, Rosling H. Konzo, an epidemic upper motor neuron disease studied in Tanzania. Brain. 1990;113 (Pt 1):223-35.
49. Mwanza JCK, Tshala-Katumbay D, Kayembe DL, Eeg-Olofsson KE, Tylleskär T. Neuro-ophthalmologic findings in Konzo, an upper motor neuron disorder in Africa. Euro J Ophthalmol. 2003;13(4):383-9.
50. Bramble MS, Vashist N, Ko A, Priya S, Musasa C, Mathieu A, et al. The gut microbiome in konzo. Nat Commun. 2021;12(1):5371.
51. Tshala-Katumbay D, Eeg-Olofsson KE, Kazadi-Kayembe T, Tylleskär T, Fällmar P. Analysis of motor pathway involvement in konzo using transcranial electrical and magnetic stimulation. Muscle Nerve. 2002;25(2):230-5.
52. Tylleskär T, Howlett WP, Rwiza HT, Aquilonius SM, Stålberg E, Lindén B, et al. Konzo: A distinct disease entity with selective upper motor neuron damage. J Neurol Neurosurg Psychiatry. 1993;56(6):638-43.
53. Bradbury JH, Lambein F. Konzo and neurolathyrism: Similarities and dissimilarities between these crippling neurodegenerative diseases of the poor. Food Chem Toxicol. 2011;49(3):537-8.
54. Cliff J, Nicala D. Long-term follow-up of Konzo patients. Trans R Soc Trop Med Hyg. 1997;91(4):447-9.
55. Okaiyeto PO, Lamidi OS. Research and development in cassava production and ruminant nutrition in Nigeria, An overview. J Engineer Appd Sci. 2006;2:117-24.

91

CHAPTER

Organophosphorus Poisoning

Dheeraj Khurana, Megha Varshney

INTRODUCTION

Organophosphates and carbamates are the two chemical groups of organophosphorus (OP) compounds commonly used worldwide as pesticides in agriculture. OP poisoning had been a common cause of hospital and intensive care unit (ICU) admission in developing countries presenting as suicidal or accidental ingestion, particularly in the young, productive age group. Due to the easy availability of these chemicals over the counter in developing agricultural countries like India, they are commonly used with suicidal intent in rural and suburban areas. The clinical features of OP poisoning in acute poisoning are characterized based on the receptor-specific involvement of muscarinic and nicotinic receptors resulting in varied manifestations. Following OP poisoning, acute symptoms commonly abbreviated SLUDGE (Salivation, Lacrimation, Urination, Defecation, Gastric cramps, and Emesis) occur within minutes to hours. It had been observed that some patients manifest delayed effects after an early period of asymptomatic or severe cholinergic symptoms and signs. Further symptoms and signs occur as a continuum involving one or more neuronal subsystems (neuromuscular symptoms/extrapyramidal). The reversibility of symptoms and signs can be predicted based on receptor-specific clinical features.

HISTORY OF ORGANOPHOSPHORUS POISONING

Pioneers in the synthesis of OP as nerve gas include two French organic chemists, Jean Louis Lassaigne and Philippe de Clermont in the 18th century with definite descriptions by the latter in 1854. It was in the early 1930s, the German scientist Willy Lange first described the toxidromes associated with exposure to nerve gas causing choking sensation and dimming of vision. These were the cholinergic effects of vapors on central nervous system (CNS). The Nazis in pre-World War II Germany realized the ability of this chemical for warfare and later on produced the G series of nerve gas during World War II, specifically sarin, tabun, soman, and other 2000 OP compounds but were not used as chemical weapons. It was after World War II, a few American companies gained access to Gerhard Schrader's work and synthesized parathion and malathion as the first OP compounds to be used as pesticides and insecticides. Recently, the use of nerve gas in chemical warfare was in Syria in 2013.[1] In 2018, an assassination attempt involving Novichok (XV), newer class of OP agents, has been perpetrated for chemical terrorism in Europe.[2] Other than the use of OP as a pesticide, another group of OP was used for industrial purposes. These are triaryl esters of phosphoric acid (e.g., triorthocresyl phosphate) and are used as plasticizing agents, lead scavengers in gasoline, and additives to hydraulic lubricants. Medical use of OP compounds includes the treatment of glaucoma and myasthenia gravis due to their ability in reversing neuromuscular blockade (neostigmine, pyridostigmine, and edrophonium).

EPIDEMIOLOGY

Organophosphorus and carbamates are used worldwide as pesticides and insecticides for >50 years. Their use declined in the last 10 years due to the occurrence of poisoning following suicidal and accidental ingestion. It is estimated that there are over 3 million cases of OP poisoning every year worldwide with approximately 10% of deaths occurring among them. As per WHO data in 2012, it was reported that >90% of fatal poisoning cases are seen in middle- and low-income countries, especially in agriculture-based developing countries.[3] The case fatality rate was nearly 20% more in developing nations as compared to developed countries.[4] Toxicity generally results from accidental or intentional ingestion or exposure to—agricultural pesticides.[5] Intentional poisoning with

OP was reported as 10–36.2% in developed countries, 40–60% in African countries, and 65–79.2% in developing countries.[6] The problems were more prevalent in rural areas of India. Chintale et al., 2016, found that organophosphate (OP) poisoning is widespread in southern and central areas of India, which results in a higher number of fatalities.[7] The percentage of people in India who commit suicide by poisoning themselves with OPs varies greatly, ranging from 10.2–43.87%.[8]

PATHOPHYSIOLOGY

Organophosphates are compounds produced by esterification between phosphorous and alcohol. Acute or chronic exposure can produce varying toxicity levels in humans. The route of exposure, amount, and specific chemical compound properties, along with the rate of metabolic degradation, determine the severity and rapidity of symptom onset. Common routes of exposure are skin, inhalation, or ingestion of the compounds. The toxidrome sets in early within a few minutes of inhalational exposure to OP compounds. In skin exposure, despite the intactness of the epidermis, the duration and volume of exposure along with the physical properties of OP being highly lipid soluble determine the symptom onset. OPs are rapidly redistributed to all body tissues with the highest concentrations found in the liver and kidneys. High-lipid solubility of OP is also responsible for crossing the blood–brain barrier producing potent effects on the CNS. The oxidative metabolites of malathion and parathion are the active form that binds to the acetylcholinesterase enzyme (AChE) and ends up in either of the three fates—endogenous hydrolysis, reactivation, or irreversible binding causing permanent inactivation of the enzyme. Irreversible binding of OP to AChE in the cholinergic synapses in the CNS and peripheral nervous system causes elevated levels of acetylcholine in the synaptic cleft causing initial excessive stimulation and later blockade of synaptic transmission. The clinical manifestation of acute OP poisoning is the result of this dysfunction; however, chronic exposure syndrome is the result of variable action on nicotinic, dopaminergic, and serotonergic receptors.

The reversibility of toxidrome depends on the reactivation of the AChE–OP complex. The process of enzyme reactivation is a slow, spontaneous aging reaction causing hydrolysis of the AChE–OP complex. As a general rule, the reactivation starts 48–72 hours after poisoning, though the rate of enzyme reactivation varies among different compounds of OP. However, pharmacological agents like oximes, which if added during the early period (48–78 hours) of poisoning, can hasten the process of enzyme reactivation.

As compared to OP agents, the carbamates–AChE complex undergoes spontaneous hydrolysis from the cholinesterase enzymatic site within 48 hours and acts as a transient cholinesterase inhibitor reducing toxidrome to a shorter duration.

CLINICAL FEATURES

Traditionally, there has been a receptor-based classification of symptoms as nicotinic and muscarinic (central and peripheral) manifestations. Early presenting cases have predominant muscarinic symptoms and usually have a characteristic "garlicky" odor. In earlier studies,[9] it was found that muscarinic symptoms are more common (84%), followed by CNS (78%) and nicotinic (17%). Time-based classification of symptoms as acute (within 24 hours), delayed (24 hours to 14 days), or late (>2 weeks) is also used to categorize clinical symptoms and signs. Most of the symptoms occur within minutes or hours following acute exposure to OP.

Acute Toxicity

Cholinergic excess: It affects the autonomic, neuromuscular junction (NMJ), and CNS. The peripheral muscarinic symptoms of SLUDGE are due to action on specifically involved glands. The onset is rapid after exposure and symptoms may last up to several days. At times, mydriasis and tachycardia can be observed due to action on sympathetic ganglia containing nicotinic receptors.

Type I paralysis is seen during the initial cholinergic phase when many muscarinic and nicotinic receptors are occupied by acetylcholine leading to persistent depolarization of the NMJ. Clinical features include fasciculations, cramps, and weakness. At this stage, the patient may require ventilatory support due to the involvement of respiratory muscles.

The central muscarinic effects though uncommon can result in a comatose mental state, depressed central respiratory drive, and convulsions rarely. These symptoms occur due to the high-lipid solubility properties of OP compounds leading to easy crossing of the blood–brain barrier.

Cardiac arrhythmias and respiratory failure due to combined effects of CNS depression, neuromuscular weakness, and excessive respiratory secretions along with bronchoconstriction are associated with case fatalities in acute OP poisoning.

Intermediate Syndrome/Type II Paralysis

Nictoninc effects, also termed "intermediate syndrome" (IS), follow the muscarinic syndrome. Approximately 10–40% of patients treated for acute toxicity develop an illness that occurs 24–96 hours after exposure to the OP compound. The onset of *type II paralysis* or IS is often rapid with the progression of limb muscle weakness centripetally over the course of 24 hours involving ocular, neck muscle, and respiratory muscles. Absent deep tendon reflexes (DTRs) are seen. Sensory impairment is not a feature of IS.

Symptoms include tachycardia and hypertension along with neuromuscular involvement. Excessive accumulation of acetylcholine at NMJ causes fasciculations initially and later progresses to muscle weakness. IS may last for several days up to 3 weeks with a maximum fatality occurring within 24 hours and those who recover usually do so within 2 weeks.

Neurological manifestations are due to nicotinic effects leading to weakness and later oropharyngeal and respiratory paralysis causing pooling of secretions and aspiration. Central depression, though a less common cause, may also lead to respiratory arrest.

Risk factors associated with IS include high-lipid solubility of OP compounds and inadequate oximes dosing.

Organophosphate-induced Delayed Peripheral Polyneuropathy/Type III Paralysis

Type III paralysis or OP-induced delayed polyneuropathy (OPIDP) is a sensorimotor axonal polyneuropathy seen after ingestion of large doses of certain OP compounds usually occurring after a latent period of 1–4 weeks of single or short-term exposures. There is distal axonal degeneration of the peripheral nerves, and in severe cases, spinal cord axonal damage may occur. The cardinal symptoms are a distal weakness of hands and feet, ataxia, and depressed DTRs often preceded by cramping calf pain and paresthesias of the distal limbs. The degree of pyramidal involvement determines the prognosis for functional recovery, and spastic ataxia may represent a permanent outcome of severe OPIDP. At the onset, the electrophysiological studies show the reduced amplitude of the compound muscle potential after supramaximal stimulation of motor nerves, increased distal latencies, and normal or slightly reduced nerve conduction velocities.[10] Further progression of the disease, usually over a few days, may lead to the nonexcitability of the nerve. Electromyography shows signs of active denervation of the affected muscles with increased insertional activity, spontaneous activity (fibrillation potentials and positive sharp waves), and reduced interference pattern.[11,12] During recovery, polyphasic motor unit potentials appear. These findings are consistent with those of distal degeneration of axons, as seen in the few cases where a biopsy of the sural nerve was performed and parallel the clinical signs of peripheral neuropathy.[13]

In addition to these classical manifestations described following acute exposure, several central CNS manifestations had also been described in the literature following low-dose chronic exposure. Chronic organophosphate-induced psychiatric disorders (COPINDs) are a term used to describe these manifestations.

LABORATORY INVESTIGATIONS

Clinical examination and history of exposure are the keys to diagnosis. Enzyme level assay (plasma butyrylcholinesterase and red cell AChE) is a useful biochemical tool for confirming exposure to OP and clinical severity is graded based on the pseudocholinesterase level, however, does not correlate well with clinical severity:

- *Mild*: 20–50% enzyme activity
- *Moderate*: 10–20% enzyme activity
- *Severe*: <10% enzyme activity

Enzyme levels are altered in patients with underlying liver disease, malnutrition, and blood disorders such as hemoglobinopathies and thalassemia.

Electrophysiological tests can be used to evaluate and characterize IS as it occurs due to failure of neuromuscular transmission. OP intoxication leads to typical endplate abnormalities that reflect the degree of acetylcholinesterase inhibition.[14] Characteristic neurophysiological abnormalities seen in OP poisoning are:

- A single supramaximal electrical stimulus-induced repetitive response
- A decrement-increment (DI) response to high-frequency (30 and 50 Hz) repetitive nerve stimulation (RNS)
- A decremental response to a high rate (30 and 50 Hz) RNS

Initial cholinergic excess produces repetitive muscle action potential following single nerve stimulation due to the persistence of acetylcholine (Ach) in the NMJ. As there is excessive Ach in the synaptic cleft, an increased contact period of the transmitter with the postsynaptic receptor leads to prolonged channel open time and prolonged end-plate potentials. Repetitive compound muscle action potentials (CMAPs) occur due to backfiring of nerve action potentials following stimulation of presynaptic Ach receptors.[15] This results in repetitive muscle membrane excitation with repetitive muscle action potentials. There could be also direct action of the OPs on the nicotinic Ach receptors channels, which increases the opening time.[16]

Reported findings of nerve conductions in OP poisoning demonstrated reduced CMAP of the peripheral nerves, while most patients' distal latencies and conduction velocities were normal.[10] The basis of the reduced amplitudes was transmission failure in the motor endplates. Diaphragmatic weakness significantly contributes to respiratory failure. Phrenic nerve conduction study with the recording of the CMAP from the diaphragm revealed the correlation between reduced CMAP and the need for mechanical ventilation.[17]

The evaluation of neuromuscular transmission using RNS at 3 Hz has shown a decremental response in a few patients, while the majority showed significant decrement with tetanic stimulation.[10,17] DI pattern was shown in milder stages of OP poisoning. The maximal decrement of the primary CMAP with the second response was seen followed by a gradual increase and accompanying disappearance of repetitive CMAP. The DI response was thought to occur due to stimulus-induced antidromic backfiring in the nerves, a presynaptic event.[18]

MANAGEMENT

It constitutes five steps:

1. Decontamination
2. Blockade of muscarinic activity
3. Reversal of cholinesterase inhibition with oxime
4. Correction of metabolic abnormalities
5. Management of complications

Decontamination includes the removal of clothes (continuous source of exposure), irrigation of skin and eyes, and gastric decontamination to minimize absorption of OP.

Blockade of muscarinic activity: The choice of treatment depends on the targeted receptor—central, peripheral, or both. Anticholinergic drugs such as atropine, glycopyrrolate, or scopolamine act on muscarinic receptors and have been found effective in reversing the effects of acute OP toxicity. However, only atropine can act on both central and peripheral cholinergic receptors due to its properties to cross the blood-brain barrier. The rest of other two have only peripheral action, hence other drugs like benzodiazepines are required. Atropine should be administered beginning at 2–5 mg intravenously and increased to double the dose if no effect is observed every 3–5 minutes until respiratory secretions are alleviated. Whenever doubt exists if OP compound had been ingested, a trial of 1 mg atropine can help to negate the diagnosis in the absence of signs or symptoms of anticholinergic effects. In some cases of mega-dose OP intoxication, there is unresponsiveness to high-dose atropine (100 mg/h) with an inadequate heart response. The addition of small doses of adrenergic agents improves heart rate with a dramatic reduction in atropine requirements.

Treatment of IS per se is mainly supportive, early recognition of the syndrome is keystone due to the high risk of death among patients with respiratory drive. No specific antidote is available to reverse IS. As the syndrome occurs following exposure to large doses of OP and persistent inhibition of AChE, prompt gastrointestinal decontamination, followed by appropriate therapy of atropine and oximes, and early assessment for ventilatory support should be helpful in ameliorating the severity and/or incidence of IS. Studies of oximes in IS as an empirical agent have shown no advantage of continuous infusion of 12 g/day for 3 days over a single dose of pralidoxime.[19] With a short half-life of oximes and difference in OP compound's susceptibility to reactivation, the exact dose of oximes required in OP poisoning needs to be individualized. The electrophysiological test objectifies the clinical findings well in acute OP poisoning and can guide oximes' dosage requirement.

The decremental response to 30-Hz RNS is a marker for the IS.[20] The amelioration of the 30-Hz decremental response, therefore, indicative of an improvement in the neuromuscular transmission with oximes can be used as a marker of improvement. The decremental response reappears later as the effects of the oxime wear off. Routine use of neuromuscular transmission studies helps to monitor the beneficial effects of oximes and to guide decisions such as the duration and dose of pralidoxime in individual cases. It is unlikely that any fixed-dose regimen of pralidoxime can be recommended. The dose, frequency, and duration of administration should be individualized and may be influenced by factors such as the individual OP agent involved, the quantity of exposure and duration of poisoning, existing cholinesterase levels, and most significantly the existing neurophysiological findings. Tailored pralidoxime administration under electrodiagnostic data guidance would be preferable rather than the administration of a fixed-dose regimen.

CONCLUSION

Organophosphorus compounds are ubiquitous as insecticides and pesticides and are a common cause of accidental/suicidal poisoning, especially in India due to their easy availability. Exposure to OPCs can lead to intoxication which carries high morbidity and mortality chiefly due to their neurotoxicity, and early recognition of the signs and symptoms of the poisoning is a key factor in limiting its harmful effects. Adequate measures should be taken to prevent accidental exposure like using protective gear while spraying. Their potential as agents of warfare and homicide still threatens humanity and cannot be ignored.

REFERENCES

1. John H, van der Schans MJ, Koller M, Spruit HET, Worek F, Thiermann H, et al. Fatal sarin poisoning in Syria 2013: forensic verification within an international laboratory network. Forensic Toxicol. 2018;36(1):61-71.
2. Chai PR, Boyer EW, Al-Nahhas H, Erickson TB. Toxic chemical weapons of assassination and warfare: nerve agents VX and sarin. Toxicol Commun. 2017;1:21-3.
3. Moebus S, Bödeker W. Mortality of intentional and unintentional pesticide poisonings in Germany from 1980 to 2010. J Public Health Policy. 2015;36(2):170-80.
4. Agrawaal KK, Karki P. Clinico-epidemiological Study on Pesticide Poisoning in a Tertiary Care Hospital in Eastern Nepal. J Nepal Med Assoc. 2014;52(196):972-6.
5. Karalliedde L, Feldman S, Henry J, Marrs T. Organophosphates and Health. London: Imperial College Press; 2001.
6. Kara IH, Güloğlu C, Karabulut A, Orak M. Sociodemographic, clinical, and laboratory features of cases of organic phosphorus intoxication who attended the Emergency Department in the Southeast Anatolian Region of Turkey. Environ Res. 2002;88(2):82-8.

7. Chintale KN, Patne SV, Chavan SS. Clinical profile of organophosphorus poisoning patients at rural tertiary health care centre. Int J Adv Med. 2016;(3):268-74.
8. Ahmed SM, Das B, Nadeem A, Samal RK. Survival pattern in patients with acute organophosphate poisoning on mechanical ventilation: A retrospective intensive care unit-based study in a tertiary care teaching hospital. Indian J Anaesth. 2014;58:11-7.
9. Lee P, Tai DY. Clinical features of patients with acute organophosphate poisoning requiring intensive care. Intensive Care Med. 2001;27:694-9.
10. Wadia RS, Chitra S, Amin RB, Kiwalkar RS, Sardesai HV. Electrophysiological studies in acute organophosphate poisoning. J Neurol Neurosurg Psychiatry. 1987;50:1442-8.
11. Moretto A, Lotti M. Poisoning by organophosphorus insecticides and sensory neuropathy. J Neurol Neurosurg Psychiatry. 1998; 64:463-8.
12. Sevim S, Aktekin M, Dogu O, Ozturk H, Ertas M. Late onset polyneuropathy due to organophosphate (DDVP) intoxication. Can J Neurol Sci. 2003;30:75-8.
13. Vasilescu C, Alexianu M, Dan A. Delayed neuropathy after organophosphorus insecticide (dipterex) poisoning: a clinical electrophysiological and nerve biopsy study. J Neurol Neurosurg Psychiatry. 1984;47:543-8.
14. Besser R, Gutmann L, Dillmann U, Weilemann LS, Hopf HC. End-plate dysfunction in acute organophosphate intoxication. Neurology. 1989;39:561-7.
15. Singh G, Mahajan R, Whig J. The importance of electrodiagnostic studies in acute organophosphate poisoning. J Neurol Sci. 1998;157:191-200.
16. Nagata K, Huang CS, Song JH, Narahashi T. Direct actions of anticholinesterases on the neuronal nicotinic acetylcholine receptor channels. Brain Res. 1997;769:211-8.
17. Singh G, Sidhu UP, Mahajan R, Avasthi G, Whig J. Phrenic nerve conduction studies in acute organophosphate poisoning. Muscle Nerve. 2000;23:627-32.
18. Besser R, Vogt T, Gutmann L, Hopf HC, Wessler I. Impaired neuromuscular transmission during partial inhibition of acetylcholinesterase: The role of stimulus-induced antidromic backfiring in the generation of the decrement-increment phenomenon. Muscle Nerve. 1992;15:1072-80.
19. Johnson S, Peter JV, Thomas K, Jeyaseelan L, Cherian AM. Evaluation of two treatment regimens of pralidoxime (1 gm single bolus dose vs 12 gm infusion) in the management of organophosphorus poisoning. J Assoc Physicians India. 1996;44:529-31.
20. Avasthi G, Singh G. Serial neuro-electrophysiological studies in acute organophosphate poisoning-correlation with clinical findings, serum cholinesterase levels and atropine dosages. J Assoc Physicians India. 2000;48:794-9.

92

CHAPTER

Snake Bite and Scorpion Sting

Himmatrao Saluba Bawaskar, Pramodinin Himmatrao Bawaskar, Parag Himmatrao Bawaskar

NEUROLOGICAL MANIFESTATIONS OF SNAKE BITE POISONING

INTRODUCTION

Snake bite is a life-threatening time-limiting medical emergency result in high morbidity and mortality if not treated in time. Though it is reported from Bangladesh, India, Nepal, Pakistan, and Sri Lanka together constitute 70% global snake bite mortality.[1] Snake bite poisoning is an occupational hazard often faced by farmers, labors, shepherds, hunters, snake rescuers, laboratory scientists milking snakes for venom, and migrating poor population of tropical and subtropical countries with heavy rainfall and high humid climate. Thus, snake bite is a disease of poverty.[2] Early diagnosis and proper management are accompanied with recovery. Elapid (*Bungarus caeruleus* and *Naja naja*) venom rich in neurotoxins results in descending neuroparalysis, delayed intervention may lead to irreversible hypoxic brain damage and lifelong vegetative stage.

EPIDEMIOLOGY

There are >2,000 snake species in the world out of which about 300 species are found in India. Total 52 species are venomous. Among these big four (*Russell's viper, Echis carinaus, Krait and Cobra*) **(Table 1)** are the most venomous species of snakes. These four result in neuroparalysis (elapid) and hematotoxicity, nephrotoxicity and severe local tissue damage result in disability (Vipers and *Cobra*).[3]

Snake bite is a century-old disease, it remains neglected though each year globally about five million people are estimated to be envenomed by snakes, of these people, 81,000 to 138,000 victims die and 400,000 victim become permanently disabled or disfigured.[1] In India each year 60,000 victims dies of snake bite.[4] Snake bite poisoning is an occupational hazard often faced by farmers, labors, shepherds, hunters, and migrating poor population of tropical and subtropical countries with heavy rain and high humid climate. Thus, snake bite is a disease of poverty.[2,5]

We analyzed the cases of venomous snake bite admitted to hospital at Mahad during 1998–2018.

Males are exposed to outside work and active farming predominately affected than females. Age group of 20–60 years is prone to this accident. Maximum cases are reported during monsoon June to December **(Table 2)**. Clinicians can identify the type of snake responsible for a bite by analyzing photographs, often image cached in mobile phone or in hospital preserved specimens. The World Health Organization (WHO) categorized snakebite as a high priority neglected tropical disease the mortality and morbidly.

TABLE 1: The incidence of snake bites and fatality from 1998 to 2018, by snake species.

	1998–2004		2005–2012		2013–2018	
Species	**Number of bites**	**Number fatal bites (%)**	**Number of bites**	**Number fatal bites (%)**	**Number of bites**	**Number fatal bites (%)**
Saw-scaled viper	15	0	108	1 (1%)	270	1 (<1%)
Russell's viper	5	0	71	6 (8%)	540	19 (4%)
Krait	48	16 (33%)	188	19 (10%)	346	42 (12%)
Naja naja	8	2 (25%)	61	5 (8%)	392	8 (2%)
All four species	76	18 (24%)	428	31 (7%)	1548	70 (5%)

TABLE 2: Monthly distribution of snakebite cases.

Month	Total	*Cobra*	*Krait*	*Russell's viper*	*Echis carinatus*	Vasculotoxic nonidentified	Pit viper
January	52	11	3	20	12	6	-
February	63	25	3	19	13	3	-
March	99	39	4	28	23	5	-
April	68	31	6	26	4	1	-
May	101	44	33	19	3	2	-
June	228	46	74	38	35	15	20
July	246	53	62	73	34	19	5
August	242	36	57	79	51	12	7
September	237	43	67	76	35	15	1
October	144	33	18	56	25	12	-
November	92	15	9	46	17	05	-
December	53	12	7	27	05	02	-
Total	1625	388	343	507	257	97	33

There has been an overall reduction in snakebite fatality, except in *krait* bite, which is difficult to treat and the most *krait* bite occurs during the night hours because of the nocturnal nature of this species. *Krait* venom causes destruction of neuromuscular receptors and can, in turn, result in descending and respiratory paralysis, which requires prolonged ventilation until receptors are regenerated. High fatality attributed to poor transportation during night hours, absence of ventilators in rural setting in addition tantric contributes a delay treatment.

India is the first country in the world to prepare the antisnake venom (ASV). Still many victims of snake bite dies due to nonadministration ASV in time or inadequate dose.[6] When Alexander the great invaded India in 327–325 BC, he was very much impressed by the arrow heads poisoned with venom from *Russell's viper* and the advanced clinical management and skill of Indian doctor. Because of regular training and Indian author's contribution to medical textbook, snake bite is no more neglected at rural setting with reduction morbidity and mortality. Real misery of snake bite is a tropical neglected disease, because of poverty tropical nation like that of India with high incidence of snake bite cannot arrange a meeting of scientists working on snake bite.

Newly posted medical office that never treated case before may not aware of clinical manifestations and management of snake bite, may neglect severe snake bite poisoning case result in death.[7] During 1998–2001 mortality due to snake bite was 36% in Mahad region,[6] with advent of training and counseling of early reporting dropped to 5% 2019–2020.[7]

BIOCHEMISTRY, PHYSIOLOGY, AND PATHOLOGY OF NEUROTOXIC ENVENOMING

Snakes are cold-blooded animals. A pair of salivary glands secrete a powerful multipurpose venom that flow at the time of envenoming through fine specific channeled or grooved teeth called fangs. It is quite clear that snake venom is not a substance evolved to attack man or any big vertebrates. Snake can bite and continue to secrete venom a number of times in succession. Venom secretion in all venomous snakes appears to vary in seasons more in warmer months with high morbidity and fatality, dark skin is poor heat conductor result in raised body temperature and in such situation, venom is more liquid form rather than more viscous, thus dark skin-colored snake injects more venom in one bite. Most snakes inject 10% of the available venom in a single strike except the *Russell's viper* which injects 75% of stored venom in one bite due to its big, long, sharp-curved fangs. Snake venom is a cocktail of twenty or more components including proteins, enzymes, nonenzymatic polypeptide toxins, lipids, free amino acids, nucleotides, carbohydrates, biogenic amines, and various activators and activates of physiological processes. *Krait* and *Cobra* venom contains acetylcholine esterase, phospholipase B, and glycerophosphatase. Phospholipase A2 is found in the majority of venom and is extensively studied. It destroys mitochondria, red blood cells, leukocytes, platelets, peripheral nerve endings, skeletal muscles, vascular endothelium, presynaptic neurotoxicity, opiate-like sedative effects, and autopharmacological release of histamine (anaphylaxis). Hyaluronidase promotes the spread of venom through the tissue. Proteolytic enzymes are responsible for local changes permeable leading to edema, blistering, blistering, and local necrosis.[8-13]

Severe, irreparable local tissue lost at the bite site of *Cobra* occurs due to myocytolysis. *Cobra* venom is rich in postsynaptic neurotoxins called alpha-bungarotoxin and *cobra* toxin. Acetylcholine receptors are primary signal transducers at neuromuscular junction. *Cobra* venom binds specially to acetylcholine receptors, prevents the interaction between acetylcholine and receptors on postsynaptic membrane result in neuromuscular blockade. Treatment with appropriate antivenom (in India polyvalent antivenom against *Krait, Cobra, Russell's viper*, and *Echis carinatus*) accelerates the dissociation of the toxin-receptors complexes and reverses the paralysis **(Figs. 1A to G)**. Cardiotoxin content of *cobra* venom has direct action on skeletal, cardiac, and smooth muscles, nerves, and neuromuscular junction; causes paralysis, circulatory and respiratory failure, and cardiac arrhythmias, venom induced sudden rise in intra myocardial calcium result in conduction defect and systolic cardiac arrest. *Cobra* venom is a smaller molecular size and rapidly absorbed in circulation. Absorption is further accelerated by threat of death and liberated catecholamine and running. This can kill the victim within 8 minutes. *Cobra* unlike the *krait* deposits its venom deeply. This in combination with hyaluronidase, allows spreading of the venom rapidly and symptoms to show abruptly. Interestingly, this rapidly of onset of symptoms prompts the rural victim in India to seek care quickly after *cobra* bite.

Common Indian *krait* (*Bungarus caeruleus*) venom content both pre- and postsynaptic beta-bungarotoxin and alpha-bungarotoxin. These toxins initially release acetylcholine at the nerve endings at neuromuscular junction and then damage it, and subsequently prevent the release of acetylcholine. As receptors get damaged and destroyed, resistant to anticholinesterase built up. Initial release of acetylcholine results in autonomic nerve stimulation in addition to release of cholecystokinin explains the acute abdominal colicky pain, vomiting, staring look, blurring of vision, gooseflesh, salivation, puling of saliva, hypertension, pulmonary edema (released of postsynaptic epinephrine stimulators),[12] and myasthenia face. Envenoming by *krait* is associated with a syndrome of neuromuscular paralysis that falls in to three distinct phases. The first phase is rapid onset of trauma leading to profound paralysis within 30–60 minutes. The second phase is a state of deep paralysis lasting for 3–4 days. The third phase is a recovery phase lasting for 2–3 weeks **(Figs. 2A to F)**. This explains the prolonged period of ventilators support and intensive care requirements essential for recovery. More insidious onset of symptoms induced by the *krait* bite, more often induce the victim to visit local traditional healer (*Mantrik or Tantrik*) for natural curatives. In spite of the fact that *krait* venom is ten times more lethal than *cobra*, victim report too late due to delayed clinical manifestations. *Krait* is a nocturnal in habit. Its fangs are small size like that of 24-size needle or like insulin needle. It injects the venom into skin, sometimes skin deep. It accidently bites to a person asleep on floor bed. Though venom is of small molecular size. It is absorbed

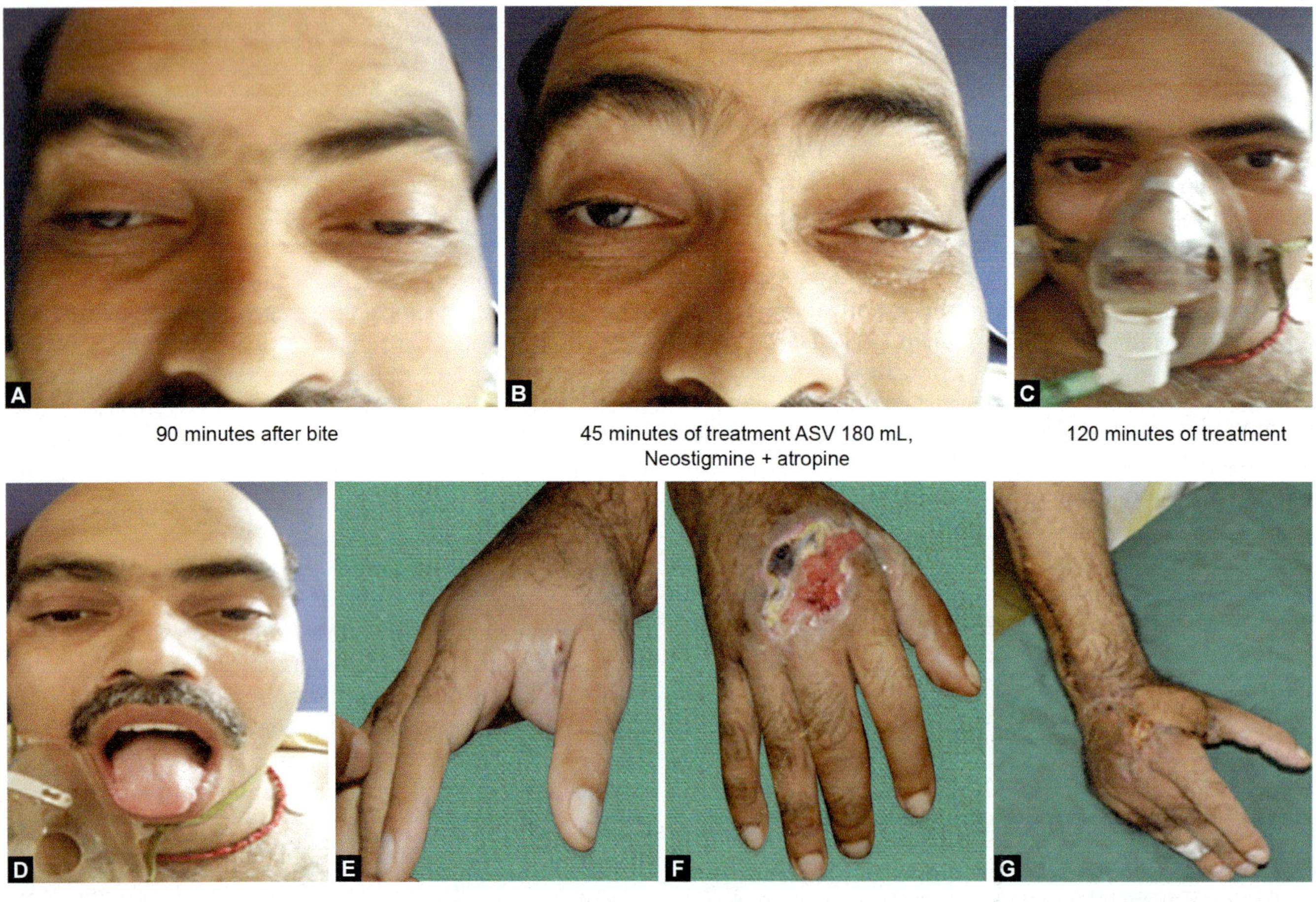

FIGS. 1A TO G: *Cobra* bite: The neurological manifestations and local effects at the bite site in *cobra* bite poisoning.

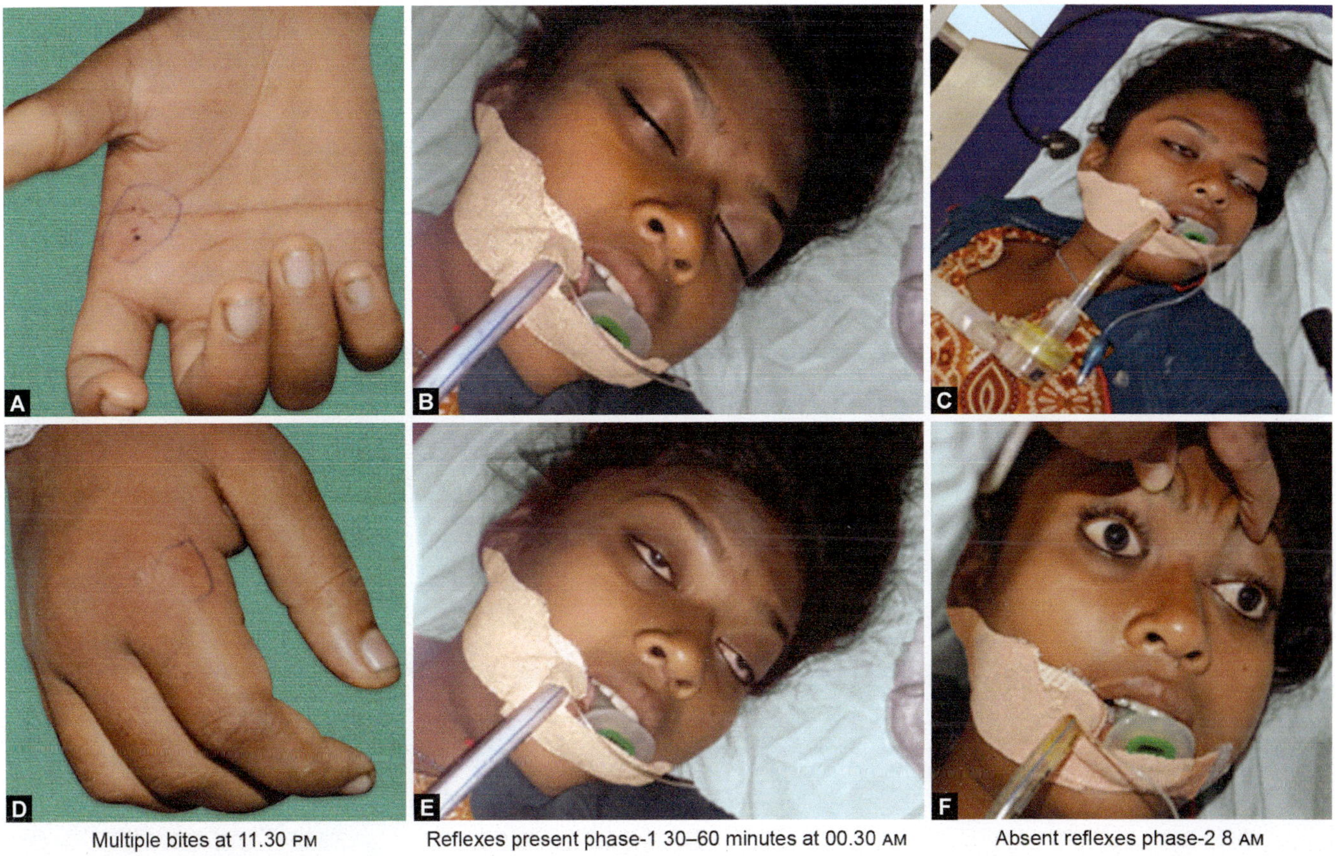

FIGS. 2A TO F: *Krait* bite clinical stages.

slowly as skin has poor circulation and reflexes are blunted during deep sleep. Neuromuscular blocked by the short-chain neurotoxin (*cobra* toxin and alpha-bungarotoxin) is more rapidly reversible than with long-chain toxin (beta-bungarotoxin). Beta-bungarotoxin in the *krait* venom bears similarity to botulinum toxin.[14]

Krait

Common Indian *krait* is *B. caeruleus*: Local names of Indian *krait* are *Kala gandait, Kala taro, Kandar, Manyar, Chitti, Kattu viriyan*, and *Vella pamboo*.

Krait is 1–4 feet long **(Figs. 3A to J)** with enlarged hexagonal vertebral scales, uniform white or red belly and narrow white crossbars on the back, more or less distinctly in pairs; the crossbars are typically absent near the head and neck region. The common *krait* resides in vicinity of human habitation, near the wattle and daub, mud, and small hut dwelling. *Krait* is a nocturnal, terrestrial snake that enters human dwellings in search of prey such as rats, mice, and lizards. It eats even the small snakes (cannibalism). The common *krait* is regarded as the most dangerous species of venomous snakes in Indian subcontinent. Most bites occur during cooler months of June to December, when snakes may during the course of hunting activity, linger on a person's bedding to take advantage of the warmth therein. Banded *krait* has head slightly broader than neck, tail is short and round tip. Body is covered with equally spaced wide, yellow/pale brown/white, and black bands. It lives in termite mounds and rodent burrows close to water. Though it is much active during night, but it is more reluctant to bite than the common *krait*. It is seen in West Bengal, Assam, Bihar, Odisha, Madhya Pradesh, and Andhra Pradesh. The greater black *krait* (*Bungarus niger*) *krait* flourished in India, Nepal, Bhutan, and Burma. In addition to neurological manifestation, there is generalized rhabdomyolysis, myalgia, odynophagia, and renal failure. Sindh *krait* (*Bungarus sindanus*) bite cases reported from Pakistan and part of India. It's venom rich in three finger toxins (3FTx), phospholipase A2, and Kunitz—type serine protease inhibitor. Other toxins proteins with restricted amount include metalloproteinase, L-amino acid oxidase, acetylcholinesterase, vespryn, and cysteine-rich secretory protein. Kappa neurotoxin and beta-bungarotoxins present the major toxins responsible for neurological effects.[1,8,13]

Clinical Manifestations of *Krait* Bite Poisoning

The majority of *krait* bite cases are reported between 11 PM and 5 AM. Victim might experience mild pain at the site of bite, paresthesia, or numbness, without any obvious local marks rarely mild swelling or bleed. In such situation, one can extensively search all over body particularly over back, axial, neck genitals, and popliteal fossa—small multiple fangs

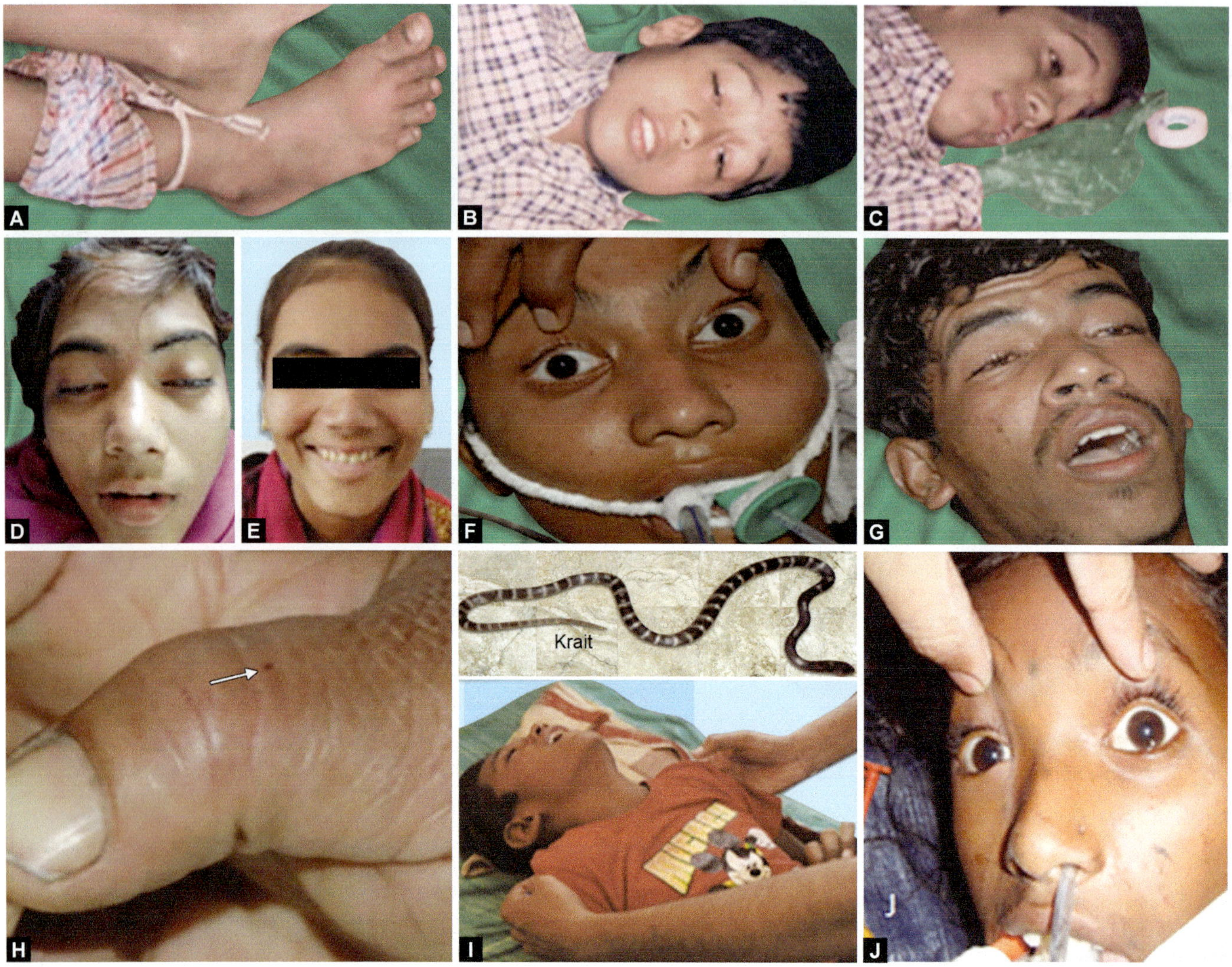

FIGS. 3A TO J: *Krait* bite. (A) *Krait* bite to right second toe. Tourniquet removed after 100 mL of ASV administered. (B) Bilateral ptosis, myastenic look; (C) Pulling of saliva; (D) *Krait* bitten to tip of nose showing swelling and bilateral ptosis; (E) Recovery after ASV, neostigmine, and calcium gluconate; (F) Ophthalmoplegia; (G) Pulling of saliva; (H) Pin head bleeding spot fangs mark at the site of *krait* bite; (I) Broken neck sign due to paralysis of neck muscles, victim unable to lift head from pillow; and (J) Dilated nonreacting pupils do not indicate the irreversible brain damage.

marks **(Figs. 2A to F)** with minimum surrounding urticaria. Because of negligible or total absence of local manifestations, envenomation is neglected and falsely initially attributed to ant or rat bite or no bite at all.

The venom stimulates the autonomic nervous system. Thus within 20–30 minutes of bite, victim wakes up due to transient abdominal colicky pain. He vomits once or twice and complains of chest pain. Relatives rarely call for doctors. Some inexperienced doctors even ignore the vital premonitory symptoms preceded to respiratory failure, may attribute to indigestion or acidity or acute attack of appendicitis and minimum T wave inversion due to ongoing hypoxia, such victims are referred and admitted to intensive coronary care units. Skillful clinical examination by some doctors may reveal bradycardia, sweating, raised blood pressure, pulmonary edema, staring look, blurring of vision, or at times photophobia. *Krait* venom has a great affinity toward presynaptic acetylcholine receptors. Thus, the tissue having high concentration of this receptors such as sphincter papillae, levator palpebral superior, neck muscles, bulbar, and subsequently limbs and diaphragm and intercostals muscles. Venom effects as early as 30 minutes or too late as 18 hours. Many times, victim says he or she had seen snake. Later on, many times the relatives might have found *krait* in bedding, pillow covers, or in a corner of the house. Bilateral ptosis, pooling of saliva, difficulty in bringing the tongue beyond teeth margin, slurred or nasal twang speech, aphasia, dysphagia, dyspnea, external ophthalmoplegia, and weakness of neck, respiratory muscles, and lastly the diaphragm are some of the symptoms. Patient complains of blurred vision, double vision, respiratory paralysis coma, and anoxic cardiac arrest. Quadriplegia with aphasia and nonreacting dilated pupils may be diagnosed as brain death or locked in syndrome or Guillain-Barré (GB) syndrome, encephalitis, meningitis, or hysteria. Patient can communicate by pelvic girdle and finger flicker. Venom-induced paralysis of pupillary muscle resulting in nonreactive dilatation of pupils is not the sign of irreversible brain damage. Few patients show signs and symptoms of peripheral neuropathy. Many times, patients succumb to iatrogenic respiratory infection or adult respiratory distress syndrome. Irrespective of quadriplegia, patient is fully conscious hence Glasgow Coma Scale is not applicable to victims of neurotoxin envenoming.[12,15]

At times, a victim bitten by *krait* brings the killed *krait*. He might not have developed any initial clinical manifestations including local fang marks urticaria indicated bite without envenoming or "dry bite". Inexperienced doctor may diagnose it as a *krait* bite even though it is a specimen of nonvenomous wolf snake. To confirm or identify the venomous *krait*, one has to look at the tail which is covered by white bands till its end. These white bands marks are absent in wolf snake **(Figs. 4A and B)**.

Thus, a person woke up from floor in midnight due to colicky pain, vomiting with or without history of snake bite subsequently developed descending neuroparalysis confirmed *krait* bite unless proved otherwise. Thus, *krait* licks the skin and bite the respiration.[12]

Management (Flowchart 1)

First aid at home or place where bite happens: If one succeeds in locating the bite on the victim's body, remove the surface venom deposited by clean cloth or cotton. Keep the bitten part below heart level. Immobilize the bitten part by apply crepe bandage or piece of cloth from distant end of bite site with pressure equal so that one can easily put and remove the finger underneath the bandage. In case of venomous bite already applied tourniquet should not be released unless full dose of antivenom is administered **(Figs. 3A to J)**. It is alright if the victim can reach a hospital within 30 minutes. If the victim is delayed in reaching to hospital for more than 4 hours, then crepe bandage has no advantage. One should not waste time in search of snake. If the snake is killed, take it to the hospital as it may help the doctor in diagnosis. Victim should not be allowed to walk. There should pilot person behind the victim if transported by bike.

At Hospital

Patient should be examined in a ventilated room. Ask the patient to show the site of snake bite and other details of history and activity at the time of bite. Initial clinical signs with timings should be noted in detail such as bulbar palsy, muscle power, tendon reflexes, respiratory rate, oxygen saturation, one minute counting, pooling of saliva, broken neck sign, blood pressure and ECG changes, serum electrolytes, and renal profile. Urine color analyzed for hemoglobin, red blood cells, and myoglobin. These signs should be closely monitored every hours till clinical improvement.

Antisnake venom—read details of referred letter regarding initial dose of ASV administered by referred doctor. On arrival and total 100 mL (10 vials) of ASV is prepared by adding 10 mL of distilled water in each powder ASV. The dissolved ASV should be clear like distilled water; if it is turbid, it indicates precipitation of protein which may lead to severe life-threatening anaphylaxis and hence should be discarded **(Fig. 5)**. About 100 mL dissolved ASV to be added to 200 mL of normal saline run over 30–50 minutes. One should sit by the side of victim for early diagnosis and treatment of anaphylaxis. Within 30 minutes after initial dose ASV, if there is no improvement of neurological manifestations one can repeat dose of ASV and no more than total 20 vials of ASV to be administered. ASV neutralizes circulating venom and it has no action once the venom is attached to the receptor (target) site. In *krait* bite, there is destruction of presynaptic receptors and thus neurological manifestation may persist for weeks till there is regeneration of receptors. At this stage administration of ASV merely wastes.

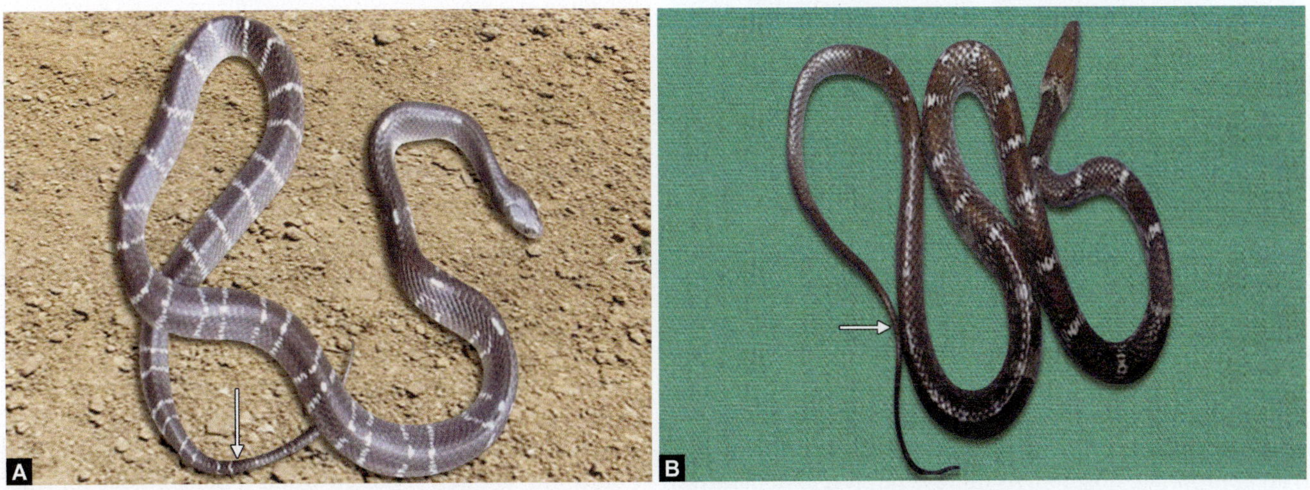

FIGS. 4A AND B: (A) Venomous *Krait* snake white bands up to the end of tail (arrow); (B) Nonvenomous wolf snake absence of white bands over tail (arrow).

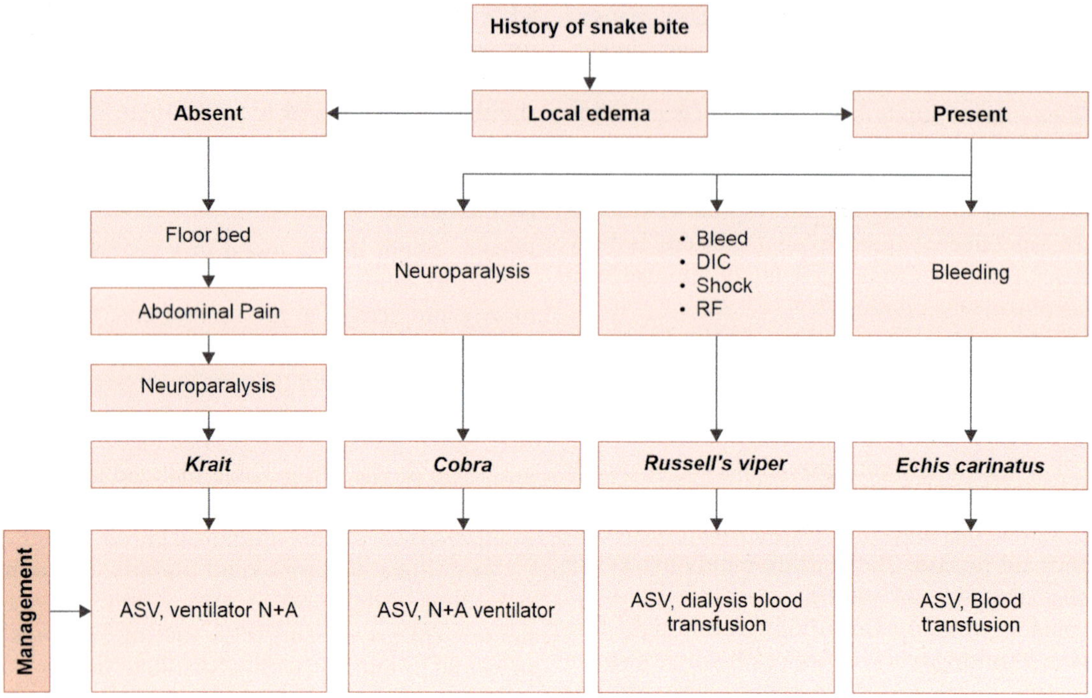

FLOWCHART 1: Clinical diagnosis of snake bite cases.
(A: atropine; ASV: antisnake venom; DIC: disseminated intravascular coagulation; N: neostigmine; RF: renal failure)

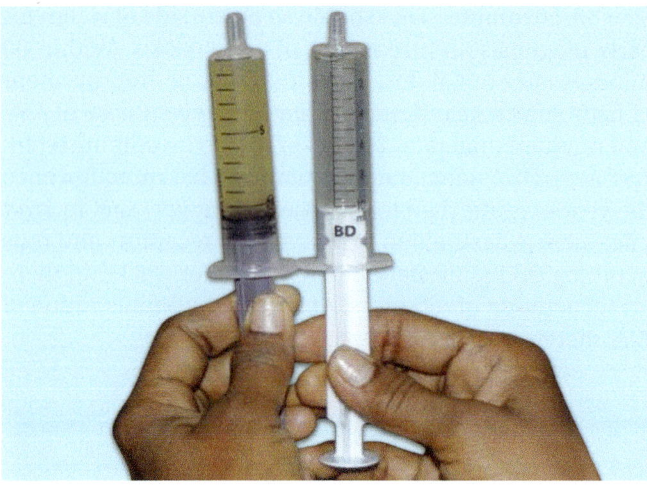

FIG. 5: Turbid-colored solution of antisnake venom should be discarded.

Ventilation: Indication of ventilator support victim has pooling of saliva, unable to lift the neck from pillow (muscle power three-fifths), reduction in SpO_2 saturation, respiratory failure (rate >24 and <5), abdominal—thoracic respiration, suffocation, and signs of cerebral hypoxia. At periphery, one can do the endotracheal intubation, if not possible a laryngeal mask can be put directly over larynx and Ambu bag (bag and valve) ventilation just to tide over emergency before reaching to an appropriate hospital. As there is rarely a total paralysis of respiration in such situation, the victim should be put on synchronized intermittent mandatory ventilation (SIMV) mode, help to wean rapidly from ventilation. Soon after extubation, the doctor should be present while giving victim first sips of water just to know the recovery of bulbar muscles **(Figs. 6A to E)**. The best way when to extubate is asked the recovering patient to remove the tube if he attempts, is the indication of extubation. Last to be recovered are ptosis and proximal muscles weakness of lower limbs. Ventilation may require >3 weeks.

Anticholinesterase inhibitor (AChEI): Indian common *krait* venom contains both pre- and postsynaptic blocker. Whether victim responds to AChEI or not can be confirmed by putting ice-filled glove figure over ptosis eyelid. Hypothermia sensitizes the acetylcholine receptors to acetylcholine. If there is little improvement in ptosis, one can try AChEI, presynaptic receptors are destroyed by *krait* venom. Neuroparalysis at time did not respond to AChEI, 10 mL calcium gluconate by intravenous route at six hourly interval improves the neuromuscular conduction and paralysis.

Cobra Bite Poisoning

Cobra (*Naja naja*): *Cobra* bite tends to occur during daytime or early darkness, when transportation is more readily available. Because of known severity of envenoming patients, relatives or bystanders make hurry to report to hospital rather than wasting time to go to the village healer. *Cobra* bite is often reported when a person goes for open toilet during night hours and children are playing near

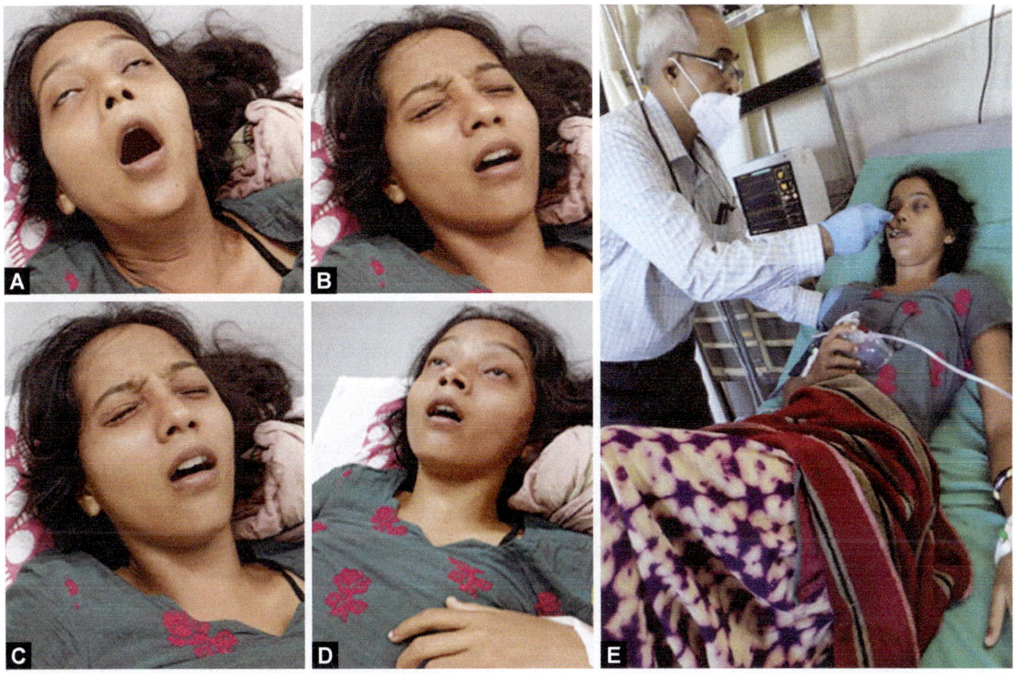

FIGS. 6A TO E: (A to D) Progressive improvement of descending neuroparlaysis; (E) Attending physician himself giving first ship of water.

loose stones or close to the basement of house or while searching ball in bushes, farmers handling the dry husk, watering the crops during night hours due to regular electric load shadings during daytime, and blindly walking through soya bean, ground nut, or gram seed crops without shoes or working at cattle shade. During holiday or weekend attempts to put hand blindly at attic to clear the rubbles.

Soon after bite the victim, experiences severe pain at the site of bite having a fang marks. While looking at bitten culprit, victim became more anxious because of threat of death rapid liberation of endogenous catecholamine result in profuse sweating, tachycardia, hypertension, and sudden death due to arrhythmias or acute myocardial infarction. Fang marks are covered with blood clots. There is rapid progression of swelling from the bittern part to the rest of limb. Skin at and around the bite site is ecchymosed. Subsequently, tense blebs and massive damage of skin and subcutaneous tissue due to myocytolysis and huge nonhealing ulcers **(Figs. 1A to G)**. If the victim had actually seen the hooded *cobra* biting him, he may die of cardiac lethal ventricular arrhythmias or cardiogenic shock due to massive myocardial infarction. As a result of massive liberation of endogenous catecholamine into circulation due to feeling or idea of threat of death. This phenomenon is absent in children having no idea of death. Sinus bradycardia, A-V block, and hypotension due to cardiodepressant action of venom and sudden respiratory arrest without any other neurological manifestations can occur resulting in anoxic cardiac arrest. Rapid ptosis and bulbar palsy accompanied with respiratory depression might occur. Rarely, hematotoxic effects are seen.[16] Blurring of vision and loss of accommodation are the earliest most sign of neurological envenoming.[17]

Management

Victim should not be allowed to walk or run and the bitten part should be kept below heart level irrespective of developing progressive swelling. No time should be wasted for applying tourniquets. If the patient is found totally unconscious with no respiration, mouth-to-mouth ventilation and chest compression should be tried. While giving mouth-to-mouth ventilation, see that chest is moving up. Reassurance and ensure the victim that medical treatment and antidote is available at hospital. Transfer the victim by available vehicle or over back of healthy person. No time should be wasted in search of snake. Killing snake is criminal. What are the first aids to snake bite victim? As early as taking victim to place where antidote is available. At primary health center 100 mL of polyvalent antivenom diluted in normal saline given by intravenous route over 30–50 minute without doing skin sensitivity test, repeat dose after 30–60 minutes not >200 mL. Use artificial ventilation by Ambu bag or ventilator. *Cobra* venom is attached reversibly to postsynaptic receptor. If in doubt, one can try short-acting AChEI or see the response of ptotic eyelid to hypothermia.[18] Neostigmine 50 µg/kg by intravenous route over first hour than 25 µg/kg in next hours preceded by atropine to counter the muscarinic action of AChEI or 0.5 mg neostigmine every 30 minutes and every third dose of neostigmine preceded by atropine. A majority of victims tend to recover within 24 hours. They may require not more than five to six doses of AChEI. In our experiences, we have noticed that victim declared dead by noting absence of respiration and nonreacting pupils by peripheral doctors recovered with ASV, ventilator, and adjuvant treatment and discharged. In case of respiratory arrest, first drug of choice is intravenous neostigmine to resuscitate or revive the paralytic respiratory muscles. Calcium gluconate by intravenous route may improve the neuromuscular conduction.

Local wound care is done by intravenous antibiotic, sterile dressing. skin grafting of all victims with nonhealing wound, one must rule out diabetes mellitus which is often forgotten by rural doctors while treating specifically snake bite cases.[19-21]

Recurrent relapse of signs and symptoms in a recovering hospitalized victim of *cobra* bite can occur.[22]

Sea Snakes (Figs. 7A to D)

Sea snake bite cases are reported from coastal region. Fishermen accidently handle sea snake resulting in envenoming. Its venom is neurotoxic, myotoxic, and hematotoxic. Soon after bite, victim complains of headache, sweating, vomiting, and tingling numbness. Foreign body sensation in throat and swelling of tongue. Within 30 minutes–3 hours after bite, the victim experiences severe muscle pain, marked tenderness all over muscles, trismus, muscle paralysis, and respiratory arrest, without local manifestations at the site of bite. Due to myotoxic effects of venom, resulting in liberation of potassium into circulation. Electrocardiogram (ECG) shows tented T weaves, widened QRS complexes, and diastolic cardiac arrest. Massive liberation of myoglobin into circulation blocks the renal tubules and acute renal shut down happens. Brown-colored urine, a diagnostic of myoglobinuria is also seen.

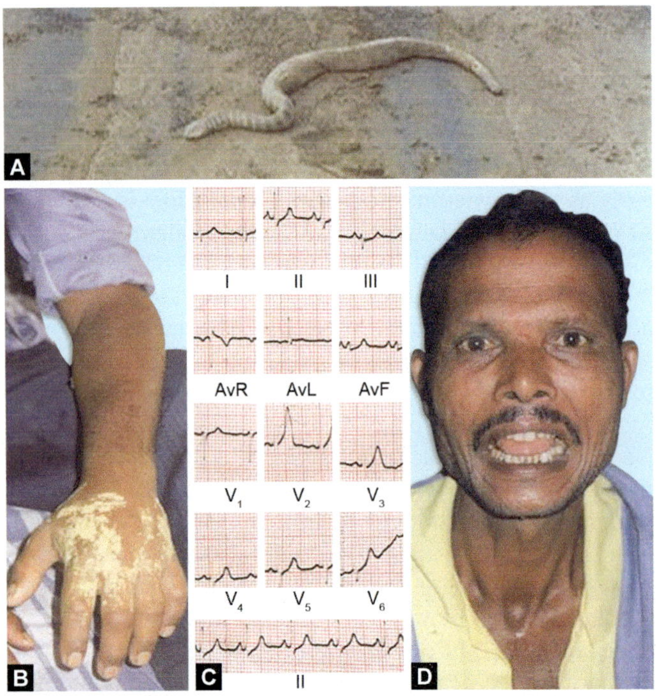

FIGS 7A TO D: Sea snake bite. (A) Sea snake—tail of snake is flattened like accelerator paddle; (B) Local edema at the bite site; (C) ECG-tented T waves due to hyperkalemia, (D) Trismus.

Management

Intravenous available polyvalent ASV 100 mL (paraspecificity of venoms), as sea snake antivenom is not available and moreover it is expensive. Ventilator for respiratory failure, correction of hyperkalemia by intravenous diuretic, calcium gluconate, insulin glucose drip, salbutamol, or dialysis. In case of resistant hyperkalemia, one can try a potassium channel drug—oral glibenclamide—provided one takes care of hypoglycemia.

Victims of neurotoxic envenoming who reported too late or there was a delay in resuscitations result in irreversible hypoxic neurological damage and in repeated convulsions; a vegetative state is an extra load to the family.

In such situation, electroencephalogram (EEG) may help reading outcome of resuscitations.

A 4-year-old boy was bitten by *cobra* over his right gluteus region while playing near basement of house. Within 1 hour had respiratory failure he rushed to hospital with no pulse, no respiration, and pupils dilated nonreacting to light. He was resuscitated by intracardiac adrenaline. Respiration and heart started functioning but brain was damaged. Magnetic resonance imaging (MRI) showed hypoxic damage to cerebrum and basal ganglion. Parents took him to tertiary care hospital and tried their best and sold out the piece of land for payment and tired and seen 3 year of bite in vegetative state. Was it worthwhile to resuscitate such child **(Figs. 8A and B)**?

Russell' s Viper (Figs. 9A to C)

Viper venom contains hematotoxins, neurotoxins (presynaptic), and thrombogenic. Envenomation may result in stroke. Neurotoxicity due to *Russell's viper* bite is not a life threatening. Moreover early antivenom did not prevent and reverse established neurotoxicity[23] snake bite induced leukoencephalopathy, pituitary dysfunctions including hypopituitarism, Sheehan's syndrome, loss of libido, amenorrhea, and growth retardation due to *Russell's viper* envenoming reported from Tamil Nadu and Kerala states.[24] Bilateral acute angle closure glaucoma, uveitis, optic neuritis, and retinal detachment are rare but can occur due venomous snake bite.[25]

Management of Anaphylaxis due to ASV

No skin test should be performed as it does not give surety regarding reaction. Antivenom should not be given intramuscular. It should be administered by a qualified person with knowledge of anaphylaxis reaction and its management. Reaction to ASV can develop within 10–180 minutes. The incidence is increased with dose of antivenom and speed of administration. Bolus dose may give rapid anaphylaxis. A turbid solution of ASV that may precipitate severe reaction should be thrown away. Earliest symptoms are hotness sensation in ears, scalp, itching over scalp, urticaria, sudden onset of intractable cough, nausea, vomiting, goose skin, giddiness often

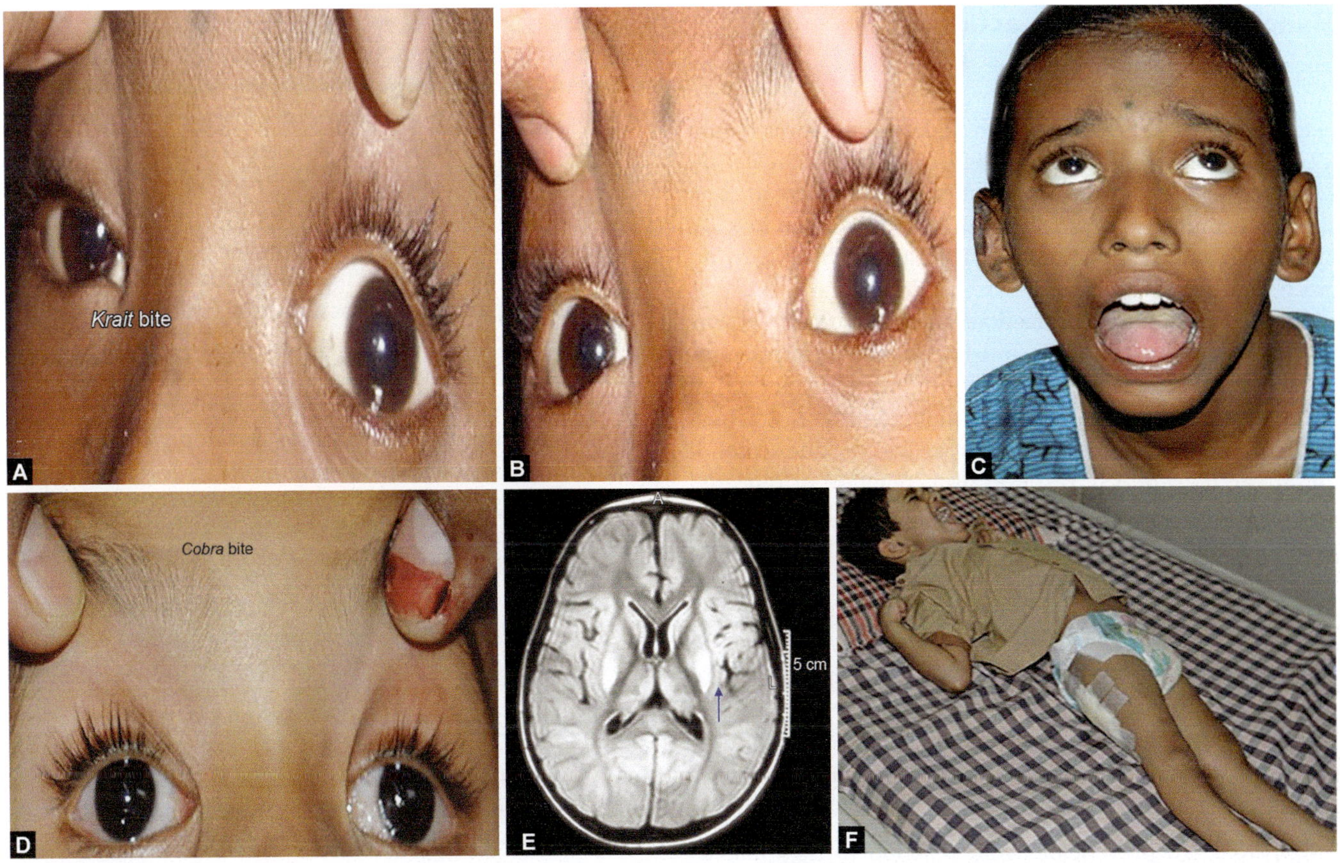

FIGS. 8A TO F: Resuscitations will be futile if victim cardiac arrest with loss of corneal luster. (A) *Krait* bite dilated non reacting pupils with healthy cornea; (B) After treatment normal size reacting pupils; (C) Total recovery without neurological deficit; (D) *Cobra* bite with lusterless corneas, dilated nonreacting pupils; (E) Extensive hypoxic brain damage; (F) Vegetative state with decerebration.

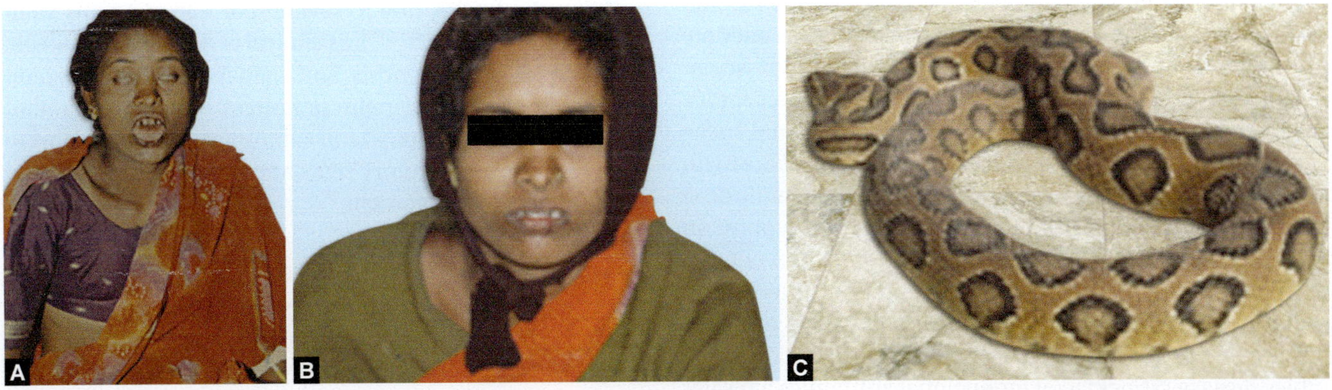

FIGS. 9A TO C: *Russell's viper*. (A) Bilateral ptosis, bleeding from mouth cavity; (B) Recovered with ASV and neostigmine; (C) Culprit *Russell' viper*.

felt as uneasiness, urinary and sub-conjunctival bleed, suffocation, and irrelevant behavior. Fever, tachycardia, and febrile reactions due to contamination of ASV with endotoxin such as compounds, rigors, vasodilatation, and hypotension occur within 1–2 hours of treatment. Children may suffer febrile convulsions. Systemic anaphylaxis: Sudden onset of projectile profound vomiting, sphincter relaxation, hypotension, bronchospasm, and angioedema. These reactions are due to complement activation by immune complexes or aggregates of immune globulin. Delayed reaction serum sickness can develop between 5 and 24 days of ASV therapy. Incidence of serum sickness depends upon dose of ASV, however, now because of extensive awareness regarding dose of ASV, such reactions clinically characterized by pyrexia of unknown origin, itching, arthralgia, and lymphadenopathy. Joint swellings, mononeuritis multiplex, albuminuria, and rarely encephalopathy are seen.

Management of ASV Reaction

Injection adrenaline 0.5 mL of 1% to be administered by intramuscular route on the lateral thigh. Dose can be repeated if anaphylaxis is not controlled. In a situation, where life is at stake that is severe hypotension and bronchospasm. Laryngeal edema, cyanosis, convulsive movement in such situation adrenaline 1,000 µg (1 mL) is to be diluted in 9 mL of normal saline, so 1 mL content 100 µg adrenaline can be given, 1 mL intravenous every 5 minutes till the reaction is reduced. In addition to intravenous aminophylline, head low position, intravenous fluids, anti-H1 blocker, chlorpheniramine maleate, intravenous methyl prednisolone, and nasal oxygen at times may be required along with endotracheal intubation and ventilation. Irrespective of due care, if administrations of ASV result in overt reaction or repeated anaphylaxis, one can select ASV from another batch of manufacturing and try. Patient should not die of reaction or due to snake bite envenoming.

One should not be afraid of administration of ASV in a severe venomous bite, provided you are fully prepared to treat the severe reaction. Many victims are referred from primary health centers without giving ASV to rural or a district hospital because of the threat of anaphylaxis, many of them die on way to hospital. One should sit by the side of the victim during treatment as if treating our own blood relatives.

Prophylaxis: To prevent or avoid reaction to ASV, subcutaneous adrenaline, antihistamine, and steroid and to be administered before ASV.

Further research: Scientist should make attempt to prepare venomous toxoid to immunize the farmers and risky population against venomous snake toxins. Toxicologists should make an attempt to prepare the pharmacological antidote to venom actions or synthetic chemical neuromuscular receptors to prevent the venom to reach to natural receptors.

To reduce the ASV dose there should be regional snake venom and antivenom bank. *Krait* beta-bungarotoxin structure is similar the rabies glycoprotein. Therapeutic dose of beta-bungarotoxin may block the action of glycoprotein of rabies virus and upgrade apoptosis and prevent the virus proliferation, maturity, and subsequent infection to surrounding neurons and arrest the progression of rabies disease and possibility of recovery of a victim from dreaded rabies disease.[26] Cocktail of monoclonal antibodies are safer and cost effective.

Prevention

Avoidance of sleeping on floor bed. Use of cot and mosquito net or net edges is properly tugged under the bedding, prevent snake bite, mosquito bite and scorpion sting alike. Wearing gum boots while walking in forest, grown of grass, plants, and crop. Use of torch and sticks while walking during night hours. Strict avoiding attending *mantrik, tantric,* or herbal remedy for snake bite. Early reporting to primary health center and administration of antisnake venom in a case of venomous bite may prevent death due to snake bite poisoning. During final years of MBBS course, there should be at least four lectures on snake bite, with spot of snake specimen, viva, and compulsory one long question and three short notes in annual papers.

A majority of cases are reported to primary health centers medical officer should be arranged regular training and workshop on snake bite poisoning and resuscitation including endotracheal intubation.

At the time of opening school after long summer holiday, the school bag to rule out possibility of snake and scorpion and the benches at school should be clean and washed. Ashram school children should be given cot and mosquito net for sleeping. Close watching and monitors the children during lunch hours. At the hospital, no stone should be left unturned to save the son of motherland.

During night hours, many relatives are accompanied with victim one should take chance and give idea of prevention of snake and scorpion sting.

SCORPION STING

INTRODUCTION

Envenomation by scorpion can result in wide range of clinical effects, including autonomic, cardiovascular, neurological, and cytotoxic effects.[27] Scientists and clinicians have studied pathophysiology of scorpion envenomation by critical observations of clinical manifestations, neurotransmitters, radioisotope, echocardiography (ECHO), and hemodynamic pattern. Since the advent of scorpion antivenom, vasodilator (prazosin), dobutamine, midazolam, and intensive care facilities, the fatality due to severe scorpion sting has been significantly reduced.[28-30] This clinical review of the available evidence on the diagnosis and management of scorpion envenoming aims to help peripheral practitioners and doctors working at tropical and subtropical countries, how to recognize the premonitory signs and symptoms of scorpion sting and their management.[31]

SCORPIONS

Scorpions belong to the large phylum of Arthropoda, which are characterized by presence of a chitin exoskeleton. Like spiders, they are part of the Chelicerata subphyla and the Arachnida class. The body of scorpions is divided into three parts: (1) the head (cephalothorax), (2) the abdomen (mesosoma), and (3) the tail (metasoma) which bears the sting (telson). Two venom glands are situated in the telson. The scorpion ejects its venom by contracting the muscle layer wrapping the glands. Scorpions are viviparous and cannibalistic. Scorpions have been able to survive in heat, drought, freezing conditions for weeks, desert condition and starvation for months, and total immersion of water for days. This remarkable power of adoption makes their survival independent of ecological condition and gives the species an unbroken continuity in adverse climatic conditions.

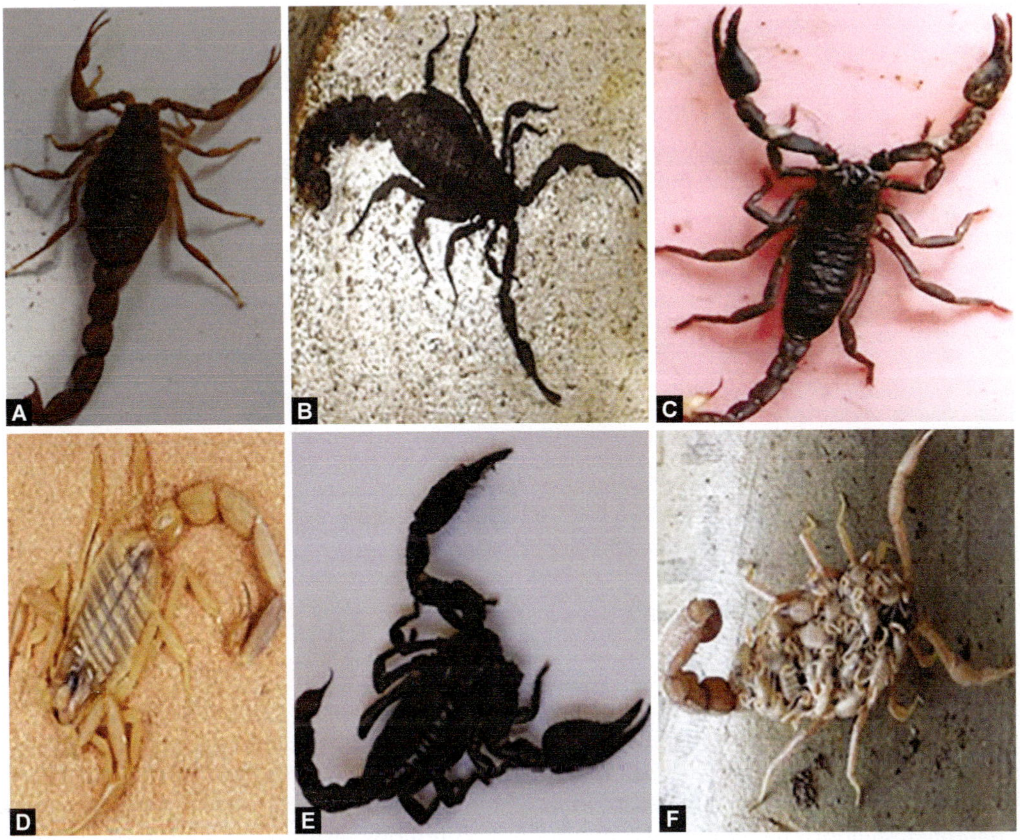

FIGS. 10A TO F: (A) An Indian red scorpion (*Mesobuthus tamulus*); (B) Indian black scorpion similar venomous like *Mesobuthus tumulus;* (C) Scorpion seen in Kerala state responsible for neurological manifestations; (D) Yellow scorpion *Leiurus quinquestriatus* from Israel similar venomous like *Mesobuthus tumulus;* (E) Big size Indian black scorpion *Palamneus gravimanus* less venomous; and (F) Scorpions are viviparous, give birth to young ones, and they nibble to their mother till she died (cannibalism).

Scorpions are generally found in dry, hot environments, although some species also occur in forests and wet savannas. All species are nocturnal, hiding during day under stones, in the piles of bricks, firewood or cow dung's, paddy husk, beddings, in the shoes left empty overnight, pockets of trousers and shirts, crevices of windows and doors, school bags, over mud walls, benches and cupboards, loose tiles of huts, and tree barks.

The annual number of scorpion stings cases exceeds 1.23 million, of which over 32,250 may be fatal.[32] Irrespective of high incidence of scorpion stings, majority experience local pain and few develop system manifestations.[33] True incidence, morbidity, and fatality are scarce because most of victim do not seek medical treatment or public health structure and prefer to consult Tantriks. Except for *Hemiscorpius lepturus*, all venomous species belong to the large family Buthidae.[32] The most notorious ones are found in the genera *Buthus* (Mediterranean Spain to the Middle East, *Parabuthus* (Western and South Africa), *Mesobuthus* (throughout Asia) **(Figs. 10A to F)**, *Hottentotta* (Southern Africa to Southeast Asia), *Tityus* (Central America, South America, and the Caribbean), *Leiurus* (Northern Africa and the Middle East), *Androctonus* (North Africa to Southeast Asia), and *Centruroides* (Southern United States, Mexico, Central America, and the Caribbean). In Mexico, hundreds of thousands stings by *Centruroides* scorpions occur each year. Similar incidence reported in other areas where scorpions are endemic in Tunisia[34] and other parts of North Africa and India.[28] Out of 1,500 scorpion species known to exit, about 30 are medical importance.[32]

VENOM AND ITS ACTIONS (FLOWCHART 2)

Scorpion venom is a cocktail several toxins, most of them are small molecular peptide toxins that target ion channels found in both mammals and insects.[35-38] Most lethal is the alpha toxins, which consist of 61 and 76 polypeptides that bind to a specific site on the mammalian voltage-gated neuronal sodium channel.[34] Delaying closing of sodium neuronal channel results in sustained depolarization and neuronal excitation, stimulating both parasympathetic and sympathetic autonomic nervous systems. As result of excitations of sodium neuronal channels, there is sudden pouring of endogenous catecholamines epinephrine and norepinephrine, and neuropeptide Y, and endothelin-1 result in "autonomic storm",[35,39] characterized by transient parasympathetic (vomiting, sweating, salivation, hypotension, bradycardia, ventricular premature contraction, and respiratory failure) and prolonged sympathetic (hypertension, tachycardia, pulmonary edema, hypotension and warm shock, and myocardial injury) stimulation.[40] Reduction

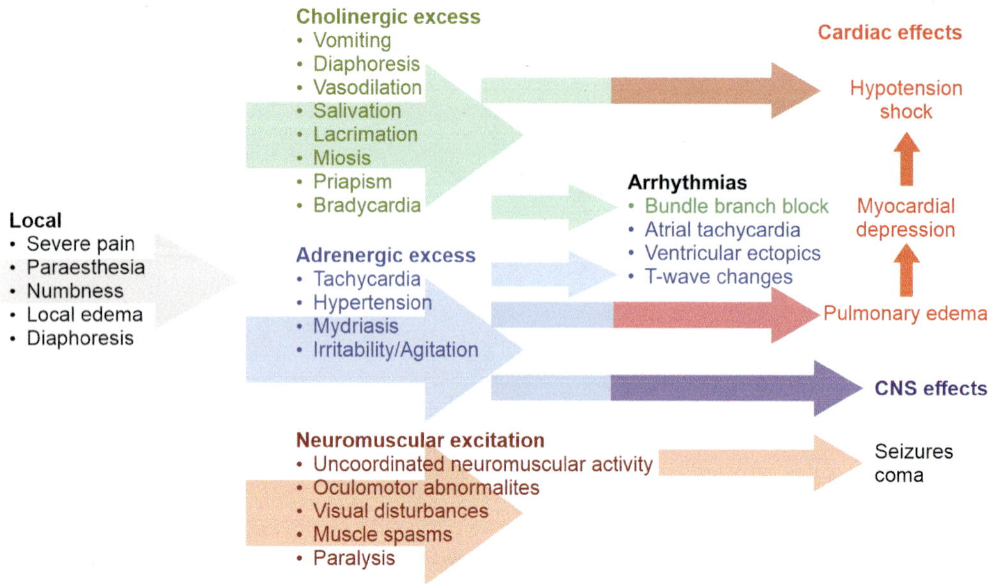

FLOWCHART 2: Showing details of pathophysiology of scorpion venom action.

in left ventricular function and hypotension is preceded by rise in blood pressure and cardiac output. Catecholamine-induced myocarditis, coronary spasm, and direct effects of toxin on heart result in stunned myocardium.[41] The direct effects of scorpion venom on the neuronal sodium channels of the somatic and cranial nervous system result in typical neuromuscular excitation observed after envenoming by *Centruroides* species in Arizona.[29] *Tityus serrulatus* from Trinidad and *Leiurus* from Israel scorpion toxin are toxic to pancreas.

DIAGNOSE OR SUSPECT SEVERE SCORPION STING (FIGS. 11A TO G)

Soon after the sting, the victim experiences severe burning and excruciating pain at the sting site. Pain radiates along with corresponding dermatomes. At the sting site, there is sweating, mild edema, and local fasciculation observed. Scorpion often searched out nearby. At times, victim brought the killed specimen. Local pain wanes within 24 hours. Victims continuously move the stung part of body in search of comfortable position for to get relief from pain but fail. Child is often agitated, confused, and continues cries and difficult to consol. Severe scorpion sting is characterized by autonomic storm. Vomiting, profuse sweating sweat literally flows all over body, cold extremities, mydriasis, and priapism **(Figs. 12A to G)** in males preceded to cardiovascular manifestations occurred.[31] Because of severe peripheral vasoconstrictions, poor peripheral circulation, hypoxia to pain conducting nerves result in decreased intensity of pain, or at time its absence indicates severe envenoming. Reappearances of pain at the sting site which was absent on arrival indicates recovery.[42]

Uncoordinated neuromuscular activity including wild flailing and thrashing of limbs, abnormal ocular movements such roving of eyes, visual disturbances and muscular fasciculation and spasm of the face, tongue, and limbs, and respiratory failure occurred in envenoming by *Centruroides* scorpions.[29] Local erythema and itching and bullous lesion with subsequently localized necrosis developed over a period hours or day occurred due to *H. leptus* scorpion sting. Victim may show minor autonomic effects at times acute renal injury with hemoglobinuria may require dialysis.[43]

The Systemic Effects of Severe Scorpion Envenoming and Grading

On the basis of clinical manifestations at the time of arrival to hospital and according to severity, they are graded in five grades.[29,44]

1. *Grade 1*: Severe excruciating local pain at the sting site radiating along with corresponding dermatomes, mild local edema with sweating at the sting site, without systemic involvement.
2. *Grade 2*: Signs and symptoms of autonomic storm characterized by acetyl choline excess or parasympathetic stimulation and sympathetic stimulation.
3. *Grade 3*: Cold extremities, tachycardia, hypotension, or hypertension with pulmonary edema (respiratory rate >24 per minute, basal rales, or crackles in lungs)
4. *Grade 4*: Massive pulmonary edema **(Figs. 12A to G)**
5. *Grade 5*: Tachycardia, hypotension with or without pulmonary edema with warm extremities (warm shock).

Cardiovascular System and Scorpion Sting

Irrespective of different species of scorpions found similar cardiovascular effects are reported. Gueron M and his colleagues from Israel studied in detail of myocardial

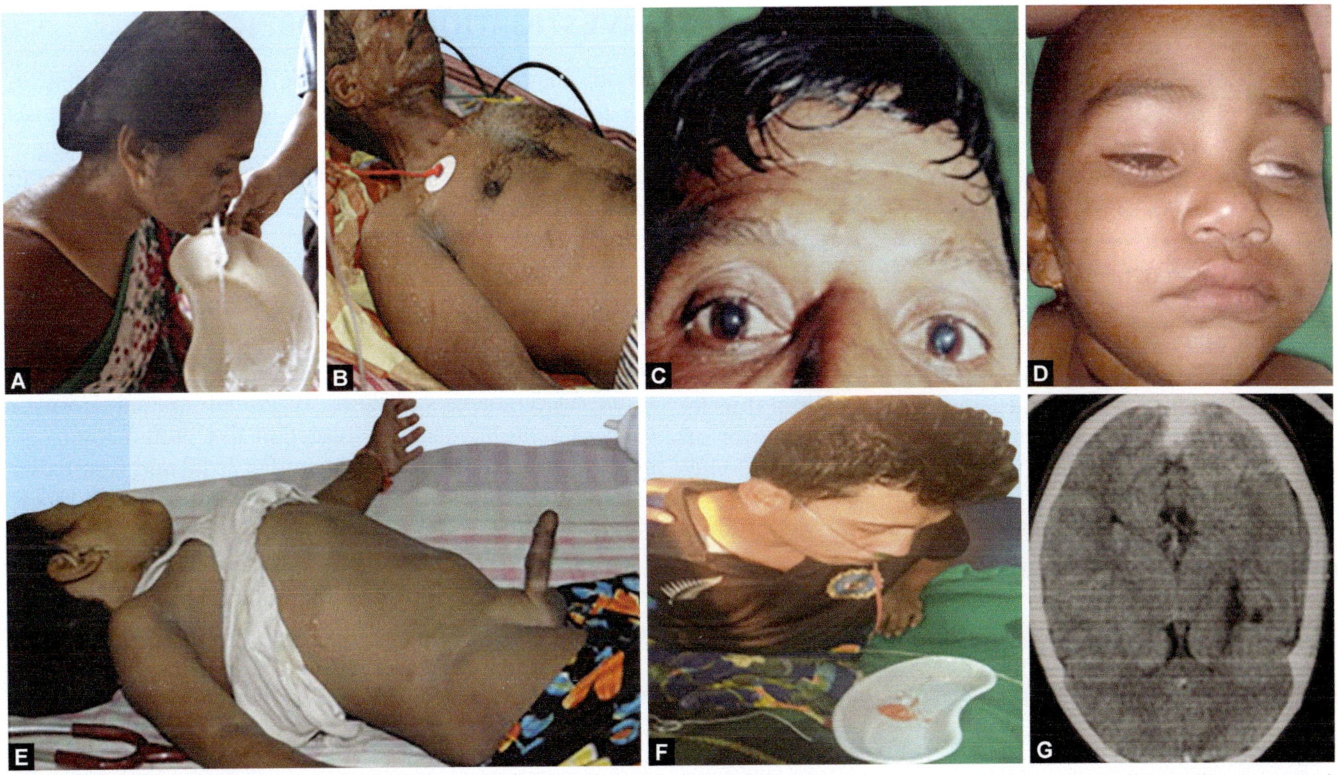

FIGS. 11A TO G: Clinical ropy manifestations. (A) Ropy salivation with sweating; (B) Profuse extensive sweating from all over body called skin diarrhea; (C) Dilated pupils due to alpha-1 receptors stimulation; (D) Oculogyric phenomenon due to autonomic storm in child; (E) Severe priapism in children; (F) Expectorating oxygenated brick red blood due to pulmonary edema due to severe left ventricular failure and ruptured of pulmonary vein; and (G) Watershed brain necrosis.

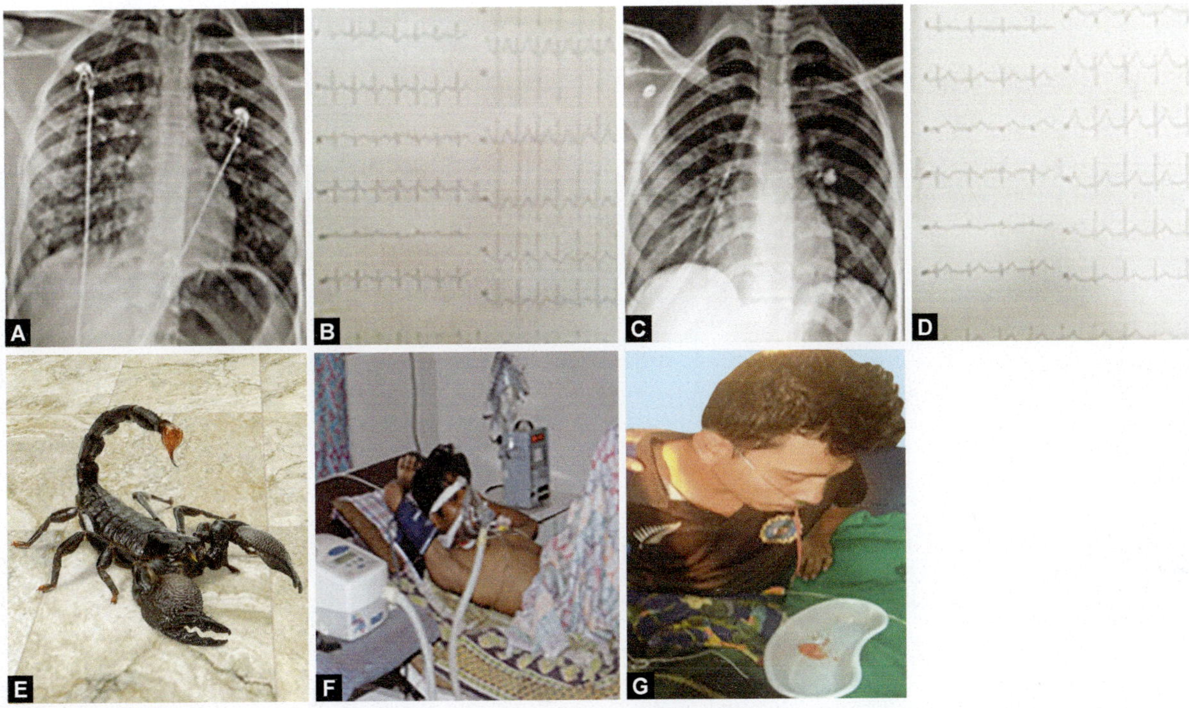

FIGS. 12A TO G: (A) Bilateral pulmonary edema; (B) Supraventricular tachycardia; (C and D) Recovered from pulmonary edema by prazosin, dobutamine; Reduction in heart rate; (E) Scorpion; (F) Noninvasive ventilator help for recovery from massive pulmonary edema addition to antiscorpion venom, dobutamine, and nitroglycerine; and (G) Expectorating brick red blood due to massive pulmonary edema.

involvement and the cardiovascular effects hypertension, heart failure, pulmonary edema, and shock-like syndrome after envenomation, 11% fatality due to cardiac complication.[45] Similar cardiovascular complication and fatality reported from India, Trinidad, Tunisia, and Brazil.[27] Sudden rise in blood pressure result in headache, chest discomfort, suffocation, and paresthesia as result ongoing vasoconstriction. Transient grade 3/6 apical systolic murmur heard over apex of heart.

Children may throw convulsions a sign of hypertensive encephalopathy with blood pressure measurements between 95 and 99 percentile for age and sex of child.[46] Up to 19% patients developed pulmonary edema due to *Mesobuthus tamulus* envenoming.[47] Similar reports of pulmonary edema recorded from Israel, Turkey, Brazil and Saudi Arabia, and Tunisia.[27]

Clinical signs may be complicated by respiratory difficulties such as tachypnea, increased bronchial secretion, refractory persistence recurrent bouts of cough with hemoptysis, inspiratory striders, expiratory rhonchi, gasping, or apneic spells. Respiratory failure or at time arrest may complicate the presence of pulmonary edema.[46,48]

INVESTIGATION OF SCORPION STING

Blood chemistry—serum glucose levels are elevated in the majority of victims on arrival to hospital. Leukocytosis ranging from 11,400 to 6,500s/mm^3 within hour of sting.[28] Cardiac enzymes, serum amylase, are raised reduction in serum insulin, serum potassium due to alpha receptors stimulation.[49,50]

Electrocardiogram Changes (Figs. 13A to F)

Not a single victim of severe envenoming has normal ECG. Initial ECG changes include hyperacute-tented T waves such as acute myocardial infarction like pattern transient nonsustained ventricular tachycardia, atrial and ventricular ectopic, coronary sinus rhythm, left bundle branch block, PQRST, T waves alternans, and prolonged QTC interval. Abnormality in ECG seen on arrival or several hours later.[48] Despite of good clinical condition of victims, the ECG may show marked changes. Progressive mark deep T waves inversion due "myocardial stunning" similar to the takotsubo cardiomyopathy.[41]

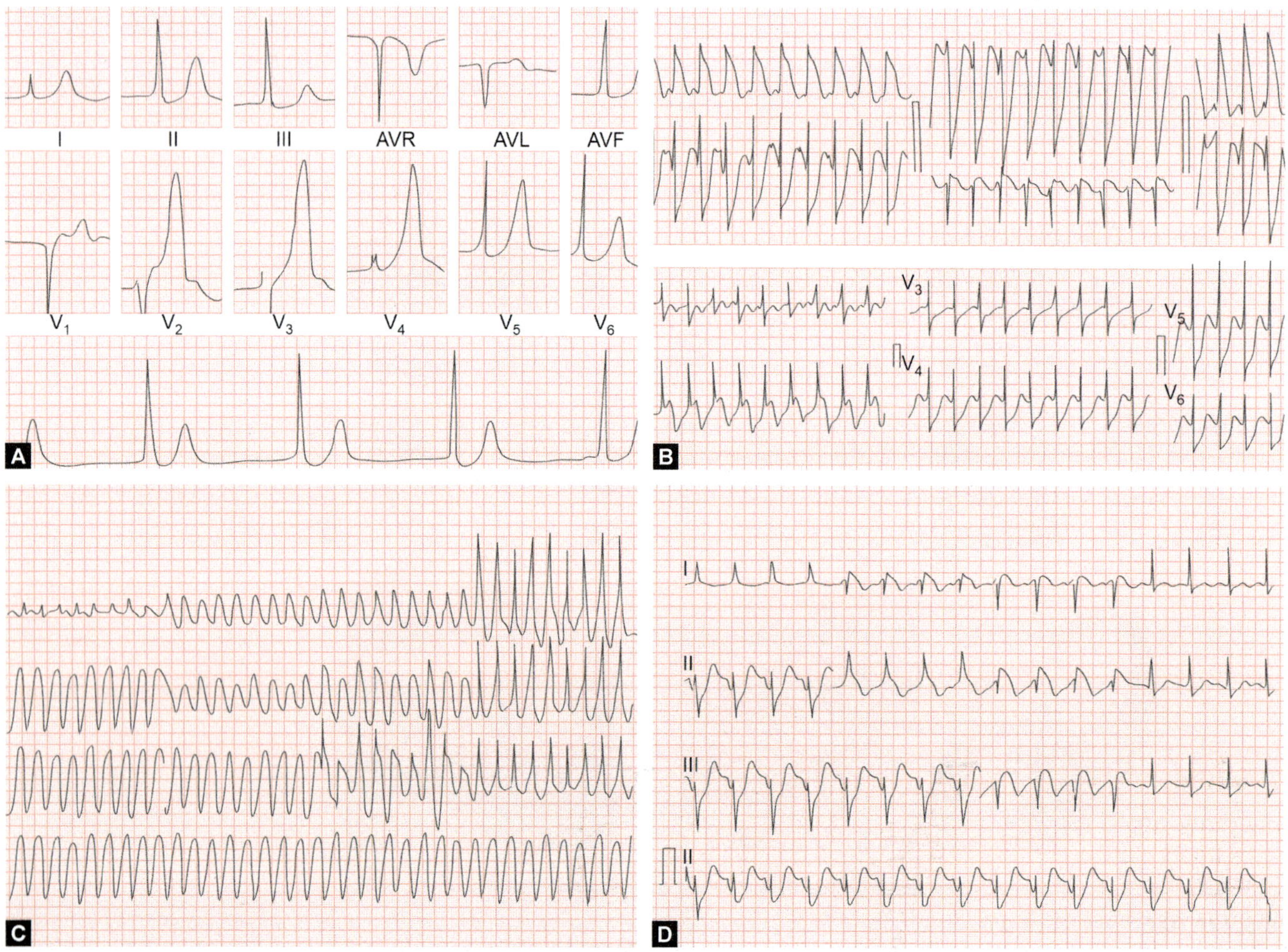

FIGS. 13A TO F: *Continued*

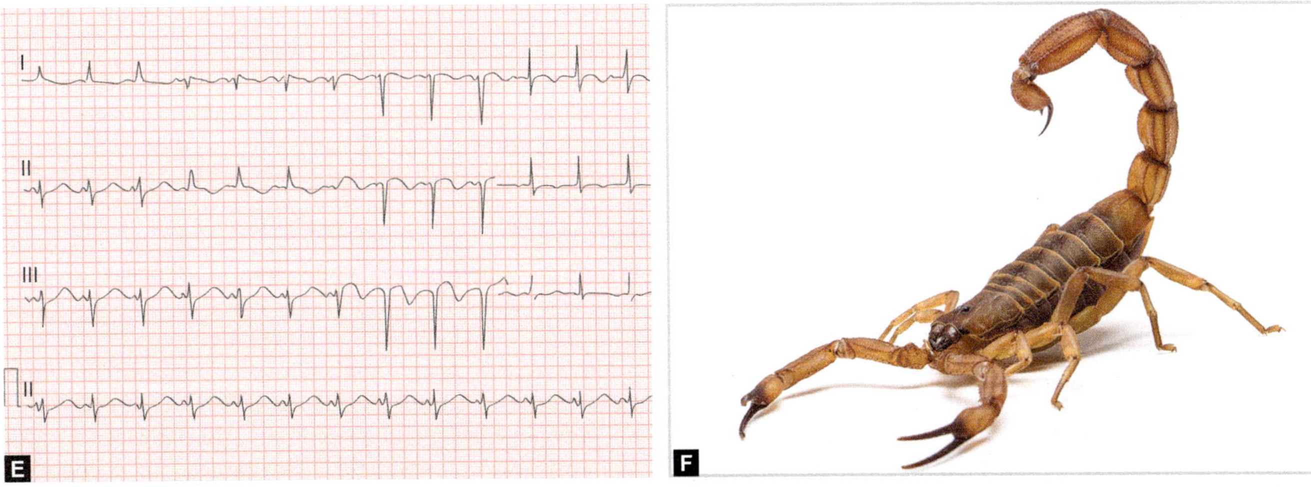

FIGS. 13A TO F: ECG Changes. (A) Tented T waves; (B) Widen QRS tachycardia with Persian helmet type QRS pattern; (C) Ventricular tachycardia resistant to repeated DC shocks; (D) Reverted by intravenous magnesium sulfate to Brugada phenocopy; (E) Regression to normal; (F) *Mesobuthus tumulus* scorpion.

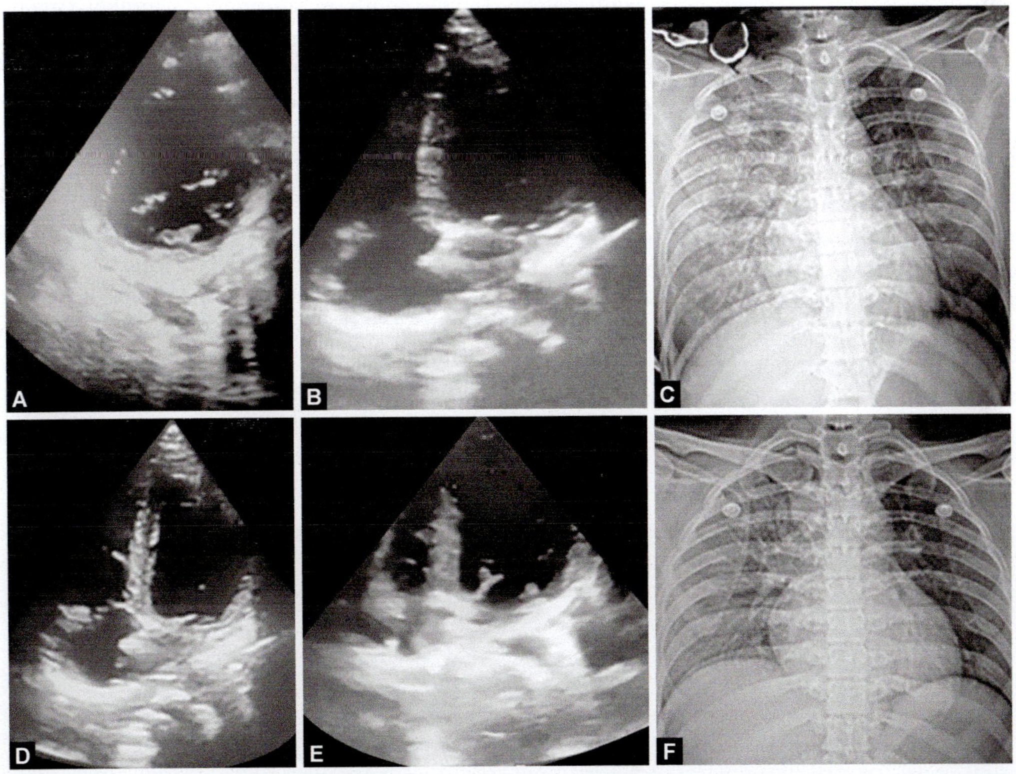

FIGS. 14A TO F: Echocardiographic changes. (A and B) Thin and noncontracting septum with ejection fraction 20%; (C and D) Recovery with contracting septum; (E) Bilateral pulmonary edema; and (F) Recovery from pulmonary edema.

Echocardiography (Figs. 14A to F)

Echocardiography shows poor global myocardial contractility 12–15 hours of sting, with low ejection fraction, decreased left ventricular performance, trivial mitral regurgitation, and abnormal diastolic filling for 5 days–4 weeks, diminished or hypokinetic left ventricular movement with reduction in systolic function. At times, systolic and diastolic frames show no change in diameter, flat septum with no systolic thickening.[51-55] There is good correlation between clinical improvement and return of the left ventricular wall motion toward normal.

Hemodynamic Changes

Karnad DR from India[55] studied hemodynamic changes in a severe ill patient due to scorpion sting. He described severe vasoconstriction and hypertension in one patient out of

11 and biventricular dysfunction with warm extremities due to vasodilatation and hyperkinetic circulation in one victim. His study was incomplete to evaluate the left ventricular diastolic function because of not assessing by the tissue Doppler measurements. Abroug F et al. from Tunisia reported dysfunction and pulmonary edema is due to reduction in left ventricular compliance and increased impendence to left ventricular emptying, makes the myocardial more susceptible and prone for failure by fluid challenge.[55,56] Elevated left ventricular filling pressure confirmed experimental data that majority of the pulmonary edema due to scorpion sting is cardiogenic in origin.[55] However, pulmonary edema could also result from isolated or associated raised pulmonary vasculature permeability produced by a vasoactive substances that might be liberated by the venom manifest a noncardiogenic pulmonary edema.[56-58] Increased systemic pressure without rise in systemic vascular resistance attributed to rise in cardiac output in such situation, vasodilators are preferred[55] Hypotension, shock, and hyperkinetic peripheral circulation due to vasodilatation, poor ventricular contractility in such situation dobutamine is preferred.[59,60]

MANAGEMENT OF SCORPION STING (FLOWCHARTS 3 TO 5)

Traditional remedies may include incisions, tourniquets, application of potassium permanganate, and herbal remedies. Most lead to local tissue damage, infection, and gangrene and should be discouraged. In the hospital for grade 2 to 5 victims, management of scorpion sting includes scorpion antivenin (SAV) therapy and supportive treatments. SAV is considered the only specific treatment for scorpion envenomation. SAV contains immunoglobulin fragments purified from immunized horses that specifically target venom toxins. While SAV therapy is widely used, its clinical efficacy has been the subject of controversy for decade.[33,61] Randomized controlled trials (RCT) have produced conflicting result and whether the SAV can reverse the cardiotoxic effects of scorpion venom or remains uncertain. A recently published meta-analysis found that old world scorpion envenomation, there was no statistical difference in clinical recovery between patients receiving SAV and those who did not.[62] In other hand, studies conducted in Arizona SAV significantly improved outcome.[29] The only randomized trial supporting SAV use for critically ill children with neurotoxicity from scorpion sting had an odds ratio of 11 and very large 94% confidence interval (CI)[2-2120] because of a very small sample size (15 patients).[29] It is therefore not considered a definitive study. In addition, conclusion can hardly be extrapolated since it dealt with *Centruroides* species which is not deadly scorpion. As against authors did an open-labeled randomized trial at general hospital situated 180 km south on Mumbai on Mumbai-Goa highway India in a severe *M. tamulus,* a most venomous scorpion from India envenomation. 70 victims were randomized to SAV plus prazosin versus prazosin alone the recovery time 8 (6.6–9.5) versus 17.7 (15.4–19.9) $p < 0.001$.[28] Similar reports from tertiary care hospital Pondicherry India,[63] since the advent of SAV and proposing the fatality's almost negligible allover India. SAV is most cost-effective treatment for scorpion sting, SAV should be administered intravenously to reach higher circulating concentration, in severely envenomed infant SAV can be administered by intraosseous route a well-established route for delivery of emergency medications. Antiscorpion antivenom is prepared by Haffkine institute Mumbai.

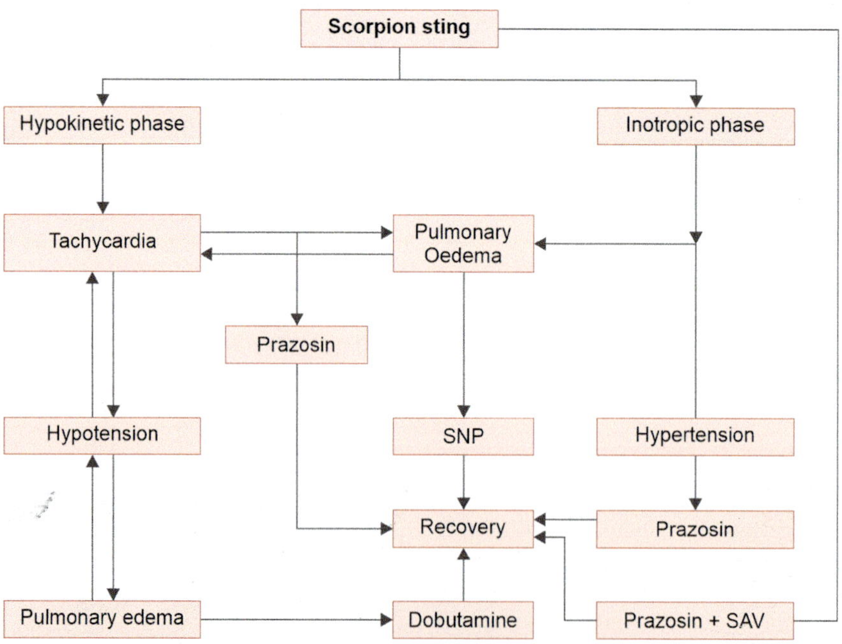

FLOWCHART 3: Management of scorpion sting.
(SAV: scorpion antivenom; SNP: sodium nitroprusside)

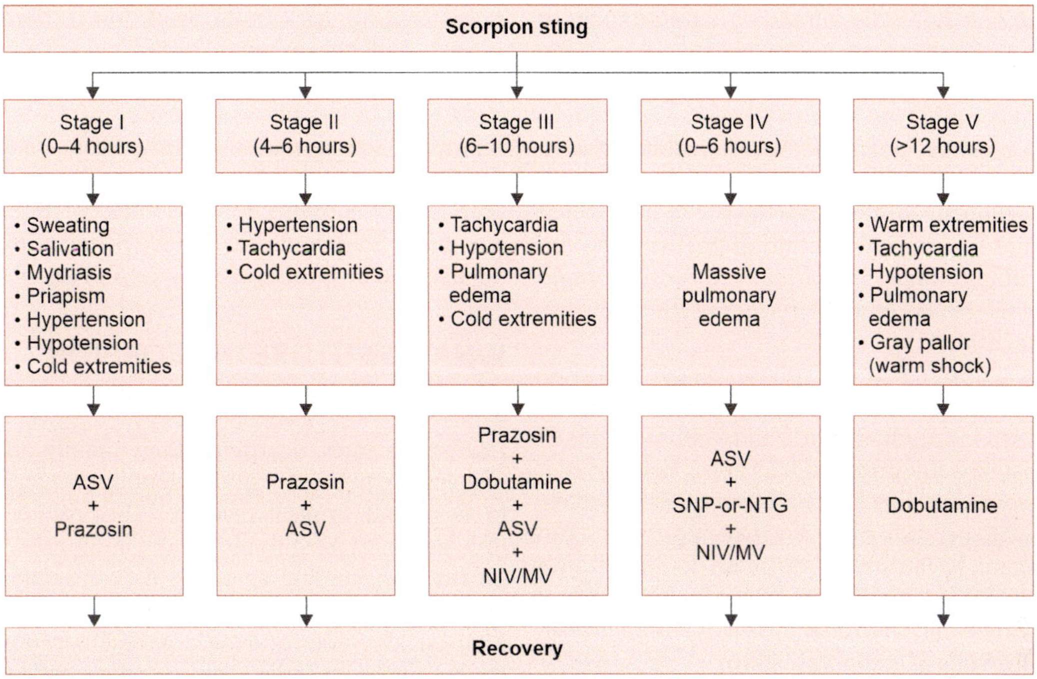

FLOWCHART 4: Final Bawaskar protocol for management.

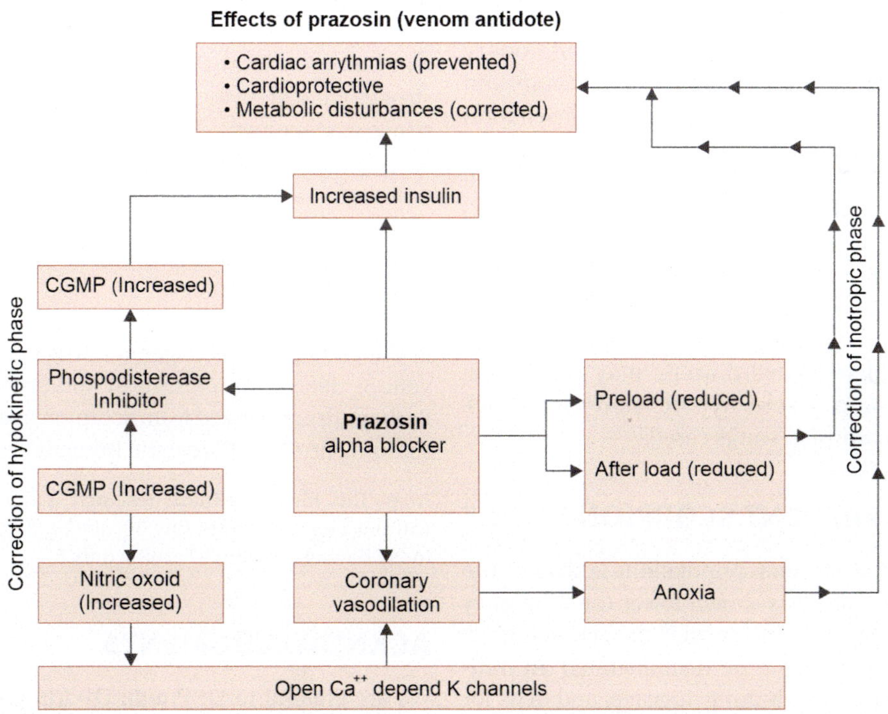

FLOWCHART 5: Action of prazosin.

Ancillary treatments are central to scorpion sting management. The most effective treatment for pain is local infiltration with anesthetics such as lidocaine. Oral medication (acetaminophen or ibuprofen) also gives good results. Victim presenting with severe envenomation class II and V warrant close monitoring in an intensive care unit. Key supportive interventions may include endotracheal intubation and noninvasive ventilators is preferred in pulmonary edema due to scorpion sting, close monitoring and treatment of myocardial ischemia, stress cardiomyopathy, and fluid therapy to correct hypovolemia. Although till date, no RCT has systematically investigated their real efficacy, vasodilators, angiotensin-converting enzyme (ACE) inhibitors, and calcium blocking agents have been used for neutralizing the cardiopulmonary manifestations of scorpion envenoming. Prazosin for instance, a postsynaptic alpha-blocker, was found to be effective in the treatment of pulmonary edema[28] **(Figs. 12A to G)**. Prazosin reduces preload and left ventricular impendence without rise in heart rate, moreover by improving peripheral circulation it enhances the venom absorption from the site of sting which acts like depot as result of this action of prazosin; venom is easily accessible to high circulating SAV result in rapid recovery. Systemic effects of alpha receptors stimulation is inhibited by prazosin.[28,63]

Prazosin is pathological and physiological anti-dote to scorpion venom action. Prazosin is oral drug, injectable not available. Attending doctor or a nurse him or herself should administered the prazosin and never hand-over it to the relatives or attendants. In a infants mother can make prazosin paste with her milk and paste it to nipple which can be sucked by infant, because taste sensation developed after the age of 4-6 months. Doctor should confirmed that oral prazosin is absorbed and started action in form of reduction in signs and symptoms of autonomic storm.

Dobutamine is also being used to manage ventricular dysfunction characterized by tachycardia, hypotension, and poor ventricular contractility with peripheral hyperkinetic circulation.[56] While others advocate the use of captopril to manage hypertension and diuretic-induced pulmonary edema due to scorpion sting.[55,64] Victims of *C. exilicauda* and *H. lepturus* commonly receive benzodiazepines for sedation and muscle spasticity in addition to SAV.[29,43]

Which are the drugs should be used with due caution in scorpion sting victim? Atropine, antihistamines add to already existing QTc prolongation due to scorpion sting, may cause sudden death, steroid enhances necrotizing effect of circulating catecholamine on the myocardium, nifedipine a calcium channel blocker may further depress the myocardium and excessive diuretic may precipitate pulmonary edema, and severe hypotension and shock should be avoided in scorpion stings cases.[27]

HOW ONE CAN PREVENT SCORPION STING?

Report of the control of scorpion populations is scarce. The use of in-door insecticides was shown lower the frequency of scorpion stings in Mexico and Brazil,[65] the actual impact on scorpion viability remains to be demonstrated. At individual level, checking shoes, clothing, luggage, and beds for scorpions are the most important preventive measure. Also stings often occur while walking barefoot or when collecting grass or lifting dry paddy husk. Wearing shoes and rubber gloves during agriculture work may therefore prevent sting. It is also recommended to keep house surroundings free from debris, logs, bricks, and other objects that would make good hiding places for scorpions. Holes and crackles also make hiding places and should be sealed whenever possible. Proper use of mosquito net during night prevents from falling scorpions from loose tiles of hut. At the time of opening schools and colleges, the benches, roof, walls, and floor should be thoroughly washed and cleaned.

WHAT IS FUTURE IN SCORPION STING STUDY?

Like snake bites, scorpion stings mainly affect the most neglected community of developing country and included in neglected tropical diseases. This community receives little attention from public health authorities, international bodies, and funding agencies. As consequences, research on scorpion envenomation is parsimonious. There are few high-quality studies and the large majority consists in animal studies and case series. This, compounded by the fact that the mechanisms underlying the clinical manifestations of scorpion envenoming are extremely complex and diverse, have hindered therapeutic progresses. Researchers in developing countries face many barriers in terms of material and human resources, and empirical schemes, rather than strong clinical evidence, have so far dictated scorpion stings management. Thousands of children die each year of scorpion envenomation, yet a safe, effective, and affordable treatment is still beyond reach. The numerous challenges which remain unaddressed, these will not only require dedicated field doctors, but far and foremost, political will and dedicated resources.

Cardiac sodium channels dysfunctions play important role in the pathogenesis congenital Brugada syndrome. Scorpion venom delays the closing of sodium neuronal channels. Perhaps drugs derived from scorpion toxin could increase the sodium current and treat the Brugada syndrome.[66]

Note: This lifetime clinical research is done since 1976 to 2023 without help of any funding agency or trust. Funding is from day today Bawaskars, family earning only.

ACKNOWLEDGMENTS

We are grateful to Dr Punde DP from Mukhed Nanded, Dr Shrikant Jaiswal Umarkhed Yavatmal Mahesh Kore, Nipani Belgaum, Dr Vinayak Hingane Buldhana, M Mahindrakar Nanded, for preparation of this chapter.

REFERENCES

1. Ralph R, Sharma SK, Faiz MB, Ribeiro I, Rijal S, Chappuis F. The timing is right to end snakebite deaths in South Asia. BMJ. 2019;364;k5317.
2. Bawaskar HS, Bawaskar PH, Bawaskar PH. Snake bite in India: a neglected disease of poverty. Lancet. 2017;390:2947-48.
3. Warrell DA. Snake bite. Lancet. 2010;375:77-88.
4. Mohapatra B, Warrell Da, Suraweera W, Bhatia P, Dhingra N, Jotkar RM, et al. Snake bite mortality in India: a nationally representative mortality survey. PLOS Negl Trop Dis. 2011;4:e1018.
5. Harrison RA, Hargreaves A, Wagstaff SC, Faragher B, Lalloo DG, et al. Snake envenoming: A disease of poverty. PLOS Negl Trop Dis. 2009;3:e569.
6. Bawaskar HS, Bawaskar PH. Profile of snakebite envenoming in western Maharashtra, India. Trans Roy Soc Trop Med Hyg. 2002;96:79-84.
7. Bawaskar HS, Bawaskar PH, Punde DP, Inamdar MK, Dongare RB, Bhoite RR. Profile of snakebite envenoming in rural Maharashtra. J Assoc Phys. 2008;56:88-95.
8. Silva A, Maduwage K, Sedgwick M, Pilapitiya S, Weerawansa P, Dahanayaka NJ, et al. Neuromuscular effects of common *krait* (*Bungarus caeruleus*) envenoming in Sri Lanka. PLOS Negl Trop Dis. 2016;10(2):e0004368.
9. Bawaskar HS, Bawaskar PH. Snake bite poisoning. J Mahatma Gandhi Inst Med Sci. 2015;20:5-14.
10. Alirol E, Sharam SK, Bawakar Hs, Kuch U, chappuis F. Snake bite in South Asia: A review. PLOS Negl Trop Dis. 2010;4:e603.
11. Bawaskar HS Bawaskar PH. Envenoming by common krait (*Bungarus caeruleus*) and Asian cobra (*Naja naja*): Clinical manifestations and their management in a rural setting. Wilderness Environ Med. 2004;15:257-66.
12. Bawaskar HS, Bawaskar PH, Bawaskr PH. Premonitory signs and symptoms of envenoming by common krait (*Bungarus caeruleus*). Trop Doct. 2014;44(2):82-5.
13. Ranawaka UK, Lalloo DG, de silva HJ. Neurotoxicity in snakebite the limit of our knowledge. PLOS Negl Trop Dis. 2013;7(10) e2302.
14. Isbister GK. Snake antivenom research: The importance of case definition. Emerg Med J. 2005;22(6):399-400.
15. Ralph R, Faiz MA, Sharma SK, Ribeiro I, Chappuis F. Managing snake bite. BMJ. 2022;376:e057926.
16. Kazandjian TD, arrahman A, Still KBM, Somsen GW, Vonk FJ, Casewell NR, et al. Anti-coagulant activity of naja nigricollis venom is mediated by phospholipase A2 Toxins and inhibited by Varespladib. Toxins. 2021;13:302.
17. Utkin YN. Three-finger toxins, a deadly weapon of elapid venom-milestone of discovery. Toxicon. 2013;62:50-5.
18. Natrajan B, Saifudheen K, Gafoor A, Jose J. Accuracy of the ice test in the diagnosis of myasthenic ptosis. Neurol India 2016;64: 1169-72.
19. Deak A, Reza MA, Hoque KMF, Deka K, Saha S, Doley R. Comparative analysis of Naja Kaouthia venom from north-east India and Bangladesh and its cross reactivity with Indian polyvalent antivenoms. Toxicon 2019;164:31-43.
20. Bawaskar HS Bawaskar PH, Punde DP, Inamdar MK, Dongare RB, Bhoite RR. Profile of snakebite envenoming in rural Maharashtra, India. J Assoc Phys India. 2008;56:88-95.
21. Warrell DA, Gutierrez JM, Calvete JJ, Williams D. New approaches and technologies of venomics to meet the challenge of human envenoming by snakebites in India. Indain J Med Res. 2013;138: 38-50.
22. Tango A, Trakulsrichai S, Putichote K, Sriapha C, Wananukul W,. Recurrent neurotoxic envenoming of cobra bite. Toxicon. 2019;167:180-3.
23. Silva AJ, Kuruppu S, Othman I, Goode RJA, Hodgson WC, Isbister GK. Neurotoxicity in Sri Lankan Russell's viper (*Daboia russelii*) envenomation is Primarily due to U1-viperitoxin-Dr1a, presynaptic neurotoxin. Neurotox Res. 2017;31:11-9.
24. Naik BN, Bhalla A, Sharam N, Mokta J, Singh S, Gupta P, et al. Pituitary dysfunction in survivors of Russell's viper snake bite: prospective study. Neurol India. 2018;68:1351-8.
25. Kumar PKV, Kumar PS, Kasturi N, Ahuja S. Ocular manifestations of venomous snake bite over a one-year period in a tertiary care hospital. Korean J opthalmol. 2015;29:256-62.
26. Bawaskar HS, Bawaskar PH, Bawaskar PAH. Rabies: Novel clinical presentation. Indian J Crit Care Med. 2017;21:872-4.
27. Bawaskar HS, Bawaskar PH. Scorpion sting: Update. J Asso Phy India. 2012;60:46-55.
28. Bawaskar HS, Bawaskar PH. Efficacy and safety of scorpion antivenom plus prazosin compared with prazosin alone for venomous scorpion (*Mesobuthus tamulus*) sting: Randomised open label clinical trial. BMJ. 2011;342:c7136.
29. Boyer LV, Theodorou AA, Berg RA, Mallie J, Chávez-Méndez A, García-Ubbelohde W; Arizona Envenomation Investigators; et al. Antivenom for critically ill children with neurotoxicity from scorpion sting. New Eng J Med. 2009;360(20);2090-9.
30. Eltrous N, Nouria S, Babes-Puanes I, Boussarsar M, Boukef R, Marghli S, et al. Dobutamine in severe scorpion envenomation: effects on standard hemodynamics: Right ventricular performance and tissue oxygen. Chest. 1999;116:748-53.
31. Bawaskar HS. Diagnostic cardiac premonitory signs and symptoms of red scorpion sting. Lancet. 1982;1(8271):552-54.
32. Chippaux JP, Goyffon M. Epidemiology of scorpionism: A global appraisal. Acta Trop. 2008;107(2):71-9.
33. Abroug F, Elatrous S, Nouria S, Haguiga H, Touzi N, Bouchoucha S, et al. Serotherapy in scorpion envenomation: A randomized controlled trial. Lancet. 1999;354(9182):906-9.
34. Bahloul M, Chabchoub I, Chaari A, Chtara K, Kallel H, Dammak H, et al. Scorpion envenomation among children: clinical manifestations and outcome (analysis of 685 cases). Am J Trop Med Hyg. 2010;83(5):1084-92.
35. Monteiro WM, Gomes J, Fe N, da Silva IM, Lacerda M, Alencar A, et al. Perspective and recommendation towards evidence-based health care for scorpion sting in the Brazil Amazon: A comprehensive review. Toxicon. 2019;169:68-80.
36. Amr ZS, Mohammad A, Baker A, AL-Sarairech M, Warrell DA. Scorpions and scorpion sting envenoming (scorpionism 0) in the Arab countries of the middle East. Toxicon. 2021;191:83-103.
37. Gwee MC, Nirthanan S, Khoo HE, Gopalakrishnakone P, Kini RM, Cheah LS. Autonomic effects of some scorpion venoms and toxins. Clin Exp Pharmacol Physiol. 2002;29(9):795-801.
38. Quintero–Hernandez V, Jimenze-Vargas JM, Gurrola GB, Valdivia HH, Possani LD. Scorpion venom components that affect ion channels function. Toxicon. 2013;76;328-42.
39. Abroug F, Nouira S, Atrous SE, Besbes L, Boukef R, Boussarsar M, et al. A canine study of immunotherapy in scorpion envenomation. Intensive care Med. 2003;29(12):2266-76.
40. Bawaskar HS, Bawaskar PH. Sting by red scorpion (*Buthotus tamulus*) in Maharashtra state, India: A clinical study. Trans Roy Soc Trop Med Hyg. 1989;83:858-60.
41. Wittstein IS, Thiemann DR, Lima JAC, Baughman KL, Schulman SP, Gerstenblith G, et al. Neurohumoral features of myocardial stunning due to sudden emotional stress. NEJM. 2005;352:539-48.
42. Bawaskar HS, Bawaskar PH. Prazosin for vasodilator treatment of acute pulmonary edema due to scorpion sting. Ann Trop Med Parsitol. 1987;81(6):719-23.

43. Pipelzadeh MH, Jalali A, Taraz M, Pourabbas R, Zaremirakabadi A. An epidemiological and a clinical study on scorpionism by the Iranian scorpion Hemiscorpius lepturus. Toxicon. 2007;50(7):984-92.
44. Khattabi A, Oulaymani–Bancheikh R, Achour S, Salmi LR; Scorpion Consensus Expert Group. Classification of clinical consequences of scorpion sting: Consensus development. Trans Roy Soc Trop Med Hyg. 2011;105:364-69.
45. Gueron M, Stern J, Cohen W. Severe myocardial damage and heart failure in scorpion sting. Am J Cardiol. 1967;19:7819-25.
46. Sofer S, Gueron M. Respiratory failure in children following envenomation by the scorpion Leiurus quinquestriatus: hemodynamic and neurological aspects. Toxicon. 1988;26(10):931-9.
47. Bawaskar HS, Bawaskar PH. Envenoming by scorpion and snakes (*Elapidae*) their neurotoxins and therapeutics. Trop Doct. 2000;30:23-5.
48. Bahloul M, Chaari A, Dammak H, Samet M, Chtara K, Chelly H, et al. Pulmonary edema following scorpion envenomation: Mechanisms, clinical manifestations, diagnosis, and treatment. Int J Cardiol. 2011;162(2):86-91.
49. Meki AR, Mohamed ZM, Mohey El. Significant of assessment of serum cardiac troponin I and interleukin-8 in scorpion envenomation in children. Toxicon. 2003;41:129-37.
50. Poon-king T. Myocarditis from scorpion sting. Br Med J. 1963;1:347-77.
51. Cupo P, Figueiredo AB, Filho AP, Pintya AO, Júnior GAT, Caligaris F, et al. Acute left ventricular dysfunction of severe scorpion envenomation is related to myocardial perfusion disturbance. Int J Cardiol. 2007;116:98-106.
52. Guerom M, Margulis G, Sofer S. Echocardiographic and radionuclide angiographic observations following scorpion envenomation by Leiurus quinquestriatus. Toxicon. 1990;28:1005-09.
53. Rahav G, Weiss AT. Scorpion sting induced pulmonary edema: scintigraphic evidence of cardiac dysfunction. Chest. 1990;97: 1478-80.
54. Bahloul M, Ben Hamida CB, Chtourou K, Ksibi H, Dammak H, Kallel H, et al. Evidence of myocardial ischemia in severe scorpion envenomation. Myocardial perfusion scintigraphy study. Intensive Care Med. 2004;30:461-7.
55. Karnad DR. Haemodynamic pattern in patients with scorpion envenoming. Heart. 1998;79:485-9.
56. Amaral CF, Barbosa SJ, Leite VH, Tafuri WL, de Rezende NA. Scorpion sting induced pulmonary edema :evidence of increased alvelo-capillary membrane permeability. Toxicon. 1994;32(8):999-1003.
57. Baseer KAA, Aboelela MG, Qubaisy HM. Echocardiographic Evaluation of the Response to Prazosin Treatment in Scorpion Sting. J Trop Pediatr. 2021 Jul 2;67(3):fmaa063.
58. Bawaskar HS, Bawaskar PH. Management of the cardiovascular manifestations of poisoning by the Indian red scorpion. Br Heart J. 1992;68:478-80.
59. Mathur A, Verma G, Gehlot RS, Ujjwal JS. Non-cardiac pulmonary oedema in scorpion bite. J Assoc Phys India. 1993;41(6):398.
60. Abroug F, Nouria S. Babes–Puanes I, Boussarsar M, Boukef R, Marghli S, et al. Dobutamine in severe scorpion envenomation. Chest. 1999;116:748-53.
61. Sofer S, Shahak E, Gueron M. Scorpion envenomation and antivenom therapy. J Pediatr. 1994(124(6):973-8.
62. Abroug F, Ouanes–baebes L, Ouanes I, Dachraoui F, Hassen MF, Haguiga H, et al. Meta-analysis of controlled studies on immunotherapy in severe scorpion envenomation. Emer Med J. 2011;28(11):963-9.
63. Pandi K, Krishnamurthy S, Srinivasaraghavan R, Mahadevan S. Efficacy of scorpion antivenom plus prazosin versus prazosin alone for Mesobuthus tamulus scorpion sting envenomation in children: A randomized controlled trial. Arch Dis Child. 2014;99: 575-80.
64. Karnad DR, Deo AM, Apte N, Lohe AS, Thatte S, Tilve GH. Captopril for correcting diuretic induced hypotension in pulmonary edema after scorpion sting. BMJ. 1989;298:1430-31.
65. Albuquerque CM, Babosa MO, Lannuzzi L. Tityus stigmurus (thorelll1876) (scorpion; Buthidae): Response to chemical control and understanding of scorpionism among the population. Rev Soc Bras Med Trop. 2009;42(3):255-9.
66. Bawaskar HS. Can scorpions be useful? Lancet. 2007;370:1664.

93

CHAPTER

Protein-energy Malnutrition, Beriberi, and Infantile Tremor Syndrome

Jayantee Kalita, UK Misra

PROTEIN-ENERGY MALNUTRITION

INTRODUCTION

Nutrition has an essential role in growth and development both during intranatal and postnatal life. Protein, carbohydrates, fat, trace elements, and vitamins are especially important for the development and maturation of different regions of the brain during intranatal, infancy, and early childhood. The effect of nutritional deficiency depends on the timing, duration, and severity of the deficit. The effect of nutritional deficiency may be mild (stage I) in which cell structure and process are normal but functionally impaired, moderate (stage II) in which there are demyelination with normal cylinder, and severe (stage III) in which there are demyelination, breakdown of axis cylinder, and cell death. Replacement of nutrients results in full recovery in stage I, and full to a partial recovery in stage II. Protein-energy malnutrition (PEM) refers to inadequate intake of protein and energy for a long time leading to depletion of body mass and fat. PEM is prevalent in Asia and Africa. It may also occur as a result of starvation and chronic illness. Generally, the body adapts to starvation with the help of hormones and adaption by reducing energy expenditure and catabolism, but at the cost of lethargy, weakness, skin, and muscle atrophy and functional disability. PEM is closely linked to socioeconomic status, political will, and natural disasters. Till 1865, there is no description of PEM. Cecile Williams in 1935 described Kwashiorkor in African children with diarrhea, edema, and wasting. These children were between 6 months and 4 years and were on maize porridge.[1] Kwashiorkor was prevalent in the whole of Africa except amongst Masai and Batussi tribes who used milk for porridge preparation.[2] World Health Organization (WHO) and Food and Agriculture Organization (FAO) described protein-calorie malnutrition as a malady. Rockefeller Foundation and the United Nations of International Children Emergency Fund (UNICEF) proposed to research with the aim of preventing PEM. Red Cross Society under the leadership of Pate surveyed 38 countries in 76 days, understood the problem and emphasized that UNICEF will serve all the children without racial and political discrimination. In 2004, about 50% of death in children was due to underlying undernutrition, and the causes of death were diarrhea in 60.7%, pneumonia in 52.3%, malaria in 57.3%, and measles in 44.8%.[3] Neonates born out of an undernourished mother may have low birth weight. Asian countries share 69% of the global burden of underweight, 58% of stunted, and 70% of wasted children.[4] Elimination of malnutrition is likely to reduce the global burden of disease by 32%.[5,6] Improper nutrition is a double-edged sword, overnutrition results in overweight and obesity, whereas undernutrition results in underweight, wasting, and stunting. There is an inverse relationship between undernutrition and overnutrition. In children, the status of nutrition is measured by height and weight against age-specific standards. Based on these parameters, the under nourished children are termed as underweight, wasted (loss of muscle mass), and stunted (both height and weight reduction). Undernutrition needs to be detected within month to 2 years for better subsequent outcome. About 3.5 million deaths occur annually due to maternal and child malnutrition.[7,8] In 2011, about 93% of 8.8% million deaths globally were from Asia and Africa.[9] Undernutrition is closely linked to mental, social, developmental, and economic burden. A neonate born out of undernourished mother is likely to have stunted growth and poor psychological development and poor immunities. In 2019, the global burden of wasting below 5 years of age was 47, and 14.3 million of them were severely wasted. More than 50% of wasted children were from Southeast Asia and 25% from sub-Saharan Africa.[10] The global burden of overweight is 5.6%—mainly in the Middle East, North Africa, Eastern Europe, Central Asia, and North America. In India, growth failure in children widely varies in different parts; prevalence of stunting is 21.3–40%, wasting 6.3–19.3%, and underweight 16.5–42.2%.[11] The global burden of malnutrition is shown in **Figures 1 and 2**.

Malnutrition may be due to the following reasons:
- Uncomplicated PEM or starvation-related malnutrition
- Chronic disease-related malnutrition—cachexia
- Acute disease-related malnutrition

Starvation-related malnutrition occurs due to prolonged inadequate food intake leading to weight loss and stunting. The severity of muscle wasting is proportional to the severity of PEM. Association of edema hinders appreciation of muscle wasting. Chronic disease-related starvation is due to chronic disease such as infection, autoimmune, hepatic, renal, cardiac, and pulmonary or malignancy. There is high catabolism resulting in fatigue, weakness, and wasting. Acute disease-related malnutrition occurs in severe sepsis, injury, and critically ill patients in intensive care. This is also due to high catabolism.

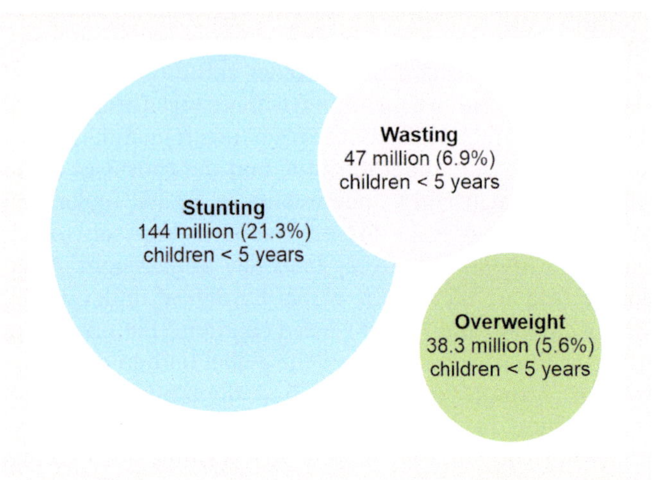

FIG. 1: Global burden of malnutrition (UNICEF/WHO/World Bank 2020).
Source: Misra UK, Kalita J. With permission from Neurological Consequences of Neurological Disorders, First edition. 2 Park Square, Milton Park, Abingdon, Oxon: CRC press; 2012.

DIAGNOSIS OF UNDERNUTRITION

Under weight, wasting and stunting, is the indicator of undernutrition in a society. Underweight refers to low weight for the age, wasting refers to low weight for height, and stunting refers to low height for age. The Indian Association of pediatrics classifies undernutrition based on standard weight for the age as—mild (70–80%), moderate (61–70%), severe (51–60%), and very severe (<50%). Mild-to-moderate undernutrition is characterized by growth failure, infection, anemia, lethargy, and hair and skin changes. The manifestations of moderate-to-severe undernutrition are marasmus **(Fig. 3)**, Kwashiorkor **(Fig. 4)**, or mixed type.

The children with marasmus are thin, no fat, and simian faces with loose and saggy skin over the buttock (haggy pant). They have good appetite, active and do not have edema. The children with Kwashiorkor manifest during 1–4 years of age with edema of hands, feet, and face. Muscle wasting occurs but hidden because of edema. Untreated children have peeling of skin with ulceration and petechiae. They have glossitis, cheilitis, angular stomatitis, and Bitot's spot due to associate other vitamin deficiencies.

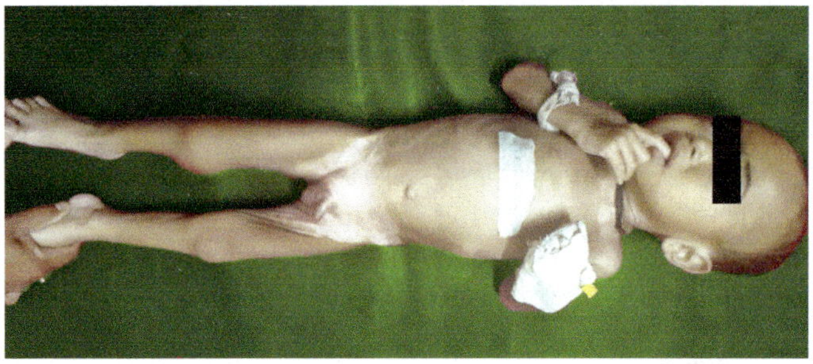

FIG. 3: A child with marasmus. He has wasting of muscles and loss of subcutaneous fat.
Image courtesy: Professor A Deka, Guwahati Medical College, Assam.

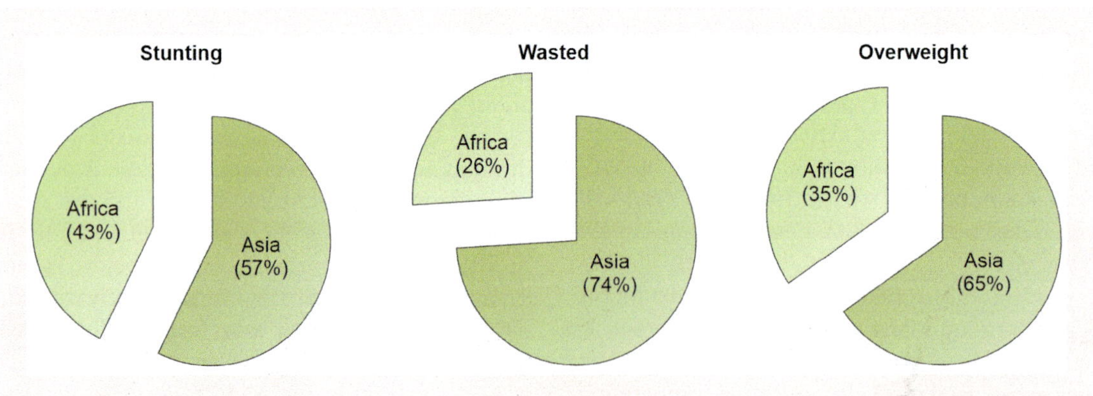

FIG. 2: Asia shares highest percentage of stunting, wasting and overweight children under 5 years of age. (UNICEF/WHO/World Bank Group—Joint Child Malnutrition Estimates 2020 edition).
Source: With permission from Misra UK, Kalita J. Neurological Consequences of Neurological disorders, First edition. 2 Park Square, Milton Park, Abingdon, Oxon: CRC press; 2012.

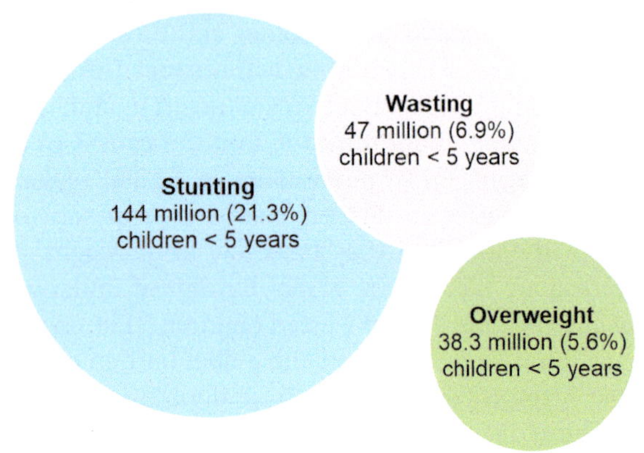

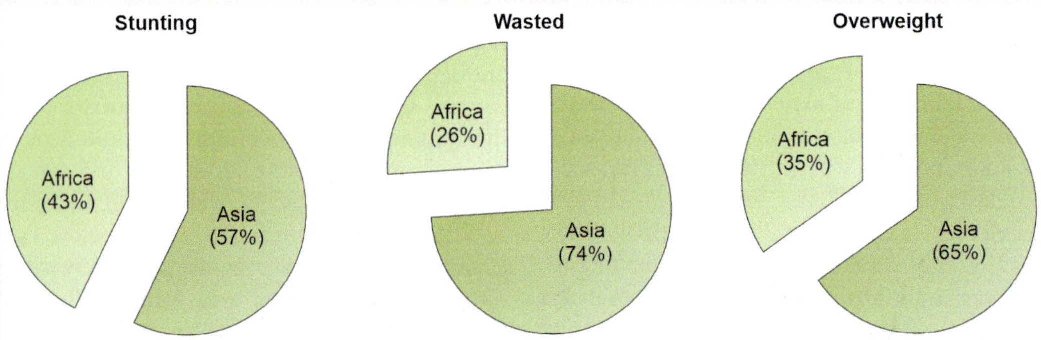

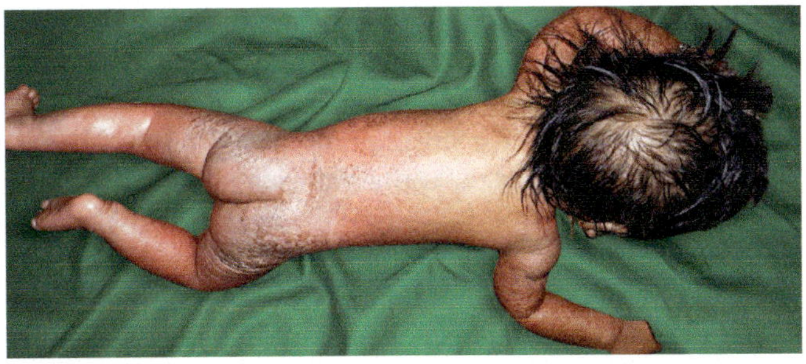

FIG. 4: A child with Kwashiorkor with edema, irritability and flaky skin lesion in his buttock.

Image courtesy: Professor A Deka, Guwahati Medical College, Assam.

DIAGNOSIS

The diagnosis of PEM is based on measurement of nutritional status: Muscle mass, subcutaneous adipose tissue, extracellular fluid volume (ECEF), body mass index (BMI), and laboratory and technical assessment.

- *Muscle mass*: Starvation-related PEM is easy to diagnose by observing the muscle bulk of the shoulder and pelvic girdle muscles. PEM in old age and chronically hospitalized patients is often missed. It is important to consider reversible cause of PEM in these patients.
- *Subcutaneous adipose tissue*: Measurement of triceps skin fold is a good indicator of fat but people on restricted diet may have preservation of fat with reduction of muscle mass.
- *Extracellular fluid volume*: Chronic undernutrition results in hypoalbuminemia leading to increased ECEF and edema.
- *Body mass index*: BMI is calculated by weight in kg/height in m^2. Normal BMI is 20–25; 25–30 overweight, more than 30 obese, less than 20 suggests loss of muscle mass, and less than 13 is incompatible with life. BMI below 17 is considered PEM but more than 17 does not rule out because of increased ECFV in Kwashiorkor. In a hospital-based study, 27.2% of stroke patients at admission were undernourished, premorbid undernourished patients had a longer hospital stay and had a worse outcome.[12] In another study, overweight females with stroke had a good outcome.[13] In old age, also frailty is an independent predictor of all-cause death. Undernutrition causes impaired innate and adaptive immunity making individuals prone to infection. Meta-analysis has shown reduction in incidence of tuberculosis by 13.5% by one point increase in BMI.[14] There is four-fold increase in tuberculosis in human immunodeficiency virus (HIV) patients having a BMI of ≤18.5.[15]
- *Muscle mass*: Assessment of muscle mass by palpation and muscle power testing is better method than ultrasound of muscle.
- *Markers of systemic inflammation*: Serum albumin and C-reactive protein are used as markers of systemic inflammation. Hypoalbuminemia occurs after several months of starvation but occurs early in acute or chronic illness due to higher catabolism. Measurement of urinary nitrogen may be used as an indicator of muscle catabolism.
- *Subjective global assessment*: Subjective global assessment is done by food intake and its component, food faddism, weight loss, systemic infection, muscle bulk, subcutaneous fat, edema, muscle strength, and mobility. This scale is helpful in defining starvation malnutrition and disease-related malnutrition.

NEUROLOGICAL EFFECT OF PEM

The neurological effect of PEM depends on the severity, associated other vitamin/mineral deficiency and age at the time of deficiency. The acute effect of PEM may be on the central and peripheral nervous system, and muscles. They may have neuropsychiatric symptoms including irritability, apathy, attention deficit, slow learning, language deficit, and poor social skill. Rarely, juvenile onset myelopathy has been reported in PEM which may be due to vitamin B12 deficiency. Soft neurological signs in rural children have correlated with the severity of malnutrition. During early childhood (<2 years), PEM may affect peripheral nerve conduction but is negligible in later life. Generalized weakness and occasional sensory and autonomic dysfunctions have also been reported. Delayed effect of PEM on neurocognitive function is difficult to assess because of simultaneous social deprivation.

Children rescued from Kwashiorkor revealed poor reasoning and organization of knowledge, memory, and perception at 8 years follow-up. These abnormalities further improved after dietary supplementation. Motor nerve conduction and motor unit potential changes are reversible sequelae of PEM, but sensory nerve action potential may not have full recovery. The cognitive evoked potential was, however, normal in children who suffered from malnutrition in infancy. The isolated effect of PEM or neurological functions is difficult to assess, because PEM is associated with multiple nutritional deficiency.

TREATMENT

The mode of treatment (oral, enteral, and parenteral) and urgency of correction depend on the severity of malnutrition. The underlying cause of malnutrition needs to be treated for a permanent cure. Conscious and cooperative patients without nausea and vomiting may be treated by oral feeding. Parenteral nutrition is given to those with a severe gastrointestinal disorder, anorexia nervosa, severe depression, and critically ill patients. There are several oral and parenteral formulas available and need to be chosen depending on clinical needs.

Nasogastric and enteral feeding may have various complications such as aspiration, diarrhea, infection, intolerance, and imbalance of volume, electrolytes, and glucose. The aim of parenteral nutrition is to provide a complete nutrition through central vein including dextrose, amino acids, triglycerides, minerals, and vitamins.

Refeeding syndrome may occur following rapid nutritional replacement during first week. There are edema and hypernatremia due to liberation of insulin and antinatriuretic peptides leading to increase in extravascular volume. Refeeding syndrome may be minimized by gradual increase in carbohydrate. During parenteral nutrition, potassium, phosphorus, zinc, and magnesium should be closely monitored. In children with PEM, caloric requirement is 150 kcal/kg/day. The requirement of protein is 3 g/kg/day, which is given in the form of milk, nuts, soy, or nonvegetarian food. Use of oil may reduce the amount of carbohydrates. PEM children should be fed at 2–3 hours internal.

PREVENTION OF MALNUTRITION

Political will and commitment of government have key role in prevention and elimination of PEM.

Improved production, attention to the supply, and distribution of food are important. Many governments including India had adopted food fortification and mid-day school meals to prevent PEM and nutritional deficiency. Community education about the nutritional value of food and false belief are important. Locally available and culturally acceptable food items having good nutritive value should be encouraged. Improvement in education especially mother may play a great role in preventing and treating malnutrition.

BERIBERI

INTRODUCTION

Beriberi is one of the neurological manifestations of thiamine deficiency, and the other manifestations are Wernicke-Korsakoff syndrome. Thiamine is an essential water-soluble vitamin of B complex group. There is no endogenous synthesis of thiamine and body stores only 30 mg, which can meet the requirement for 8–9 days only, hence, a regular intake is necessary. The clinical presentation of thiamine deficiency is quite variable, and there is no easily available laboratory test leading to often delayed diagnosis. Thiamine deficiency is common in low-income, rice (polished) eating Asian countries with high carbohydrate intake and in alcoholics. Thiamine deficiency in developed countries occurs because of food faddism, isolation, addiction, depression, and critically ill patients. Early clinical diagnosis and treatment are necessary to reduce mortality and full functional recovery.

Beriberi was first described in 2600 BC in Chinese literature. In Sinhalese language Beriberi means "I cannot" or "weak". Beriberi like illness (weakness, numbness, and swelling of feet) was described in 3rd century and in 1580, Portuguese priest reported beriberi who was unaware about the slippers coming out of his feet. Eijkman through his chick experiment proposed that this disease is due to nutrient in rice which has been lost during milling.[16] This hypothesis was ignored because of the influence of rice mill industry in Asia and Europe. In 1935, Grijns confirmed the etiology of beriberi.[17] Pure crystals of nutrient were isolated in 1926,[18] and the chemical structure of thiamine was discovered in 1935 by Robert William.[19] Eijkman and Hopkins were awarded the Nobel Prize in 1929 for their contribution in the discovery of thiamine.

Thiamine is a colorless organosulfur compound, and it consists of an aminopyrimidine and a thiazolium ring linked by methylene bridge. The thiazole is substituted by methyl-hydroxyethyl side chain. Thiamine triphosphate acts as a coenzyme in various intracellular reactions.

PATHOPHYSIOLOGY

Adult male requires 1.2 mg thiamine and female 1.1 mg daily. The requirement increases to 1.4 mg/day during pregnancy and 1.5 mg/day in lactating mothers. There is no thiamine toxicity in high doses as it is excreted in the urine. Thiamine is rich in whole grains, yeast, legumes, nuts, and meat. It is absorbed in the lower intestine through thiamine transporter 1, which is an adenosine triphosphate (ATP)-dependent active process. About 90% thiamine is present in red blood cell (RBC) and white blood cell (WBC). Thiamine di-phosphate works as a cofactor in multiple enzymatic processes such as pyruvate dehydrogenase, α-ketoglutarate dehydrogenase complex, α-transketolase, and α-ketoacid dehydrogenase. Due to reduced α-ketoglutarate dehydrogenase activity in thiamine deficiency, there is reduced energy metabolism and increased glutamate and free radical formation in mitochondria. Thiamine mainly distributed through RBCs to various cells of the body. Intracellular thiamine acts at cytosol, mitochondria, and peroxisome enzymatic reactions.

CLINICAL FEATURES

Beriberi is common in East Asia, East Africa, and South America. High carbohydrate, low protein, and fat diet predispose Beriberi. Beriberi has a diverse clinical presentation, and mainly can be classified as wet beriberi, dry beriberi, and mixed types. These are also known as thiamine deficiency disorders. The age-wise presentation of beriberi includes:

- Infantile beriberi
- Beriberi in older infants and children
- Beriberi in adults

Infantile Beriberi

Infantile beriberi occurs in poor socioeconomic strata, when infant depends on thiamine deficient mother's milk.[20] Infantile beriberi occurs by 4 months but not in neonatal period. These infants have shrill cry, irritability, refusal to feed, and vomiting. The infants may be tachypneic, dyspneic, and cyanosed due to heart failure. Sometime, infantile beriberi may be triggered by infection. If not treated, they have a fatal outcome.[21] Often these infants are misdiagnosed as having malaria, typhoid, or pneumonia.

Beriberi in Older Infants and Children

Beriberi in older infant and children manifests with nystagmus, ophthalmoplegia, and altered sensorium. These children may have anorexia and bulging fontanel.[22,23] The clinical features simulates meningoencephalitis. Older children and adolescences may have tingling, numbness, pain, paresthesia, weakness, and hypo or areflexia suggestive of neuropathy.

Beriberi in Adults

In children and adults, symptoms and signs of beriberi are mainly neuropathic and are known as dry beriberi. Untreated patients develop foot drop, wrist drop, muscle tenderness and weakness, and loss of tendon reflexes along with sensory symptoms. Patients with severe beriberi may have dysphagia, dysphonia, or even deafness due to vagal and cochlear nerves involvement.[24,25]

Beriberi neuropathy is usually subacute or chronic, and rarely may it present like Guillain–Barré syndrome. In a study on 13 patients with beriberi neuropathy, two had acute and 11 had chronic presentation. These patients had anorexia, recurrent vomiting, and alcohol consumption as underlying risk factors. Their clinical features included weakness in 12, dysautonomia in six, and bulbar weakness in four and nystagmus in three patients. Cerebrospinal fluid analysis was normal and nerve conduction studies were suggestive of axonal sensory-motor neuropathy. Thiamine treatment resulted in improvement in 11 and 2 had sequelae. One patient died of a pulmonary embolism.[26]

PATHOLOGY OF BERIBERI

Nerve biopsy in early stage reveals segmental demyelination, and in late stage reveals axonal degeneration. Beriberi due to alcohol intake may reveal both demyelination and axonal changes.

TREATMENT AND PREVENTION

The patients with beriberi are treated with vitamin-rich high-calorie diet and thiamine 5–25 mg thrice daily. Thiamine >50 mg/day has no advantage.[27] About 50% patients with beriberi neuropathy improve completely. Mildly symptomatic patients have recovery within weeks but severely affected patients may take months to years to improve. Thiamine is a water-soluble vitamin; therefore, needs to supply on regular basis using thiamine-rich diet or by injection in critically ill patients.

INFANTILE TREMOR SYNDROME

INTRODUCTION

Infantile tremor syndrome (ITS) is characterized by four classical clinical features:

1. Palor
2. Developmental delay
3. Skin pigmentation
4. Brown scanty scalp hair

This disorder has been reported in many terminologies such as nutritional dystrophy and anemia,[28] infantile meningoencephalitis syndrome,[29] vitamin B12 deficiency in Indian infants,[30] megaloblastic anemia of infancy and vitamin B12,[31] syndrome of tremor in infants,[32] mental and physical retardation, mental regression and anemia,[33] and light-colored hair and anemia in malnourished children.[34] This syndrome is popularly known as infantile tremor syndrome because of the predominant occurrence of tremors in children below 2 years of age.[35]

Infantile tremor syndrome mainly described from Indian subcontinent. About 0.7–2.5% admission in pediatric ward is due to ITS.[33,36] A study of 25 infants with ITS was reported from Hyderabad in 1957. Subsequently, similar cases have been reported from Maharashtra, Karnataka, Andhra Pradesh, Tamil Nadu, Rajasthan, Gujarat, New Delhi, Uttar Pradesh, Chandigarh, Bihar, Madhya Pradesh, and West Bengal. Although the cases are reported throughout the year, but clustering has been noted during summer, post monsoon, and winter.

Infantile tremor syndrome mainly occurs from 6 to 24 months. There is male preponderance. Most of the children are from poor socioeconomic strata. The children are usually born out of a poor nourished vegetarian mother who is deprived of the dairy products either due to lack of availability, ignorance, or religious reasons. Some studies have reported pernicious anemia in mother,[30] and others have shown multiple nutritional deficiency in mothers.[34,37,38]

NUTRITIONAL STATUS OF THE INFANTS

Typically ITS infants are plump with preserved subcutaneous fat, but they are pale, apathetic with lusterless skin, and hair simulating Kwashiorkor.[1,3,4] Some infants fail to thrive and have marasmic features.[36,39,40] Growth indices of ITS remain normal till 5–6 months. Later, growth is affected because of dependence on exclusive breast feeding, intercurrent infection, and lack of transition to solid food. Moreover, children with ITS exhibit clinically feature of undernutrition including calorie, vitamins, and minerals. Hyper pigmentation of skin over hands, feet, and knuckles are common, which may have a honeycombing or reticulate pattern. Hairs on the other hand are sparse, brittle, depigmented, and lusterless.

NEUROLOGICAL MANIFESTATIONS

There may be a slowing in neurodevelopment or even regression of milestones after 5–6 months of the initial normal course. These children are less active, lethargic, and less reactive. Tremors are the cardinal neurological presentation of ITS, which are coarse and jerky looking like myoclonus. The onset of tremor may be focal affecting upper limb, then become generalized. The onset may be sudden or gradually progressive, and at times it may be multifocal. Voice tremor sometime may simulate "bleating of goat".[33,35] To begin with, tremor is intermitted and gets aggravated during crying, excitement, and stimuli, but later it becomes continuous. Tremor disappears during sleep tremor thus distinguishing it from seizures. Sometimes, there may be coexistent myoclonus or chorea.[33,41] There are reports of aggravation of tremors following vitamin B12 treatment).[28,42] Children may have dysphagia, hypotonia, and weakness with normal tendon reflexes. The sensation is usually preserved.

SYSTEMIC FINDING

Mild hepatosplenomegaly and congestive heart failure have been reported in some ITS.[3,40]

DIAGNOSIS OF INFANTILE TREMOR SYNDROME

The diagnosis of ITS is based on typical clinical tetrad and ruling out other nutritional and metabolic abnormalities. Blood counts are usually low to normal unless there is infection. Hemoglobin level may be low to normal. There may be megaloblastic RBC. Blood glucose and electrolytes are normal but have hypoalbuminemia. Low level of iron and magnesium has been reported in some studies.[43,44] There is no urinary amino acid excretion. [44] There are low serum vitamin B12 in infants as well as in the mothers.[32,37] Cranial CT scan reveals diffuse cortical atrophy. MRI may reveal diffuse cortical atrophy, [32,37] and delayed myelination.[37,45] Subdural effusion has also been reported which may be an effect of cortical atrophy. Electroencephalogram reveals nonspecific changes. Changes in nerve conduction and evoked potentials are not explored.

TREATMENT AND OUTCOME

Treatment of ITS is symptomatic including a nutritive diet and supplementation of vitamins and minerals. The correction of anemia and control of infection are important. Supplementation of vitamin B12 to lactating mother is another option to correct vitamin B12 deficiency in infants. Within 3 days of treatment, children become altered, agile, reactive, and playful. The tremor disappears by 1–4 weeks times. Skin pigmentation resolves by 2–4 weeks and normalization of hair changes takes months to year. Propranolol, sedatives, and carbamazepine have been used to treat tremor but its role is difficult to assess in view to uncontrolled studies. There is no mortality although mild neurocognitive deficit may persist.

CONCLUSION

Protein-energy malnutrition, beriberi, and ITS are important treatable neurological disorders and have complete recovery if diagnosed and treated early. Political will and commitment of government have key role in prevention and elimination of PEM. Nutritional education about the values of locally available foods is important especially to the mothers. Consumption of unpolished rice and thiamine rich diet, and avoiding alcohol intake may be able to prevent thiamine-related complications. In ITS children, a trial of vitamin B12 treatment may beneficial.

ACKNOWLEDGMENT

We thank Mr Shakti Kumar for his secretarial help.

REFERENCES

1. Williams CD, Oxon BM, Lond H. Kwashiorkor: a nutritional disease of children associated with a maize diet. 1935. Bull World Health Organ. 2003;81(12):912-3.
2. Brock JF, Marcel A, World Health Organization. (1952). Kwashiorkor in Africa / J. F. Brock, M. Autret. [online] Available from https://apps.who.int/iris/handle/10665/40717 [Last accessed February, 2023].
3. Caulfield LE, de Onis M, Blössner M, Black RE. Undernutrition as an underlying cause of child deaths associated with diarrhea, pneumonia, malaria, and measles. Am J Clin Nutr. 2004;80(1):193-8.
4. Kliegman RM, Stanton BMD, Geme JS, Schor NF. Nelsons Text book of Pediatrics. Philadelphia: Elsevier Health Sciences; 2019.
5. WHO. (2020). Malnutrition. [online] Available from https://www.who.int/news-room/fact-sheets/detail/malnutrition [Last accessed February, 2023].
6. World Health Organization (WHO). (2020). Nutrition 2020. [online] Available from: https://www.who.int/nutrition/topics/2_background/en/ [Last accessed February, 2023].
7. World Health Organization. Management of severe malnutrition: a manual for physicians and other senior health workers. Geneva: World Health Organization; 1999.
8. Black RE, Allen LH, Bhutta ZA, Caulfield LE, de Onis M, Ezzati M, et al. Maternal and child undernutrition: global and regional exposures and health consequences. Lancet (London, England). 2008;371(9608):243-60.
9. Walton E, Allen S. Malnutrition in developing countries. Paediatr Child Health. 2011;21(9):418-24.
10. UNICEF. (2020). UNICEF-WHO-World Bank: Joint Child Malnutrition Estimates 2020 edition—interactive dashboard. [online] Available from https://data.unicef.org/resources/joint-child-malnutrition-estimates-interactive-dashboard-2020/ [Last accessed February, 2023].

11. India State-Level Disease Burden Initiative Malnutrition Collaborators. The burden of child and maternal malnutrition and trends in its indicators in the states of India: the Global Burden of Disease Study 1990-2017. Lancet Child Adolesc Health. 2019;3(12): 855-70.
12. Pandian JD, Jyotsna R, Singh R, Sylaja PN, Vijaya P, Padma MV, et al. Premorbid nutrition and short term outcome of stroke: a multicentre study from India. J Neurol Neurosurg Psychiatry. 2011;82(10):1087-92.
13. Bembenek JP, Karlinski M, Niewada M, Kurkowska-Jastrzębska I, Członkowska A. . Measurement of Nutritional Status Using Body Mass Index, Waist-to-Hip Ratio, and Waist Circumference to Predict Treatment Outcome in Females and Males with Acute First-Ever Ischemic Stroke. J Stroke Cerebrovasc Dis. 2018;27(1):132-9.
14. Lönnroth K, Williams BG, Cegielski P, Dye C. A consistent log-linear relationship between tuberculosis incidence and body mass index. Int J Epidemiol. 2010;39(1):149-55.
15. Van Rie A, Westreich D, Sanne I. Tuberculosis in patients receiving antiretroviral treatment: incidence, risk factors, and prevention strategies. J Acquir Immune Defic Syndr. 2011;56(4):349-55.
16. Eijkman C. Beri-beri: Zur Abwehr. Arch Schiffs Tropen Hyg. 1898;2:103.
17. Grijns G. Researches on Vitamins. 1901–1911. Gorinchem, Holland: J. Noorduyn en Zoon; 1935.
18. Jansen BCP, Donath WF. On the isolation of the anti-beriberi vitamin. Proc Konink Akad van Wetensch Amsterdam. 1926;107:1390-400.
19. Williams RR, Cline JK. Synthesis of vitamin B1. J Am Chem Soc. 1936;58:1504-5.
20. Whitfield KC, Smith G, Chamnan C, Karakochuk CD, Sophonneary P, Kuong K, et al. High prevalence of thiamine (vitamin B1) deficiency in early childhood among a nationally representative sample of Cambodian women of childbearing age and their children. PLoS Negl Trop Dis. 2017;11(9):e0005814.
21. Luxemburger C, White NJ, ter Kuile F, Singh HM, Allier-Frachon I, Ohn M, et al. Beri-beri: the major cause of infant mortality in Karen refugees. Trans R Soc Trop Med Hyg. 2003;97(2):251-5.
22. Harel Y, Zuk L, Guindy M, Nakar O, Lotan D, Fattal-Valevski A. The effect of subclinical infantile thiamine deficiency on motor function in preschool children. Matern Child Nutr . 2017;13(4):e12397.
23. Wani NA, Qureshi UA, Ahmad K, Choh NA. Cranial ultrasonography in infantile encephalitic beriberi: A useful first-line imaging tool for screening and diagnosis in suspected cases. AJNR. Am J Neuroradiol. 2016;37(8):1535-40.
24. McCandless DW. Thiamine Deficiency and Associated Clinical Disorders. Contemporary Clinical Neuroscience Series. New York, NY: Humana Press; 2009. pp. 31-46.
25. Duce M, Escriba JM, Masuet C, Farias P, Fernandez E, de la Rosa O. Suspected thiamine deficiency in Angola. Field Exch. 2003;20:25.
26. Saini M, Lin W, Kang C, Umapathi T. Acute flaccid paralysis: Do not forget beriberi neuropathy. Journal of the peripheral nervous system: JPNS. 2019;24(1):145-9.
27. Whitfield KC, Bourassa MW, Adamolekun B, Bergeron G, Bettendorff L, Brown K. Thiamine deficiency disorders: diagnosis, prevalence, and a roadmap for global control programs. Ann N Y Acad Sci. 2018;1430(1):3-43.
28. Dikshit AK. Nutritional dystrophy with anemia. Indian J Child Health. 1957;6:132-6.
29. Pohowalla JN, Kaul KK, Bhandari NR, Singh SD. Infantile "meningo-encephalitic" syndrome. Indian J Pediatr. 1960;27:49-54.
30. Jadhav M, Webb JK, Vaishnava S, Baker SJ. Vitamin B12 deficiency in Indian infants. A clinical syndrome. Lancet. 1962;2:903-7.
31. Srikantia SG, Reddy V. Megaloblastic anaemia of infancy and Vitamin B12. Br J Haematol. 1967;13:949-53.
32. Kaul KK, Prasan N, Chowdhry RM. Some clinical observations and impressions on a syndrome of tremors in infants from India. J Pediatr. 1963;63:1158-66.
33. Sachdev KK, Manchanda SS, Lal H. The syndrome of tremors, mental regression and anaemia in infants and young children: A study of 102 cases. Indian Pediatr. 1965;2:239-51.
34. Mathur GP, Dayal RS, Prasad R, Mathur S. Tremors, mental and physical retardation, light coloured hairs and anaemia in malnourished children. Indian Pediatr. 1969;6:483-7.
35. Bajpai PC, Tandon PN, Sharma NL, Misra PK. Infantile tremor syndrome. Acta Neurol Scand. 1965;41:473-86.
36. Ramakumar L, Pandove SP. Infantile tremor syndrome. Indian J Pediatr. 1975;42:215-25.
37. Goraya JS, Kaur S. Infantile tremor syndrome—down but not out. Indian Pediatr. 2015;52:249-50.
38. Gupte S, Pal M. Infantile tremor syndrome (Observations from North India). Indian Pract. 1979;32:369-75.
39. Sirolia V, Arya S. Study of clinical profile and estimation of Vitamin B12 level in infantile and pre-infantile tremor syndrome. J Evol Med Dent Sci. 2014;3:10134-7.
40. Deshpande TV, Ingle VN. Tremor syndrome in children. Indian Pediatr. 1969;6:550-6.
41. Goraya JS, Kaur S, Mehra B. Neurology of nutritional Vitamin B12 deficiency in infants: Case series from India and literature review. J Child Neurol. 2015;30:1831-7.
42. Mahajan CM, Walia BN, Perkash A. Anemia in infantile tremor syndrome. Indian J Pediatr. 1971;38:362-4.
43. Agarwal R, Singh RN, Gupta BD, Agarwal DK, Arora AK. Serum magnesium, calcium, zinc in infantile tremor syndrome. Indian Pediatr. 1993;30:374-6.
44. Ingle VN, Hatwalne BV. Urinary aminoacids in the syndrome of tremors. A study of 12 cases. Indian J Pediatr. 1967;34:235-7.
45. Thora S, Mehta N. Cranial neuroimaging in infantile tremor syndrome (ITS). Indian Pediatr. 2007;44:218-20.

94

CHAPTER

The Important Role of Neurology in Oncology

Wolfgang Grisold, Anna Grisold

NEURO-ONCOLOGY

Introduction

Neuro-oncology is developing due to the increased needs, as cancer is a frequent disease and there is increased awareness of neurological symptoms and signs. Due to modern therapies, the survival and the number of long-term survivors are progressively increasing.

Historically, neuro-oncology was dedicated to primary brain tumors (BTs), e.g. glioblastoma, and also to direct, indirect, and therapy-related effects of cancer. As cancer is the second most frequent cause of death globally the need for neurological care is obvious (https://www.who.int/news-room/fact-sheets/detail/cancer). Cancer is much more frequent in primary BTs. Yet the variety of neoplastic, toxic, and other causes needs specialization. For this chapter, the primary BTs will not be discussed and the focus will be cancer and neurology.

Cancer is usually treated by oncologists, surgeons, and radiotherapists, and other organ-specific specialists. The present therapeutic results are very encouraging and range from curable cancers to highly therapy-resistant types and in countries with available oncological services and access, survival increases. Neurologists are classically involved in observing the function of the central nervous system (CNS) and peripheral nervous system (PNS) and help to define localize and analyze neurological dysfunction at various sites and stages of the disease. Traditionally neurologists were required when neurologic symptoms appeared at the time of diagnosis, or in the further course of the tumor disease. Most frequently the call was to find, prove or exclude neoplastic involvement in the brain, spinal cord, or nerve plexus **(Box 1)**.

At the onset of the tumor, or before, heralding the disease, the detection of symptoms such as paraneoplastic, humoral, or metabolic effects could appear.

The World Federation of Neurology (WFN) has a specialty group on neuro-oncology which is chaired by Professor Tracey Batchelor. This specialty group is composed of members of several regions of the world and tries to enhance and foster neuro-oncology worldwide.

BOX 1 **A tentative shortlist of the role of neurologists in oncology.**

- Awareness of common neurological symptoms in cancer patients
- Diagnosis, localization, and causes of neurological symptoms in cancer patients
- Awareness of the wide range of non-neoplastic causes such as endocrine, humoral, paraneoplastic, metabolic, inflammatory, and toxicities
- Neuro-oncological specific therapies
- Integration in multidisciplinary tumor therapy
- Symptomatic therapy
- Oncorehabilitation
- Palliative care

For many regions of the world, the practical tools needed for neurosurgery, imaging, and histology are not available. It will be most important to set worldwide standards for the neurological care of patients with either primary BTs and effects of cancer on the nervous system. It can be assumed that the increase in the average age expectancy will also induce more neurological complications in cancer patients. Equal access to care and treatment of patients is important.

Another important task of neurology is the symptomatic therapy of neuropathic pain, seizures, and miscellaneous other neurological symptoms, including general muscle weakness, and cachexia.

Neurorehabilitation is important and should be available increasingly for cancer patients with neurological symptoms. This is important, due to modern therapies the number of cancer survivors increases, and this brings forward also the issues of long-term therapy and therapy-related symptoms.[1]

Several symptomatic treatments for higher cognitive, sensory, and motor function, as well as neuropathic pain syndromes need neurological expertise.

Developments in the Field of Neuro-oncology

The past years have shown several developments. For many disease entities, oncologic therapies are effective and influence the quality of life and survival. Often the "natural" history of the tumor entity is changing. This is an emerging trend, as new therapies need health resources, and also improved availability, and wider access. In a large survey, it has been shown, that the 5-year survival times are increasing (https://ourworldindata.org/grapher/five-year-cancer-survival-in-usa?country=~All+races%2C+total).

However, in many countries of the world, neither access nor availability of neurology is available[2] and large out-of-pocket[3] expenses may lead to catastrophic consequences.[4]

The classical neurological assessment and neurospecific investigations are important in neuro-oncology. In addition, modern tools such as imaging detect small lesions. Staging as well as target-oriented imaging has added new dimensions. Molecular and liquid biopsy is increasingly emerging and will change procedures. In primary tumors, the pathological spectrum is shifting toward genetics and molecular diagnosis.[5]

Cancer therapies are increasingly effective and in several circumstances, the effects of therapy must be thoroughly recognized and distinguished from the effects of cancer.

New and different therapies will be needed.

In addition to radiotherapy (RT), classical chemotherapy and now immune therapies, among others add to the spectrum of toxicity, which can appear immediately or with a variable delay. Involvement of the brain and spinal cord can also dramatically influence the quality of life or reduced survival.

In addition to neoplastic and toxic conditions, there are also other effects such as paraneoplastic syndromes, and humoral and endocrine side effects. In addition to developing aspects such as chemobrain,[6] chemofog, radiation fibrosis syndrome,[7] and other rarer side effects **(Table 1)**.[8]

TABLE 1: Effects of different causes on the brain, spinal cord, and the neuromuscular system.

Type	Brain	Spinal cord	Neuromuscular
Surgery	+		+
Neoplastic	+++	++	+
Toxic including RT	++	+	+++
Cryotherapy, hyperthermia	+		
Metabolic	++		
Infection	+		+
Humoral/endocrine	++		+
Paraneoplastic	++	+	++

(RT: radiotherapy)

Mechanisms

Neoplastic

Metastasis into brain parenchyma occurs in several types of cancer and can be single or multiple. Depending on the cancer type, appearing is an early sign of cancer or in its course.[9] Recent advances in targeted therapies and immune checkpoint inhibitor (ICI) have changed the fate and prognosis of many patients, where these drugs are available.

In addition to well-known brain metastasis, several other types of CNS spread can occur, in particular leptomeningeal carcinomatosis (LC),[10] the base of the skull tumors,[11] cancer in the skull[12] and soft tissue,[12] and in spinal metastasis and local metastasis in the NM system. In addition to this, we are also experiencing the spread of cancer as neurolymphomatosis in the peripheral nerves and the brachial plexus.

Yet in individual cases, the differential diagnosis needs to include other potential issues such as posterior reversible encephalopathy syndrome (PRES),[13] "brain fog", cognitive changes, possible late effects of prior radiotherapy, and other toxic effects.

In a newly diagnosed patient with suspected brain metastasis, the search for a primary should be conducted by excluding the most frequent sources. If not positron emission tomography-computed tomography (PET-CT) might be helpful. Yet cancer of unknown primary (CUP) remains[14] often enigmatic.

Imaging and tissue analysis remain the gold standard of diagnosis, yet increasingly also immunological, biological, and molecular markers are identified and liquid biopsy might even replace histology in the future.[15]

Toxicity and Side-effects[16,17]

Surgical intervention can cause isolated painful mononeuropathies (e.g., intercostobrachial or accessory nerve) **(Fig. 1)** or nerve plexus lesions.

Toxicity includes a wide spectrum of mechanisms for example in peripheral nerves **(Fig. 2)** or cranial nerves.[18] In the classical setting, RT has a spectrum of time-related side effects, chemotherapy has substance-dependent toxicities and so have hormonal therapies as steroid treatment. In addition to CNS toxicity which can be induced by chemo- and radiotherapy[19] and also recent therapies such as targeted therapies and immune therapies such as immune checkpoint inhibitors and chimeric antigen receptor (CAR) T-cell therapies have opened a new spectrum of side effects with both unusual effects and often delays.

Chemotherapy-induced neuropathy[20] is an example of toxicity, which can present as acute, chronic cumulative and late toxicity, and is strongly substance and time dependent. As the number of cancer survivors increases, also late effects appear.

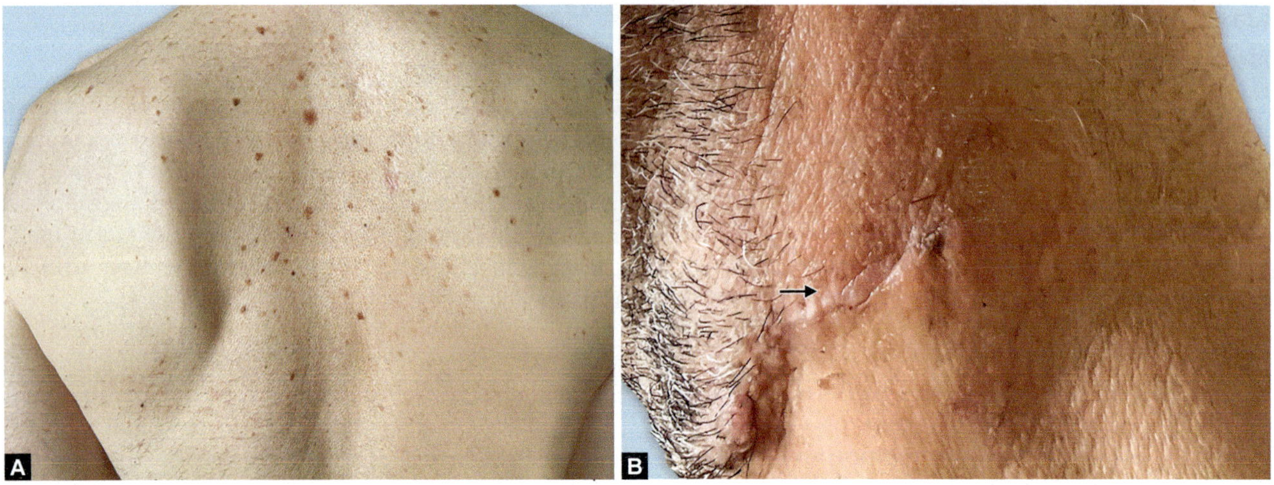

FIGS. 1A AND B: Iatrogenic accessory nerve lesion in neck dissection. (A) Left: Winging of the scapula; and (B) Right: Scar behind the sternocleidomastoid muscle/arrow.

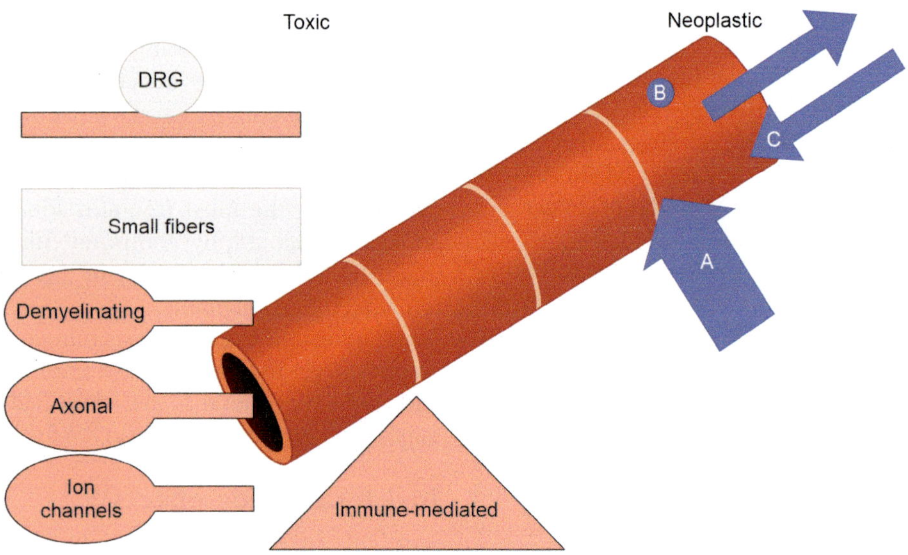

Notes:

- Cartoon to illustrate various influences on the peripheral nerve in neuro-oncology.
- *Toxic*: Effects can be directed toward the dorsal root ganglia (DRG), myelin, axons, ion channels, and potentially small fibers.
- Immune-mediated effects as caused by immune checkpoint inhibitor (ICI) have different mechanisms.
- Neoplastic can be caused by nerve compression and invasion (A), intranerval metastasis (B), or perineural spread (C).

FIG. 2: Different effects on peripheral nerves in neuro-oncology.

Image courtesy: JD Widdicombe 227.

Metabolic

Metabolic effects in cancer patients are numerous and can be tumor-related or therapy-induced. An example of CNS toxicity is Wernicke encephalopathy following hypovitaminosis and malnutrition in patients with gastrointestinal tumors or resections. Other examples are humoral, endocrine, and electrolyte disorders, often in association with neuroendocrine tumors, and also in association with some paraneoplastic syndromes. Amyloid deposition in myeloma can cause mono-, polyneuropathies, autonomic neuropathies, or myopathies.

Humoral

Humoral and endocrine effects are often associated with neuroendocrine neoplasm (NEN), yet the effects of humoral syndromes, and paraendocrine substances are important.[21]

One of the most frequent side effects is those from steroid therapies which usually induce weakness and atrophy of proximal thigh muscles[21,22] among other symptoms. Many of these effects are avoidable.

Antiestrogen therapies in breast cancer can cause an increase in incidence of carpal tunnel syndrome, as well as may induce mental changes in particular depressive states.[23]

Infections

Infections are often due to immune compromise. Typical examples are swallowing disorders due to oral mucosal infections, and frequent but not specific, herpes zoster is often associated with cancer and often needs pain management. Progressive multifocal leukoencephalopathy is a rare and serious complication.[24]

Paraneoplastic

Paraneoplastic neurological syndromes (PNS) are rare, yet attract interest for several reasons. They may indicate or reveal tumors, they can have severe effects on neurological function and in particular, the immunologically mediated syndromes can point to important interactions between the tumor and the immune system. Presently immune-mediated, humoral, and endocrine and several frequent but unresolved PNS are considered. The classifications and relations of onconeuronal and surface autoantibodies[25] have been updated in 2021. The number of antibodies associated with PS is increasing over time[26] and several terminologies are used.

Search for tumors in suspected PNS should be based on the clinical phenotype and the likely tumor association. Work-up may need PET-CT and whole body MRI in individual cases. The diagnosis is based on the phenotype of presentation.

Differential Diagnosis

Although the diagnosis of focal neoplastic lesions as brain and spinal metastasis can be often well defined, the differential diagnosis for symptoms and signs in cancer patients is wide and includes treatment effects and toxicity, metabolic effects, seizures, and infections. PS mainly appears at the time of tumor presentation. Immune therapies and ICIs can have overlapping features.

Symptomatic Therapy

Many neurological symptoms can appear, depending on the site and cause of the injury. For examples, treatment of seizures and cancer pain need to be in the extended repertoire of neuro-oncologists. Also acute interventions for brain edema, metabolic syndromes, and hypercalcemia need to be available.

CONCLUSION

Neurology has an important role in multidisciplinary and multiprofessional cancer therapy and needs to be included in oncological tumor boards to be an integral part of cancer therapy.

Symptomatic therapy for neurological symptoms such as seizures, or neuropathic pain is an important help in patient management. Cancer, metastasis, and also side effects can cause cancer pain, which often has neuropathic components.[27] Although pain is the primary concern with other effects on cognition and it also affect the quality of life and it has to be considered.

In the past years increasingly, possibly also due to longer survival, cancer rehabilitation has been introduced,[28] which has many components of neurology as cognitive rehabilitation, motor and functional rehabilitation, seizure control, preservation of movement and motility, and pain therapy among others.

One important future task is also palliative care for BT patients[29] and patients with neurological symptoms in cancer patients. In these situations, the quality of life, pain control, and control of neurological symptoms are important.

Conflict of interest: The authors declare no conflict of interest, the chapter is not sponsored and upon invitation.

REFERENCES

1. de Moor JS, Mariotto AB, Parry C, Alfano CM, Padgett L, Kent EE, et al. Cancer survivors in the United States: prevalence across the survivorship trajectory and implications for care. Cancer Epidemiol Biomarkers Prev. 2013;22(4):561-70.
2. Brain GBD, Other CNSCC. Global, regional, and national burden of brain and other CNS cancer, 1990-2016: a systematic analysis for the Global Burden of Disease Study 2016. Lancet Neurol. 2019;18(4):376-93.
3. Iragorri N, de Oliveira C, Fitzgerald N, Essue B. The Out-of-Pocket Cost Burden of Cancer Care: A Systematic Literature Review. Curr Oncol. 2021;28(2):1216-48.
4. Ahmed S, Ahmed MW, Hasan MZ, Mehdi GG, Islam Z, Rehnberg C, et al. Assessing the incidence of catastrophic health expenditure and impoverishment from out-of-pocket payments and their determinants in Bangladesh: evidence from the nationwide Household Income and Expenditure Survey 2016. Int Health. 2022;14(1):84-96.
5. Louis DN, Perry A, Wesseling P, Brat DJ, Cree IA, Figarella-Branger D, et al. The 2021 WHO Classification of Tumors of the Central Nervous System: a summary. Neuro Oncol. 2021;23(8):1231-51.
6. El-Agamy SE, Abdel-Aziz AK, Esmat A, Azab SS. Chemotherapy and cognition: comprehensive review on doxorubicin-induced chemobrain. Cancer Chemother Pharmacol. 2019;84(1):1-14.
7. DiFrancesco T, Khanna A, Stubblefield MD. Clinical Evaluation and Management of Cancer Survivors with Radiation Fibrosis Syndrome. Semin Oncol Nurs. 2020;36(1):150982.
8. Kwakman JJM, Elshot YS, Punt CJA, Koopman M. Management of cytotoxic chemotherapy-induced hand-foot syndrome. Oncol Rev. 2020;14(1):442.
9. Franchino F, Ruda R, Soffietti R. Mechanisms and Therapy for Cancer Metastasis to the Brain. Front Oncol. 2018;8:161.
10. Wang N, Bertalan MS, Brastianos PK. Leptomeningeal metastasis from systemic cancer: Review and update on management. Cancer. 2018;124(1):21-35.
11. Karlin JN, Krauss HR. Ophthalmic and orbital considerations in the evaluation of skull base malignancies. J Neurooncol. 2020;150(3):483-91.
12. Grisold W, Grisold A. Cancer around the brain. Neurooncol Pract. 2014;1(1):13-21.

13. How J, Blattner M, Fowler S, Wang-Gillam A, Schindler SE. Chemotherapy-associated Posterior Reversible Encephalopathy Syndrome: A Case Report and Review of the Literature. Neurologist. 2016;21(6):112-7.
14. Balestrino R, Ruda R, Soffietti R. Brain Metastasis from Unknown Primary Tumour: Moving from Old Retrospective Studies to Clinical Trials on Targeted Agents. Cancers (Basel). 2020;12(11):3350.
15. Poulet G, Massias J, Taly V. Liquid Biopsy: General Concepts. Acta Cytol. 2019;63(6):449-55.
16. Grisold W, Soffietti R, Oberndorfer S, Cavaletti G. Effects of Cancer Treatment on the Nervous System, 1st edition. UK: Cambridge Scholars Publishing; 2020.
17. Grisold W, Soffietti R, Oberndorfer S, Cavaletti G. Effects of Cancer Treatment on the Nervous System, 1st edition. UK: Cambridge Scholars Publishing; 2021.
18. Chong V. Imaging the cranial nerves in cancer. Cancer Imaging. 2004;4 Spec No A:S1-5.
19. Thomas A, Laurenge A, Psimaras D, Bompaire F, Hoang-Xuan K, Ricard D. Radiotherapy including hyperthermia and brain toxicity. In: Grisold W, Soffietti R, Oberndorfer S, Cavaletti G (Eds). Effects of Cancer Treatment on the Nervous System, 1st edition. UK: Cambridge Scholars Publishing; 2021. pp. 31-71.
20. Staff NP, Grisold A, Grisold W, Windebank AJ. Chemotherapy-induced peripheral neuropathy: A current review. Ann Neurol. 2017;81(6):772-81.
21. Kaltsas G, Androulakis, II, de Herder WW, Grossman AB. Paraneoplastic syndromes secondary to neuroendocrine tumours. Endocr Relat Cancer. 2010;17(3):R173-93.
22. Guilmette J, Nose V. Paraneoplastic syndromes and other systemic disorders associated with neuroendocrine neoplasms. Semin Diagn Pathol. 2019;36(4):229-39.
23. Yusufov M, Nathan M, Wiley A, Russell J, Partridge A, Joffe H. Predictors of increased risk for early treatment non-adherence to oral anti-estrogen therapies in early-stage breast cancer patients. Breast Cancer Res Treat. 2021;185(1):53-62.
24. Cortese I, Reich DS, Nath A. Progressive multifocal leukoencephalopathy and the spectrum of JC virus-related disease. Nat Rev Neurol. 2021;17(1):37-51.
25. Graus F, Vogrig A, Muniz-Castrillo S, Antoine JG, Desestret V, Dubey D, et al. Updated Diagnostic Criteria for Paraneoplastic Neurologic Syndromes. Neurol Neuroimmunol Neuroinflamm. 2021;8(4):e1014.
26. Jitprapaikulsan J, Paul P, Thakolwiboon S, Mittal SO, Pittock SJ, Dubey D. Paraneoplastic neurological syndrome: an evolving story. Neurooncol Pract. 2021;8(4):362-74.
27. Yoon SY, Oh J. Neuropathic cancer pain: prevalence, pathophysiology, and management. Korean J Intern Med. 2018;33(6):1058-69.
28. Smith SR, Zheng JY, Silver J, Haig AJ, Cheville A. Cancer rehabilitation as an essential component of quality care and survivorship from an international perspective. Disabil Rehabil. 2020;42(1):8-13.
29. Pace A, Dirven L, Koekkoek JAF, Golla H, Fleming J, Ruda R, et al. European Association for Neuro-Oncology (EANO) guidelines for palliative care in adults with glioma. Lancet Oncol. 2017;18(6):e330-e40.

95

CHAPTER

Neurology of Pregnancy

Sureshkumar Kamalakannan, Bindu Menon

INTRODUCTION

Pregnancy is a unique time in which a fetus develops inside a womb or uterus of a woman. It usually lasts for about 40 weeks from the time of the last menstrual period to delivery.[1] From a neurological perspective, these 40 weeks of pregnancy present with specific physiological conditions that may predispose certain diseases and health conditions or worsen them.[2] These diseases or health conditions, predisposed or worsened during pregnancy, could be neurological in nature and can present with varying degrees of severity.[2] This topic has become more important in recent days because of two reasons. Firstly, the diagnoses and prevalence of neurological conditions have substantially increased in the past few decades. Secondly, there is a delay in childbearing by women of reproductive age worldwide.[3,4] It is not just these two reasons that make it important to understand the neurology of pregnancy but also the impact that each of these reasons could have on each other.[4] The impact of pregnancy on the course of neurological diseases such as epilepsy, multiple sclerosis (MS), myasthenia gravis, and cerebrovascular diseases, as well as the impact of the neurological diseases on the entire course of pregnancy starting from prenatal, antenatal, labor, and delivery as well as the postnatal course, has raised several important implications for practice, policy, capacity building, and research.[4,5]

These implications are heavily interconnected. Neurological as well as reproductive child health practitioners rely on evidence for the effects of neurological conditions on pregnancy, childbirth, and lactation.[6] There is a huge demand for evidence on medications and their optimization during pregnancy to prevent those at risk of neurological complications.[7] Such evidence could influence practice and might demand a policy related to it in public health and primary care.[8] It could also support the training needs of those practitioners involved in the care and ensure there is sufficient capacity for addressing the needs of those with neurological issues during pregnancy or those pregnant women who are at risk of neurological diseases.[9] Additionally, the growth of research and availability of evidence in this field of practice particularly in low- and middle-income countries (LMICs) context including India needs to be assessed.[10] This is especially because, we could hardly find intersectoral/interdisciplinary practice of practitioners with expertise in neurology, reproductive child health, and disability working together globally, let alone LMICs.[11]

This chapter is aimed to raise awareness and enable an understanding of these aspects of neurology during pregnancy. It will include epidemiology, pathophysiology, clinical presentation, diagnosis, and treatment perspectives of specific neurological conditions that are closely related to pregnancy. Importantly, this chapter will also highlight the importance of this topic in an Indian context with special reference to the health systems and policies. This chapter will additionally include aspects related to implications for practice, policy, and research on this topic. These learning outcomes are expected to enable an understanding of the paucity of evidence on this topic in India and enhance the capacity of the readers to pragmatically utilize the learning from this chapter for practice in the Indian context with a biopsychosocial perspective.

EPIDEMIOLOGY OF NEUROLOGICAL CONDITIONS DURING PREGNANCY

Neurological disorders have been an important contributor to mortality and morbidity during pregnancy globally.[12] Women with neurological disorders accounted for 37 out of 87 maternal deaths arising from pregnancy and childbirth in the UK.[13] Epilepsy and stroke have been the major neurological contributors to these deaths.[13] In India, epilepsy has been reported as a top prevalent neurological condition during pregnancy with a cumulative incidence of 3–5 per 1,000 births.[14] It is also very similar to the findings from a study conducted in Africa.[15] Additionally, other common neurological conditions during pregnancy include myasthenia gravis, stroke, headache, peripheral neuropathies, MS, and brain tumor.[16]

However, measuring the burden of neurological conditions during pregnancy has been challenging.[17] There are hardly any reviews exclusively focusing on the neurological conditions during pregnancy globally.[18] Key challenges in measuring the burden could be the availability of diagnostics and the assessment protocols in various countries as well as heterogeneity in the approach to the measurement of various kinds of neurological disorders, particularly during pregnancy worldwide.[19] This is especially true when a comparison is made in relation to high-income countries (HICs) and LMICs where resources for even getting a computerized tomography (CT) scan for everyone who needs it could be an issue.[20] The other common issue could be that neurological conditions may present both medical and obstetric challenges to health professionals especially, those unfamiliar with practice protocols for management within the context of pregnancy.[21] This implies the need for measuring the global as well as the national burden of neurological conditions related to pregnancy to bridge this paucity of evidence in this area.

PATHOLOGY AND PATHOPHYSIOLOGY

Understanding the physiological changes during pregnancy, particularly among those with neurological conditions or at its risk, could help us to contextualize the pathology and pathophysiology of neurological conditions experienced during pregnancy.[22] These changes occur predominantly to protect the mother and child from any risks and negative consequences during pregnancy and childbirth.[23] Cardiac output increases by 25–50% during pregnancy through increased heart rate and stroke volume, especially during the third trimester.[24] This increased cardiac output may cross the threshold and might subsequently lead to hypertension during pregnancy causing pre-eclampsia, epilepsy, stroke, and sometimes rare condition such as arteriovenous malformations.[24] More details are available in **Table 1**.[25-30]

Conditions such as iron deficiency anemia during pregnancy increase the volume of red blood cells and proportional increase in the plasma volume.[31] This could lead to a rise in levels of fibrinogen, factor VIII, IX, and X, and increased risk of thrombus formation and stroke in these instances.[31] There is evidence that changes in cytokine levels and reduced immune response to cytotoxic substances could result in autoimmune disorders such as MS and rheumatoid arthritis during pregnancy.[32]

The pharmacological prescriptions for the prevention and management of these above-mentioned conditions could sometimes increase the glomerular filtration rate, reduce albumin concentration, and alter the pharmacokinetics of pregnant women leading to abnormal metabolic processes

TABLE 1: Neurological disorders and their attack patterns during pregnancy and postpartum.[7,25-30]

Neurological disorders	Attack during pregnancy	Attack during postpartum
Leg muscle cramps	Increase	Decrease
Chorea gravidarum	Increases	Decreases
Restless leg syndrome	Increases	Not known
Multiple sclerosis	Decreases during last trimester	Increases
Myasthenia gravis	Increases in first trimester	Increases
Migraine	Decreases in >80%	Decreases
Migraine without aura	Decreases in 80%	Decreases
Menstrual migraine	Increases	Increases
Idiopathic intracranial hypertension	Increases	Reduces
Epilepsy	Increases in focal seizures noted. Frontal lobe epilepsy increases	Frontal lobe epilepsy increases

and related complications.[33] More details are provided in **Table 2**.[25-35]

Therefore, it is highly important to understand the pathophysiology of neurological conditions during pregnancy from a pharmacological management point of view. Especially, because pregnancy alters body physiology automatically, those with or at risk of neurological conditions must be cautious when they are on medication for neurological disease conditions.[35]

NEUROLOGICAL CONDITIONS RELATED TO PREGNANCY

Epilepsy

The majority of women with epilepsy (WWE) will have an uneventful pregnancy and give birth to healthy children. However, the teratogenic potential of antiseizure medication (ASM) is a cause of concern. The aim of epilepsy treatment during pregnancy will aim to ensure a balance between the most effective seizure control versus avoiding the risk of teratogenicity to the developing fetus.[36]

Effect of Pregnancy on Seizures

Pregnancy also raises concern about the recurrence of seizures where one-third of women may experience increased seizure frequency.[36,37] European and International Registry of Antiepileptic Drugs and Pregnancy (EURAP) epilepsy pregnancy registry and the Maternal Outcomes and Neurodevelopmental Effects of Antiepileptic Drugs (MONEAD) Study did not report a higher frequency of

TABLE 2: Impact of medications for neurological disorders on pregnancy and breastfeeding.[7,25-35]

S. No.	Medications for neurological disorders	Condition	Teratogenic effect	Impact on breastfeeding
A	• Lamotrigine • Lacosamide • Levetiracetam • Oxcarbazepine	Epilepsy	Risk to humans has not been excluded	Can be considered safe for baby
B	• Carbamazepine • Phenobarbitone • Phenytoin • Valproate • Clonazepam • Topiramate		Unsafe	
C	Glatiramer acetate	Multiple sclerosis	Safe during conception	Incomplete evidence
D	Beta interferons		Risk to humans has not been excluded	
E	Dimethyl fumarate		Risk to humans has not been excluded	
F	Teriflunomide		Highly teratogenic	
G	Fingolimod		Risk to humans has not been excluded	
H	Natalizumab		Risk to humans has not been excluded	
I	Rituximab/ocrelizumab		Risk to humans has not been excluded	
J	Alemtuzumab		Risk to humans has not been excluded	
K	Glatiramer acetate		Safer	
L	Mitoxantrone		Highly teratogenic	
M	Preventive pharmacotherapy	Migraine	To be avoided	Address risk–benefit ratio
N	Opioids	Chronic use for pain	Fetal defects and preterm delivery	Avoid
O	Naproxen sodium	Occasional single dose	Relatively safe	Safe
P	Ergotamine and dihydroergotamine	Migraine	Avoid	Avoid
Q	NSAIDs	Migraine	Avoiding NSAIDs after 30 weeks' gestation	Safe
R	Triptans	Migraine	• Inconclusive • Low teratogenic • Probable increased rates of spontaneous abortions	Cautious use
S	Azathioprine and cyclosporine	Myasthenia gravis	• Avoid • Cyclosporine can be used during pregnancy in standard doses • Azathioprine drug of choice in pregnancy after steroids	Avoid
T	Mycophenolate		Avoid	Avoid
U	Rituximab		Relatively contraindicated	Avoid
V	Pyridostigmine		Safe	Safe
W	Plasmapheresis		Safe with careful monitoring	Safe
X	Corticosteroids		Safe but increase the risk for gestational diabetes and pre-eclampsia, cleft lip	Safe
Y	Intravenous human immunoglobulin		Safe with careful monitoring	Safe
Z	Aspirin	Stroke	Safe at low-dose acetylsalicylic acid	Safe at low-dose acetylsalicylic acid

(NSAIDs: nonsteroidal anti-inflammatory drugs)

seizures in pregnant women as compared to nonpregnant controls.[38,39] Monitoring of serum drug concentration with adjustment of doses of ASM and ensuring strict compliance could be an elective method to manage seizures.[40,41] Lamotrigine, levetiracetam, and oxcarbazepine particularly show a decline in serum concentration during pregnancy. Ensuring a seizure-free interval 9 months before conception has more chances of remaining seizure-free during pregnancy.[42]

Effect of Seizure/s on Pregnancy

Generalized seizures can lead to trauma to the mother and fetus during an epileptic attack. A tenfold increased mortality risk was reported in WWE.[42] Consideration for increased risk of pre-eclampsia, postpartum hemorrhage, and preterm labor leading to increased maternal injury and death is warranted.[43] Apart from seizure-related death, Sudden Unexpected Death in Epilepsy (SUDEP) has been increasingly reported.[44] Recurrent seizures can be associated with premature delivery and intrauterine growth retardation.

Teratogenic Risk

Monotherapy is recommended to reduce the malformation rate and long-term cognition changes. The risk for major congenital malformation (MCM) predominantly occurs during the first trimester of pregnancy. But effects on behavior and cognition extend all through the pregnancy.[44] A rational selection of ASM should be done in women of childbearing potential. The maximum risk of MCMs is associated with valproate, intermediate risk with phenobarbital and topiramate, and the lowest risk with lamotrigine and levetiracetam. Lamotrigine, carbamazepine, phenobarbital, and valproate have been associated with dose-dependent teratogenicity. 4 mg of folic acid for all women of childbearing age on ASMs is recommended, as it reduces the risk of fetal neural tube defects.[44]

Hypertensive Disorder of Pregnancy

Pre-eclampsia and eclampsia are one of the four categories of hypertensive disorders of pregnancy (HDPs) with neurological implications that pose a major risk for the mother and the fetus.[10] Pre-eclampsia as the name suggests is before eclampsia, marked by a new-onset of hypertension with systolic blood pressure ≥140 mm Hg and diastolic blood pressure ≥90 mm Hg after 20 weeks of gestation presenting with end-organ dysfunction including that of the central nervous system.[10] Eclampsia can be defined as the new onset of generalized seizures (tonic-clonic) in women with pre-eclampsia.[45] Despite the advances in neurological investigation, the causes are still unclear and it is assumed that there is increased permeability of blood-brain barriers which disturbs autoregulation and impairs cerebral blood flow.[45]

Women experiencing eclampsia usually present with tonic-clonic seizures that may last for 60–90 seconds with a postictal state following the seizure.[36] They also complain of headaches, abdominal pain, and visual problems before they experience seizures. Blood pressure is a primary concern and hence the evaluation primarily will be on hypertension, especially around 20 weeks of pregnancy. Since there is potential end-organ dysfunction, the additional evaluation will include blood protein level, liver and kidney function, pulmonary edema, and nervous system examination related to headache and visual problems.[37] Differential neurological diagnosis includes primary seizure disorders, thrombotic thrombocytopenic purpura, ruptured aneurysm, brain tumor, stroke, and intracranial hemorrhage (ICH).[36,37]

Eclamptic seizures are a serious medical emergency, and they must be promptly diagnosed and treated at the earliest.[38] Eclamptic seizures are treated with magnesium sulfate at a loading dose of 4–6 g intravenously followed by a maintenance dose of 2 g per hour for at least 24 hours. This could prevent morbidity and mortality of the mother and the child.[36-39] The airway must be secured for those who are actively convulsing and conservatively managed by positioning and sufficient ventilation.[39] Given that this condition requires obstetric and neurologic support, interdisciplinary team working is very crucial for the management of the problem.[45]

Stroke

Stroke is a leading cause of death and disability globally. A recent review reported that the cumulative incidence of stroke is 30 per 100,000 pregnancies which is three times more compared to those women who are not pregnant at their reproductive age (15–44 years).[46] The peripartum and postpartum periods carry the maximum risk for stroke corresponding to the increased risk of hypertension and hypercoagulability. About 14% of the fatality was due to hemorrhagic stroke (HS) and 3.5% was due to ischemic stroke (IS).[46,47] Disability following HS was 50% compared to an IS of 33%. ICH was the most common cause of maternal deaths in this review. Intracerebral bleed accounts for 60% of all types of strokes in pregnancy. Vascular malformations, hypertension, pre-eclampsia, and coagulopathy are the predisposing factors for intracerebral bleed.[48] Increased bleed due to arteriovenous malformation has not been documented in studies with a reported incidence of around 2.6%.[48]

The risk factors for stroke identified in this review were gestational diabetes [odds ratio (OR) 26.8], preexisting hypertension (OR 8.5), migraine (OR 8.5), pre-eclampsia and eclampsia (OR 7.7), and maternal age (OR 2.3).[46] Most strokes occurring in pregnancy are due to hemostatic, hormonal, and metabolic factors. Pregnancy is associated with increasing levels of estrogen, and progesterone, doubling of cardiac output, and water retention by the last trimester. High estrogen leads to increased procoagulants and high progesterone causes vasodilation, which are risk factors for stroke. IS, ICH, subarachnoid hemorrhage (SAH), and cerebral venous thrombosis are seen in pregnancy. The conventional risk factors could be a contributing factor to stroke; however, there are few specific risk factors in pregnancy though less common.[46-48]

Hypertensive disorder of pregnancy, especially pre-eclampsia and eclampsia, has been associated with increased risk for stroke accounting for around 25–57% of strokes in pregnancy.[49] HDP has also been associated with double the risk of stroke in later life. HDP carries a higher risk for stroke in pregnancy compared to conventional risk factors.[50] History of migraine with aura (MA) produces an increased risk of maternal stroke. The association between HDP and migraine has been explored and has been suggested in studies.[51-53] The increased prevalence of patent foramen ovale (PFO) with migraine further increases the risk of maternal stroke.[51-53]

Treatment of a high-risk state like an IS, which would require anticoagulation outside pregnancy, would include LMWH twice daily or adjusted dose UFH subcutaneously till the 13th week when it is substituted with VKA nearing delivery when the treatment is again shifted to LMWH or UFH. Low-risk conditions needing antiplatelet treatment outside pregnancy might not be considered for any treatment or a low-dose aspirin after the first trimester of pregnancy depending on the clinical situation.[54] There is a lack of guidelines for the treatment of acute stroke with reperfusion therapy in pregnancy. However, intravenous alteplase might be considered in select patients with moderate-to-severe stroke where the benefits overweigh the risk of uterine bleeding.[55]

Headaches

Headaches can be primary or secondary during pregnancy. Migraine, tension-type headache (TTH), cluster headache, and trigeminal autonomic cephalgia are the primary headaches. There is also a tendency for a migraine to change in pattern from migraine without aura (MO) to MA or vice versa from MO to TTH.[56] Migraine is more frequently seen in the first trimester.[57] Patients with MA are noted to have more frequent fluctuations with almost half of the patients continuing to have headaches during pregnancy.[58] Menstrual migraine patients tend to have poor remissions of headaches during pregnancy. TTH is not known to increase during pregnancy. The most common secondary headaches during pregnancy are due to stroke, cerebral venous thrombosis, SAH, pituitary tumor, choriocarcinoma, eclampsia, pre-eclampsia, idiopathic intracranial hypertension, and reversible cerebral vasoconstriction syndrome (RCVS).[54]

Headache due to IIH is seen in any trimester of pregnancy. There are considerations in the treatment of IIH in pregnancy.[59] Acetazolamide, which is the drug of choice, is classified as a class C in pregnancy. A lumbar puncture can improve headaches and vision loss; however, the procedure can be difficult in obese women. Optic nerve fenestration is reserved for patients with progressive and severe loss of vision.[60] Pituitary apoplexy should be considered in pregnant women who present with thunderclap headaches. Other manifestations of raised intracranial pressure accompanied by visual symptoms and hypopituitarism should alert the clinician to distinguish from other causes of thunderclap headache.

Early diagnosis of the disease manifested by headache is important to protect the life of the mother and the fetus from any red flags suggesting that headache is a symptom of a disease.[61] During pregnancy and breastfeeding, nonpharmacological treatment should be the preferred therapeutic strategy for the treatment of primary headaches. However, poorly managed headaches could lead to sleep deprivation, stress, and anxiety, which could have a bad prognosis on the fetus and mother.[55] Mild and moderate headaches can be managed with paracetamol and nonsteroidal anti-inflammatory drugs (NSAIDs) in the first trimester; however, NSAIDs should be avoided in the third trimester. Triptans are to be considered if the benefits overweigh the risk. Prophylactic therapy with tricyclic antidepressants, divalproex, and antidepressants has a high risk of teratogenicity. Calcium channel blockers, beta-blockers, and antihistamines are probably safer alternatives.[62]

Peripheral Nerve Diseases

Peripheral nerve diseases (PND) are common during pregnancy and postpartum. The most common peripheral neuropathies during pregnancy are Bell's palsy, carpal tunnel syndrome (CTS), and lower extremity neuropathies. Nerve compression is the usual pathophysiology for PND during pregnancy.[63] CTS is most commonly present in the third trimester; it has to be distinguished from other forms of pain that are bilateral in nature and do not involve the median nerve. Like CTS, Bell's palsy is also common during the third trimester and the first 2 weeks after delivery.[57] Hypertensive disorders and obesity during pregnancy seem to be risk factors for Bell's palsy during pregnancy. Most neuropathies are reversible; however, the disabilities imposed might affect the functioning and require therapeutic rehabilitation.[63,64]

Movement Disorder

The most common movement disorder arising during pregnancy is restless leg syndrome (RLS) and chorea gravidarum. The prevalence of RLS is estimated to be between 10 and 25% during the third trimester of pregnancy.[65] Counseling and dopaminergic drugs have been used for treating RLS; however, the treatment must consider preexisting RLS and the worsening of its symptoms during pregnancy, unlike secondary RLS where symptoms may appear even earlier than the third trimester.[66] Women with a history of rheumatic fever, systemic lupus erythematosus (SLE), antiphospholipid antibody syndrome (APLS), syphilis, and encephalitis are known to develop chorea gravidarum. The abnormal movements begin after the first trimester in half of the patients and spontaneously remit before delivery in one-third, with most of the remaining patients experiencing remission after delivery. While chorea gravidarum once had significant mortality due to resultant rhabdomyolysis, it is now thought to be manageable with medication in most cases. However, the need for medications to prevent complications to the mother or fetus must be balanced against possible side effects, but haloperidol is generally preferred among neuroleptics in pregnancy.[65,66]

Vasculopathies

Reversible cerebral vasoconstriction syndrome can lead to both ischemic and HS. RCVS is a clinicoradiological syndrome characterized by reversible vasoconstriction of medium- and large-size cerebral arteries.[67] The presentation is often with thunderclap headache and focal deficits and might progress to IS, ICH, or SAH in severe cases leading to permanent disability. It is also termed postpartum angiopathy or angiitis. Imaging shows multifocal stenosis of intracranial vessels with reversal usually in 12 weeks.[68]

Moyamoya disease (MMD) is a rare progressive disorder of the carotid vessels leading to narrowing and/or occlusion. MMD can lead to IS due to embolus from the stenotic site or intracerebral hemorrhage due to raised blood pressure and blood volume. 2.6–3 per 100,000 pregnancies.[69] Hormonal and hemodynamic changes are probable attributing factors. Valsalva-induced intima injury with hematoma formation during labor could trigger thromboembolic stroke.[70]

Hypercoagulable and Prothrombotic States

Antiphospholipid antibody syndrome (APS) is an autoimmune disorder with an increased predisposition to arterial and venous stroke. Thrombosis is presumed to cause many of the pregnancy complications associated with APS. Sickle cell disease (SCD) is also associated with both arterial and venous stroke.[71] Women with SCD should be closely monitored for neurological complaints, especially headaches. Acute-onset severe headache should undergo imaging to rule out intracerebral bleed. Hypertension during pregnancy in SCD could be an added risk for IS. Exchange transfusion is also indicated for acute stroke with SCD.[72]

Choriocarcinoma is a rare neoplasm type of trophoblastic disease. It tends to metastasize to the brain early. Patients present with signs of raised intracranial tension.[73] The presentation is with intracerebral bleed due to the highly vascular nature of the tumor. Thrombosis of vessels can cause IS.[74] Another pregnancy-related rare complication in multiparous older women is amniotic fluid embolism. This occurs due to the disruption of the barrier between maternal circulation and amniotic fluid. Cardiac, respiratory, and coagulopathy symptoms predominate.[75] Seizures and paradoxical cerebral embolism are other presenting manifesting symptoms. Thrombosis in the dural sinuses is more likely in the puerperium due to venous stasis, a hypercoagulable prothrombotic state. Presentation is with headache particularly supine, seizures, and signs of raised intracranial pressure and venous infarction.[76] Neuroimaging with magnetic resonance imaging (MRI) is sensitive in the diagnosis **(Figs. 1A and B)**.

Myasthenia Gravis

Myasthenia gravis is a complex autoimmune disorder that causes antibodies to destroy the connections between nerves and muscles at the neuromuscular junctions. It affects women twice as much as men, particularly during their childbearing age.[77] The condition could affect just the ocular muscles or their entire body. If the myasthenia gravis is generalized, then it could be further categorized into mild,

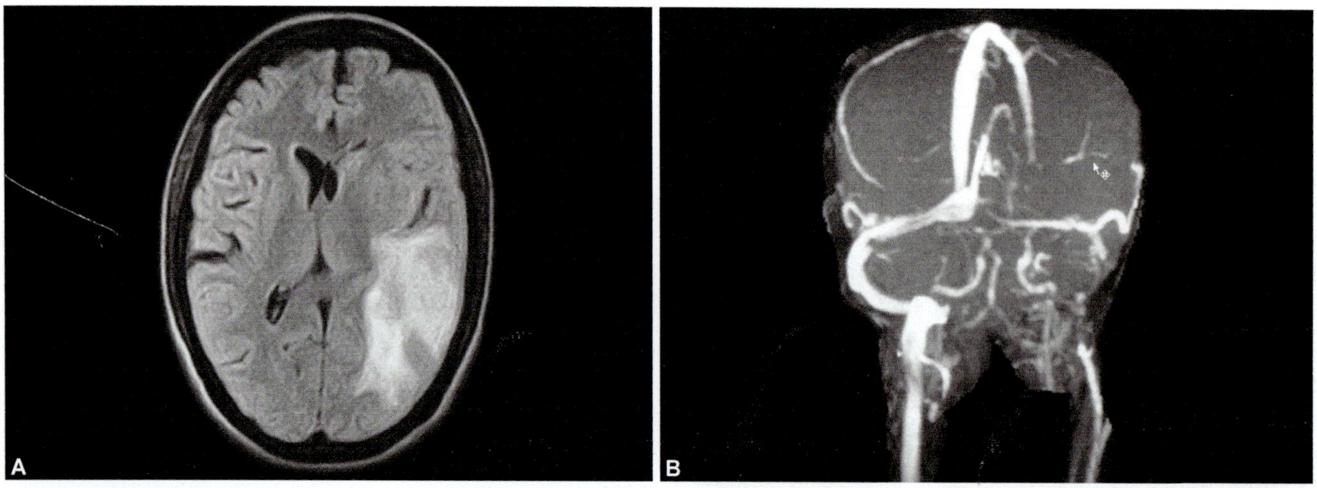

FIGS. 1A AND B: (A) MRI FLAIR shows cortical and subcortical hyperintense signals involving left temporal cortex with mild mass effect on left lateral ventricle. (B) MRV shows absent flow-related enhancement in left transverse sinus.
(FLAIR: fluid-attenuated inversion recovery; MRI: magnetic resonance imaging; MRV: magnetic resonance venography)

moderate, and severe depending on their weakness. The primary problem in those experiencing myasthenia gravis is muscle weakness.[78] One of the main causes of exacerbation of myasthenia gravis during pregnancy is hypoventilation due to weakness of respiratory muscles. Given that this condition affects women of childbearing age, the evidence from research suggests that the symptoms of myasthenia gravis worsen during the first trimester and improve during the second and third trimester due to pregnancy-induced immune suppression during these times.[79] However, pregnancy does not determine the severity of onset and long-term outcomes of myasthenia gravis. It is also evident that myasthenia gravis does not affect pregnancy to a large extent.

Myasthenia gravis is caused by polyclonal immunoglobulin G (IgG) antibodies that negatively impact on nicotinic acetylcholine receptor present in the skeletal muscles of the human body causing muscle weakness, fatigue, ptosis, diplopia, dysphagia, and dysarthria in addition to respiratory muscle weakness described earlier.[78,79] This disease is also associated with thyroid disease and thymoma. Pregnant women requiring medical treatment for myasthenia gravis may be taking anticholinesterases such as neostigmine and pyridostigmine. These drugs prevent the breakdown of neurotransmitters.[78,79]

The first line of treatment is oral pyridostigmine and prednisolone for immunosuppression. As the effect of thymectomy takes time, the procedure should not be planned during pregnancy. Chest CT should be preferably postponed due to the radiation risk to the fetus. In the setting where pyridostigmine and prednisolone do not relieve the symptoms, cyclosporine and azathioprine might be considered. Intravenous immunoglobulin (IVIg) and plasmapheresis are considered when an urgent short-term response is needed. The risk and benefits need to be weighed carefully.[80]

However, methotrexate is absolutely contraindicated in pregnancy and mycophenolate is teratogenic and should be avoided in these cases.[69] Neuromuscular blocking agents like magnesium sulfate are contraindicated for eclampsia in pregnancy.[81] As for any neurological conditions during pregnancy, management of myasthenia gravis does not stop only with pharmacological management. The treatment starts with prenatal counseling, antenatal care, delivery, and neonatal considerations in addition to the pharmacological strategies mentioned above.[81]

Multiple Sclerosis

Demyelinating diseases of the nervous system affect the myelin with relative sparing of the axons. The common disorders are MS, acute disseminated encephalomyelitis, and neuromyelitis optica spectrum disorders, which occur as part of inflammation. Pregnancy is an immune tolerant condition that, once disturbed, leads to adverse outcomes.[82]

Multiple sclerosis is an autoimmune disorder that affects the central nervous system of the human body.[83] About 1 in 1,000 people is said to experience MS in the United States. It affects women more than men and it is usually diagnosed during reproductive and childbearing age.[83] The common signs and symptoms of MS include muscle weakness, tingling, numbness, pain, tremor, loss of balance, mobility issues, speech problems, visual impairment, fatigue, bladder/bowel problems, cognitive-perceptual problems, particularly thinking, and memory issues as well as depression.[84] Relapsing-remitting form of MS affects 85% of patients. One of the earliest prospective studies noted that the relapses decreased during pregnancy to increase 3 months postpartum to the prepregnancy rates.[85] This has been attributed to the neuroprotective effects of estrogen and other sex hormones, which remain high in pregnancy, especially in the last trimester.

Disease-modifying treatment (DMT) must be given with caution to avoid teratogenicity. Relapses in the second and third trimesters can be treated with a short course of high-dose methylprednisolone, however, should be avoided in the first trimester.[86] Injectable glatiramer and interferon-beta may be continued till pregnancy and during pregnancy in more active cases. Dimethyl fumarate and teriflunomide are contraindicated during pregnancy.[87,88] Fingolimod needs to be stopped 2 months prior to conception and bridging with another DMT should be done. Pregnancy is safe after 6 months after the last dose of cladribine.[89]

Natalizumab can be stopped with a positive pregnancy, however, the reactivation of the disease is very high. In patients with high activity, the dose can be modified to the 8th weekly injection. Most pregnant women will have a good outcome; hence, physicians should give updated information on the teratogenicity. Women should be encouraged to take folate and vitamin D supplements.[87-89]

Posterior Reversible Encephalopathy Syndrome

Posterior reversible encephalopathy syndrome (PRES) is a clinicoradiological distinct syndrome consisting of a group of symptoms with classical imaging features. Patients present with acute or subacute symptoms, which include headache, seizures, visual dysfunction, and altered sensorium. PRES is seen in classical diseases and situations such as accelerated hypertension, renal failure, patients undergoing dialysis and on immunosuppressants or chemotherapeutic agents, sepsis, autoimmune disease, and pre-eclampsia. Symptoms of PRES have been reported in the second and third trimesters with the rapid development of symptoms within 12–48 hours.[90] Preeclamptic patients presenting with visual loss should be suspected of PRES even in the absence of seizures.[91] The presentation is essentially similar in nonpregnant women; however, altered sensorium was reported less in pregnant women.[92] MRI is characteristic with vasogenic edema in the occipital and parietal white matter **(Figs. 2A and B)**.

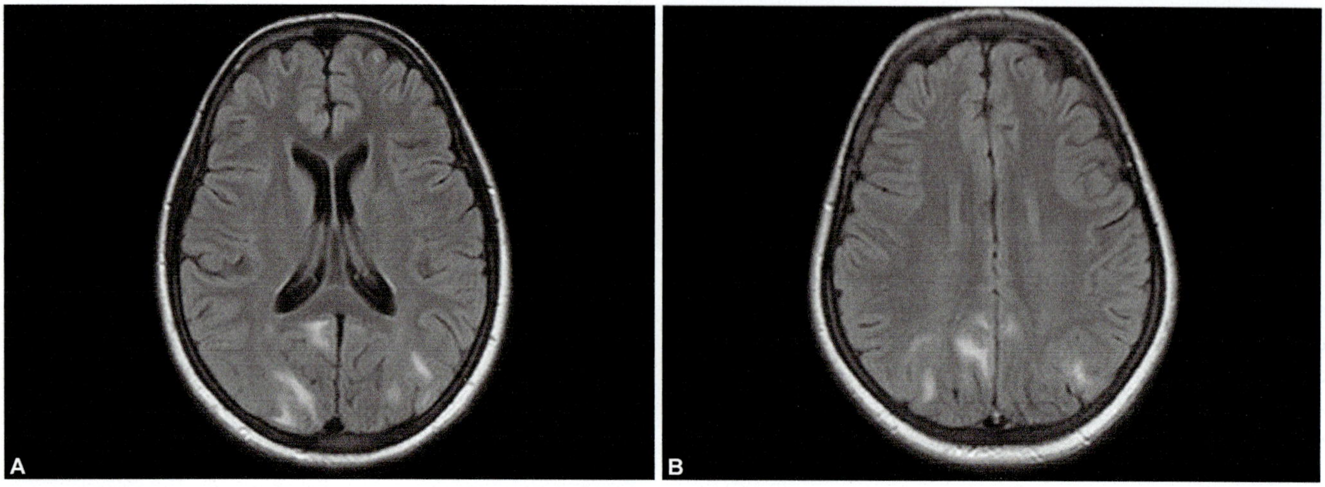

FIGS. 2A AND B: MRI FLAIR shows cortical subcortical hyperintensities involving bilateral parieto-occipital cortex suggestive of posterior reversible encephalopathy syndrome.
(FLAIR: fluid-attenuated inversion recovery; MRI: magnetic resonance imaging)

Though there is a paucity of literature on the outcome, patients with PRES from pre-eclampsia have a better outcome as compared to other causes. The treatment of PRES is targeted to the underlying cause. Eclampsia should be treated with magnesium sulfate which will treat the seizure and the accelerated hypertension.[93]

Wernicke's Encephalopathy

Wernicke's encephalopathy is caused by thiamine deficiency. The condition is frequently encountered in alcoholics, however, also seen in malnutrition induced by gastric surgery, malignancies, and hyperemesis.[94] The requirement for thiamine in pregnancy increases threefold. Apart from the high demand, thiamine deficiency is precipitated by hyperemesis gravidarum and poor dietary intake.

Wernicke's encephalopathy is an acute reversible neuropsychiatric condition. The classical presentation is ataxia, altered sensorium, and ocular dysfunction. However, all patients may not have the classical triad. MRI is the imaging modality of choice. MRI shows symmetrical high-signal intensities in the thalamus, periaqueductal area, and mammillary bodies. Timely replacement with thiamine will result in reversal of symptoms within hours to days depending on the disease severity. Untreated Wernicke's can progress to Wernicke-Korsakoff syndrome (WKS).[95] Hence, a high index of suspicion should be there to recognize and institute timely treatment to prevent maternal and fetal morbidity.

NEUROLOGICAL DISABILITY DURING PREGNANCY

Neurological conditions are mostly disabling. Compared to musculoskeletal impairments, neurological impairments are more disabling because these conditions affect the central nervous system, which helps to control body movements and functions.[96] The impairments are expected to be diverse affecting the sensory-motor, cognitive-perceptual, psychological, and social-emotional aspects of body function. As defined by the International Classification of Functioning (ICF), these impairments are just one aspect of disability.[97] Impairments often limit an affected individual to participate in his everyday activities such as self-care, mobility, communication, etc. These activity limitations can subsequently restrict social participation and productive contribution to one family and society. In addition, the physical and psychosocial environments in which a person experiences these impairments, activity limitations, and participation restrictions pose an additional burden. Architectural barriers, as well as attitudinal barriers such as social stigma and discrimination, increase the burden of disability.[98]

Neurological disability during pregnancy is much more important to consider because pregnancy alters the physiology of the human body on its own and neurological disability during pregnancy can impose risk to both pregnant women as well as the fetus.[99] The synergistic effects of both could exponentially increase the risk to the mother and fetus.[99] Disability can affect pregnant women with neurological diseases during the prenatal, natal, and postnatal stages of pregnancy.[99] During the prenatal stage, disability impacts the performance of activities of daily living (ADLs). Pregnant women with neurological conditions require a substantial amount of energy, muscle power, and endurance to independently perform their ADLs.[100] They are also at risk of falls, malnutrition, depression, and other kinds of disabilities that might hamper the experience of a normal pregnancy that one without a neurological disability could have. Comprehensive, evidence-based, client-centered rehabilitation for the management of neurological disability is absolutely essential to those pregnant women with neurological conditions. In most cases, the disability caused by these neurological conditions is permanent and hence rehabilitation must be continuous and consistent.[101]

Supportive treatment and a continuum of rehabilitation and care are very critical to pregnant women with neurological disabilities.[102] Enabling independence in ADLs, providing rehabilitation based on the needs of the pregnant women and their families, provision, and training for the use of assistive devices that can enhance independence in their family and social roles, remediating the impairments, improving communication skills, supporting bowel and bladder management, and environmental modification are some of the core principles that need to be focused during the rehabilitation of pregnant women with neurological disability, particularly during the prenatal phase.[103]

The benefits of such care and rehabilitation become essential and even more important during labor because pregnant women with these kinds of neurological problems cannot have the sensation of pelvic movements and feel pain during contractions. Additionally, their muscle power and voluntary motor control will be weak and uncontrolled to facilitate the delivery.[104]

Any problems during labor can be detrimental to the health of the pregnant women and the fetus. This could lead to hypoxic brain damage and other disabling conditions such as cerebral palsy, limb dislocation, and infantile stroke in the baby.[105] Neurological conditions will make pregnancy harder as well as the labor and delivery of the baby difficult. Therefore, in addition to medical, surgical, and pharmacological management of those pregnant women with neurological conditions, due attention must be provided to neurological disability and its impact on pregnancy, labor, and delivery.[106]

THE INDIAN CONTEXT

India, the second-most populous country in the world, caters to the health needs of 1.3 billion people.[107] The country has a state-led public health system in each of its 38 states and union territories which are centrally managed by the national health systems through the National Health Mission (NHM) initiatives.[108] One of India's oldest and most heavily invested health programs is called the Reproductive, Maternal, Newborn, Child and Adolescent Health (RMNCH+A).[109] This program particularly focuses on pregnant women in the reproductive age group. All pregnant women receive three antenatal visits, 100 iron and folic acid (IFA) tablets, and two tetanus toxoid injections. There is health insurance covering pregnant women too under the Ayushman Bharat scheme (National Health Insurance Scheme).[108] However, the treatment and management of neurological conditions experienced by pregnant women in their own community or outside the hospital setting are not covered by national insurance.[79] Neurological disability as defined by ICF, experienced by any individual, is also not covered by the national insurance scheme.[109,110] Overall, if pregnant women with neurological conditions require medical help, they pay for it and access it from private hospitals which cover 80% of the healthcare market in India. The government programs and schemes are often underutilized even by those living in rural areas where private healthcare access is very minimal.[111]

On the contrary, the epidemiology of neurological diseases has substantially raised over the past few decades in India. The contribution of noncommunicable neurological disorders was 8% in 2019 compared to 4% in 1990.[112] Although increasing, these are considered underestimates because the data as reported by the global burden of disease team are still not available from all the Indian states.[112] Additionally, there are also several challenges to measure the epidemiological burden of neurological diseases and injuries to estimate the true magnitude of the problem in India.[113]

Neurological disability is poorly understood by the health system as well as healthcare providers in both government and private sectors in India.[114] There is no system for the management of disability and provision of rehabilitation services in general, let alone neurological rehabilitation.[114] Noncomprehensive, unidisciplinary services led by neurologists or physiotherapists, predominantly in private tertiary care hospitals in urban cities are the only kind of rehabilitation services that are available for people with disabilities.[115] Access to comprehensive and consistent rehabilitation services from multidisciplinary teams is hardly available even in urban contexts. Even if available, they are not affordable.[115]

Given this context, there are not any specific pathways and protocols for the comprehensive management of pregnant women with neurological conditions in most healthcare facilities in India.[116] There are several implications for practice, policy, and research which will be dealt with next in this chapter.

IMPLICATIONS FOR PRACTICE, POLICY, AND RESEARCH

Neurological conditions during pregnancy have several practice implications. First and foremost is the evidence for medical and surgical management of pregnant women with neurological diseases.[117] Although evidence for clinical management of pregnant women with neurological conditions is available in HICs, translating the evidence for LMICs like India is highly challenging. This is particularly because of the difference in access to the medicines between HICs and LMICs as well as the affordability of these medicines in LMICs.[118] Additionally when there is not a system in place for disability management and rehabilitation in a country like India, it is not pragmatically possible to translate evidence related to rehabilitation from HICs. Even if we try translating such evidence, it may not be as intensive and comprehensive as that implemented in HICs.[118]

Secondly, the implications relate to the skills and competencies of the health workforce to cater to the needs of pregnant women with neurological conditions. Although there are specialists like neurologists and obstetricians/gynecologists available in India, it is expected that the competencies and skills may not be consistent among all healthcare providers. Especially because there is hardly a common pathway and protocol for practice.[104-116] Thirdly, the awareness and knowledge of disability management among health professionals involved management of pregnant women with neurological disabilities. In many LMICs including India, disability is not conceptualized from an ICF perspective. Disability is only approached from a charity perspective where disability is only sympathized with, and people believe that disability can only be alleviated through charity.[98]

The implications for practice inform the need for research in this area of neurological science. The paucity of evidence on the questions related to neurology in pregnancy specific to LMICs and India is an important implication.[117] Understanding the magnitude of the problem, developing complex interventions, and scaling it up require data and information at all levels. Even estimation of the problem is not possible without reliable and consistent data. Hence, documenting data related to practice as well as the research questions on this topic starting from the epidemiological burden of neurology in pregnancy is very pertinent.[116-118] These kinds of systematic data collection and optimization of the available data can help in gathering affirmative evidence on this topic and enable the generation of evidence that are relevant to the context.

The above implications give plausible opportunities for policy change related to this topic in a context like India. If practice could be standardized and research evidence can inform practice, it could potentially help in developing and ratifying existing policies related to antenatal care for women with a neurological disorder, access to medicines, and coverage of insurance for medical as well as rehabilitation management of pregnant women with neurological disabilities.[116-118] The current context of LMICs, including in India, requires policy and programmatic change to provide safe, effective, and good quality care for those requiring support during their pregnancy, specifically with neurological diseases and disabilities.

CONCLUSION

The global burden of morbidity and disability experienced by pregnant women experiencing neurological conditions is becoming a potential silent epidemic. This implies the importance of looking at this issue as a public health issue rather than a clinical problem. In the world's most populous country like India, it is absolutely crucial to understand the magnitude of this problem and identify strategies to address it. The efforts to reduce maternal mortality and morbidity through national and state-led programs have been immense in the context of India. A significant proportion of financial allocation has been to these programs. However, it is unfortunate that scientific global evidence of preventing and promoting the health of pregnant women, particularly those experiencing neurological problems is not integrated with the existing national programs in India to reduce the burden of this problem. Therefore, developing interventions to bridge this implementation gap and integrate these newly developed interventions within the national and state-led programs for sexual and reproductive health must be a public health priority. These could strengthen the health and social care system in India to bridge the implementation gaps as well as address the unmet needs of pregnant women with neurological problems in India.

REFERENCES

1. Fowler JR, Mahdy H, Jack BW. (2022). Pregnancy. [online] Available from ncbi.nlm.nih.gov/books/NBK448166/. [Last accessed March, 2023].
2. Toscano M, Thornburg LL. Neurological diseases in pregnancy. Curr Opin Obstet Gynecol. 2019;31(2):97-109.
3. GBD 2016 Neurology Collaborators. Global, regional, and national burden of neurological disorders, 1990-2016: a systematic analysis for the Global Burden of Disease Study 2016. Lancet Neurol. 2019;18(5):459-80.
4. Sawle GV, Ramsay MM. The neurology of pregnancy. J Neurol Neurosurg Psychiatry. 1998;64(6):711-25.
5. Anheim M. Neurology and pregnancy: The delivery. Rev Neurol (Paris). 2021;177(3):166-7.
6. Brussé IA, Kluivers ACM, Zambrano MD, Shetler K, Miller EC. Neuro-obstetrics: A multidisciplinary approach to care of women with neurologic disease. Handb Clin Neurol. 2020;171:143-60.
7. Dathe K, Schaefer C. The use of medication in pregnancy. Dtsch Arztebl Int. 2019;116(46):783-90.
8. Andermann A; CLEAR Collaboration. Taking action on the social determinants of health in clinical practice: a framework for health professionals. CMAJ. 2016;188(17-18):E474-E483.
9. Kalinowska A, Kułakowska A, Adamczyk-Sowa M, Czajkowski K, Kurowska K, Pietrzak B, et al. Recommendations for neurological, obstetrical and gynaecological care in women with multiple sclerosis: a statement by a working group convened by the Section of Multiple Sclerosis and Neuroimmunology of the Polish Neurological Society. Neurol Neurochir Pol. 2020;54(2):125-37.
10. Miller EC, Vollbracht S. Neurology of preeclampsia and related disorders: An update in neuro-obstetrics. Curr Pain Headache Rep. 2021;25(6):40.
11. Jaglal SB, Guilcher SJT, Bereket T, Kwan M, Munce S, Conklin J, et al. Development of a Chronic Care Model for Neurological Conditions (CCM-NC). BMC Health Serv Res. 2014;14:409.
12. Hosley CM, McCullough LD. Acute neurological issues in pregnancy and the peripartum. Neurohospitalist. 2011;1(2):104-16.
13. French JA, Meador K. Risks of Epilepsy During Pregnancy: How Much Do We Really Know? JAMA Neurol. 2015;72(9):973-4.

14. Thomas SV. Managing epilepsy in pregnancy. Neurol India. 2011;59(1):59-65.
15. Menon S, Siewe Fodjo JN, Weckhuysen S, Bhwana D, Njamnshi AK, Dekker M, et al. Women with epilepsy in sub-Saharan Africa: A review of the reproductive health challenges and perspectives for management. Seizure. 2019;71:312-7.
16. Haider B, von Oertzen J. Neurological disorders. Best Pract Res Clin Obstet Gynaecol. 2013;27(6):867-75.
17. Kaddumukasa M, Mugenyi L, Kaddumukasa MN, Ddumba E, Devereaux M, Furlan A, et al. Prevalence and incidence of neurological disorders among adult Ugandans in rural and urban Mukono district; a cross-sectional study. BMC Neurol. 2016;16:227.
18. Kass JS, Rose RV. Legal and ethical challenges in the care of the pregnant patient after brain death. Continuum (Minneap Minn). 2022;28(1):180-5.
19. Christyn E, Guidon AC. Neuromuscular disorders in pregnancy. Semin Neurol. 2017;37(06):643-52.
20. Platz T, Giorgio S. Specialty Grand Challenge for NeuroRehabilitation Research. Front Neurol. 2020;11:349.
21. Ahmed R, Apen K, Endean C. Epilepsy in pregnancy—a collaborative team effort of obstetricians, neurologists and primary care physicians for a successful outcome. Aust Fam Physician. 2014;43(3):112-6.
22. Thomas SV. Neurological illness in pregnancy. Indian J Med Res. 2018;148(3):355-6.
23. Lopez-Leon S, Geissbühler Y, Sabidó M, Turkson M, Wahlich C, Morris JK. A systematic review and meta-analyses of pregnancy and fetal outcomes in women with multiple sclerosis: a contribution from the IMI2 ConcePTION project. J Neurol. 2020;267:2721-31.
24. Sanghavi M, Rutherford JD. Cardiovascular physiology of pregnancy. Circulation. 2014;130(12):1003-8.
25. Harvey S, King MD, Gorman KM. Paroxysmal movement disorders. Front Neurol. 2021;12:659064.
26. Varytė G, Zakarevičienė J, Ramašauskaitė D, Laužikienė D, Arlauskienė A. Pregnancy and multiple sclerosis: An Update on the Disease Modifying Treatment Strategy and a Review of Pregnancy's Impact on Disease Activity. Medicina (Kaunas). 2020;56(2):49.
27. Weimer LH. Neuromuscular disorders in pregnancy. Handb Clin Neurol. 2020;172:201-18.
28. Goadsby PJ, Goldberg J, Silberstein SD. Migraine in pregnancy. BMJ. 2008;336(7659):1502-4.
29. Petrovski BÉ, Vetvik KG, Lundqvist C, Eberhard-Gran M. Characteristics of menstrual versus non-menstrual migraine during pregnancy: a longitudinal population-based study. J Headache Pain. 2018;19:27.
30. Tomson T, Battino D, Perucca E. Teratogenicity of antiepileptic drugs. Curr Opin Neurol. 2019;32(2):246-52.
31. Breymann C. Iron Deficiency Anemia in Pregnancy. Semin Hematol. 2015;52(4):339-47.
32. Piccinni MP, Lombardelli L, Logiodice F, Kullolli O, Parronchi P, Romagnani S. How pregnancy can affect autoimmune diseases progression? Clin Mol Allergy. 2016:14;11.
33. Feghali M, Venkataramanan R, Caritis S. Pharmacokinetics of drugs in pregnancy. Semin Perinatol. 2015;39(7):512-9.
34. Daroff R, Bradley W, Jankovic J. Bradley and Daroff's Neurology in clinical practice, 8th edition. Philadelphia: Elsevier; 2021. pp. 1614-63.e14.
35. Kazma JM, van den Anker J, Allegaert K, Dallmann A, Ahmadzia HK. Anatomical and physiological alterations of pregnancy. J Pharmacokinet Pharmacodyn. 2020;47(4):271-85.
36. Thomas SV, Syam U, Devi JS. Predictors of seizures during pregnancy in women with epilepsy. Epilepsia. 2012;53(5):e85-8.
37. Battino D, Tomson T, Bonizzoni E, Craig J, Lindhout D, Sabers A, et al. Seizure control and treatment changes in pregnancy: Observations from the EURAP epilepsy pregnancy registry. Epilepsia. 2013;54(9):1621-7.
38. Pennell PB; EURAP Study Group. Seizure control and treatment in pregnancy: observations from the EURAP epilepsy pregnancy registry. Neurology. 2006;66(3):354-60.
39. Pennell PB, French JA, May RC, Gerard E, Kalayjian L, Penovich P, et al.; MONEAD Study Group. Changes in Seizure Frequency and Antiepileptic Therapy during Pregnancy. N Engl J Med. 2020;383(26):2547-56.
40. Harden CL, Hopp J, Ting TY, Pennell PB, French JA, Hauser WA, et al.; American Academy of Neurology; American Epilepsy Society. Practice parameter update: management issues for women with epilepsy--focus on pregnancy (an evidence-based review): obstetrical complications and change in seizure frequency: report of the Quality Standards Subcommittee and Therapeutics and Technology Assessment Subcommittee of the American Academy of Neurology and American Epilepsy Society. Neurology. 2009;73(2):126-32.
41. Adab N, Kini U, Vinten J, Ayres J, Baker G, Clayton-Smith J, et al. The longer term outcome of children born to mothers with epilepsy. J Neurol Neurosurg Psychiatry. 2004;75(11):1575-83.
42. MacDonald SC, Bateman BT, McElrath TF, Hernández-Díaz S. Mortality and Morbidity During Delivery Hospitalization Among Pregnant Women with Epilepsy in the United States. JAMA Neurol. 2015;72(9):981-8.
43. Edey S, Moran N, Nashef L. SUDEP and epilepsy-related mortality in pregnancy. Epilepsia. 2014;55(7):e72-4.
44. Thomas SV, Indrani L, Devi GC, Jacob S, Beegum J, Jacob PP, et al. Pregnancy in women with epilepsy: preliminary results of Kerala registry of epilepsy and pregnancy. Neurol India. 2001;49(1):60-6.
45. Magley M, Hinson MR. (2022). Eclampsia. [online] Available from https://www.ncbi.nlm.nih.gov/books/NBK554392/. [Last accessed March, 20123].
46. Karjalainen L, Tikkanen M, Rantanen K, Laivuori H, Gissler M, Ijäs P. Pregnancy-associated stroke—a systematic review of subsequent pregnancies and maternal health. BMC Pregnancy Childbirth. 2019;19(1):187.
47. Camargo EC, Feske SK, Singhal AB. Stroke in Pregnancy: An Update. Neurol Clin. 2019;37(1):131-48.
48. Liu S, Chan WS, Ray JG, Kramer MS, Joseph KS. Stroke and cerebrovascular disease in pregnancy. Stroke. 2019;50(1):13-20.
49. Lv X, Liu P, Li Y. The clinical characteristics and treatment of cerebral AVM in pregnancy. Neuroradiol J. 2015;28(3):234-7.
50. Cantu-Brito C, Arauz A, Aburto Y, Barinagarrementeria F, Ruiz-Sandoval JL, Baizabal-Carvallo JF. Cerebrovascular complications during pregnancy and postpartum: clinical and prognosis observations in 240 Hispanic women. Eur J Neurol [Internet]. 2011;18(6):819-25.
51. Wu P, Haththotuwa R, Kwok CS, Babu A, Kotronias RA, Rushton C, et al. Preeclampsia and Future Cardiovascular Health: A Systematic Review and MetaAnalysis. Circ Cardiovasc Qual Outcomes [Internet]. 2017;10(2):e003497.
52. Elgendy IY, Nadeau SE, Bairey Merz CN, Pepine CJ. Migraine Headache: An Under-Appreciated Risk Factor for Cardiovascular Disease in Women. J Am Heart Assoc. 2019;8:e014546.
53. Bandoli G, Baer RJ, Gano D, Pawlowski LJ, Chambers C. Migraines during pregnancy and the risk of maternal stroke. JAMA Neurol. 2020;77(9):1177-9.
54. Bates SM, Greer IA, Middeldorp S, Veenstra DL, Prabulos AM, Vandvik PO. VTE, thrombophilia, antithrombotic therapy, and pregnancy: Antithrombotic Therapy and Prevention of Thrombosis, 9th edition; American College of Chest Physicians Evidence-Based Clinical Practice Guidelines. Chest. 2012;141(suppl):e691S-736S.
55. Powers WJ, Rabinstein AA, Ackerson T, Adeoye OM, Bambakidis NC, Becker K, et al.; American Heart Association Stroke Council. 2018 Guidelines for the Early Management of Patients with Acute Ischemic Stroke: A Guideline for Healthcare Professionals from the American Heart Association/American Stroke Association. Stroke. 2018;49(3):e46-110.

56. Negro A, Delaruelle Z, Ivanova TA, Khan S, Ornello R, Raffaelli B, et al.; European Headache Federation School of Advanced Studies (EHF-SAS). Headache and pregnancy: a systematic review. J Headache Pain. 2017;18(1):106.
57. Maggioni F, Alessi C, Maggino T, Zanchin G. Headache during pregnancy. Cephalalgia. 1997;17(7):765-9.
58. Granella F, Sances G, Pucci E, Nappi RE, Ghiotto N, Napp G. Migraine with aura and reproductive life events: a case control study. Cephalalgia. 2000;20(8):701-7.
59. Evans RW, Friedman DI. Expert opinion: the management of pseudotumor cerebri during pregnancy. Headache. 2000;40(6): 495-7.
60. Kesler A, Kupferminc M. Idiopathic intracranial hypertension and pregnancy. Clin Obstet Gynecol. 2013;56(2):389-96.
61. Robbins MS. Headache in Pregnancy. Continuum (Minneap Minn). 2018;24(4, Headache):1092-107.
62. Saldanha IJ, Roth JL, Chen KK, Zullo AR, Adam GP, Konnyu KJ, et al. Management of Primary Headaches in Pregnancy [Internet]. Rockville (MD): Agency for Healthcare Research and Quality (US); 2020. (Comparative Effectiveness Review, No. 234.) [online] Available from https://www.ncbi.nlm.nih.gov/books/NBK564853/?report=classic. [Last accessed March, 2023].
63. Klein A. Peripheral nerve disease in pregnancy. Clin Obstet Gynecol. 2013;56(2):382-8.
64. Rosier C, Camdessanché JP. Neuropathy and pregnancy: An overview. Rev Neurol (Paris). 2021;177(3):220-4.
65. Miyasaki JM, Aldakheel A. Movement disorders in pregnancy. Continuum (Minneap Minn). 2014;20(1 Neurology of Pregnancy): 148-61.
66. Kranick SM, Mowry EM, Colcher A, Horn S, Golbe LI. Movement disorders and pregnancy: a review of the literature. Mov Disord. 2010;25(6):665-71.
67. Bezerra AS, Andrade AAAJ, Polimanti AC, Fürst RVC, Criado PR, Corrêa JA. Livedoid vasculopathy: diagnosis and treatment in pregnant women. J Vasc Bras. 2020;19:e20190093.
68. Rocha EA, Topcuoglu MA, Silva GS, Singhal AB. RCVS2 score and diagnostic approach for reversible cerebral vasoconstriction syndrome. Neurology. 2019;92(7):e639-47.
69. Maragkos GA, Ascanio LC, Chida K, Boone MD, Ogilvy CS, Thomas AJ, et al. Moyamoya disease in pregnancy: a systematic review. Acta Neurochir (Wien). 2018;160(9):1711-9.
70. Manasewitsch NT, Hanfy AA, Beutler BD, Antwi-Amoabeng D, Taha M, Elnaggar M, et al. Postpartum vertebral artery dissection: case report and review of the literature. Thrombosis J. 2020;18:30.
71. Ohene-Frempong K, Weiner SJ, Sleeper LA, Miller ST, Embury S, Moohr JW, et al. Cerebrovascular accidents in sickle cell disease: rates and risk factors. Blood. 1998;91:288-94.
72. Oakley LL, Mitchell S, von Rege I, Hadebe R, Howard J, Robinson SE, et al. Perinatal outcomes in women with sickle cell disease: a matched cohort study from London, UK. Br J Haematol. 2022;196(4):1069-75.
73. Bishop BN, Edemekong PF. (2021). Choriocarcinoma. [online] Available from https://www.ncbi.nlm.nih.gov/books/NBK535434/. [Last accessed March, 2023].
74. Mas JL, Lamy C. Stroke in pregnancy and the puerperium. J Neurol. 1998;245(6-7):305-13.
75. Clark SL. Amniotic fluid embolism. Clin Obstet Gynecol. 2010;53(2):322-8.
76. McBride AM. Clinical Presentation and Treatment of Amniotic Fluid Embolism. AACN Adv Crit Care. 2018;29(3):336-42.
77. Hamel J, Ciafaloni E. An Update: Myasthenia Gravis and Pregnancy. Neurol Clin. 2018;36(2):355-65.
78. Grover KM, Sripathi N. Myasthenia gravis and pregnancy. Muscle Nerve. 2020;62(6):664-72.
79. Chaudhry SA, Vignarajah B, Koren G. Myasthenia gravis during pregnancy. Can Fam Physician. 2012;58(12):1346-9.
80. Manu P, Rogozea LM, Roman-Filip C. Pharmacological management of myasthenia gravis: A century of expert opinions in Cecil Textbook of Medicine. Am J Ther. 2021;28(6):e631-7.
81. Sanders DB, Wolfe GI, Benatar M, Evoli A, Gilhus NE, Illa I, et al. International consensus guidance for management of myasthenia gravis: Executive summary. Neurology. 2016;87(4):419-25.
82. Tsui A, Lee MA. Multiple sclerosis and pregnancy. Curr Opin Obstet Gynecol. 2011;23(6):435-9.
83. Varytė G, Arlauskienė A, Ramašauskaitė D. Pregnancy and multiple sclerosis: an update. Curr Opin Obstet Gynecol. 2021;33(5):378-83.
84. Li H, Hu F, Zhang Y, Li K. Comparative efficacy and acceptability of disease-modifying therapies in patients with relapsing-remitting multiple sclerosis: a systematic review and network meta-analysis. J Neurol. 2020;267(12):3489-98.
85. Christian C, Michael H, Marie HM, Patricia CT, Thibault M. Rate of Pregnancy-Related Relapse in Multiple Sclerosis. N Engl J Med. 1998;339:285-91.
86. Park-Wyllie L, Mazzotta P, Pastuszak A, Moretti ME, Beique L, Hunnisett L, et al. Birth defects after maternal exposure to corticosteroids: prospective cohort study and meta-analysis of epidemiological studies. Teratology. 2000;62:385-92.
87. Hellwig K, Neudorfer O, Melamed-Gal S, Qassem S, Baruch P. Pregnancy outcomes in patients with multiple sclerosis and exposure to branded glatiramer acetate during all three trimesters. Paris, France: ECTRIMS-ACTRIMS; 2017.
88. Hellwig K, Geissbuhler Y, Sabido M, Popescu C, Adamo A, Klinger J, et al. Pregnancy outcomes in interferon-beta-exposed patients with multiple sclerosis: results from the European Interferon-beta Pregnancy Registry. J Neurol. 2020;267:1715-23.
89. Hellwig K, Thiel S, Ciplea AI, Galazka A, Schick R, Hubschen M. Pregnancy of MS patients treated with cladribine tablets. Toronto, Canada: AAN; 2020.
90. Edlow JA, Caplan LR, O'Brien K, Tibbles CD. Diagnosis of acute neurological emergencies in pregnant and post-partum women. Lancet Neurol. 2013;12:175-85.
91. Ural UM, Balik G, Sentürk S, Ustüner I, Cobanoğlu U, Sahin FK. Posterior Reversible Encephalopathy Syndrome in a Postpartum Preeclamptic Woman without Seizure. Case Rep Obstet Gynecol. 2014;2014:657903.
92. Liman TG, Bohner G, Heuschmann PU, Scheel M, Endres M, Siebert E. Clinical and radiological differences in posterior reversible encephalopathy syndrome between patients with preeclampsia-eclampsia and other predisposing diseases. Eur J Neurol. 2012;19(7):935-43.
93. Postma IR, Slager S, Kremer HP, de Groot JC, Zeeman GG. Long-term consequences of the posterior reversible encephalopathy syndrome in eclampsia and preeclampsia: a review of the obstetric and non-obstetric literature. Obstet Gynecol Surv. 2014;69:287-300.
94. Chataway JE, Hardman EL. Thiamine in Wernicke's syndrome—how much and how long? Postgrad Med J. 1995;71:249.
95. Yoon CK, Chang MH, Lee DC. Wernicke-Korsakoff syndrome associated with hyperemesis gravidarum. Korean J Ophthalmol. 2005;19(3):239-42.
96. Wade DT. Epidemiology of disabling neurological disease: how and why does disability occur? J Neurol Neurosurg Psychiatry. 1997;63:S11-8.
97. Kostanjsek N. Use of The International Classification of Functioning, Disability and Health (ICF) as a conceptual framework and common language for disability statistics and health information systems. BMC Public Health. 2011;11:S3.
98. Krahn GL. WHO World Report on Disability: a review. Disabil Health J. 2011;4(3):141-2.
99. Andersen JB, Wandall-Holm MF, Andersen PK, Sellebjerg F, Magyari M. Pregnancy in women with MS: Impact on long-term disability accrual in a nationwide Danish Cohort. Mult Scler. 2022;28(8):1239-47.

100. Redshaw M, Malouf R, Gao H, Gray R. Women with disability: the experience of maternity care during pregnancy, labour and birth and the postnatal period. BMC Pregnancy Childbirth. 2013;13:174.
101. Tarasoff LA, Ravindran S, Malik H, Salaeva D, Brown HK. Maternal disability and risk for pregnancy, delivery, and postpartum complications: a systematic review and meta-analysis. Am J Obstet Gynecol. 2020;222(1):27.e1-27.e32.
102. Tarasoff LA, Murtaza F, Carty A, Salaeva D, Hamilton AD, Brown HK. Health of newborns and infants born to women with disabilities: A meta-analysis. Pediatrics. 2020;146(6):e20201635.
103. Malouf R, Henderson J, Redshaw M. Access and quality of maternity care for disabled women during pregnancy, birth and the postnatal period in England: data from a national survey. BMJ Open. 2017;7:e016757.
104. Bohren MA, Hofmeyr GJ, Sakala C, Fukuzawa RK, Cuthbert A. Continuous support for women during childbirth. Cochrane Database Syst Rev. 2017;7(7):CD003766.
105. Carter AM. Placental Gas Exchange and the Oxygen Supply to the Fetus. Compr Physiol. 2015;5(3):1381-403.
106. Heideveld-Gerritsen M, van Vulpen M, Hollander M, Oude Maatman S, Ockhuijsen H, van den Hoogen A. Maternity care experiences of women with physical disabilities: A systematic review. Midwifery. 2021;96:102938.
107. Kochhar AS, Bhasin R, Kochhar GK, Dadlani H, Mehta VV, Kaur R, et al. Lockdown of 1.3 billion people in India during Covid-19 pandemic: A survey of its impact on mental health. Asian J Psychiatr. 2020;54:102213.
108. Prinja S, Sharma A, Nimesh R, Sharma V, Madan Gopal K, Badgaiyan N, et al. Impact of National Health Mission on infant mortality in India: An interrupted time series analysis. Int J Health Plann Manage. 2021;36(4):1143-52.
109. Black RE, Walker N, Laxminarayan R, Temmerman M. Chapter 1. Reproductive, Maternal, Newborn, and Child Health: Key Messages of This Volume. In: Black RE, Laxminarayan R, Temmerman M, Walker N (Eds). Reproductive, Maternal, Newborn, and Child Health: Disease Control Priorities, 3rd edition (Volume 2). Washington (DC): The International Bank for Reconstruction and Development/The World Bank; 2016.
110. Ali B, Dhillon P, Mohanty SK. Inequalities in the utilization of maternal health care in the pre- and post-National Health Mission periods in India. J Biosoc Sci. 2020;52(2):198-212.
111. Bagchi T, Das A, Dawad S, Dalal K. Non-utilization of public healthcare facilities during sickness: a national study in India. J Public Health (Berl.) 2022;30:943-51.
112. India State-Level Disease Burden Initiative Neurological Disorders Collaborators. The burden of neurological disorders across the states of India: the Global Burden of Disease Study 1990-2019. Lancet Glob Health. 2021;9(8):e1129-44.
113. Gourie-Devi M. Epidemiology of neurological disorders in India: review of background, prevalence and incidence of epilepsy, stroke, Parkinson's disease and tremors. Neurol India. 2014;62(6):588-98. Erratum in: Neurol India. 2016;64(5):1110-1.
114. Das A, Botticello AL, Wylie GR, Radhakrishnan K. Neurologic disability: a hidden epidemic for India. Neurology. 2012;79(21):2146-7.
115. Pal HR, Saxena S, Chandrashekhar K, Sudha SJ, Murthy RS, Thara R, et al. Issues related to disability in India: a focus group study. Natl Med J India. 2000;13(5):237-41.
116. Senjam SS, Singh A. Addressing the health needs of people with disabilities in India. Indian J Public Health. 2020;64(1):79-82.
117. Birbeck G, Meyer AC, Ogunniyi A. Nervous system disorders across the life course in resource-limited settings. Nature. 2015;527:S167-71.
118. Howard LM, Khalifeh H. Perinatal mental health: a review of progress and challenges. World Psychiatry. 2020;19(3):313-27.

96
CHAPTER

Neurocutaneous Syndromes

Maya Thomas, Sangeetha Yoganathan, Dharshini Sathishkumar

INTRODUCTION

Neurocutaneous disorders, also referred to as Phakomatoses earlier, have their origin in the Greek word phakos, meaning "mother spot" or birthmark. These include a diverse group of disorders with predominant involvement of the skin and central nervous system tissues, owing to their common origin from the ectoderm. They are now believed to be disorders of neural crest tissue and are also called neurocristopathies. The disorders that are categorized under neurocristopathies include tuberous sclerosis complex (TSC), neurofibromatosis type 1 (NF1), neurofibromatosis type 2 (NF2), epidermal nevus syndrome, neurocutaneous melanocytosis, incontinentia pigmenti, and hypomelanosis of Ito. Additional disorders that are considered under phakomatosis are Sturge-Weber syndrome, von Hippel-Lindau syndrome, and ataxia telangiectasia, to mention a few. Recognizing and being familiar with these skin lesions is important as they provide a clue to the underlying neurological disorder. Four major disorders will be discussed, and the salient features of the rest are represented in **Table 1**.[1]

TABLE 1: Other neurocutaneous disorders.

Syndrome	Neurologic features	Non-neurologic features	Inheritance/Gene
Schwannomatosis	Multiple schwannomas	Subcutaneous schwannomas	Autosomal dominant, *INI1/ SMARCB1* on chromosome 22
Epidermal nevus syndrome **(Fig. 1)**	Hemimegalencephaly, epilepsy, intellectual disability, and focal motor deficits	Linear verrucous lesions in craniofacial distribution, precocious puberty, renal anomalies, colobomas	Sporadic
Von Hippel–Lindau disease	Retinal, cerebellar and spinal hemangioblastomas	Tumors of the pancreas, kidney, epididymis, and endolymphatic sac tumors	Autosomal dominant. *VHL* gene on chromosome 3p25-26
Neurocutaneous melanosis **(Fig. 2)**	Hydrocephalus, seizures, behavioral abnormalities	Giant hairy pigmented nevi, multiple hyperpigmented cutaneous nevi	Sporadic
Pigmentary mosaicism[2] **(Fig. 3)**	Intellectual disability, seizures, ocular features such as strabismus, myopia, and optic nerve hypoplasia	Linear streaks or whorls of hypo- or hyperpigmentation along lines of Blaschko	Sporadic
Incontinentia pigmenti **(Fig. 4)**	Intellectual disability, seizures, pyramidal tract dysfunction, ocular abnormalities such as retinal detachment	Hyperpigmented brown macular lesions along lines of Blaschko that evolve through 3 stages of vesiculobullous lesions, verrucous lesions, and the final brown lesions	X-linked dominant, *NEMO* gene

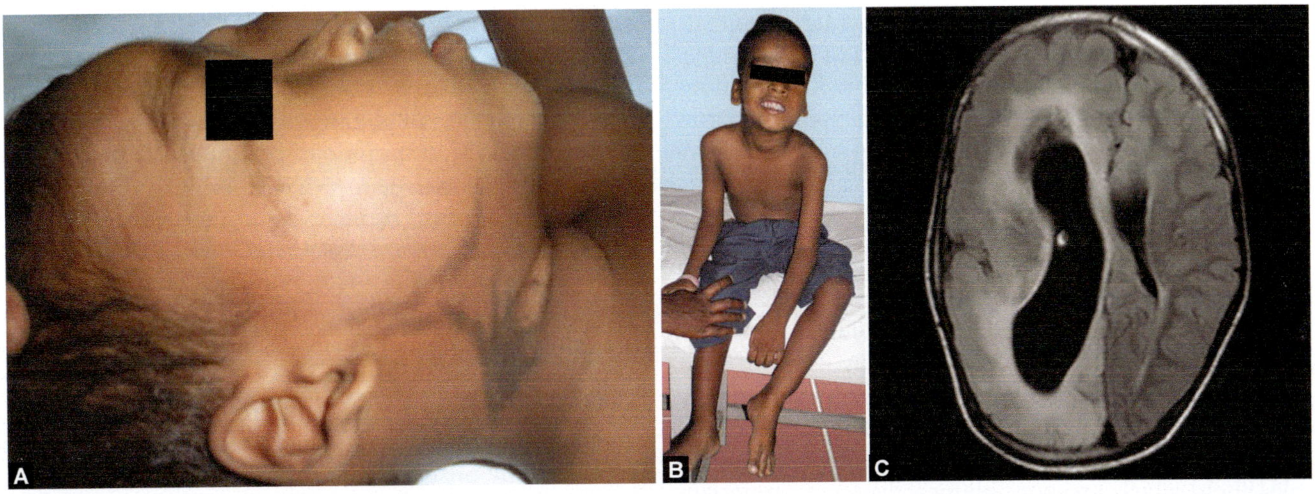

FIGS. 1A TO C: Linear verrucous lesions along the right side of neck and face in a child with epidermal nevus syndrome. T2-FLAIR axial image of the brain shows flat and thick gyri involving the entire right cerebral hemisphere suggestive of hemimegalencephaly causing left hemiparesis and refractory epilepsy.

(FLAIR: fluid-attenuated inversion recovery)

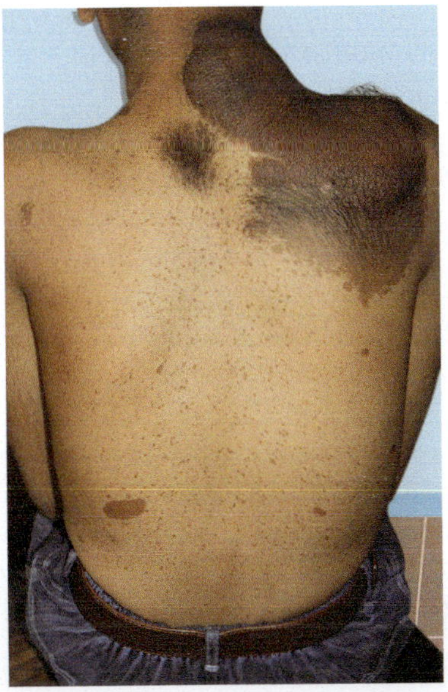

FIG. 2: Giant hairy pigmented nevi and multiple hyperpigmented cutaneous nevi over the back seen in neurocutaneous melanosis.

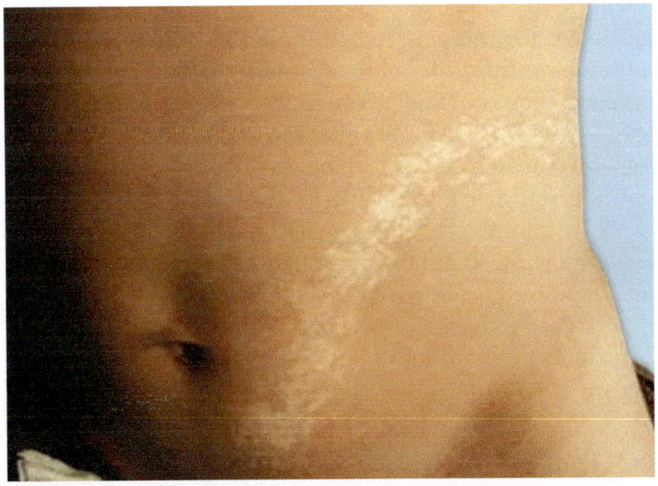

FIG. 3: Linear streak of hypopigmentation along the lines of Blaschko in a child with pigmentary mosaicism.

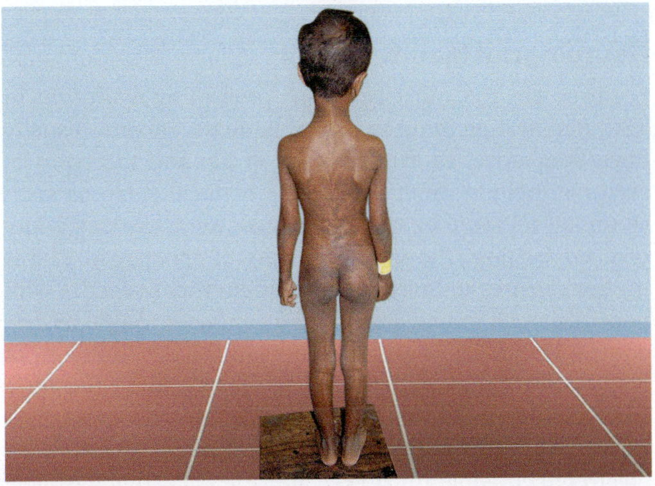

FIG. 4: Extensive hyperpigmented brown macular lesions along lines of Blaschko, the final stage of cutaneous lesion in a child with incontinentia pigmenti.

TUBEROUS SCLEROSIS COMPLEX

Tuberous sclerosis complex is a disorder that can affect multiple organ systems of varying severity and hence has differing clinical expression. It is also called Bourneville's disease, who is credited with the first detailed description of cerebral lesions. Birth incidence is estimated to be 1 in 5,800 live births.[3]

Etiology

It is an autosomal dominant disorder with complete penetrance but variable expressivity. Only one-third of cases are inherited, the rest are sporadic and occur due to spontaneous mutation. Current molecular diagnostic methods detect mutation in either the *TSC1* or *TSC2* gene in 85% of TSC patients, both inherited and sporadic. Mutations in *TSC2* are five times more common in sporadic cases whereas in inherited cases, the proportion of mutations in *TSC1* and *TSC2* is equal.

Pathogenesis

The *TSC1* gene on chromosome 9q34 encodes hamartin and *TSC2* gene on chromosome 16p13.3 encodes tuberin. Hamartin and tuberin complexes normally work together and through a cascade of downstream reactions stimulate protein translation, cell growth, and proliferation. The complex inhibits the GTPase Ras homolog enriched in the brain (Rheb), which is responsible for activating an important intracellular regulator of cell growth and metabolism known as the mammalian target of rapamycin complex 1 (mTORC1). Thus, mutations of hamartin or tuberin in TSC lead to hyperactivation of the downstream mTOR pathway resulting in unchecked cell growth and proliferation. This has led to the use of mTORC1 inhibitors such as sirolimus and everolimus for the treatment of several clinical manifestations of TSC like cerebral subependymal giant cell astrocytoma (SEGA) and renal angiomyolipomas (AMLs). Rapamycin also used in TSC makes the dysregulated mTOR pathway return to normal in cells that lack *TSC1* or *TSC2*.

The brain lesions found in TSC include cortical tubers, subependymal nodules, and SEGA. Heterotopic neurons are commonly scattered in the deep white matter. Cortical tubers are characterized by the proliferation of glial and neuronal cells, and loss of the six-layered structure of the cortex.

Clinical Features

The clinical features of TSC depend on the location of the tubers, which are predominantly located in the brain, skin, eyes, heart, kidneys, and lungs.

Neurological Manifestation

Seizures are the most common presenting symptom in TSC, manifesting in up to 85% of patients. Seizures usually have their onset in the first year of life and the types of seizures include infantile spasms or focal seizures such as unilateral tonic or clonic seizures, tonic eye deviation, or head turning. The natural history of epilepsy in TSC is for the seizures to increase in frequency and severity with poor response to antiseizure medications. Prompt seizure control is important and can prevent the development of epileptic encephalopathy and improve cognitive outcomes. Unfavorable prognostic factors include the onset of seizures in infancy, multiple seizure types, multifocal spikes on electroencephalogram (EEG), and the occurrence of new EEG foci during evolution. Cortical tubers act as epileptic foci and epileptogenesis within these dysplastic neurons is caused by diminished neuronal inhibition, secondary to molecular changes of gamma-aminobutyric acid (GABA) receptors, and enhanced excitation, which is secondary to molecular changes of glutamate receptors. Vigabatrin, an inhibitor of GABA transaminase, through this mechanism can control spasms in up to 95% of children.

Tuberous sclerosis complex-associated neuropsychiatric disorders (TANDs) are associated with cognitive and behavioral manifestations like profound cognitive impairment in about 30% of individuals. This includes attention-deficit hyperactivity disorder (ADHD) and an autistic spectrum disorder. More than 50% have average intelligence but could have specific impairments in memory, attention, or executive skills. The risk for developing autism includes early onset infantile spasms with EEG changes, tubers in the temporal lobe, and a mutation in the *TSC2* gene.

In about 10% of cases, the subependymal nodules transform slowly into SEGAs which are of mixed glioneuronal lineage. Growth of these lesions at the foramen of Monro can block the circulation of the cerebrospinal fluid (CSF), leading to progressive lateral ventricular dilatation and increased intracranial pressure.

Cutaneous Manifestation

Cutaneous lesions are seen in up to 96% of patients with TSC, the most common being facial angiofibroma, also called adenoma sebaceum. These are pink or red papules that appear between 1 and 4 years of age in a butterfly distribution over the nose and cheeks **(Fig. 5)**. The lesions increase in number and size through adolescence. Other skin includes hypomelanotic macules known as ash-leaf macules **(Fig. 6)**, gingival fibromas, thickened, firm areas of subcutaneous tissue often at the lower back called as shagreen patch **(Fig. 7)**, and fibrous plaques on forehead and face **(Fig. 8)**.

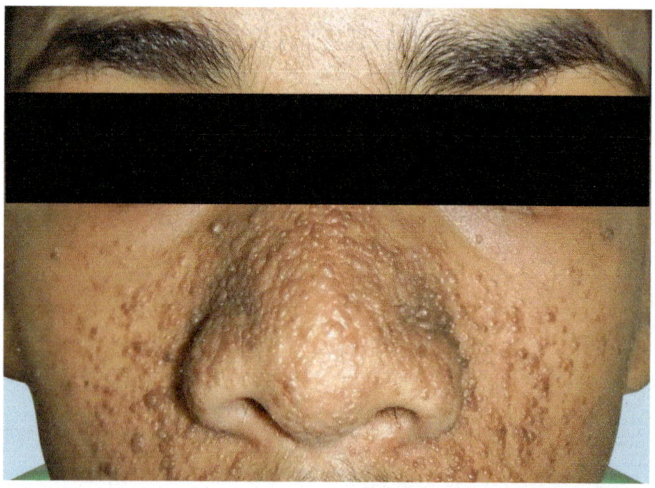

FIG. 5: Adenoma sebaceum, papular lesions in a butterfly distribution over the nose and cheeks.

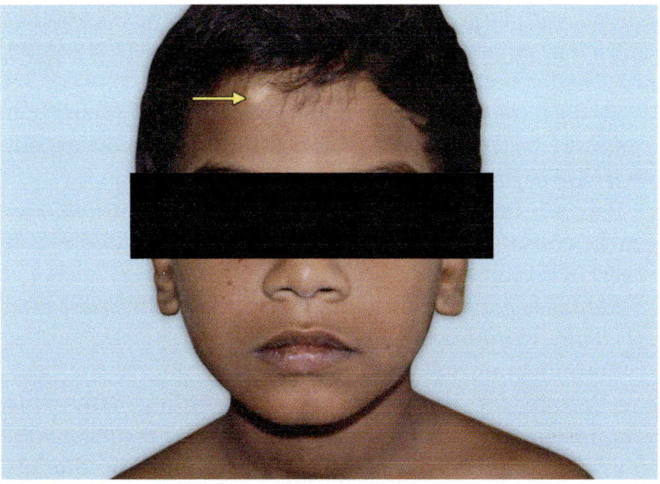

FIG. 6: Hypomelanotic macule or ash leaf macule (arrow) over the forehead.

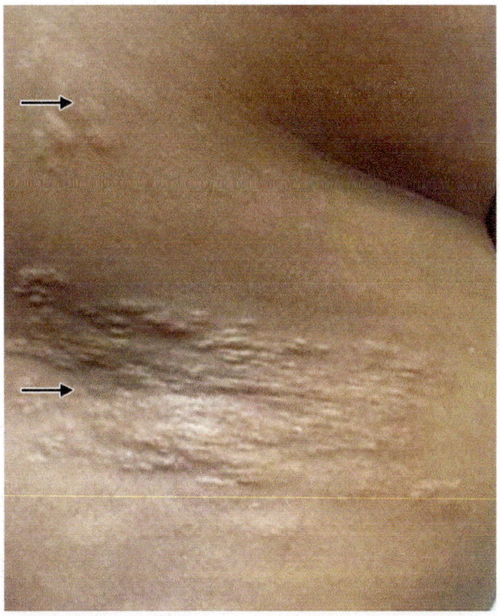

FIG. 7: Shagreen patch (arrow) seen over low back is firm area of subcutaneous tissue.

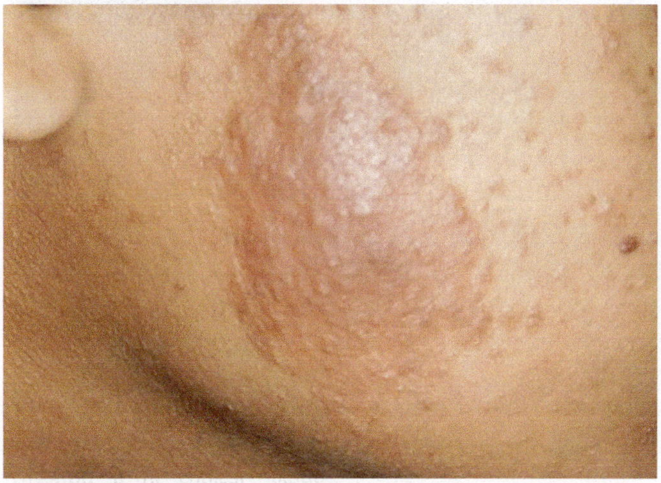

FIG. 8: Fibrous plaque on face.

Other Manifestations

Renal manifestations of TSC are the third most common clinical feature. The lesions seen are AMLs, isolated renal cyst, autosomal dominant polycystic kidney disease (PKD), and renal cell carcinoma. AMLs observed in as many as 80% of individuals with TSC are usually detected after the 3rd year of age. They are usually picked up incidentally but can also cause nonspecific flank pain. The AMLs potentially carry a risk of life-threatening hemorrhage from rupture of the dysplastic feeding blood vessel.

Cardiac involvement is usually in the form of rhabdomyomas, seen in 50–60% of patients with TSC. They are benign tumors that develop during intrauterine life and usually undergo spontaneous regression in the first few years of life. They produce symptoms predominantly through outflow tract obstruction, interference with valvular function or they can disrupt electrical conductivity and cause arrhythmias.

Ophthalmic manifestation is mainly in the form of retinal hamartomas present in about 50% of patients and can be found at any age. They appear as rounded, nodular, or lobulated areas on funduscopic examination and cause no symptoms. Rarely do they affect visual acuity when it impinges on the fovea or optic nerve.

Pulmonary involvement occurs in three forms mainly in adult women and is symptomatic only in 1% of them. These are seen as multifocal micronodular pneumocytes hyperplasia, pulmonary cysts, and lymphangioleiomyomatosis (LAM).

Approach to Diagnosis

Cutaneous lesions of TSC are unmistakable and provide the single main clue to the diagnosis. The diagnostic criteria are given in **Table 2**. Diagnosis is made when two major features, or one major and two minor ones are present. However, identification of a pathogenic variant in *TSC1* or *TSC2* is sufficient for the diagnosis or prediction of TSC as clinical manifestations appear at various ages. Genetic testing and counseling should be offered to individuals with TSC when they reach reproductive age and to first-degree relatives of affected individuals.

Management

Current management guidelines are based on the recommendations of the 2021 International Tuberous Sclerosis Complex Consensus Conference. Once a diagnosis of TSC is made, a complete baseline investigative workup should be carried out to determine the extent of involvement of each of organ system. This includes neuroimaging **(Fig. 9)**, ophthalmologic examination, echocardiogram, and renal ultrasound. An EEG needs to be done in case of suspected seizures and when seizure occurrence is unclear such as in unexplained sleep disturbances, behavioral changes or when other alterations in cognitive or neurological function are present. Chest computed tomography (CT) is required in women during adulthood.

Epilepsy in TSC is treated with antiseizure medication depending on the seizure type. Vigabatrin is especially effective in treating infantile spasms in TSC. Adrenocorticotropic hormone (ACTH) can be used if treatment with vigabatrin is unsuccessful.

Tuberous sclerosis complex-associated neuropsychiatric disorders require comprehensive neuropsychological evaluation and appropriate treatment.

Cortical tubers and subependymal nodules require no treatment. SEGA, if asymptomatic, may be left alone but requires periodic neuroimaging to ensure there is no growth.

TABLE 2: Diagnostic criteria for tuberous sclerosis.

Major features	Minor
Hypomelanotic macules (≥3; at least 5 mm diameter)	Confetti skin lesions
Angiofibromas (>3) or fibrous cephalic plaque	Dental enamel pits (≥3)
Ungual fibroma (≥2)	Intraoral fibromas (≥2)
Shagreen patch	Retinal achromic patch
Multiple retinal hamartomas	Multiple renal cysts
Multiple cortical tubers and/or radial migration lines	Nonrenal hamartomas
Subependymal nodule (2)	Sclerotic bone lesions
Subependymal giant cell astrocytoma	
Cardiac rhabdomyoma	
LAM (lymphangiomyomatosis)	
Angiomyolipomas (≥2)	

Note: Definite tuberous sclerosis complex (TSC): Two major features or one major feature with two minor features. *Possible TSC*: Either one major feature or two minor features.

Patients with large or growing SEGA, or with SEGA causing ventricular enlargement, should undergo surgical resection and CSF diversion.

Medical treatment with mammalian target of rapamycin complex (mTOR) inhibitors may be used for growing but otherwise asymptomatic SEGA.

If skin lesions are rapidly changing or disfiguring, they may be considered for excision, laser, or topical application of mTOR inhibitors.

Retinal lesions are left alone, and reevaluation is required only if any symptoms arise.

Embolization followed by corticosteroids is the first-line therapy for angiomyolipoma presenting with acute hemorrhage. Nephrectomy is to be avoided. Treatment with an mTOR inhibitor is the recommended first-line therapy for asymptomatic, growing angiomyolipoma measuring >3 cm in diameter.

Women who develop LAM with moderate-to-severe lung disease will require mTOR inhibitors. They may even be candidates for lung transplantation.

NEUROFIBROMATOSIS TYPE 1

Introduction

Neurofibromatosis type 1 was also known as von Recklinghausen's disease until the end of the 20th century after von Recklinghausen, who in the latter part of the 19th century described tumors arising from the endoneurium of peripheral nerves as "neurofibromas" in two patients.[4]

Currently, neurofibromatosis includes at least three distinct disorders, referred to as NF1, NF2, and schwannomatosis.

Neurofibromatosis type 1 is the most common type of the neurofibromatoses, affecting approximately 1 in 3,000 individuals worldwide.

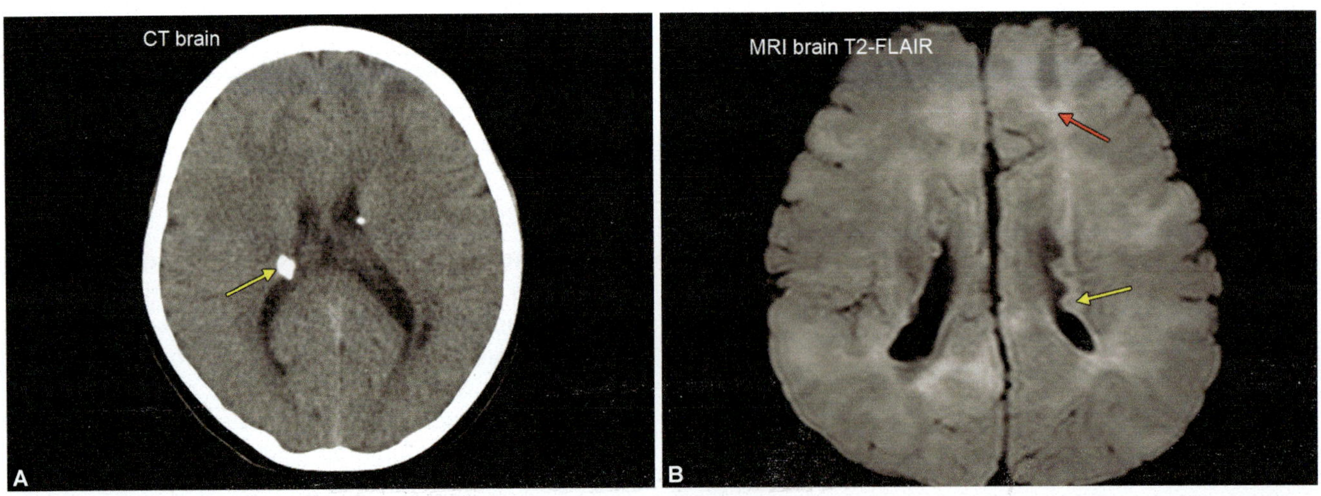

FIGS. 9A AND B: Plain CT brain showing calcified subependymal calcifications (arrow) and MRI brain T2-FLAIR axial image showing subependymal nodules (yellow arrow) seen as projections into the lateral ventricles and high-signal intensities involving the cortex which represent cortical tubers (red arrow).

(CT: computed tomography; FLAIR: fluid-attenuated inversion recovery; MRI: magnetic resonance imaging)

Etiology

Neurofibromatosis type 1 is inherited as an autosomal dominant disorder that affects males and females and all ethnic groups equally. It occurs due to a mutation in the *NF1* gene localized to chromosome 17q11.2 and spans over 350 kb of genomic DNA.

Pathogenesis

The *NF1* gene encodes for the NF1 protein called neurofibromin, which functions as a negative regulator of Ras. Loss of neurofibromin results in high levels of activated Ras. In many cell types, activated Ras is a potent driver of cell proliferation and may be sufficient for tumor formation. In glial cells, through downstream intermediates, Ras regulates cell growth through the Akt/mTOR pathway. Neurofibromin is also a positive regulator of intracellular cyclic adenosine monophosphate (cAMP) levels. Initial studies in Drosophila revealed that learning and memory defects in NF1 mutant flies reflect reduced cAMP generation. Understanding of these pathways has led to clinical trials for new therapeutic drugs.

Clinical Features

Neurofibromatosis type 1 principally affects the skin, bone, and peripheral nervous system and is characterized by multiple café-au-lait spots (CLSs), although CLSs are not specific to NF1 alone.

Café-au-lait macules are flat, pigmented spots that are usually visible in room light regardless of background skin pigmentation **(Fig. 10)**.

Skinfold freckling **(Fig. 11)** is observed in 85% of NF1 individuals after the age of 3 years, and is noticeable in the axillae, groins, at the base of the neck, on the upper eyelids, and under the breasts.

Neurofibromas **(Fig. 12)** are benign tumors that arise from Schwann cells and may occur anywhere in the body and involve a discrete region of an individual nerve. If it involves multiple nerve fascicles and extends over a length of a nerve and its branches, it is called plexiform neurofibroma (PN). Neurofibromas increase in number after puberty.

Iris Lisch nodules are melanocytic hamartomas, which are highly specific to NF1. They appear as dome-shaped pigmented hamartomas on the iris in late childhood, remain asymptomatic, and require a slit-lamp examination to be visualized.

Optic glioma **(Figs. 13A to C)** occurs in approximately 15% of individuals with NF1, usually beginning in the early years of life. The tumors are pilocytic astrocytomas that may involve the optic nerve, chiasm, and/or hypothalamus. Most are asymptomatic, but some may interfere with vision or cause hypothalamic disturbance such as precocious puberty, or other neurological symptoms.

Skeletal dysplasia associated with NF1 includes long bone dysplasia and dysplasia of the sphenoid wing. Long

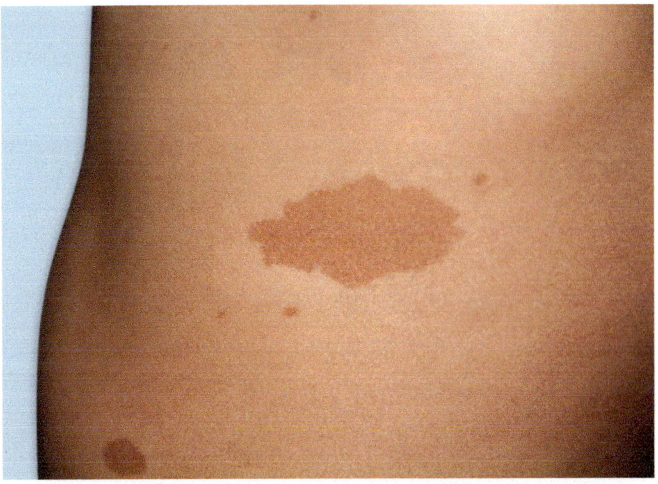

FIG. 10: Café-au-lait macule, hallmark of neurofibromatosis, is a flat, hyperpigmented spot.

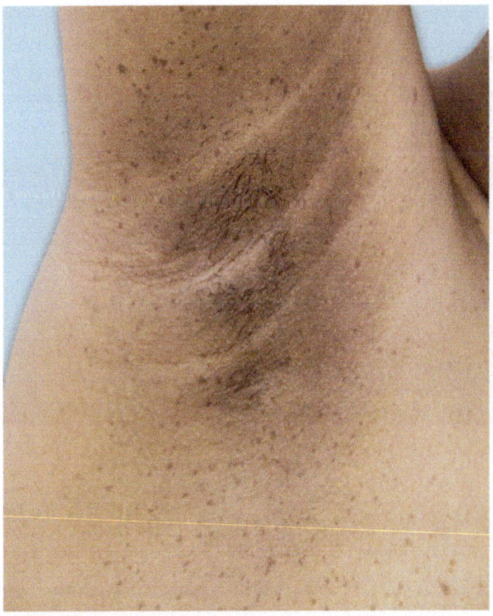

FIG. 11: Axillary freckling (Crowe sign) is clusters of concentrated melanin appearing as flat light brown macules.

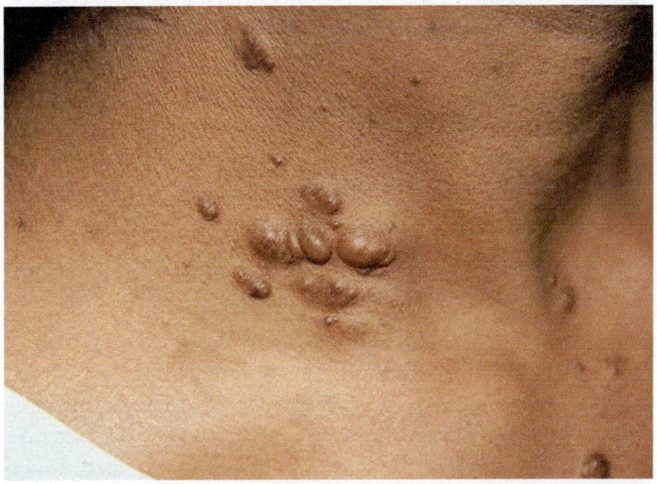

FIG. 12: Cutaneous neurofibromas are fleshy sessile skin lesions that arise from nerves in the skin.

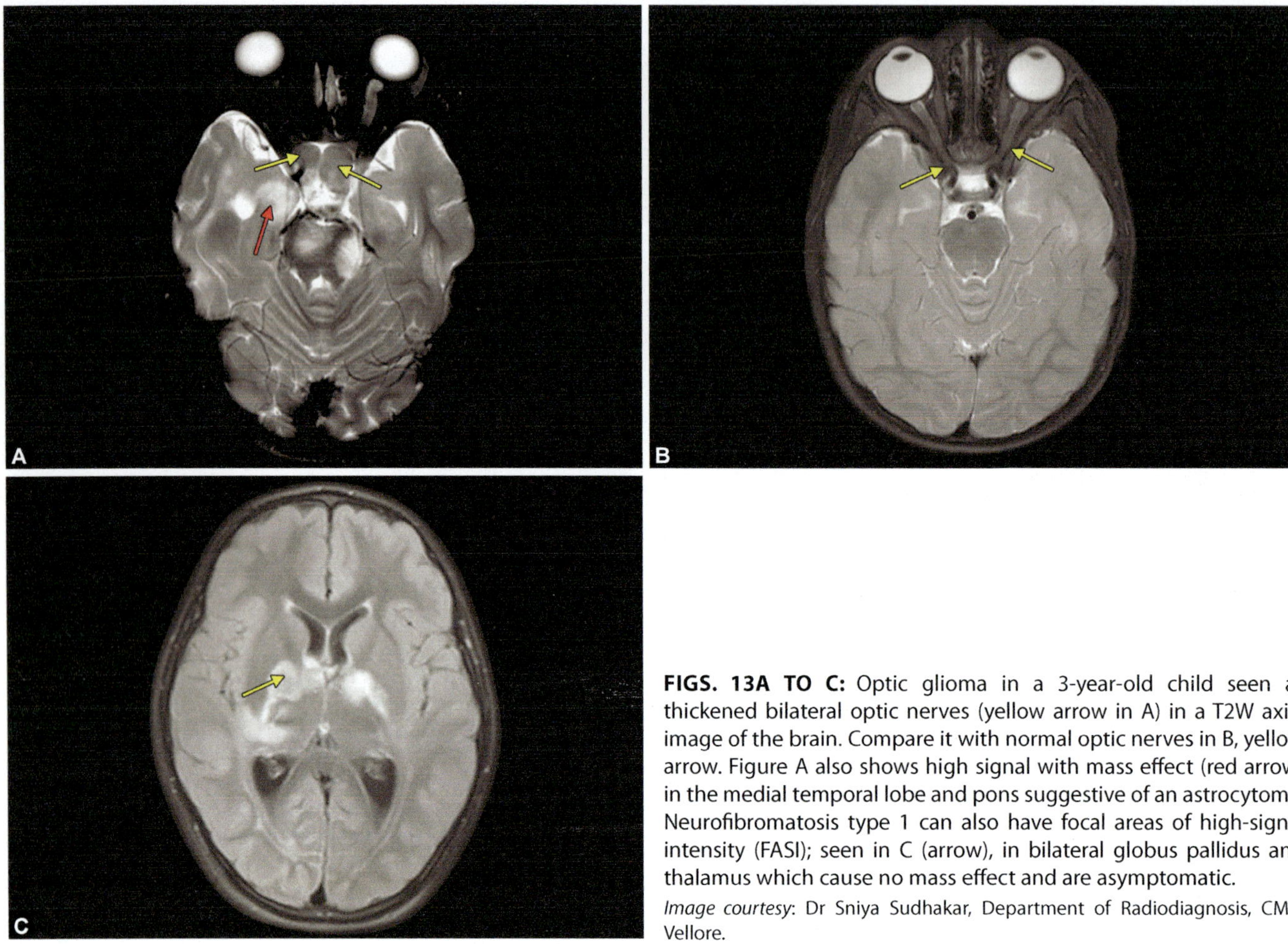

FIGS. 13A TO C: Optic glioma in a 3-year-old child seen as thickened bilateral optic nerves (yellow arrow in A) in a T2W axial image of the brain. Compare it with normal optic nerves in B, yellow arrow. Figure A also shows high signal with mass effect (red arrow) in the medial temporal lobe and pons suggestive of an astrocytoma. Neurofibromatosis type 1 can also have focal areas of high-signal intensity (FASI); seen in C (arrow), in bilateral globus pallidus and thalamus which cause no mass effect and are asymptomatic.

Image courtesy: Dr Sniya Sudhakar, Department of Radiodiagnosis, CMC, Vellore.

bone dysplasia involving the tibia is usually visible in early childhood as the bowing of the leg. It may also involve other long bones such as the fibula, radius, and ulna.

The final diagnostic criterion is the occurrence of a first-degree relative with NF1. Being an autosomal dominant disorder with complete penetrance and variable expression, many parents are first diagnosed when a child is referred for evaluation. Approximately 50% of affected individuals have no affected parent and represent new mutations of the *NF1* gene. Some parents of sporadically affected children may have germline mosaicism, so recurrence is possible, though rare.

Complications seen in NF1 are many and are listed in **Table 3** along with the age and frequency of occurrence.

Approach to Diagnosis

Diagnostic criteria for NF1 are given in **Box 1**. Neuroimaging is warranted in the case of neurological manifestations. Magnetic resonance imaging (MRI) T2 hyperintensities **(Figs. 13A to C)** occur in the majority of NF1 children, particularly in the brainstem, cerebellum, and basal ganglia, but also in the hippocampi, thalami, and cerebral hemispheres. They are thought to represent abnormal myelination and gliosis. Echocardiogram, CT of the abdomen, and chest are required only if there is clinical suspicion of underlying involvement.

Management

Management of NF1 currently consists of surveillance, surgical treatment of progressive lesions, targeted genetic treatment, and genetic counseling.[5] Surveillance involves monitoring for complications and appropriate management of the same. Dermal neurofibromas can be removed by plastic surgery, the use of the CO_2 laser, or electrodessication for cosmesis. Debulking of PNs is sometimes necessary both for cosmesis and to relieve pressure on the airway or spine. Optic gliomas usually do not require treatment, but progressive symptomatic lesions usually are treated with chemotherapy (vincristine and carboplatin). Radiation therapy is best avoided in young children due to vascular complications and malignancies in the radiation field. Surgical removal of tumors is indicated when they cause pressure symptoms.

It is important to educate parents about the possibility of cognitive impairment and to provide the neuropsychological assessment.

TABLE 3: System-wise complications seen in NF1.

Clinical feature	Age of onset (years)	Frequency
Neurological:		
Aqueduct stenosis	Lifelong	1.5%
Chiari I malformation	Lifelong	1.5%
Glioma—brain and spinal cord	Lifelong	2–3%
Optic pathway glioma	Birth to 7	15%
Dysembryoplastic neuroepithelial tumor	Lifelong	<5%
Cognitive impairment IQ <70 (learning problems)	Birth	4–8%
Epilepsy	Lifelong	6–7%
Multiple sclerosis	Adulthood	<5%
Cerebrovascular disease	Lifelong	2.5–6%
Peripheral nervous system:		
Neurofibromatous neuropathy	Adulthood	1.3%
Eye:		
Congenital glaucoma	Birth	0.7%
Bone:		
Scoliosis	Birth to 18	10%
Bone dysplasia with or without pseudoarthrosis	Birth to 3	2%
Osteoporosis	Childhood onwards	Not known
Short stature 10th–25th percentile	Birth	30%
Cardiovascular disease:		
Congenital heart disease—pulmonary stenosis	Birth	2%
Respiratory system:		
Restrictive lung defect	Childhood onwards	<5%
Gastrointestinal:		
Stromal tumor	Adulthood	6%
Carcinoid	Adulthood	1.5%
Other tumors:		
Pheochromocytoma	>10	2%
Breast carcinoma	Adulthood in women <50	Fivefold increase
Rhabdomyosarcoma	Lifelong	<5%

(NF1: neurofibromatosis type 1)

The Neurofibromatosis Clinical Trials Consortium, established in 2006, conducts collaborative trials for the therapeutic management of NF1 and NF2. Sirolimus, an mTOR pathway inhibitor, delays PN progression and pain. Imatinib, a tyrosine kinase inhibitor, has shown tumor regression in PN. Mitogen-activated protein kinase kinase (MEK) inhibitors, involved in the cell proliferation pathway, have also been tried for PN, of special note include selumetinib. Cabozantinib, a multiple tyrosine kinase inhibitor, is also an option for inoperable PN.

BOX 1 Diagnostic criteria for neurofibromatosis type 1 (NF1).

- Six or more café-au-lait spots measuring at least 5 mm before puberty or 15 mm after puberty
- Skin-fold freckling
- Two or more neurofibromas or one plexiform neurofibroma
- Two or more iris Lisch nodules
- Optic glioma
- Characteristic skeletal dysplasia (long bone or sphenoid wing)
- Affected first-degree relative

Note: NF1 is diagnosed in an individual fulfilling two or more of these criteria.

NEUROFIBROMATOSIS TYPE 2

Introduction

Neurofibromatosis type 2 was considered a separate entity from the more common NF1 after a consensus conference at the National Institute of Health in 1987.[6] With advanced neuroimaging, recent studies have suggested that the prevalence is approximately 1 in 60,000.

Etiology

Neurofibromatosis type 2 is an autosomal dominant condition with complete penetrance and variable expression characterized by multiple tumors of the nervous system and meninges as well as lesions of the eyes and skin. It results from a defect in the NF2 tumor suppressor gene situated on chromosome 22q11. Around 50–60% of patients have no family history, and these represent new mutations.

Pathogenesis

The *NF2* gene encodes the protein Merlin (moesin-ezrin-radixin-like protein), also called schwannomin. Merlin is localized to the cell membrane/cytoskeletal interface and influences downstream regulation of cell proliferation.

Clinical Features

Neurofibromatosis type 2 usually presents in early adulthood although milder phenotypes can present much later. Children more frequently present with visual disturbance, skin tumors, mononeuropathy, or symptoms related to other, nonvestibular intracranial or spinal tumors whereas adults most often present with symptoms related to vestibular schwannomas.

Vestibular schwannomas **(Figs. 14A and B)** are the most common tumors to occur in NF2 and the clinical presentation is usually with hearing loss, which starts unilaterally and becomes bilateral with time. The second most common tumor type encountered is meningioma, which usually

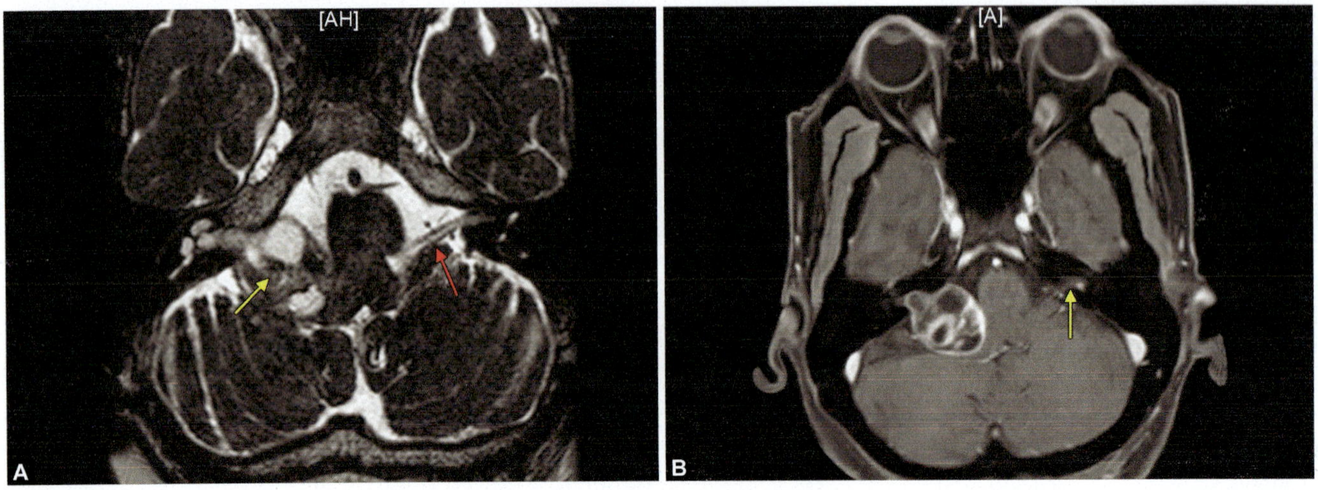

FIGS. 14A AND B: T2 drive sequence (A) and postgadolinium (B) axial images of the brain of an adult with bilateral vestibular schwannoma. The tumor on the right is large causing mass effect on the cerebellopontine angle. Compare it with the normal looking seventh eight nerve complex on the left which on the postgadolinium image (B) shows an enhancing lesion also suggestive of a schwannoma.

Image courtesy: Dr Sniya Sudhakar, Department of Radiodiagnosis, CMC, Vellore.

occurs on the cerebral convexities. Extramedullary spinal tumors such as meningioma or schwannoma may also develop, causing symptoms of myelopathy.

Neurofibromatosis type 2 can also cause neuropathy with no evidence of tumor infiltration. Children could present with mononeuropathy affecting the facial nerve or unilateral wasted limb. In adulthood, 3–10% of patients may develop severe polyneuropathy although up to 40% of adults show evidence of polyneuropathy in nerve conduction studies. The pathogenesis of the neuropathy is unclear but may be due to Schwann cell proliferation among the axons of nerves in the absence of frank tumor, the local toxic effect of tumor cells, or cellular dysfunction due to Merlin deficiency.

Up to 80% of them can have ophthalmological lesions in the form of posterior subcapsular cataracts or cortical wedge opacities.

Cutaneous lesions are few and include intracutaneous, plaque-like lesions that are usually slightly hyperpigmented and may be covered in excess hair.

BOX 2 Diagnostic criteria for neurofibromatosis type 2 (NF2).

- Bilateral vestibular schwannomas (VS)
- A first-degree relative with NF2 *and*—
  - Unilateral VS *or*
  - *Any two* of the following: Meningioma, schwannoma, glioma, neurofibroma, cataract in the form of posterior subcapsular lenticular opacities or cortical wedge cataract
- Unilateral vestibular schwannoma *and any two* of the following: Meningioma, schwannoma, glioma, neurofibroma, cataract in the form of posterior subcapsular lenticular opacities or cortical wedge cataract
- Multiple meningiomas *and*—
  - Unilateral vestibular schwannoma *or*
  - *Any two* of the following: Schwannoma, glioma, neurofibroma, cataract in the form of posterior subcapsular lenticular opacities or cortical wedge cataract

Note: NF2 is diagnosed in an individual if any one of the criteria is present.

Approach to Diagnosis

Diagnostic criteria for NF2 are given in **Box 2**. Diagnosis is often delayed due to the paucity of cutaneous lesions. Depending on the clinical presentation, neuroimaging either of the brain or spinal cord will help to identify the tumor. Genetic testing will detect 90% of mutations.

Mosaicism can lead to segmental or unilateral involvement or milder disease.

Management

Tumors associated with NF2 require surgical excision. Timing and extent of surgery depend on tumor size and the involvement of adjacent structures. Stereotactic radiation therapy is also effective in treating tumors, but there is concern about the later occurrence of malignant tumors in the radiation field. Recently, bevacizumab, an anti-vascular endothelial growth factor (anti-VEGF) monoclonal antibody that inhibits the angiogenic effects of VEGF, has been used in the treatment of vestibular schwannomas. The neuropathy associated with NF2 is not responsive to any form of therapy.

STURGE-WEBER SYNDROME

Sturge-Weber syndrome or encephalofacial angiomatosis is a sporadic disorder occurring due to early embryological malformation of the vascular system with a failure of the primitive cephalous venous plexus to regress and properly mature in the first trimester.[7]

It is characterized by a facial capillary malformation (port-wine stain) in the ophthalmic distribution of the

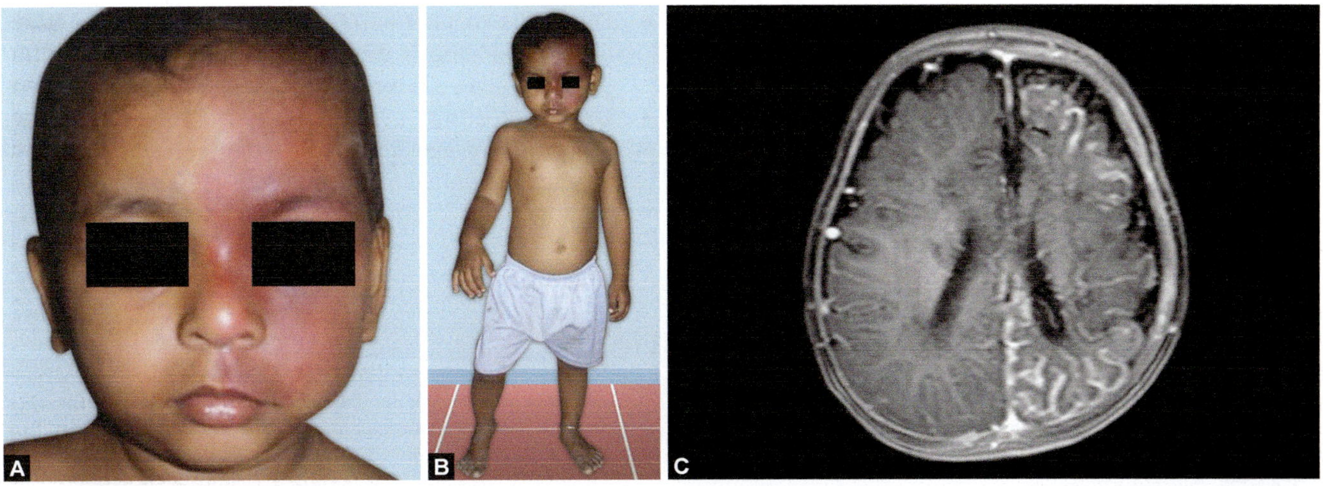

FIGS. 15A TO C: Child with Sturge–Weber syndrome (SWS) showing the classic port wine stain involving the left half of the face with contralateral hemiplegia. Postgadolinium axial images of the brain show ipsilateral leptomeningeal enhancement which represent the angiomatosis and underlying left cerebral hemiatrophy.

trigeminal nerve, with ipsilateral vascular glaucoma and vascular malformation of the eye, and vascular malformation of the brain (leptomeningeal angioma).

The port-wine stain or facial angioma could be unilateral or bilateral and might extend to involve regions of the maxillary and mandibular divisions of the trigeminal nerve and in a few patients to the thorax, abdomen, and upper and lower limbs **(Fig. 15)**.

Neurological manifestations include epilepsy, focal neurological deficit, and psychomotor delay. Seizures that occur in 75–85% of patients are related to leptomeningeal angioma. They are usually focal motor contralateral to the leptomeningeal angioma but can be of other types including infantile spasms. Focal neurological deficits include hemiplegia and hemianopsia. Headaches and migraines are also common in SWS, which may result from an increased vasogenic leakage of plasma and neuropeptides into the subarachnoid space.

Ocular involvement may include eyelid hemangioma, glaucoma, conjunctival and episcleral hemangiomas, diffuse choroidal hemangiomas, and heterochromia of the iridis.

Magnetic resonance imaging brain with gadolinium is the neuroimaging of choice which will show leptomeningeal angioma and ipsilateral cerebral volume reduction **(Fig. 15)**. CT scan is superior to conventional MRI for demonstration of the characteristic calcification seen in SWS. It is seen as a double-lined gyriform pattern of calcification paralleling cerebral convolutions referred to as the railroad track sign **(Fig. 16)**.

Management of SWS involves anticonvulsants for seizures, symptomatic and prophylactic medications for headache, glaucoma treatment, and laser therapy for facial angioma if they persist. Seizures are resistant to medications in about half the patients and they respond well to resective or disconnective epilepsy surgery like hemispherotomy.

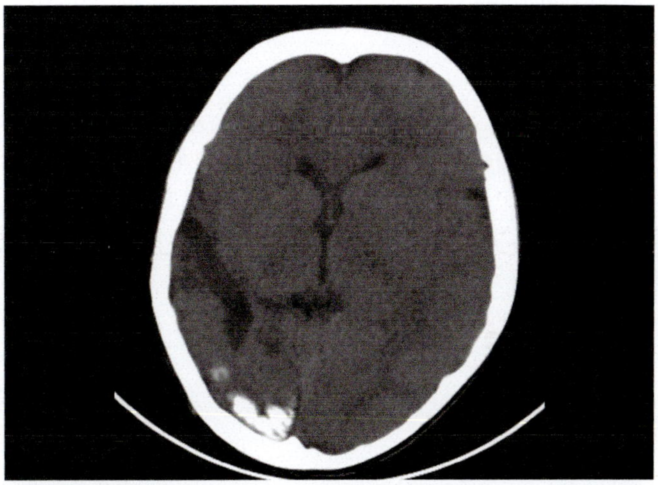

FIG. 16: Plain CT brain of a child with SWS who underwent right posterior quadrantectomy for refractory epilepsy showing gyriform pattern of calcification over the right occipital lobe.
(CT: computed tomography; SWS: Sturge–Weber syndrome)

CONCLUSION

- Neurocutaneous disorders are a diverse group of disorders with predominant involvement of the skin and nervous system tissues.
- Tuberous sclerosis complex is an autosomal dominant disease, though only one-third of cases are inherited. In 85%, it occurs due to a mutation in tumor suppressor gene *TSC*. It is characterized by hypomelanotic macules, facial angiofibroma, facial plaque, and shagreen patch. The predominant complications are seizures and intellectual disability.
- Neurofibromatosis type 1 is autosomal dominantly inherited with 50% representing a new mutation. Diagnosis is clinical, based on presence of CLSs and

neurofibroma. It can lead to number of complications that require surveillance.
- Neurofibromatosis type 2 is characterized by presence of bilateral vestibular schwannomas and inheritance is autosomal dominant.
- Sturge-Weber syndrome is a sporadic disorder with port wine stain and cerebral leptomeningeal angiomatosis causing seizures and focal neurological deficits.
- Diagnosis of all neurocutaneous disorders is based on clinical criteria and once diagnosed, they require periodic follow-up for evolution of complications.
- Genetic testing is offered when individuals reach reproductive age and to first-degree relatives of the affected individual.
- Management requires multidisciplinary care and is based on the clinical presentation.

REFERENCES

1. Gupta P, Menon PSN, Ramji S, Lodha R. PG Textbook of Pediatrics, 1st edition. New Delhi: Jaypee Brothers Medical Publishers; 2015.
2. Schaffer JV. Pigmentary mosaicism. Clin Dermatol. 2022;40(4): 322-38.
3. Islam MP, Roach ES. Tuberous sclerosis complex. Handb Clin Neurol. 2015;132:97-109.
4. Anderson JL, Gutmann DH. Neurofibromatosis type 1. Handb Clin Neurol. 2015;132:75-86.
5. Wilson BN, John AM, Handler MZ, Schwartz RA. Neurofibromatosis type 1: New developments in genetics and treatment. J Am Acad Dermatol. 2021;84(6):1667-76.
6. Evans DG. Neurofibromatosis type 2. Handb Clin Neurol. 2015;132: 87-96.
7. Comi AM. Sturge-Weber syndrome. Handb Clin Neurol. 2015;132: 157-68.

97

CHAPTER

Mitochondriopathies

Bhagyadhan Patel, Ninad Desai, Satish V Khadilkar

INTRODUCTION

Mitochondrial disorders (MDs) present with a wide variety of clinical features involving one or more organs. Although many organs can be affected by MDs, they usually tend to affect the nervous system as they are highly dependent on mitochondrial oxidative phosphorylation. Both central and peripheral nervous systems can be affected in varying proportions by mitochondrial dysfunction. MDs are clinically heterogeneous, can occur at any age, and can manifest with a wide range of clinical symptoms. This heterogeneity in the clinical presentation can make a diagnosis of MDs extremely difficult. However, there are certain clinical features that are sine qua non for the diagnosis of mitochondrial cytopathies and should be considered "tell-tale signs" for suspecting underlying mitochondrial cytopathies. The presence of such "tell-tale" signs should arouse the possibility of mitochondrial cytopathies and they should be considered as a first differential diagnosis in such cases. Recently, it has been found that MDs are not only caused by abnormalities in mitochondrial DNA (mtDNA) but also by mutations in nuclear DNA (nDNA). Although histochemical and biochemical analysis of tissue biopsies and laboratory features can be helpful, genetic testing is considered diagnostic. The management of MDs is aimed to reduce morbidity and mortality, prevent end-organ damage and definitive treatment, whenever available.[1,2]

EPIDEMIOLOGY

In the 1950s, the nomenclature of MDs was initially based on eponyms or clinicopathological correlations, e.g., Leigh syndrome or chronic progressive external ophthalmoplegia (CPEO). By the 1980s, based on clinical and pathology findings, many well-defined syndromes had been described. With the advent of genetics, various mutations in nDNA and mtDNA coding for mitochondrial proteins have been detected. Mitochondrial DNA depletion syndromes (MDS) are due to defects in mtDNA maintenance caused by mutations in nuclear genes that function in either mitochondrial nucleotide synthesis or mtDNA replication, e.g., mitochondrial neurogastrointestinal encephalopathy (MNGIE) syndrome and POLG mutations.

Due to vast heterogeneity among clinical features and the spectrum of genetic mutations in both mtDNA and nDNA, the exact worldwide incidence and prevalence of MDs are unknown. However, mtDNA mutations seem to cause 80% of adulthood MDs, while nDNA mutations seem to be more common (up to 80%) in childhood (<16 years) onset MDs. According to some studies, the prevalence of childhood-onset MDs can range from 5 to 15 per 100,000 population in the world namely England, Spain, Finland, Ireland, and Sweden. Similar data on the prevalence of MDs have been published from Australia but they seem to be more common in the Australian Lebanese population (up to 71 per 100,000). In a Japanese study, the estimated prevalence of MDs was 2.9 per 100,000 population. Among the childhood-onset MDs, Leigh syndrome, MELAS (mitochondrial encephalomyopathy, lactic acidosis and stroke-like episode), and POLG mutations are the most common disorders reported in various literature. Due to its large phenotypic variability and constraints in resources, reporting from Asian countries, particularly the Indian subcontinent is very less. Isolated case reports of MDs such as MNGIE, MELAS, MERRF (myoclonic epilepsy and ragged-red fiber syndrome), Kearns–Sayre syndrome (KSS), myopathy, and Leigh syndrome have been reported.[1,3] In a case series of 14 patients, KSS, MERRF, and MELAS were suspected based on clinical and laboratory features but final genetic diagnosis could not be achieved.[4] Till now, there are 15 case reports of genetically proven mitochondrial diseases from India namely MELAS, Leigh syndrome, cystic leukoencephalopathy, MNGIE, and mtDNA depletion syndromes.[3-6]

PATHOLOGY AND PATHOPHYSIOLOGY

Inheritance: Mitochondria are a complex structure that requires around 1,200–1,500 proteins for its maintenance and smooth functioning. Except for a small proportion of mitochondrial proteins that are coded by mDNA, most of them are encoded by nDNA. As compared to nDNA, mDNA is small in size, circular, and located in the mitochondria itself. MDS are a genetically and clinically heterogeneous group of autosomal recessive disorders that are characterized by a severe reduction in mtDNA content leading to impaired energy production in affected tissues and organs. MDS are due to defects in mtDNA maintenance caused by mutations in nuclear genes that function in either mitochondrial nucleotide synthesis. Till now, human mitochondrial diseases have been linked to *37 mtDNA* and *350 nDNA* genes. The rules that govern mtDNA transmission differ from that of mendelian inheritance. During fertilization, only the nucleus of spermatozoa enters the ova and the paternal mitochondrial structure is excluded. Consequently, all mtDNA and mitochondrial proteins are of maternal origin. Hence, diseases with mtDNA mutations have exclusive maternal inheritance while those with nDNA mutations follow mendelian inheritance. **Table 1** summarizes the type of genetic defects, inheritance, and common mutations in MDs.

Biochemistry: Out of these many proteins, only 100 are required for oxidative phosphorylation, which is the primary function of mitochondria. In this process, the mitochondrial structure oxidizes nutrients to release energy in the form of adenosine triphosphate (ATP). Although ATP is generated through a series of chemical reactions in the glycolysis and citric acid cycle pathway, it requires the final step, i.e., oxidative phosphorylation. The various proteins involved in this final process are:

- Complex I [nicotinamide adenine dinucleotide hydrogen (NADH): coenzyme Q oxidoreductase] oxidizes NADH with the reduction of coenzyme Q10 (also known as CoQ) from its ubiquinone (CoQ; Q) form to ubiquinol (QH2), generating an electrochemical gradient across the inner mitochondrial membrane.
- Complex II (succinate-CoQ oxidoreductase) intricately links the Krebs cycle [also known as the tricarboxylic acid (TCA) cycle] to the respiratory chain. Complex II oxidizes succinate with the reduction of CoQ from its ubiquinone (CoQ; Q) form to ubiquinol (QH2).
- Complex III (ubiquinol-cytochrome c oxidoreductase) catalyzes the reduction of cytochrome c by oxidation of ubiquinol with the generation of an electrochemical gradient.
- Complex IV (cytochrome c oxidase) is responsible for the terminal enzymatic reaction of the respiratory chain that transfers electrons (e^-) to molecular oxygen and generates an electrochemical gradient.
- Complex V converts transmembrane electrochemical proton (H^+) gradient energy into mechanical energy, which catalyzes the chemical bond energy between ADP and phosphate (P) to form ATP.

TABLE 1: Types of genetic defects, common mutations, and syndromes in mitochondrial disease.[1,7-9]

Type of genetic defect and inheritance	Genes affected and common mutations	Clinical syndromes
mtDNA (maternal)	*Complex I genes*: *G11778A*, *G3460A*, and *T14484C*	Leber hereditary optic neuropathy (LHON)
	tRNA^{Leu} gene: *m.A3243G* (80%), *m.T3271C* (7%), *A3260G* (about 5%), and *m.A3252G* (<5%)	MELAS
	tRNA^{Lys}: *m.A8344G* (80%), *m.T8256C*, *m.G8363A*, *m.G8361A*, and others	MERRF
	Complex I and *IV* genes and *ATP6* gene (complex V)	NARP
	ATP6 gene (*mT8993G* and *mT8993C*)	Leigh syndrome (childhood-onset) and NARP (adult onset)
	Point mutations in the mtDNA, such as *m.A3243G*	CPEO and CPEO plus (a small proportion of cases)
nDNA (Mendelian inheritance)	PC (pyruvate carboxylase deficiency), *PDHC* (pyruvate dehydrogenase deficiency), and *SURF1*, *SCO1*, *SCO2*, *COX10*, *COX15*, *SERAC1* mutations	Leigh syndrome (childhood-onset) and NARP (adult onset)
MDS	In all cases, deletion and depletion result in an inadequate amount of wild mtDNA to support the production of normal levels of mtDNA-encoded proteins, tRNAs, or rRNAs, e.g., mitochondrial nucleotide synthesis (*TK2, SUCLA2, SUCLG1, RRM2B, DGUOK*, and *TYMP*) or mtDNA replication (*POLG* and *C10orf2*)	• Clinical presentations may be myopathic, encephalomyopathic, hepatocerebral, or neurogastrointestinal • *Following syndromes can occur*: ○ CPEO ○ CPEO plus ○ KSS ○ Pearson syndrome ○ MNGIE

(CPEO: chronic progressive external ophthalmoplegia; DNA: deoxyribonucleic acid; KSS: Kearns–Sayre syndrome; MNGIE: mitochondrial neurogastrointestinal encephalopathy; MELAS: mitochondrial encephalomyopathy, lactic acidosis and stroke-like episode; MDS: mitochondrial DNA depletion syndromes; MERRF: myoclonic epilepsy and ragged-red fiber syndrome; mtDNA: mitochondrial DNA; NARP: neuropathy, ataxia, and retinitis pigmentosa; nDNA: nuclear DNA)

Structure: The mitochondrion consists of a double membrane, rod-like structure which consists of an inner membrane, outer membrane, and gel-like structure called matrix. Most of the biochemical reactions such as the citric acid cycle occur in the matrix. The inner mitochondrial membrane is electrochemically charged where the process of oxidative phosphorylation takes place. The outer membrane is a bilayer structure that is composed of two-tailed phospholipids that include phosphatidylcholine, phosphatidylethanolamine, and phosphatidylinositol and the four-tailed phospholipid cardiolipin. It is designed in such a way that it provides the chemical milieu to hold the electron transport chain supercomplexes in place. As a part of normal oxidative phosphorylation, some electrons escape as oxidative-free radicals.

In primary mitochondrial diseases, mutations in genes responsible for oxidative phosphorylation lead to impaired ATP production and excess oxidative-free radicals which lead to impaired cellular function. Secondary mitochondrial dysfunction can result from ischemia and neurodegeneration leading to impaired energy production.[8]

CLINICAL PRESENTATIONS

Mitochondrial diseases exhibit diverse clinical manifestations that may overlap with other neurological and non-neurological conditions. This heterogeneity is due to the fact that different genetic causes of mitochondrial disease may produce similar phenotypes, while the same genetic cause may result in different clinical presentations.

Organs that are most reliant on energy, such as the brain, heart, skeletal muscles, and endocrine pancreas, are commonly affected by mitochondrial disease as they are most vulnerable to dysfunction in oxidative ATP production.

Common neurological and overlap symptoms and signs observed in patients with MDs are summarized in **Figure 1**. Although migraine, exercise intolerance, parkinsonism, epilepsy, ataxia, and dementia may occur in patients with mitochondrial disease, they are infrequent when present in isolation. Common non-neurological symptoms include dyspnea on exertion and syncope from cardiac disease, malaise from hepatic failure, constipation

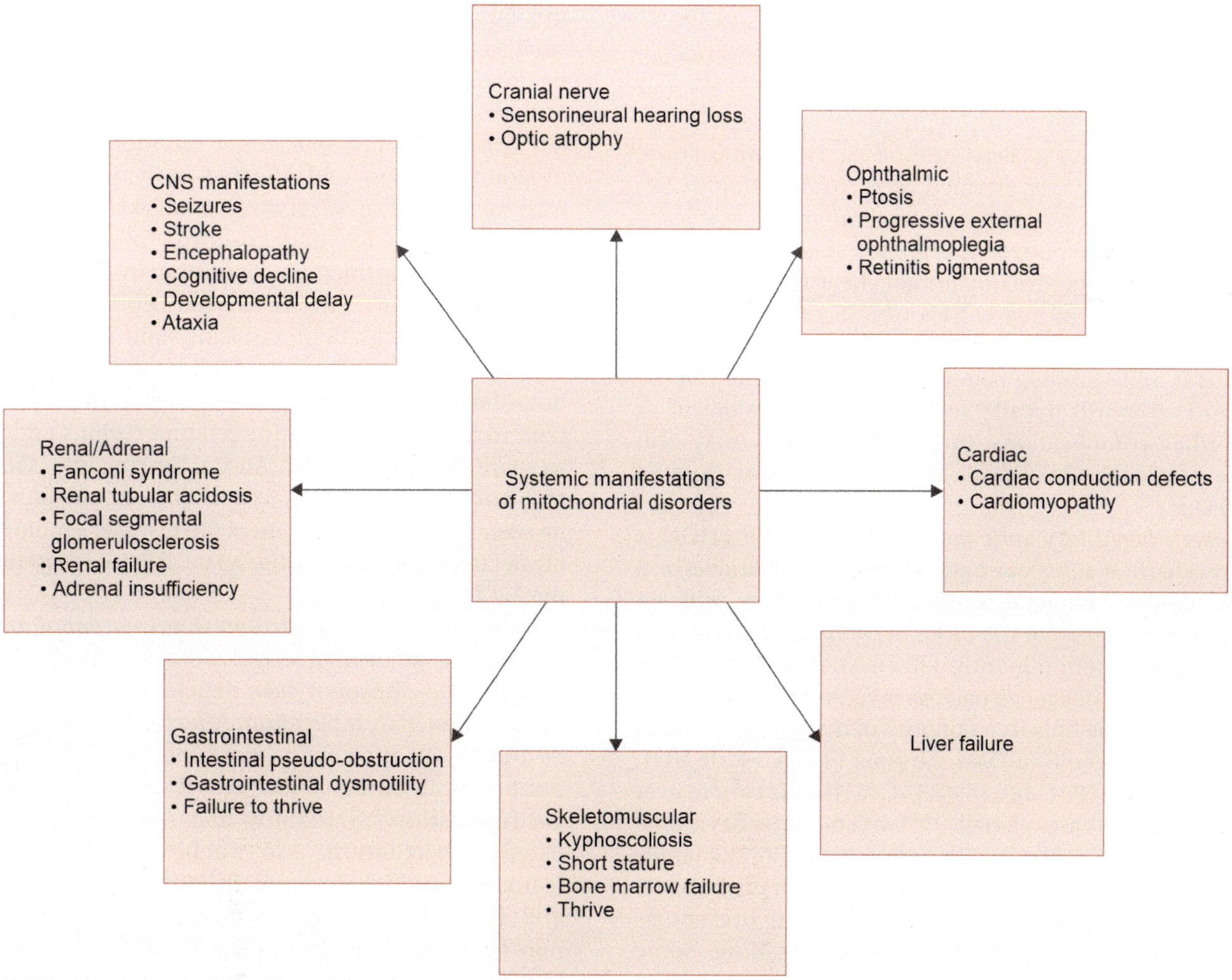

FIG. 1: Neurological and multisystem involvement in MDs.
(MD: mitochondrial disorder)

and/or acute abdomen from gastrointestinal dysmotility, and short stature.

Multisystem involvement is often seen in adult patients with classic mitochondrial syndromes, but these classic syndromes are less prevalent in young children with mitochondrial disease, except for Alpers–Huttenlocher syndrome and Leigh syndrome. Detailed clinical features of commoner MDs are described below.

Common clinical syndromes:

- *Chronic progressive external ophthalmoplegia*: CPEO is one of the myopathy manifestations of mitochondrial disease. Patients with this condition present with progressive impairment of extraocular movements, generally accompanied by ptosis but only occasionally by diplopia, most commonly in the third or fourth decade of life.[10,11]
- The majority of the cases are a result of a sporadic mtDNA mutation,[12] but it can also be inherited in an autosomal dominant or recessive fashion, in which case there can be multiorgan involvement with associated visual impairment (cataracts and pigmentary retinopathy), hearing impairment, movement disorders (ataxia, tremor, and parkinsonism), rhabdomyolysis, and hypogonadism.[12]
- *Kearns-Sayre syndrome*: KSS is defined by the presence of progressive external ophthalmoplegia (PEO) and pigmentary retinopathy with onset before the age of 20 years, and at least one of: cardiac conduction, cerebellar ataxia, or elevated cerebrospinal fluid (CSF) protein (>100 mg/dL). Other commonly associated abnormalities reported include short stature, intellectual disability or cognitive impairment, hearing loss, anemia, and diabetes. In nearly 80% of KSS cases, there is a sporadic, single large-scale mtDNA deletion present. This is a life-limiting condition with death often in the third or fourth decade secondary to neurological or cardiac complications. Proximal myopathy may also be present in individuals with either KSS or isolated PEO.[12]
- *Leber's hereditary optic neuropathy (LHON)*: LHON is an inherited subacute optic neuropathy characterized by painless, bilateral, sequential vision loss, with an inter-eye interval in the order of weeks to months. This condition predominantly affects males, between 15 and 35 years of age. Visual loss is central or centrocecal, and reversible only in a minority of the patients. One of three pathogenic mtDNA variants (3460G>A in ND1, 11778G>A in ND4, and 14484T>C in ND6) is seen in over 90% of LHON cases globally,[13,14] with the latter having the best recovery potential. There may be additional family members with cardiac, neurological, or orthopedic abnormalities. Occasionally, LHON can present as multiple sclerosis-like syndromes, leading some researchers to postulate mitochondrial dysfunction as a disease mechanism in MS.[15]
- *Leigh syndrome*: Leigh syndrome is a subacute necrotizing encephalopathy with onset in infancy in the majority of cases, although adult forms have been recognized.[16,17] The clinical picture is one of stepwise psychomotor delay or regression in the setting of intercurrent illnesses and other metabolic stresses manifesting with ataxia, dystonia, stroke-like episodes and seizures, along with lactic acidosis and vomiting. Classical histological features include symmetrical necrotizing lesions with spongy changes and microcyst formation in the basal ganglia, thalami, brainstem, and spinal cord.[17] There is a corresponding T2 and T2 fluid-attenuated inversion recovery (FLAIR) hyperintense signal on MR imaging in these regions.[18] A number of different causative mtDNA and nDNA mutations with maternal, autosomal, or sex-linked patterns of inheritance have been described. Natural history is one of relentless progressions, leading to death in early childhood. This condition should be strongly considered in patients with lactic acidosis and episodic metabolic decompensation manifesting with features suggestive of brainstem/spinal cord dysfunction. The term "Leigh-like syndrome" is employed when individuals exhibit atypical or non-neurologic symptoms such as diabetes, short stature, hypertrichosis, cardiomyopathy, anemia, or renal failure.
- *Mitochondrial encephalopathy, lactic acidosis, stroke-like episode*: MELAS falls under the spectrum of encephalomyopathies, and affected individuals manifest with symptoms of short stature, stroke-like episodes and seizures which may co-occur, migraines, lactic acidosis, and intractable vomiting in childhood or early adulthood. The stroke-like episodes can be transient or permanent, clinically and radiologically, and characteristically do not follow vascular territory boundaries. Additionally, these stroke-like episodes tend to involve the posterior cerebral regions and tend to spare the white matter. Ataxia, hearing loss, skeletal and cardiac myopathy, as well as diabetes mellitus may be seen with the progression of the disease. Around 80% of affected individuals harbor an m.3243A>G mutation in the *MTTL1* gene.
- *Mitochondrial neurogastrointestinal encephalopathy*: MNGIE is an autosomal recessive disorder resulting from a thymidine phosphorylase deficiency, which causes impaired mtDNA replication. Affected individuals may be healthy in their early years but typically develop symptoms in the late teenage years,[19] consisting of gastrointestinal dysmotility and resultant intestinal pseudo-obstruction and cachexia. Neurological features may include optic atrophy, PEO with ptosis, and demyelinating polyneuropathy. Investigations may reveal lactic acidosis, ragged red fibers on muscle biopsy, and leukoencephalopathy on MR imaging, which are out of proportion to the clinical symptoms.[20]

This is also a life-limiting illness, with most patients dying before the age of 40 years.[21]

- *Myoclonic epilepsy with ragged-red fibers*: MERRF is another maternally inherited encephalomyopathy, which has an onset in childhood or young adulthood, commonly after normal early development. Stimulus-sensitive myoclonic epilepsy typically heralds the onset of this condition, which is followed by ataxia, myopathy, and intellectual impairment. Other reported features include visual loss in the setting of optic atrophy and pigmentary retinopathy, sensorineural hearing loss, and cardiomyopathy with conduction defections including Wolff–Parkinson–White syndrome. A distinctive feature is the development of cutaneous lipomas. Lactic acidosis may be present. The clinical course in MERRF is variable, but it is typically progressive. The vast majority of the patients with this MERRF have an mtDNA point mutation, m.8344A>G.[22]
- *Neuropathy, ataxia, and retinitis pigmentosa* (NARP): NARP is another disorder that tends to present in late childhood or early adulthood. The characteristic features, in addition to NARP, can include developmental delay or regression, myopathy, and epilepsy. This results from maternally inherited point mutations (m.8993T>G/C) in the mitochondrial *MT-ATP6* gene. The same mutation at a higher load (mutated mtDNA>90%) results in a more severe phenotype of maternally inherited Leigh syndrome (MILS).

Some less common MDs are summarized in **Table 2**.

While this discussion has focused on the common syndromes of mitochondrial disease and their most common genetic abnormalities, special mention must be made of the spectrum disorders resulting from mutations in the *POLG* gene given its wide phenotypic diversity. The *POLG* gene encodes the protein mitochondrial DNA polymerase, which plays a crucial role in mitochondrial replication. *POLG* mutations are the most common cause of inherited MDs and can result in childhood-onset mtDNA depletion syndromes, or later-onset mtDNA deletion syndromes.[11] The POLG spectrum disorders include, but are not limited to, Alpers syndrome, Leigh disease in infancy, MNGIE, MIRAS (mitochondrial recessive ataxia syndrome), MEMSA (myoclonic epilepsy, myopathy, sensory ataxia), SCAE (spinocerebellar ataxia with epilepsy) in childhood or early adolescence, MELAS, PEO, SANDO (sensory ataxic neuropathy, dysarthria, and ophthalmoparesis) in adulthood, and parkinsonism in the elderly.

TABLE 2: Uncommon mitochondrial disorders presenting in adult life.

Syndrome	Core features	Variable features
ADOA	Optic atrophy	SNHL, SANDO-like disorder
ADPEO	PEO, myopathy	SNHL, neuropathy, ataxia, depression, parkinsonism, cataracts
AHS	Childhood-onset, progressive encephalopathy, intractable epilepsy, and liver failure	
ARPEO	Same as ADPEO	
CMT-2A	Polyneuropathy	
MEMSA	Epilepsy, myopathy, and ataxia without ophthalmoplegia	
MIDD	Insulin deficiency, SNHL	Maculopathy, cardio-myopathy, FSGS
Pearson	Anemia and pancreatic dysfunction	Beyond childhood may resemble KSS
SANDO	Sensory ataxic neuropathy dysarthria and ophthal-moplegia	

(ADOA: autosomal dominant optic atrophy; ADPEO: autosomal dominant progressive external ophthalmoplegia; AHS: Alpers–Huttenlocher syndrome; ARPEO: autosomal recessive progressive external ophthalmoplegia; CMT-2A: Charcot–Marie–Tooth 2A; FSGS: focal segmental glomerulosclerosis; MEMSA: myoclonic epilepsy, myopathy, and sensory ataxia; MIDD: maternally inherited diabetes and deafness; SANDO: sensory ataxic neuropathy, dysarthria, and ophthalmoparesis; SNHL: sensorineural hearing loss)

DIAGNOSIS AND DIFFERENTIAL DIAGNOSIS

Diagnosing MDs is challenging. Some of the prevalent clinical features such as diabetes mellitus, epilepsy, migraine-like headache, peripheral neuropathy, or sensorineural hearing loss have low specificity. Patients can present oligo symptomatically rather than with a classic syndromic phenotype involving multiple affected organ systems, requiring further evaluation over time or through detailed family history. Additionally, the inheritance pattern of mitochondrial disease, which is often maternally inherited or transmitted through autosomal dominant or recessive patterns, but can also arise spontaneously, adds to the complexity of diagnosis, as mtDNA point mutations may also be heteroplasmic, varying between individuals and generations in the maternal line and potentially not causing symptoms in close maternal relatives. Lastly, the natural history of many mitochondrial diseases is not known and some like Leigh's disease have a fluctuating clinical course. The following observations should lead to the consideration of an MD in the differential diagnosis and can be considered as tell-tale signs for MDs **(Box 1)**.

Other clues favoring MDs:

- A presentation consistent with one of the better-recognized MDs like MELAS, as described in the previous section.
- Prominent symptom deterioration in the setting of acute febrile illnesses or metabolic stressors.
- Familial disease with the maternally transmitted mode of inheritance.

The differential diagnosis of commonly encountered MDs with their key distinguishing features is detailed in **Table 3**.

INVESTIGATIONS

The diagnostic algorithm of suspected MDs begins with the clinical phenotype, and every effort must be made to characterize it accurately. In patients with presentations typical for a common MD with well-defined mtDNA or nDNA mutations, it may be worthwhile directly proceeding with focused genetic testing for confirmation of the diagnosis. In others, following certain basic screening tests, further investigations are determined based on the clinical concern of specific organ system(s) being involved.

BOX 1 Tell-tale signs in MDs.

- Progressive external ophthalmoplegia with or without ptosis; pigmentary retinopathy and optic atrophy
- Early onset SNHL with coexistent other neurological involvement such as stroke, myopathy, peripheral neuropathy, etc.
- Epilepsy, especially with symptomatology suggestive of occipital lobe origin and/or presentation with epilepsia partialis continua, myoclonic jerks, and worsening with sodium valproate
- Cerebral stroke-like lesions in the nonvascular territory
- Cerebellar ataxia with peripheral neuropathy, pigmentary retinopathy, and myopathy
- Early onset cognitive decline

(MD: mitochondrial disorder; SNHL: sensorineural hearing loss)

Screening Tests

The conventional biomarkers that are used to support a diagnosis of MD are either end-products of anaerobic metabolism, metabolic intermediaries, and/or specific enzymes involved in the electron transport chain.[1] The screening tests recommended by the Mitochondrial Medicine Society[23] in cases of suspected MDs are summarized in **Table 4**.

Unfortunately, the screening tests in general have low sensitivity and specificity, are prone to errors with sample collection and transport, do not help to differentiate between primary and secondary mitochondrial dysfunction, and with certain tests, there is no clear cutoff between normal and abnormal values. Biomarkers fibroblast growth factor 21 (FGF21) and growth/differentiation factor-15 (GDF15) are gaining popularity for purportedly improved sensitivity and specificity over the more traditional ones.[27,32]

Histology and Immunohistochemistry

Despite the advent of genetic testing, tissue analysis (typically performed on a biopsied muscle sample) remains a core modality in the diagnosis of MDs. This helps to provide supportive evidence for MDs based on certain characteristic findings (see below), validate the pathogenicity of variants

TABLE 3: Differential diagnosis of common mitochondrial disorders.

Mitochondrial syndromes	Differential diagnosis	Key distinguishing features
CPEO	Myasthenic syndrome	Slowly progressive, symmetrical, nonfluctuating, and nonfatigable ptosis, and ophthalmoparesis without diplopia or bulbar involvement. The presence of ataxia, retinal degeneration, and cardiac involvement favors mitochondrial cytopathy
Peripheral neuropathy (NARP syndrome)	CMT2, ganglionopathy	Sometimes, mitochondrial diseases can present with an axonal type of peripheral neuropathy. Mitofusin (*Mfn*) gene mutations can lead to peripheral neuropathy plus phenotype (optic atrophy, hearing impairment, and pyramidal dysfunction). Associated ophthalmoparesis, ataxia, and retinitis pigmentosa favor mitochondrial disorder
MERRF	Progressive myoclonic epilepsy (PME)	• The presence of myopathy, ataxia, hearing loss, ptosis, and multiple lipomatosis favors mitochondrial cytopathy • Pigmentary retinopathy and optic atrophy can occur in other PME. Lafora body disease (cognitive decline and visual disturbances)
Optic atrophy	Primary optic atrophy; optic neuritis	Bilateral, subacute, progressive, painless vision diminution in young males with disk edema followed by disk atrophy in LHON
Pigmentary retinopathy (PR)	Usher's syndrome	It usually occurs as a part of the syndrome—NARP and KSS. The presence of PR and hearing impairment can occur with Usher's syndrome
Stroke-like episodes (MELAS)	CNS vasculitis, CADASIL	Episodic, less acute, bilateral parieto-occipital cortex involvement (not confined to arterial territory), seizures, CSF (raised lactate, normal proteins), and associated hearing impairment favor MELAS
Cerebellar ataxia	Inherited ataxias	Cerebellar ataxia is usually associated with peripheral neuropathy, myopathy, ophthalmoparesis, seizures, and PR in mitochondrial disorders while isolated cerebellar ataxia points toward causes other than mitochondrial cytopathy

(CMT: Charcot–Marie–Tooth; CNS: central nervous system; CPEO: chronic progressive external ophthalmoplegia; CSF: cerebrospinal fluid; LHON: Leber hereditary optic neuropathy; MERRF: myoclonic epilepsy and ragged-red fiber syndrome; NARP: neuropathy, ataxia, and retinitis pigmentosa; KSS: Kearns–Sayre syndrome)

TABLE 4: Routine biochemical findings in MDs.

Sample	Test	Comment
Blood	Complete blood count	
	Albumin and amino acids	An altered redox state results in elevations of alanine, glycine, proline, threonine etc.[24]
	Creatine kinase	Significant elevations (esp. > 1,000 U/L) unusual in MDs *Exception*: TK2D
	Lactate	• *Lactate elevations in MDs*:[25-27] ○ *Specificity*: 34–62% ○ *Sensitivity*: 83–100% • Low sensitivity in Leigh, KSS, POLG-spectrum[23] • Postprandial levels more sensitive than fasting
	Pyruvate	Elevated in pyruvate metabolism enzymatic defects[28]
	Lactate to pyruvate ratio	• Useful if lactate is elevated • Helps to differentiate ETC disorders from pyruvate metabolism disorders[29]
	Acylcarnitine	*Impaired fatty acid oxidation*: Low free carnitine and elevated acyl/free carnitine ratio
	Uric acid, 3-methylgluticonic acid	Uric acid in patients with myopathic symptoms
Urine	Organic acids	Malate and fumarate have best correlation with MDs[30]
	3-methylgluticonic acid	
CSF (avoided in the absence of CNS symptoms)	Lactate and pyruvate	See above
	Amino acids	See above
	5-methyltetrahydrofolate	Correlates with cerebral folate deficiency states seen in various MDs[31]

(CNS: central nervous system; CSF: cerebrospinal fluid; KSS: Kearns–Sayre syndrome; MD: mitochondrial disorder)

of unknown significance, and importantly can establish a diagnosis for non-MD etiologies. The vastus lateralis is preferred for sampling. Besides muscle, other tissues amenable for histological and biochemical analysis include skin fibroblasts, liver, and heart.[33] The stains utilized in the study of biopsied muscle tissue are listed in **Table 5**.

If no pertinent abnormalities are noted and suspicion for MD with muscle involvement remains high, electron microscopy (EM) should be performed, especially in children in whom histological findings are often limited. EM can detect mitochondrial inclusions and ultrastructural abnormalities.

Biochemical Analysis

This comprises biochemical analysis of enzyme activity of various respiratory enzyme complexes and is generally performed on muscle but can also be assessed on liver, fibroblast, or buccal swab samples. Oxidative phosphorylation analysis by polarography measures integrated mitochondrial function and needs to be performed on freshly isolated tissue.[34] ETC enzymology (spectrophotometry) enables measurement of the function of individual complex, and needs to be performed on snap-frozen tissue or freshly isolated mitochondria.[23] As with most other investigation modalities, biochemical testing does not help to differentiate primary from secondary MDs.

TABLE 5: Muscle histology findings in mitochondrial disorders (MDs).

Stain	Findings
Hematoxylin and eosin	Basic muscle histology
Modified Gomori trichrome	• "Ragged-red fibers (RRF)"—proliferated mitochondria (red) in subsarcolemmal and intermyofibrillar regions (blue) • *RRF*: >2% at age <50 and >5% at age >50 is abnormal[33]
NADH	Can detect "ragged-blue fibers (RBF)"
Succinate dehydrogenase	• Reflects activity of complex II which is entirely DNA encoded • Can detect "ragged-blue fibers (RBF)" perivascular/endothelial mitochondrial proliferation
Cytochrome C oxidase	• Reflects activity of complex IV (mtDNA and nDNA encoded) • RRF/RBF + COX-negative fibers: mtDNA defects • RRF/RBF + COX-positive fibers: mtDNA defects sparing COX subunits in complex IV
Periodic acid–Schiff	Glycogen deposits
Oil red O	Increased lipid droplets

(COX: cytochrome oxidase; NADH: nicotinamide adenine dinucleotide hydrogen)

Imaging

Brain MR imaging is helpful in the evaluation of stroke-like episodes, which show diffusion and/or FLAIR changes that classically do not follow major vascular territories, and may be fully reversible. Symmetric deep gray matter lesions are seen in Leigh's disease, and cerebral/cerebellar atrophy can be seen in mtDNA deletion disorders.[35] MR spectroscopy may show increased lactate in an otherwise normal-appearing brain parenchyma.[36,37]

Neurophysiology

Electromyography (EMG)/nerve conduction study (NCS) testing is helpful for the evaluation of lower motor neuron disorders; in patients with neuropathy, a demyelinating pattern is seen in MNGIE and only rarely in some other disorders such as MELAS, MERRF, and Leigh's syndromes.[38] The utility of electroencephalogram (EEG) is similar to that in non-MDs.

Genetic Testing

Genetic testing is now the gold standard in the diagnosis of MDs. Given the increasing affordability and availability, targeted next-generation sequencing (NGS) is now the testing modality of choice.

While the mtDNA genome has been mapped and all known pathogenic mutations have been linked to specific mitochondrial phenotypes, the same is not true for nDNA mutations. New disease-associated genes are being reported regularly, and new pathogenic alleles within known disease-causing genes are being identified continuously.

For mtDNA analysis, massively parallel sequencing and/or NGS are preferred over other genetic testing modalities, owing to their ability to detect low-level mutations, deletions, and heteroplasmy down to the 1% level, thus providing a single test to accurately diagnose mtDNA disorders[39] Patients in whom an mtDNA mutation is strongly suspected but have negative testing in blood should have mtDNA analysis performed in another tissue taking into consideration the possibility of tissue-specific mutations or low levels of heteroplasmy in blood. For nDNA analysis, NGS panel testing of all known nuclear genes is preferred over that of individual genes; if nondiagnostic, whole-exome sequencing should be performed. It is worth noting that a genetic diagnosis can be made in only 50–70% of the cases. Additional testing is necessary when variants of uncertain significance are encountered.

Prior to performing genetic testing, obtaining informed consent is essential, and the involvement of a genetic counselor may help to navigate the intricacies of the process. Once a diagnosis of MD has been made, screening of family members can be done less invasively, using buccal, urine, or blood DNA samples.

MANAGEMENT

General Measures

In spite of the advances in our understanding of the MDs in the last three decades, management remains primarily supportive. Listed below are certain commonly encountered neurological disorders in patients with mitochondrial disease, while those affecting other organ systems are elaborated in **Table 6**. In general, the treatment approach is similar to that in nonmitochondrial neurological disorders, with certain special considerations:

- *Headache*: Patients with MDs with headaches can have concurrent seizures and stroke-like episodes; acute-onset or worsening severity of headaches. Certain medications employed as abortive or prophylactic headache treatments would need to be used cautiously.
- *Movement disorders*: Botulinum toxin has the potential to exacerbate weakness in MD patients with muscle involvement.
- *Myopathy*: In patients with recurrent rhabdomyolysis and myoglobinuria, fatty acid oxidation disorders should be considered; acylcarnitine and urine organic acid testing is indicated in them.
- *Neuropathy*: The increased prevalence, often with early onset, of diabetes mellitus in patients with certain MDs puts them at increased risk of developing polyneuropathy.
- *Seizures and epilepsy*: As with other underlying etiologies, epilepsia partialis continua in patients with MDs can be refractory to treatment, and may be a pointer toward a concurrent stroke-like episode. It is important to suspect MDs and confirm the diagnosis, as sodium valproate needs to be avoided in such patients with myoclonic jerks.
- *Stroke-like episodes*: Emergent administration of intravenous (IV) arginine hydrochloride[40] should be instituted for the treatment of stroke-like episodes in patients with MELAS with *MTTL1* gene m.3243A>G mutation, and may also be beneficial in stroke-like episodes associated with other MDs. Continuous administration for 3 days prior to reassessment is recommended. Daily oral arginine supplementation may help stroke prophylaxis in MELAS patients.[40]

Special circumstances:

- *Acute illness*: In the setting of an acute illness, treatment must be focused on optimizing nutrition, avoiding potentially mitochondrial toxic exposures, correction of metabolic disturbances, and avoidance of fasting. IV fluids, with added dextrose in the absence of contraindications (patients on a ketogenic diet, known or suspected disorder of pyruvate metabolism, poor tolerance to prior glucose loads), should be utilized as clinically indicated to avoid a catabolic state.[23]

TABLE 6: Non-neurological disorders in mitochondrial disease and their management.

Organ system	Potential disorders	Management
Cardiovascular	Arrhythmia, cardiomyopathy, fatigue, and exercise intolerance	Pharmacotherapy, ablation/defibrillator implantation, pacemaker placement, cardiac assistive devices/heart transplant
ENT	Sensorineural hearing loss	Loud noise avoidance, hearing aids, cochlear implantation
Endocrinology	Adrenal insufficiency, diabetes mellitus, GH deficiency, hypoparathyroidism, hypothyroidism, osteopenia, short stature	Pharmacotherapy, hormone replacement
Gastroenterology	Constipation, dysphagia, dysmotility/pseudo-obstruction, hepatic dysfunction, malnutrition, pancreatic dysfunction, pancreatic dysfunction	Pharmacotherapy and enzyme replacement therapy, macro- and micronutrient supplementation, gastrostomy/jejunostomy, liver transplant
Hematology	Iron deficiency, pancytopenia, sideroblastic anemia	Iron supplementation, transfusions
Immunology	Recurrent infections	Prophylactic antibiotics, immunoglobulin supplementation, G-CSF
Nephrology	Glomerulopathy, tubulopathy	Electrolyte management, renal replacement therapy
Ophthalmology	Cataracts, ophthalmoparesis, optic atrophy, ptosis, retinopathy	Low-vision aids, strabismus surgery, eyelid crutches/oculoplastic surgery
Orthopedic	Contractures, fractures, kyphoscoliosis	Surgical intervention
Pulmonary	Aspiration, hypoventilation, sleep-disordered breathing	Noninvasive ventilation, tracheostomy

(G-CSF: granulocyte colony-stimulating factor; GH: growth hormone)

- *Anesthesia*: There are several important considerations in the management of MD patients being administered anesthesia. These patients may be hypersensitive to the effects of volatile anesthetics and muscle relaxants.[41,42] Isoflurane and propofol may result in mitochondrial dysfunction,[43] and MD patients are at an increased risk of developing propofol-related infusion syndrome.[44] IV fluids, if indicated, should preferably be lactose-free. Perioperative hypoglycemia is to be avoided, with precautions as stated above. Local anesthesia is generally well tolerated in these patients.

Immunization

There is no scientific evidence to indicate vaccination is associated with deleterious effects in patients with MDs, and in general, their use is advocated in the absence of other contraindications.[45] The risk of decompensation from serious, potentially life-threatening infections far outweighs the risks associated with vaccination itself.[46] Although not specifically investigated, vaccine administration individually or in small batches may reduce the metabolic stress in MD patients.[45]

Supplements

Mitochondrial diseases are associated with increased oxidative stress from reactive oxygen species,[47] which cause cellular damage by membrane lipid peroxidation. This is the basis for the use of antioxidants in mitochondrial disease.[48] Supplementation of electron transport chain enzymes is done to replenish known or suspected deficient states.[49] The commonly used supplements, their roles, and commonly used dosages are listed in **Table 7**.

Exercise

Physical activity appears to be safe and effective, and overall has a positive impact on those with MDs. Studies have linked aerobic exercise with improvements in peak work performance, improvement in exercise tolerance and in muscle weakness.[50,51] The optimal approach for these patients is a combination of aerobic and resistance exercises, which are considered safe when gradually introduced under supervision. An appropriate cardiovascular evaluation is indicated in high-risk patients prior to recommending structured exercise.

Diet

Patients with different MDs can have specific energy, protein, and micronutrient requirements, and input from a trained dietician is often warranted to ensure adequate nutrition. These may need to be further tailored if dysphagia, gastrointestinal dysmotility, or cognitive impairment is present. In general, fasting is to be avoided and small, frequent meals are recommended. Fluid intake should be increased in the setting of acute illnesses.

There is no "one-size-fits-all" macronutrient profile that can be used in patients with mitochondrial disease. The use of the ketogenic diet in MDs remains a controversial topic. While it may help in patients with drug-resistant epilepsy and in patients with pyruvate dehydrogenase deficiency,[48] it is often poorly tolerated,[52] and patients with MDs often

TABLE 7: Supplements used in mitochondrial disorders (MDs).

	Role	Adult dose	Pediatric dose	Comment
Alpha-lipoic acid	Antioxidant cofactor for mitochondrial alpha-keto acid dehydrogenases	50–200 mg	50–200 mg	
L-arginine	Precursor of nitric oxide that stimulates vasodilation	150–300 mg/kg		Used for stroke prophylaxis in MELAS[40]
L-carnitine	Removal of toxic acetyl coenzyme A metabolites	1 g	50 mg/kg	Potentially curative in carnitine transporter deficiency; cautious use in coronary artery disease
Coenzyme Q10	Antioxidant that transfers electrons from complex I to II and III	400 mg	10–20 mg/kg	Ubiquinol (reduced form) has best bioavailability and is the preferred form
L-citrulline	Stimulates vasodilation			
Creatine	Regenerates ATP	5–10 g	0.1 g/kg	Titrate slowly to avoid cramps
Folinic acid	Increases brain 5-MTHF levels; believed to reduce white matter demyelination	2.5–25 mg	0.5–1.5 mg/kg	Indicated in mitochondrial disease patients with known/suspected CNS folate-deficient states (can be seen in KSS, NARP, Leigh's, etc.)
Niacin	Increased NAD+ and NADH; increase complex I function	Highly variable	Highly variable	Nicotinamide better tolerated than niacin
Riboflavin	Component of electron carriers flavin adenine dinucleotide and flavin mononucleotide	50–400 mg	50–400 mg	Multiple acyl-CoA dehydrogenase deficiency (MADD), for use in riboflavin transporter deficiency
Thiamine	Coenzyme in oxidative decarboxylation		50–100 mg	
Vitamin C	Antioxidant	50–200 mg	5 mg/kg	
Vitamin E	Antioxidant	100–200 IU	1–2 IU/kg	

(ATP: adenosine triphosphate; CNS: central nervous system; CoA: coenzyme A; KSS: Kearns–Sayre syndrome; MELAS: mitochondrial encephalomyopathy, lactic acidosis and stroke-like episode; NADH: nicotinamide adenine dinucleotide hydrogen; NARP: neuropathy, ataxia, and retinitis pigmentosa)

have secondary fatty acid oxidation dysfunction,[53] which may be exacerbated by ketogenic diets.

Toxin Avoidance

It is imperative to exercise caution when administering medication to patients suffering from MDs, as some pharmaceutical agents have been known to exacerbate organ dysfunction. The associated risks of these drugs must be thoroughly evaluated and weighed against their expected benefits when considering their use as summarized in **Table 8**.

In addition to the medications listed in the table, several other medications particularly immunosuppressants and immunomodulators (corticosteroids, hydroxychloroquine, and interferon-α), chemotherapeutics (bortezomib, trastuzumab, and doxorubicin), and certain diuretics have been associated with the development of mitochondrial toxicity and/or metabolic acidosis. The interested reader is referred to the work by Mancuso et al. for an exhaustive list.[43]

Specific Management of Individual Disorders

Patients with several MDs can have a meaningful response to vitamin supplementation. High-dose riboflavin supplementation can help in ACAD9 deficiency,[58] Brown-Vialetto-Van Laere[59] and Fazio-Londe diseases, and multiple acyl-coenzyme A (CoA) dehydrogenase deficiency syndrome,[60] among others. Biotin replacement in biotinidase deficiency,[61] and additionally thiamine in biotin-thiamine-responsive basal ganglia disease,[62] can help a proportion of patients with these conditions; the latter can mimic Leigh disease.

High-dose coenzyme Q10 deficiency can help patients with primary or secondary deficiency states. Oral deoxynucleoside supplementation can help in patients with thymidine kinase 2 deficiency.[63] Allogeneic hematopoietic stem cell transplantation and orthotopic liver transplantation can help to restore thymidine phosphorylase activity.[64] Idebenone has been approved in Europe for the treatment of vision loss in adolescent and adult LHON patients.[65]

For information on rarer MDs responsive to specific treatments, the interested reader is referred to the work of Distelmaier et al.[66]

Reproductive Counseling

Given the differences in patterns of inheritance for mtDNA versus nDNA defects, appropriate reproductive counseling depends on an accurate genetic diagnosis. For patients with nDNA defects, the options are similar to those with other autosomal or sex-linked genetic disorders. mtDNA disorders

TABLE 8: Medications that can potentially worsen MDs.

Class	Agent(s)	Toxicity	Comment
Antiseizure medications	Valproate[43]	Liver failure, seizure worsening	POLG mutation carriers most susceptible
	Carbamazepine, phenytoin, phenobarbital	Seizure worsening	
	Topiramate, zonisamide[54]	Metabolic acidosis	
	Vigabatrin		mtDNA depletion syndromes
Antibacterials	Aminoglycosides[43]	Hearing loss	Certain mtDNA mutations susceptible, especially the m.1555A>G.109
	Chloramphenicol	Acute hepatitis, marrow suppression	Avoid in mtDNA depletion and Pearson syndromes
	Linezolid[55]	Lactic acidosis	
Antivirals[43]	Antiretrovirals	Myopathy, peripheral neuropathy	NRTIs implicated, zidovudine considered most toxic
	Clevudine	Myopathy	
Antihyperglycemics	Metformin[56]	Lactic acidosis	
Lipid-lowering agents	Statins[57]	Myopathy	Atorvastatin preferred over simvastatin
Antipyretics	Acetaminophen	Hepatic failure	Frequent/chronic use to be avoided

(MD: mitochondrial disorder; NRTI: nucleoside reverse transcriptase inhibitor)

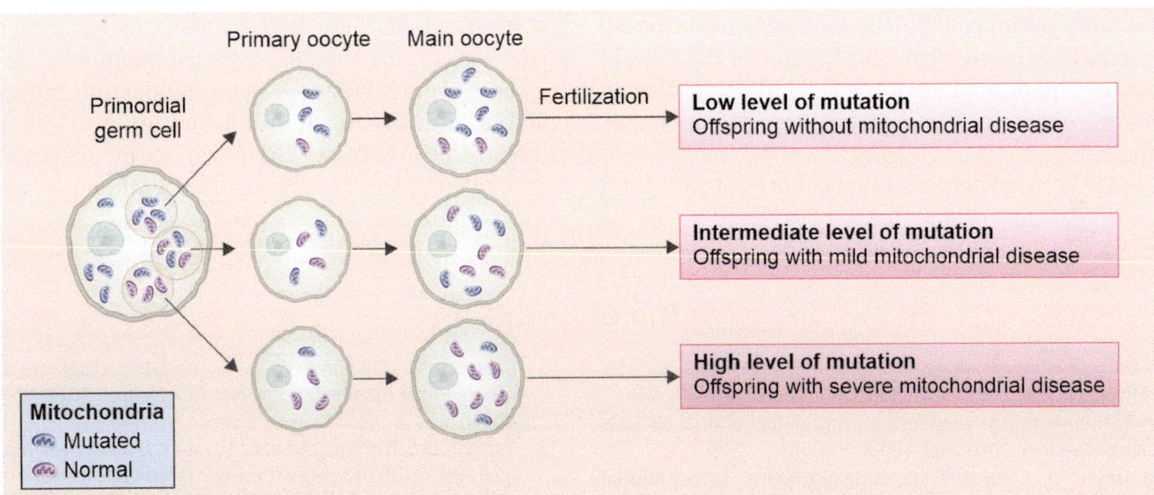

FIG. 2: Genetic bottleneck phenomenon.

bring with them an altogether different set of challenges.[67] The mtDNA is almost completely maternally inherited, and the "bottleneck phenomenon" **(Fig. 2)** affecting carriers of heteroplasmic mutations means that different oocytes can have widely varying levels of mutated mtDNA, and the outcome of fertilization can be impossible to predict. Options available for women include:[68]

- Normal reproduction with the associated risk of having a child with mtDNA disease.
- Planned childlessness
- Adoption
- In vitro fertilization with donor eggs

In recent years, prenatal testing and preimplantation genetic diagnosis (PIGD) have become available. Prenatal testing, done via chorionic villus sampling or amniocentesis, is an option in women with a low-mtDNA disease transmission risk, and in whom pregnancy termination can be considered. PIGD involves in vitro fertilization and egg collection with the development of embryos to the blastocyst (eight cell) stage, followed by the selection of an embryo with the lowest level of mtDNA mutations for implantation.[69]

In some women with mtDNA mutations known to have a high likelihood of defective mtDNA transmission, the above options may not be feasible. In such cases, the use of a donor egg or mitochondrial replacement therapy (selective use of donor woman mtDNA) is option.[70] Legal and ethical constraints limit the use of these techniques in certain countries.

FUTURE THERAPIES

In addition to further research into optimal diet, supplements, and exercise regimens, the ongoing developments are focused on pharmacological interventions to improve mitochondrial function using one or more of the following strategies:[63,71]

- Increasing the level of mitochondrial mass in cells with mitochondrial dysfunction
- Increasing mitochondrial content of NAD^+ as cells with mitochondrial dysfunction have reduction in NAD^+ and NAD^+/NADH ratio
- Preventing mitochondrial toxicity
- Inducing chronic, low-level hypoxia which has been observed to slow disease progression
- Increasing mitophagy by elective removal of defective mitochondria in heteroplasmic mtDNA diseases
- Restoring mtDNA homeostasis via enzyme replacement therapy, allogeneic stem cell transplantation, etc.

Additionally, genetic engineering approaches being explored include vector-based wild-type gene delivery of defective genes, manipulation of the level of heteroplasmy (gene shifting), and use of mitochondrial-targeted nucleases among others.[72,73]

Lastly, near-infrared light-emitting diode (NIR-LED) and transcranial direct current stimulation (TDCS) are two of the several emerging device-based treatments used for primary mitochondrial diseases.[74]

CONCLUSION

Mitochondrial disorders have a myriad of clinical presentations. This has been aptly summed up by Munnich and Rustin[75]—*any symptom, in any organ or tissue, at any age, with any mode of inheritance.* Neurologists need to be aware of the common symptoms and syndromic presentations of MDs, as well as of common nonneurological clinical features. Timely diagnosis can enable the institution of appropriate treatments early on, and also ensure appropriate precautions are taken to prevent iatrogenic mitochondrial toxicity.

We have made remarkable progress in our understanding of mitochondrial physiology and pathology in recent years. At the same time, the advent of NGS has substantially improved the ability to make a genetic diagnosis, and this will help to overcome one of the many hurdles in designing clinical trials, where standardization has been limited by a lack of objectivity. Recognition of the role of secondary mitochondrial dysfunction in many commoner neurological disorders (Alzheimer's, Parkinson's, Huntington's, etc.) as well as non-neurological disorders has spurred both clinical and commercial interest with the goal of developing effective, targeted treatments.

The rarity of MDs necessitates multicentric, international collaboration for the funding, design, and execution of clinical trials with well-defined, clinically meaningful outcome measures in order to discover therapies with a real impact on the lives of these patients.

REFERENCES

1. Gorman GS, Chinnery PF, DiMauro S, Hirano M, Koga Y, McFarland R, et al. Mitochondrial diseases. Nat Rev Dis Primers. 2016;2:16080.
2. Parikh S. The neurologic manifestations of mitochondrial disease. Dev Disabil Res Rev. 2010;16(2):120-8.
3. Hettiarachchi D, Lakmal K, Dissanayake VHW. Mitochondrial diseases in South Asia – A systematic review. Mitochondrion. 2022;62:24-30.
4. Mehndiratta MM, Agarwal P, Tatke M, Krishnamurthy M. Neurological mitochondrial cytopathies. Neurol India. 2002;50:162.
5. McFarland R, Taylor RW, Turnbull DM. A neurological perspective on mitochondrial disease. Lancet Neurol. 2010;9(8):829-40.
6. Satishchandra P, Sinha S. Progressive myoclonic epilepsy. Neurology India. 2010;58(4):514.
7. Chinnery PF. Mitochondrial Disorders Overview. Seattle: University of Washington; 2014. [online] Available from https://www.ncbi.nlm.nih.gov/books/NBK1224/. [Last accessed March, 2023].
8. Cohen BH. Mitochondrial and Metabolic Myopathies. Continuum (Minneap Minn). 2019;25(6):1732-66.
9. El-Hattab AW, Scaglia F. Mitochondrial DNA depletion syndromes: review and updates of genetic basis, manifestations, and therapeutic options. Neurotherapeutics. 2013;10(2):186-98.
10. DiMauro S, Schon EA, Carelli V, Hirano M. The clinical maze of mitochondrial neurology. Nat Rev Neurol. 2013;9(8):429-44.
11. Rahman S, Copeland WC. POLG-related disorders and their neurological manifestations. Nat Rev Neurol. 2019 Nov 19;15(1):40-52.
12. Yamashita S, Nishino I, Nonaka I, Goto Y. Genotype and phenotype analyses in 136 patients with single large-scale mitochondrial DNA deletions. J Hum Genet. 2008;53(7):598-606.
13. Baracca A, Solaini G, Sgarbi G, Lenaz G, Baruzzi A, Schapira AH, et al. Severe Impairment of Complex I–Driven Adenosine Triphosphate Synthesis in Leber Hereditary Optic Neuropathy Cybrids. Arch Neurol. 2005;62(5):730-6.
14. Piotrowska A, Korwin M, Bartnik E, Tońska K. Leber hereditary optic neuropathy—Historical report in comparison with the current knowledge. Gene. 2015;555(1):41-9.
15. Matthews L, Enzinger C, Fazekas F, Rovira A, Ciccarelli O, Dotti MT, et al. MRI in Leber's hereditary optic neuropathy: the relationship to multiple sclerosis. J Neurol Neurosurg Psychiatry. 2015;86:537-42.
16. Sofou K, De Coo IFM, Isohanni P, Ostergaard E, Naess K, De Meirleir L, et al. A multicenter study on Leigh syndrome: disease course and predictors of survival. Orphanet J Rare Dis. 2014;9:52.
17. Lee HF, Tsai CR, Chi CS, Lee HJ, Chen CC. Leigh syndrome: clinical and neuroimaging follow-up. Pediatr Neurol. 2009;40(2):88-93.
18. Wei Y, Cui L, Peng B. Mitochondrial DNA mutations in late-onset Leigh syndrome. J Neurol. 2018;265(10):2388-95.

19. Nishino I, Spinazzola A, Papadimitriou A, Hian LS, Afroze B. Mitochondrial neurogastrointestinal encephalomyopathy: an autosomal recessive disorder due to thymidine phosphorylase mutations. Ann Neurol. 2000;47(6):792-800.
20. Hirano M, Silvestri G, Blake DM, Lombes A, Minetti C, Bonilla E, et al. Mitochondrial neurogastrointestinal encephalomyopathy (MNGIE): Clinical, biochemical, and genetic features of an autosomal recessive mitochondrial disorder. Neurology. 1994;44(4):721-1.
21. Garone C, Tadesse S, Hirano M. Clinical and genetic spectrum of mitochondrial neurogastrointestinal encephalomyopathy. Brain. 2011;134(11):3326-32.
22. Velez-Bartolomei F, Lee C, Enns G. (2003). MERRF. In: Adam MP, Everman DB, Mirzaa GM, Pagon RA, Wallace SE, Bean LJH, Gripp KW, Amemiya A (Eds). GeneReviews® [Internet]. Seattle (WA): University of Washington, Seattle; 1993-2023. [online] Available from https://www.ncbi.nlm.nih.gov/books/NBK1116/. [Last accessed March, 2023].
23. Parikh S, Goldstein A, Koenig MK, Scaglia F, Enns GM, Saneto R, et al. Diagnosis and management of mitochondrial disease: a consensus statement from the Mitochondrial Medicine Society. Genet Med. 2015;17(9):689-701.
24. Mitochondrial Medicine Society's Committee on Diagnosis; Haas RH, Parikh S, Falk MJ, Saneto RP, Wolf NI, et al. The in-depth evaluation of suspected mitochondrial disease. Mol Genet Metab. 2008;94(1):16-37.
25. Tarnopolsky M, Stevens L, MacDonald JR, Rodriguez C, Mahoney D, Rush J, et al. Diagnostic utility of a modified forearm ischemic exercise test and technical issues relevant to exercise testing. Muscle Nerve. 2003;27(3):359-66.
26. Suomalainen A, Elo JM, Pietiläinen KH, Hakonen AH, Sevastianova K, Korpela M, et al. FGF-21 as a biomarker for muscle-manifesting mitochondrial respiratory chain deficiencies: a diagnostic study. Lancet Neurol. 2011;10(9):806-18.
27. Davis RL, Liang C, Edema-Hildebrand F, Riley C, Needham M, Sue CM. Fibroblast growth factor 21 is a sensitive biomarker of mitochondrial disease. Neurology. 2013;81(21):1819-26.
28. Patel KP, O'Brien TW, Subramony SH, Shuster J, Stacpoole PW. The spectrum of pyruvate dehydrogenase complex deficiency: clinical, biochemical and genetic features in 371 patients. Mol Genet Metab. 2012;106(3):385-94.
29. Debray FG, Mitchell GA, Allard P, Robinson BH, Hanley JA, Lambert M. Diagnostic accuracy of blood lactate-to-pyruvate molar ratio in the differential diagnosis of congenital lactic acidosis. Clin Chem. 2007;53(5):916-21.
30. Barshop BA. Metabolomic approaches to mitochondrial disease: correlation of urine organic acids. Mitochondrion. 2004;4(5-6): 521-7.
31. Ramaekers V, Sequeira JM, Quadros EV. Clinical recognition and aspects of the cerebral folate deficiency syndromes. Clin Chem Lab Med. 2013;51(3):497-511.
32. Yatsuga S, Fujita Y, Ishii A, Fukumoto Y, Arahata H, Kakuma T, et al. Growth differentiation factor 15 as a useful biomarker for mitochondrial disorders. Ann Neurol. 2015;78(5):814-23.
33. Bernier FP, Boneh A, Dennett X, Chow CW, Cleary MA, Thorburn DR. Diagnostic criteria for respiratory chain disorders in adults and children. Neurology. 2002;59(9):1406-11.
34. Barrientos A, Fontanesi F, Díaz F. Evaluation of the mitochondrial respiratory chain and oxidative phosphorylation system using polarography and spectrophotometric enzyme assays. Curr Protoc Hum Genet. 2009;Chapter 19:Unit19.3.
35. Haas RH, Parikh S, Falk MJ, Saneto RP, Wolf NI, Darin N, et al. Mitochondrial disease: a practical approach for primary care physicians. Pediatrics. 2007;120(6):1326-33.
36. Majoie CB, Akkerman EM, Blank C, Barth PG, Poll-The BT, den Heeten GJ. Mitochondrial encephalomyopathy: comparison of conventional MR imaging with diffusion-weighted and diffusion tensor imaging: case report. AJNR Am J Neuroradiol. 2002; 23(5):813-6.
37. Castillo M, Kwock L, Green C. MELAS syndrome: imaging and proton MR spectroscopic findings. AJNR Am J Neuroradiol. 1995;16(2):233-9.
38. Clarke C, Howard R, Rossor M, Shorvon S. Neurology: A Queen Square Textbook, 2nd edition. Hoboken: Wiley-Blackwell; 2016.
39. McCormick E, Place E, Falk MJ. Molecular genetic testing for mitochondrial disease: From one generation to the next. Neurotherapeutics. 2013;10(2):251-61.
40. Koenig MK, Emrick L, Karaa A, Korson M, Scaglia F, Parikh S, et al. Recommendations for the management of stroke-like episodes in patients with mitochondrial encephalomyopathy, lactic acidosis, and stroke-like episodes. JAMA Neurol. 2016;73(5):591-4.
41. Padmanabhan U, Leslie K. Australian Anaesthetists' Practice of Sedation for Gastrointestinal Endoscopy in Adult Patients. Anaesth Intensive Care. 2008;36(3):436-41.
42. Cohen PJ. Effect of anesthetics on mitochondrial function. Anesthesiology. 1973;39(2):153-64.
43. Mancuso M, Orsucci D, Filosto M, Simoncini C, Siciliano G. Drugs and mitochondrial diseases: 40 queries and answers. Expert Opin Pharmacother. 2012;13(4):527-43.
44. Finsterer J, Frank M. Propofol is mitochondrion-toxic and may unmask a mitochondrial disorder. J Child Neurol. 2016;31(13): 1489-94.
45. Klein NP, Aukes L, Lee J, Fireman B, Shapira SK, Slade B, et al. Evaluation of immunization rates and safety among children with inborn errors of metabolism. Pediatrics. 2011;127(5):e1139-46.
46. Shahni R, Cale CM, Anderson G, Osellame LD, Hambleton S, Jacques TS, et al. Signal transducer and activator of transcription 2 deficiency is a novel disorder of mitochondrial fission. Brain. 2015;138(10):2834-46.
47. Esposito LA, Melov S, Panov A, Cottrell BA, Wallace DC. Mitochondrial disease in mouse results in increased oxidative stress. Proc Natl Acad Sci U S A. 1999;96(9):4820-5.
48. Finsterer J. Clinical therapeutic management of human mitochondrial disorders. Pediatr Neurol. 2020;113:66-74.
49. DiMauro S, Hirano M, Schon EA. Approaches to the treatment of mitochondrial diseases. Muscle Nerve. 2006;34(3):265-83.
50. Jeppesen TD, Schwartz M, Olsen DB, Wibrand F, Krag T, Dunø M, et al. Aerobic training is safe and improves exercise capacity in patients with mitochondrial myopathy. Brain. 2006;129(12): 3402-12.
51. Cejudo P, Bautista J, Montemayor T, Villagómez R, Jiménez L, Ortega F, et al. Exercise training in mitochondrial myopathy: A randomized controlled trial. Muscle Nerve. 2005;32(3):342-50.
52. Pitceathly RD, Viscomi C. Effects of ketosis in mitochondrial myopathy: potential benefits of a mitotoxic diet. EMBO Molecular Medicine. 2016;8(11):1231-3.
53. Peracha H, Sawamoto K, Averill L, Kecskemethy H, Theroux M, Thacker M, et al. Molecular genetics and metabolism, special edition: Diagnosis, diagnosis and prognosis of Mucopolysaccharidosis IVA. Mol Genet Metab. 2018;125(1-2):18-37.
54. Mirza NS, Alfirevic A, Jorgensen A, Marson AG, Pirmohamed M. Metabolic acidosis with topiramate and zonisamide: an assessment of its severity and predictors. Pharmacogenet Genomics. 2011;21(5):297-302.
55. Zuccarini NS, Yousuf T, Wozniczka D, Rauf AA. Lactic acidosis induced by linezolid mimics symptoms of an acute intracranial bleed: a case report and literature review. J Clin Med Res. 2016;8(10):753-6.
56. Protti A, Russo R, Tagliabue P, Vecchio S, Singer M, Rudiger A, et al. Oxygen consumption is depressed in patients with lactic acidosis due to biguanide intoxication. Crit Care. 2010;14(1):1-9.

57. Schirris TJ, Renkema GH, Ritschel T, Voermans NC, Bilos A, van Engelen BG, et al. Statin-induced myopathy is associated with mitochondrial complex III inhibition. Cell Metab. 2015;22(3): 399-407.
58. Gerards M, Van Den Bosch BJ, Danhauser K, Serre V, van Weeghel M, Wanders RJ, et al. Riboflavin-responsive oxidative phosphorylation complex I deficiency caused by defective ACAD9: new function for an old gene. Brain. 2011;134(1):210-9.
59. Green P, Wiseman M, Crow YJ, Houlden H, Riphagen S, Lin JP, et al. Brown-Vialetto-Van Laere syndrome, a ponto-bulbar palsy with deafness, is caused by mutations in c20orf54. Am J Hum Genet. 2010;86(3):485-9.
60. Olsen RKJ, Koňaříková E, Giancaspero TA, Mosegaard S, Boczonadi V, Mataković L, et al. Riboflavin-responsive and-non-responsive mutations in FAD synthase cause multiple acyl-CoA dehydrogenase and combined respiratory-chain deficiency. Am J Hum Genet. 2016;98(6):1130-45.
61. Jay AM, Conway RL, Feldman GL, Nahhas F, Spencer L, Wolf B. Outcomes of individuals with profound and partial biotinidase deficiency ascertained by newborn screening in Michigan over 25 years. Genet Med. 2015;17(3):205-9.
62. Zeng WQ, Al-Yamani E, Acierno JS, Slaugenhaupt S, Gillis T, MacDonald ME, et al. Biotin-responsive basal ganglia disease maps to 2q36. 3 and is due to mutations in SLC19A3. Am J Hum Genet. 2005;77(1):16-26.
63. Tinker RJ, Lim AZ, Stefanetti RJ, McFarland R. Current and emerging clinical treatment in mitochondrial disease. Mol Diagn Ther. 2021;25(2):181-206.
64. Bax BE. Mitochondrial neurogastrointestinal encephalomyopathy: approaches to diagnosis and treatment. J Transl Genet Genom. 2020;4:1-16.
65. Carelli V, Carbonelli M, Irenaeus F, Kawasaki A, Klopstock T, Lagrèze WA, et al. International consensus statement on the clinical and therapeutic management of Leber hereditary optic neuropathy. J Neuroophthalmol. 2017;37(4):371-81.
66. Distelmaier F, Haack TB, Wortmann SB, Mayr JA, Prokisch H. Treatable mitochondrial diseases: cofactor metabolism and beyond. Brain. 2017;140(2):e11.
67. Stewart JB, Chinnery PF. The dynamics of mitochondrial DNA heteroplasmy: implications for human health and disease. Nat Rev Genet. 2015;16(9):530-42.
68. Gorman GS, McFarland R, Stewart J, Feeney C, Turnbull DM. Mitochondrial donation: from test tube to clinic. Lancet. 2018;392 (10154):1191-2.
69. Hellebrekers DM, Wolfe R, Hendrickx AT, de Coo IF, de Die CE, Geraedts JP, et al. PGD and heteroplasmic mitochondrial DNA point mutations: a systematic review estimating the chance of healthy offspring. Human Reprod Update. 2012;18(4):341-9.
70. Greenfield A, Braude P, Flinter F, Lovell-Badge R, Ogilvie C, Perry ACF, et al. Assisted reproductive technologies to prevent human mitochondrial disease transmission. Nat Biotechnol. 2017;35(11): 1059-68.
71. Russell OM, Gorman GS, Lightowlers RN, Turnbull DM. Mitochondrial diseases: hope for the future. Cell. 2020;181(1):168-88.
72. Tachibana M, Amato P, Sparman M, Woodward J, Sanchis DM, Ma H, et al. Towards germline gene therapy of inherited mitochondrial diseases. Nature. 2013;493(7434):627-31.
73. Yu-Wai-Man P. Genetic manipulation for inherited neurodegenerative diseases: myth or reality? Br J Ophthalmol. 2016;100(10): 1322-31.
74. Anderson L, Antkowiak P, Asefa A, Ballard A, Bansal T, Bello A, et al. FDA regulation of neurological and physical medicine devices: access to safe and effective neurotechnologies for all Americans. Neuron. 2016;92(5):943-8.
75. Munnich A, Rustin P. Clinical spectrum and diagnosis of mitochondrial disorders. Am J Med Genet. 2001;106(1):4-17.

98

CHAPTER

Headache Disorders

Debashish Chowdhury

INTRODUCTION

Patients with headaches are commonly encountered in routine clinical practice. People usually seek medical attention when their headaches become recurrent and disabling. Sometimes, an episode of headache heralds an acute catastrophic event. There are many causes of headaches and only a minority of people with headache disorders are diagnosed appropriately. Multiple studies have shown that headache disorders have been underestimated, under-recognized, and undertreated worldwide.

Headache disorders significantly burden the individual, society, and the country. Migraine ranks second in disability among all the disorders of the world. An exceptionally high economic burden has been recognized for patients with recurrent headaches. This is due to indirect economic costs such as absenteeism and poor performance at work and the direct costs of multiple consultations, investigations, and medications. This has led to considerable research and progress in the understanding and management of various headache disorders in the last two decades. The present chapter aims to describe these advancements regarding diagnosing and managing common headache disorders seen in clinical practice.

CLASSIFICATION OF HEADACHE DISORDERS

The first attempt at headache classification was undertaken by the Ad-Hoc Committee in 1962 and was sponsored by the National Institute of Health. For the last 30 years, the International Headache Society (IHS) has published four editions of the International Classification of Headache Disorders (ICHD)—ICHD-1, 2, 3β, and 3 editions. ICHD-3 is now being in use since 2018.[1]

International Classification of Headache Disorders-3 divides headache disorders into three broad parts **(Table 1)**. Part 1 consists of primary headaches; part 2 consists of

TABLE 1: International Classification of Headache Disorders 3rd edition (ICHD-3) classification of headache disorders.

ICHD groups	Headache disorders
Part one: The primary headaches	
1	Migraine
2	Tension-type headache
3	Trigeminal autonomic cephalalgias
4	Other primary headache disorders
Part two: The secondary headaches	
5	Headache attributed to trauma or injury to the head and/or neck
6	Headache attributed to cranial or cervical vascular disorder
7	Headache attributed to nonvascular intracranial disorder
8	Headache attributed to a substance or its withdrawal
9	Headache attributed to infection
10	Headache attributed to disorder of homeostasis
11	Headache or facial pain attributed to a disorder of the cranium, neck, eyes, ears, nose, sinuses, teeth, mouth or other facial or cervical structure
12	Headache attributed to psychiatric disorder
Part three: Painful cranial neuropathies, other facial pains, and other headaches	
13	Painful lesions of the cranial nerves and other facial pain
14	Other headache disorders
	Appendix

Source: Headache Classification Committee of the International Headache Society (IHS) (2018).[1]

secondary headaches; and part 3 consists of painful cranial neuropathies, other facial pains, and other headaches. An "Appendix group" is incorporated in the last to accommodate the research criteria for novel entities, alternative diagnostic criteria for some of the existing entities, and for eliminating a few entities which have been historically included in the previous classification but still lack sufficient evidence. It is important to note that to diagnose primary headaches, the patients should have no red flags for secondary headaches, normal neurological examination, and normal investigations (if done). Occasionally some abnormalities can be found on clinical examination or investigations in patients with primary headaches. However, these should not be temporally related to or be able to explain the headache syndrome. Primary headaches constitute about 85% of all headache disorders in routine clinical practice. In this chapter, we shall be dealing with headache disorders enlisted in parts 1 and 2.

EPIDEMIOLOGY OF HEADACHE DISORDERS

According to a global burden of diseases study, the estimated global prevalence of active headache disorder was 52.0% [95% confidence interval (CI) 48.9–55.4]. About 15.8% of the world's population has headaches each day. Of the primary headaches, migraine 14.0% (12.9–15.2), tension-type headache (TTH) 26.0% (22.7–29.5), and headaches on ≥15 days per month (signifying chronic daily headaches) were reported in 4.6% (3.9–5.5).[2] About 5% of global ill health, quantified as years lived with disability, results from migraine. Hence, it is a disorder of high public health importance. Migraine occurs more commonly in females than in males. Based on a meta-analysis of 16 population-based studies, the pooled lifetime prevalence of cluster headaches (CHs) was found to be 0.12%.[3] Earlier, CH was considered a predominantly male disease. However, recent studies have shown the male: female ratio to be around 4.3:1. Data regarding the epidemiology of other trigeminal autonomic cephalalgias (TACs) and other primary and secondary headaches are limited. It is noteworthy that even the data about migraine and TTH were primarily derived from high-income countries and may not reflect global prevalence. For example, a population-based survey from Karnataka state in India reported that 63.9% of subjects had a headache in the preceding year.[4] The age-standardized 1-year prevalence of migraine was 25.2%; prevalence was higher among women than men [odds ratio (OR) 2.1 (1.7–2.6)] and among those from rural areas than urban [OR 1.5 (1.3–1.8)]. The age-standardized 1-year prevalence of TTH was 35.1%. The estimated prevalence of all headaches on ≥15 days per month was 3.0%. These estimates were higher than the global prevalence estimates.

PRIMARY HEADACHES

Primary headaches are classified into four groups, namely migraine, TTH, TACs, and other primary headaches.

Migraine

Migraine is the most common primary headache disorder seen in clinics. It is a complex neurovascular disorder characterized by recurrent attacks of moderate-to-severe intensity headaches with multiple neurological and systemic accompaniments.

Classification

In the ICHD-3 classification, migraine is in group 1 of the primary headaches. It is further subdivided into six groups: (i) migraine without aura, (ii) migraine with aura, (iii) chronic migraine, (iv) complications of migraine, (v) probable migraine, and (vi) episodic syndrome that may be associated with migraine **(Box 1)**. Migraine with aura is subdivided into four groups: typical aura that can last up to 5–60 minutes (with or without headache), brainstem aura [brainstem symptoms include dysarthria, vertigo, tinnitus, hyperacusis, diplopia, ataxia not attributable to sensory deficit, and decreased level of consciousness (Glasgow Coma Scale ≤13)], hemiplegic migraine (motor weakness), and retinal migraine (monocular vision loss). The last three groups necessitate the fulfilment of migraine with aura as the qualifying condition. Hemiplegic migraine can be familial or sporadic, and the familial ones can be further subclassified into identifiable genetic abnormalities.

BOX 1 Subtypes of migraine.

- Migraine without aura
- *Migraine with aura*:
  - Migraine with typical aura
    - Typical aura with headache
    - Typical aura without headache
  - Migraine with brainstem aura
  - Hemiplegic migraine:
    - Familial hemiplegic migraine (FHM):
      - Familial hemiplegic migraine type 1 (FHM1)
      - Familial hemiplegic migraine type 2 (FHM2)
      - Familial hemiplegic migraine type 3 (FHM3)
      - FHM, other loci
    - Sporadic hemiplegic migraine (SHM)
  - Retinal migraine
- Chronic migraine
- *Complications of migraine*:
  - Status migrainosus
  - Persistent aura without infarction
  - Migrainous infarction
  - Migraine aura-triggered seizure
- *Probable migraine*:
  - Probable migraine without aura
  - Probable migraine with aura
- *Episodic syndromes*:
  - Recurrent gastrointestinal disturbance
    - Cyclical vomiting syndrome
    - Abdominal migraine
  - Benign paroxysmal vertigo
  - Benign paroxysmal torticollis

Source: Headache Classification Committee of the International Headache Society (IHS) (2018).[1]

Chronic migraine is defined as a headache occurring on ≥15 days per month for more than 3 months and having features of migraine headache on at least 8 days per month. Complications of migraine include entities such as status migrainosus, persistent aura without infarction, migrainous infarction, and migraine aura-triggered seizure. Episodic syndromes, seen mainly in children, can occur in association with typical migraine with or without aura or the child may develop migraine in later years. These include gastrointestinal disturbances (cyclical vomiting and abdominal migraine), paroxysmal vertigo, and paroxysmal torticollis.

Diagnostic Features: Core Concepts

Migraine headaches are long-lasting (lasting 4–72 hours without treatment in adults). The headaches are unilateral, throbbing, moderate-to-severe intensity, and aggravated by routine physical activity, suggesting motion sensitivity. Patients avoid physical activities during the attack. Of these four headache characteristics, *at least two* must be fulfilled. Migraine headaches are associated with nausea, vomiting, photophobia (increased sensitivity to normal light), and phonophobia (increased sensitivity to normal sound). Of these four systemic features, ICHD-3 requires fulfillment of either nausea *or* vomiting or photophobia and phonophobia. A patient with a typical migraine phenotype with severe headache usually cannot carry out her/his activity, retires to a dark, quiet room, and lies down. Many variations from the typical phenotype are seen in clinical practice, and milder migraines are not uncommon. Two other clinical features help in diagnosis. First is a consistent set of migraine triggers that precipitate migraine attacks **(Table 2)** and the second is the presence of family history. These should be routinely enquired during clinical evaluation.

From a diagnostic point of view, migraine should be better conceptualized as a syndrome consisting of four phases with a timeline.[5] The first phase is that of premonitory symptoms, which precede the headache by hours to days and consist of altered mood, irritability, depression or euphoria, fatigue, yawning, excessive sleepiness, craving for a particular food (e.g., chocolate), stiff muscles (especially in the neck), constipation or diarrhea, and increased urination. The second phase consists of aura. It is a transient brain dysfunction that usually precedes the headache. Visual aura is the most common type seen in migraine. Classically, the patient develops a visual disturbance in the form of flashes of black and white or multicolored zigzag lines at the periphery and a central scotoma. These develop and expand slowly over 5–20 minutes, usually lasting less than 60 minutes. Many other visual phenomena have been described such as "foggy" vision, small bright dots, and "like looking through heat waves or water" and rarely metamorphopsias. Sometimes other forms of the aura are reported, such as sensory symptoms (like auditory or olfactory hallucinations, tingling, pins and needles sensation in arms, legs, and face), language symptoms (difficulty in speaking, finding words, naming), and motor symptoms (weakness of limbs). The aura is often followed by an intense headache lasting from 4 hours to 3 days. This constitutes the third phase. The headache usually builds up in severity over time, although the severities and frequency of attacks are highly variable. In most patients, the headache intensifies on activity, and most prefer to retire in a dark, quiet room. Thus, many patients become vegetative during headaches. An abnormal sensitivity to pain develops in many patients where even an innocuous stimulus is perceived as painful (called "allodynia", the other pain). For example, combing hair may give rise to painful scalp sensations or using a pillow to support the head may give rise to excruciating painful sensations over the side of the contact. The fourth phase is that of postdrome when even though the patient recovers from headache, general malaise and exhaustion persist for a variable time. Not all these phases need to be present in all patients or in all attacks for a migraine diagnosis.

TABLE 2: Common triggers for migraine stratified by sex.

Triggers	Female	Male
Menstruation	78.1	–
Stress	76.7	69.2
Bright (sun) light	68.5	63.2
Sleep deprivation	67.7	60.3
Skipping meals	47.9	42.4
Alcoholic beverages	45.0	45.5
Physical exercise/sexual activity	41.7	45.8
Weather changes	45.9	38.7
Certain food/nonalcoholic beverages	28.6	31.9
Mild head trauma	24.5	21.9
High altitudes	18.0	11.5

Source: van Casteren DS, Verhagen IE, Onderwater GL, MaassenVanDenBrink A, Terwindt GM. Sex differences in prevalence of migraine trigger factors: A cross-sectional study. Cephalalgia. 2021;41(6):643-8.

Pathophysiology

The pathophysiology of migraine is not fully understood. A patient with migraine is believed to have a hyperexcitable brain that lacks habituation with repeated sensory stimuli. Migraine patients also have a strong positive family history. Various triggers can initiate hypothalamic activation in migraine patients resulting in premonitory symptoms. Hypothalamic activation leads to an alteration of parasympathetic and sympathetic tone in intracranial vessels including those supplying the dura.[5,6] A sterile neurogenic inflammation in the dural vessels leads to the activation of the trigeminal ganglion. Multiple neuropeptides such as calcitonin gene-related peptide (CGRP) and pituitary adenylate cyclase-activating polypeptide (PACAP) are released during this sterile inflammation. This trigeminovascular activation leads to the activation of the so-called trigeminocervical complex in the upper neck, followed by activation of various brainstem nuclei and the pain pathway up to the thalamus and thence to the cortex for the conscious perception of pain. About 25–30% of patients with migraine have a history of aura which is believed to occur due to the phenomenon of "cortical spreading depression", resulting in a wave of oligemia that moves from the posterior regions of the brain anteriorly and leads to transient neurological dysfunctions in the visual, sensory, language, or motor systems.

Treatment

Treating migraine aims to abort acute attacks and prevent future attacks by instituting appropriate management strategies. These include pharmacological as well as nonpharmacological treatments. Patient education, lifestyle modifications, behavioral and physical therapies, yoga, meditation, and optimum pharmacological treatment ensure good outcomes.

Acute Treatment

The goal of acute treatment of migraine includes rapid and consistent freedom from pain and associated symptoms without recurrence and restoration of the ability to function. There should be shared decision-making with the patient regarding acute treatment strategies. Three models, namely, stratified care [prescribing milder drugs such as nonsteroidal anti-inflammatory drugs (NSAIDs) for milder or less disabling attacks], stepped care across migraine attacks (treating milder attacks with NSAIDs and severe attacks with triptans), or stepped care within a migraine attack (treating initially with NSAIDs and adding triptans for nonresponding attacks) have been advocated. Three important points should always be discussed with the patients: the need to take an appropriate dose, the need to take the acute medicines early during the attack (before central centralization occurs), and the potential for medication overuse if the medicines are taken indiscriminately. Various options are available to treat acute migraine attacks with a sound evidence base **(Tables 3 and 4)**.[7] NSAIDs though nonspecific, are helpful for mild-to-moderate attacks. Ergot preparations are no longer favored due to many adverse effects, including high chances of medication overuse. Since the mid-1990s, triptans (5HT1B/1D receptor agonists) have become the mainstay for moderate-to-severe migraine attacks. However, they are contraindicated for persons with cardiovascular risk factors such as uncontrolled hypertension and peripheral artery disease. Triptans can also cause medication overuse headaches (MOHs). The latest drugs for acute migraine treatment include ditans (5HT1F receptor agonists) and small molecule CGRP antagonists called gepants. A significant advantage of the ditans and gepants is their safety profile regarding cardiovascular risk factors (in contrast to triptans). However, their efficacy is lower regarding pain freedom at 2 hours compared to triptans.[8] Besides the oral routes, alternative routes of administration of acute migraine drugs have been developed for quicker response and to bypass absorption problems due to nausea, vomiting, and gastric stasis which are common systemic accompaniments during acute migraine attacks.

Patients should also be prescribed at-home rescue medications if the first-line acute treatment fails. These may include a combination of NSAIDs and a triptan, other acute drugs from the drug basket, and dopamine antagonists. Opioids should be avoided. Many patients with a severe

TABLE 3: Common first-line established acute treatments for migraine.

Drug	Route	Recommended dose	Number needed to treat	Therapeutic gain (%)
Paracetamol	Oral	1,000 mg	12	7
Acetyl-salicylic acid	Oral	1,000 mg	8.1	12
Diclofenac	Tablet powder	50 mg	7.4	14
Ibuprofen	Oral	400–600 mg	7.2 (for 400 mg) 6.3 (for 600 mg)	12–15
Naproxen	Oral	500–850 mg	11–15	9

TABLE 4: Triptans, ditans, and CGRP antagonists for acute treatment of migraine.

Drug	Route	Recommended dose	Number needed to treat	Therapeutic gain (%)
Sumatriptan	SC Oral IN TDP	SC: 3, 4, 6 mg PO: 50–100 mg IN: 10–20 mg TDP: 6.5 mg	2.3 4.7–6.1 4.7	22
Rizatriptan	Oral	5–10 mg	3–5	32
Zolmitriptan	Oral IN	2.5, 5 mg 2.5, 5 mg	4.8–5 4.6	21
Eletriptan	Oral	20, 40, 80 mg	3.7–9.9	25
Frovatriptan	Oral	2.5 mg	11.9	19
Naratriptan	Oral	2.5 mg	8.2	22
Almotriptan	Oral	12.5 mg	5.2	26
Lasmiditan	Oral	50, 100, and 200 mg	5.9–13.7	15–17%
Ubrogepant	Oral	50, 100 mg	10.7–13.3	9
Rimegepant	Oral	75 mg	9.4	8

Note: Triptans are contraindicated in coronary heart disease, cerebrovascular disease, uncontrolled hypertension, peripheral vascular disease; subcutaneous (SC) sumatriptan has highest bioavailability. Eletriptan, frovatriptan, and naratriptan suitable for attacks of longer duration. Although all triptans are superior to placebo, highest likelihood of consistent success has been reported with rizatriptan (10 mg), eletriptan (80 mg), and almotriptan (12.5 mg).

(CGRP: calcitonin gene-related peptide; IN: intranasal; TDP: transdermal patch)

attack of migraine fail to respond to acute therapies and visit the emergency department.[9] Some of these attacks may last for more than 72 hours, and this condition has been called "status migrainosus". These patients are very anxious, highly disabled, and seek quick relief from pain. Reassurance, liberal fluid replacement, injectable sumatriptan (if not already taken), injection metoclopramide, or prochlorperazine are the evidence-based treatment options for these patients **(Table 5)**. Diphenhydramine is usually added to prevent the extrapyramidal side effects of metoclopramide and prochlorperazine. Alternatively, an injection of diclofenac or ketorolac can be given. Second-line treatment includes dihydroergotamine (DHE) and valproate. A single shot of dexamethasone has been shown to prevent headache recurrence.

Preventive Treatment

Various classes of drugs are now available for migraine prevention. Preventive treatment should be offered to any patient with a significant disability that interferes with daily routines, despite acute treatment. It should also be offered irrespective of disability in patients with hemiplegic migraine, basilar migraine, migraine with prolonged aura, or migrainous infarction (to prevent neurological damage). In general, preventive therapy aims to reduce the attack frequency, severity, and duration; improve responsiveness to acute treatment; improve function and reduce disability; and prevent the evolution of episodic headaches into chronic daily headache.[9]

While prescribing preventive therapy, the first step is to maximize compliance by discussing with the patient the rationale for prevention, when and how to use these drugs, and common adverse effects. The patient's expectations need to be addressed. Expected benefits and the need for an adequate drug trial must be emphasized before therapy starts. For most oral medications, at least a 4–6 weeks trial should be given; the dose should be escalated stepwise until improvement occurs or the side effects develop. When a successful dose is found, tapering should be considered in 6–12 months, if the headache has been controlled. Headache diaries are an essential element of all preventive programs.

Migraine preventives with good evidence base can be classified into five groups: established oral medications, small-molecule oral CGRP antagonists and monoclonal antibodies (mAbs) against CGRP receptors (or ligands) (anti-CGRP-mAbs), toxins, peripheral blocks, and neuromodulation devices.

Among the established oral medications, beta-blockers (such as propranolol and metoprolol), calcium channel blockers like flunarizine, angiotensin receptor blockers such as candesartan, antidepressants such as amitriptyline and venlafaxine and antiseizure medicines such as divalproex and topiramate are useful in episodic migraine **(Table 6)**. The choice of a particular agent is determined by the patient's profile, contraindications, and preferences. The problem with these agents includes their nonspecific mechanism of action for migraine, slow dose titration, slow onset of action, lack of adherence, and adverse effects. Along with these established oral agents, many nutraceuticals such as riboflavin, coenzyme Q10, magnesium, and vitamin D have been found to have modest efficacy for migraine prevention. Mostly these agents are combined with the standard oral drugs in patients who fail to respond to monotherapy, and in children **(Table 7)**.

TABLE 5: Drugs for treating migraine in emergency department (ED).

Drug	Dose	Adverse effect
Sumatriptan	6 mg SC	Triptan symptoms (chest pressure or heaviness, flushing, weakness, drowsiness, dizziness, malaise, a feeling of warmth, and paresthesias)
Prochlorperazine*	10 mg IV	Extrapyramidal side effects such as acute dystonic reactions and akathisia
Metoclopramide*	10–20 mg IV	Extrapyramidal side effects such as acute dystonic reactions and akathisia
Chlorpromazine*	0.1 mg/kg (or 12.5 mg) single dose or as a slow IV infusion (maximum rate 1 mg/min); maximum cumulative dose 25 mg	Extrapyramidal side effects such as acute dystonic reactions and akathisia; arrhythmia from QT-segment prolongation on ECG, drowsiness, and postural hypotension
Dihydroergotamine combined with metoclopramide	1 mg +10 mg IV	Contraindicated in ischemic vascular disease involving cardiac, cerebrovascular, or peripheral circulations
Ketorolac	30 mg IV or 60 mg IM	Renal dysfunction
Sodium valproate**	500–100 mg IV	Reaction at the injection site, and nausea, somnolence, vomiting, dizziness, taste perversion, and rarely hematologic complications such as bleeding
Dexamethasone***	8–24 mg IM or IV	Hypersensitivity, mood changes, fluid retention

*Intravenous (IV) diphenhydramine (12.5–25 mg) is usually added to prevent extrapyramidal side effects when using parenteral antiemetics.

**Valproate is the second-line agent.

***Dexamethasone is used to prevent headache recurrence.

(ECG: electrocardiogram; IM: intramuscular; SC: subcutaneous)

TABLE 6: Established oral drugs for preventive treatment of migraine.

Drug	Starting dose	Maximum dose	Adverse event	Contraindication
Propranolol	40 mg	240 mg	Bradyarrhythmias, bronchospasm, insomnia, memory impairment, sexual dysfunction, masking hypoglycemia	Bradycardia, uncompensated heart failure, cardiogenic shock, bronchial asthma, hypersensitivity
Atenolol	25 mg	100 mg		
Metoprolol	50 mg	200 mg		
Bisoprolol	5 mg	10 mg		
Topiramate	25 mg	200 mg	Dizziness, cognitive dysfunction, psychiatric disturbances, paresthesia, metabolic acidosis, nephrolithiasis, acute myopia with secondary angle closure glaucoma, maculopathy, hyperthermia, weight loss	Hypersensitivity, recent alcohol intake, pregnancy
Valproic acid/divalproex	500 mg	1,500 mg	Dizziness, cognitive dysfunction, cytopenia, hepatotoxicity, hyperammonemia, hypersensitivity reactions, pancreatitis	Women with childbearing potential, hypersensitivity
Candesartan	4 mg	16 mg	AKI, hypotension	Hypersensitivity
Amitriptyline	10 mg	150 mg	Anticholinergic effects, bleeding risk, cardiac conduction abnormalities, CNS depression, fragility fractures, hyponatremia, acute angle closure glaucoma, orthostatic hypotension, serotonin syndrome,	Hypersensitivity, MAO-B inhibitors, cisapride, acute recovery phase of MI
Flunarizine	5 mg	10 mg	Drowsiness, psychiatric disturbances, extrapyramidal syndrome, weight gain, galactorrhea	Hypersensitivity, Parkinson's disease, depression

(AKI: acute kidney injury; CNS: central nervous system; MAO-B: monoamine oxidase B)

TABLE 7: Nutraceuticals for migraine prevention.

Nutraceuticals	Dose per day	Route	Adverse effects	Contra-indication
Riboflavin	400 mg	Oral	Diarrhea, polyuria	Hyper-sensitivity
Magnesium	600 mg	Oral	Diarrhea	
Coenzyme Q-10	300 mg	Oral	Cutaneous allergy	
Vitamin D	2,000 IU	Oral	Hyper-vitaminosis D	

Small molecule CGRP antagonists such as atogepant have recently been approved for migraine prevention.[10] Similarly, another gepant called rimegepant, which has been approved for acute treatment, has shown modest benefit for migraine prevention when given on alternate days.[11] Another recent advancement in migraine prevention has been the development of four anti-CGRP-mAbs, namely erenumab, galcanezumab, fremanezumab, and eptinezumab.[12] The first three can be given subcutaneously every month, whereas eptinezumab can be given intravenously every 3 months. These drugs are helpful for the prevention of both episodic and chronic migraines. Longitudinal data of more than 5 years have shown that these drugs retain their efficacy and are generally safe and well tolerated. Some longitudinal studies have noted rash, constipation, and systolic hypertension as side effects **(Table 8)**. The major limiting factor of these agents is the cost.

Botulinum toxin A (BOTA) is efficacious for preventing chronic migraines but ineffective for episodic migraines. The Phase III Research Evaluating Migraine Prophylaxis Therapy (PREMEPT) paradigm recommends 155–195 units of the toxin to be injected into 31 areas in the head, neck, and shoulders every 3 months.[13] It is devoid of any significant side effects. The effect of BOTA accrues over time, and hence at least two to three cycles of BOTA need to be tried before considering it ineffective. Again, the cost is a limiting factor for its wider use. An alternative investigated in recent years is greater occipital nerve blocks (GONBs) and multiple peripheral nerve blocks in chronic migraine;[14] however, more evidence is needed to recommend their routine use.

Food and Drug Administration (FDA) has recently approved many devices for acute and preventive treatment of migraine. These include transcutaneous supraorbital and supratrochlear stimulation (Cefaly™), noninvasive vagal nerve stimulation (GammaCore™), and single-pulse transcranial magnetic stimulation (sTMS mini™).[15] These devices are attractive options for patients who do not want to use drugs, pregnant patients, or as a supplement to established in treatment **(Table 9)**. About 2–3% of chronic migraine patients remain refractory to all currently available preventives and may need invasive neurostimulation, like occipital nerve stimulation (ONS), for relief.

TABLE 8: Calcitonin gene-related peptide (CGRP)-targeted drugs for migraine prevention.

Name	Starting dose	Maximum dose	Route	Adverse event	Contraindication
Monoclonal antibody against CGRP receptor or ligand					
Erenumab	70 mg/month	140 mg/month	SC	Constipation, hypertension, injection site reaction	Hypersensitivity, recent cardio/cerebrovascular events
Fremanezumab	225 mg/month	675 mg/3 months	SC	Injection site reaction	
Galcanezumab	240 mg first dose and then 120 mg/month	240 mg/month	SC	Injection site reaction	
Eptinezumab	100 mg/3 months	300 mg/3 months	IV	Injection site reaction, visual blurring	
Small molecule CGRP antagonists (Gepants)					
Rimegepant	75 mg alternate day	75 mg alternate day	Oral	Abdominal pain, hypersensitivity	Hypersensitivity
Atogepant	10 mg	60 mg	Oral	Weight loss, constipation	

(IV: intravenous; SC: subcutaneous)

TABLE 9: Neurostimulation devices for acute and preventive treatment of migraine.

Stimulation site	Device	Acute treatment paradigm	Preventive treatment paradigm	Adverse effects	Contraindications
Transcutaneous trigeminal stimulation targeting supraorbital and supratrochlear nerves	Cefaly™ device	Activated for 60 minutes to eliminate or reduce acute migraine pain at a high impulse frequency (100 Hz), with a pulse width of 250 μs with a maximum intensity of 16 mA	Daily 20-minute sessions at a low impulse frequency (60 Hz) with a pulse width of 250 μs with a maximum intensity of 16 mA	Forehead paresthesia, sleepiness, fatigue, insomnia, and headache	Recent facial trauma, metallic head implants, or intracardiac lines or pacemaker devices
• Noninvasive transcutaneous vagal nerve stimulation • Targeting vagus nerve	GammaCore™ device	Two stimulations applied at headache onset (within 20 minutes), followed by two more after 20 minutes and after 2 hours if needed	Two stimulations (each 2-minute long) thrice a day	Stiff neck, frequent urination, lip/facial droop, mild confusion, and dizziness	Active devices near the site of stimulation (such as pacemakers, defibrillators), as well as carotid atherosclerosis, history of cervical vagotomy, significant hypertension, hypotension, bradycardia, or tachycardia
Single pulse transcranial magnetic stimulation of cerebral cortex	STMS mini™ device	Three sequential pulses can be given at the onset of the migraine attack, followed by additional pulses at 15-minute intervals if needed.	Twice daily treatment with 4 pulses (two consecutive pulses, wait 15 minutes, then repeat another two consecutive pulses	Lightheadedness, tingling, and tinnitus	• History of stroke or seizure; those with a cardiac pacemaker/defibrillator, vagus stimulator, or other implanted medical device • Dental implants and fillings are not affected by the device
Remote electrical of the upper arm at the onset of migraine pain or aura	Nerivio Migra™ device	Activate with smartphone app for 45 minutes	--------------------	Warm sensation, arm/hand numbness, itching, pain, tingling, and muscle spasms	Congestive heart failure, uncontrolled epilepsy, and active implantable medical device (pacemakers, hearing aid implant, etc.)

Tension-type Headache

Many terms, such as psychogenic headache, stress headache, psychomyogenic headache, and muscle contraction headache, were previously used for tension-type headaches. The term "tension-type headache" was chosen by ICHD-1 and has been retained since then. The words "tension" and "type" underscore its uncertain pathogenesis and indicate that mental or muscular tension may play a causative role. It is the most common form of primary headache seen in the general population, but most subjects with acute TTHs never consult a doctor. Sometimes, however, these can be frequent or chronic (as well as severe), causing major health problems and significant suffering.

Classification

Tension-type headache has been divided into two forms: episodic TTH (ETTH) and chronic TTH (CTTH) (first-digit classification). The ETTH has been divided into two groups: infrequent and frequent (second-digit classification). All three types of TTH share similar clinical features except for frequency. It is also suggested that on clinical examination, clinicians should look for pericranial tenderness in patients with TTH and subclassify them as associated or not associated with pericranial tenderness (third-digit classification) **(Box 2)**.

Diagnostic Features: Core Concepts

Tension-type headaches are recurrent episodes of headache lasting minutes to weeks. The pain in TTH is typically pressing or tightening in quality, of mild-to-moderate intensity, and bilateral in location, and does not worsen with routine physical activity. Nausea and vomiting are usually absent, but photophobia or phonophobia may be present. Because of the paucity of florid symptoms (contrasting migraine and TACs patients), TTH has been termed a "featureless" headache.[16]

Pathophysiology

Despite numerous clinical and neurophysiological studies, the exact cause of TTH remains elusive. It has been suggested that pericranial myofascial mechanisms are crucial in ETTH. In contrast, sensitization of pain pathways in the central nervous system resulting from prolonged nociceptive stimuli from pericranial myofascial tissues seems responsible for converting episodic to CTTH.[17]

BOX 2 Subtypes of tension-type headache.

- *Infrequent episodic tension-type headache*:
  - Infrequent episodic tension-type headache associated with pericranial tenderness
  - Infrequent episodic tension-type headache not associated with pericranial tenderness
- *Frequent episodic tension-type headache*:
  - Frequent episodic tension-type headache associated with pericranial tenderness
  - Frequent episodic tension-type headache not associated with pericranial tenderness
- *Chronic tension-type headache*:
  - Chronic tension-type headache associated with pericranial tenderness
  - Chronic tension-type headache not associated with pericranial tenderness
- *Probable tension-type headache*:
  - Probable infrequent episodic tension-type headache
  - Probable frequent episodic tension-type headache
  - Probable chronic tension-type headache

Source: Headache Classification Committee of the International Headache Society (IHS) (2018).[1]

Treatment

Acute Treatment

Most patients of infrequent ETTH do not report to the physician and self-medicate with over-the-counter analgesics. For patients with frequent ETTH, simple analgesics and NSAIDs are the mainstays of acute management. Aspirin (500 or 1,000 mg) and acetaminophen (1,000 mg) are both effective for acute pain management and superior to placebo. NSAIDs such as ibuprofen (200–400 mg) and naproxen sodium (375–550 mg) can be used and have been demonstrated to be more effective and better tolerated than other NSAIDs. Frequent intake of NSAIDs and simple analgesics (≥10 days per month) and combination analgesics should be avoided to prevent the development of MOHs. Some patients with ETTH may also have associated migraine, which may respond to triptans. These patients need careful education to identify their attack phenotype and to take the appropriate drug.

Preventive Treatment

Preventive pharmacotherapy should be considered in all patients with CTTH, those with frequent ETTH (more than 8 headache days per month), and those with headache-related disabilities. Amitriptyline is the most extensively used and efficacious drug for the preventive treatment of TTH. Since 1964, it has been the mainstay in treating CTTH patients, and several studies support its use. It is generally well tolerated, though some side effects such as dry mouth, drowsiness, and weight gain can be seen. The treatment should be started at a low dose (10–25 mg/day) and titrated by 10–25 mg weekly until a therapeutic effect or side effects appear. Mirtazapine, a noradrenergic and serotonergic antidepressant, is efficacious in situations where amitriptyline is either ineffective or contraindicated. The usual dose is 15–30 mg/day and has been shown to reduce the headache index by 34% more than a placebo in difficult-to-treat patients. Centrally-acting muscle relaxants like tizanidine (6–18 mg/day) may have some benefit, though not recommended routinely. A randomized study has shown that a combination of tizanidine (4 mg/day) and amitriptyline (20 mg/day) during the first 3 weeks of treatment gave faster relief of head pain than amitriptyline alone. As pharmacological interventions are not optimally effective in TTH, nonpharmacologic interventions are essential in their management. Behavioral treatments such as regulation of sleep, exercise, and meals, cognitive behavioral therapy, relaxation, biofeedback, and combinations of the above have been advocated. The improvement seen after behavioral treatment might appear slowly compared with tricyclics; however, it is maintained for extended periods. Physical therapy includes positioning, exercise program, hot and cold packs, massage, ultrasound, and transcutaneous electrical nerve stimulation (TENS). Adding craniometrical training to classical physiotherapy might be better than physiotherapy alone.

Trigeminal Autonomic Cephalalgias

Trigeminal autonomic cephalalgias, a term first coined by Goadsby and Lipton, is now considered a broad rubric under which four types of primary headache disorders are included. They have two features in common: unilateral extremely severe headache attacks and typical ipsilateral cranial autonomic symptoms (CASs). Functional neuroimaging has shown the involvement of the posterior hypothalamus in these headaches, which is taken as supportive evidence for grouping them and linking them pathophysiologically.[18]

Classification

Four phenotypes of TACS have been described **(Box 3)**. These include CH, paroxysmal hemicrania (PH), short-lasting unilateral neuralgiform headache attacks with conjunctival injection and tearing (SUNCT), and short-lasting unilateral headache attacks with autonomic features (SUNA) [under short-lasting unilateral neuralgiform headache attacks (SUNHA)] and hemicrania continua (HC). All four phenotypes can occur in episodic (or remitting in case of HC) and chronic forms (or unremitting in case of HC). Episodic CH (ECH) is seen in about 80% of CH patients, while chronic forms of the disease are typical for the other types. All TACs patients should undergo neuroimaging to rule out secondary causes.

BOX 3 **Subtypes of trigeminal autonomic cephalalgias.**

- *Cluster headache*:
  - Episodic cluster headache
  - Chronic cluster headache
- *Paroxysmal hemicrania*:
  - Episodic paroxysmal hemicrania
  - Chronic paroxysmal hemicrania
- *Short-lasting unilateral neuralgiform headache attacks*:
  - Short-lasting unilateral neuralgiform headache attacks with conjunctival injection and tearing (SUNCT):
    - Episodic SUNCT
    - Chronic SUNCT
  - Short-lasting unilateral neuralgiform headache attacks with cranial autonomic (SUNA) symptoms:
    - Episodic SUNA
    - Chronic SUNA
- *Hemicrania continua*:
  - Hemicrania continua, remitting subtype
  - Hemicrania continua, unremitting subtype
- *Probable trigeminal autonomic cephalalgia*:
  - Probable cluster headache
  - Probable paroxysmal hemicrania
  - Probable short-lasting unilateral neuralgiform headache attacks
  - Probable hemicrania continua

Source: Headache Classification Committee of the International Headache Society (IHS) (2018).[1]

Diagnostic Features: Core Concepts

The subtypes are described individually later in the section. However, certain general remarks about the core concepts may be helpful. The first three subgroups, namely, CH, PH, and SUNHA, differ on two main attributes: attack duration and attack frequency. All these are short-duration headaches (<3 hours) in contrast to migraine (which requires an attack duration of at least 4 hours when untreated in adults). Between the groups, however, CH can have an attack duration between 15 and 180 minutes, PH 2–30 minutes, and SUNHA 1–600 seconds. The attack frequency per day varies inversely, being 1–8 in CH, more than five in PH, and 1–600 in SUNHA. This increased propensity of attacks per day is also in contradiction to migraine. Overlaps in headache duration and attack frequency may sometimes cause diagnostic confusion. Other clinical features will be helpful in that situation among the TACs subtypes. The second core feature is the presence of CASs and signs. For diagnosis, only one out of the following five groups is sufficient:

1. conjunctival injection and/or lacrimation
2. nasal congestion and/or rhinorrhea
3. eyelid edema
4. forehead and facial sweating
5. miosis and/or ptosis ipsilateral to headache

The third important feature of TACs is the occurrence of restlessness during the attack. TACs patients are unable to lie down or sit still during the attacks. Although ICHD-3 included restlessness as a diagnostic feature in CH and HC, it is seen in all the groups of TACs. This feature distinguishes TACs from migraine in which the patient generally refrains from movement or activity. The fourth important core feature in two of these TACs, namely PH and HC, is the inclusion of absolute response to indomethacin. The word "absolute" is important to emphasize.

Pathophysiology of Trigeminal Autonomic Cephalalgias

The pathophysiological model of CH can be considered a general model for explaining three cardinal features of TACs, namely the trigeminal distribution of pain, ipsilateral CASs and signs, and circadian/circannual periodicity (most prominent in CH but occurs also in PH).

The critical pathways involved in headaches include the trigeminocervical and trigeminovascular systems. The trigeminocervical complex receives the pain-producing innervations of the cranium (branches of trigeminal and upper cervical nerves) and projects the nociceptive pathways to the higher centers. The trigeminal ganglion has bipolar cells which synapse peripherally with pain-sensitive large intracranial vessels (internal carotid and middle cerebral artery) and have central connections in the brain stem and upper cervical cord. Activation of afferents releases vasodilator peptides such as CGRP, substance P, and neurokinin A during an acute attack and leads to flushing in trigeminal distribution.

It has been proposed that the trigeminal-autonomic reflex is responsible for the CAS. The trigeminal-autonomic reflex pathway involves trigeminal afferents; the brainstem connections between the trigeminal nucleus and superior salivatory nucleus, and its cranial parasympathetic outflow through the facial nerve. It has been proposed that central disinhibition of this reflex causes cranial parasympathetic activation and sympathetic hypofunction.

Circadian/circannual periodicity has been attributed to perturbations in the functioning of posterior hypothalamic structures. Clues to the involvement of the posterior hypothalamus as a key substrate in the pathophysiology of CH have come from various sources. Functional imaging studies, including positron emission tomography (PET) and functional magnetic resonance imaging (fMRI), have shown hypothalamic involvement in CH. MR morphometry showed increased posterior hypothalamic gray matter, and proton magnetic resonance spectroscopy (MRS) showed a reduction in N-acetylaspartate (NAA) content. Neuroendocrine changes during cluster bouts also suggest hypothalamic dysfunction. Finally, hypothalamic deep brain stimulation (DBS) in refractory CH patients has shown a good response, confirming its key role in the pathophysiology of CH. However, some researchers argued that hypothalamic activation might be an epiphenomenon, as such activations have also been seen in patients with migraine and hypnic headaches (HHs).

Trigeminal Autonomic Cephalalgias Types

Cluster Headache

- *Clinical features*: Cluster headache has also been called "suicide headache" because of extremely severe pain intensity. 80% of sufferers had a headache intensity of 10 (maximum) as measured by the CH rating scale and 8–10 on the visual analog scale (VAS). Characteristically, CH patients have abrupt onset of severe unilateral short-lasting pain lasting 15–180 minutes with restless and ipsilateral CAS. The average attack duration is 30–45 minutes. The headache peaks early in most attacks, 5–10 minutes in more than 76% of cases. Usually, it also subsides rapidly. In contrast, a typical migraine attack takes longer to peak and abates slowly.

  Premonitory symptoms in the form of blurred vision, watering from the eyes, localized pain, anxiety, and yawning have been reported in CH. Aura has been reported in 6–23% of patients. Headache is side-locked in more than 80% of cases; however, it may be side-shifting in 15–20% of cases. The orbit-temporal region is affected most often. The character of pain may be variable; many patients describe their pain as being neuralgic (stabbing, sharp, dull, burning), while others may describe it as throbbing or pulsating. Typically, some patients describe that pain would drill and blow out their eyes on the affected side. The frequency of attacks varies from 1 to 8 per day. Migrainous features such as nausea, vomiting, photophobia, and phonophobia can occur, although uncommon and lateralized. The most characteristic feature is the "clustering of attacks", for which it bears its name. The headache attack occurs in bouts or periods, usually lasting for weeks or months, followed by periods of complete remission. These are called cluster periods (CPs) and remission periods, respectively. The cluster headache attacks and the CP have strict circadian and circannual periodicity roughly in about 50% of cases. Predominant nocturnal attacks may occur in 40–70% of patients. Alcohol (during CP), change in ambient temperature (hot), sleep, emotional stress, insomnia, relaxation, odors (especially of solvents and oil-based paints), smoking, fatigue, altitude, menstruation, flashing lights, histamine, and nitroglycerin have been noted as triggers in various studies. The majority of CH patients are smokers.
- *Treatment*: Acute (abortive), transitional, and preventive treatments are available for CH. Patients should be educated about their headaches, especially clustering, and triggers. They should be informed about avoiding specific triggers such as afternoon naps, high-altitude travel, alcohol intake, and exposure to paints and solvents.
  - Acute treatment: Three main options include inhaling 100% oxygen (oxygen inhalation therapy), subcutaneous sumatriptan, and zolmitriptan nasal spray. Oxygen inhalation therapy is the safest and most effective treatment. Its efficacy has been confirmed in double-blind studies. About 70% of attacks are aborted within 10 minutes and 90% within 20 minutes. The equipment consists of C (large) or E (portable) tank containing 100% oxygen, a rebreathable facial mask, tubing, and a regulator. Recent studies have suggested higher flow rate (12–15 L/min) is better. The patient should assume a sitting posture, leaning slightly forward. Oxygen therapy should not be used in patients with chronic obstructive airway disease.

    Sumatriptan 6 mg subcutaneously, sumatriptan 20 mg intranasal, and zolmitriptan 5 mg intranasal effectively treat CH. Intranasal forms are less efficacious than subcutaneous injections. Intranasal forms should be used on the contralateral nose. Up to two doses of sumatriptan and three doses of zolmitriptan in 24 hours are acceptable. Dihydroergotamine (DHE) 1 mg intramuscular (IM) is effective in the relief of acute attacks of CH. The intranasal DHE has not proved to be very effective. Topical lidocaine nasal drop given ipsilaterally may be used to treat acute attacks of CH. The patient lies supine with the head tilted back toward the floor at 30° and turned to the side of the headache. A nasal dropper may be used and the dose (1 mL of 4–10% lidocaine) is repeated once after 15 minutes. Octreotide 100 μg subcutaneously was modestly effective in one trial.

General principles of preventive therapy in CH: The options for preventive treatment in CH are mainly determined by the CP. Verapamil is considered the first-line preventive treatment of choice. However, for some patients with short CPs, limited courses of oral corticosteroids or greater occipital nerve injection may be sufficient. These short-term approaches can also be employed as transitional therapy till the dose of the preventive drug such as verapamil are built up adequately for optimal response. Some CH patients will require more than one preventive.

- *Transitional preventives*: Four days of corticosteroids (prednisone 1 mg/kg up to 60 mg) followed by tapering of the dose over 3 weeks can be an option. GONBs may result in remission lasting up to 2 months. GONBs can be very helpful in shorter CPs, in reducing the burden in more prolonged CPs, in chronic CH (CCH), and during pregnancy.
- *Long-term preventives*: Verapamil is more effective than a placebo. Large doses are needed in CH. After obtaining a baseline electrocardiogram (ECG), adult patients can be started on 80 mg three times daily; after that, the total daily dose is increased in increments of 80 mg every 10–14 days. An ECG should be performed prior to each increment and at least 10 days after the dose change to look for heart blocks. The dose is increased until the cluster attacks are suppressed, side effects appear, or the maximum dose of 960 mg/day is achieved. Other side effects include constipation, leg swelling, and gingival hyperplasia. The effect of verapamil is usually evident in 2–3 weeks. Lithium carbonate can be used in both ECH and CCH. The usual dose of lithium is 600–900 mg/day in divided doses. Lithium levels should be obtained within the first week and periodically after that with target serum levels of 0.4–0.8 mEq/L. Patients must be monitored for short-term neurotoxic and long-term effects such as hypothyroidism and nephrogenic diabetes insipidus. Topiramate is helpful in the prevention of CH attacks. Typical doses are 100–200 mg daily, with the same adverse events as seen with its use in migraine. Melatonin (9 mg daily) may be helpful in CH as a preventive. Other preventive agents include gabapentin (up to 3,600 mg daily), methysergide (3–12 mg daily), oral pizotifen (3 mg/day), repeated ipsilateral intranasal capsaicin, ergotamine with caffeine as a rectal suppository in nocturnal CH and longer-acting oral triptans such as naratriptan and frovatriptan. An occasional patient may respond to indomethacin (>225 mg/day). A recent study has shown that subcutaneous galcanezumab 300 mg can be an effective treatment for ECH.[19]
- *Neuromodulation*: The sphenopalatine ganglion (SPG) and DBS in the posterior hypothalamic gray matter region have been successfully tried in medically refractory cases. In noninvasive methods, vagal nerve stimulation has shown encouraging results in ECH.

Paroxysmal Hemicrania

- *Clinical features*: The clinical features are precisely the same as CH except that the attack duration is much briefer, between 2 and 30 minutes, and the attack frequency is more, being more than 5 per day in at least 50% of the attacks when the disease is active. The average duration of attacks is 13–21 minutes. Although paroxysmal, mild interictal pain may persist (30%). Restlessness is seen in 47–80% of cases. Verbal aggression may be seen in one-fourth. The majority has side-locked headaches; only a minority has side-shifting hemicranial headaches. Headaches are reported to be excruciating in 97% of cases. The character of pain is described as neuralgic in two-thirds and vascular in one-third. The most common trigger in adults has been the rotation of head and neck movements; in children, it is the physical effort. Other triggers include alcohol and change in ambient temperature. Unlike CH, periodicity is a less striking feature in PH, seen in less than 50% of cases. Also, the attacks do not have nocturnal preponderance like CH.
- *Treatment*: The treatment of PH is preventive. Absolute response to indomethacin is one of the diagnostic features of PH. Most patients have complete remission of headaches after starting indomethacin at 150–225 mg/day in three divided doses within 2–7 days. As indomethacin has a t1/2 of 4 hours, it should be given in divided doses. The minority will require a trial of more than 1 week for a complete response to become evident. In the clinic, for rapid diagnosis of PH (and HC), an "Indotest" has been suggested by giving an IM injection of indomethacin. Responders usually have complete remission of headaches within the mean duration of 11–13 hours. As most patients of PH have chronic PH (CPH) subtypes, long-term treatment is necessary. This becomes problematic in many because of gastritis due to indomethacin. A proton-pump inhibitor is usually given in addition. In CPH patients, a few weeks after remission of headaches, the dose should be reduced to a minimum maintenance dose and continued. In general, an attempt should be made to withdraw the drug after 6 months, although many patients have a prompt recurrence of headaches following withdrawal attempts.

In episodic PH (EPH) patients, indomethacin can be given longer than the usual bout period and then withdrawn. Tachyphylaxis with indomethacin has not been noted. Alternatives to indomethacin include cyclooxygenase 2 (COX2) inhibitors such as rofecoxib and celecoxib, verapamil, flunarizine, and nicardipine. Recently, topiramate has been found to be helpful in PH. GONBs have also been tried with success in PH.

Short-lasting Unilateral Neuralgiform Headache Attacks

- *Clinical features*: The attacks are typically characterized by sharp lancinations and electric shock-like stabs or jabs, typical of neuralgic pain centering on the ocular, orbital, and retro-orbital area. A minority also complains of a throbbing sensation. Interictal dull pain may persist in one-fifth of SUNA and half in SUNCT cases. Analysis of large cohorts has revealed three patterns that can be distinguished clinically, namely, groups of stabs (most common), sawtooth pattern, and single stabs (least common). The pain begins abruptly and abates abruptly. The duration varies from 1 to 600 seconds. Frequency varies from 1 to 300 per day or even more. An important feature is the lack of a refractory period between the attacks in 90% of cases. Headaches are side-locked in >90%. More than 80% of SUNCT patients report severe pain (10 on the VAS scale) compared to 33% in SUNA cases.[20] Like trigeminal neuralgia, 65–85% of patients of SUNCT/SUNA report triggers. The most common are cutaneous triggers, including chewing/eating (54%), touching (52%), wind (35%), washing face (33%), brushing teeth (31%), and brushing hair (10%). Other triggers are neck movements, emotional stress, talking, coughing, alcohol intake, and smoking. Some authors noted an increased occurrence of triggers in those who have sawtooth pattern of attacks. Attacks occur both during day and night. Restlessness, though not included as a diagnostic criterion in SUNCT/SUNA, has been reported in 50–60% of patients.
- *Treatment*: Early literature suggested that SUNHA was challenging to treat, and many patients remained refractory to treatment. However, currently, many therapeutic options are available for SUNHA. Treatment of SUNHA is preventive; however, like CH, transitional treatment may be offered for immediate relief of persistent SUNCT/SUNA attacks.[20]
  - Transitional treatment: For quick and complete remission of frequent attacks of SUNHA, intravenous lidocaine infusion is beneficial. Some patients of SUNCT may have continuous and incessant attacks called "SUNCT status". Lidocaine infusion is also beneficial to them. The recommended dose is 1.3-3.3 mg/kg/h for 7–10 days, with infusion speed from 15 to 30 mL/h. Another option for these patients is GONB which may ameliorate the attacks for weeks to months. This may, thus, buy time for the preventives to act.
  - Preventive treatment: There are no controlled trials for SUNHA. The effective drugs in case series and reports include lamotrigine, topiramate, and gabapentin.[21] Lamotrigine is the drug of the first choice but needs to be escalated slowly. The usual dose is 200–400 mg/day. Topiramate (up to 400 mg/day) and gabapentin (up to 900 mg/day) are also helpful.
  - Surgery and neuromodulation: The benefits of surgical procedures involving trigeminal ganglion were neither consistent nor long-lasting. Few medically refractory patients of SUNHA reported improvement after ONS and posterior hypothalamic DBS. However, these procedures need to be further evaluated. Those with neurovascular conflict on the symptomatic side may benefit dramatically from microvascular decompression. In one report involving 16 patients, the responder rate was 75%.[21] Results are sustained for up to 3 years. However, long-term data are needed.

Hemicrania Continua

- *Clinical features*: Unlike the other groups in TACs, the headache is continuous in HC. It is side-locked in almost all patients. In the background of continuous pain, which is usually mild, moderate-to-severe exacerbations may occur. The exacerbation occurs daily in almost half of the patients and may last hours. Hence, many HC patients are initially diagnosed with side-locked migraine if the background headache history is missed. This mistake is compounded because HC patients may have other migraine-like clinical features such as throbbing headaches, photophobia and phonophobia (usually ipsilateral), and motion sensitivity during exacerbations. Common triggers are relaxation after rest, alcohol intake, and irregular sleep. Behavioral restlessness occurs in about two-third of patients. Verbal aggression is noted. Premonitory symptoms have not been noted, and aura has been reported rarely. Insomnia is a common comorbidity. The diagnostic delay noted in some studies ranges between 5 and 7 years.
- *Treatment*: Just like PH, complete response to indomethacin is one of the diagnostic features of HC as per ICHD 3. Most patients have complete remission of headaches after starting indomethacin at a smaller dose of 100–200 mg/day in three doses. Topiramate has emerged as a good alternative, and GONB is also helpful.

Symptomatic (Secondary) Trigeminal Autonomic Cephalalgias

All four TAC subtypes of TACs are known to occur in patients with a secondary intracranial and very rarely extracranial pathology. These are called symptomatic or secondary TACs. These patients may have typical or atypical features of respective headache types. Hence, it is recommended that all patients of TACs must have a neuroimaging (MRI brain) and other appropriate investigations to rule out a secondary pathology before labeling them as primary headaches.[22]

Other Primary Headache Disorders

This group contains heterogeneous primary headache disorders, which are relatively uncommon but can pose diagnostic and treatment challenges **(Box 4)**.[23] Further,

BOX 4 Other primary headaches.

- Primary cough headache
- Primary exercise headache
- Primary headache associated with sexual activity
- Primary thunderclap headache
- Cold-stimulus headache
- External pressure headache
- Primary stabbing headache
- Nummular headache
- Hypnic headache
- New daily persistent headache (NDPH)

Source: Headache Classification Committee of the International Headache Society (IHS) (2018).[1]

they can only be diagnosed if the physicians know about the entities and ask relevant questions.

This group's first three headache disorders have specific activity-related triggers such as cough, exercise, and sexual activity. *Cough headaches* are not only triggered by cough but may also be triggered by other Valsalva maneuvers such as sneezing, laughing, and straining. It is important to recognize that the common primary headaches such as migraine and CH can worsen due to cough but are not triggered by it. The cough headaches are usually bilateral, short-lasting, and can be severe. Secondary cough headaches due to Chiari malformations, posterior fossa lesions, spontaneous intracranial hypotension (SIH), and subdural hematoma can occur and must be excluded. Treatment options for primary cough headaches include indomethacin, beta-blockers, acetazolamide, and topiramate. *Primary exercise headache* occurs after sustained nonsexual physical exertion. Headache is bilateral, throbbing, and long-lasting. Hence migraine, which can be triggered or worsened by physical activity, must be ruled out. Secondary causes also need to be excluded. An important secondary cause in the elderly is cardiac cephalalgia. Avoiding or limiting strenuous physical activity and prophylactic use of indomethacin, beta-blockers, and flunarizine helps. *Headaches during sexual activity* usually have thunderclap onset that reaches a peak at orgasm and then gradually subsides within 1–4 hours. Secondary causes such as subarachnoid hemorrhage (SAH), reversible cerebral vasoconstriction syndrome (RCVS), and arterial dissections must be ruled out. For the primary disorder, short-term prophylactic (1–2 hours before the sexual activity) such as indomethacin, and for recurrent headaches, long-term prevention with propranolol or topiramate may be helpful.

Primary thunderclap headaches are those headaches that present with a thunderclap onset, and extensive investigations for a secondary cause are negative. Sequence and the timing of the investigations are important to rule out secondary causes of thunderclap headaches.

The next group of disorders, *external stimulus headaches,* are triggered by *cold stimuli* and *external pressure* over the head. Application of cold stimuli to the head or ingestion or inhalation of cold substance and sustained compression or traction of the soft tissue of the cranium trigger these headaches. These headaches resolve upon cessation of exposure to the stimulus. These headaches are more commonly complained of by migraine patients.

The last group consists of epicranial headache disorders. The *primary stabbing headaches* are short-lasting stabs lasting up to 5 seconds, occurring multiple times a day, and do not have associated CASs or signs (unlike SUNHA) or specific cutaneous or spontaneous triggers (unlike trigeminal neuralgia). Although stabs can occur at any area of the head, the area supplied by the first division of the trigeminal nerve is predominantly affected. These headaches are commonly associated with migraine and respond well to indomethacin. Headache in a small, rounded circumscribed area (4–6 cm) over the scalp characterizes a *nummular headache*. It is possibly due to affliction of the terminal branches of the trigeminal nerves over a specific area of the scalp, primarily seen in the parietal region. Paresthesia, dysesthesia, or hyperesthesia in the area may be noted. Secondary causes need to be ruled out by local examination and imaging.

The last two entities in this group include: *HHs* and *new daily persistent headaches* (NDPHs). HH are sleep-related recurrent short-lasting headaches (from 15 minutes to 4 hours) that awaken patients during early hours (usually 2–4 AM) in an alarm-clock fashion. These headaches are more commonly reported by the elderly (over 50 years). Characteristically the patient gets up, moves around, makes himself/herself a cup of tea or coffee, and goes off to sleep again after remission. There are no CASs. Lithium and indomethacin are the treatment of choice.[24] NDPH is an enigmatic headache disorder. Patients remember the headache onset clearly (in terms of date, day, and time) and complain that the headache has become unremitting within 24 hours of its onset. NDPH occurs de novo and does not become persistent in the background of a previous primary headaches disorder such as migraine or TTH. However, the phenotype after their development may resemble migraine or TTH. Management of NDPH is complex and is based on headache phenotype.[25]

SECONDARY HEADACHES

General Diagnostic Considerations

The causes of secondary headaches are numerous and have been classified in ICHD-3 from groups 5 to 12 **(Box 5)**. These headaches develop under two settings. Some of these headaches develop in close temporal association with a disorder that can cause headaches (and can have a phenotype mimicking a primary headache disorder). In such a situation, the headaches are classified as secondary even if the phenotype is that of a primary headache. Contrarily, a preexisting primary headache disorder at times, can become chronic or significantly worse due to the occurrence of

BOX 5 Secondary headache groups (5–12).

- Headache attributed to trauma or injury to the head and/or neck
- Headache attributed to cranial and/or cervical vascular disorder
- Headache attributed to nonvascular intracranial disorder
- Headache attributed to a substance or its withdrawal
- Headache attributed to infection
- Headache attributed to disorder of homeostasis
- Headache or facial pain attributed to a disorder of the cranium, neck, eyes, ears, nose, sinuses, teeth, mouth, or other facial or cervical structure
- Headache attributed to psychiatric disorder

Source: Headache Classification Committee of the International Headache Society (IHS) (2018).[1]

another disorder that can cause headaches. In this situation, both the primary and the secondary diagnoses are given.[1] A general description of each group with a few common conditions is detailed below.

Headache Attributed to Trauma or Injury to the Head and Neck

These headaches occur in close temporal relationship with the head and neck trauma, lack characteristic features, and can have migraine, TTH, or "mixed" phenotypes. They are classified *as acute* if seen during the first 3 months after trauma and *persistent* if the headache continues beyond 3 months. Axonal injury, changes in cerebral metabolism or blood flow, genetic factors, medication overuse, and patient psychopathology are believed to be involved in its pathogenesis. These headaches may occur in isolation or may be a part of postconcussion syndrome. Further, these headaches may be perpetuated by post-traumatic sleep, mood disturbances, and stressors. Treatment of these headaches includes medications appropriate for the phenotype, regulated NSAIDs, and management of psychological and behavioral complaints. Medication overuse can cause the persistence of post-traumatic headaches and hence needs to be ruled out and treated if present.

Headache Attributed to a Cranial and Cervical Vascular Disorder

Many causes of cranial and cervical vascular disorder-related headaches are potentially life-threatening and present acutely, sometimes as "thunderclap headaches". These need to be evaluated, diagnosed, and treated promptly. Examples include acute stroke, SAH, cerebral sinovenous thrombosis, reversible vasoconstriction syndrome, and intracranial dissections. Many other vascular conditions can cause acute, subacute, or persistent headaches. Examples include acute subdural hemorrhage, transient ischemic attacks, arterio-vascular malformations, dural arteriovenous (AV) fistulas, Sturge-Weber syndrome, and headaches attributable to arteritis, including giant cell arteritis (GCA). GCA should always be considered in patients more than 50 years with a new onset headache. Other chronic intracranial vasculopathies, many with a genetic basis can cause headaches and migraine aura-like symptoms. Examples include headaches attributed to cerebral autosomal dominant arteriopathy with subcortical infarcts and leukoencephalopathy (CADASIL), mitochondrial encephalomyopathy, lactic acidosis, and stroke-like episodes (MELAS), moyamoya angiopathy, retinal vasculopathy with cerebral leukoencephalopathy and systemic manifestations (RVCLSMs) and migraine-like aura attributed to cerebral amyloid angiopathy (CAA).

Headache Attributed to Nonvascular Intracranial Disorder

This group contains diverse intracranial conditions that can cause headaches. Both high and low cerebrospinal fluid (CSF) pressures can cause headaches. Headache attributed to increased CSF pressure can be idiopathic or secondary to many conditions such as metabolic, toxic, or hormonal causes, chromosomal disorders, and hydrocephalus. Headache attributed to low CSF pressure can be due to post-dural puncture, CSF fistula headache, and headache attributed to SIH. *Postdural puncture headache* occurs within 5 days of a lumbar puncture due to CSF leakage through the dural puncture site. It usually accompanies neck stiffness and subjective hearing symptoms with orthostatic headache features. It remits spontaneously within 2 weeks or after sealing the leak with an autologous epidural lumbar patch. SIH patients classically present with orthostatic headaches (headaches occurring on assuming an upright position and relieved on recumbency). The typical history of orthostatic headaches may disappear in chronic cases. The basic problem is CSF hypovolemia rather than hypotension. The diagnostic investigation is a contrast-enhanced MRI of the brain which shows diffuse meningeal involvement and evidence of sagging of the brain and crowding of the brainstem. A search for a dural leak or fistula must be done by performing a heavily T2-weighted MRI of the spine. Exceptional cases may require digital subtraction myelography. Treatment involves conservative management (bed rest, fluids, caffeine), epidural blood patches, and surgical leak correction.[26] *Idiopathic intracranial hypertension* (IIH) is defined by clinical criteria that include symptoms and signs related to increased intracranial pressure (ICP) (e.g., headache, papilledema, vision loss), normal CSF composition and raised pressure (>250 mm), and no other cause of intracranial hypertension evident on neuroimaging or other evaluations. Headache is the most common symptom of IIH, complained by more than 80% of patients. Pulsatile tinnitus and transient visual obscurations are other common symptoms. Classically, a raised ICP headache is considered positional, with nocturnal awakening, worse on waking and aggravated by the Valsalva maneuver. However, headache phenotype in IIH can mimic episodic migraine, chronic migraine, and TTH. Many patients of IIH have been described without papilledema. CSF pressure measurement and MRI brain will clinch the diagnosis in most patients. Headaches are managed as per the phenotype. Treatment options include weight reduction, carbonic anhydrase inhibitors, serial lumber puncture, optic nerve sheath fenestrations, and CSF shunting, depending on severity, refractoriness, and impending visual loss.[27] Many noninfectious inflammatory intracranial diseases, such as neurosarcoidosis, aseptic (noninfectious) meningitis, and lymphocytic hypophysitis, can cause headaches. A rare but exciting disease called the *syndrome of transient headache and neurological deficits with cerebrospinal fluid lymphocytosis* (HaNDL) can cause headaches, especially in children. Finally, headaches caused by intracranial neoplasia, epileptic seizures, intrathecal injections, and Chiari malformations are also included in this group.

Headache Attributed to a Substance or Its Withdrawal

An important entity in this group is MOH, possibly, the most common cause of secondary headaches. Medication overuse is common in frequent or chronic primary headache disorders such as migraine and TTHs. It can result from overuse of ergot compounds, triptans, ditans, NSAIDs including paracetamol, opioids, and combination analgesics overuse. Management strategies include withdrawing the offending medication either on an outpatient or inpatient basis and optimizing preventive treatment.[28]

Headache Attributed to Infection

Headache is a common symptom of both intracranial and systemic infection and 60% of the general population may have experienced headaches during an infection. Headache attributed to infection is classified as *acute* when it resolves within 3 months of successful treatment of causative infection and *chronic* if the infection persists beyond 3 months. Intracranial bacterial, viral, fungal, or other parasitic infections, brain abscesses, and subdural empyemas can cause headaches. In all these infections, accompanying features of meningeal irritation or focal neurological deficit give away the diagnosis; occasionally, headache can be the sole presenting symptom, and the diagnosis is suspected based on subtle signs on examination or by the exclusion process. Imaging and CSF analysis usually help confirm the diagnosis in this setting. The headache usually resolves with appropriate antimicrobial therapy. In about 30% of cases, headache may persist even 3 months after successful infection treatment and is called *persistent;* other causes such as vasculitis, vasospasm, and septic thrombosis of dural sinuses and cortical veins, worsening hydrocephalus, or drug-induced headache must be excluded.

Headache Attributed to Disorder of Homeostasis

Headaches can be caused by hypoxia and hypercapnia. Headache secondary to hypoxia begins within 24 hours after acute onset of hypoxia with arterial partial pressure of oxygen (PaO_2) <70 mm Hg or in chronically hypoxic patients with PaO_2 persistently <70 mm Hg. Headache is the most common neurologic symptom and complication arising from ascent to altitudes >2,500 m. Headache starts within 24 hours of reaching a height, often awakening patients from sleep, usually lasts less than 1 day, and in most cases, is bilateral, generalized, frontal in location, dull pressure-type or pulsatile bursting-type pain. It may be exacerbated by bending, coughing, or sneezing, suggesting the possibility of raised ICP as a contributing factor. It usually resolves within 24 hours of descent. In severe cases, high-altitude headaches may be associated with impaired judgment and signs that suggest cerebral edema (acute mountain sickness) or progress to an acute encephalopathy or high-altitude cerebral edema (HACE). Preventative strategies include allowing 2 days of acclimatization before engaging in strenuous exercise at high altitudes, avoiding alcohol, liberalizing fluid intake, prophylactic use of acetylsalicylic acid or NSAIDs, and dexamethasone. *Headache attributed to airplane travel* is a stereotyped short-lasting severe jabbing, stabbing, or pulsatile headache that is usually unilateral and periocular, without autonomic symptoms caused by airplane travel. It occurs exclusively on airplane travel, worsens during ascent (15%) or descent (85%), and remits within 30 minutes of ascent or landing. It is thought to occur due to the squeeze effect on the frontal sinus wall, when air trapped inside it contracts producing a negative pressure leading to mucosal edema, transudation, and intense pain. Prophylactic therapy includes simple analgesics, NSAIDs, antihistamines, and nasal decongestants administered 30 minutes to 1 hour before travel. *Diving headache* is classically caused by diving below 10 m and occurs during the dive, often intensifies on resurfacing, and occurs in the absence of decompression illness. It occurs due to carbon dioxide intoxication and is usually relieved spontaneously within 72 hours but can be quickly remitted by oxygen inhalation. *Sleep apnea headache* is a recurrent morning headache that is usually bilateral, mild, or moderate in intensity and lasts for <4 hours on >15 days a month. In obstructive sleep apnea, (OSA) patients, sleep apnea headaches may occur in up to 12%. Proper sleep history must be elicited in all headache patients. Appropriate treatment for OSA usually alleviates the headache. *Hemodialysis headache* occurs in 30–70% of hemodialysis patients, especially during the second half. It resolves spontaneously within 72 hours after the hemodialysis session. It also remits after successful kidney transplantation. *Hypertension* is probably overemphasized as a cause of headaches. Mild-to-moderate arterial hypertension (<180/100 mm Hg) does not appear to cause headaches though some reports have found a significant correlation between blood pressure levels and headaches. However, disorders that cause abrupt, severe, and paroxysmal elevations in blood pressure are associated with headaches. *Headache attributed to hypertension* is, often bilateral and pulsating, usually caused by an acute rise in systolic (>180 mm Hg) and diastolic (>120 mm Hg) blood pressure and remits after normalization of blood pressure. Causes include pheochromocytoma, posterior reversible encephalopathy syndrome (PRES), autonomic dysreflexia due to spinal cord injury, baroreceptor reflex failure (after carotid endarterectomy, irradiation of the neck, bilateral lesions of the nucleus of the solitary tract, familial paraganglioma syndrome or surgical resection of the glossopharyngeal nerves and Page syndrome). Headache in preeclampsia and eclampsia is usually described as a bilateral, pulsating headache aggravated by activity, but thunderclap headaches associated with RCVS and PRES may also occur. *Headache attributed to hypothyroidism* is more common in females, mimicking TTH, lasting >72 hours, and responds well to salicylate therapy. *Fasting* and hypoglycemia are one of the most common migraine triggers but can also cause headaches in people without a history of migraine or headaches. This is often seen in prolonged religious fasting and has been documented as "Yom Kippur headache" and "first of Ramadan headache" or with fasts for *Navratri* and after *Karvachauth* in India. The typical headache mimics TTH, though migrainous features may be seen in those with a prior history of migraine. The term *cardiac cephalalgia* is used for a migraine-like headache usually aggravated by exercise, occurring during an episode of myocardial ischemia with or without accompanying chest pain. It subsides with rest or with antianginal treatment. The headache of cardiac cephalalgia can be differentiated from other exertional headaches by its gradual onset with exertion in contrast to the more explosive onset in primary exertional headache and primary sexual headache.

Headache or Facial Pain is Attributed to a Disorder of the Cranium, Neck, Eyes, Ears, Nose, Sinuses, Teeth, Mouth, or Other Facial or Cervical Structures

Although disorders of the cervical spine and other head and neck structures are commonly implicated as causing headaches, an actual causative effect has not been delineated in most cases. A cervical spine disorder, however, can cause *cervicogenic headaches.* It is usually accompanied by neck pain, with a prevalence of 0.4–4% in the general population. The headache is a dull aching nonthrobbing, nonlancinating pain of moderate-to-severe intensity that is fluctuating or continuous, predominantly in the occipital and unilateral, and may radiate to parietal, temporal, and frontal regions and upper limbs. Movements of the head can increase the headache. There may also be restriction of neck movements. *Neck-tongue syndrome* due to posterior subluxation of the lateral atlantoaxial joint on the rapid turning of the head causes ipsilateral occipital pain because of tension in the joint capsule and numbness of the tongue due to compression of the C2 spinal nerve. *C2 neuralgia* is characterized by intermittent, lancinating pain into the occiput, which may be accompanied by lacrimation and ciliary injection. *Occipital neuralgia* results in paroxysms of stabbing or shooting pain in the distribution of the greater, lesser, or third occipital nerve. There may be sensory loss and tenderness along the nerve.

It is a misconception in the general population that headaches are often the result of eye disease or refractory error. Pain from eye diseases is usually localized to the offending eye and often associated with a red eye, thereby causing little diagnostic confusion. *Acute primary angle closure glaucoma* and some forms of secondary glaucoma, associated with either inflammation or neovascularization can cause severe, boring pain located in and around the eye along with nausea and vomiting. *Refractive errors* are usually overemphasized as a cause of headaches but can worsen a preexisting primary headache. *Trochleitis* can lead to unilateral eye pain and frontal headache that is increased by movements of the eye involving the superior oblique muscle. Trochleitis may be due to a primary or secondary inflammatory disorder that can mimic the phenotype of NDPHs or HC.

Sinus headache is an older term often erroneously used for migraines without aura with prominent autonomic symptoms in the nose. Most patients with self-diagnosed "sinus headaches" have migraine headaches because of the mistaken belief that pain over the sinuses must be related to sinusitis. The headache in sinusitis is relatively nonspecific, worsens in the morning, may vary with head movement, and demonstrates sinus tenderness. Sphenoid sinusitis can cause pain in the vertex, often without a purulent discharge, and may cause thunderclap headaches or NDPHs.

Temporomandibular disorders (TMDs) significantly cause nondental pain in the orofacial region and are frequently associated with headaches.[29] TMDs include musculoskeletal and neuromuscular conditions that involve the temporomandibular joints (TMJs), the masticatory muscles, and all associated tissues. The TMJ, masticatory muscles, and associated orofacial structures may act as triggering or perpetuating factors for primary headaches and vice versa. The pain of TMD is described as a unilateral facial pain that may radiate to the ear, temporal and periorbital regions, angle of the mandible, and posterior neck. It is a dull, constant ache that waxes and wanes in intensity with intermittent paroxysmal episodes of sharper, more intense pain. The pain is often worsened by jaw motion. Patients may complain of fatigue and heaviness in jaw muscles after meals, which need to be differentiated from GCA claudication. For most patients with TMD, initial conservative treatment is recommended. It may include patient education and self-care, cognitive behavioral interventions, pharmacotherapy (NSAIDs, centrally-acting skeletal muscle relaxants, long-acting benzodiazepines), physical therapy, and orthopedic appliances. TMJ surgery should only be considered when conservative nonsurgical therapy has proved ineffective.

Headache Attributed to Psychiatric Disorder

The presence of headaches in a psychiatric disorder can be purely a chance occurrence because of their high prevalence. Evidence supporting psychiatric causes of headaches remains scarce and most evidence supports a bidirectional association rather than a causative relationship.

CONCLUSION

Headache disorders have emerged as one of the topmost conditions that are amenable to treatment in neurological practice. Increasing awareness and further research will pave the way to remove multiple barriers to their correct diagnosis and treatment.

REFERENCES

1. Headache Classification Committee of the International Headache Society (IHS). The International Classification of Headache Disorders, 3rd edition. Cephalalgia. 2018;38(1):1-211.
2. Stovner LJ, Hagen K, Linde M, Steiner TJ. The global prevalence of headache: an update, with analysis of the influences of methodological factors on prevalence estimates. J Headache Pain. 2022;23:34.
3. Fischera M, Marziniak M, Gralow I, Evers S. The incidence and prevalence of cluster headache: A meta-analysis of population-based studies. Cephalalgia. 2008;28:614-8.
4. Kulkarni GB, Rao GN, Gururaj G, Stovner LJ, Steiner TJ. Headache disorders and public ill-health in India: Prevalence estimates in Karnataka State. J Headache Pain. 2015;16:67.
5. Dodick DW. A Phase-by-Phase Review of Migraine Pathophysiology. Headache. 2018;58(Suppl 1):4-16.
6. Puledda F, Silva EM, Suwanlaong K, Goadsby PJ. Migraine: from pathophysiology to treatment. J Neurol. 2023.
7. VanderPluym JH, Halker Singh RB, Urtecho M, Morrow AS, Nayfeh T, Torres Roldan VD, et al. Acute Treatments for Episodic Migraine in Adults: A Systematic Review and Meta-analysis. JAMA. 2021;325:2357-369.
8. Eigenbrodt AK, Ashina H, Khan S, Diener HC, Mitsikostas DD, Sinclair AJ, et al. Diagnosis and management of migraine in ten steps. Nat Rev Neurol. 2021;17:501-14.
9. Yang CP, Liang CS, Chang CM, Yang CC, Shih PH, Yau YC, et al. Comparison of New Pharmacologic Agents With Triptans for Treatment of Migraine: A Systematic Review and Meta-analysis. JAMA Netw Open. 2021;4(10): e2128544.
10. Ailani J, Lipton RB, Goadsby PJ, Guo H, Miceli R, Severt L, et al; ADVANCE Study Group. Atogepant for the Preventive Treatment of Migraine. N Engl J Med. 2021;385:695-706.
11. Blair HA. Rimegepant: A Review in the Acute Treatment and Preventive Treatment of Migraine. CNS Drugs. 2023;37:255-65.
12. Vandervorst F, Van Deun L, Van Dycke A, Paemeleire K, Reuter U, Schoenen J, et al. CGRP monoclonal antibodies in migraine: an efficacy and tolerability comparison with standard prophylactic drugs. J Headache Pain. 2021;22:128.
13. Dodick DW, Turkel CC, DeGryse RE, Aurora SK, Silberstein SD, Lipton RB, et al; PREEMPT Chronic Migraine Study Group. OnabotulinumtoxinA for treatment of chronic migraine: pooled results from the double-blind, randomized, placebo-controlled phases of the PREEMPT clinical program. Headache. 2010;50: 921-36.
14. Chowdhury D, Mundra A. Role of greater occipital nerve block for preventive treatment of chronic migraine: A critical review. Cephalalgia Reports. 2020;3:1-20.
15. Reuter U, McClure C, Liebler E, Pozo-Rosich P. Non-invasive neuro-modulation for migraine and cluster headache: a systematic review of clinical trials. J Neurol Neurosurg Psychiatry. 2019;90:796-804.
16. Chowdhury D. Tension type headache. Ann Indian Acad Neurol. 2012;15(Suppl 1):S83-8.
17. Bhoi SK, Jha M, Chowdhury D. Advances in the Understanding of Pathophysiology of TTH and its Management. Neurol India. 2021;69(Suppl):S116-23.
18. Chowdhury D, Chopra R. Trigeminal autonomic cephalalgia. In: Arabinda Mukherjee (Ed). IAN Textbook of Neurology, 1st edition. New Delhi: Jaypee Brothers Medical Publishers (P) Ltd; 2018. pp. 31-43.
19. Goadsby PJ, Dodick DW, Leone M, Bardos JN, Oakes TM, et al. Trial of Galcanezumab in Prevention of Episodic Cluster Headache. N Engl J Med. 2019;381:132-41.
20. Duggal AK, Chowdhury D. SUNCT and SUNA: An Update. Neurol India. 2021;69(Suppl):S144-59.
21. Lambru G, Rantell K, O'Connor E, Levy A, Davagnanam I, Zrinzo L, et al. Trigeminal neurovascular contact in SUNCT and SUNA: a cross-sectional magnetic resonance study. Brain. 2020;143:3619-28.
22. Chowdhury D. Secondary (Symptomatic) Trigeminal Autonomic Cephalalgia. Ann Indian Acad Neurol. 2018;21(Suppl 1):S57-69.
23. Ravishankar K. Uncommon (Group 4.0) Primary Headaches: Less Familiarity and More Missed Diagnosis. Neurol India. 2021;69(7):168-72.
24. Silva-Néto RP, Santos PEMS, Peres MFP, Hypnic headache: A review of 348 cases published from 1988 to 2018. J Neurol Sci. 2019;401:103-9.
25. Yamani N, Olesen J. New daily persistent headache: a systematic review on an enigmatic disorder. J Headache Pain. 2019;20:80.
26. Schievink WI. Spontaneous intracranial hypotension. N Engl J Med. 2021;385:2173-8.
27. Mollan SP, Davies B, Silver NC, Shaw S, Mallucci CL, Wakerley BR, et al. Idiopathic intracranial hypertension: consensus guidelines on management. J Neurol Neurosurg Psychiatry. 2018;89:1088-100.
28. Ashina S, Terwindt GM, Steiner TJ, Lee MJ, Porreca F, Tassorelli C, et al. Medication overuse headache. Nat Rev Dis Primers. 2023;2;9:5.
29. Yakkaphan P, Smith JG, Chana P, Renton T, Lambru G. Temporo-mandibular disorder and headache prevalence: A systematic review and meta-analysis. Cephalalgia Reports. 2022;5.

99

CHAPTER

Sleep and Its Disorders

Joy D Desai

INTRODUCTION

Unraveling the functions and value of physiological sleep has been the Holy Grail of neuroscience research for over a century. The advent of animal models and single-cell neurophysiology propelled insights into mechanisms and cellular bases of sleep with a rewarding clarity and a heady euphoria. The discovery of the glymphatic system, an exclusive sleep-dependent neurochemical brain housecleaning paradigm, forced new questions that spawned an exciting era of research into sleep health and neurodegeneration/neuroprotection. This sleep chapter is an integrative attempt at incorporating current ideas at the frontiers of sleep research with clinical disorders of sleep and general neurology.

NEUROPHYSIOLOGIC BASIS OF SLEEP

Sleep and wakefulness are cyclical alternating states of differing manifestations of the level of awareness and responsiveness of the brain to its environment. During wakefulness, the brain engages with the environment in a unique manner of productivity utilizing physiologic resources to fuel these activities. During sleep, there is a progressive drop in these engagement abilities resulting in a temporary immobile, disengaged state. Innate physiologic processes vital for survival persist albeit at a different metabolic rate while cellular, metabolic, and organ-specific rejuvenation occurs, allowing a restored ability to engage again with the environment on awakening.[1] Sleep and wakefulness are biologically spontaneous and the urge to shift from one to another is driven by numerous physiologic processes including a circadian rhythm (process *C*) and a cumulative daytime effort/work exhaustion (homeostatic)-driven process (process *S*) driven by the accumulation of adenosine in the basal forebrain.[2] Adenosine receptors are antagonized by coffee, explaining the ability of caffeine to prolonged wakefulness. Reciprocally, when sleep deprived due to work pressures, adenosine receptors get upregulated as a compensatory mechanism to garner sleep pressure.

Sleep architecture physiologically consists of stereotyped, repetitive cycles of sleep-related brain changes [assessable via a polysomnogram (PSG)] with each epoch of the hypnogram lasting from 90 to 100 minutes. Four to five such hypnographic cycles can be assessed/observed in a typical 7–8-hour period of sleep. The initial stages are called non-rapid eye movement (NREM), subdivided into *N1* to *N3*, followed by a period of REM (Rapid Eye Movement) sleep. The duration of the REM period gradually increases as time is spent asleep with the longest REM period occurring just before awakening.[3] Spontaneous and very transient awakening occurs about twice in an 8-hour sleep period in normal healthy adults. In a healthy young adult, NREM sleep constitutes 75–90% of sleep time while REM constitutes 10–25% of sleep. A full-term newborn's sleep cycle lasts 60 minutes with 50% each spent in alternating NREM and REM sleep, alternating through a 3–4-hour interfeeding period. A full-term newborn baby sleeps approximately 16–20 hours a day and this declines to about 10 hours in childhood.[3] The electroencephalogram (EEG) undergoes signature changes in each sleep stage. The awake EEG is characterized by a low amplitude, high-frequency rhythm, which progressively slows down as the brain transits from awake to drowsiness in stage N1 and further deeper drowsiness in stage N2. In N2 sleep, the EEG manifests sleep spindles and K complexes, while in the further deep sleep of the N3 stage, delta waves predominate. During REM sleep, the EEG seemingly paradoxically becomes fast wherein a high-frequency low amplitude rhythm again dominates. During REM sleep, the eyes move rapidly, breathing is deep and effortful, while the rest of the body muscles are atonic. In contrast to NREM sleep and similar to wakefulness, REM sleep is marked by intense cholinergic activity from the basal forebrain and pontine nuclei, which activate cortical activity.

This combination of phenomena, a cholinergically "wakeful" cortex fused with skeletal muscle paralysis, allows the brain to perform a critically important function, the consolidation of emotionally laden memories.[4] REM sleep is, therefore, also called paradoxical sleep.

In summary, slow-wave sleep (NREM) is physiologically characterized by a progressive reduction in heart rate, blood pressure, and spinal reflexes. The brain blood flow and the temperature drop, while growth hormone secretion peaks. Parasympathetic tone increases while sympathetic tone decreases during NREM sleep. The EEG has now synchronized to a slow rhythm.[1] In REM sleep, spinal reflexes are absent, somatic muscles barring those of respiration are atonic, eyes move rapidly, brain blood flow and temperature increase, and the phenomenon of dreaming dominates. The EEG is a desynchronized low-amplitude fast rhythm with a spiky morphology.[1]

It appears that the brain hums with an electrical symphony in sleep that has numerous physiological functions, e.g., memory consolidation, emotional equilibration, autonomic tone recalibration, and energy revitalization. During NREM sleep, electrical changes occur hierarchically. Hippocampal ripples (80–120 Hz) are followed by slow-wave oscillations (<1.25 Hz) that couple with sleep spindles (12–16 Hz). In this phase, memories held in temporary storage in the hippocampus during the day get transferred to the lobar neocortices for permanent storage. Relevant memories get consolidated while irrelevant ones get wiped out.[5] If sleep health is impaired in any manner, this process can be hampered. Two distinct cortical states oscillate during NREM sleep alternating every 3–6 seconds. The first is a state of high synchrony, where coupled slow wave oscillations and sleep spindle complexes engage the mesial temporal lobe and trigger hippocampal ripples. The second is a state of low synchrony, where information flow from mesial temporal lobes to the neocortices is maximal but no prominent oscillatory activity is present. This two-step organization might reflect an endogenous timing mechanism that ensures that new information arrives at the neocortex when processing capabilities are maximized.[6]

It is the integrity and anatomical robustness of the prefrontal cortices that determine the efficiency of this nocturnal memory consolidatory process. With increasing age, it has been shown that prefrontal atrophy leads to disrupted NREM slow-wave synchrony and coupling in sleep, resulting in impaired hippocampal-dependent memory in the elderly.[7] Walker and colleagues showed that REM sleep is associated with an intense amygdala-prefrontal cortex exchange that serves to depotentiate the emotional burden of memories.[8] Very simply, good sleep hygiene results in an enhanced capability of coping with emotionally traumatizing experiences, especially when sleep is REM replete. This is of great relevance in the understanding and management of post-traumatic stress disorder (PTSD). It has also been shown that insomniacs are haunted by their past, as old distressing memories remain salient in them when compared to individuals who slept well.[9]

The synaptic homeostasis hypothesis (SHY) postulates that the key function of sleep is to prune and sculpt synapses acquired during daytime cerebral experiences and functioning from a large collection of all data to a molded and useful archive of synapses which will constitute relevant memories of the daytime experiences. These memories to be archived and stored are selected by a process being understood as based on thresholds of synaptic frequency and intensity. The actual regulatory processes are not fully understood.[10] This process occurs in both NREM and REM sleep. This process integrates restoration and repair of central nervous system (CNS) architecture.

Sleep is promoted and maintained by a complex set of neural circuitry and chemical mechanisms. The daily rhythm of sleep and arousal is regulated by the suprachiasmatic nucleus (SCN) in the hypothalamus, with its phasic entrainment determined by light. Light is considered a *"zeitgeber"* (a German word meaning timekeeper) for promoting wakefulness, while secretion of melatonin by the pineal gland approximately 3–4 hours after sunset sets the tone for induction of sleep onset.[1] The neural circuitry underlying the regulation of sleep and wakefulness is discrete yet interdependent. Arousal systems are inhibited by sleep-promoting neural networks/neurons, which in turn are suppressed by the arousal network to return to wakefulness. This works like a biological flip-flop switch[1] **(Figs. 1A and B)**.

A pontomesencephalic pathway mediates wakefulness and arousal via an ascending network that innervates the thalamus and independently the posterior hypothalamus and forebrain. The key cell populations that constitute this ascending arousal/wakefulness pathway are *acetylcholine*-secreting neurons of the pedunculopontine and laterodorsal tegmental nuclei, *noradrenaline*-secreting neurons of the locus coeruleus, *serotonin*-secreting neurons from the dorsal and median raphe nuclei, *dopamine*-secreting neurons of the periaqueductal gray matter, and *histamine*-secreting neurons of the tuberomamillary nucleus. A modest number of cells in the lateral hypothalamus are the sole source of hypocretin or orexin, wakefulness-promoting peptide. These orexinergic neurons project to a sprawling network of all wakefulness-promoting regions including the locus coeruleus and tuberomammillary nucleus. Orexinergic neurons fire during wakefulness and are silent during NREM and REM sleep.[11] In summary, cholinergic and monoaminergic cell populations form one pontomesencephalic ascending arousal/wakefulness-promoting network to the thalamus. This is paralleled by a second peptidergic arousal system of orexin-/hypocretin-secreting nuclei in the lateral hypothalamus. They discharge in a coordinated and stereotyped manner to promote arousal, each making unique and overlapping contributions to wakefulness maintenance.[11]

During sleep, these networks are suppressed by the ventrolateral preoptic neurons (VLPO). Neurons of the VLPO form a dense cluster that innervates the arousal

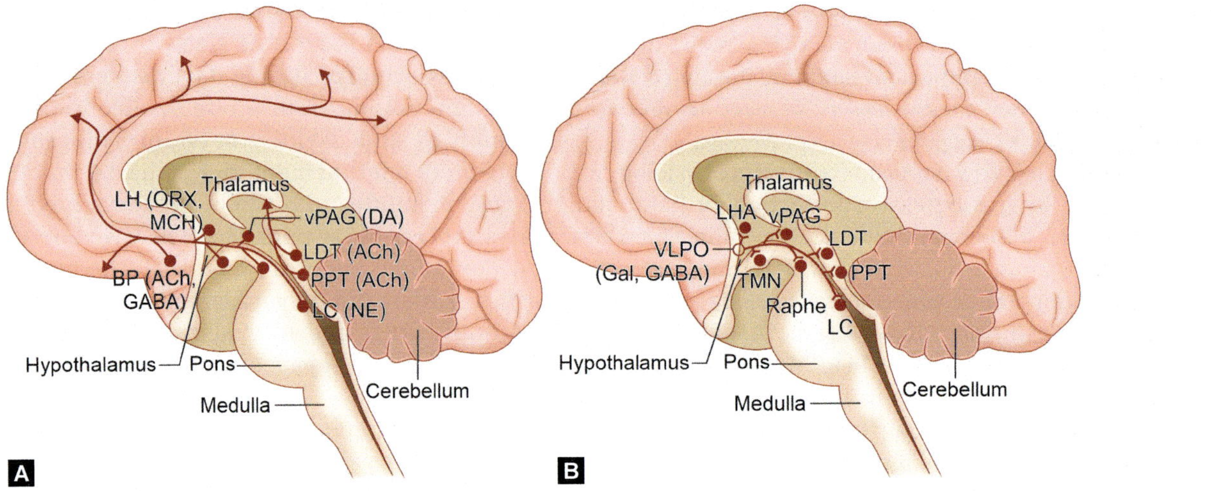

FIGS. 1A AND B: Ascending and descending sleep pathways.
(ACh: acetylcholine; GABA: γ-aminobutyric acid; LC: locus coeruleus; LDT: laterodorsal tegmentum; LHA: lateral hypothalamic area; MCH: melanin-concentrating hormone; ORX: orexin; PPT: pedunculopontine tegmentum; TMN: tuberomammillary nucleus; VLPO: ventrolateral preoptic neurons)

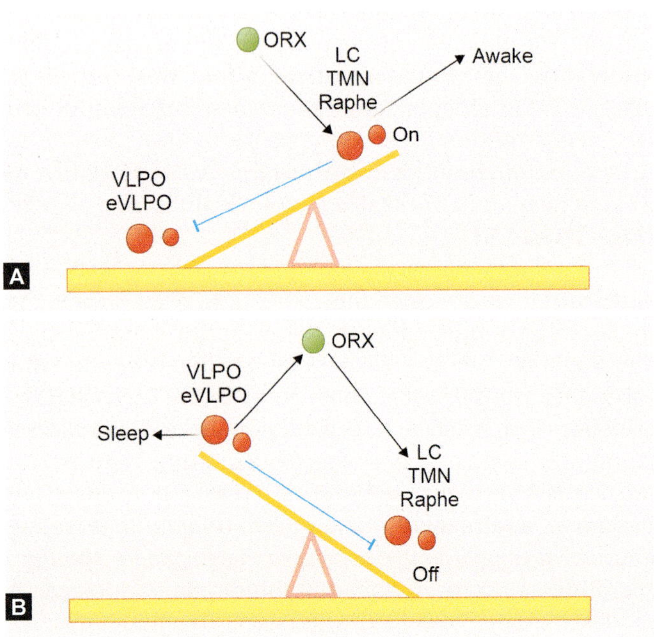

FIGS. 2A AND B: Sleep flip-flop switch.
(LC: locus coeruleus; ORX: orexin; TMN: tuberomammillary nucleus; VLPO: ventrolateral preoptic neurons)

network. The VLPO neurons secrete γ-aminobutyric acid (GABA) and galanin. These two neurotransmitters promote sleep by suppressing the arousal network. These two reciprocal inhibitory systems are understood as a fast bistable, flip-flop switch that is either rapidly and fully "on" or rapidly and fully "off". Intermediate states that are partially on or off are resisted. This explains the mammalian trait of quickly falling asleep or coming awake, as the time spent in transition states is only 1–2% per day[1,11] **(Figs. 2A and B)**.

The neural circuitry for REM sleep is complex. The laterodorsal, pedunculopontine, and sublaterodorsal nuclei appear to the REM on neurons (promoters) that trigger and maintain REM sleep and are counterbalanced by the locus coeruleus neurons that are "REM off" inhibitors of REM sleep when active. During REM sleep, pontine sublaterodorsal fibers activate the magnocellular reticular formation in the medulla, which subsequently descends and inhibits spinal motor neurons. This is the currently accepted explanation of physiological somatic muscle atonia during REM sleep.[12]

Humans have evolved to have these sleep/wake changes occur bihemispherically as a norm. However, in some species, e.g., whales, porpoises, manatees, sea lions, and migratory birds like the arctic tern and frigate birds, sleep occurs physiologically as a unihemispheric phenomenon. One-half of the brain is awake while to opposite half is asleep and vice versa. This is perhaps an evolutionary adaptation to avoid predation and sustain survival, both in the skies and in the oceans.[13] In humans, this phenomenon has been observed when sleeping in a novel environment with the dominant hemisphere maintaining a night watch of wakeful rhythms while the nondominant brain sleeps with a traditional slow rhythm, so to speak.[14] Such sleep-associated slow-wave inter-hemispheric asymmetry on a first night at a new place illustrates that sleep physiology is constantly modulable and adaptive to needs.

The circadian influence on sleep and wake propensities and vulnerabilities deserves some understanding. The loss of ambient light at sunset stokes a special signal via the retinal ganglion cells to the pineal gland to initiate the secretion of melatonin. It begins between 9 and 11 PM, peaks between 1 and 3 AM and falls to baseline by 7 AM at sunrise. Chronotype is the behavioral expression of the set point of an individual's circadian rhythm. It describes their sleep-wake cycle about time, and the two ends of the chronotype spectrum are called "morningness" (*lark*) and "eveningness" (*owl*). Morningness is characterized by early morning waking, with mental and physical performance peaking in the first half of the day and going to sleep relatively early; eveningness is the opposite, with late awakening and working late into the night during the traditional sleeping period.[15] The eveningness chronotype has been associated with a predisposition to diabetes, metabolic syndrome, high body mass index and sarcopenia, as well as depressive disorders.[16] It is understood that every bodily organ has a circadian clock with the master being the *SCN*. The master clock within the SCN functions a bit like the "kapellmeister" of a symphony orchestra, regulating all the peripheral organ clocks to function in a smooth circadian rhythm. Circadian clocks are formed through transcription-translation feedback loops (TTFLs) that are gene driven.[15] The following genes[15] have a cardinal role to play in circadian rhythm equilibrium:

- *CLOCK (circadian locomotor output cycles kaput)*: A gene encoding protein that affects the length and persistence of a circadian cycle.
- *BMAL1 (brain and muscle aryl hydrocarbon receptor nuclear translocator-like protein 1)*: A basic helix-loop-helix transcription factor
- *PER1, PER2, and PER3 (period)*: A negative element in the circadian transcription loop by interacting with other circadian regulatory proteins and transporting them to the nucleus
- *CRY1 and CRY2 (cryptochrome)*: A negative element inhibiting CLOCK-mediated transcription in maintaining period length and circadian rhythmicity
- *Rev-ErbA (orphan nuclear receptor)*: An alpha thyroid receptor splice variant that regulates CLOCK and BMAL1 expression

Melatonin is part of a complex circadian network regulatory process that harmonizes the synchrony with which the master clock in the SCN regulates the peripheral clocks in all organ systems.

When circadian harmony of sleep (sleep onset at 4 hours after sunset and waking with sunrise) is disrupted due to lifestyle or sociological factors, circadian misalignment is bound to occur. A pattern of sleep behavior has emerged in urban settings that have been implicated in numerous health disorders. Urban residents now predominantly work on weekdays late into the night, usually beyond midnight, and wake early by six in the morning to go to work. Thus, they are sleep deprived on weekdays. On weekends, they sleep in late and wake after ten in the morning. The analysis of this pattern of lifestyle is that bodily mechanisms behave as if jet lagged. This pattern has been called social jetlag.[16,17] Persistent social jetlag is now implicated in a host of medical disorders that include hypertension, diabetes, metabolic syndrome, cyclothymic mood disorders, polycystic ovarian syndrome, and some autoimmune conditions.[17]

NEUROBIOLOGY OF SLEEP

Neurons with the classical teaching of being electrically active from depolarization shifts of ion channels and associated with neurotransmitter release at synapses were thought to be the prototypic components of functioning neural networks. The word "neuroglia" was derived from the Latin word for glue as originally astrocytes and microglia were thought to be scaffolding cells of brain architecture holding together neurons like a brain glue. However, with the advent of cell studies involving calcium ion movements in the 1990s, it became clear that astrocytes have an intimate network within themselves (both locally and at a distance) and with neurons. This led to the elucidation of calcium cation shifts across astrocyte membranes leading to the release of gliotransmitters at astrocyte synapses both within astrocytes and from astrocyte to neurons. Haydon proposed that a dominant part of this interaction occurred at night in sleep and coined the term "tripartite synapse" to describe the unique manner in which an astrocyte could regulate functions across both pre- and postsynaptic neurons.[18] He confirmed that there were multiple roles that the astrocyte played in maintaining neurotransmitter and energy balance, many occurring essentially at night (in sleep)[19] **(Fig. 3)**.

The close association of the astrocytic process with the presynaptic and postsynaptic terminals exerts a crucial contribution in clearing K^+ ions that accumulate following neuronal activity. The second contribution of the tripartite synapse is in the uptake of the synaptic transmitter glutamate by the activity of plasma-membrane glutamate transporters. Additionally, neurotransmitter release from presynaptic terminals can activate astrocytic receptors that induce Ca^{2+} elevations which in turn triggers the release of gliotransmitters from these cells. These are D-serine, glutamate, and adenosine triphosphate (ATP), which in turn have feedback modulatory effects on neurons.[18,19] Astrocytes

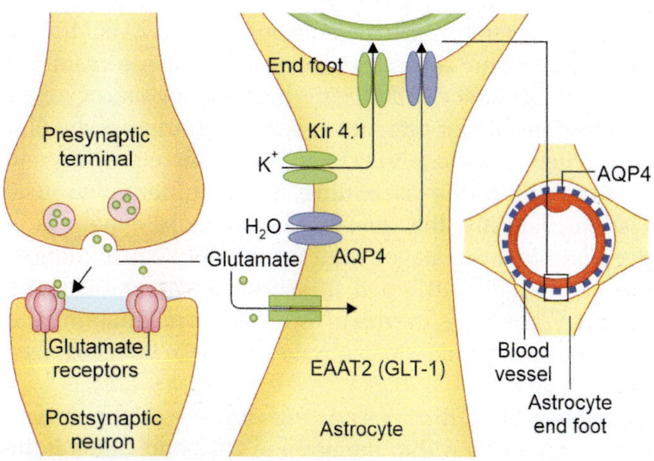

FIG. 3: Astrocyte functions in sleep.

(AQP4: aquaporin-4; EAAT2: excitatory amino acid transporter 2; GLT-1: glutamate transporter-1)

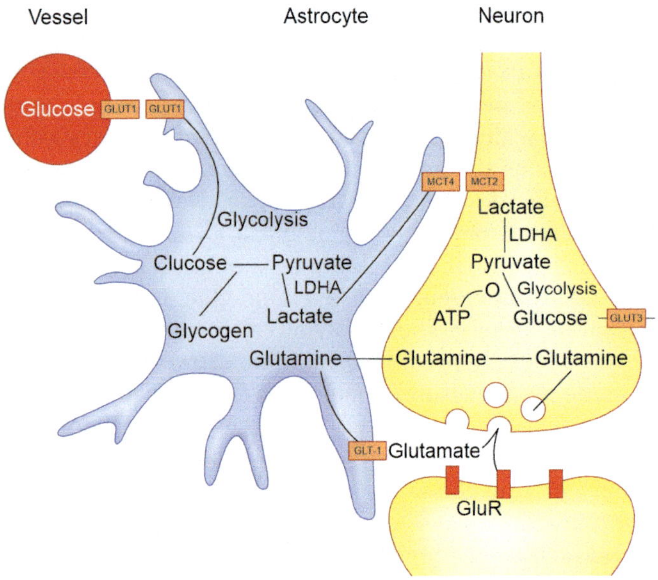

FIG. 4: Astrocyte neuron lactate shuttle.

(ATP: adenosine triphosphate; GLT-1: glutamate transporter-1; GLUT1: glucose transporter 1; GluR: glutamate receptors; LDHA: lactate dehydrogenase A; MCT2: monocarboxylate transporter 1)

take up glucose from the neurovascularly coupled vessel. Astrocytes metabolize this glucose to lactate. Thus, the astrocyte derives energy for itself. It then shuttles the lactate to the neuron via a monocarboxylate transporter (MCT). In the neuron, lactate is converted to pyruvate as an aerobic energy source. A source of lactate is pivotal for memory consolidation in sleep and hippocampal neurogenesis. This is known as the astrocyte-neuron lactate shuttle (ANLS). A large part of this energy-restorative exercise occurs during sleep[20] **(Fig. 4)**.

Once released from neurons and astrocytes, ATP is rapidly converted into adenosine monophosphate (AMP) and then into adenosine by extracellular nucleotidases. The reuptake of adenosine occurs through equilibrative nucleoside transporters, and phosphorylation by the astrocyte-specific enzyme adenosine kinase *(*ADK*)* breaks down adenosine and clears excess adenosine from the extracellular space. Adenosine build-up by astrocytes is also responsible for pressure to sleep, as it triggers the flip-flop switch to activate VLPO neurons to secrete GABA and galanin, inhibiting ascending monoaminergic arousal systems.[21] Lastly, the slow-wave oscillatory dynamics of deep NREM sleep stages, vital for memory consolidation, are now largely attributed to astrocytic cation-regulated activity.[22] Therefore, the role of astrocytes in maintaining and harmonizing optimal sleep physiology has to be recognized as being pivotal.

Nedergaard discovered the unique sleep-driven excretory system within the brain in 2013 and called it the glymphatic system after combining the words "glial" and "lymphatic".[23] She and others proposed that this solely nocturnal, unidirectional gentle flow of cerebrospinal fluid (CSF) across the interstitium of the brain was propelled by the rhythmic pulsatory effects of respiration, vascular pulsations synchronous with the heart rate, and slow wave oscillations of N2 and N3 sleep.[24] The glymphatic system ceases to function on awakening and this is attributed to the increase in adrenergic tone. Glymphatic drainage is responsible for the excretion of β-amyloid and tau in normal healthy humans.[25] The directionality of the CSF from arterial to the venous side was attributed to aquaporin-4 polarization in the foot processes of the astrocytes. Sleeping supine and laterally optimizes glymphatic drainage, while a prone posture in sleep decreases glymphatic efficiency by 40%.[26] Voluntary exercise, low doses of alcohol, and intermittent fasting improve glymphatic drainage, perhaps by optimizing aquaporin-4 polarization in the foot processes.[27] Thus, the astrocyte is a true star of nocturnal neurobiology revitalizing, cleaning, and stabilizing neuronal reserves.[28]

NEW HORIZONS IN SLEEP PHYSIOLOGY: LOCAL AND SEGMENTAL SLEEP

Sleep is considered a global cerebral phenomenon that affects the whole brain uniformly and simultaneously. Sleep and wakefulness are considered two distinct mutually exclusive behavioral states with no gray zones in-between. This all or none view of sleep dominates traditional research and has led to the formulation of the sleep architectural hypnogram as a concept. Undeniably, sleep and wakefulness have distinct EEG signatures. Can sleep occur locally, can sleep and wakefulness occur simultaneously in regional brain parts, and what is the cognitive fallout of such an occurrence? Intriguing insights into the potential answers to these research questions have emerged from recent studies.[29] Slow waves, the hallmark of NREM sleep, are not uniformly distributed across the cortical surface during sleep but occur locally and asynchronously across variable brain regions. The regional distribution and amplitude of slow waves are determined by brain maturation, and time spent awake, and are mediated in part by experience-dependent variation in synaptic strength. Local low-frequency oscillations (<8 Hz) can also occur in REM sleep and during wakefulness, leading to region-specific cognitive errors when awake.

A motor learning task involving the right parietal region produced a local increase in slow-wave activity (SWA) during subsequent NREM sleep.[30] After prolonged audiobook listening, subjects displayed an increase in SWA in subsequent sleep in the left frontal brain derivations and after playing a driving simulator game SWA activity increased in the right parietal regions in subsequent sleep.[31]

It appears that such local and segmental asynchrony of SWA distribution occurs in wakeful times too following periods of sleep deprivation (SD). This intrusion of SWA in wakeful periods is regional anatomy specific. It increased predominantly over the left frontal region during a language-based task producing SD, and over the posterior parietal region during a visuomotor task. This was naturally associated with performance errors in cognition.[32] The cerebral anatomical location of SWA appears to be dependent on cognitive tasks being performed during the period of SD. Local and segmental SWA intrusions during periods of wakefulness may also occur in individuals who have a sleep disorder like obstructive sleep apnea (OSA) (almost always associated with physiological SD when untreated). The conceptualization is that regional intrusions of SWA while awake may occur subclinically, or as manifest episodes of microsleep or lapses in attention.[33] The physiological and lifestyle-associated factors leading to frequent such occurrences are not well elucidated. Poor sleep hygiene and sleep disorders such as sleep apnea and periods of SD from any cause are contributors.

Sleep–wake transitions are also now thought to be asynchronous regionally within the brain leading to phenomena such as sleep inertia, hypnagogic or hypnopompic hallucinations, sleep paralysis, and sleep onset amnesia. Sleep transitions are characterized by a regionally asynchronous process of electrical phenomena which are signatures of the state of consciousness: asleep or awake.[34] Falling asleep exhibits an anteroposterior gradient of SWA and is preceded by hippocampal spindle activity. This explains the phenomenon of anterograde and retrograde amnesia that often accompanies sleep onset. Awakening likewise is also a regionally asynchronous process, with a persistent posteriorly dominant delta rhythm producing sleep inertia.[34] The coexistence of local sleep-like and wake-like activity in regional brain parts is characteristic of several sleep disorders labeled "sleep arousal disorders," e.g., somnambulism, NREM parasomnias like sexsomnia, somniloquy, sleep-related eating disorder, confusional arousals, and sleep terrors. These NREM parasomnias are understood as disorders of sleep-state dissociations.[35] In older adults, the existence of neurodegenerative disorders may unmask such phenomenology. REM sleep behavioral dysfunction (RBD), characterized by the absence of physiological REM-associated limb muscle atonia in degenerative diseases like dementia with diffuse Lewy bodies and multiple system atrophy (MSA), reflects such a regional disruption of sleep-associated electrical harmony/synchronization. This leads to the stricken patient developing sometimes catastrophic dream enactment behavior.[36]

CLINICAL APPLICATIONS OF SLEEP PHYSIOLOGY AND NEUROBIOLOGY

The evaluation of patients who seek medical attention due to a "sleep disorder" hinges on the rational understanding of sleep physiology, neurobiology, and laboratory hallmarks. Medical assistance is sought when patients are either too sleepy in the daytime or unable to initiate, or maintain nocturnal sleep continuity resulting in daytime fatigue, and loss of productivity (often associated with mood and memory dysfunction). Rarely, those who struggle to maintain healthy circadian entrainment of individual sleep cycles for myriad reasons may also require assistance. In essence, at the bedside, one may have to evaluate a sleepy, sleepless, or fragmentarily sleep-interrupted individual. Some may have other neurological and/or systemic ailments. The neurologist has to be able to assess the cardinal tenets of sleep hygiene and its practice concerning the patient's activities of daily living.

THE SLEEPY PATIENT

Excessive daytime sleepiness (EDS) is defined as the inability to stay awake and alert during the major waking episodes of the day, resulting in periods of irrepressible need for sleep or unintended lapses into drowsiness or sleep. This may affect about one-fourth of the population.[37] The common causes of such excessive daytime drowsiness have been summarized in the **Box 1**.

Like other neurological disorders, the evaluation of the excessively sleepy patient hinges on a meticulous history and a diligent physical examination. An average person needs to sleep at least 7 hours daily, preferably in good circadian harmony with sleep onset about four and a half hours after sunset and awakening within an hour of sunrise. The most common causes of EDS are poor sleep habits and/or hygiene. It is useful to interview the patient's spouse or sleeping partner to ascertain salient information about snoring in sleep, apneic snorts while asleep, erratic breathing rhythms in sleep, irregular leg movements, vocalization in sleep, symptoms of dream enactment, nocturia, dryness of mouth, and headaches or giddiness on awakening. Attention has to be paid to the lifestyle habits of

BOX 1 Common causes of EDS.

Primary sleep disorders:
- Behaviorally induced insufficient sleep syndrome
- *Sleep-disordered breathing*: Obstructive and central
- Circadian rhythm disorders
- Periodic limb movement disorder
- Idiopathic hypersomnia
- Narcolepsy (type 1 and type 2)
- Klein–Levin syndrome (recurrent hypersomnia)

Accompanying neurological diseases:
- Traumatic brain injury
- Migraine
- Multiple sclerosis
- MND/ALS
- Alzheimer's disease
- Parkinson's disease
- Stroke
- Epilepsy

(ALS: amyotrophic lateral sclerosis; EDS: excessive daytime sleepiness; MND: motor neuron disease)

such patients, e.g., the amount and timing of consumption of caffeinated drinks and alcohol. A holistic evaluation includes a diligent assessment of systemic disorders that could have a bearing on sleep-related breathing, i.e., chronic obstructive pulmonary disease (COPD) or congestive heart failure (CHF). Assessment of the Mallampati score and an evaluation of the alignment of the upper jaw with the lower one are useful (for the assessment of retrognathia) when one suspects OSA.

The traditional understanding of OSA is that it occurs in obese individuals due to an increase in soft tissue density in the oropharynx and neck resulting in the collapse of the airway during breathing in sleep.[38] This in turn results in hypoxia, hypercarbia, and an exaggerated/abrupt respiratory excursion to obviate this. This apnea-induced snort re-establishes breathing, allowing the cycle to be repeated. Physicians attribute adult hypertension, diabetes, cardiac arrhythmias, congestive cardiac failure, and obesity despite dieting and exercise to OSA. Moderate-to-severe OSA results in frequent nocturnal respiratory arousals with a failure of accrual of the physiological benefits of sleep. This in turn produces lethargy and difficulty in awakening, daytime drowsiness, and a sense of fatigue. Regular and frequent alcohol and sedative consumption can worsen OSA. Clinical questionnaire-related scales have been devised to screen for OSA. The most often used ones are the Epworth Sleepiness Scale[39] and The STOP-BANG Scale.[40] Limitations of some aspects of these scales have led to the development of alternatives such as the Berlin Questionnaire and the Stanford Sleepiness Scale.

The Epworth Sleepiness Scale[39] requests patients to answer and grade the chance of dozing off while performing routine activities of daily living graded from 0 to 4:

- *No chance of dozing = 0*
- *Slight chance of dozing = 1*
- *Moderate chance of dozing = 3*
- *High chance of dozing = 4*

The following activities are then rated by the patient:

- Sitting and reading
- Watching television
- Sitting inactive in a public place—theater or meeting
- As a passenger in a car for an hour without a break
- Lying down in the afternoon after a meal
- Sitting and talking to someone
- Sitting quietly after lunch without alcohol
- In a car, while stopped for a few minutes in traffic
  0–7 = normal; 8–9 = mild sleepiness; 10–15 = moderate sleepiness; 16–24 = severe sleepiness

The *STOP-BANG* questionnaire[40] on the other hand utilizes age, gender, BMI, neck circumference, hypertension, snoring, tiredness, and observed nocturnal apneas with a single point being appointed for each parameter. The understanding is that male gender, age over 50 years, a neck circumference over 17 inches, and a BMI of 35 kg/m^2 are risk factors for OSA when there is a history of snoring, tiredness, and hypertension.

When OSA is clinically suspected, a sleep study has to be performed either as an unsupervised home study or as a technician-supervised in-hospital assessment within a polysomnographic laboratory. The fundamental concept is the documentation of sleep-associated breathing efficiency or disturbance. To evaluate the diagnosis of OSA, several respiratory signals are assessed, including nasal pressure, nasal-oral thermistor, respiratory effort, pulse oximetry, and snoring signal. The currently accepted norms for this have been laid down within the manual of the American Academy of Sleep Medicine (AASM).[41] An obstructive apnea is defined as a reduction of at least 90% in thermistor-based airflow for at least 10 seconds with ongoing inspiratory effort. For reference, a central apnea is of similar length but has an absent inspiratory effort. Hypopnea is a more complex respiratory event with multiple definitions. The AASM-recommended definition for hypopnea is a 30% reduction in nasal pressure or airflow for 10 seconds in combination with a 3% or more oxygen desaturation and/or EEG-based arousal from sleep.[41] The AASM alternative hypopnea definition is a 30% reduction in nasal pressure or airflow for 10 seconds in combination with a 4% or greater oxygen desaturation. OSA severity is assessed primarily by the number of apneas and hypopneas divided by the hours of sleep during the sleep study; this score is defined as the apnea-hypopnea index (AHI). An AHI <5 events per hour is defined as normal breathing for an adult, mild OSA is 5–14.99/hour, moderate OSA is 15–29.99/hour, and 30 or more per hour are considered severe OSA.[42] In some sleep laboratories in the UK, an AHI of over 25/hour of sleep is considered severe OSA.

The frequency of respiratory events (AHI) is not the only mechanism to assess the severity of sleep-disordered breathing (although it is the most common), other options include the oxygen desaturation index or the time below 90%, which has been associated with 3-year mortality in patients with cardiovascular disease. The occurrence of moderate-to-severe OSA sets into motion numerous physiological derangements with far-reaching, disease-accelerating repercussions within almost any organ system. Patients need counseling and initiation of titrated continuous positive airway pressure (CPAP) therapy via a nasal or full face mask and tubing connected to a CPAP device.[43] The advent of nasal pillows and nasal cradles has made compliance and adherence to CPAP therapy better.

Solriamfetol is the only drug that has successfully undergone a randomized controlled trial for the treatment of excessive sleepiness in OSA. It is a selective dopamine and norepinephrine reuptake inhibitor that exhibits wakefulness-promoting effects. In 459 patients studied, doses of Solriamfetol at 75, 150, and 300 mg successfully improved daytime sleepiness in patients with OSA and there were no major adverse effects.[44] In a subgroup analysis, it was demonstrated that this clinical benefit was regardless of adherence to primary OSA therapy with CPAP, and that Solriamfetol did not affect CPAP therapy in any way.[45] Currently, it is not available in the Indian markets.

> *"Sleep that knits up the ravell'd sleave of care, The death of each day's life, sore labor's bath, Balm of hurt minds, great nature's second course, Chief nourisher in life's feast."*
>
> **—William Shakespeare in Macbeth**

The functions of sleep have been suspected to be essentially brain restorative in numerous ways as conjectured by William Shakespeare in his play "Macbeth." Sleep functions have been the focus of research for the last century and numerous observant lay persons have suspected that it is vital for mental health too. Allan Rechtschaffen (1927–2021), a sleep researcher at the University of Chicago Sleep Laboratory, said—"If sleep does not serve an absolutely vital function, then it is the biggest mistake the evolutionary process has ever made." "I've always envied people who sleep easily. Their brains must be cleaner, the floorboards of the skull well swept, all the little monsters closed up in a steamer trunk at the foot of the bed." This quote by David Benioff in his 2008 novel "City of Thieves" is ahead of its time as it antedates the Maiken Nedergaard discovery of the glymphatic system in 2013.

The functions of sleep as we know it include memory consolidation, emotional equilibrium maintenance, autonomic system recalibration, immune competence, harmonizing glycemic profile, optimizing fat stores, controlling senescence, and glymphatic-driven deep cleaning of the brain.[46] Sleep-disordered breathing leads to accelerated endothelial dysfunction and is associated with an independent higher risk of precipitating strokes, especially lacunar and/or subcortical infarcts. According to the Wisconsin study, an AHI of more than 20 increased the stroke by more than three times independent of hypertension, diabetes, and BMI dysregulation.[47] A Korean study demonstrated that moderate-to-severe sleep apnea conferred an independent and higher risk for the development of white matter disease in middle-aged and older individuals.[48] A Japanese study correlated severe OSA with an independent risk of accelerated carotid artery intimal thickness.[49] An Italian American collaborative study implied that white matter integrity compromised due to OSA could be reversed with CPAP therapy.[50] A recent contemplative proposal has suggested that subcortical ischemic strokes are a disorder of aberrant glymphatic function ("glymphopathy"), wherein OSA may be a major player contributing to glymphatic dysfunction.[51] The fact that OSA impairs the efficiency of the glymphatic system has been the focus of research from alternative standpoints too, especially in the realm of cognition and the risk of Alzheimer's disease.[52]

The relationship of OSA to cognition and cognitive reserve is more complex. Forgetfulness for names and immediate events is now included in the symptom complex associated with OSA. An NYU study proposed that sleep-disordered breathing advances cognitive decline in the elderly.[53] Others demonstrated that CPAP therapy could retard the trajectory of decline in patients with Alzheimer's disease who had OSA.[54] A neuropsychological assessment and Pittsburgh compound positron emission tomography (PET) scanning performed on patients who attended a sleep clinic for moderate and severe OSA found that they had a higher burden of amyloid in the brain in a distribution similar to that observed in Alzheimer's disease.[55] A New York study by Bubu demonstrated a similar longitudinal change in AD biomarkers in patients with OSA in older age.[56] The hypothesis proposed to explain these observations is that OSA impairs the efficiency of glymphatic clearance of amyloid and tau in patients frequently enough to impart a higher vulnerability for amyloid and tau accumulation. Claudio Liguori asked the question—"Is it time to consider OSA as a risk factor for Alzheimer's disease?" in a thought-provoking editorial.[57] The same authors were able to demonstrate that patients with OSA mimic glucose consumption and biomarker trajectories, reminiscent of Alzheimer's disease when studied early in the course of biological consequences resulting from OSA. In some patients, these changes reverse after CPAP therapy for OSA.[58] A 2018 study from Houston found that 28/31 patients with idiopathic normal pressure hydrocephalus (iNPH) had undiagnosed sleep abnormalities compatible with OSA.[59] The authors hypothesized that the severe increase in negative intrathoracic pressure required to overcome apneic spells in OSA leads to repetitive though transient arrests in CSF absorption leading to its accumulation over time.[60] These insights into the poorly recognized association between OSA in the elderly and dementia are worthy of more diligent research confirmation. Beth Malow showed that in older onset epilepsy with worsening seizure control, OSA plays an important contribution.[61] Since then, the relationship between seizure vulnerability and OSA is well recognized. In some patients, the treatment of OSA brings about rewarding seizure control.[62] Patients with OSA at times present with isolated nocturnal seizures in the REM replete periods of sleep between 2 and 6 AM when apnea is maximal. Many such patients have under-recognized/ill-reported symptoms of EDS.

Similarly, some patients with unrecognized OSA present to the clinic with recurrent and unexplained syncope.[63] It is useful to take a diligent sleep history and screen for OSA when routine investigations for syncope have not yielded a positive result. Neurologists need to be vigilant and aware of the numerous ways in which OSA may be relevant to the clinical assessment of their patients.

NARCOLEPSY AND IDIOPATHIC HYPERSOMNIA

The diagnosis of hypersomnia has to be made in the context of having ruled out excessive sleepiness due to a medical condition, e.g., cirrhosis of the liver, consumption of sedation-inducing medications, a psychiatric condition, and poor sleep hygiene. In the community, the two non-sleep disordered breathing-related causes of excessive daytime somnolence with a pressure/compulsion to sleep in the daytime are narcolepsy and idiopathic hypersomnia. The five core clinical features of narcolepsy type-1 are EDS, cataplexy, sleep paralysis, sleep-associated visual hallucinations (hypnogogic or hypnopompic), and disrupted nocturnal sleep.[64] Many patients will not exhibit all five features. Classically, people with narcolepsy type 1 experience sudden "attacks" of a need to sleep, while people with idiopathic hypersomnia more often describe their sleepiness as a state of persistently low vigilance. Cataplexy is the sudden loss of muscle tone induced by emotion, most commonly strong positive emotions and especially laughter. It is thought to represent the intrusion of REM-sleep muscle atonia into wakefulness.[65] Consciousness is maintained in these episodes. Sleep paralysis is the term for brief, persistent REM atonia on awakening. The narcolepsy type-1 tetrad of EDS, cataplexy, sleep paralysis, and sleep-related hallucinations occur in only 45% of patients with narcolepsy. Typically, all may not be present when the patient seeks medical attention. In idiopathic hypersomnia, the core clinical symptoms are long sleeping hours and sleep inertia. People with idiopathic hypersomnia experience long nocturnal sleep of >10–11 hours, along with very long daytime naps. This extended duration of sleep is typically not refreshing.[66] On awakening, they feel a compulsion to continue sleeping, are lethargic, and are often confused with some degree of being cognitively dysfunctional. They may require another person to awaken them and may take a long time to become alert. This is known as sleep drunkenness.[67] Narcolepsy type-2 is the designation for those who do not have cataplexy. The other features are identical to narcolepsy type-1. Klein–Levin syndrome is an idiopathic disorder that manifests as prolonged, recurrent hypersomnolence, associated with cognitive dysfunction, altered perception, altered eating habits, and disinhibition (often sexual).[68]

Narcolepsy is strongly believed to be autoimmune and has an association with specific HLA alleles especially DQB1*06:02.[69] In others, it is believed to be caused by a mutation in the gene-regulating orexin integrity. Correlations have been made in canine genetic models with orexin deficiency/dysregulation and narcolepsy.[70,71] There are some cases that have been precipitated after H1N1 infection or vaccinations for it.[72] The cause or causes of idiopathic hypersomnia also remain unknown. One theory involves abnormal activation of the sleep-promoting GABAergic system. CSF from people with hypersomnia disorders (primarily idiopathic hypersomnia and narcolepsy type 2), applied to $GABA_A$ receptors in vitro, resulted in greater potentiation of receptor activity than did CSF from controls, implying the presence of a positive allosteric modulator of $GABA_A$ receptors in patients with hypersomnia.[73] However, these findings were not replicated by others.[74] The diagnosis of Klein–Levin syndrome is clinical and evaluation of both narcolepsy and idiopathic hypersomnolence requires the patient to undergo a PSG first followed by a multiple sleep latency test (MSLT). The overnight polysomnography aims to achieve the following: Rule out sleep-disordered breathing as a cause of EDS, establish a routine latency to REM sleep, and exclude sleep restriction which can alter MSLT results. The MSLT is a daytime test in which patients are given five nap opportunities, spaced 2 hours apart and beginning 1.5 hours after waking in the morning. During each nap opportunity, patients are asked to lie in bed, close their eyes, and try to fall asleep. Two main diagnostic measures are obtained from the MSLT: (i) the mean sleep latency and (ii) a number of sleep-onset REM periods. The mean sleep latency is the average time to the first epoch of sleep across all five nap periods during the test. A mean sleep latency of ≤8 minutes is specific and sensitive for narcolepsy type-1.[75] A sleep-onset REM period (SOREMP) is the onset of REM sleep within 15 minutes of falling asleep. The presence of two or more sleep-onset REM periods supports the diagnosis of either kind of narcolepsy. It also excludes the diagnosis of idiopathic hypersomnia. Ideally, patients should not be on a selective serotonin reuptake inhibitor and should not be using any recreational drug. Narcolepsy type-1 may be diagnosed by testing orexin (hypocretin) levels within CSF. Orexin (hypocretin) levels are low or absent (<110 pg/mL) in people with narcolepsy type-1 but normal (>200 pg/mL) in those with other hypersomnias. Together with sleepiness, orexin (hypocretin) deficiency is sufficient to diagnose narcolepsy type-1, even in the absence of other clinical features or MSLT findings.

PHARMACOTHERAPY OF EXCESSIVE DAYTIME DROWSINESS

Modafinil

The therapy of hypersomnolence hinges on the modulation of wake-promoting neurotransmission systems in the brain. Modafinil is a racemic mix of two enantiomers. Though debated, it is believed that it modulates dopaminergic, glutamatergic, and orexinergic systems to produce clinical efficacy.[76] In a meta-analysis of narcolepsy studies, modafinil reduced ESS scores, prolonged MSLT latencies, improved wakefulness, and enhanced quality of life when compared to placebo.[77] Armodafinil is the R-enantiomer of modafinil. Unlike modafinil, which better controls sleepiness when prescribed in two divided doses, armodafinil is prescribed as a single morning dose. The common side effects are headaches and anxiety. Serious side effects of modafinil and armodafinil include Stevens–Johnson syndrome and other related conditions, angioedema, psychosis, mania, hallucinations, suicidal ideation, and dependency or abuse. Traditional psychostimulants such as methylphenidate, dextroamphetamine, and amphetamine are often used to treat narcolepsy and idiopathic hypersomnia. Randomized controlled study data justifying such usage is lacking.

Sodium Oxybate

Sodium oxybate is the sodium salt of gamma-hydroxy-butyrate and is approved for the treatment of both sleepiness and cataplexy in narcolepsy type-1. It is taken at bedtime and again after a period of 2.5–4 hours. It promotes deep sleep and sleep consolidation. In a meta-analysis of narcolepsy studies, it improved the ability to stay awake in the maintenance of wakefulness test and reduced the frequency of cataplexy attacks (by a mean of 8 attacks per week).[78] In a non-randomized smaller study, it was effective in reducing sleep drunkenness in patients with idiopathic hypersomnia.[79] Common adverse effects include nausea, bed-wetting, and dizziness. Serious adverse effects include depression, dependence, abuse potential, psychosis, and suicidal ideation.

Solriamfetol

It is a dopamine and norepinephrine reuptake inhibitor. In phase-3 randomized controlled trial of solriamfetol for narcolepsy, daily doses of 75 mg, 150 mg, and 300 mg all significantly decreased Epworth Sleepiness Scale scores (by 2.2 points, 3.8 points, and 4.8 points more than placebo, respectively), and daily doses of 150 mg and 300 mg significantly improved the ability to remain awake during the maintenance of wakefulness test (by 7.7 minutes and 10.2 minutes more than placebo, respectively).[80] Common side effects include headache, nausea, anxiety, suppression of appetite, and insomnia. Serious adverse effects include elevation of the heart rate and blood pressure. It is recommended to be used in a dosage of 75–150 mg per day only.

Pitolisant

It is a histamine H3 inverse agonist/antagonist that enhances wakefulness by increasing CNS histaminergic transmission. A phase-three randomized controlled study demonstrated its efficacy in reducing daytime sleepiness and cataplexy in patients with narcolepsy.[81] It is also used in idiopathic hypersomnia based on one study.[82] Its common side effects include insomnia, nausea, and anxiety. Venlafaxine and fluoxetine are also used in narcolepsy on perceived experiential benefits in some patients.

The therapy of Klein–Levin syndrome is challenging. Medications such as methylphenidate are often used but the efficacy is limited. In a single-center cohort of 130 patients (a national referral center for Klein–Levin syndrome), 71 patients who chose lithium treatment and 49 patients who opted for no treatment were followed for nearly 2 years on average. The patients treated with lithium showed a shorter duration, reduced number, and severity of hypersomnolence.[83] Carbamazepine, valproate, phenytoin, and methylprednisolone have been tried with variable results in a smaller number of anecdotal studies. The outcome of therapy in Klein–Levin syndrome is regrettably suboptimal and many patients continue to struggle with symptoms despite well intentioned therapy.

RESTLESS LEGS SYNDROME

Restless legs syndrome (RLS) is a disorder characterized by abnormal sensations in the legs leading to an irresistible urge to move the legs, essentially when patients are at rest or in the evening/night. It is usually accompanied by difficulty in initiating and maintaining sleep. This leads to fatigue, lethargy, and somnolence on awakening. Many systemic medical conditions may accompany this constellation of symptoms and signs. Iron deficiency anemia, pregnancy, polyneuropathy, chronic kidney disease, Parkinson's disease, multiple sclerosis, depression and anxiety, and attention-deficit hyperactivity disorder often accompany RLS.[84] Periodic leg movements in sleep constitute the main motor signs observed in this condition. These are observed by the sleeping partners of the affected individuals and during the objective assessment of the patient during a polysomnographic evaluation.[85] RLS is common during pregnancy and in individuals with RLS, pregnancy may worsen symptoms. Some associative studies have implied that RLS may lead to an increase in coronary and cerebro-vascular thrombotic events.[86] More than 50% of affected patients have one first-degree relative with similar symptoms. Several polymorphisms have been identified that could pose a risk of developing RLS.

Patients with RLS require higher peripheral ferritin levels than controls and do to obtain equivalent CSF ferritin levels. It is suggested that impaired transport of ferritin across the blood–brain barrier is an integral part of the pathophysiology leading to RLS.[87,88] Strategic loci within the nervous system demonstrate a deficiency in central iron stores, implying an abnormality of iron transport across the blood–brain barrier and aberrant regional accumulation into critical neuronal cells, e.g., neuromelanin cells of the substantia nigra.[89] Therefore, central iron deficiency constitutes the best documented biological abnormality in RLS. The two key abnormalities in neurotransmitter systems serving as putative therapeutic targets in RLS are: (1) increased dopaminergic function in the peripheral nerves leading to aberrant sensations and periodic leg movements in sleep, and (2) increased central glutamatergic dysfunction leading to hyperarousal and sleep loss and secondary periodic leg movements in sleep.[90] The laboratory evaluation of RLS must include a complete blood cell count and a biochemical assessment of iron metabolism, transport, and storage.

The following five criteria have to be met to establish a diagnosis of RLS:

1. An urge to move the legs usually but not always accompanied by or caused by unpleasant sensations in the legs
2. The urge to move the legs and accompanying unpleasant sensations worsen or start during periods of inactivity such as resting or lying down or sitting
3. The urge to move the legs and accompanying unpleasant sensations are partially or relieved by movement such as walking or stretching
4. The urge to move the legs and accompanying unpleasant sensations during rest or inactivity only occur or are worse in the evening or night (diurnal circadian variation)
5. The above features cannot solely be accounted for by myalgia, polyneuropathy, venous stasis, leg edema, leg cramps, or arthritis.

The diagnosis of RLS is essentially clinical. Polysomnography is not a mandatory investigation for the RLS diagnosis to be confirmed; however, it can be useful because it allows for objectification and quantification of periodic leg movements in sleep, a motor sign of this disorder. During polysomnography, periodic leg movements in sleep are quantified by using tibialis anterior surface electromyography (EMG), giving an indirect index of RLS severity. Periodic leg movements in sleep are found in 24–48% of patients with OSA.[91]

Iron replacement is indicated in patients with RLS if transferrin saturation is <45% and the serum ferritin level is <300 ng/mL (to minimize iron overload risk).[92] Adjunctive therapies include moderate exercise, improvement in sleep hygiene, reduction of caffeine-containing beverages, hot leg baths, massage, and acupuncture/yoga.

The symptomatic therapies to ameliorate RLS hinge on the nocturnal consumption of dopamine agonists such as pramipexole and ropinirole.[93] The other class of medications that have been deployed is α2-delta ligand modulators like gabapentin enacarbil. Sometimes, using a dopamine agonist to treat RLS results in augmentation.[93] Classical features of augmentations are breakthrough episodes during the daytime, shorter duration of treatment effect, an increase in symptom frequency or intensity, worsening sleep quality, increased frequency of periodic leg movements in sleep, and in general an overall decrease in treatment effects. It helps to keep the dosage of dopamine agonist therapy at a minimum. Other attempts at treating RLS have relied on the knowledge of the modulatory role of adenosine in RLS. A novel study assessed the treatment of RLS using dipyridamole. Dipyridamole is an inhibitor of nucleoside equilibrative transporters which are the main presynaptic reuptake system for extracellular adenosine and, therefore, increase tonic A1 receptor activation, implicated in the pathogenesis of RLS. In this study, dipyridamole showed significant improvement in RLS symptoms, periodic leg movements in sleep, and sleep.[94] Regular cardiovascular exercise, moderating caffeine and alcohol intake, maintenance of sleep hygiene, and especially the avoidance of SD help in reducing the severity of RLS.[95]

REM SLEEP BEHAVIOR DISORDER

In 1953, Aserinsky and Kleitman coined the term REM sleep to describe their observation of a sleep phase characterized by low-amplitude, high-frequency EEG signature, skeletal muscle paralysis, profound autonomic fluctuations with a high heart rate, paroxysmal changes in respiration, tidal volume, and core body temperature accompanied by REMs. When awakened, these individuals recalled vivid visual imagery and the association of REM sleep with dreaming was cemented.[4] The key function of REM sleep is the depotentiation of the emotional burden of traumatizing life experiences, as a process of emotion-stabilizing synaptic homeostasis, essential for daytime emotional salience.[8] In 1986, Carlos Schenck evaluated a 68-year-old man who had been for years kicking and punching violently while enacting his dreams in sleep, injuring both himself and his wife. Polysomnography confirmed the REM sleep-related manifestation of his physical movements. After assessing five other such patients, Schenck and Mahowald coined the term REM sleep behavior dysfunction (RBD) to describe their findings.[96]

We now know that RBD is a prodromal symptom of α-synuclein pathology in the brain with a majority of patients ultimately developing a neurodegenerative disorder. When followed up over >5 years, patients develop features of either nontremor-dominant Parkinson's disease, diffuse Lewy body dementia (DLBD), or MSA.[97-99] The trajectory of Parkinson's disease that follows RBD is faster with a preponderance of gait dysfunction and cognitive impairment. Patients who have RBD with comorbid hyposmia and constipation but who are not taking an antidepressant are at high risk of phenoconversion to a neurodegenerative disorder.[100] Unlike the earlier misperception, recent insights suggest that antidepressants do not induce RBD but unmask dream enactment in an individual already burdened with subclinical α-synuclein pathology in the brain.

Low-dose clonazepam (0.25-1 mg) at bedtime and melatonin are standard therapies utilized to treat RBD. Melatonin can be initiated in a dose of 3 mg and gradually increased to 12 or 18 mg as required.[101] In patients who have DLBD, donepezil or rivastigmine are prescribed in the daytime to augment their cholinergic deficit. Since patients who have RBD are at risk of developing a neurodegenerative brain disorder, they require empathy and patient counseling to confront this challenging condition.

NREM PARASOMNIAS

The NREM parasomnias are nomenclature wise classified as disorders of arousal. As discussed in the section earlier on *local* and *dissociated* sleep, these parasomnias are characterized by *dissociated* sleep, with wake and sleep phenomena intermingling, and *local* sleep, in which different areas of the brain exist simultaneously in different states of wakefulness or sleep.[35] Sleepwalking (somnambulism), sleep talking (somniloquy), night terrors, confusional arousals, sleep-related eating disorders, and sexomnia are typified by incomplete awakenings from slow-wave sleep, limited recall of imagery, and partial or complete amnesia. Most occur in childhood and adolescence.

The typical phenomenology of these disorders is that they occur in the early hours of sleep when NREM sleep dominates. Individuals may appear to waken partially and perform a complex task, e.g., walking, eating, talking, and sexually charged physical movements. They may appear confused or bewildered and are unable to respond when questioned or restrained. Usually, they have no recall of the event when fully wakened. Occasionally, they may accrue an injury but as a rule violent behavior is rare in NREM parasomnia. The lifetime prevalence of sleepwalking is 7% though 20% of childhood sleepwalkers may sleepwalk in adulthood too. Precipitating factors for such disorders of arousal are those that deepen slow-wave sleep, e.g., SD, shift work, some sedative, and those that worsen sleep fragmentation, e.g., noise, stress, alcohol, and OSA. The diagnosis of NREM parasomnias is usually clinical, but in some cases, video-EEG and polysomnography may be required to rule out suspicions of nocturnal seizures and/or OSA.

Management of disorders of arousal includes reassurance, correction of precipitating factors, addressing safety, behavioral therapies, and medications. Parents of children with arousal disorders can often be reassured once they understand the benign and usually self-limiting nature of the condition.[102] They need to be informed that it is usual for the children to be unresponsive to their comforting words and actions. Improvement in home safety is important and should be based on the clinical features of the individual patient. Stairways and windows may need to be protected and doors to the outside adequately secured. Weapons should be removed from the bedroom, and sometimes bed or door alarms are needed. In adults, sodium oxybate and zolpidem have been reported to produce NREM parasomnias usually ones associated with nocturnal eating.[103] Sometimes, it is associated with RLS.

Patients with exploding head syndrome experience an auditory hallucination of sudden loud noise or a perception of a painless explosion in their heads. The sound may sometimes be described as that made by an object falling to the ground from a height or a clash of cymbals.[104] It is sometimes accompanied by a flash of light or occasionally a myoclonic jerk. In most patients, it is associated with a sense of fright. Sometimes, it is associated with insomnia. The etiology is unknown, and most patients improve with attempts at improving sleep hygiene.

INSOMNIA

Insomnia is the most common sleep complaint for which medical attention is sought. Its definitions and classification have undergone recent changes. The division into primary and secondary insomnia is now discarded as is the terminology of psychophysiology, idiopathic, and paradoxical insomnia. Simply understood, if an individual confesses to having sustained difficulty in initiating and maintaining sleep, despite the presence of appropriate opportunity and circumstances to do so, which results in a daytime negative consequence, one can diagnose insomnia. If these symptoms persist at least three times a week for at least 3 months, the designation is "chronic insomnia disorder". Individuals who confess to no daytime consequences are excluded from this reckoning. Those who suffer from chronic pain, psychiatric dysfunction, or an established or suspected sleep disorder (like OSA or RLS) are also excluded from this definition. The symptoms necessary for this diagnosis are difficulty in initiating or maintaining sleep, earlier and/or frequent awakening from sleep, resistance in going to bed at the desired time, and difficulty in sleeping without parent/caregiver attention. The daytime symptoms include fatigue, lethargy, mood and memory disturbances, impaired social, vocational, or academic performance, impaired attention or concentration leading to performance errors/accidents, and concerns regarding these features.

A typical physiologically normal person has a circadian rhythm that warrants sleeping at 11 AM and waking by 7 AM. Patients with circadian misalignment of these normal timing either from habitual precipitation or from frequent travel zone timing changes require assessment for circadian sleep-wake disorders. Polysomnography in a sleep laboratory or home sleep apnea testing is not routinely indicated for circadian rhythm sleep-wake disorders except when suspicion exists for a comorbid sleep disorder such as OSA or RLS. The primary goal of the treatment of circadian rhythm sleep-wake disorders is to realign the circadian timing of sleep and wake with the desired or required sleep-wake period. After the due assessment, therapeutic approaches typically include intentional altering of bedtimes and awakening times, appropriately timed melatonin, melatonin receptor agonists, and light therapy.

Chronic insomnia disorder remains a clinical diagnosis and polysomnography is usually not warranted. Assessment of a sleep diary/log, actigraphy, and clinical sleep surveys at the bedside are usually helpful. Cognitive behavioral therapy for insomnia, a structured and personalized nonpharmacologic program, generally conducted by a sleep behavioral psychologist who guides individuals to modify their cognitive processes and sleep behaviors to improve their sleep, remains the gold standard therapy for insomnia. The lack of such trained personnel in India has led to the irrational usage of anxiolytic and hypnotic prescriptions from family physicians. The cardinal therapy for insomnia is patient counseling on the value and functions of sleep, an introduction to sleep circadian rhythms and its benefits, guidance on avoiding evening caffeinated drinks and/or strenuous exercise, avoiding using the bed for purposes other than sleep and sexual activity, decreasing nocturnal screen time, and the use of adjuvants like melatonin. Patients are advised that if they cannot fall asleep in bed beyond 20 minutes, they could go to another room and read or listen to music in low light until they feel sleepy again. Such patients are also advised not to nap in the daytime. Many of these facets are incorporated in cognitive behavioral therapy either physically by trained psychologists or online.

Hypnotics are not usually recommended in the therapy of chronic insomnia disorder. Traditional hypnotic agents are benzodiazepine receptor agonists and target the GABA pathway in the descending sleep-inducing network. Eszopiclone (2 mg or 3 mg), zaleplon (5 mg or 10 mg), and zolpidem (5 mg or 10 mg) are the currently prescribed hypnotics. The quality of evidence for their usage is low but their benefits probably outweigh the potential harm. Some patients on these medications, especially zolpidem, develop sleep-related eating disorders like NREM parasomnia. The benzodiazepine receptor agonists carry a risk of worsening pre-existent or inducing a de novo sleep-disordered breathing in these vulnerable patients. A new class of medications, the dual orexin receptor antagonists (DORAs), have paved the way for alternative rational therapy. Suvorexant, lemborexant, and daridorexant are currently approved in this category. Of these, lemborexant (5–10 mg at bedtime) is available in the Indian pharmaceutical industry. Melatonin in doses from 3 to 10 mg can be used 2 hours before bedtime in those who manifest sleep fragmentation from poor sleep hygiene and those with a perceived circadian rhythm disorder. Ramelteon (in doses of 8 mg and 16 mg) is an alternative medication that is a specific agonist of the melatonin M1 and M2 receptors in the brain.

The following measures are useful in guiding patients with chronic insomnia disorder.

- Maintain a regular sleep schedule
- Understand that the human brain is wired to sleep from 10:30 PM to 6:30 AM
- Avoid daytime naps
- Exercise is preferred in the morning hours and avoided within 3 hours of bedtime
- Remove laptops, cell phones, and TVs from the bedroom
- Restrict screen time after 9:30 PM.
- Avoid caffeinated drinks after 3 PM and alcohol within 2 hours of bedtime
- Ensure low light, a pleasant aroma, and a comfortable ambient temperature in the bedroom
- If vulnerable to anxiety, meditation and mindfulness are adjuncts to good sleep.

The value of sustained and healthy sleep physiology across the human lifespan cannot be overemphasized. A large body of research on human SD has led to insights that are thought provoking.[105] SD leads to impairment of attention, memory processing, emotional stability, risk-reward assessment (and value judgments within this domain), and cardiovascular autonomic harmony. This has implications for many facets of brain-related health paradigms including stroke risk and neurodegeneration. The understanding that sleep health and hygiene across the human lifespan have a large contribution to health maintenance and longevity has to be emphasized in the public domain as an imperative health advocacy measure.

CONCLUSION

As can be easily seen, tremendous advances have occurred in the understanding of normal sleep and the pathophysiology of sleep disorders. These have helped the development of medications and strategies to reduce the impact of these common neurological diseases.

Disclaimer: Dr Joy D Desai has written the entire manuscript of this chapter independently. Dr Vaibhav Mathur, MD, DM, a fellow at the Jaslok Hospital, has contributed to the digital diagram configurations within the text material.

REFERENCES

1. Schwartz JRL, Roth T. Neurophysiology of sleep and wakefulness: basic science and clinical implications. Curr Neuropharmacol. 2008;6:367-78.
2. Basheer R, Strecker RE, Thakkar MM, McCarley RW. Adenosine and sleep wake regulation. Prog Neurobiol. 2004;73:379-96.
3. Li J, Vitiello MV, Gooneratne N. Sleep in normal aging. Sleep Med Clin. 2018;13(1):1-11.
4. Aserinski E, Kleitman N. Regularly occurring periods of eye motility, and concomitant phenomena, during sleep. Science. 1953;118:273-4.
5. Staresina BP, Bergmann TO, Bonnefond M, van der Meij R, Jensen O, Deuker L, et al. Hierarchical nesting of slow oscillations, spindles, and ripples in the human hippocampus during sleep. Nat Neurosci. 2015;18(11):1679-86.
6. Helfrich RF, Lendner JD, Mander BA, Guillen H, Paff M, Mnatsakanyan L, et al. Bidirectional prefrontal-hippocampal dynamics organize information transfer during sleep in humans. Nat Commun. 2019;10:3572.
7. Mander BA, Rao V, Lu B, Saletin JM, Lindquist JR, Ancoli-Israel S, et al. Prefrontal atrophy, disrupted NREM slow waves, and impaired hippocampal dependent memory in aging. Nat Neurosci. 2013;16(3):357-64.
8. Van der Helm E, and Walker MP. Overnight therapy? The role of sleep, in emotional brain processing. Psychol Bull. 2009;135(5): 731-48.
9. Wassing R, Schalkwijk F, Lakbila-Kamal O, Ramautar JR, Stoffers D, Mutsaerts HJMM, et al. Haunted by the past: old emotions remain salient in insomnia disorder. Brain. 2019;142(6):1783-96.
10. Tononi G, Cirelli C. Sleep and the price of plasticity. From synaptic and cellular homeostasis to memory consolidation and integration. Neuron. 2014;81(1):12-34.
11. Rothschild AE, Appelbaum L, de Lecea L. Neuronal mechanisms for sleep/wake regulation and modulatory drive. Neuropsychopharmacology. 2018;43:937-52.
12. Park SH, Weber F. Neural and homeostatic regulation of REM sleep. Front Psychol. 2020;11:1662.

13. Rattenborg NC, Amlaner CJ, Lima SL. Behavioural, neurophysiological, and evolutionary perspectives on unihemispheric sleep. Neurosci Biobehav Rev. 2000;24(8):817-42.
14. Tamaki M, Bang JW, Watanabe T, Sasaki Y. Night watch in one brain hemisphere during sleep associated with the first-night effect in humans. Curr Biol. 2016;26(9):1190-4.
15. Rosenwasser AM, Turek FW. Neurobiology of circadian rhythm regulation. Sleep Med Clin. 2015;10:403-12.
16. Knutson KL, von Schantz M. Associations between chronotype, morbidity, and mortality in the UK biobank cohort. Chronobiol Int. 2018;35(8):1045-53.
17. Caliandro R, Streng AA, van Kerkhof LWM, van der Horst GTZ, Chaves I. Social jet lag and related risks for human health. A timely review. Nutrients. 2021;13(12):4543.
18. Halassa MM, Fellin T, Haydon PG. The tripartite synapse: roles for gliotransmission in health and disease. Trends Mol Med. 2007;13(2):54-63.
19. Haydon PG. Astrocytes and the modulation of sleep. Curr Opin Neurobiol. 2017;44:28-33.
20. Weber B, Barros LF. The astrocyte: powerhouse and recycling centre. Cold Spring Harb Perspect Biol. 2015;7(12):a020396.
21. Schmitt LI, Wimmer RD. Astrocytic regulation of sleep processes. Curr Sleep Med Rep. 2015;1:9-19.
22. Bellot-Saez A, Cohen G, van Schaik A, Ooi L, W Morley J, Buskila Y. Astrocytic modulation of cortical oscillations. Nature Sci Rep. 2018;8:11565.
23. Nedergaard M. Garbage truck of the brain. Science. 2013;340(6140): 1529-30.
24. Iliff JJ, Wang M, Zeppenfeld DM, Venkataraman A, Plog BA, Liao Y, et al. Cerebral arterial pulsation drives paravascular CSF-interstitial fluid exchange in the murine brain. J Neurol Sci. 2013;33(46): 18190-9.
25. Xie L, Kang H, Xu Q, Chen MJ, Liao Y, Thiyagarajan M, et al. Sleep drives metabolite clearance from the adult brain. Science. 2013;342:373-7.
26. Jessen NA, Munk ASF, Lundgaard I, Nedergaard M. The glymphatic system—A beginner's guide. Neurochem Res. 2015;40(12): 2583-99.
27. Benveniste H, Liu X, Koundal S, Sanggaard S, Lee H, Wardlaw J, et al. The glymphatic system and waste clearance with brain aging: A review. Gerontology. 2019;65:106-19.
28. Camandola S. Astrocytes, emerging stars of energy homeostasis. Cell Stress. 2018;2(10):246-52.
29. Siclari F, Tononi G. Local aspects of sleep and wakefulness. Curr Opin Neurobiol. 2017; 44:222-7.
30. Huber R, Ghilardi MF, Massimini M, Tononi G. Local sleep and learning. Nature. 2004;430:78-81.
31. Hung CS, Sarasso S, Ferrarelli F, Riedner B, Ghilardi MF, Cirelli C, et al. Local experience-dependent changes in the wake EEG after prolonged wakefulness. Sleep 2013;36:59-72.
32. Bernardi G, Siclari F, Yu X, Zennig C, Bellesi M, Ricciardi E, et al. Neural and behavioral correlates of extended training during sleep deprivation in humans: evidence for local, task-specific effects. J Neurosci. 2015;35:4487-500.
33. Morrone E, D'Artavilla Lupo N, Trentin R, Pizza F, Risi I, Arcovio S, et al. Microsleep as a marker of sleepiness in obstructive sleep apnoea patients. J Sleep Res. 2020; 29(2):e12882.
34. Siclari F, Bernardi G, Riedner BA, LaRocque JJ, Benca RM, Tononi G, et al. Two distinct synchronization processes in the transition to sleep: A high density electroencephalographic study. Sleep. 2014;37(10):1621-37.
35. Castelnovo A, Lopez R, Proserpio P, Nobili L, Dauvilliers Y. NREM Parasomnias as disorders of sleep-state dissociation. Nat Rev Neurol. 2018;14(8):470-81.
36. Olson EJ, Boeve BF, Silber MH. Rapid eye movement sleep behaviour disorder: demographic, clinical, and laboratory findings in 93 cases. Brain. 2000;123:331-9.
37. Slater G, Steier J. Excessive daytime sleepiness in sleep disorders. J Thorac Dis. 2012;4(6):608-16.
38. Gottlieb DJ, Punjabi NM. Diagnosis and management of obstructive sleep apnoea: A review. JAMA. 2020;323(14):1389-400.
39. Johns MW. A new method for measuring daytime sleepiness: The Epworth Sleepiness Scale. Sleep. 1991;14(6):540-5.
40. Chung F, Abdullah HR, Liao P. STOP-Bang Questionnaire: A practical approach to screen for obstructive sleep apnoea. Chest. 2016;149(3):631-8.
41. Berry RB, Albertario CL, Harding SM, Lloyd RM, Plante DT, Quan SF, et al. The AASM manual for the scoring of sleep and associated events: rules, terminology, and technical specifications. Version 2.5. Darien, IL: American Academy of Sleep Medicine; 2018.
42. American Academy of Sleep Medicine Task Force. Sleep-related breathing disorders in adults: recommendations for syndrome definition and measurement techniques in clinical research. The Report of an American Academy of Sleep Medicine Task Force. Sleep. 1999;22(7):667-89.
43. Patil SP, Ayappa IA, Caples SM, Kimoff RJ, Patel SR, Harrod CG, et al. Treatment of adult obstructive sleep apnoea with positive airway pressure: an American Academy of Sleep Medicine Systematic Review, Meta-Analysis, and GRADE Assessment. J Clin Sleep Med. 2019;15(2):301-34.
44. Schweitzer PK, Rosenberg R, Zammit GK, Gotfried M, Chen D, Carter LP, et al. Solriamfetol for excessive sleepiness in obstructive sleep apnoea (TONES3). A randomized controlled trial. Am J Respir Crit Med. 2019;199(11):1421-31.
45. Schweitzer PK, Mayer G, Rosenber R, Malhotra A, Zammit GK, Gotfried M, et al. Randomized controlled trial of Solriamfetol for excessive daytime sleepiness in OSA: An analysis of subgroups adherent and anon-adherent to OSA treatment. Chest. 2021;160(1):307-18.
46. Assefa FZ, Diaz-Abad M, Wickwire EM, Scharf SM. The functions of sleep. AIMS Neuroscience. 2015;2(3):155-71.
47. Young T, Palta M, Dempsey J, Peppard PE, Nieto FJ, Hla KM. Burden of sleep apnoea: Rationale, design, and major findings of the Wisconsin Sleep Cohort Study. WMJ. 2009;108(5):246-9.
48. Kim H, Yun CH, Thomas RJ, Lee SH, Seo HS, Cho ER, et al. Obstructive sleep apnoea as a risk factor for cerebral white matter change in a middle-aged and older general population. Sleep. 2013;36(5):709-15.
49. Minoguchi K, Yokoe T, Tazaki T, Minoguchi H, Tanaka A, Oda N, et al. Increased carotid intima-media thickness and serum inflammatory markers in obstructive sleep apnoea. Am J Respir Crit Care Med. 2005;172:625-30.
50. Castronovo V, Scifo P, Castellano A, Aloia MS, Iadanza A, Marelli S, et al. White matter integrity in obstructive sleep apnoea before and after treatment. Sleep. 2014;37(9):1465-75.
51. Benveniste H, Nedergaard M. Cerebral small vessel disease: A glymphopathy? Curr Opin Neurobiol. 2022;72:15-21.
52. Roy B, Nunez A, Aysola RS, Kang DW, Vacas S, Kumar R. Impaired glymphatic system actions in obstructive sleep apnoea adults. Front Neursci. 2022;16:884234.
53. Osorio RS, Gumb T, Pirraglia E, Varga AW, Lu SE, Lim J, et al. Sleep disordered breathing advances cognitive decline in the elderly. Neurology. 2015;84(19):1964-71.
54. Richards KC, Gooneratne N, Diccico B, Hanlon A, Moelter S, Onen F, et al. CPAP adherence may slow one-year cognitive decline in older adults with mild cognitive decline and apnoea. J Am Geriatr Soc. 2019;67(3):558-64.
55. Jackson ML, Cavuoto M, Schembri R, Doré V, Villemagne VL, Barnes M, et al. Severe obstructive sleep apnoea is associated with higher brain amyloid burden: A preliminary PET imaging study. Alzheimers Dis. 2020;78(2):611-7.
56. Bubu OM, Pirraglia E, Andrade AG, Sharma RA, Gimenez-Badia S, Umasabor-Bubu OQ, et al. Obstructive sleep apnoea and longitudinal Alzheimer's disease biomarker changes. Sleep. 2019;42(6): zsz048.

57. Liguori C, Placidi F. Is it time to consider obstructive sleep apnoea syndrome a risk factor for Alzheimer's disease? Am J Respir Crit Care Med. 2018;197(7):855-56.
58. Fernandes M, Mari L, Chiaravalloti A, Paoli B, Nuccetelli M, Izzi F, et al. 18F-FDG-PET, cognitive functioning, and CSF biomarkers in patients with obstructive sleep apnoea before and after continuous positive airway pressure treatment. J Neurol. 2022;269(10):5356-5367.
59. Roman GC, Verma AK, Zhang YJ, Fung SH. Idiopathic normal pressure hydrocephalus and obstructive sleep apnoea are frequently associated: a prospective cohort study. J Neurol Sci. 2018;395:164-8.
60. Roman GC, Jackson RE, Fung SH, Zhang YJ, Verma AK. Sleep disordered breathing and idiopathic normal pressure hydrocephalus: recent pathophysiological advances. Curr Neurol Neurosci Rep. 2019;19(7):39.
61. Malow BA, Levy K, Maturen K, Bowes R. Obstructive sleep apnoea is common in medically refractory epilepsy patients. Neurology. 2000;55(7):1002-7.
62. Malow BA, Foldvary-Schaefer N, Vaughn BV, Selwa LM, Chervin RD, Weatherwax KJ, et al. Treating obstructive sleep apnoea in adults with epilepsy: a randomized pilot trial. Neurology. 2008;71:572-7.
63. Willis FB, Isley AL, Geda YE, Shaygan A, Quarles L 4th, Fredrickson PA. Resolution of syncope with treatment of sleep apnoea. J Am Brd Fam Med. 2008;21(5):466-8.
64. Peacock J, Benca RM. Narcolepsy: Clinical features, co-morbidities, and treatment. Indian J Med Res. 2010;131:338-49.
65. Dauvilliers Y, Siegel JM, Lopez R, Torontali ZA, Peever JH. Cataplexy: clinical aspects, pathophysiology, and management strategy. Nat Rev Neurol. 2014;10(7):386-95.
66. Khan Z, Trotti LM. Central disorders of hypersomnolence: focus on the narcolepsies and idiopathic hypersomnia. Chest. 2015;148(1):262-73.
67. Roth B, Nevsimalova S, Rechtschaffen A. Hypersomnia with "sleep drunkenness." Arch Gen Psychiatry. 1972;26(5):456-62.
68. Arnulf I, Groos E, Dodet P. Kleine-Levin syndrome: a neuropsychiatric disorder. Rev Neurol (Paris). 2018;174(4):216-27.
69. Bassetti CLA, Adamantidis A, Burdakov D, Han F, Gay S, Kallweit U, et al. Narcolepsy: clinical spectrum, aetiopathophysiology, diagnosis and treatment. Nat Rev Neurol. 2019;15(9):519-39.
70. Thannickal TC, Moore RY, Nienhuis R, Ramanathan L, Gulyani S, Aldrich M, et al. Reduced number of hypocretin neurons in human narcolepsy. Neuron. 2000;27(3):469-74.
71. Lin L, Faraco J, Li R, Kadotani H, Rogers W, Lin X, et al. The sleep disorder canine narcolepsy is caused by a mutation in the hypocretin (orexin) receptor 2 gene. Cell. 1999; 98(3):365-76.
72. Ahmed SS, Schur PH, MacDonald NE, Steinman L. Narcolepsy, the 2009 A (H1N1) pandemic influenza, and pandemic influenza vaccinations: what is known and unknown about the neurological disorder, the role for autoimmunity, and vaccine adjuvants. J Autoimmun. 2014;50:1-11.
73. Rye DB, Bliwise DL, Parker K, Trotti LM, Saini P, Fairley J, et al. Modulation of vigilance in the primary hypersomnias by endogenous enhancement of GABAA receptors. Sci Transl Med. 2012;4(161):161ra151.
74. Dauvilliers Y, Evangelista E, Lopez R, Barateau L, Jaussent I, Cens T, et al. Absence of γ-aminobutyric acid-a receptor potentiation in central hypersomnolence disorders. Ann Neurol. 2016;80(2): 259-68.
75. Arand D, Bonnet M, Hurwitz T, Mitler M, Rosa R, Sangal RB. The clinical use of the MSLT and MWT. Sleep. 2005;28(1):123-44.
76. Murillo-Rodriguez E, Barciela Veras A, Barbosa Rocha N, Budde H, Machado S. An overview of the clinical uses, pharmacology, and safety of modafinil. ACS Chem Neurosci. 2018;9(2):151-8.
77. Golicki D, Bala MM, Niewada M, Wierzbicka A. Modafinil for narcolepsy: systematic review and meta-analysis. Medical Sci Monit. 2010;16(8):RA177-86.
78. Alshaikh MK, Tricco AC, Tashkandi M, Mamdani M, Straus SE, BaHammam AS. Sodium oxybate for narcolepsy with cataplexy: systematic review and meta-analysis. J Clin Sleep Med. 2012;8(4): 451-8.
79. Leu-Semenescu S, Louis P, Arnulf I. Benefits, and risk of sodium oxybate in idiopathic hypersomnia versus narcolepsy type 1: a chart review. Sleep Med. 2016;17:38-44.
80. Thorpy MJ, Shapiro C, Mayer G, Corser BC, Emsellem H, Plazzi G, et al. A randomized study of solriamfetol for excessive sleepiness in narcolepsy. Ann Neurol. 2019;85(3):359-70.
81. Dauvilliers Y, Bassetti C, Lammers GJ, Arnulf I, Mayer G, Rodenbeck A, et al. Pitolisant versus placebo or modafinil in patients with narcolepsy: a double-blind, randomised trial. Lancet Neurol. 2013;12(11):1068-75.
82. Leu-Semenescu S, Nittur N, Golmard JL, Arnulf I. Effects of pitolisant, a histamine H3 inverse agonist, in drug-resistant idiopathic and symptomatic hypersomnia: a chart review. Sleep Med. 2014;15(6):681-7.
83. Leu-Semenescu S, Le Corvec T, Groos E, Lavault S, Golmard JL, Arnulf I. Lithium therapy in Klein-Levin syndrome: an open-label, controlled study in 130 patients. Neurology. 2015;85(19): 1655-62.
84. Trenkwalder C, Allen R, Högl B, Paulus W, Winkelmann J. Restless legs syndrome associated with major diseases: a systematic review and new concept. Neurology. 2016;86(14):1336-43.
85. Ferri R, Koo BB, Picchietti DL, Fulda S. Periodic leg movements during sleep: phenotype, neurophysiology, and clinical significance. Sleep Med. 2017;31:29-38.
86. Winkelman JW, Shahar E, Sharief I, Gottlieb D. Association of restless legs syndrome and cardiovascular disease in the Sleep Heart Health Study. Neurology. 2008;70(1):35-42.
87. Sun ER, Chen CA, HoG, Earley CJ, Allen RP. Iron and the restless legs syndrome. Sleep. 1998;21(4):371-7.
88. Mizuno S, Mihara T, Miyaoka T, Inagaki T, Horiguchi J. CSF iron, ferritin, and transferrin levels in restless legs syndrome. J Sleep Res. 2005;14(1):43-7.
89. Earley CJ, Barker PB, Horská A, Allen RP. MRI-determined regional brain iron concentrations in early- and late-onset restless legs syndrome. Sleep Med. 2006;7(5):458-61.
90. Ferré S, García-Borreguero D, Allen RP, Earley CJ. New insights into the neurobiology of restless legs syndrome. Neuroscientist. 2019;25(2):113-25.
91. Al-Alawi A, Mulgrew A, Tench E, Ryan CF. Prevalence, risk factors and impact on daytime sleepiness and hypertension of periodic leg movements with arousals in patients with obstructive sleep apnoea. J Clin Sleep Med. 2006;2(3):281-7.
92. Allen RP, Picchietti DL, Auerbach M, Cho YW, Connor JR, Earley CJ, et al. Evidence-based and consensus clinical practice guidelines for the iron treatment of restless legs syndrome/Willis-Ekbom disease in adults and children: an IRLSSG task force report. Sleep Med. 2018;41:27-44.
93. Garcia-Borreguero D, Silber MH, Winkelman JW, Högl B, Bainbridge J, Buchfuhrer M, et al. Guidelines for the first-line treatment of restless legs syndrome/Willis-Ekbom disease, prevention and treatment of dopaminergic augmentation: a combined task force of the IRLSSG, EURLSSG, and the RLS-foundation. Sleep Med. 2016;21:1-11.
94. Garcia-Borreguero D, Guitart X, Garcia Malo C, Cano-Pumarega I, Granizo JJ, Ferré S, et al. Treatment of restless legs syndrome/ Willis-Ekbom disease with the non-selective ENT1/ENT2 inhibitor dipyridamole: testing the adenosine hypothesis. Sleep Med. 2018;45:94-7.
95. Aukerman MM, Aukerman D, Bayard M, Tudiver F, Thorp L, Bailey B. Exercise and restless legs syndrome: a randomized controlled trial. J Am Board Fam Med. 2006;19(5):487-93.
96. Schenck CH, Bundlie SR, Ettinger MG, Mahowald MW. Chronic behavioural disorders of human REM sleep: a new category of parasomnia. Sleep. 1986;9:293-308.

97. Schenck CH, Mahowald MW. Delayed emergence of a parkinsonian disorder in 38% of 29 older males initially diagnosed with idiopathic REM sleep behaviour disorder. Neurology. 1996;46: 388-93.
98. Boeve BF, Silber MH, Ferman TJ, Kokmen E, Smith GE, Ivnik RJ, et al. REM sleep behaviour disorder and degenerative dementia: an association likely reflecting Lewy body disease. Neurology. 1998;51:363-70.
99. Tison F, Wenning GK, Quinn NP, Smith SJM. REM sleep behaviour disorder as the presenting symptom of multiple system atrophy. J Neurol Neurosurg Psychiatry. 1995;58:379-80.
100. Postuma RB, Iranzo A, Hu M, Högl B, Boeve BF, Manni R, et al. Risk and predictors of dementia and parkinsonism in idiopathic REM sleep behaviour disorder: a multicentre study. Brain. 2019;142(3):744-59.
101. Jung Y, and St Louis EK. Treatment of REM sleep behaviour disorder. Curr Treat Options Neurol. 2016;18(11):50.
102. Attarian H, Zhu L. treatment options for disorders of arousal: a case series. Int J Neurosci. 2013;123(9):623-5.
103. Morgenthaler TI, Silber MH. Amnestic sleep related eating disorder associated with zolpidem. Sleep Med. 2002;3(4):323-7.
104. Frese A, Summ O, Evers S. Exploding head syndrome: six new cases and review of the literature. Cephalalgia. 2014;34(10):823-7.
105. Krause AJ, Simon EB, Mander BA, Greer SM, Saletin JM, Goldstein-Piekarski AN, et al. The sleep deprived human brain. Nat Rev Neurosci. 2017;18(7):404-18.

100

CHAPTER

Diseases of Cerebrospinal Fluid Circulation

Vedantam Rajshekhar

INTRODUCTION

Cerebrospinal fluid (CSF) is present in the cerebral ventricles and the subarachnoid spaces around the brain and spinal cord. The total amount of CSF in an average adult is estimated to be around 150 mL. CSF is produced mainly by the choroid plexus which is present in the lateral, third, and fourth ventricles. About 500 mL of CSF is produced daily.

Cerebrospinal fluid that is produced in the ventricles of the brain exits through the outlets of the fourth ventricle, namely the foramen of Magendie (which is located in the midline) and the foramina of Luschka which are located laterally, one on either side. These foramina connect the ventricular system to the basal subarachnoid spaces (cisterns). The foramen of Magendie opens into the cisterna magna (cerebellomedullary cistern) and the foramina of Luschka opens into the cerebellopontine angle cisterns.

Cerebrospinal fluid travels down into the dorsal spinal subarachnoid space up to the lower end of the thecal sac in the sacral spine and then up again mostly in the ventral spinal subarachnoid space to reach the cranial subarachnoid spaces. Finally, the CSF reaches the cerebral subarachnoid spaces over the cerebral convexities to be absorbed mainly through the arachnoid granulations (Pacchionian granulations) which are small projections of the arachnoid membrane, measuring a few millimeters, into the dural venous sinuses .

Figure 1 shows CSF circulation in detail in a schematic diagram. Disorders of CSF circulation often lead to an increase in the volume of CSF in the cranial cavity and

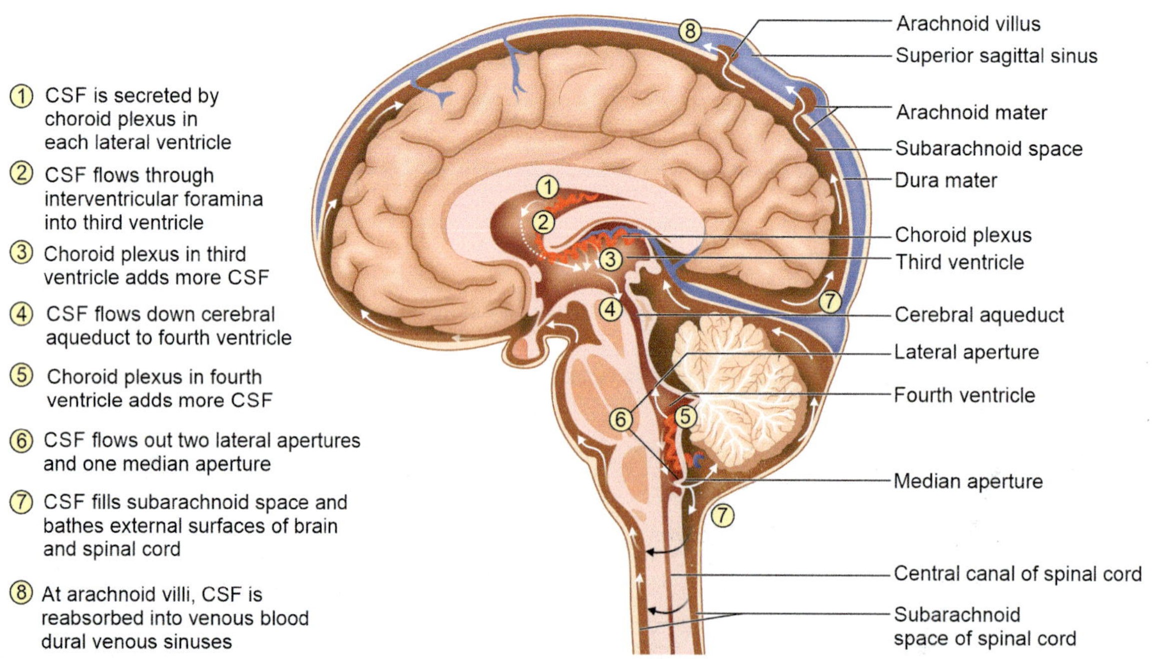

FIG. 1: Schematic diagram of CSF circulation.

cause raised intracranial pressure (ICP). An increase in the intracranial CSF volume is usually accommodated by enlargement of the ventricles (hydrocephalus). However, not all patients with hydrocephalus have increased ICP [normal pressure hydrocephalus (NPH)]. Conversely, not all patients with raised ICP have hydrocephalus [idiopathic intracranial hypertension (IIH)]. Infrequently, a decrease in CSF volume in the cranial and spinal compartments can lead to a decrease in the ICP [intracranial hypotension (IH)].

EPIDEMIOLOGY

Hydrocephalus can be seen in patients of all ages and both sexes.

Congenital hydrocephalus manifests almost always in infants or early childhood whereas some forms of communicating hydrocephalus such as NPH occur most often in elderly patients. Obstructive hydrocephalus due to tumors can occur in all age groups.

Infectious causes of hydrocephalus are more often seen in underdeveloped countries where infections such as neonatal meningitis and tuberculous meningitis are more common than in developed countries.

Posthemorrhagic hydrocephalus (PHH) is commonly seen in premature neonates but can also be seen in full-term newborns.

Idiopathic intracranial hypertension is usually seen in middle-aged women who are obese and might be taking drugs such as oral contraceptives.

Idiopathic NPH (iNPH) is more often diagnosed in patients in developed countries and might be attributed to the higher proportion of elderly persons in the population. The incidence increases with increasing age beginning from about 60 years. Patients who have had a head injury, previous intracranial surgery for brain tumors or other pathologies, or aneurysmal subarachnoid hemorrhage can also present with NPH-like symptoms [secondary NPH (sNPH)].

Spontaneous IH is often seen in middle-aged individuals of both sexes. Iatrogenic IH can occur in any patient following a lumbar puncture (LP) or following a thecoperitoneal shunt (TP shunt).

PATHOLOGY AND PATHOPHYSIOLOGY

The pathophysiology of CSF circulation-related disorders is presented in **Box 1**. In general, disorders of CSF production, circulation, and absorption manifest as hydrocephalus (enlargement of the cerebral ventricles or ventriculomegaly).

Overproduction of CSF occurs in almost all patients with meningitis. This in itself rarely causes hydrocephalus unless there are other abnormalities such as obstruction to the CSF pathways or reduction in CSF absorption. However, overproduction associated with choroid plexus papillomas often causes hydrocephalus.

BOX 1 Pathophysiology of CSF-related disorders.

CSF production disorders (overproduction):
- Choroid plexus papillomas
- Leptomeningitis (pyogenic, tuberculous, fungal, etc.)

CSF circulation disorders:
- Obstruction to ventricular pathways and fourth ventricle outlets:
  - Congenital
  - Tumors
  - Ependymal infections
- Obstruction to subarachnoid pathways:
  - Arachnoiditis (infectious, neoplastic)
  - Following subarachnoid hemorrhage (aneurysmal, traumatic, and surgical)
- CSF absorption disorders:
  - Infectious (tuberculous, neoplastic)
  - Increased protein in CSF (Froin's syndrome)
  - Following subarachnoid hemorrhage (aneurysmal, traumatic, and surgical)

(CSF: cerebrospinal fluid)

The ventricular pathways are most susceptible to obstruction at points where they are the narrowest such as the foramen of Monro (connection between the lateral and third ventricle) and the cerebral aqueduct (connecting the third to the fourth ventricle) and at the outlets of the fourth ventricle. The obstruction can occur due to congenital anomalies such as stenosis or the presence of membranes. Congenital hydrocephalus often refers to hydrocephalus seen in neonates or infants and is frequently caused by aqueductal stenosis. It can also be acquired later in life due to narrowing and distortion by a mass lesion such as a tumor adjacent to the pathways or within the pathways. Finally, scarring due to infections in the subarachnoid space or of the ependymal lining (ependymitis) can also obstruct the ventricular pathways and the fourth ventricular outlet. Obstruction at any point in the ventricular pathways will lead to dilatation of the upstream ventricular system. Obstruction at the level of a foramen of Monro will lead to dilatation of the ipsilateral lateral ventricle, at the level of both foramina to bilateral lateral ventricular dilatation, at the level of the aqueduct to dilatation of both lateral and third ventricles and at the level of the fourth ventricular outlets to dilatation of all four ventricles.

Obstruction to the flow of CSF in the basal subarachnoid cisterns occurs as a result of arachnoiditis due to infections such as tuberculous meningitis or following hemorrhage such as in PHH, causing scarring and closing off of the pathways and can lead to dilatation of all four ventricles. Less frequently, the subarachnoid spaces can also be choked by too many cells in the CSF such as in carcinomatous meningitis.

Absorption defects occur due to the choking of the arachnoid granulations by either too many inflammatory or neoplastic cells in the subarachnoid space or too much protein in the CSF. This can also lead to dilatation of all four ventricles.

The concept of obstructive or communicating hydrocephalus is derived from the absence or presence of communication between the lateral ventricles and the spinal subarachnoid space. Thus, obstruction to the ventricular pathways will lead to obstructive hydrocephalus whereas obstruction to the basal subarachnoid spaces in the brain, overproduction of CSF, or defects in the absorption of CSF will all lead to communicating hydrocephalus.

The cause of IIH is poorly understood.[1] A combination of increased CSF production, decreased absorption, and venous sinus obstruction (partial or complete) has been postulated as a possible cause. Partial or complete stenosis of the transverse sinuses is often noted in patients with IIH. But whether this is the cause or consequence of the raised ICP is unclear.

Idiopathic NPH is supposedly caused by poor venous compliance in the superior sagittal sinus which reduces CSF pulsations and CSF absorption through arachnoid granulations.[2] Another theory for ventriculomegaly is reduced compliance of the ventricles due to ischemia-related changes to the subependymal periventricular white matter. sNPH is possibly due to the reduced flow of CSF through the subarachnoid spaces which are obstructed by the adhesions due to bleeding and reduced absorption of the CSF through the arachnoid granulations which are obstructed by the cellular debris in the CSF.

Intracranial hypotension is usually caused by a defect in the spinal thecal sac (dura) (spontaneous or iatrogenic) through which CSF leaks out.[3] The site of the dural defect in spontaneous IH is usually in the thoracic region. The leak is worsened by an upright posture. In the case of IH associated with a TP shunt, the drainage of CSF from the thecal sac into the peritoneal cavity is the cause of hypotension.

CLINICAL PRESENTATION

Raised Intracranial Pressure

Patients with raised ICP have symptoms such as headache, vomiting, blurring of vision, papilledema, diplopia, and alteration of sensorium.

Patients with IIH present with headaches, blurring of vision, diplopia, and tinnitus. Papilledema is a constant feature. One unusual presentation of patients with IIH, which is being increasingly recognized, is spontaneous CSF rhinorrhea.[4] CSF rhinorrhea will lead to a reduction in the CSF pressure and hence these patients might not have clinical features of raised ICP such as headache and papilledema.

Intracranial Hypotension

Patients with IH usually present with postural headache which worsens on standing or sitting, nuchal pain and vomiting associated with the upright posture, and rarely with altered sensorium or focal deficits due to chronic subdural hematoma (CSDH) in the supratentorial compartment. The headache also worsens with any kind of straining such as coughing, sneezing, or straining while passing stools. Rare symptoms include tinnitus, hearing loss, dizziness, and diplopia. In some patients, fever may accompany these symptoms.

Normal Intracranial Pressure

Patients with NPH (iNPH or sNPH) present typically with a triad of gait ataxia, urinary incontinence, and cognitive impairment. However, early symptoms may only include gait ataxia with or without urinary incontinence and minimal memory disturbances.

INVESTIGATIONS

Raised Intracranial Pressure

Neuroimaging

Any patient with clinical features of raised ICP should undergo neuroimaging [computed tomography (CT) or magnetic resonance imaging (MRI)] even if an acute neurological illness such as meningitis or encephalitis is suspected. Ideally, a contrast-enhanced study should be performed. In patients with disorders of CSF circulation causing raised ICP, there will usually be hydrocephalus.

Special MR sequences will be needed in some patients to determine the cause of obstruction. For example, patients with cystic lesions in the ventricles might need heavily T2 weighted [constructive interference in steady state (CISS) or DRIVE sequences] to distinguish the cyst from the CSF surrounding it.

Magnetic resonance venography might be needed in patients suspected to have IIH.

Lumbar Puncture

Lumbar puncture may be performed in patients with raised ICP once the CT/MR has not revealed a mass lesion or hydrocephalus. LP is done to measure the CSF pressure and also to obtain CSF to study its composition (sugar, protein, cells, cytology, and microbiological studies). A diagnosis of IIH can only be confirmed with the measurement of the lumbar puncture opening pressure (LPOP).

Visual Testing

In patients with IIH and any patient with raised ICP who has visual symptoms, formal visual testing for visual acuity and visual field testing with Humphrey's field analyzer (HFA) should be done. It is important to document baseline function to monitor the effect of therapy.

Intracranial Hypotension

Contrast-enhanced MR imaging of the head is the ideal investigation for a patient with spontaneous IH.

Spinal imaging with MR myelography or CT myelography will be needed to determine the site of the dural defect. Invasive MR myelography with injection of gadolinium is reportedly more sensitive than CT myelography.

A LP may be done to document the low CSF pressure (<5 cm of water) but is not necessary.

Normal Pressure Hydrocephalus

Patients with suspected NPH should undergo contrast-enhanced MR imaging of the brain.

Additional investigations such as LP may be done to measure the CSF pressure and also as a therapeutic test (Tap test) to determine the possible benefit of a ventriculoperitoneal (VP) shunt.

DIAGNOSIS

Raised Intracranial Pressure

Computed tomography or MR will show hydrocephalus in most patients with features of raised ICP due to disorders of CSF circulation.

Table 1 shows how to determine the level of obstruction in the ventricular system in patients who have hydrocephalus.

It is important to note that dilatation of all four ventricles with a large cisterna magna does not necessarily indicate communicating hydrocephalus. Dilatation of all four ventricles with a large communication between the fourth ventricle and the cisterna magna might indicate communicating hydrocephalus. However, the only method to confirm the diagnosis of communicating hydrocephalus is to perform a dynamic study wherein a contrast agent is injected into one lateral ventricle and a CT scan is done to determine the flow of the contrast agent (CT ventriculography). If the contrast agent is seen in the basal subarachnoid spaces such as the prepontine, ambient, and interpeduncular cisterns then a diagnosis of communicating hydrocephalus is confirmed.

The common causes of obstructive and communicating hydrocephalus are listed in **Box 2**.

TABLE 1: Determining level of obstruction in patients with hydrocephalus.

Imaging findings	Level of obstruction
One lateral ventricle dilated	Ipsilateral foramen of Monro
Both lateral ventricles dilated	• Bilateral foramen of Monro • Anterior third ventricle
Both lateral ventricles and third ventricle dilated	• Posterior third ventricle • Aqueduct
Both lateral ventricles, third ventricle, and aqueduct dilated	• Lower end of aqueduct • Mass filling fourth ventricle
All four ventricles dilated*	Fourth ventricular outlet

*Do not confuse with communicating hydrocephalus (see text).

BOX 2 Common causes of hydrocephalus.

Children:
- *Obstructive*:
  - Aqueductal stenosis
  - Dandy–Walker malformation
  - Craniopharyngiomas
  - Optic chiasmatic-hypothalamic glioma
  - Arachnoid cysts
  - Intraventricular tumors (glioma)
  - Tectal glioma
  - Cerebellar tumors (medulloblastoma, pilocytic astrocytoma, and ependymoma)
  - Cerebellar tuberculoma
- *Communicating*:
  - Posthemorrhagic hydrocephalus (PHH)
  - Postpyogenic meningitis
  - Tuberculous meningitis (TBM) hydrocephalus
  - Choroid plexus papilloma

Adults:
- *Obstructive*:
  - Colloid cyst of the third ventricle
  - Intraventricular tumors (glioma, central neurocytomas, and meningioma)
  - Pineal region tumors (pineal parenchymal tumor, epidermoid, and teratoma)
  - Tectal glioma
  - Posterior fossa tumors (vestibular schwannoma, meningioma, epidermoid, and hemangioblastoma)
  - Neurocysticercosis (intraventricular and subarachnoid)
  - Cerebellar tuberculoma
- *Communicating*:
  - TBM hydrocephalus
  - Post-aneurysmal subarachnoid hemorrhage (SAH)
  - Post head injury

Elderly:
- *Communicating*:
  - Normal pressure hydrocephalus
  - Carcinomatous meningitis

In some patients with raised ICP, CT/MR might not reveal any mass lesions or hydrocephalus. These patients can be presumed to have possible IIH. However, for a definitive diagnosis of IIH, patients will need to fulfill certain criteria **(Box 3)**. As mentioned above most patients with IIH who present with spontaneous CSF rhinorrhea may not fulfill several criteria for the diagnosis of IIH such as LPOP of >25 cm of water and the presence of papilledema as the rhinorrhea itself reduces the ICP. Therefore, diagnosis of IIH in such patients is difficult and a modification of the existing criteria for IIH has been proposed **(Box 4)**.

Intracranial Hypotension

A diagnosis of iatrogenic IH is straightforward. However, the diagnosis can be difficult in patients with spontaneous

BOX 3 Diagnostic criteria for IIH.

Definite IIH:

A. Papilledema or unilateral/bilateral sixth nerve palsy

B. Normal neurological examination except cranial nerve deficits

C. No hydrocephalus or mass lesions or enhancement of the meninges on gadolinium-enhanced MR or contrast-enhanced CT

D. Normal CSF composition

E. Elevated LPOP of >250 mm CSF in adults and >280 mm CSF in children

Probable IIH:

i. When A to D are fulfilled but LPOP is lower than the threshold value.

ii. When papilledema and sixth nerve palsy are absent, B to E of definite IIH criteria are fulfilled, and the MR reveals three of the following:

   a. Empty sella
   b. Flattening of the posterior globe
   c. Optic nerve sheath is enlarged with or without tortuosity
   d. Transverse sinus stenosis

(CSF: cerebrospinal fluid; CT: computed tomography; IIH: idiopathic intracranial hypertension; LPOP: lumbar puncture opening pressure; MR: magnetic resonance)

Source: Friedman DI, Liu GT, Digre KB. Revised diagnostic criteria for the pseudotumor cerebri syndrome in adults and children. Neurology. 2013;81(13):1159-65.

BOX 4 Proposed diagnostic criteria for IIH in patients presenting with spontaneous CSF rhinorrhea.

Mandatory criteria:

- Diagnosis of spontaneous CSF rhinorrhea
- Absence of mass lesion, hydrocephalus, and meningeal enhancement on MRI
- Normal CSF composition

Definite IIH:

- Mandatory criteria + any one of the following criteria:
  - Empty sella (Yuh grades IV and V) with any one of the following MR features:
    - Flattened posterior globe
    - Enlarged Meckel's cave with or without meningocele
  - Papilledema or unilateral/bilateral sixth nerve paresis/palsy
  - LPOP of >25 cm of CSF

Probable IIH:

- Mandatory criteria +
  - Empty sella (Yuh grades IV and V) with any one or both of the following MR features:
    - Enlarged optic nerve sheath
    - Optic nerve tortuosity

    Or
  - Partial empty sella (Yuh grade III) with any one or both of the following MR features:
    - Flattened posterior globe
    - Enlarged Meckel's cave with or without meningocele

(CSF: cerebrospinal fluid; IIH: idiopathic intracranial hypertension; LPOP: lumbar puncture opening pressure; MRI: magnetic resonance imaging)

Source: Rupa V, et al (2022).[4]

IH. A high index of suspicion is needed to make a clinical diagnosis. Gadolinium-enhanced MR imaging of the brain in these patients will reveal sagging of the brain with or without tonsillar herniation and diffuse enhancement of the meninges. The pituitary gland may be enlarged. Occasionally, sizable CSDH in the frontal and parietal regions, either unilateral or bilateral, might be present.

Pinpointing the site of the dural defect in patients with spontaneous IH can be difficult even with MR or CT myelography as the size of the leak can be very small and consequently, the leak is slow or intermittent and small.

Normal Pressure Hydrocephalus

Diagnosis of NPH is also straightforward if a patient presents with classical triad of symptoms. However, a clinical diagnosis may not be clear in the early stages of the disease when only one or two of the symptoms are present.

On MRI imaging the presence of dilated ventricles does not necessarily indicate NPH as age-related loss of cortical and white matter leads to dilatation of the ventricles (ex vacuo dilatation). There are several measurements of the ventricular structures on MR imaging that have been proposed to differentiate NPH from age-related dilatation. The presence of periventricular CSF seepage, seen as hyperintensities around the ventricular walls (particularly the frontal horns and occipital horns) on T2 weighted or fluid-attenuated inversion recovery (FLAIR) MR images is another indicator of NPH rather than age-related dilatation of the ventricles.

There are several quantitative measurements and qualitative changes in the ventricles on the MR which indicate ventriculomegaly. These include Evan's index >0.3, widening of the temporal horns of the lateral ventricles >6 mm, acute callosal angle, upward bowing of the corpus callosum, and dilated Sylvian fissures with narrowed cortical sulci close to the midline. A combination of the dilated ventricles and Sylvian fissures with narrowed high cortical sulci is termed disproportionately enlarged subarachnoid space hydrocephalus (DESH). Cingulate sulcus sign, where the cingulate sulcus is narrower posteriorly compared to the anterior half is another indicator of NPH.

DIFFERENTIAL DIAGNOSIS

Raised Intracranial Pressure

The combination of clinical features with imaging findings usually provides a definite diagnosis of hydrocephalus. Most often the cause of the hydrocephalus is also evident on the imaging but the etiology may not be confirmed without further investigations such as pathological examination of abnormal tissue causing obstruction of the ventricular pathways or examination of the CSF.

Patients with venous sinus thrombosis may have features of IIH but as mentioned above it is difficult to determine whether the narrowing of the transverse sinus is a consequence of the raised ICP in patients with IIH.

Intracranial Hypotension

Presence of the characteristic clinical features of orthostatic headache with the MR findings of diffuse pachymeningeal enhancement should confirm the diagnosis of IH. But because patients with IH may have associated fever differential diagnosis of chronic meningitis may be considered. Hypertrophic cranial pachymeningitis, which might be idiopathic or secondary to infections such as tuberculosis, fungal, or syphilis may be considered in the differential diagnosis. Carcinomatous meningitis is another differential diagnosis. Finally, autoimmune disorders such as systemic lupus erythematosus may be associated with diffuse meningeal enhancement.

The enlarged pituitary gland has been mistaken for a pituitary adenoma.

It may be impossible to suspect IH in patients in whom CSDH are noted on MR or CT imaging especially if they present with altered sensorium. Most such patients will be diagnosed with CSDH.

Normal Pressure Hydrocephalus

Ventriculomegaly in the presence of the classical triad of symptoms of NPH does not always imply that the diagnosis of iNPH is confirmed. In patients who are >60 years of age, Alzheimer's dementia, Parkinson's disease, and normal aging brain must be considered.

Secondary NPH is easier to diagnose when the predisposing condition such as prior cranial surgery or aneurysmal SAH is recognized.

MANAGEMENT

Raised Intracranial Pressure

Hydrocephalus

As far as possible the treatment of hydrocephalus should be directed toward the cause of the hydrocephalus. For example, in patients with obstructive hydrocephalus due to a cerebellar tumor, excision of the tumor will often relieve the hydrocephalus. But in several instances, the cause of the hydrocephalus might not be amenable to therapy, or if there is a delay in the resolution of the etiology it could lead to irreversible harm to the patient. In such situations, the hydrocephalus itself has to be treated.

Temporary Measures

In situations where there could be a delay in the treatment or resolution of the cause of the hydrocephalus, temporary procedures can be utilized to relieve the raised ICP caused by the hydrocephalus. Temporary procedures are usually performed in an emergency situation to save the patient's life while preparing for a more permanent treatment.

Ventricular Puncture

This procedure is usually an emergency bedside procedure performed using a twist drill. The drill is used to make a small opening in the skull (usually in the frontal region). A ventricular puncture (VP) needle which is blunt tipped and graduated is then inserted into the frontal horn to tap the ventricle and let out CSF which will be under pressure. However, the needle cannot be left in situ and therefore, the CSF pressure will rise again over a period of a few hours. A common indication for this procedure is not for treatment of hydrocephalus but to obtain CSF for diagnosis of leptomeningeal infections when there is obstructive hydrocephalus and to rule out infection prior to insertion of a shunt in a patient with suspected postmeningitic hydrocephalus.

External Ventricular Drain

For more prolonged drainage, an external ventricular drain (EVD) is inserted after the VP to continue to drain CSF from the lateral ventricle (usually the frontal horn). It is brought out through a short subcutaneous tunnel in the scalp to drain into a closed drainage system. An EVD can be maintained for a maximum duration of about 5 days as a longer duration increases the risk of infection.

When an EVD has to be in place for a longer duration (such as hydrocephalus associated with active meningitis), then the length of the subcutaneous tunnel is increased and the drain is brought out through the abdominal wall—long-tunnel EVD. This can be maintained for several weeks as the risk of infection is less than the traditional EVD.

Definitive Surgery

A shunt from the lateral ventricle to the peritoneal cavity (VP shunt) is the most frequently employed shunt in the treatment of hydrocephalus. The CSF which is drained into the peritoneal cavity is absorbed there. The earliest indwelling shunt systems introduced in the 1960s were ventriculoatrial (VA) shunts which were placed in the right atrium. However, VP shunts are safer and have less risk of infection, and almost completely replaced VA shunts. VA shunts were also sometimes associated with a complication known as shunt nephritis. Shunts being foreign bodies can be associated with several complications including infection, extrusion, erosion of skin over the shunt components, blockage, and migration which can occur even several years after the surgery. Overdrainage leading to subdural hygromas or hematomas and slit ventricle syndrome are other possible shunt-related complications.

In order to avoid the placement of a foreign body, endoscopic third ventriculostomy (ETV) was introduced in the 1990s. However, ETV is not a panacea for patients suffering from hydrocephalus. It can only be used when the obstruction is distal to the posterior third ventricle. It is most useful in patients with obstruction at the level of the aqueduct.

Idiopathic Intracranial Hypertension

Treatment of IIH starts with weight reduction and acetazolamide. Acetazolamide is usually started at 250 mg twice daily. In patients with impending visual loss or rapidly declining visual function, a TP shunt might be indicated. Although optic nerve sheath fenestration through an endoscopic route has been suggested, results with TP shunt are better.

Stenting of a partially blocked transverse sinus has also been suggested as therapy for IIH.

In patients presenting with spontaneous CSF rhinorrhea, endoscopic repair of the dural fistula (usually located in the cribriform plate or roof of the ethmoid sinus) should be performed. Simultaneous TP shunt may be done to lower the CSF pressure and help the repair heal. If a TP shunt is not done, then patients with definite IIH on the modified diagnostic criteria for IIH should be carefully followed up after the repair of the dural fistula to look for symptoms and signs of raised ICP. Once the CSF leak is stopped, patients might develop raised ICP which will require treatment.

Intracranial Hypotension

Iatrogenic IH responds well to bed rest of 2–3 days with consumption of plenty of fluids such as coffee which lead to an increase in the CSF production and reduction in the leak of CSF from the dural opening.

Spontaneous IH responds to the abovementioned conservative management in about 30% of patients but most will need other therapy.

An epidural blood patch applied through an epidural catheter inserted at the lumbar level with bed rest for a few days in the Trendelenburg position provides a cure in nearly two-thirds of patients. A large blood patch of >20 mL is recommended.

If all these conservative measures fail, then surgery will be required to repair the dural defect. However, surgical exploration should be preceded by definite identification of the site of the dural defect.

Patients with IH who present with CSDH will invariably be treated for the CSDH with burr hole drainage with or without subdural drain for 2–3 days. However, these patients will not respond to the drainage of CSDH as expected but instead may continue to deteriorate in their sensorium. Postoperative CT scan will reveal a large pneumocephalus in the frontal regions with the re-collection of the SDH. A careful examination of the CT will reveal sagging of the brain at the tentorial hiatus. It is important to recognize this unusual presentation of IH as multiple attempts to drain the "recurrent" CSDH will not help the patient. Unless the site of the spinal dural defect is treated, the patient will not improve.

Normal Pressure Hydrocephalus

A VP shunt is the treatment of choice in patients with NPH. Although TP shunt and ETV have been proposed as alternatives to VP shunt, most surgeons prefer VP shunt.

Patients with sNPH respond very well to the surgery with over 85% of them having a good outcome.

However, not all patients with iNPH respond well to the shunt surgery. This might be because the diagnosis of NPH is not correct or because the disease itself has progressed too far to be reversed.

Prognostic features predicting a good outcome with a shunt are:
- Symptom duration of <6 months
- Lack of significant dementia
- Response to the CSF tap test (drainage of 40 mL of CSF through a LP leading to an improvement in gait parameters)
- Aqueductal flow void on MR imaging

However, it is suggested that patients should be given the benefit of doubt as VP shunt is not a major surgery and even if there is a small chance of improvement then surgery should be done.

SPECIAL FEATURES IN THE INDIAN CONTEXT

Tuberculous Meningitis with Hydrocephalus

Tuberculous meningitis (TBM) with hydrocephalus (TBMH) is a very common cause of hydrocephalus in India. Patients with TBMH should be graded for prognostication and for deciding their management **(Table 2)**.[5] The management of TBMH has been rationalized since the 1990s but there are still some unanswered questions especially regarding the utility of shunts in patients in poor grade TBM.

TABLE 2: Vellore grading of TBMH.

Grade	Features
1	GCS 15; no neurological deficit
2	GCS 15; neurological deficit present
3	GCS 9–14; with or without neurological deficit
4a	GCS 7, 8; no basal ganglia or brainstem infarcts on neuroimaging
4b	GCS 7, 8; basal ganglia or brainstem infarcts present on neuroimaging Or GCS 3–6

(GCS: Glasgow coma score; TBMH: tuberculous meningitis with hydrocephalus)
Source: Rajshekhar V, (2021).[5]

CONCLUSION

Disorders of CSF circulation can lead to an increase, decrease, or no change in ICP. While features of increased ICP are well recognized by most clinicians, those caused by IH may be missed. Similarly, features of NPH may be mistaken for those of degenerative conditions. Imaging plays a major role in the diagnosis of disorders of CSF circulation. While the changes in ICP may be managed medically or surgically, the ultimate prognosis depends on the etiology.

REFERENCES

1. Mollan SP, Davies B, Silver NC, Shaw S, Mallucci CL, Wakerley BR, et al. Idiopathic intracranial hypertension: consensus guidelines on management. J Neurol Neurosurg Psychiatry. 2018;89:1088-100.
2. Vibha D, Tripathi M. Normal-Pressure Hydrocephalus - Patient Evaluation and Decision-Making. Neurol India. 2021;69:S406-S412.
3. D'Antona L, Jaime Merchan MA, Vassiliou A, Watkins LD, Davagnanam I, Toma AK, et al. Clinical Presentation, Investigation Findings, and Treatment Outcomes of Spontaneous Intracranial Hypotension Syndrome: A Systematic Review and Meta-analysis. JAMA Neurol. 2021;78(3):329-37.
4. Rupa V, Jasper A, Abraham L, Rajshekhar V. MR findings suggestive of idiopathic intracranial hypertension in 117 patients with spontaneous cerebrospinal fluid rhinorrhea. Neuroradiology. 2022;64(5):949-58.
5. Rajshekhar V. Three Decades of Vellore Grading for Tuberculous Meningitis with Hydrocephalus: A Reappraisal. Neurol India. 2021;69:S569-S574.

101

CHAPTER

Anoxic Encephalopathy

Thomas Mathew, Raghunandan Nadig, Sharath Kumar GG

INTRODUCTION

Anoxia is a complete lack of oxygen, while hypoxia is a partial lack of it. Neurons are absolutely dependent on blood flow and oxygen for their survival and function. In most cases of anoxia, there is a total lack of blood supply to brain as occurs in postcardiac arrest situations and hence anoxic encephalopathy in this context is better called anoxic-ischemic encephalopathy. The degree of brain damage depends on the acuteness of the onset and the time period for which oxygenation and blood supply is cut off. The longer the time period of anoxia, the greater is the damage and more severe the neurological sequel. The common causes of anoxic encephalopathy are cardiac arrest, hanging, strangulation, near-drowning, and carbon monoxide (CO) poisoning.[1]

EPIDEMIOLOGY

The exact incidence of anoxic encephalopathies is not known, especially in India. The incidence rate is proportionate to the incidence of cardiac arrests that happen due to coronary artery diseases or arrhythmias. Based on prospective studies from North America, Europe, and Asia, the incidence of cardiac arrest is estimated to be somewhere between 50 and 100 per 100,000 in the general population.[2] About 82% of in-hospital cardiac arrests and 91–98% of out-of-hospital arrests will either die or will suffer brain injury.[3] Due to the improvement in pre-hospital emergency care, the prevalence of patients surviving resuscitation and suffering from severe hypoxic brain damage is increasing.[1]

PATHOPHYSIOLOGY

Anoxia for 2–4 minutes initiates various molecular and biochemical events which results in irreversible neuronal damage. The normal human brain is highly dependent on blood oxygen and glucose. Neuronal metabolism is predominantly aerobic and 92% of the adenosine triphosphate (ATP) in the brain comes from the oxidative metabolism of glucose. The adult human brain needs about 3.3 mL O_2/100 g/min and 8 mg glucose/100 g/min under basal cerebral conditions at a blood flow of an average of 55 mL/100 g/min. Blood flow to gray matter is 4–5 times higher (70–80 mL/100 g/min) than that of white matter (15–20 mL/100 g/min). The neuronal oxygen stores are depleted within 20 seconds of cardiac arrest. If the blood flow is totally cut off for 4–5 minutes, it may lead to irreversible damage of neurons. The cortical pyramidal neurons in the layers 3, 4, 5, neurons in the CA1 region of hippocampus, neurons in the corpus striatum, and Purkinje cells of cerebellum are extremely susceptible to hypoxic injury. The damage to the layers 3, 4, 5, of neocortex is pathologically seen as "laminar necrosis". An explanation of the selective vulnerability of these neurons is that, they are the ones that produce more glutamate and have more receptors for excitatory neurotransmitters like glutamate, predisposing them for more excitotoxicity. The neurons in these areas also have high metabolic rate. Ischemia lasting longer leads to irreversible damage to thalamus and to the brainstem. Spinal cord remains unaffected for longer periods, even after the rest of the central nervous system is severely damaged. In pure ischemic injury due to hypoperfusion, border zone infarcts occur in the water shed territories between major cerebral arteries.[4]

The molecular events following hypoxic injury evolves in three phases, especially in the newborns: initial phase called primary energy failure, followed by a latent period and the third phase called secondary energy failure. In primary energy failure, a reduction of cerebral blood flow or oxygen will result in loss of ATP production. The reduced ATP levels cause dysfunction of cell membrane ion pumps, especially ATP-dependent Na^+/K^+ pump. When the Na^+/K^+ pumps fail, there occurs an excess influx of the positively charged sodium ions causing massive depolarization of neurons. This triggers the release of glutamate which binds to glutamate receptors, especially N-methyl-D-aspartate (NMDA) receptors causing excitotoxicity. The inhibitory neurotransmitters such as glycine and gamma-aminobutyric acid (GABA) are decreased concomitantly.[3] Activation of NMDA receptors by glutamate leads to an influx of calcium into the intracellular space. Total intracellular calcium increases by approximately 25% due to calcium influx during anoxic depolarization.[5] Increased intracellular calcium activates a series of second messengers, which amplifies injury by increasing calcium permeability and further glutamate release. Elevated calcium levels also increases oxygen-free radicals by interfering with the mitochondrial respiratory chain and also activates carbolic enzymes, endonucleases, and caspases. These events produce significant detrimental effects resulting in cerebral edema and microvascular injury, leading on to necrosis and/or apoptosis. Most of the effects of the primary energy failure lead to cellular necrosis through impaired cellular integrity, disruption of the cytoskeleton and cell membrane. The necrosed cells release their cellular contents initiating additional inflammation. This results in an influx of microglia to the area, causing further release of inflammatory mediators. If the insult is less severe, the cells may recover or progress to apoptosis or programmed cell death. Apoptosis causes cell shrinkage and general preservation of the cellular membranes with no associated inflammation. The apoptosis can occur days following the initial injury. Once blood flow is restored, there is a brief period of recovery called the latent period. This period is characterized by normal cerebral metabolism. The latent period is thought to vary depending on the extent of the severity of the hypoxic-ischemic insult. The more severe the insult, the shorter the latent period is. The latent period is considered as the optimum time period for therapeutic interventions. The exact timing of when the primary energy failure phase, the latent period, and the secondary energy failure phase begin and end remains unknown.[4] The secondary energy failure phase is due to reperfusion injury and occurs 6–48 hours after the initial insult. The exact mechanisms of secondary energy failure remain unclear, but appear to be related to oxidative stress, excitotoxicity, and inflammation. There is massive production of reactive oxygen species (ROS) in the forms of a superoxide anion (O_2^-), H_2O_2, and hydroxyl radical (OH^-).[5] During a hypoxic-ischemic state, the iron bound to proteins is released, which makes the free iron (Fe^{2+}) available to react with peroxides and form free radicals. The peroxidative action of ROS hinders activation of enzymes of glucose metabolism. Other free radicals, such as reactive nitrogen species (RNS) produced by reaction of nitric oxide (NO), can also disrupt cell homeostasis. These ROS/RNS cause variable oxidative damage of the mitochondria to the cell membrane through lipid peroxidation, protein oxidation, and deoxyribonucleic acid (DNA) fragmentation. The pathological features of neuroinflammation at the cellular level include activation of microglia and infiltration of inflammatory cells from the peripheral circulation, which further exacerbates cell damage.[4] The cellular events after hypoxic-ischemic insult is summarized in **Table 1**.

TABLE 1: Cellular events after hypoxic-ischemic insult.

Hypoxic-ischemic insult		
Primary energy failure →	Latent period →	Secondary energy failure
Decrease in oxygen/glucose	Restoration of blood flow	Reperfusion
		Reoxygenation
Decrease ATP production		
Na^+/K^+ pump failure		
Massive Na^+ influx/depolarization		
Increase calcium influx		Oxidative stress
Increase extracellular glutamate/activation of NMDA/AMPA receptors		
Mitochondrial injury		
Activation of caspases/calpains		Excitotoxicity
Increase NO/ROS		
Fragmentation of cellular DNA		
Disruption of protein synthesis		Inflammation
Cell death		

(AMPA: alpha-amino-3-hydroxy-5-methyl-4-isoxazolepropionic acid; DNA: deoxyribonucleic acid NMDA: N-methyl-d-aspartate; NO: nitric oxide; ROS; reactive oxygen species)

ETIOLOGY

The common causes of anoxic encephalopathy are:

- Hypoxia from drowning, strangulation, hanging, choking, suffocation, general anesthesia accidents, and sedative drug overdose
- Global cerebral hypoperfusion from cardiac arrest due to myocardial infarction, ventricular arrhythmia, aortic dissection, hypovolemic shock due to blood loss, and septic shock
- Neuromuscular weakness caused by Guillain–Barré syndrome, amyotrophic lateral sclerosis, and myasthenia gravis
- Carbon monoxide poisoning [Gas geyser syndrome (GGS)] and cyanide intoxication

CLINICAL FEATURES

A good history should be taken from relatives or friends who have witnessed the event. This may reveal the context of hypoxic brain injury. A phone call to the witness or a video footage of the event may also help to understand the sequence of events more vividly. One should ask about the time of onset, duration of cardiopulmonary resuscitation (CPR), prodromal symptoms, presence of cardiovascular disorders, arrhythmias, medications used, and exposure to substances of abuse. A focused clinical and neurological examination should be done, particularly looking for motor response to pain, pupillary reflexes, eye movements, brainstem reflexes, focal neurological deficits, and presence of myoclonus.

Hypoxic encephalopathy can cause transient or permanent neurological dysfunction based on the degree and duration of hypoxia. Mild degrees of hypoxia may result in headache, inattentiveness, confusion, abnormal behavior, poor judgment, and incoordination. Patients with mild-to-moderate hypoxic injury may recover with varying degrees of neurological disability.[6] Patients with moderate-to-severe degrees of hypoxia can enter a persistent vegetative state (PVS), a form of "eyes-open permanent unconsciousness" with loss of cognitive function and awareness of the environment but with preservation of sleep-wake cycles, thermoregulation, and digestion. Some people enter what is described as a minimally conscious state (MCS) that is characterized by inconsistent but clearly discernible behavioral evidence of consciousness and can be distinguished from PVS in that, the patients in MCS may follow, from time to time, specific commands, gestural or verbal, yes/no responses, and have some degree of purposeful movements.[7] Patients can also develop varying degrees of dementia with or without extrapyramidal syndromes. Parkinsonian syndromes are more common after CO poisoning as it predominantly affects basal ganglia. Patients with moderate-to-severe hypoxic injury may develop choreoathetosis and cerebellar ataxia. As hippocampus is a favored site for hypoxic injury, its involvement may result in an amnestic state. Seizures in the form of myoclonus can occur after severe hypoxic injury. This posthypoxic myoclonus (PHM) can be either acute or chronic. Acute PHM, also called posthypoxic myoclonic status epilepticus (MSE), occurs soon after a hypoxic insult in patients who are deeply comatose and is characterized by continuous and vigorous jerking movements involving the facial muscles, limbs, and abdominal muscles including diaphragm.[8] These myoclonic jerks can be elicited and aggravated by either touch or sound. MSE usually begins within the first 72 hours after cardiac arrest and usually stops after a few days.[9] The chronic type of PHM, also known as Lance-Adams syndrome (LAS), is characterized by action myoclonus that begins days to weeks after CPR and persists in patients who have recovered consciousness.[10,11] Severe degrees of hypoxia can cause altered sensorium, coma, absent pupillary, and brainstem reflexes. Patient may decerebrate spontaneously or in response to painful stimuli. Death may happen in 1–2 days due to deepening coma, high temperature, and circulatory collapse. Some patients may enter a state of brain death characterized by irreversible coma, absence of brainstem reflexes, and apnea. The posthypoxic neurological syndromes are summarized in **Box 1**.

BOX 1 Posthypoxic neurological syndromes.

- Brain death
- Persistent vegetative state (PVS)
- Minimally conscious state (MCS)
- Dementia
- Parkinsonism
- Choreoathetosis
- Cerebellar ataxia
- Myoclonus intention or action [posthypoxic myoclonic status epilepticus (MSE) and Lance–Adams syndrome (LAS)]
- Korsakoff amnestic state
- Balint syndrome and cortical blindness
- Proximal arm and shoulder/hip weakness ("man-in-the-barrel syndrome")

Delayed Posthypoxic Leukoencephalopathy

Delayed posthypoxic leukoencephalopathy (DPHL) is a rare condition in which patients appear to make a complete clinical recovery after an episode of anoxia or hypoxia followed by development of a neuropsychiatric syndrome. The incidence of DPHL is unclear but has been reported to range from less than 1 to 28 per 1,000 in patients who have suffered hypoxic or anoxic events.[12] The exact etiopathogenesis remains unknown. DPHL is characterized by acute onset of apathy, confusion, irritability, agitation, mania and/or progressive neurologic deficits days to weeks following apparent recovery from coma. Other causes of delirium should be ruled out. The diagnosis can be supported by magnetic resonance imaging (MRI) brain which may reveal hemispheric demyelination, sparing cerebellar and brainstem white matter tracts **(Fig. 1)**. Cerebrospinal fluid (CSF) analysis may show elevated CSF myelin basic protein (MBP). Standard or hyperbaric oxygen following CO poisoning may reduce the likelihood of DPHL or other neurological sequel. Bed rest and avoidance of stressful procedures for the first 10 days following any prolonged hypoxic event may also lower the risk of DPHL. Gradual recovery over a 3–12-month period is common, but impaired attention or executive function, parkinsonism, or corticospinal tract signs may persist. Amantadine or levodopa may be considered for persisting cognitive or parkinsonian symptoms. Anticipation and recognition of DPHL should lead to earlier and more appropriate utilization of healthcare services.[13]

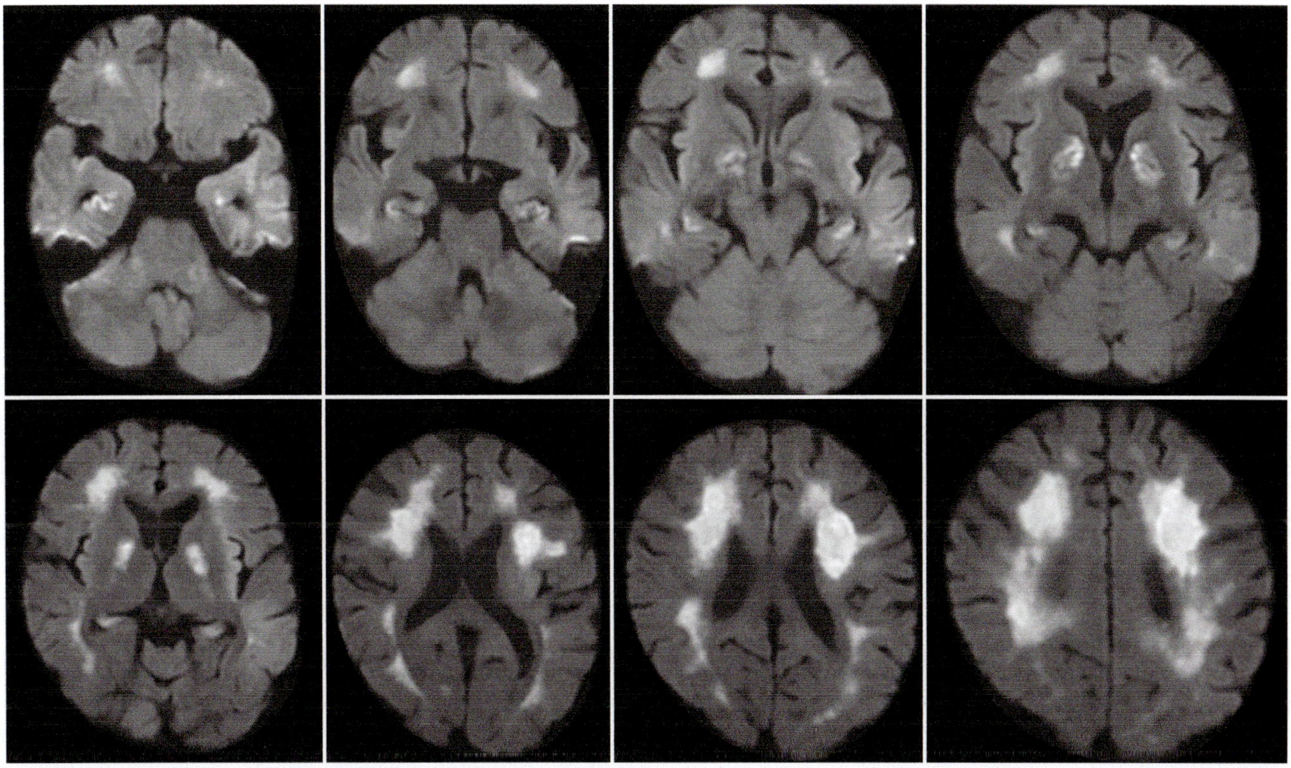

FIG. 1: Diffusion-weighted images (DWI) showing bilateral symmetrical signal changes involving hippocampi and globus pallidus consistent with Hypoxic-ischemic lesions. More brighter symmetrical confluent white matter signal changes are noted in supratentorial lobar white matter and posterior limb of internal capsule suggestive of delayed posthypoxic leukoencephalopathy (DPHL).
Image courtesy: Dr Sharath Kumar G G, Sr Consultant Neuroradiologist.

Carbon Monoxide Poisoning

Carbon monoxide has more than 200 times affinity to hemoglobin than oxygen. It is a colorless, odorless gas which is toxic to humans. Once inhaled it reduces the oxygen content of blood and subjects the brain to prolonged hypoxia and acidosis. The causes of CO poisoning are exposure to car exhaust in a closed garage, faulty furnace, and in our country, the Gas geyser syndrome (GGS). The manifestations are similar to hypoxic injury postcardiac arrest but delayed neurological deterioration is more common in CO poisoning.

Gas Geyser Syndrome

Gas geyser syndrome is a classic example of anoxic encephalopathy due to CO poisoning. GGS is usually noted in winter months in countries like India, especially northern regions, where liquefied petroleum gas (LPG) geysers are used very frequently for heating water due economic reasons and erratic electrical supply. Gas geysers are preferred to electric geysers as it heats up the water faster, are cheaper to operate, and saves electricity.[14] GGS is usually reported in young to middle aged individuals without any significant risk factors. GGS occurs in those individuals who spend long time in the poorly ventilated bathrooms fitted with gas geysers. Most of the cases reported are in females, probably due to the fact that they spend longer time taking bath. Patients may present with seizure like episodes and can develop altered sensorium or coma due to CO poisoning. Most patients recover but few may have a sequel in the form of cognitive deficits and extrapyramidal syndromes like parkinsonism. In a study by Correia et al., three out of 26 (11.5%) patients had memory deficits and early parkinsonian features as a consequence to GGS.[14] In the case series by Mehta et al., two out of 24 died.[15] MRI brain is usually normal but may show symmetrical signal abnormalities in basal ganglia particularly globus pallidus and also in other areas such as hippocampi, bilateral occipital regions, and cerebellar cortex.[16,17] These lesions are usually hyperintense on T2-weighted (T2W) and fluid-attenuated inversion recovery (FLAIR) images and also show restricted diffusion **(Fig. 2)**.

DIAGNOSIS

The confirmation of diagnosis of anoxic encephalopathy needs detailed history, thorough clinical examination and neuroimaging findings supported by appropriate neurophysiologic tests such as electroencephalogram (EEG) and somatosensory evoked potentials (SSEPs). Laboratory tests should include a comprehensive metabolic workup including serum electrolytes, hepatic function tests including ammonia and blood gas analysis for acid-base disturbances.

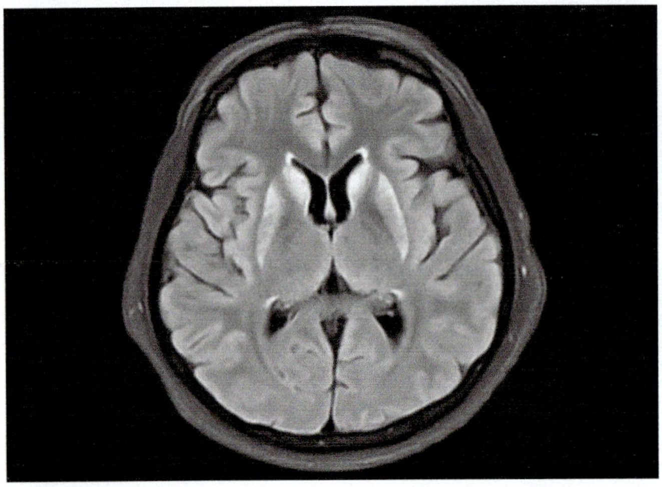

FIG. 2: Magnetic resonance imaging (MRI) brain fluid-attenuated inversion recovery (FLAIR) image showing hyperintensities in putamen and caudate nucleus in a 19-year-old lady with gas geyser syndrome.

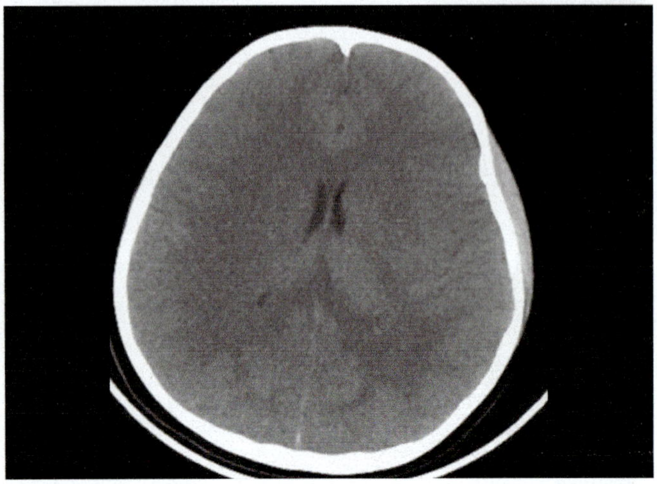

FIG. 3: Computed tomography (CT) brain showing diffuse cerebral edema and loss of gray white differentiation in the cortex and basal ganglionic regions in an 8-year-old after partial hanging.

BOX 2 Differential diagnosis for anoxic encephalopathy.

- Hypoglycemia
- Hyponatremia
- Acute hepatic failure
- Acute renal failure
- Nonketotic hyperosmolar state
- Brainstem stroke
- Creutzfeldt–Jakob's disease (CJD), especially for postanoxic myoclonus
- Pontine and extrapontine myelinolysis
- Viral encephalitis
- *Drug-induced coma*: Sedating medications, anesthetic agents, and anticholinergics

Potential causes such as infection or drug overdose should be considered and excluded using cultures and drug and toxicology screens. If the precipitating event was cardiac arrest, a cardiac evaluation, including EKG, echocardiogram, and cardiac biomarkers, could be considered. A lot of medical and neurological conditions may mimic anoxic encephalopathy. The differentials of anoxic encephalopathy are given in **Box 2**.

INVESTIGATIONS

Computed Tomography Brain

Computed tomography (CT) imaging of the brain is frequently normal. A repeat CT imaging taken 3–5 days after the event will often show manifestations of anoxic injury such as cerebral edema, loss of gray-white matter differentiation and decreased bilateral basal ganglia attenuation **(Fig. 3)**. One may find the classically described signs associated with a bad prognosis the "reversal" sign or "white cerebellum" sign **(Fig. 4)**.[18]

Magnetic Resonance Imaging Brain

Magnetic resonance imaging of the brain is the best imaging tool in suspected cases of anoxic encephalopathy. The most important sequence in MRI is the diffusion-weighted imaging (DWI). DWI shows changes within hours after the event compared to T2W and FLAIR images. DWI is particularly sensitive to ischemia **(Fig. 5A)** and apparent diffusion coefficient (ADC) values **(Fig. 5B)** can provide a quantitative measure of injury. DWI, FLAIR, and T2W images may show diffuse hyperintense signals in cerebral cortices, basal ganglia, hippocampi, and cerebellar hemispheres. This pattern of hypoxic injury is seen in older children and adults. Severe hypoxia-ischemia in both preterm and term neonates preferentially damages the deep gray matter, while perirolandic involvement is more frequently seen in term neonates. Less profound insults result in intraventricular hemorrhages and periventricular white matter injury in preterm neonates and parasagittal watershed territory infarcts in term neonates. In the postnatal period, severe insults result in diffuse gray matter injury, with relative sparing of the perirolandic cortex and the structures supplied by the posterior circulation. In adults, these abnormalities pseudonormalize by end of first week. Magnetic resonance spectroscopy (MRS) is more sensitive and more indicative of injury severity in first 24 hours after hypoxic injury. Increase in lactate >1.3 ppm after 24 hours portends poor neurologic outcome. N-acetylaspartate (NAA) is usually normal in acute setting and declines 48 hours after acute injury. T2*gradient and susceptibility-weighted imaging (T2*GRE/SWI) is helpful to detect petechial or subarachnoid hemorrhage. Patterns associated with poor clinical outcome are diffuse cortical and deep gray matter pattern, medial occipital with perirolandic involvement, precentral gyrus involvement, diffuse white matter involvement, brainstem, and cerebellar with or without hippocampal involvement.

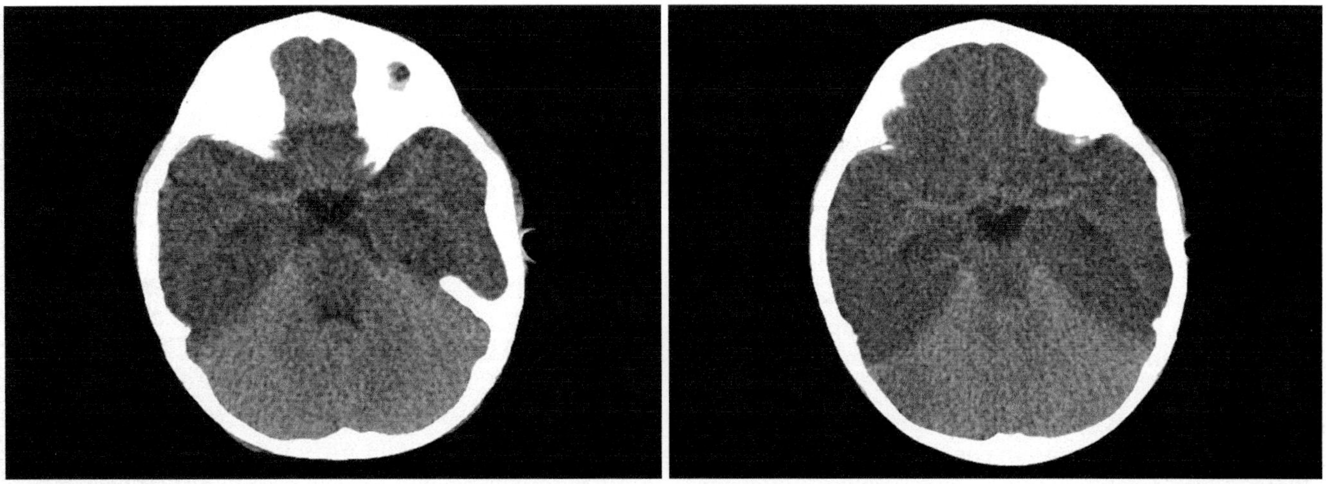

FIG. 4: Plain computed tomography (CT) head at temporal lobe level shows diffuse bilateral supratentorial hypodensity with loss of gray white differentiation and relative sparing of cerebellar hemispheres suggestive of white cerebellar sign also know reversal sign or dense cerebellar sign.

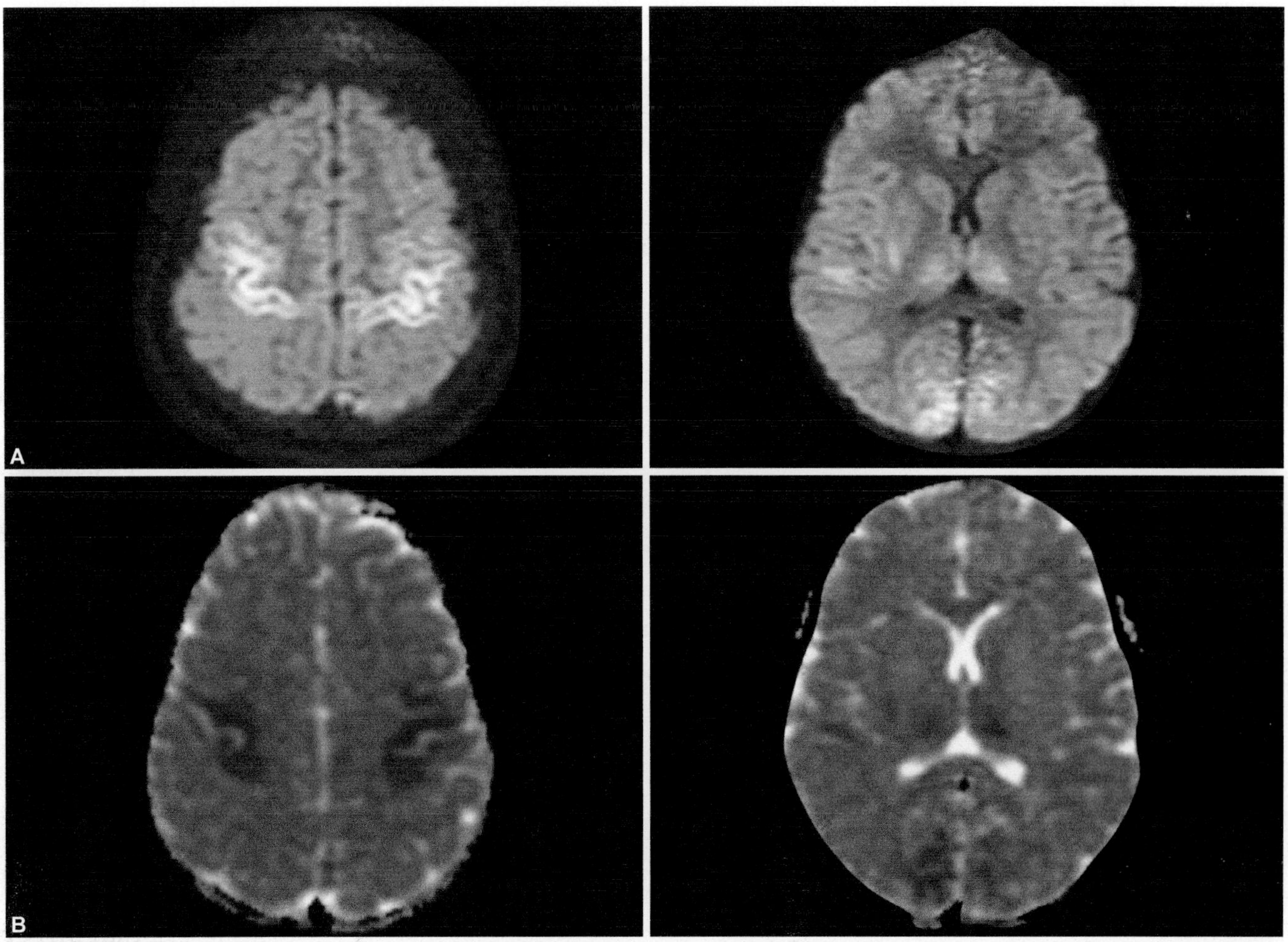

FIGS. 5A AND B: (A) Magnetic resonance imaging (MRI) brain diffusion-weighted image (DWI) showing perirolandic, thalamic, occipital cortex, and post putamen hyperintensities in an 8-year-old patient with Guillain–Barré syndrome (GBS), postresuscitation, after respiratory arrest and (B) Apparent diffusion coefficient (ADC) showing reversal in the corresponding areas.

Electroencephalogram

The utility of EEG is in providing some information regarding prognostication. However, the role of EEG in the routine diagnosis of anoxic encephalopathy is uncertain due to the potential for interpretation variability due to sedative drug use, metabolic abnormalities, or sepsis. There are findings that may suggest the presence of anoxic injury such as alpha-theta pattern, intermittent or continuous seizures, burst-suppression, generalized periodic complexes, complete or near-complete suppression, as well as generalized or focal low voltage output.[19,20] The so called malignant EEG patterns are burst suppression **(Fig. 6)**, nonreactive alpha coma and isoelectric EEG. The burst suppression pattern consists of medium to high voltage, mixed frequency slow wave activity, sometimes intermixed with spikes with intervening periods of severe voltage suppression. These bursts may be accompanied by massive myoclonic jerks. The alpha comma pattern is characterized by monorhythmic alpha activity which is generalized, with frontal dominance and nonreactive to external stimuli. The postanoxic periodic pattern consists of generalized spikes or sharp waves that occur at a frequency of 1–2 per second. It can occur independently over each hemisphere and may be accompanied by myoclonic jerks of the limbs or the whole body.

Knowing the limitations, there are EEG classification systems for anoxic encephalopathy that have been proposed. One system classifies the encephalopathy into four different grades utilizing global waveform patterns seen on EEG. Grade I anoxic encephalopathy has the most favorable prognosis and consists of alpha wave activity. Grade II anoxic encephalopathy consists of predominantly theta wave activity on EEG. For grade III, a predominant delta wave pattern is typical, and this extends into grade IV, where the low amplitude delta waves approach an isoelectric EEG.[21] A delta wave pattern is associated with a worse prognosis, and the isoelectric EEG is suggestive of a poor outcome. In order to fully evaluate these findings, monitoring using continuous EEG is preferred to single static EEG. Continuous EEG monitoring should be done with therapeutic hypothermia and rewarming as nonconvulsive seizures and nonconvulsive status epilepticus (NCSE) can occur. The malignant changes observed during rewarming are associated with poor prognosis.[19]

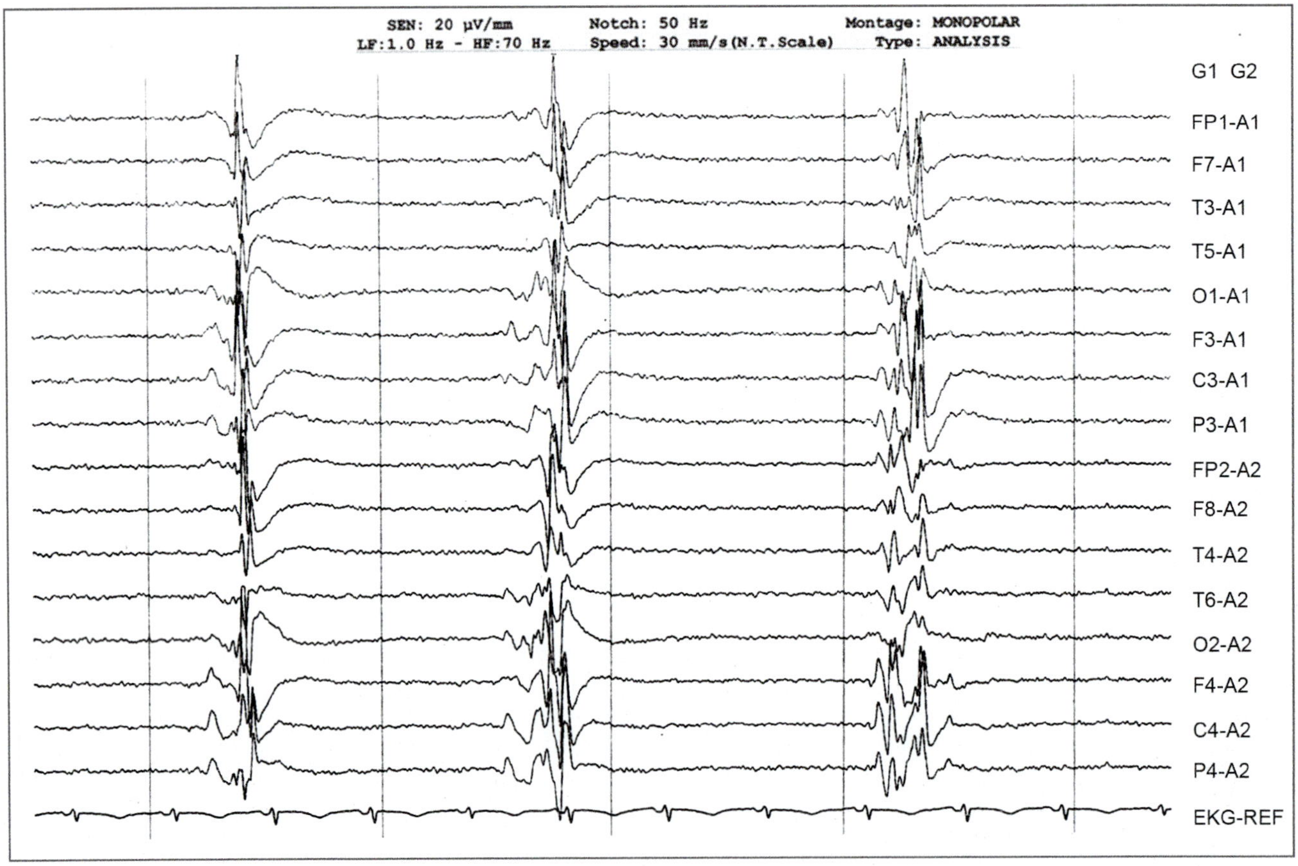

FIG. 6: Electroencephalogram (EEG) showing burst of sharp wave complexes (arrow) followed by suppression in an 8-year-old patient with Guillain–Barré syndrome (GBS), postresuscitation, after respiratory arrest.

Image courtesy: Professor GRK Sarma.

MANAGEMENT

The initial course of management is the stabilization of the patient upon presentation. This includes correction of metabolic abnormalities, initiation of antibiotics if septic, stabilization of hemodynamics, as well as a reversal of any possible toxic ingestions or overdose. As hypothermia improves the tolerability of hypoxia, potential interventions include targeted temperature management. Targeted temperature management is the process of maintaining the temperature at or below 36°C, whereas therapeutic hypothermia involves maintaining the temperature within the range of 32–34°C. Historically, the suggested temperature range was 32–34°C.[22] However, newer trials suggest similar benefits at 36° when compared to 33° giving rise to targeted temperature management.[23] While temperature management may be accomplished using external cooling, therapeutic hypothermia may require the use of invasive cooling measures. There are no standard treatment guidelines or large clinical trials for treatment of myoclonic jerks associated with MSE or LAS. Response to treatment is largely based on anecdotal evidence and the presumed origin (cortical or subcortical). Antiepileptic drugs, benzodiazepines, anesthetic agents, and serotonergic drugs [5-hydroxytryptophan (5-HTP), methysergide] have been used for both conditions.[9] One may use antimyoclonic agents such as levetiracetam, brivaracetam, clonazepam, valproate, or perampanel. It is also essential to counsel the family members regarding the potential of anoxic insult to cause permanent brain damage or brain death.

PROGNOSIS

The prognosis may be favorable in case of mild hypoxia of very short duration. Postcardiac arrest recovery can be complete if CPR is done within 3–5 minutes. Beyond 5 minutes there is usually permanent injury. However, some individuals may recover even after 8–10 minutes as some amount cardiac function might have been there. But prognosis is unfavorable in severe cases of anoxic-ischemic encephalopathy. The presence of fixed dilated pupils 6 hours after CPR is a sign of poor prognosis. One should be aware that use of intravenous atropine during CPR may also cause dilated pupils. Sustained upward gaze indicates a significant global cerebral injury with involvement of thalamus. Posthypoxic MSE is a poor prognostic sign. Persisting coma 24 hours after CPR, is also a bad sign with a mortality rate of 87%. The presence of EEG background nonreactivity and discontinuity may predict bad neurological outcome. But this may be difficult to interpret when sedative drugs and anesthetic agents are administered and in the context of therapeutic hypothermia. MRI patterns associated with poor outcomes include diffuse and persistent cortical DWI abnormalities, the combination of cortical and deep gray matter DWI/FLAIR abnormalities and severe global ADC reduction. But the prognostic value of MRI patterns is indeterminate as 20–50% of patients with good outcomes can have diffusion abnormalities. Bilateral absence of N20 response on SSEPs and neuron-specific enolase (NSE) above >33 μg/L at any time also predict poor outcome.[24]

PREVENTION

As the most common cause of anoxic encephalopathy is cardiac arrest, prevention of sudden cardiac deaths may prevent anoxic encephalopathy. Management of cardiovascular risk factors and early identification and management of cardiac arrhythmias may prevent sudden cardiac deaths. Awareness regarding CO intoxication due to usage of ill-fitted, ill-ventilated gas geyser is necessary as they are entirely preventable conditions. GGS can be prevented by avoiding the use of gas geysers in bathrooms. Flueless gas water heaters are considered dangerous if used to supply hot water to a bath or shower, because the products of combustion contain CO and discharge directly into the room, and may build up to dangerous levels. They are now obsolete and banned in countries such as Hong Kong and Canada.[14] In Hong Kong, the ordinance specifies that even a flueless (sink) gas water heater for the kitchen must provide a warning label and should not be used for more than 5 minutes continuously. In the United Kingdom, the gas safety (installation and use) regulations have prescribed specific criteria of ventilation for flueless gas appliances. People should follow the guidelines developed by regulatory agencies for the use of these geysers, including the use of timers, site of installations and dimensions, and ventilation requirements of the room in which they are fitted.[25]

CONCLUSION

Anoxic encephalopathy is an unfortunate and devastating sequel of abrupt cessation of oxygen and blood supply to the brain. The most common cause is postcardiac arrest hypoxic-ischemic injury. An early CPR within 5–10 minutes may avoid permanent neurological sequel but few people are fortunate to have an early CPR. Majority of people may sustain varying degrees of hypoxic brain injuries. The prognosis depends on the abruptness of onset and duration of the hypoxic event. Prognostication is difficult but involves data generated from clinical examination, neuroimaging, EEG, and biomarkers. GGS is an important preventable cause of anoxic encephalopathy due to CO poisoning in our country.

REFERENCES

1. Heinz UE, Rollnik JD. Outcome and prognosis of hypoxic brain damage patients undergoing neurological early rehabilitation. BMC Res Notes. 2015;8:243.
2. Rao BH. Global burden of Sudden Cardiac Death and insights from India. Indian Heart J. 2014;66 Suppl 1(Suppl 1):S18-23.
3. Geocadin RG, Koenig MA, Jia X, Stevens RD, Peberdy MA. Management of brain injury after resuscitation from cardiac arrest. Neurol Clin. 2008;26(2):487-506, ix.
4. Allen KA, Brandon DH. Hypoxic Ischemic Encephalopathy: Pathophysiology and Experimental Treatments. Newborn Infant Nurs Rev. 2011;11(3):125-33.
5. Wang Z, Mascarenhas C, Jia X. Positron Emission Tomography After Ischemic Brain Injury: Current Challenges and Future Developments. Transl Stroke Res. 2020;11(4):628-42.
6. Ropper AH, Samuels MA, Kliein JP. The acquired metabolic disorders of the nervous system. In: Ropper AH, Samuels MA, Kliein JP, Prasad S (Eds). Adams and Victor's Principles of Neurology, 10th edition. New York: McGraw-Hill Medical Publishers Division; 2005. pp. 1133-8.
7. Giacino JT, Ashwal S, Childs N, Cranford R, Jennett B, Katz DI, et al. The minimally conscious state: definition and diagnostic criteria. Neurology. 2002;58:349-53.
8. Fugate JE, Wijdicks EFM. Anoxic-ischemic encephalopathy. In: Daroff RB, Jankovic J, Mazziotta JC, Pomeroy SL, (Eds). Bradley's Neurology in Clinical Practice, 7th edition. New York: Elsevier; 2016. pp. 1201-8.
9. Acharya JN. Post-hypoxic myoclonus: The good, the bad and the ugly. Clin Neurophysiol Pract. 2017;2:105-6.
10. Lance JW, Adams RD. The syndrome of intention or action myoclonus as a sequel to hypoxic encephalopathy. Brain. 1963;86:111-36.
11. English WA, Giffin NJ, Nolan JP. Myoclonus after cardiac arrest: Pitfalls in diagnosis and prognosis. Anaesthesia. 2009;64:908-11.
12. Custodio CM, Basford JR. Delayed postanoxic encephalopathy: a case report and literature review. Arch Phys Med Rehabil. 2004;85(3):502-5.
13. Shprecher D, Mehta L. The syndrome of delayed post-hypoxic leukoencephalopathy. Neuro Rehabilitation. 2010;26(1):65-72.
14. Correia P, Agrawal C, Ranjan R. Gas geyser syndrome: An important preventable cause of disabling neurological events. Ann Indian Acad Neurol. 2013;16(2):245-8.
15. Mehta A, Mahale R, John AA, Abbas MM, Javali M, Acharya P, et al. Odorless inhalant toxic encephalopathy in developing countries household: Gas geyser syndrome. J Neurosci Rural Pract. 2016;7(2):228-31.
16. Patil VA, Lovhale NS, Jaggi ST, Tandel SV. A Case of Gas Geyser Syndrome with Peculiar Findings on MRI Brain. Neurol India. 2021;69:772-3.
17. Correia P, Agrawal C, Ranjan R. Gas geyser syndrome: An important preventable cause of disabling neurological events. Ann Indian Acad Neurol. 2013;16(2):245-8.
18. Zingler VC, Krumm B, Bertsch T, Fassbender K, Pohlmann-Eden B. Early prediction of neurological outcome after cardio-pulmonary resuscitation: a multimodal approach combining neurobiochemical and electrophysiological investigations may provide high prognostic certainty in patients after cardiac arrest. Eur Neurol. 2003;49(2):79-84.
19. Freeman WD. Continuous EEG in therapeutic hypothermia after cardiac arrest: prognostic and clinical value. Neurology. 2013;81(9):855.
20. Rossetti AO, Logroscino G, Liaudet L, Ruffieux C, Ribordy V, Schaller MD, et al. Status epilepticus: an independent outcome predictor after cerebral anoxia. Neurology. 2007;69(3):255-60.
21. Bateman RM, Sharpe MD, Jagger JE, Ellis CG, Solé-Violán J, López-Rodríguez M, et al. 36th International Symposium on Intensive Care and Emergency Medicine: Brussels, Belgium. 15-18 March 2016. Crit Care. 2016;20(Suppl 2):94.
22. Arrich J, Holzer M, Havel C, Müllner M, Herkner H. Hypothermia for neuroprotection in adults after cardiopulmonary resuscitation. Cochrane Database Syst Rev. 2016;2:CD004128.
23. Nielsen N, Wetterslev J, Cronberg T, Erlinge D, Gasche Y, Hassager C, et al. Targeted temperature management at 33°C versus 36°C after cardiac arrest. N Engl J Med. 2013;369(23):2197-206.
24. Zandbergen EG, Hijdra A, Koelman JH, Hart AA, Vos PE, Verbeek MM, et al. Prediction of poor outcome within the first 3 days of postanoxic coma. Neurology. 2006;66(1):62-8.
25. Mehta A, Mahale R, John AA, Abbas MM, Javali M, Acharya P, et al. Odorless inhalant toxic encephalopathy in developing countries household: Gas geyser syndrome. J Neurosci Rural Pract. 2016;7(2):228-31.

102
CHAPTER

Neurocritical Care

UK Misra, Jayantee Kalita, Boby Varkey Maramattom

INTRODUCTION

Neurocritical care unit (NICU) is a specialized facility in the hospital with advanced life support and monitoring facilities, providing care to the patients with life-threatening neurological illnesses by a team of specially trained doctors and nurses. Acute neurologic illnesses (ANIs) are key determinates of global disability and death and affect populations in low-income and middle-income countries (LMICs) where access to critical care and neurologic expertise is constrained.[1] Several disease conditions are associated with this high burden of ANI in LMICs, such as stroke, traumatic brain injury (TBI), epilepsy, neurological infections, etc., compared to affluent countries. There is a higher frequency of central nervous system (CNS) infections (meningitis, encephalitis, and parainfectious disorders), stroke, and venous sinus thrombosis compared to the western world. Neuromuscular conditions such as myasthenia gravis (MG) and Guillain-Barré syndrome (GBS) are also found in large numbers. These patients have a better outcome if they get proper NICU care. The organization and management of patients in NICU have special issues in LMIC such as resource crunch, paucity of intensive care unit (ICU) and ventilators, lack of trained manpower and a disproportionately large number of critically ill patients, poorly developed medical insurance, and limited support by the Government for care of patients. This calls for proper and rational use of limited resources for optimal management. Some basic clinical issues in NICU are discussed in this chapter and for specific conditions, the readers are referred to the respective chapters.

There should be a clear policy for admission to NICU, based on the likely outcome and benefit in quality-of-life of the patient. An increasing requirement for organ support in itself should not be a reason for admission of a patient who is suffering their terminal illness, and is unlikely to recover. Presence of comorbidities and physiological reserve also influences the decision for ICU admission. The admission in ICU should not be prejudged by age or socioeconomic status. Patient's stated or written preference for or against intensive care must also be considered.

NURSING CARE AND PHYSICAL THERAPY

Neurocritical care in the NICU requires teamwork and excellent cooperation among nurses, technicians, neurologists, and other physicians who take care of critically ill patients.

Care of eye, skin, chest physiotherapy, preventing infection, and care of fluid electrolytes and nutrition are important components.

Neurological patients, if not on mechanical ventilation (MV), should be nursed in a lateral position **(Figs. 1A and B)** and two hourly turning should be maintained. Most ICUs

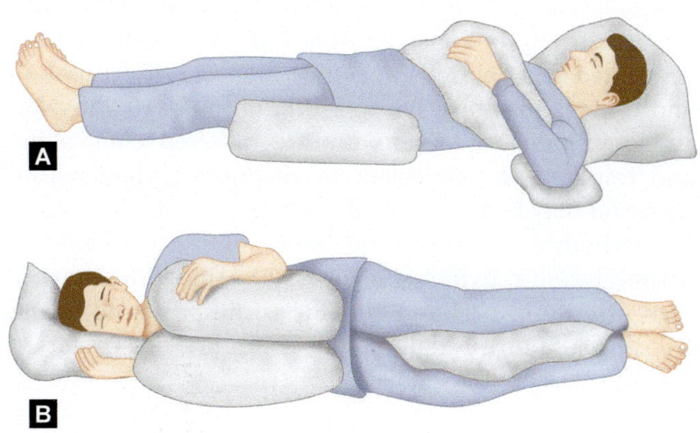

FIGS. 1A AND B: Position of lying down in ICU: (A) Supine and (B) lateral position patients who are not on mechanical ventilation should preferably lie in lateral position.

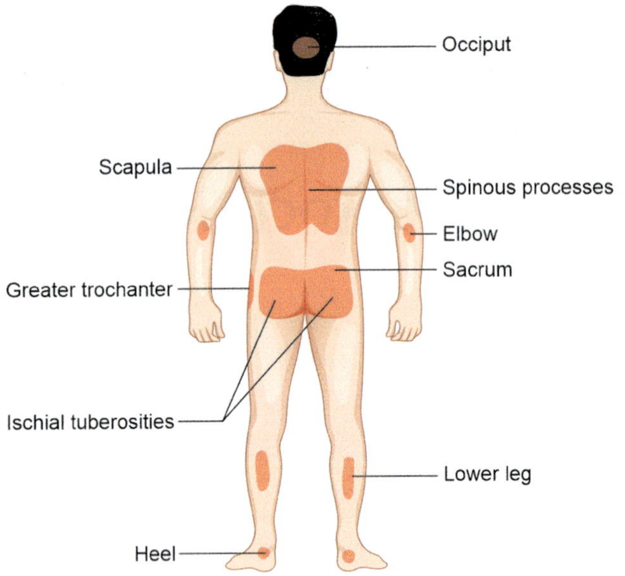

FIG. 2: Schematic diagrams showing the common sites of pressure sore.

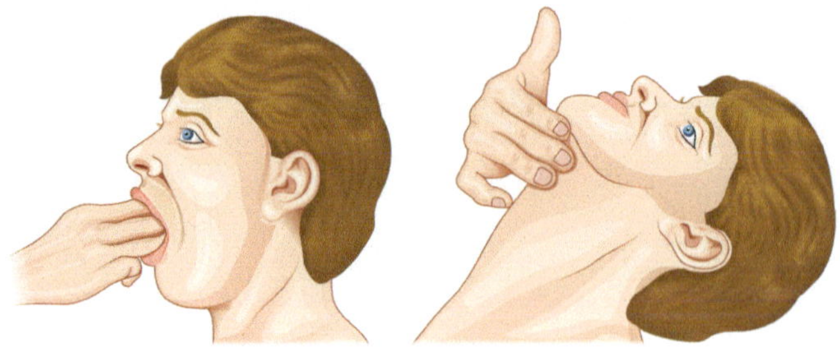

FIG. 3: Bedside estimates of difficult intubation: Inability to insert three fingers in the oral cavity and to place three fingers between the thyroid bone and the mandible when the head is extended.

recommend 45° elevation of the head to reduce intracranial pressure (ICP), but we feel that the lateral position is ideal in nonintubated patients, because it prevents aspiration and tongue fall. One should be aware of pressure sites and take care of the skin to avoid pressure sore **(Fig. 2)**. Chest physiotherapy and incentive spirometry should be regularly performed.

Communication with the patient and family is important. The discussion should be honest, fair, and clear. Overestimation or unduly optimistic comments should be avoided. The need for invasive monitoring, therapy, and MV should be discussed in light of the patient's condition.

Analgesia and Sedation

Analgesia and sedation are commonly used in NICU. Many neurologists generally avoid sedation as it interferes with the assessment of consciousness. However, if the patient is agitated and delirious, it could result in self-extubation and removal of lines. For sedation propofol (0.1 mg/kg) and lorazepam (1-2 mg 4 hourly) are preferred to morphine and fentanyl, which result in respiratory depression. Agitation may be due to alcohol withdrawal, beta-blocker, antiarrhythmic drugs, and metabolic abnormalities (hyperglycemic hyperosmolar state). Analgesics have a high priority in ICU and codeine is the preferred agent. Nonsteroidal anti-inflammatory drugs are not preferred because of gastrointestinal bleeding risk.

Endotracheal Intubation

Endotracheal intubation is indicated in the following group of patients:

- Suffer from hypoventilation and hypoxia leading to hypoxia, hyperpnea, or metabolic alterations.
- Who cannot protect their airway.
- Are not fully alert and are prone to aspiration of gastric contents.

Nasal intubation has several advantages, including improved patient comfort, tighter tube fixation, rare laryngeal damage, and the possibility of proper mouth care. However, in patients with a head injury and potential cerebrospinal fluid leak, nasal intubation may lead to infection and transient bacteremia. Prolonged nasotracheal intubation (>5 days) may lead to bacterial sinusitis.

The difficulty in intubation is likely if there is an inability to visualize oral structures such as soft palate, tonsillar fossa, and uvula—when the mouth is wide open, significant facial trauma, cervical spine fracture, mandibular hypoplasia, history of rheumatoid arthritis, ankylosing spondylitis, obesity, and short thick neck. Important bedside estimates are the ability to insert three fingers in the oral cavity and to place three fingers between the thyroid bone and the mandible when the head is extended **(Fig. 3)**. Patients with long-standing insulin-dependent diabetes mellitus have reduced cervical spine mobility.

Elective Intubation

Elective intubation is usually done in the patient, who is fasting for at least 6 hours. Endotracheal intubation should be accompanied by cricoid pressure (Sellick maneuver). Movement of this circle of cartilage posteriorly occludes the esophagus and may prevent regurgitation.

The patient is placed in the "sniffing position" (achieved by tilting the head backward) **(Fig. 4A)** and 100% oxygen is administered through a bag and mask. For laryngoscopy, the patient's head is extended carefully, and the laryngoscope is introduced into the patient's mouth with the left hand taking care not to injure the patient's teeth and lips.

During the laryngoscopy, the base of the tongue is seen first. As the laryngoscope is advanced, the epiglottis appears. If the Miller blade is used, the tip is placed under the epiglottis to lift it up and out of the way. At this point, the laryngoscope is lifted in the direction of its handle. Pivoting the instrument back onto the upper incisor will injure the patient's teeth. Lifting the laryngoscope brings the arytenoids, at the most posterior part of the larynx, into view. Further lifting exposes the cords **(Fig. 4B)**. External pressure on the thyroid

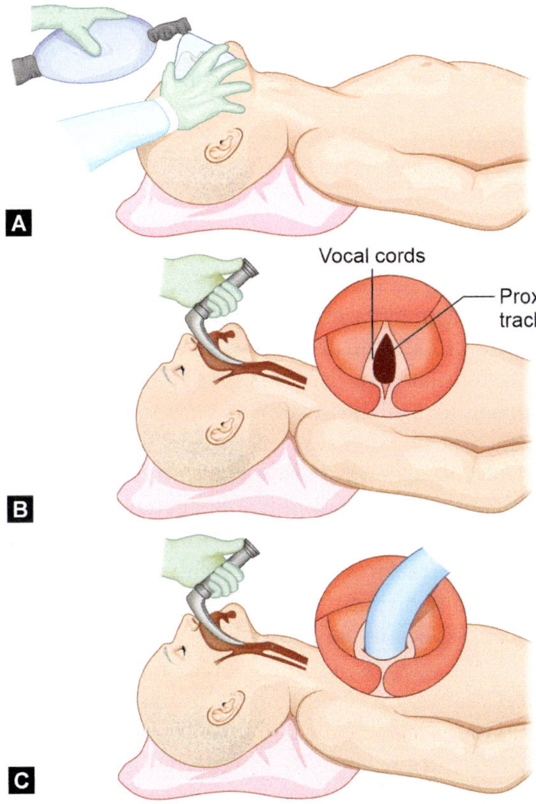

FIGS. 4A TO C: Technique of endotracheal intubation.

cartilage or cricoid cartilage by an assistant might help to bring the laryngeal structures into view. As the endotracheal tube is advanced, it passes between the cords **(Fig. 4C)**. After the cuff has passed the cords, advancement of only 3 cm is needed for proper placement. The cuff is inflated up to 10–15 cmH_2O or more when a leak is still heard. Both lungs are auscultated for breath sounds. The gastric area is also auscultated to rule out esophageal ventilation. The location of the tube may be confirmed by a chest radiograph, which identifies the tip of the endotracheal tube 5–7 cm above the carina at T-6 level.

Laryngeal Mask Ventilation

It may be used in an emergency by less trained doctors or in patients with difficult airways. The mask has been modified to facilitate tracheal intubation with a tracheal tube **(Fig. 5)**. It is useful if visualization of the larynx is obscured by blood or secretions or if there is a potential for spinal cord damage when neck injuries have not been fully assessed. Laryngeal mask ventilation may be a useful bridging device to more traditional use of a cuffed tracheal tube in acute trauma care, but it is not particularly useful in the NICU.

Indications for Mechanical Ventilation

These can be discussed with reference to hemispheric and brainstem lesions, peripheral effector organs, and primary pulmonary causes of inadequate ventilation.

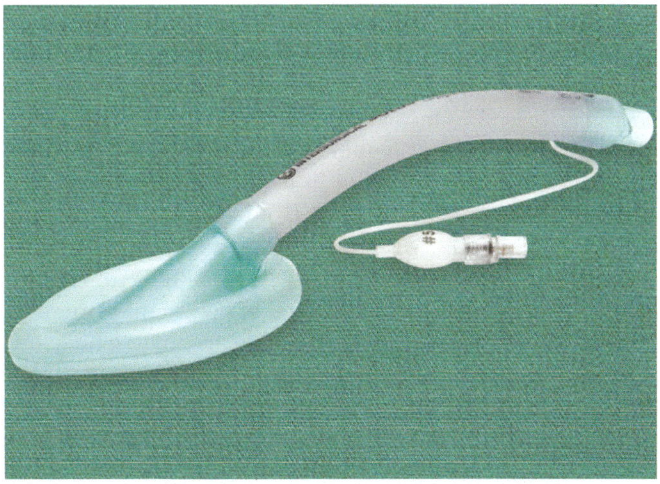

FIG. 5: Laryngeal masks for ventilation without intubation.

Central nervous system dysfunction: Following acute insult to CNS, respiratory drive may be reduced especially in the first few hours, resulting in hypoventilation. In some patients, hyperventilation may be a mechanism to compensate for hypoxia. Prolonged hyperventilation can be managed by assisted ventilation with mild sedation. In other patients, tachypnea compensates for metabolic acidosis, which needs to be concurrently corrected.

Intubated patients with acute CNS pathology are generally able to maintain efficient gas exchange which can be monitored by pulse oximeter and arterial blood gas (ABG). However, patients with abnormal breathing patterns that result in inadequate oxygen delivery and hypercapnia need MV. Hemispheric ischemic stroke needing MV may have pulmonary edema or heart failure.

Brain edema may manifest with impairment of consciousness and is a common cause for intubation and MV in ischemic stroke. Aneurysmal subarachnoid hemorrhage may be associated with apnea and may require MV.

Viral encephalitis: Endotracheal intubation is mandatory in patients with reduced alertness, seizures, or hypoxemia. Most patients have normal respiratory drive and mechanics and breathe spontaneously on a T-piece only, but continuous positive airway pressure (CPAP) (5–10 cmH_2O) can be added.

In tuberculous meningitis (TBM), patients who require MV have a poorer prognosis.[2] High mortality in MV patients in TBM may be due to multiple complications such as celebrities, granuloma, stroke, drug-induced hepatitis, hyponatremia, or hydrocephalus.

Status epilepticus (SE): In ICU, patients with refractory and super-refractory SE are admitted.[1] If the patient with SE is refractory to benzodiazepine and one more antiepileptic drug (AED), it is recommended to prescribe intravenous (IV) anesthetics and MV may be needed. There is no randomised controlled trial to favor this treatment strategy.

A retrospective study of SE patients revealed that mortality was three times higher and higher proportion of infectious complications in SE patients receiving anesthetic drugs compared to those who did not. This study provides Class III evidence that patients with SE receiving IV AEDs have a higher proportion of infection, an increased risk of death and poor outcome as compared to patients not receiving IV AEDs.[3]

Undergoing burst suppression has led to ethical concerns and the cost-effectiveness of ICU management of SE. However, it has been suggested that acceptable recovery is possible following less aggressive treatment.

NEUROCRITICAL CARE IN PERIPHERAL NERVOUS SYSTEM AND MUSCLE DISORDERS

Neuromuscular Respiratory Failure

Clinical features that suggest the possibility of neuromuscular respiratory failure are listed in **Box 1**.

Guillain–Barré Syndrome

About one-third of patients develop respiratory failure needing MV, and 3.5–12% of patients die of complications during the acute stage.[4,5] Autonomic dysfunction usually is associated with severe GBS, and contributes to mortality in about 3–10% of patients.

Patients with acute motor axonal neuropathy (AMAN) need MV more frequently than acute demyelinating polyradiculoneuropathy (AIDP) (47.4% *vs.* 33.8%).[5] Several studies have reported predictors of MV, and include rapidly progressive disease course needing hospitalization, bulbar or facial weakness, dysautonomia, severe weakness of neck flexor or arm abduction, vital capacity, maximum inspiratory pressure, and maximum expiratory pressure.[5]

Kalita et al. evaluated the role of single breath count (SBC) at 2 Hz using a 2-Hz auditory clicking sounds. None of the patients with an SBC of 7 or above had ABG abnormality ruling out need of ABG and MV in 14 days of admission. An SBC of 5 or less could rule in MV with 90% sensitivity and specificity.[6] SBC at 2 Hz is easily trainable and patients could do self-scoring and any drop in SBC by >20%, or if 7 or below should be informed to duty doctors immediately.

BOX 1 **The clinical signs of neuromuscular respiratory failure.**

Dyspnea at rest or minimal exertion:
- Restlessness
- Pulse rate >100/min
- Respiratory rate >20/min
- Use of accessory respiratory muscle [sternocleidomastoid, scalene (by palpation alone)]

Forehead sweating:
- Staccato speech
- Asynchronous (paradoxical) breathing

Myasthenia Gravis

Admission to neurocritical care is needed in the patients with impending respiratory failure or in myasthenic crisis (MC).

The triggering factors of MC include infection, use of contraindicated medications, surgery, physical or mental stress, insomnia, extreme or weather, premature withdrawal of immunomodulator, or drug default **(Table 1)**.

The predictors of noninvasive ventilation (NIV) are hypercarbia [partial pressure of carbon dioxide ($PaCO_2$) >45 mm Hg], hypoxemia ($PaCO_2$ < 60 mm Hg), and bicarbonate concentration >30 mmol/L. Repeated measurement of vital capacity, however, has been found not useful as a predictor of MC (facial and bulbar weakness may result in erroneous findings on pulmonary function tests). The bedside predictors of respiratory failure and MV are the recruitment of accessory muscles (inspiratory muscle weakness), weak cough, and inability to count up to 20 in a single breath. Once the patient is intubated, a little higher tidal volume (8–10 mL/kg) and pressure (8–15 cmH_2O) are used in the initial period to prevent atelectasis. Acetylcholinesterase inhibitors (AChEIs) should be discontinued.[7] The management of MG in ICU is presented in **Flowchart 1**.

PHYSIOLOGIC PRINCIPLES AND MODES OF MECHANICAL VENTILATION

Settings of the Ventilator

The initial tidal volume delivered by the ventilator is usually set to be relatively large, ranging from 12 to 15 mL/kg (based on ideal, not actual, body weight). A tidal volume of >15 mL/kg may significantly increase the risk of barotrauma. Patients with underlying pulmonary disease may need smaller tidal volumes (9–10 mL/kg). In some ventilators (e.g., Hamilton Veolar), the tidal volume is controlled by an independently adjustable knob. In others (e.g., Siemens Servo), the minute volume is dialed in. (The minute volume is determined by respiratory rate times tidal volume.) The respiratory rate usually ranges from 8 to 12 breaths/minute.

TABLE 1: The laboratory criteria for weaning.

Criteria	Requirement
PaO_2	>60 mm Hg
Tidal volume	>5 mL/kg
Vital capacity	15 mL/kg
Min ventilation	<10 L//kg
Negative inspiratory pressure	–30 mm Hg

(PaO_2: partial pressure of oxygen in the arterial blood)

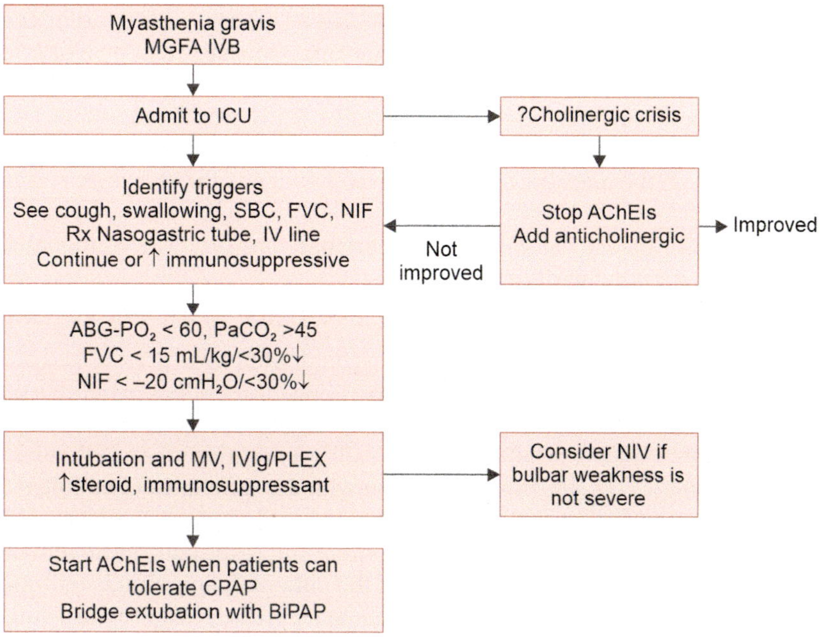

FLOWCHART 1: Management of myasthenia gravis.

(AChEIs: acetylcholinesterase inhibitors; FVC: forced vital capacity; ICU: intensive care unit; IVIg: intravenous immunoglobulin; MV: mechanical ventilation; NIV: noninvasive ventilation; $PaCO_2$: partial pressure of carbon dioxide; SBC: single breath count)

The respiratory rate must be chosen at the lowest possible setting to reduce the phenomenon of intrinsic positive end-expiratory pressure (PEEP) or gas trapping. When rapid rates are set, intrinsic PEEP is created when the time for expiration is diminished. This phenomenon is harmful as it increases the work of breathing, increases the proximal airway pressures, and may cause hypotension. Flow rate is set by the inspiratory time in most ventilators, usually through selection by the ratio of inspiration to expiration. This ratio is determined by inspiratory time, pause time, and expiratory time, and is expressed in percentages of the total ventilatory cycle. Commonly, the inspiratory time is set for 20% and the pause time for 5%, with the remaining 75% allowed for expiration (an inspiration:expiration ratio of 1:3). An important setting is a fraction of inspired oxygen (FiO_2), which is based on the arterial PO_2. High FiO_2 values, those exceeding 0.8 for at least 2 days, are considered toxic (these increase the chance of lung injury in animal experiments). Efforts should be made to reduce FiO_2 in patients on MV. However, if reduction of FiO_2 is not tolerated, adequate gas exchange is possible by increasing PEEP. PEEP refers to a setting that increases the end-expiratory pressure to produce a larger functional residual capacity. It maintains alveolar patency throughout respiration, recruits previously collapsed alveoli, and improves ventilation-perfusion matching. Most often, PEEP is indicated when the PO_2 remains <60 mm Hg despite an FiO_2 of 0.8. As indicated in cardiogenic pulmonary edema, adult respiratory distress syndrome (ARDS), and diffuse bilateral pneumonia, PEEP is often added to ventilation.

TABLE 2: Typical ventilator setting.

Mode	Intermittent mandatory ventilation
FiO_2	0.4–0.9
Respiratory rate	8–12 bpm
Tidal volume	10–15 mL/kg
PEEP	2–5 cmH_2O
IE ratio	1:3

(E: expiration; FiO_2: fraction of inspired oxygen; I: inspiration; PEEP: positive end-expiratory pressure)

Most mechanical ventilators have the capability of producing a breath of large volume (sigh) in an attempt to prevent alveolar collapse, but whether this function should be used routinely is unresolved. A typical ventilation parameter in a critically ill neurologic patient is shown in **Table 2**.

Controlled Mechanical Ventilation

Controlled mode ventilation should be used in patients who do not have a breathing drive as in acute basilar artery occlusion, rebleeding after subarachnoid hemorrhage, pontine-medullary stage of herniation, damage to the high cervical cord, and high barbiturates for the management of SE, or brain death. More often, controlled ventilation mode is used in MV combative patients treated with neuromuscular blockade, particularly in patients with polytrauma and significant respiratory distress. Its principle is a preset tidal volume with a dialed-in frequency without any effort by the patient. The timing mechanism determines the delivery of breaths, and the patient is completely dependent on the ventilator. Controlled MV has many disadvantages, mainly related to the use of sedation and neuromuscular blockade. Important risks are disconnection from the machine and the inability to perform any spontaneous breathing. In addition, prolonged controlled MV may cause disuse atrophy and asynchrony of respiratory muscles, resulting in difficulty in weaning.

Assist-control Ventilation

Assist-control ventilation is a frequent initial mode of ventilation in patients with acute neurologic catastrophes. In this mode, the patient is dominant and the ventilator takes over if the patient fails to trigger the ventilator. Patients trigger the ventilator by creating a pressure drop in the system, which in turn starts inspiration. The assist control ventilatory mode is often poorly tolerated in awake patients and acutely confused ones may lead to patient-ventilator dyssynchrony that can be overcome by sedating the patient. Excessive work by the patient, if the ventilatory drive is increased, may result in inadequate peak flow. The most common side effect of assist-control ventilation is respiratory alkalosis.

Intermittent Mandatory Ventilation

This mode is a combination of ventilator-initiated breathing at a fixed rate and spontaneous ventilation. Intermittent mandatory ventilation (IMV) is chosen for most patients in the NICU after initial stabilization. In IMV, a preset number of positive pressure breaths is available to the patient, which is interrupted by spontaneous breaths. The major limitation of positive pressure ventilation is that ventilator breaths are out of phase with spontaneously generated breaths (stacking). Stacking can be eliminated by synchronization. This mode is widely used for weaning, but comparative studies with other regimens (e.g., increasing T-piece circuit intervals) are not available. The major theoretical disadvantage is that because spontaneous breaths are not assisted, the mode is not responsive to the patient's needs, therefore, may rapidly lead to inadequate ventilation.

Pressure Support Ventilation

This mode supplies a pressurized breath during spontaneous breathing. The patient generates each breath by triggering the ventilator, by opening the valve that delivers the breath by creating a negative pressure similar to that in the IMV mode, but with the difference of cut off at a certain flow threshold. This mode decreases the work of breathing, but the tidal volume and respiration cycle remain controlled by the effort of the patient. Inspiration is terminated when a certain flow threshold is reached. Pressure support ventilation (PSV) is often used to overcome the resistance of the endotracheal tube and in combination with the IMV mode.

Continuous Positive Airway Pressure

This mode assists in spontaneous breathing and may improve oxygenation remarkably. The CPAP mode is often used in patients with sleep apnea, but in the medical ICU, its major goal is to prevent MV. The range of CPAP varies from 0 to 30 cmH_2O. The modes of MV are shown in **Figure 6**.

Noninvasive Ventilation

Noninvasive bi-level positive pressure airway ventilation (BiPAP) is an established alternative mode of MV. The major objective of BiPAP is to maintain adequate gas exchange

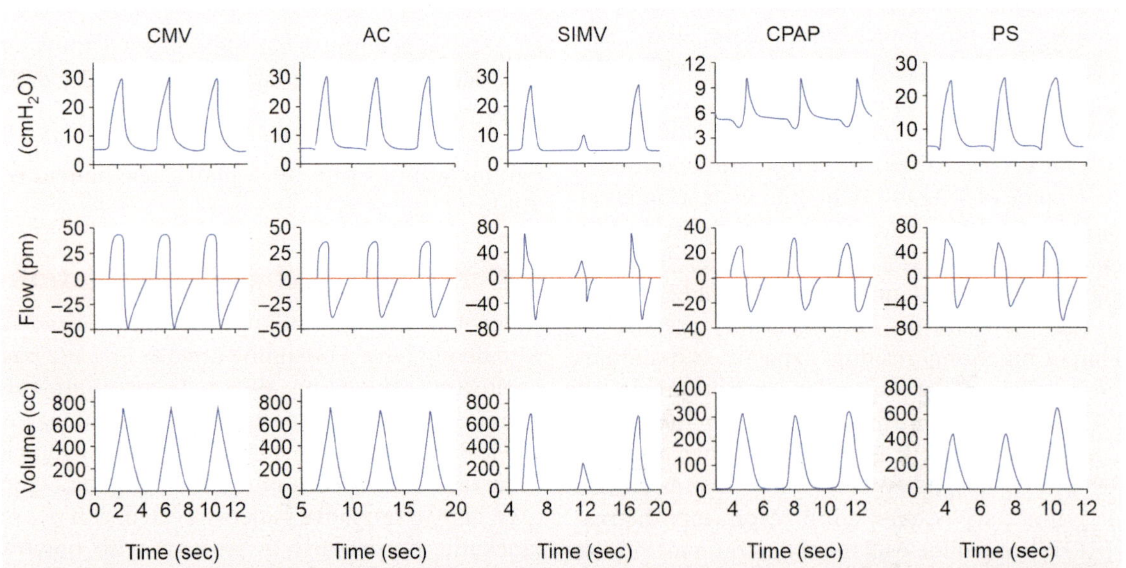

FIG. 6: Modes of mechanical ventilation: Three breaths with pressure curves and corresponding flow and volume waveforms are shown in commonly used modes.

without intubation. In ICU, BiPAP is typically used in patients with exacerbations of chronic obstructive pulmonary disease (COPD) and in patients with acute neuromuscular disease. Its place in chronic neuromuscular diseases, such as amyotrophic lateral sclerosis (ALS) or muscular dystrophy, has been established. The role of BiPAP in deteriorating GBS is limited because of upper airway collapse and increased secretions; however, it is useful in MG. In 18 patients, with MG, intubation was prevented in 7 and reintubation in 2 using BiPAP and it may have a role in selected patients with MG.[8] Major limitations of NIV include discomfort from the close-fitting mask, difficulty with rest and sleep, leaks, and gastric distension. Patients can be given BiPAP ventilation only if their BP is normal without vasopressors, are alert and cooperative, can protect the airway, and have hypoxemia requiring $FiO_2 > 50\%$, or hypercapnia (> 50 mm Hg).

Tracheostomy

Early tracheostomy should be considered if prolonged MV is likely; however, the timing of tracheostomy placement is controversial. The potential serious complications and cosmetic disfiguration following tracheostomy influence this decision. The important complications of tracheostomy are massive hemorrhage and tracheal stenosis at the stoma site, though these are very rare. The potential advantages of early tracheostomy are the comfort of the patient and more effective tracheal suctioning, but at a considerable risk of tracheolaryngeal stenosis following prolonged intubation. The prevalence of tracheal stenosis is nearly 10% within 2 weeks after endotracheal intubation.

Weaning from a Ventilator

Discontinuation from MV is an important part of ICU care. There is a paucity of studies on weaning criteria in patients with CNS and neuromuscular injury, and the results of prolonged MV may not apply to the majority of patients with acute brain injury. The criteria for weaning can be easily assessed at the bedside **(Table 1)**. In addition, weaning should not be attempted in patients who still require PEEP for adequate oxygenation and those who have significantly abnormal chest radiographs and do not show considerable remission and if general anesthesia is planned within 1 or 2 days for surgery or neurologic condition is worsening. Weaning from the ventilator also includes important adjunctive measures, such as correction of electrolyte imbalance, adequate hydration and nutrition, patient in an upright position, proper care of secretions, and adequate sleep. Weaning should be gradual, because a sudden transition may be stressful to patients with underlying cardiovascular disease.

In most patients with acute CNS pathology who have been intubated for a short time, weaning can be done by gradual T-tube weaning. Before the weaning is tried, it is useful to observe the patient for 5 minutes after placing a T piece and check for signs of discomfort, an increase in respiratory rate (>25 breaths/min), a decrease in tidal volume (not below 300 mL), a change in BP (increase or decrease), increase in heart rate (>20 beats/min), or development of ventricular ectopic or bigeminy. The T piece can remain in place for 30 minutes, with incremental increases in duration twice a day. ABG values are determined regularly. It is recommended to begin with T piece trial of 30 minutes, and subsequently, the duration can be rapidly increased to 1–2 hours. Extubation is performed when the ABG values remain satisfactory and rapid shallow breathing is not present. If the T-piece trial fails, the patient is given at least 24 hours of rest with full ventilation, before another attempt. Another approach for weaning is to change the settings of the IMV mode. The frequency is reduced in gradual steps. ABG determinations are used to recognize potential trends of respiratory acidosis. IMV weaning is fairly simple, consisting of gradual reduction with 3 breaths/minute starting three times a day. It is prudent to add pressure support at low levels (5–10 cmH_2O) for further comfort. Pressure support weaning may be preferred to other weaning regimens and may increase synchrony. Pressure support is set at a level that is comfortable to the patient, usually 15–40 cmH_2O, followed by decrements of 3 cmH_2O. When the pressure support level of 5 cmH_2O is tolerated (pressure just enough to overcome the resistance of the tube) and the laboratory criteria are fulfilled, extubation can be undertaken. It has been suggested that rapid shallow breathing diagnosed by the ratio of respiratory rate to tidal volume predicts weaning failure. Patients with a frequency-volume ratio of >100 had a 95% likelihood of failure in a weaning trial. Patients with a frequency-volume ratio of <100 had an 80% likelihood of successful weaning. Nonetheless, the use of the frequency-volume ratio may be very helpful as a clinical guide after extubation. Even if extubation is well tolerated, but one should watch for inspiratory stridor up to 1 hour after extubation. Most patients have transient hoarseness following extubation. Topical epinephrine into the hypopharynx may be helpful, but reintubation is often necessary. Laryngospasm though is less common but may be life-threatening. It is much more common in children and young adults. Typically, the crowing sound of stridor is absent and strenuous efforts are seen, with significant desaturation. Succinylcholine (0.1 mg/kg IV) or lidocaine (2 mg/kg IV) may also significantly reduce laryngospasm if used several minutes before extubation.[9]

HYDRATION AND FLUID THERAPY

The volume status of the patient can be assessed by history and examination. Generally, most patients admitted to NICU are dehydrated. Overlooking reduced thirst, altered sensorium, vomiting, and fever may lead to underestimation of dehydration. An initial fluid intake of 150–200 mL/h is appropriate. The crystalloid of choice is 0.9% sodium chloride; glucose-based solutions are not preferred in patients with acute neurologic disorders unless there is severe hypernatremia. In a patient having a head injury or ischemic stroke, glucose infusions may worsen hyperglycemias and anaerobic cerebral glucose metabolism. In a study on ischemic stroke, blood glucose >144 mg/dL reduced penumbral salvage and increased the final infarct size.[10] Normoglycemia improved tissue salvage.

Optimal intravenous fluid (IVF) is not well defined, but a patient in shock is recommended to be given fluid challenge or a bolus of IVF. Fluid bolus refers to a therapeutic intervention in which 500 mL of fluid is administered in 15 minutes to correct hypotensive shock. Fluid challenge refers to a diagnostic infusion of 500–1000 mL crystalloid or 500 mL colloid in 30 minutes to evaluate the effect of fluid in optimizing tissue perfusion. About 300 mL blood is present in leg veins and passive leg rising introduces 300 mL without increasing the blood volume and helps in assessing fluid responsiveness. In a patient with septic shock, it is recommended to administer 30 mL/kg/h IVF to get a central venous pressure (CVP) of 8–12 cmH_2O, mean arterial blood pressure of >65 mm Hg, and urine output of >0.5 mL/kg/h. The effect of fluid challenge can be monitored by static or dynamic measures. The static parameters of fluid responsiveness include CVP and pulmonary artery occlusion pressure (cardiac filling pressure). The dynamic markers of fluid responsiveness are available in patients who are on MV. During positive pressure, inspiration increases intrathoracic pressure, resulting in decreased preload and stroke volume. During expiration, the intrathoracic pressure decreases with increased venous return, preload, and stroke volume. These dynamic changes in stroke volume in response to the respiratory cycle may be used to assess fluid responsiveness.

Intravenous fluid therapy:

- *Crystalloids*: Several electrolyte solutions are used such as Ringer lactate, Plasma-Lyte, and other fluids. There are concerns about the other physiological ions in addition to sodium (such as potassium, calcium, magnesium, bicarbonate, and phosphate) and their effect on renal perfusion. A large amount of 0.9% saline may result in extracellular potassium shift leading to hyperkalemia. The chloride-rich solution can result in renal vasoconstriction and acute kidney injury, hyperchloremic metabolic acidosis, and gastrointestinal dysfunction. The comparative usefulness of isotonic crystalloids for fluid resuscitation of critically ill patients is based on a few observational studies and a single-center study. These studies demonstrated the association of balanced fluid like lactated Ringer's solution with reduced incidence of acute kidney injury and mortality and better outcome compared to normal saline.[11] In septic shock, balanced fluid improved survival rates. A recent study compared normal saline with Plasma-Lyte 148 in ICU fluid therapy (SPLIT) trial. This trial did not reveal any difference with respect to acute kidney injury, need for renal replacement therapy, or mortality in the patients receiving normal saline or balanced salt solution. However, these patients were of mild severity—mostly surgical patients with few comorbidities, and the fluid received was only 2 L, which may be insufficient to demonstrate the effect of chloride-restrictive fluid therapy on renal functions. Moreover, the incidence of acute kidney injury was <10%.[12]
- *Colloids*: Colloids comprise a group of high-molecular-weight compounds suspended in a carrier vehicle. Colloids are retained in the intravascular compartment and provide oncotic pressure, thereby increasing plasma volume. Albumin and starch compounds are commonly used colloids. Albumin is available as 4–5% (iso-oncotic) and 20–25% (hyperoncotic) formulations, and is widely used as a volume expander. The Saline versus Albumin Evaluation (SAFE) study randomized 6,997 patients to 4% albumin or 0.9% saline. There was no difference in 28-day mortality; however, 492 (7%) head injury patients had higher death in the albumin arm compared to saline (OR 1.62, 95% CI 0.12–2.34; p = 0.009) and mortality was attributed to coagulopathy following albumin.[13] In ALBIOS trial in sepsis, 20% albumin did not result in a reduction in mortality, length of hospitalization, and degree of organ dysfunction, but there was no harm attributed to albumin.[14] Owing to high cost and lack of convincing reproducible benefit, Surviving Sepsis Campaign recommends albumin to those selected patients who have received substantial crystalloids.
- *Starch*: Semisynthetic colloids prepared by hydroxylation of amylopectin from sorghum, corn, or potatoes may be iso-oncotic (6%) or hyperoncotic (10%). Hydroxyethyl starch (HES) is the third-generation starch that has a low-molecular weight (130 KD), lower substitution, and is cheaper and easier to procure than albumin. Several trials have proven its safety and efficacy compared to crystalloids. Crystalloid versus HES Trial (CHEST) compared 6% HES with normal saline in 7,000 critically ill patients requiring resuscitation. There was no difference in 90-day mortality. HES patients had double the adverse events compared to crystalloid arm, including skin rash, itching, and requirement for renal replacement therapy (7% vs. 5.6%, p = 0.004).[15] A comparison of volume-expanding agents is presented in **Table 3**.

NUTRITIONAL CARE IN NICU

Critically ill patients have special nutritional requirements. Daily nutrition is aimed at countering the effects of hypermetabolism, acute gastroparesis, and preventing the complications associated with enteral nutrition. Early feeding prevents gastrointestinal mucosal atrophy, whereas delay in nutritional support may result in weakness, poor cough, and a predisposition to infections. In severe head injury and stroke, early nutritional support has been reported to reduce mortality and frequency of nosocomial infections.

TABLE 3: Comparisons of volume-expanding agents.

Agent	Na	Cost	T/2	Toxicity
Isotonic saline	154	D	Min	None
5% albumin	130–160	20D	5–6	Anaphylaxis, pulmonary edema
25% albumin	130–160	20D	5–6	Anaphylaxis, pulmonary edema
Ringer lactate	130	2D	Min	Hypo-osmolar state
Hypertonic saline	130	D	Min	Hypernatremia, hyperchloremia, hypokalemia, pulmonary edema
Fresh frozen plasma	170	30D	5–6 h	Hepatitis, HIV, anaphylaxis
Dextran 70	154	10D	6 h	Renal failure, anaphylaxis, pseudo-hyperglycemia, coagulopathy
Hetastarch	130	10D	12 h	Coagulopathy, congestive heart failure, vomiting, mild hepatotoxicity

Note: D = Hospital-based price

In contrast, early nasogastric (NG) tube feeding in patients with acute gastroparesis increases the risk of aspiration, mortality, ventilator-associated pneumonia (VAP), and *Clostridium difficile* infection.[16]

The main goals of nutritional support are to preserve muscle mass and to provide adequate fluids, vitamins, minerals, and fats. The patients can tolerate extended periods of semistarvation because the body responds to reduced energy intake by reduction of the basal metabolic rate (BMR) and using body fat as the primary fuel. Proteins stored from lean body mass are rapidly mobilized. Fever, leukocytosis, hyperglycemias, hypoalbuminemia, and uremia contribute to a hypermetabolic state. Malnutrition in ICU patients adversely affects pulmonary function by weakening respiratory muscles, decreasing ventilatory drive, and reducing lung defense mechanisms, which hamper weaning. However excess carbohydrate calories (>3,000 kcal/day) lead to hypercapnia, which also results in weaning difficulty.

Caloric needs of the patients have been estimated as 25–30 kcal/kg/day. Nutritional needs in patients with neurologic critical illness should be calculated using the Harris-Benedict equation to obtain the basal energy expenditure (BEE) in calories. The Harris-Benedict formulas are based on kilograms of weight (W), centimeters of height (H), and years of age (A). For men, the formula is:

$$BEE = 66.5 + 13.8W + 5H - 6.8A$$

And, for women, the formula is:

$$BEE = 65.5 + 9.6W + 1.8H - 4.7$$

It is reasonable to add a "stress factor" in patients with an acute CNS event and marked sympathetic manifestations, such as profuse sweating, hyperthermia, hypertension, and tachycardia. Total calories are then calculated by BEE + 20%. In obese patients, 75% of the basal Harris-Benedict calculation seems reasonable.

The estimated energy expenditure is divided into proteins of 1.5 g/kg per day, and the remaining calories are evenly divided between carbohydrates and lipids. Blood glucose should be maintained at a range of 80–110 mg/dL, blood urea nitrogen <100 mg/dL, and triglyceride <500 mg/dL. Measurement of body weight is the simplest way to monitor nutritional status. A severe catabolic state can also be monitored by nitrogen balance which is calculated if the renal function is not changing. Urinary nitrogen is measured in a 24-hour urine collection. The nitrogen balance is calculated as follows: nitrogen balance (g) = (protein intake/6.25) – (urinary nitrogen + 4). Increased nitrogen secretion results in a negative nitrogen balance and more protein must be prescribed.

Aspiration Risk

Swallowing mechanisms can be impaired in CNS infection, head injury, stroke, and in patients with acute neuromuscular disease. Other important risk factors are impaired level of consciousness, vomiting, seizures, obesity, NG feeding, and diabetes-associated gastrointestinal motility disorder.

Aspiration risk is also increased following emergency intubation or extubation or following anesthesia. Aspiration pneumonia can be prevented if patients with abnormal swallowing mechanisms are identified early.

Enteral Nutrition

The integrity of the gut is maintained by enteral feeding and is greatly compromised in parenteral nutrition. The timing of enteral nutrition is not known. However, enteral nutrition is probably required early in patients who are hypermetabolic from the ictus.

Nasogastric tube feeding: It should be given to most patients. NG tube placement may be facilitated by flexion of the neck, lubrication of the tube, Cooling the tube to increase rigidity, the Jarmon technique (filling the nostril with Lidocaine jelly, which enters the posterior pharynx and relaxes the nasal constrictors), and, as a last resort, direct visualization with a laryngoscope and advancement with a forceps. Auscultation of a gurgling sound after pushing air through the tube may not be always reliable and aspiration of the gastric contents confirms the location of the tube in the stomach. Correct placement of the NG tube should be checked by radiography before starting the feeding. Complications of placement of the NG tube are rare. One may consider postpyloric feeding in patients with CNS disorders because gastric atony increases the risk of aspiration. In such patients, nasoduodenal or nasojejunal tubes may reduce the risk of aspiration. Duodenal placement can be tried by inserting a coiled tube that is at least 10 cm more than the calculated length into the stomach and then waiting 24 hours to allow spontaneous advancement past the pylorus. The right lateral decubitus position may facilitate the motion. Another helpful bedside technique, with a 75% success rate, is air insufflation. A 50-mL syringe is used to pump 500 mL of air into the stomach. Tubes that fail to pass may be placed fluoroscopically, and this technique is very successful. Additionally, metoclopramide or erythromycin elixir facilitates transpyloric passage of the tube. Erythromycin (200 mg) given intravenously in patients with a gastric feeding tube may improve nutritional intake, similar to that in patients fed through a tube placed transpylorically, and could be considered in appropriate patients. Enteral feeding should preferably be done by continuous infusion with a volumetric pump. Continuous tube feedings have been associated with a positive nitrogen balance and weight gain more often than intermittent tube feedings. A recent successful protocol started feeding at 25 mL/h and increased the volume by 25 mL/h every 4 hours until the goal of nutrition was achieved. When a gastric residual volume of >250 mL is detected, feeding is held for 4 hours and restarted at the same rate but with a slower increase. A prokinetic agent (metoclopramide or domperidone) may be tried. If this approach is not tolerated and residuals are significant, the tube should be relocated into the jejunum. This can be done on a tilting fluoroscopic table with placement beyond the ligament of Treitz. Continuous administration is essential in jejunal feeding because a rapidly formed bolus of a hyperosmolar solution may cause cramps and diarrhea.

Feeding gastrostomy: The percutaneous endoscopic gastrostomy (PEG) is performed in patients who cannot tolerate NG tubes, who frequently extubate themselves, or who may need long-term enteral feeding. However, NG tubes can be tolerated for months by most patients. PEG placement is much less attractive in patients with a high probability of death or who are severely disabled or if a withdrawal of support is anticipated. Complications of PEG are rare but include bleeding from submucosal vessels of the stomach, local infection, and necrotizing fasciitis, but the morbidity associated with this procedure is low (<10%).

INVESTIGATIONS AND MONITORING

A large number of laboratory tests such as blood counts, culture, chemistry, ABG, radiography, and ultrasonography are regularly done as clinically indicated. Other monitoring tools include Doppler studies, intracranial pressure monitoring, invasive BP monitoring, jugular vein oximetry, brain tissue oximetry, microdialysis, electroencephalography (EEG), and evoked potential monitoring. Many of these have a theoretical basis but have not been validated. The investigations should be considered for their results altering the management, cost, and complications. If the results of a test do not offer clear answer, it should be avoided unless part of a research protocol.

CONCLUSION

Paucity of resources and scarcity of neurocritical care facility necessitate rational and cost-effective approach in LMIC. The admission policy to NICU should be clear and based on probable outcome. In NICU, a teamwork involving neurologists, intensivists, and various medical and surgical specialist nurses and technologist is crucial. The communication in ICU should be clear, honest, and without overoptimism or exaggeration. Care of eye, skin, chest physiotherapy, and prevention of bedsores are crucial. Where indicated, analgesia and sedation should be carefully administered and monitored. Nasal or oral intubation or laryngeal mask ventilation is performed as indicated. Neuromuscular disorders, e.g., GBS, may be considered for MV based on SBC. Stroke, encephalitis, SE meningitis, and encephalopathies are commonly managed in NICU. Burst suppression in refractory SE needs EEG monitoring and is not of proven value. Management of hydration is crucial and N saline is generally recommended. Calories should be maintained as far as possible by enteral feeding through NG tube or feeding gastrostomy. Investigations and monitoring in NICU are crucial and should be rationalized to have a cost-effective approach.

ACKNOWLEDGMENT

We thank Mr Shakti Kumar for secretarial help.

REFERENCES

1. Dewan MC, Rattani A, Gupta S, Baticulon RE, Hung YC, Punchak M, et al. Estimating the global incidence of traumatic brain injury. J Neurosurg. 2018:1-18. Online ahead of print.
2. Misra UK, Kalita J, Betai S, Bhoi SK. Outcome of tuberculous meningitis patients requiring mechanical ventilation. J Crit Care. 2015;30(6):1365-9.
3. Sutter R, Marsch S, Fuhr P, Kaplan PW, Rüegg S. Anesthetic drugs in status epilepticus: risk or rescue? A 6-year cohort study. Neurology. 2014;82(8):656-64.
4. Wijdicks EF, Klein CJ. Guillain-Barré Syndrome. Mayo Clin Proc. 2017;92:467-79.

5. Kalita J, Ranjan A, Misra UK. Outcome of Guillain-Barre syndrome patients with respiratory paralysis. QJM. 2016;109(5):319-23.
6. Kalita J, Kumar M, Misra UK. Serial single breath count is a reliable tool for monitoring respiratory functions in Guillain-Barré Syndrome. J Clin Neurosci. 2020;72:50-6.
7. Kalita J, Kohat AK, Misra UK. Predictors of outcome of myasthenic crisis. Neurol Sci. 2014;35(7):1109-14.
8. Misra UK, Kumar S, Singh VK, Dubey D, Kalita J. Noninvasive ventilation in myasthenia gravis. Neurol India. 2020;68(3):648-51.
9. Wijdicks, Eelco FM. Clinical Practice of Critical Care Neurology, 2nd edition. New York: Oxford University Press; 2003.
10. Parsons MW, Barber PA, Desmond PM, Baird TA, Darby DG, Byrnes G, et al. Acute hyperglycemia adversely affects stroke outcome: a magnetic resonance imaging and spectroscopy study. Ann Neurol. 2002;52(1):20-8.
11. Misra UK, Kalita J. Water as nutrient in health and disease. Neurological Consequences of Nutritional Deficiency, 1st edition. Boca Raton: CRC Press; 2021. pp. 142-64.
12. Young P, Bailey M, Beasley R, Henderson S, Mackle D, McArthur C, et al.; SPLIT Investigators; ANZICS CTG. Effect of a Buffered Crystalloid Solution vs Saline on Acute Kidney Injury Among Patients in the Intensive Care Unit: The SPLIT Randomized Clinical Trial. JAMA. 2015;314(16):1701-10.
13. Finfer S, Bellomo R, Boyce N, French J, Myburgh J, Norton R; SAFE Study Investigators. A comparison of albumin and saline for fluid resuscitation in the intensive care unit. N Engl J Med. 2004;350(22):2247-56.
14. Caironi P, Tognoni G, Masson S, Fumagalli R, Pesenti A, Romero M, et al.; ALBIOS Study Investigators. Albumin replacement in patients with severe sepsis or septic shock. N Engl J Med. 2014;370(15):1412-21.
15. Myburgh JA, Mythen MG. Resuscitation fluids. N Engl J Med. 2013;369(13):1243-51.
16. Ibrahim EH, Mehringer L, Prentice D, Sherman G, Schaiff R, Fraser V, et al. Early versus late enteral feeding of mechanically ventilated patients: results of a clinical trial. JPEN J Parenter Enteral Nutr. 2002;26(3):174-81.

103 CHAPTER

Tumors of the Spine and the Spinal Cord

Tobin George, Ganesh Divakar, Prakash Nair, Easwer HV, Sanjay Behari

INTRODUCTION

Tumors and other space-occupying lesions within the spinal canal can be divided into: (1) those that arise within the substance of the spinal cord, either as a primary neural neoplasm or as metastasis (*intramedullary*), (2) those arising outside the substance of the spinal cord but confined within the dura (*intradural extramedullary*), and (3) those arising from vertebral bodies and epidural tissues (*extradural*). In general, roughly 60% of spinal tumors are extradural, 30% intradural-extramedullary, and 10% intramedullary.[1] A majority of the extradural tumors are metastatic cancers.

EPIDEMIOLOGY

Extradural neoplasms of the spinal canal arise either from primary tumors of the vertebral column or due to metastatic lesions. Primary tumors of the vertebral column may be benign or malignant and account for less than 10% of all spinal tumors and 4–13% of all primary bone tumors.[2] The common benign primary tumors of the spinal column include hemangioma, osteoid osteoma, osteoblastoma, aneurysmal bone cyst, osteochondroma, chondroma, chondroblastoma, and giant cell tumor. The common malignant primary tumors of the spine include chondrosarcoma, Ewing sarcoma, osteosarcoma, and chordomas.

Metastatic tumors of the spine occur more commonly than primary tumors affecting the spine, and may be seen in up to 90% of all cancer patients.[3] Spinal metastases most commonly involve the thoracic spine. The metastatic disease commonly arises from primary cancers of the prostate, breast, lung, kidney, and thyroid cancers. Spinal tumors are uncommon in patients younger than 30 years of age and are typically benign, with the exceptions of Ewing sarcoma and osteosarcoma. In patients older than 30 years of age, they tend to be malignant. Various parts of the vertebra are affected by different tumor types. The vertebral body may be involved by metastatic lesions, multiple myeloma, Langerhans cell histiocytosis, chordoma, giant cell tumor, and hemangioma. Spinal tumors commonly involving the posterior elements of the spine include benign tumors such as aneurysmal bone cyst, osteoblastoma, osteochondroma, and osteoid osteoma. Malignant bony tumors commonly affect the anterior rather than the posterior spinal elements.

Intradural extramedullary (IDEM) tumors constitute around 4–8% of the primary tumors of the spine.[4] Nerve sheath tumors (schwannomas and neurofibromas) and meningiomas are the most common types of IDEM tumors. These tumors account for about 60% of all IDEM tumors, with myxopapillary ependymomas (10%); and rare tumors, including metastases, sarcomas, chordomas, paragangliomas, hemangioblastomas, arachnoid cysts, lipomas, dermoid and epidermoid cysts, teratomas, hemangiopericytomas, and hemorrhages accounting for the remaining 10–15% of IDEM tumors.[5]

Primary intramedullary spinal cord tumors make up 5–10% of spinal tumors in adults and about 35% of spinal tumors in children.[6] Over 80% of these intramedullary tumors are tumors of glial origin. The most common include astrocytomas and ependymomas, along with less common neoplasms such as gangliogliomas, oligodendrogliomas, and subependymomas. In adults, ependymomas account for 50–70% of intramedullary tumors.[7] Astrocytomas, on the other hand, occur more frequently in children under the age of 10 years. The average age at presentation of intramedullary tumors is about 35–39 years, with a slight male preponderance. Other intramedullary tumors of the spinal cord include lipomas, epidermoids, dermoids, teratomas, hemangiomas, hemangioblastomas, chordomas, schwannomas, and intraspinal metastatic carcinomas.

Secondary tumors involving the spinal cord tumors can either be extramedullary or intramedullary in location. Metastases (carcinoma, lymphoma, and myeloma) may affect the spinal cord. They arise from hematogenous deposits or extension of tumors of the vertebral bodies or extensions of paraspinal tumors traversing through the intervertebral foramina. Intradural extramedullary tumors of secondary origin could be due to either meningeal carcinomatosis or lymphomatosis, or rarely, due to spread of primary melanoma of the meninges. Intramedullary metastases are most common due to bronchogenic carcinoma. Imaging with magnetic resonance imaging (MRI) with gadolinium shows extensive contiguous edema.

CLINICAL FEATURES

Patients with spinal cord tumors are likely to present with one of three clinical syndromes which include: (1) compression/destruction of the spinal cord, (2) compression of both the spinal cord and exiting roots, or (3) syringomyelia-like syndrome in intramedullary tumors.

Patients with a spinal tumor most frequently present with back pain. Pain occurs due to the effect of the tumor on nociceptors within the spine. Pain may be worse at night and in recumbency. This phenomenon is due to venous congestion caused by the distension of the epidural venous plexus, which occurs on lying down. Sudden pain which exacerbates on standing and while walking may suggest a pathological fracture. 80–90% of patients with metastatic spinal cord compression have pain as their earliest symptom.[8] More than 75% of primary bone tumors of the spine present with pain, and about half with no other symptoms. About 50% of patients with intradural tumors present with pain which rises to over 80%, for tumors below the conus.[9]

Symptoms caused by compression and less frequently by invasion and destruction of the spinal cord consist of a mixture of (1) an asymmetrical spastic weakness involving the lower limbs in thoracolumbar lesions and both the upper and lower limbs with cervical lesions, (2) a sensory level on the trunk below which sensation of pain and temperature is reduced or lost, (3) dorsal column signs, and (4) a spastic bladder with impaired voluntary control. The onset of the compressive symptoms is usually gradual and occurs over weeks and months, often with back pain. Extradural tumors can present with paralysis that develops over a short period. The initial presentation may involve motor or sensory function, and the distribution may be asymmetrical. High cervical lesions or foramen magnum lesions produce an "around the clock" progression of weakness beginning in one limb and proceeding to the adjacent one in a clockwise or counterclockwise direction. The quadriparesis is associated with weakness and atrophy of the hands and dorsal neck muscles, marked imbalance, and inconsistent sensory changes. There may be signs of cerebellar and lower cranial nerve involvement with lesions. With thoracic lesions, one leg usually becomes spastic before the other one. Posterior column (tingling paresthesias) sensations also assume similar distributions. Pain and thermal senses are more likely to be affected than touch, vibration, and joint position. The bladder and bowel may also be involved with paralysis of the legs. If the compression is relieved, the recovery of sensory and motor symptoms occur in the reverse order of their appearance, where the first part affected is the last to recover, and sensory symptoms tend to improve before motor ones. Lesions at the level of the lowermost thoracic and the first lumbar vertebrae may result in mixed cauda equina and spinal cord symptoms. A Babinski sign indicates that the spinal cord is involved above the fifth lumbar segment.

Spinal cord compression in combination with compression of the sensory nerve root causes radicular pain. The discomfort is described as knife-like with superimposed sharp stabs of pain, which radiates away from the spine, and is intensified by coughing, sneezing, or straining. In addition, there may also be segmental sensory changes (paresthesias, impaired perception of pinprick and touch) or motor disturbances (cramp, atrophy, fascicular twitching, and loss of tendon reflexes) and backache. Tenderness of the spinous processes over the tumor can also be found. Sensory symptoms often precede the signs of spinal cord compression. Rarely, intramedullary tumors of the thoracolumbar cord are associated with hydrocephalus, which is associated with markedly elevated cerebrospinal fluid (CSF) protein. Less often, these tumors are associated with a pseudotumor cerebri syndrome.

Intramedullary tumors, especially those arising from the filum terminale, present with pain. Central cord syndrome or syringomyelia syndrome may occur when the intramedullary tumor involves the central gray matter. The main features are segmental or dissociated sensory loss, amyotrophy, early incontinence, and late corticospinal weakness. Sacral sparing of sensations may be found. Dissociation of the loss of hot and cold sensations and touch sensation over several adjacent segments on the trunk is a consistent sign of an intramedullary lesion. Rarely, an extramedullary tumor may give rise to a syringomyelic sensory syndrome, possibly by causing vascular insufficiency in the central portion of the cord.

BENIGN INTRADURAL EXTRAMEDULLARY TUMORS

Nerve Sheath Tumors

Nerve sheath tumors have an annual reported incidence of 0.3–0.4/100,000 and account for 40% of all intradural spinal cord tumors.[10] In contrast to intracranial and peripheral sites, adult spinal nerve sheath tumors are more common in males. Their peak incidence is in the fourth to sixth decades. These tumors are broadly categorized into schwannomas and neurofibromas. Schwannomas are more common than neurofibromas. These tumors commonly arise from the dorsal nerve roots, though occasionally they arise from the ventral nerve roots as well. Nerve sheath tumors are more commonly intradural in location. They may also present as "dumbbell" tumors that occupy both intradural and extradural compartments. Schwannomas and neurofibromas are difficult to distinguish on neuroimaging. Both are isointense on T1-weighted images, have a high

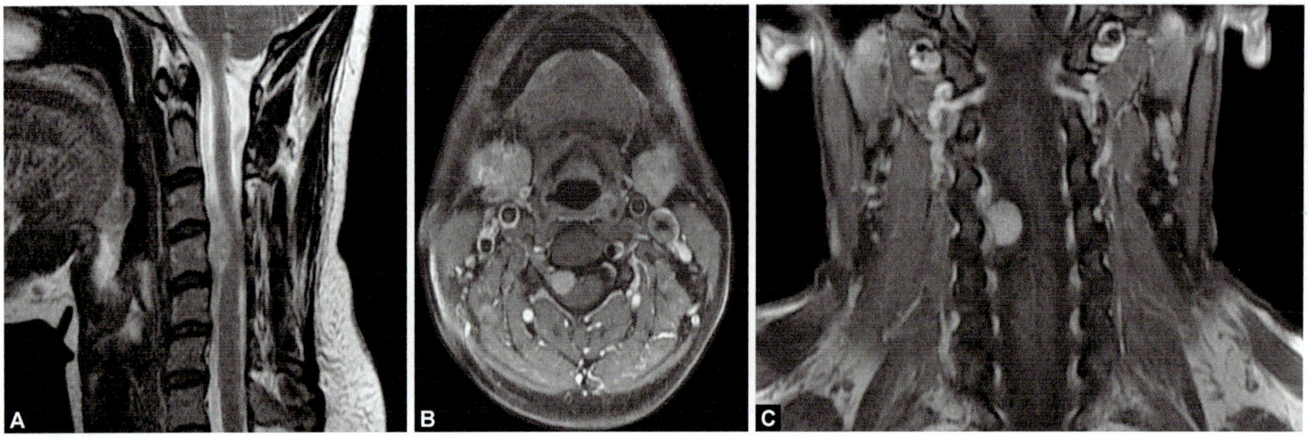

FIGS. 1A TO C: An intradural extramedullary cervical schwannoma that is well-defined with T2-weighted (T2W) hyperintensity, homogenous contrast enhancement and extension into the right neural foramen.

signal on T2-weighted images, and enhance with gadolinium **(Fig. 1)**. Schwannomas are more commonly associated with fatty degeneration, hemorrhage, and cystic change compared to neurofibromas.[11] Occasionally, neurofibromas on T2-weighted images show a "target sign" characterized by a hyperintensity surrounding the lesion's periphery with central hypointensity.

Schwannomas are well-encapsulated lesions that tend to displace the nerve root rather than engulf it. Schwannomas are seen in both patients with neurofibromatosis (NF-2) as well as in patients without neurofibromatosis. *NF-2* gene encodes for a protein called merlin. The loss of expression of this protein results in multiple cranial and spinal schwannomas.[12] Microscopically, these lesions display a bimodal pattern of cellularity with compact, cellular Antoni A areas with palisading Verocay bodies, and less cellular Antoni B areas. Schwannomatosis is a clinical condition in which patients present with multiple schwannomas without vestibular schwannomas. Asymptomatic or minimally symptomatic patients and poor surgical candidates who have spinal tumors with imaging features characteristic of a schwannoma can be followed by interval imaging. Patients with significant or progressive symptoms will need surgical excision of the lesion.

Neurofibromas arising as a result of neurofibromatosis 2 (NF-2) are encapsulated lesions but tend to arise from within the nerve, engulfing it and causing a fusiform enlargement. Plexiform neurofibromas involve multiple nerve roots and have a greater chance for progression in size. Though benign, they have a potential for malignant degeneration. Though they commonly arise from the dorsal nerve roots, they more frequently arise from the ventral roots than schwannomas. They occupy the intervertebral foramina more regularly, giving rise to dumbbell lesions. Two-thirds of these tumors arise in patients with NF-1. The presence of the NF-1 mutation also acts as a risk factor for malignant degeneration.[13] Patients with plexiform neurofibromas should be screened for optic nerve gliomas in addition to NF-1. Histologically, neurofibromas contain all elements of peripheral nerves, namely, Schwann cells with wire-like collagen fibrils, mast cells, Wagner–Meissner corpuscles, Pacinian corpuscles, axons, fibroblasts, and collagen, within a fibromyxoid stroma. The absence of Antoni A areas, along with cytological atypia, differentiates neurofibromas from schwannomas, an exception being ancient schwannomas, which are hypocellular in nature. Indications and modalities of treatment and adjuvant therapy for these lesions are the same as for schwannomas.

Meningiomas

Spinal meningiomas account for 12% of all meningiomas and generally occur between the fifth and eighth decades.[14] They are more common in women (3:1 ratio) as compared to men.[15] These lesions occur more commonly in the thoracic region and infrequently in the lumbosacral region. Incidence of cervical meningiomas is more common in men than in women. NF-2, exposure to radiation and trauma are known to predispose to the formation of spinal meningiomas. Spinal meningiomas in patients younger than 50 years portend a poorer prognosis.[16] Spinal meningiomas are located at the intradural site in 95% of cases. Dural attachment is most common ventrolaterally. Pure ventral and dorsal attachments are rarer. These meningiomas arise from neoplastic changes in the arachnoid cap cells surrounding the spinal cord and nerves, especially the exit zones of nerves and the entry zones of arteries. Histologically, they are similar to intracranial meningiomas, with the psammomatous variety being the most common. Pial penetration is uncommon. On MRI, they show iso- to hypointense signal on T1-weighted images, hyperintense signal on T2-weighted imaging and intense contrast enhancement **(Fig. 2)**. They show a characteristic dural tail and can show calcification.

Complete surgical resection is the primary modality of treatment with adjuvant therapy being reserved for aggressive or recurrent tumors that have only been incompletely excised. Patients with a prior neurological deficit and/or pia/arachnoid invasion seen during surgery

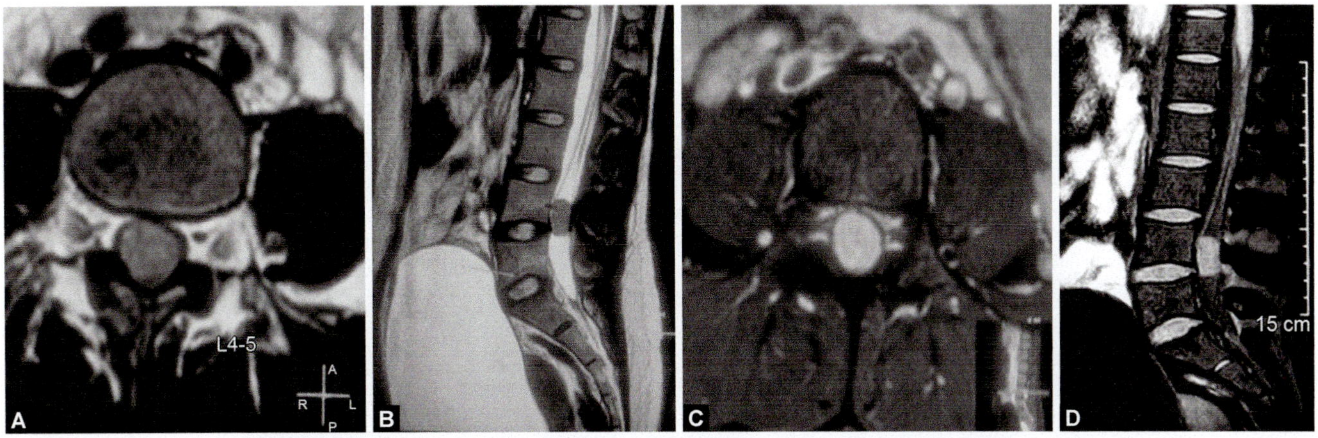

FIGS. 2A TO D: An intradural extramedullary meningioma appearing as a round, dorsal dural based mass with a low signal on T2-weighted (T2W) imaging and homogenously enhancing with contrast.

and those with a long duration of symptoms have worse outcomes.

Myxopapillary Ependymomas

Ependymomas are neoplastic lesions that arise from the ependymal cells lining the ventricles, spinal canal, filum terminale, and the cauda equina. Fifty percent of these ependymomas occur in the intraspinal compartment. The majority of the ependymomas are intramedullary. Myxopapillary ependymoma constitutes around 40% of all ependymomas and occurs in the conus medullaris, cauda equina, and the filum terminale. Myxopapillary ependymomas are World Health Organization (WHO) grade 2 tumors. When myxopapillary ependymomas involve the sacral roots, they can be extradural in location. They are more common in males and occur in the third decade.[17] These tumors tend to recur and disseminate via CSF following resection.

Histologically, the tumor displays a papillary arrangement of cuboidal cells, along with pools of extravasated mucin in the fibrovascular cores. On immunohistochemistry, these cells show positivity for glial fibrillary acidic protein (GFAP) and vimentin. Gross total excision is the gold standard of treatment. These tumors do not respond well to radiation and have a higher rate of recurrence in children.[18]

INTRAMEDULLARY TUMORS

The vast majority of intramedullary spinal cord tumors are ependymomas (60–70%) and astrocytomas (30–40%). Hemangioblastoma (3–8%), metastasis, ganglioglioma, epidermoid, lymphoma, germinoma, and melanoma are other relatively rare intramedullary spinal cord tumors.[19]

Ependymoma

The most common intramedullary spinal cord tumor in adults is the ependymoma, a slow-growing tumor with regular margins, originating from the ependymal cells lining the central canal of the spinal cord. One-third of CNS ependymomas are seen in the spine, of which 40% are extramedullary and arise from the filum terminale. The updated fourth edition of the WHO classification of CNS tumors (2016) enlisted three WHO grades for different types of ependymomas (1) subependymoma (WHO grade 1), (2) myxopapillary ependymoma (WHO grade 2), (3) classic ependymoma with its histological subtypes— (a) cellular, (b) papillary, (c) clear cell, and (d) tanycytic (WHO grade 2), (4) anaplastic ependymoma (WHO grade 3), and (5) ependymoma, RELA fusion-positive (WHO grade 2/3).[20]

The recent fifth edition of the WHO classification of CNS tumors (WHO 2021) has incorporated significant changes by including the molecular characteristics of ependymal tumors, as there was a poor association between the existing tumor grading system and outcome.[21] Methylome profiling data allows further separation of ependymal tumors based on anatomic site, viz., posterior fossa, supratentorial, and spinal cord ependymomas with distinct clinicopathological outcomes and therapeutic strategies. Accordingly, spinal cord ependymomas are divided into myxopapillary (most common type), classic, and rare subependymomas. A rarer, aggressive type characterized by early dissemination throughout the neuraxis, an anaplastic morphology and MYCN amplification with the poor outcome has also been reported. In contrast to the older classification, myxopapillary ependymomas are designated WHO grade 2 based on clinical behavior; and subtypes cellular, papillary, clear cell, and tanycytic are no longer included in the classification of classic ependymoma.[22]

On MRI, ependymoma appears hyperintense on T2 and hypo- to isointense to the cord on T1-weighted images with heterogenous contrast enhancement and occasional areas of cystic change, hemorrhage, necrosis, and/or calcification **(Fig. 3)**. Most often, they are centrally located, causing focal symmetric expansion of the cord with intramedullary polar cysts rostral and caudal to the lesion. In about a third of cases, T2-weighted imaging may show a cap sign due to a hypointense rim caused by hemosiderin deposition.

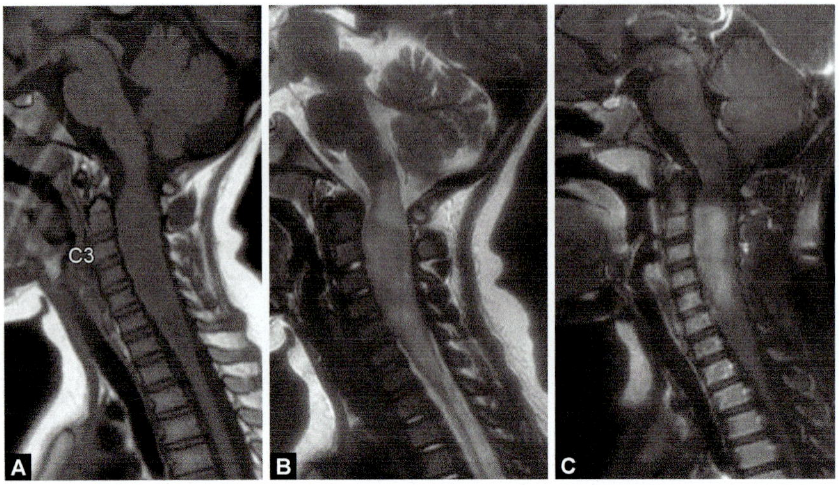

FIGS. 3A TO C: Intramedullary ependymoma (A) sagittal T1, (B) T2, and (C) contrast-enhanced images showing a well-defined cervical intramedullary lesion with homogenous contrast enhancement and expansion of the cord. Note the polar cysts located rostral and caudal to the enhancing lesion.

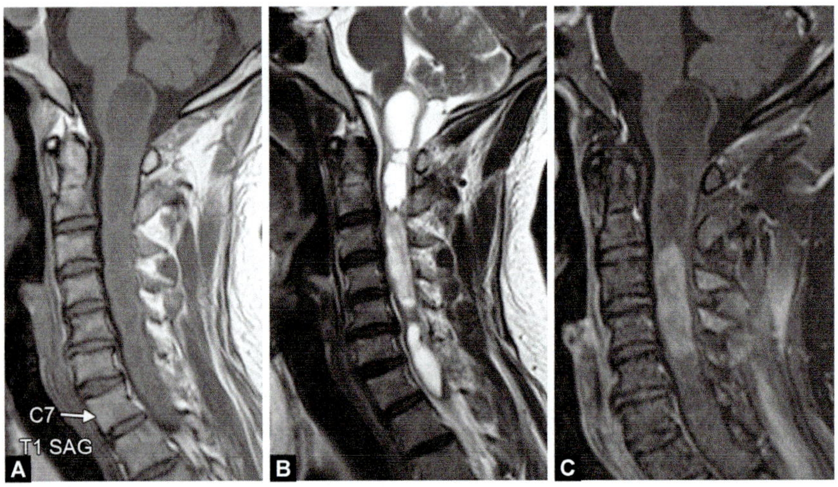

FIGS. 4A TO C: Intramedullary astrocytoma (A) sagittal T1, (B) T2, and (C) contrast enhanced images showing a diffuse irregular lesion with nonhomogenous contrast enhancement and focal expansion of the cord.

Complete surgical excision of the tumor is the treatment of choice and except for rare anaplastic variants, spinal cord ependymomas follow a benign predictable course.[23] Even though complete excision cannot be achieved in some cases due to the presence of a poor plane with the surrounding spinal cord, in general, these tumors have a prolonged progression-free and overall survival (82 and 180 months respectively). The prognosis depends on the extent of resection and the histological type. Fractionated external-beam radiotherapy to a cumulative dose of 54 Gy is indicated for subtotally resected or malignant tumors; craniospinal irradiation can be considered for patients with rare disseminated or metastatic disease.[24]

The role of chemotherapy in spinal ependymomas is unclear. It may be used in recurrent cases as salvage therapy when both surgery and radiotherapy fail. Few studies have reported the usage of carboplatin and etoposide in such cases.

Astrocytoma

Astrocytomas constitute 40% of adult spinal intramedullary tumors of which the majority (75%) are low-grade astrocytomas with 5-year survival rates exceeding 70%. High-grade gliomas are less common and are associated with a poor survival. Astrocytomas are the most common intramedullary spinal cord tumors seen in children (60%) and tend to be pilocytic astrocytomas (WHO grade 1), which are well-circumscribed and often cystic with an indolent pattern of growth.[19]

Magnetic resonance imaging shows the fusiform expansion of the cord with an irregular lesion, which is hypointense to isointense on T1, and hyperintense on T2-weighted images, with variable and often patchy contrast enhancement **(Fig. 4)**. Sometimes, there may be an intratumoral cystic component, associated edema or syrinx;

hemorrhage is seen less often than in ependymomas. Juvenile pilocytic astrocytomas are usually well-circumscribed solid enhancing lesions; or, cystic with an enhancing mural nodule.

As most spinal cord astrocytomas are infiltrative lesions, complete excision is often not feasible except for pilocytic astrocytomas. There is controversy regarding the optimal extent of resection and adjuvant therapy. Generally, adjuvant radiotherapy is given for high-grade histology, tumors that have been partially resected or only biopsied, and those with disease progression following surgery.

Adjuvant radiotherapy should be avoided in pilocytic astrocytoma as it is not found to improve overall survival rates. It is recommended that other low-grade astrocytomas be treated up to a total dose of 5,040 cGy in 180 cGy fractions over 28 treatment days; and, high-grade astrocytomas treated to a total dose of 5,400 cGy in 180 cGy fractions. In those patients with disease progression following radiotherapy, chemotherapy may be considered though its utility is not substantial. Temozolomide is the chemotherapeutic agent used most often, other agents being lomustine, carboplatin, and vincristine.[24]

Hemangioblastoma

Hemangioblastomas are the most common nonglial intramedullary spinal cord tumors. Around 15–25% of patients with hemangioblastoma of the spinal cord have the von Hippel–Lindau (VHL) syndrome, an autosomal dominant disorder caused by a deletion in chromosome 3p.[25] These WHO grade 1 tumors can be found throughout the central nervous system (CNS) and, apart from the spinal cord, are most frequently encountered in the cerebellum. These tumors are predominantly found in males and occur during the fourth decade of life. In addition to the usual symptomatology of intramedullary tumors, they may also rarely present with subarachnoid hemorrhage or hemorrhage into the substance of the spinal cord causing acute onset paraparesis. On MRI, spinal hemangioblastomas are hypointense on T1-weighted imaging and are T2 iso- to hyperintense with an associated cyst, syrinx, or peritumoral edema due to venous hypertension. They are usually seen on the dorsal aspect of the cord and usually show avid homogenous contrast enhancement. Spinal angiography shows enlarged feeding arteries, intense nodular stains and early draining veins. Hemangioblastoma can be differentiated from ependymoma by the vascular markings on MRI and the presence of tumor hypervascularity with feeding arteries and draining veins on spinal angiogram. It is differentiated from a spinal cord vascular malformation by the presence of associated syrinx and tumor enhancement on MRI.

Surgical resection is the primary treatment modality for these tumors. The presence of well-defined margins permits for total resection and thus surgical cure in these patients. Patients with VHL-associated hemangioblastomas have poorer outcomes, mostly because of multifocal CNS or extra-CNS manifestations of the disease. Excessive intraoperative bleeding, obscuring the operative field, may result in subtotal resections. Though preoperative embolization may be considered to reduce intraoperative blood loss, it may not be feasible in most cases due to the close proximity of feeders to the anterior spinal artery. There is a limited role for radiotherapy and experience with chemotherapy is minimal. Stereotactic radiosurgery is an option for patients with recurrent, unresectable, or multiple tumors, especially in the setting of VHL.

Ganglioglioma

Spinal intramedullary gangliogliomas are exceedingly rare WHO grade 1 tumors. They are slow-growing, glial-neuronal tumors and are almost exclusively seen in children. On MRI, they appear as T1 hypointense; and are heterogeneously hyperintense on T2 images with variable, often patchy contrast enhancement, and may be associated with tumor cysts, scoliosis, and bone scalloping due to long-standing nature of these lesions.

The optimal treatment is maximal surgical resection, and this carries excellent long-term survival with minimal morbidity. Postoperative radiotherapy is not recommended, even in patients who undergo subtotal resection. Rare case reports of anaplastic transformation have been documented. At recurrence, reoperation should be considered, and though radiotherapy is also an option, it is not usually given as these lesions predominantly affect children.

Lymphoma

Primary intramedullary spinal cord lymphoma is a rare lesion especially seen in immunocompromised patients as in human immunodeficiency virus (HIV) infection or in the setting of organ transplant. The most common subtype is the diffuse B-cell type.

On MRI, lymphoma appears as a single or multifocal enhancing lesion. Being a diffuse disease with significant morbidity following surgery, aggressive surgical resection should not be undertaken and treatment should include intravenous or intrathecal methotrexate and radiotherapy.

Germinoma

Primary intramedullary spinal cord germinoma is an extremely rare lesion. Imaging of the entire neuraxis and CSF cytology should be obtained to assess for other sites of the disease. Since germinoma is usually radiosensitive and chemosensitive, surgical treatment is limited to biopsy for histopathological diagnosis, which is followed by radiotherapy in combination with cisplatin or etoposide-based chemotherapy.

TABLE 1: Intramedullary tumors, differential diagnosis, radiological types, and treatment.

Tumors	Incidence	MRI	Treatment
Ependymoma	Most common intramedullary spinal cord tumor in adults	Hyperintense on T2 and hypo- or isointense on T1 with heterogenous contrast enhancement and the presence of polar cysts	• Surgery is treatment of choice • Radiotherapy for recurrent or malignant tumors • Chemotherapy (etoposide and carboplatin) for recurrence–the following radiotherapy
Astrocytoma	Most common pediatric intramedullary spinal cord tumor	• Fusiform expansion with irregular margins • Hypo- to isointense on T1, hyperintense on T2, with variable contrast enhancement	• Maximal safe surgical resection followed by observation or radiotherapy • Radiotherapy is not indicated for pilocytic variant usually seen in children
Hemangioblastoma	Rare, common in patients with von sydrome Hippel–Lindau	Homogenously enhancing, may be having a mural nodule with associated cyst or syrinx	• Total resection is treatment of choice • Preoperative embolization may be considered. There is no role for radiotherapy and experience with chemotherapy is limited • Stereotactic radiosurgery is an option for recurrent or unresectable tumors
Ganglioglioma	Rare, low grade, seen in the pediatric population	• The mixed signal on T1, hyperintense on T2, with variable patchy enhancement • Bony deformity and/or bone erosion/ scalloping may be seen	Maximal surgical resection. Postoperative radiotherapy is not recommended, even in patients with subtotal resection
Lymphoma	Rare, seen in immunocompromised patients	Single or often multifocal, ill-defined T2 hyperintense lesions with homogenous contrast enhancement	Intravenous or intrathecal methotrexate-based chemotherapy
Germinoma	Extremely rare	Uniform contrast enhancing	Radiotherapy alone or in combination with chemotherapy

Melanoma

Melanoma can rarely arise in the substance of the spinal cord. On MRI, the tumor is usually hyperintense on T1-weighted images, iso- or hypointense on T2-weighted images with mild contrast enhancement. Intratumoral hemorrhage is common at presentation, leading to a misdiagnosis of cavernous angioma or other vascular malformations. The skin, squamous mucosa, and eyes should be thoroughly examined as it is difficult to distinguish between primary and metastatic tumors. Total surgical resection is curative but often not possible and hence adjuvant radiotherapy is given for most cases. Novel biologics and targeted therapies are promising and have a favorable side effect profile and may be preferable to the administration of cytotoxic chemotherapeutic agents.

Other Rare Tumors

Other rare primary spinal cord intramedullary tumors include teratoma, neurocytoma, dermoid cyst, epidermoid cyst, lipoma, and metastasis **(Table 1)**.

CONCLUSION

A variety of brain tumors affect the spinal cord and their clinical manifestations are varied.

Based on the clinical features and radiological appearance, the histology could be predicted. An early detection and prompt management of these diseases are important in improving the overall prognosis and quality of life.

REFERENCES

1. Van Goethem JWM, van den Hauwe L, Ozsarlak O, De Schepper AMA, Parizel PM. Spinal tumors. Eur J Radiol. 2004;50(2):159-76.
2. Ciftdemir M, Kaya M, Selcuk E, Yalniz E. Tumors of the spine. World J Orthop. 2016;7(2):109-16.
3. Delank KS, Wendtner C, Eich HT, Eysel P. The treatment of spinal metastases. Dtsch Arztebl Int. 2011;108(5):71-9.
4. Mehta AI, Adogwa O, Karikari IO, Thompson P, Verla T, Null UT, et al. Anatomical location dictating major surgical complications for intradural extramedullary spinal tumors: a 10-year single-institutional experience. J Neurosurg Spine. 2013;19(6):701-7.
5. Engelhard HH, Villano JL, Porter KR, Stewart AK, Barua M, Barker FG, et al. Clinical presentation, histology, and treatment in 430 patients with primary tumors of the spinal cord, spinal meninges, or cauda equina. J Neurosurg Spine. 2010;13(1):67-77.
6. Mechtler LL, Nandigam K. Spinal cord tumors: new views and future directions. Neurol Clin. 2013;31(1):241-68.

7. Duong LM, McCarthy BJ, McLendon RE, Dolecek TA, Kruchko C, Douglas LL, et al. Descriptive epidemiology of malignant and nonmalignant primary spinal cord, spinal meninges, and cauda equina tumors, United States, 2004-2007. Cancer. 2012;118(17):4220-7.
8. Cole JS, Patchell RA. Metastatic epidural spinal cord compression. Lancet Neurol. 2008;7(5):459-66.
9. Wu YL, Chang CY, Hsu SS, Yip CM, Liao WC, Chen JY, et al. Intraspinal tumors: analysis of 184 patients treated surgically. J Chin Med Assoc. 2014;77(12):626-9.
10. Seppälä MT, Haltia MJ, Sankila RJ, Jääskeläinen JE, Heiskanen O. Long-term outcome after removal of spinal schwannoma: a clinicopathological study of 187 cases. J Neurosurg. 1995;83(4): 621-6.
11. Wein S, Gaillard F. Intradural spinal tumours and their mimics: a review of radiographic features. Postgrad Med J. 2013;89(1054): 457-69.
12. Neurofibromatosis. Conference statement. National Institutes of Health Consensus Development Conference. Arch Neurol. 1988;45(5):575-8.
13. Seppälä MT, Haltia MJ, Sankila RJ, Jääskeläinen JE, Heiskanen O. Long-term outcome after removal of spinal neurofibroma. J Neurosurg. 1995;82(4):572-7.
14. Gottfried ON, Gluf W, Quinones-Hinojosa A, Kan P, Schmidt MH. Spinal meningiomas: surgical management and outcome. Neurosurg Focus. 2003;14(6):e2.
15. Preston-Martin S. Descriptive epidemiology of primary tumors of the spinal cord and spinal meninges in Los Angeles County, 1972-1985. Neuroepidemiology. 1990;9(2):106-11.
16. Cohen-Gadol AA, Zikel OM, Koch CA, Scheithauer BW, Krauss WE. Spinal meningiomas in patients younger than 50 years of age: a 21-year experience. J Neurosurg. 2003;98(3 Suppl):258-63.
17. Landriel F, Ajler P, Tedesco N, Bendersky D, Vecchi E. Multicentric extramedullary myxopapillary ependymomas: Two case reports and literature review. Surg Neurol Int. 2012;3:102.
18. Al-Habib A, Al-Radi OO, Shannon P, Al-Ahmadi H, Petrenko Y, Fehlings MG. Myxopapillary ependymoma: correlation of clinical and imaging features with surgical resectability in a series with long-term follow-up. Spinal Cord. 2011;49(10):1073-8.
19. Grimm S, Chamberlain MC. Adult primary spinal cord tumors. Expert Rev Neurother. 2009;9(10):1487-95.
20. Louis DN, Perry A, Reifenberger G, von Deimling A, Figarella-Branger D, Cavenee WK, et al. The 2016 World Health Organization Classification of Tumors of the Central Nervous System: a summary. Acta Neuropathol. 2016;131(6):803-20.
21. Louis DN, Perry A, Wesseling P, Brat DJ, Cree IA, Figarella-Branger D, et al. The 2021 WHO Classification of Tumors of the Central Nervous System: a summary. Neuro Oncol. 2021;23(8):1231-51.
22. Ellison DW, Aldape KD, Capper D, Fouladi M, Gilbert MR, Gilbertson RJ, et al. cIMPACT-NOW update 7: advancing the molecular classification of ependymal tumors. Brain Pathol. 2020;30(5):863-6.
23. Hussain I, Parker WE, Barzilai O, Bilsky MH. Surgical Management of Intramedullary Spinal Cord Tumors. Neurosurg Clin N Am. 2020;31(2):237-49.
24. Tobin MK, Geraghty JR, Engelhard HH, Linninger AA, Mehta AI. Intramedullary spinal cord tumors: a review of current and future treatment strategies. Neurosurg Focus. 2015;39(2):E14.
25. Lee DK, Choe WJ, Chung CK, Kim HJ. Spinal cord hemangioblastoma: surgical strategy and clinical outcome. J Neurooncol. 2003;61(1): 27-34.

104

CHAPTER

Brain Tumors

Prakash Nair, George C Vilanilam, Easwer HV, Sanjay Behari

INTRODUCTION

The diverse spectrum of human brain tumors extends across more than 100 histological subtypes, with a plethora of clinical features, epidemiological profiles, and prognostic outcomes.[1-3] Over the last two decades, newer imaging techniques have hastened the diagnosis of brain tumors and immunogenetic profiling has offered better prognostication. The incidence of central nervous system (CNS) tumors in India ranges from 5 to 10 per 100,000 population with an increasing trend and accounts for 1.5–2% of all malignancies. The incidence of primary malignant brain tumors worldwide is 3.7 per 100,000 for males and 2.6 per 100,000 for females.[1,2]

The most recent World Health Organization (WHO) classification of CNS tumors (2021, 5th edition) describes a hierarchical taxonomic classification with a site, category, family, type, and subtype for each tumor's unique histogenetic-immunological profile.[3] In the year 2022 as the world's population touches 7.9 billion, the number of people living with brain tumors would also be proportionately higher than ever before. 5-year relative survivals for malignant brain tumors have increased from 23% (1975–1977) to 36% (2009–2015), thereby suggesting better treatment outcomes and survival over the decades[1,4,5] **(Fig. 1)**.

EPIDEMIOLOGY

An uncontrolled proliferation of neural or glial tissue cells within the brain is the hallmark of all primary brain tumors.

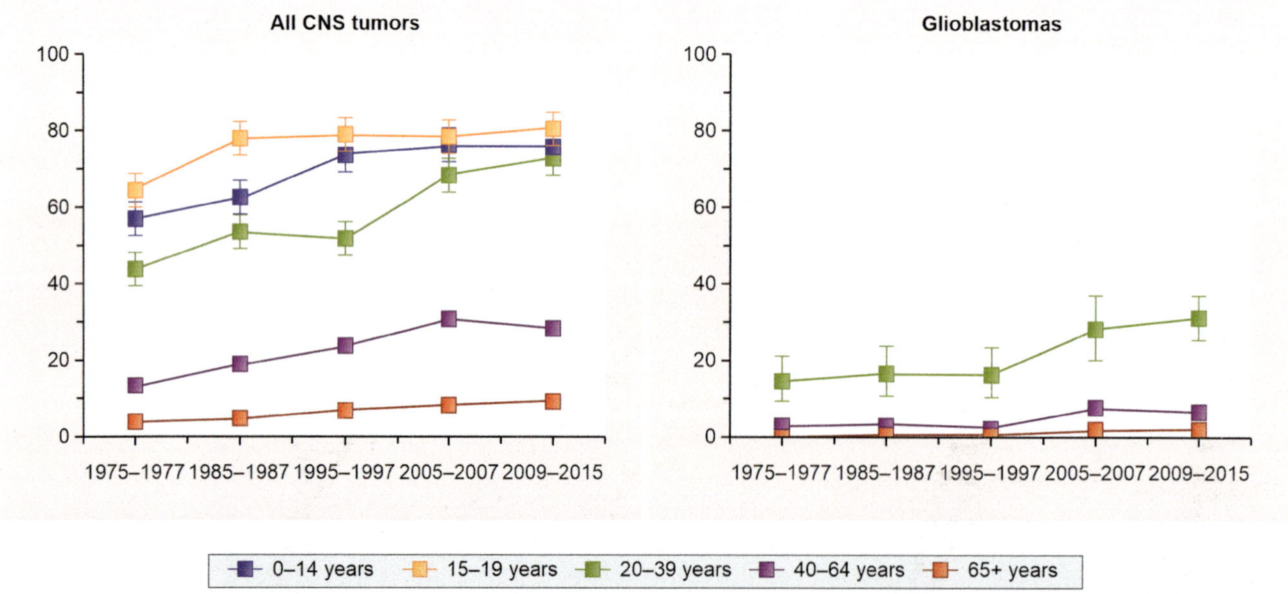

FIG. 1: Trends in 5-year and 3-year relative survival for all malignant brain and other central nervous system (CNS) tumors.

Most are localized tumors, while some disseminate throughout the CNS and become multicentric, they rarely spread outside the neuraxis.

An incidence of 5–10 per 100,000 population of primary brain tumors in India is less than the average incidence in developed countries but slightly above the world average.[5,6] Malignant brain tumors account for approximately 1–2% of all invasive cancer cases in the world, and are the most commonly diagnosed solid tumor in children and adolescents. Brain tumors are the leading cause of cancer death among males aged <40 years. Incidence rates of brain tumors appear to be higher in more developed countries (males, 5.8 and females, 4.1 per 100,000) than in less developed countries (males 3.0 and females 2.1 per 100,000). About 29.7% of primary brain tumors are malignant while 70.3% are benign **(Fig. 2)**. Among the malignant tumors, glioblastoma is most common (48.6%) and meningiomas are most common among the benign tumors (53%) **(Fig. 3)**.[1,5,7]

In India, astrocytomas (38.7%) are the most common primary tumors with the majority being high-grade gliomas (59.5%) **(Fig. 3)**. The median age of glial tumors was seen to be at least a decade earlier than reported in the Western population, which could be partially explained by the lower life expectancy and a higher proportion of the younger population in India Data.[8] The Swedish cancer registry and the Central Brain Tumor Registry of the United States (CBTRUS) suggest that medulloblastoma (MB) (23.5%) and low-grade glioma (31.7%) are the most common type of tumors in pediatric cases aged 15 years and younger **(Fig. 4)**.[1,2]

The WHO classification of brain tumors (2021) assigns brain tumors into one of the following among 13 subgroups—(1) gliomas, glioneuronal tumors, and neuronal tumors, (2) choroid plexus tumors, (3) embryonal tumors, (4) pineal tumors, (5) cranial nerve tumors, (6) meningioma, (7) mesenchymal, nonmeningothelial tumors involving the CNS, (8) melanocytic tumors, (9) hematolymphoid tumors involving the CNS, (10) germ cell tumors, (11) tumors of the sellar region, (12) metastasis to the CNS, and (13) genetic tumor syndromes involving the CNS.[3]

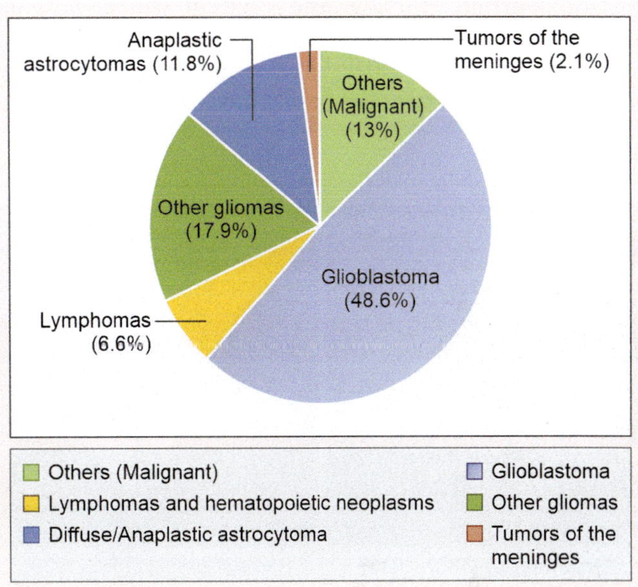

FIG. 3: Malignant brain tumors: Incidence and pathological spectrum.

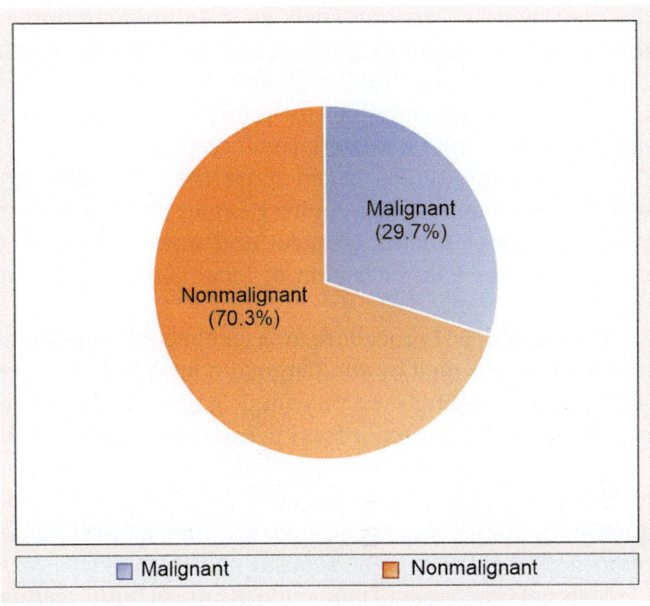

FIG. 2: Brain tumors incidence and pathological spectrum.

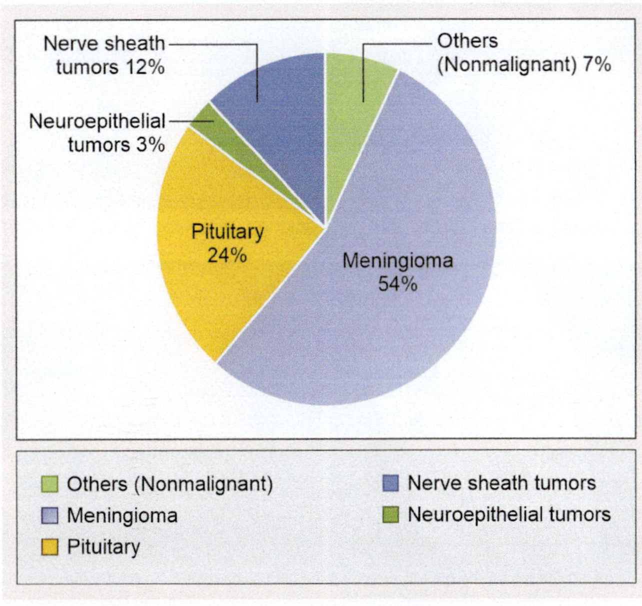

FIG. 4: Benign brain tumors: Incidence pathological spectrum.

HISTORY OF BRAIN TUMOR SURGERY

Since antiquity, brain tumors were considered a sacrosanct territory and thus major developments in this field happened only over the last 150 years. William Macewen of Scotland is considered to have performed the first successful brain tumor resection in 1879 in a young woman with a meningioma.[9,10] On November 25, 1884, Mr Rickman J Godlee performed the first recognized resection of a primary intrinsic brain tumor **(Fig. 5)**. This operation was carried out at the behest of Dr A Hughes Bennett, a neurologist at the hospital for Epilepsy and Paralysis, Regents Park, London. Jackson, Ferrier, Horsley, and Charcot will always be remembered for their contributions to cerebral localization. Harvey Cushing known to be father of modern neurosurgery is credited with advancing brain tumor surgery by using new anesthetic methods, motor-driven suction, and electrosurgical devices.

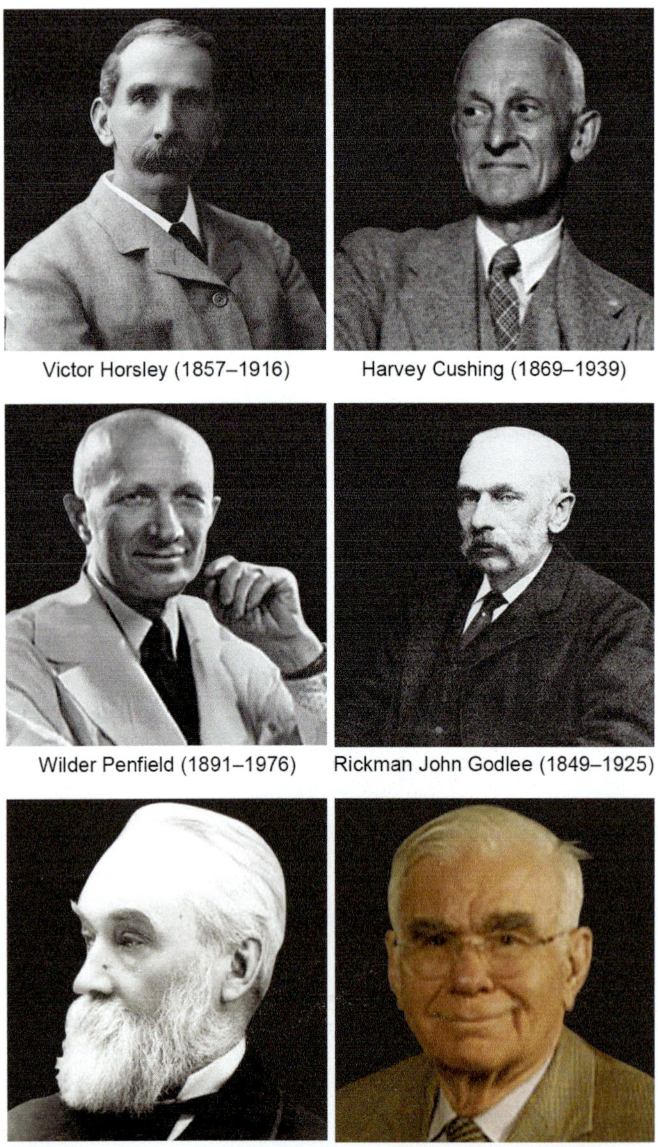

Victor Horsley (1857–1916) | Harvey Cushing (1869–1939)

Wilder Penfield (1891–1976) | Rickman John Godlee (1849–1925)

Hughlings Jackson (1835–1911) | Mahmut Gazi Yaşargil

FIG. 5: Giants from the history of brain tumor surgery.

Dandy's ventriculography aided to better understand brain tumor anatomy and distortions from normal. Egas Moniz's cerebral angiography also helped the diagnosis of brain tumors immensely in the precomputed tomography (CT) scan era. Elsberg, Frazier, and Allen Starr also contributed immensely to developing various aspects of brain tumor surgery.[10]

In 1926, the completed monograph by Bailey and Cushing, "A Classification of the Tumors of the Glioma Group on a Histogenetic Basis with a Correlated Study of Prognosis", was published. This book revolutionized the understanding of neuro-oncology and for nearly a century, the classification of brain tumors has been based on concepts of histogenesis which is the idea that tumors can be classified according to their microscopic similarities with putative cells of origin and their developmental differentiation states. The new edition of the WHO book on "Histological Typing of Tumours of the Central Nervous System" reflects the progress in brain tumor classification which has been achieved since publication of the first edition in 1979. The 2000, 2007, 2016, and 2021 editions of the WHO classifications have further enhanced the understanding of these lesions.[3,9]

Hermann Schloffer of Austria reported the first successful resection of a pituitary tumor via a transsphenoidal approach in 1907. Harvey Cushing further refined the transsphenoidal sublabial approach to the sella and it was further refined by Norman Dott, Gerard Guiot and Jules Hardy subsequently augmented this with the incorporation of the operating microscope paving the way for safe and effective resection of primary suprasellar tumors in the setting of a normal-sized sella, while preserving the healthy pituitary gland. This approach has revolutionized the treatment of lesions such as craniopharyngioma, tuberculum sellae meningiomas, and Rathke cleft cysts. Oldfield, Kato, Laws, Jho, Frank, de Divitiis, Kassam, and Cappabianca further modified the procedure and expanded the spectrum of transsphenoidal endoscopy.

Awake craniotomies began more than 50 years ago when Wilder Penfield and André Pasquet published their landmark paper on the surgical and anesthetic aspect of surgery after administration of local and intermittent sedation with analgesia.[9]

The first surgical procedure for a cerebellopontine angle tumor was performed by von Bergmann in 1890. It was not until Harvey Cushing's era that surgical techniques for the exploration of the posterior fossa became standardized and acoustic tumor excision was associated with an acceptable level of complications and mortality. In 1969, Lars Leksell and Bjorn Meyerson performed the first gamma knife radiosurgical ablation for an acoustic neurinoma.[9,10]

Mahmut Gazi Yaşargil pioneered the use of the operating microscope, popularized the Sylvian fissure dissection and enhanced the safety profile of contemporary brain tumor surgery.[9] Oertel *et al.* found that the perioperative morbidity and mortality rates for brain tumors especially gliomas, as well as the time from diagnosis to treatment have been remarkably reduced over the last 30 years **(Fig. 5)**.[9-12]

RISK FACTORS

Primary brain tumors account for approximately 1% of new cancer cases and approximately 2% of cancer deaths.[11,12] Epidemiological studies have explored numerous potential risk factors, and thus far the only validated associations for brain tumors are ionizing radiation (which increases risk in both adults and children) and history of allergies (which decreases risk in adults). Studies of genetic risk factors have identified 32 germline variants associated with increased risk for these tumors in adults (25 in glioma, 2 in meningioma, 3 in pituitary adenoma, and 2 in primary CNS lymphoma), and further studies are currently under way for other histologic subtypes, as well as for various childhood brain tumors. Though most gliomas are sporadic, about 5% of them are familial and approximately 1–2% of adult and 4% of pediatric brain tumors are due to known neurocutaneous syndromes **(Table 1)**.

The hereditary syndromes associated with brain tumors include neurofibromatosis (NF) type 1 and 2, tuberous sclerosis complex, von Hippel Lindau disease, and the less frequently encountered Cowden's disease, Li-Fraumeni, Turcot's, and Gorlin's syndrome.[13] Demographic factors associated with brain tumor incidence include age, gender, race/ethnicity, and socio economic status. Incidence of brain tumors increases with age and malignant tumors are more frequent in males. They are less common in low socio economic strata and certain ethnic groups.[14]

History of atopic conditions (including asthma, hay fever, eczema, and allergies) leads to reduced glioma risk. The primary hypothesis is that allergic conditions may lead to a heightened state of immune-surveillance, discouraging abnormal cell growth which is responsible for development of a brain tumor. Moderate-to-high doses of radiation are the strongest and most consistently documented environmental risk factor for brain tumors having been independently observed in atomic bomb survivor studies.

The epidemiological evidence does not support an association between nonionizing radiation as in cellular phone use and risk of brain tumors. Nonradiation occupational exposures, dietary habits, and smoking confer no additional risk. A recent meta-analysis found that regular use of aspirin was associated with significantly decreased risk of all gliomas (WHO grades II/III glioma) and glioblastoma. Three studies suggest that regular use of statins may confer a slight reduction in glioma risk.[14]

PATHOLOGICAL SPECTRUM AND TOPOGRAPHICAL DISTRIBUTION

Primary neoplasms of the CNS account for approximately 9% of all primary tumors in the human body. In children, the CNS is the second most common site of primary tumors, and 70% of all intracranial tumors in children are infratentorial.[12] The WHO grading of tumors has been

TABLE 1: Neurocutaneous syndromes.

Type	Gene involved	Inheritance	Common clinical manifestation	Brain tumors
Neurofibromatosis 1	*NF1* gene *Chr17q11.2*	Autosomal dominant	Café au lait spots, neurofibromas, axillary freckling, optic path gliomas, lisch nodules, sphenoid dysplasias, and thinning of long bone cortices	Optic pathway tumors, other brain tumors
Neurofibromatosis 2	*NF2* gene *Chr22q12*	Autosomal dominant	Bilateral vestibular schwannoma, meningioma, glioma, spinal schwannomas, and posterior subcapsular lens opacity	Vestibular schwannoma, meningioma, and ependymoma
Tuberous sclerosis	*TSC1 Chr9q34* *TSC2 Chr16p13*	Autosomal dominant	Cortical tuners/hamartomas, subependymal nodules, SEGA, ash leaf macules, shagreen patch, adenoma sebaceum, mental retardation, and subependymal calcifications	Astrocytoma, cortical tubers, ependymoma, and ganglioneuroma
Sturge–Weber syndrome	*GNAQ* gene *Chr9q21*	Somatic mosaic mutation	Facial angioma/port wine stain, ipsilateral localized cerebral cortical atrophy and calcifications, and tram track calcifications	
Von Hippel–Lindau disease	*VHL* gene *Chr3p25*	Autosomal dominant	Hemangioblastoma (cerebellum/retina/brainstem/cord), pancreatic and renal cysts, RCC, pancreatic NET or serous cystadenoma, and pheochromocytoma	Hemangioblastoma
Ataxia telangiectasia	*ATM* gene *Chr11q22-23*	Autosomal recessive	Multiple capillary telangiectasias, progressive cerebellar atrophy, demyelination, and gliosis	

(NET: neuroendocrine tumor; RCC: renal cell carcinoma; SEGA: subependymal giant cell astrocytoma)

used primarily for gliomas though extended to certain other tumors as well. Grade I lesions are generally tumors with less proliferative potential and the possibility of cure after complete surgical resection. Grade II lesions are usually infiltrative in nature and often recur, in spite of having low levels of proliferative activity. Grade II diffuse astrocytoma holds the risk of transformation to grade III anaplastic astrocytoma and glioblastoma. They also have a clear histological evidence of malignancy, including nuclear atypia and sometimes brisk mitotic activity. The grade IV designation is applied to cytologically malignant, mitotically active, necrosis-prone neoplasms that are often associated with rapid pre- and postoperative disease evolution and poorer outcomes.[3,11,12] Glioblastoma and most embryonal neoplasms are examples of grade IV lesions. Infiltration of surrounding tissues and a propensity for craniospinal dissemination characterize many grade IV neoplasms, although these features are not essential. Among gliomas, the frontal lobe is the most predominant site of involvement (30%) with the temporal lobe being the next common site (23%) **(Fig. 6)**. Other histological variants like oligodendroglioma and anaplastic astrocytoma also affect the frontal lobe more often.

CLINICAL PROFILE

A long symptom-diagnosis time is often characteristic of brain tumors affecting the noneloquent cortex and benign brain tumors. Often, benign lesions due to their indolent nature may present with gradual progression of symptoms **(Fig. 7)**.[15-17]

At an initial stage, especially in low-grade tumors, most symptoms are focal depending on the localization of the lesion. More generalized symptoms including headache, nausea and vomiting develop when tumor size increases and results in increased intracranial pressure.

In a large series of brain tumors (Alther et al.), seizures were the most common initial symptom (33%), followed by headaches (19%), sensory disturbances (10%), cognitive impairment (10%), ataxia (6%), visual disturbances (6%),

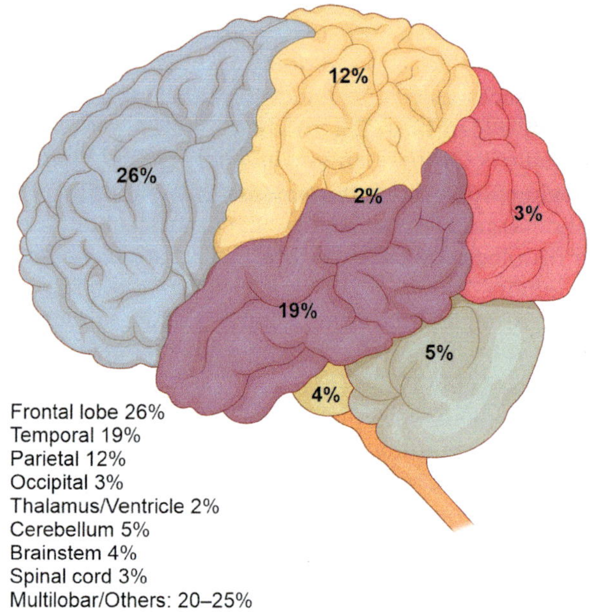

FIG. 6: Topographic distribution of gliomas.

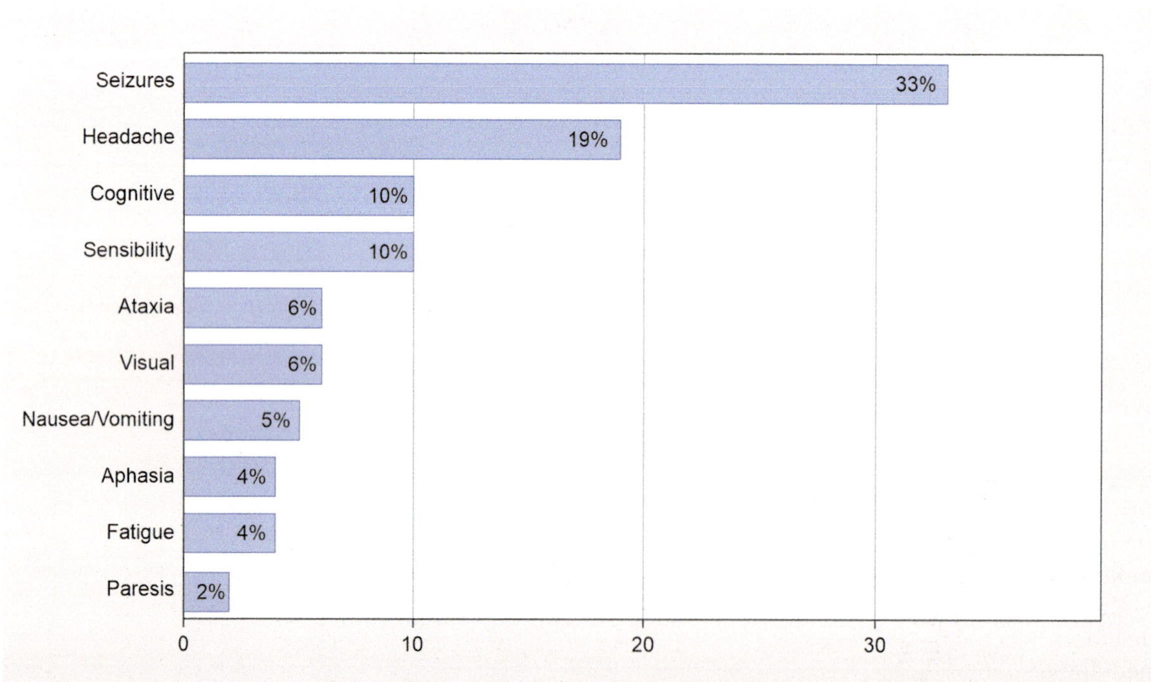

FIG. 7: Frequency of initial and subsequent signs and/or symptoms of primary brain tumors.

and nausea/vomiting (5%). During the time course until diagnosis, the most common symptoms were headaches (28%), cognitive loss/personality change (28%), sensory disturbances (27%), and nausea/vomiting (25%), followed by seizures (20%), visual disturbances (18%), ataxia (17%), fatigue (15%), aphasia (7%), motor weakness (6%), and appetite loss (4%) **(Fig. 7)**.[15]

The positive predictive value of headache for adult patients with brain tumors is low (0.09% overall but 0.12% in 60- to 69-year olds) as compared to new-onset seizure (1.2%). Headaches associated with brain tumors are frequently of "tension" type or mimic migraine and the "red flags" include increasing frequency and severity of headache (e.g., worsening with cough or bending, nocturnal headaches, or headaches on awakening). Compared to seizures and nausea, the time to diagnosis interval remains relatively long for headaches as first symptom (59 days). With the advent of newer magnetic resonance imaging (MRI) sequences and more frequent imaging for unrelated symptoms, several incidental brain tumors are being diagnosed in the contemporary era.[16,17]

INVESTIGATIONS

Imaging Modalities

Computerized Tomography

Computerized tomography (CT) is often used as the initial imaging modality when raised intracranial pressure is suspected. CT imaging has advantages of rapid image acquisition, and is the modality of choice in cases of suspected intracranial hemorrhage or hydrocephalus. Presence of calcification may also give clues for suspecting certain brain tumors like oligodendroglioma.

Magnetic Resonance Imaging (Table 2)

The imaging modality of choice for evaluating a brain tumor is the MRI with gadolinium used as a contrast agent. MRI provides anatomical information about the location of the lesion as well as to extension into adjacent spaces. Certain MRI sequences like the diffusion-weighted sequence (DWI), MR perfusion, and MR spectroscopy can be used to understand aspects like the tumor cellularity, blood flow, and tumor vascularity as well as metabolism and cell turnover within the tumor **(Figs. 8 and 9)**. This information can be used to distinguish neoplastic lesions from non-neoplastic lesions, inflammatory, or infective conditions. For instance, an epidermoid in the intracranial compartment shows diffusion restriction, an imaging characteristic that can be used to distinguish it from other tumors like schwannomas, which do not show diffusion restriction. MRI also aids in planning biopsies, especially when stereotactic biopsy is being planned. For malignant tumors like the medulloblastoma or an anaplastic ependymoma, craniospinal MRI can be performed to identify tumor dissemination in the spinal subarachnoid space (drop metastasis) **(Figs. 10A to C)**. In patients who have undergone cranial irradiation, MRI provides an imaging basis for assessing response to treatment. Post-treatment changes like radiation necrosis can be differentiated from tumor progression using MR spectroscopy **(Figs. 11A to C)**.

In cases where imaging diagnosis is a metastatic tumor, systemic screening for a primary should be performed. This includes a detailed physical examination, as well a chest and abdomen CT should be done.

Functional MRI imaging can be used for preoperative localization of eloquent cortex (speech and motor activity) provides invaluable information about the relationship of a tumor with the eloquent areas, this information can be used to planning the surgical procedure and the extent of resection.

Systemic Imaging

Positron Emission Tomography Scan

Positron emission tomography (PET) scan is based on the principle that fluorodeoxyglucose (FDG) which like glucose can be transported into brain tissue but only partially metabolized. FDG, hence, accumulates in the brain and its rate of uptake can be used to assess the metabolic function of brain tissue. For instance, malignant brain tumors have increased glucose metabolism compared to normal brain tissue and show greater FDG uptake compared to normal brain tissue. This information can be used to target certain high uptake areas for stereotactic biopsy, diagnose tumor recurrence, and differentiate tumor progression from radiation necrosis **(Figs. 11A to C)**.

MANAGEMENT BASED ON TUMOR TYPE

Pilocytic Astrocytomas

Microsurgical resection remains the primary modality of treatment for pilocytic astrocytomas. Radical resection in cases where it is feasible is recommended. Patients in whom gross total tumor resection is possible, 5-year overall survival is in the range of 90–95%.[18] This may not always be possible, especially in areas like the brainstem or the optic pathway, when compared to a gross total resection. Due to the circumscribed nature of pilocytic astrocytomas, imaging follow-up is recommended for the residual tumor.

Low-grade Gliomas

Low-grade gliomas are divided into diffuse fibrillary astrocytomas and oligodendrogliomas. Early and maximal safe resection is the initial treatment for those patients. The 2021 WHO update classifies low grade gliomas into three subgroups based on isocitrate dehydrogenase (IDH)1/2 mutation and 1p/19q codeletion status.[19] IDH mutant and 1p/19q codeleted tumors (oligodendrogliomas) hold the

TABLE 2: MRI features of brain tumors.

Lesion	T1	T2	Contrast	Spectroscopy	Perfusion (rCBV values)	DWI
Grade 1 astrocytoma	Cystic—hypointense	Cystic—hyperintense	Only wall of cyst	NA	Reduced	
	Solid—isointense	Solid—hyperintense	Heterogeneous enhancement	Reduced NAA and choline peak	Normal or reduced	
Grade 2 astrocytoma	Hypointense	Hyperintense	Nil	Reduced NAA and choline peak	Normal or reduced	
Grade 3 astrocytoma	Hypointense	Heterogeneous hyperintense	Heterogeneous enhancement	Reduced NAA and high choline peak	Increased	
Grade 4 astrocytoma	Hypointense	Hyperintense	Heterogeneous enhancement	Marked reduction of NAA and high choline peak	Marked increase	
Gliomatosis cerebri	Hypointense	Hyperintense	Nil or minimal enhancement	Reduced NAA and increased myoinositol peak	Low	
Tumor necrosis	Hypointense	Hyperintense	Nil	Reduced NAA and lipid-lactate peaks	Low	
Tumefactive demyelination	Hypointense	Hyperintense	Open ring enhancement[1]	Reduced NAA, increased choline, increased beta, gamma glutamate/glutamine (β, γ-Glx)	Low	
Oligodendroglioma	Hypointense	Heterogeneous hyperintense	Heterogeneous enhancement	High choline	Increased (irrespective of grade)	
Ependymoma[2]	Iso/hypointense	Iso/hyperintense	Heterogeneous	Reduced NAA and increased choline	Increased	Patchy restriction
Meningioma[1]	Iso/hypointense	Variable	Early, diffuse, and marked	Alanine peak and Absent NAA peak	Increased	Nil
Primary CNS lymphoma	Immunocompetent					
	Iso/hypointense	Iso/hypointense	Homogenous	Increased choline and lipid peak	Increased (but lesser values than glioma)	Present
	Immunocompromised[3]					
	Iso/hypointense	Iso/hypointense	Peripheral enhancement	Increased choline and lipid-lactate peak	Peripheral increase	Peripheral
Central neurocytoma	Isointense	Hyperintense with bubble like appearance	Variable enhancement	Strong choline peak and glycine peak	Normal or mild increase	Present (solid part)
Metastasis	Iso/hypointense	Heterogeneous hyperintense	Ring like	Choline peak	Increased	Nil

(CNS: central nervous system; MRI: magnetic resonance imaging; NAA: N-acetylaspartate; rCBV: relative cerebral blood volume; DWI: diffusion-weighted imaging)

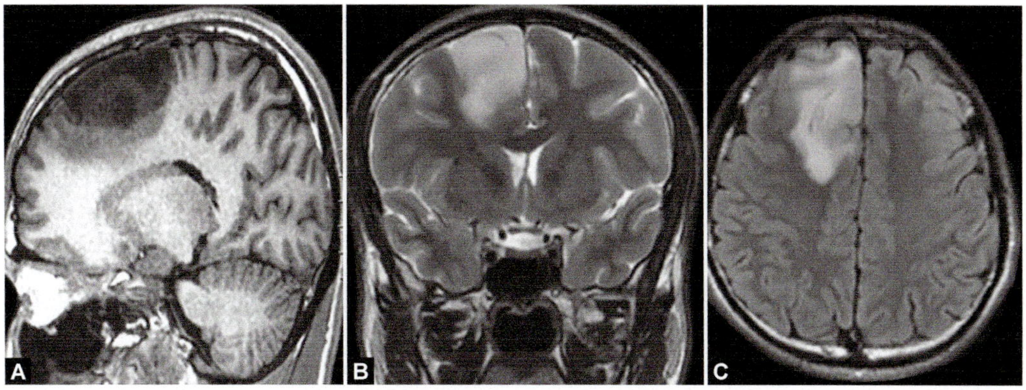

FIGS. 8A TO C: Right medial frontal glioma—(A) sagittal T1, (B) coronal T2, and (C) axial T2 fluid-attenuated inversion recovery (FLAIR).

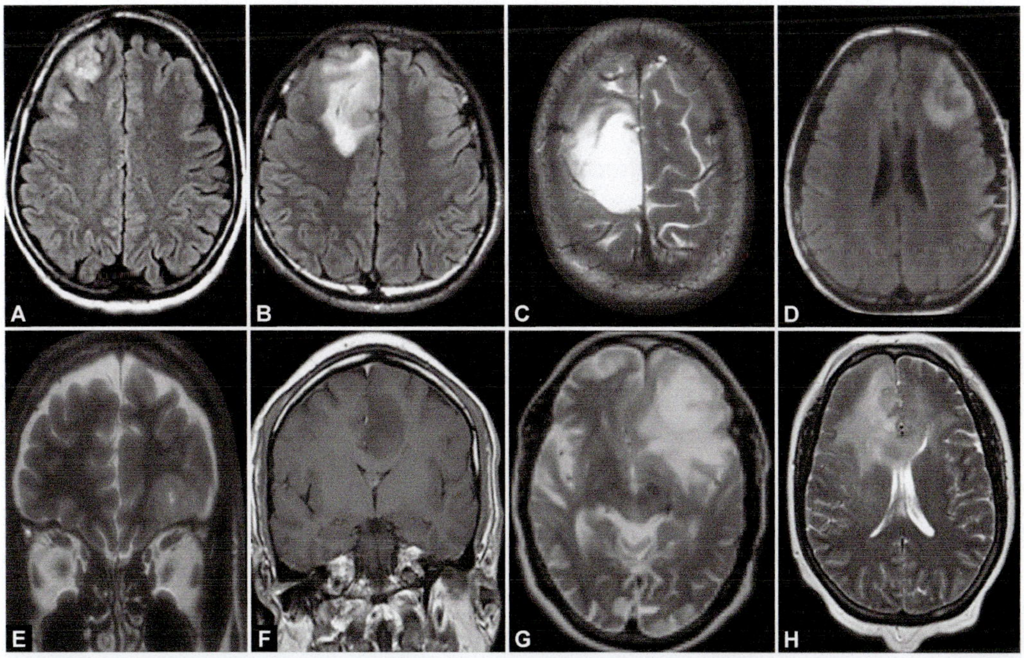

FIGS. 9A TO H: Various types of brain involvement in glioma—(A) right frontal polar, (B) right medial frontal, (C) right motor cortex (Rolandic), (D) left perisylvian, (E) left basifrontal, (F) left cingulate, (G) diffuse (frontoinsular), and (H) diffuse callosal (Butterfly).

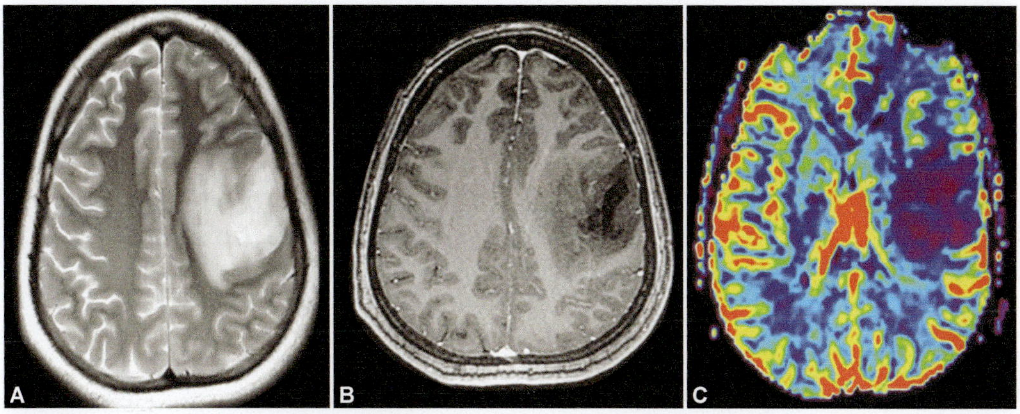

FIGS. 10A TO C: 25-year old male (left frontoparietal glioma)—(A) axial T2, (B) axial contrast, (C) MR perfusion (indicating the blood flow into the tumor).

best prognosis, followed by IDH mutant and 1p/19q intact tumors, and by IDH wild-type tumors.[20] Gliomas which are IDH wild type are now considered high-risk tumor and are classified as IDH wild-type glioblastoma.[19]

Diffuse high-grade gliomas which include WHO grade 3 anaplastic astrocytomas and anaplastic oligodendrogliomas and WHO grade 4 tumors are treated with maximal safe surgical resection followed by radiation and chemotherapy. In patients with good performance status [Karnofsky Performance Status (KPS) ≥60], radiation dose of 60 Gy over 6 weeks with concurrent daily temozolomide, followed by at least six cycles of adjuvant temozolomide (5 days over 21 days cycle) is usually administered. In glioblastoma patients aged older than 70 years who may not tolerate the conventional 6 week radiotherapy regimen, hypofractionated radiation doses over a 3 week course with concurrent and adjuvant temozolomide was recently shown to be superior to hypofractionated radiotherapy alone. The European Organization for Research and Treatment of Cancer/National Cancer Institute of Canada trial demonstrated a survival benefit for glioblastoma patients who received concurrent temozolomide with postoperative radiation (Stupp protocol), with median survival of 14.6 months for those receiving concurrent therapy versus 12.1 months for those who received radiotherapy alone **(Table 3)**.

Brain Metastasis

Brain metastasis develops in nearly 30% of patients with solid tumors, the incidence has increased over the past two decades with longer patient survival, increased access to healthcare, and improved brain imaging techniques. The most common metastasis to the brain, include cancers of the lung, breast, and malignant melanoma. Metastasis from melanomas, choriocarcinomas, thyroid cancers, and renal cell carcinoma (RCC) have a greater incidence of hemorrhage within the metastasis. Patients with cerebral metastasis may present with clinical features of mass effect, local brain edema, and seizures or may be detected incidentally during CNS imaging. Corticosteroids and antiepileptics are used to treat a patient who has brain edema or seizures. Steroids can be tapered over 10–14 days to avoid medical issues related to steroid overuse. Surgery relieves mass effect due to large metastasis and also establishes the histology of the lesion. In patients with good KPS where the extracranial disease is controlled, resection of a single

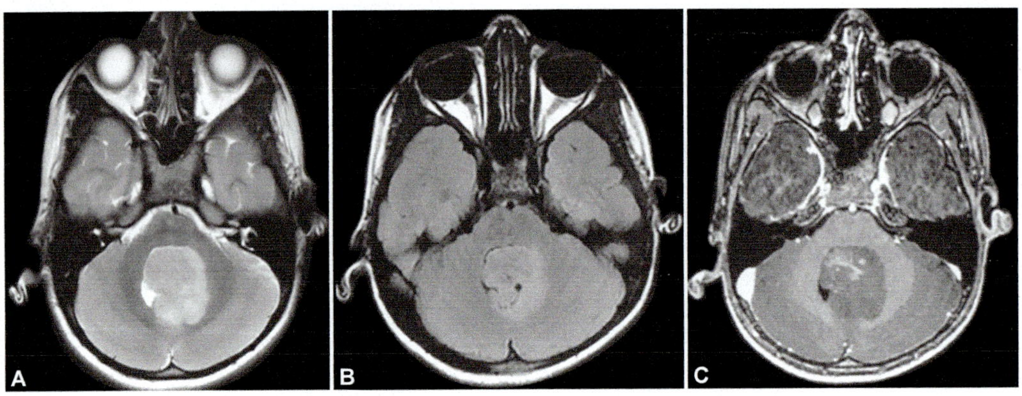

FIGS. 11A TO C: 4-year-old male presenting with a posterior fossa vermian medulloblastoma—(A) MRI T2 axial, (B) MRI T2 FLAIR axial, and (C) MRI axial contrast.

TABLE 3: Primary brain tumors: Survival statistics.

	5-year relative survival rate		
	Age		
Type of tumor	**20–44**	**45–54**	**55–64**
Low-grade (diffuse) astrocytoma	73%	46%	26%
Anaplastic astrocytoma	58%	29%	15%
Glioblastoma	22%	9%	6%
Oligodendroglioma	90%	82%	69%
Anaplastic oligodendroglioma	76%	67%	45%
Ependymoma/anaplastic ependymoma	92%	90%	87%
Meningioma	84%	79%	74%

brain metastasis improves the overall survival of the patient. In brain metastasis that have a clear plane of demarcation between tumor and normal tissue, an en-bloc resection of the capsule is usable possible, however, this may not be feasible in eloquent areas of the brain or in the skull base where the tumor may have to resected piecemeal. Adjuvant whole-brain radiotherapy (WBRT) following surgical resection decreases the risk of local recurrence and intracranial disease progression following surgery. WBRT is also associated with the risk of long-term complications such as cognitive decline, amnesia, and leukoencephalopathy.

Ependymoma

The primary treatment modality for ependymoma is surgical resection. Grade I ependymomas are noninfiltrative and are curable by gross total resection. In cases where the resection is sub-total, close imaging follow up is needed.

Postoperative radiotherapy is usually employed in adult patients with subtotally resected intracranial grade II ependymomas. For intracranial grade III ependymomas (irrespective of the extent of resection), radiation is needed to decrease the risk of recurrence. Spinal ependymomas that have undergone subtotal resection usually require radiation.

Meningioma

Surgical resection remains the modality of choice for treatment of meningiomas. The incidence of recurrence of meningiomas following surgical resection is influenced by the extent of resection, site of occurrence of the meningioma, and the grade of the tumor. The extent of surgical resection is graded using the Simpson's grade. Overall tumor recurrence rates for Simpson resection grades I, II, III, and IV were 5%, 22%, 31%, and 35%.[21] Skull base meningiomas or parasagittal meningiomas that involve the wall of the sagittal sinus are difficult to resect completely and have a greater incidence of recurrence following surgery when compared to convexity meningiomas **(Figs. 12A and B)**. The histological grade of the meningioma also determines the risk of long-term recurrence, WHO grade 2 meningiomas which include atypical, choroid, and clear cell meningiomas and WHO grade 3 meningiomas which include anaplastic, rhabdoid, and papillary meningioma all have a greater incidence of recurrence following surgery.[19]

Adjuvant Treatment for Meningiomas

Adjuvant radiation therapy following surgical resection of an intracranial meningioma is indicated for WHO grade 2 and grade 3 meningiomas or following partial resection of a meningioma where radical resection may be associated with significant morbidity or in recurrent tumors when repeat surgery may be associated with greater morbidity. Stereotactic radio surgery (SRS) is utilized following surgery to address residual tumors <3 cm or in areas that are difficult to access like the cavernous sinus.

Pituitary Adenomas

Pituitary adenomas may be either nonfunctioning tumors (without features of hormone hypersecretion) or may secrete hormones and present with clinical features of hormonal excess (acromegaly and Cushing's disease). Prolactin secreting pituitary adenoma demonstrates elevated prolactin levels and responds dramatically to pharmacological treatment with dopaminergic agonists like cabergoline and bromocriptine. Other functional tumors (acromegaly, Cushing's disease, and thyrotropinoma) need to be resected to normalize hormonal excess and minimize the physiological morbidity that results from the hypersecretion of hormones. Nonfunctioning pituitary adenomas (NFPA) need surgical resection to relieve mass effect on optic chiasm (bitemporal hemianopia) **(Figs. 13A to C)**. In some patients, a pituitary adenoma may develop acute apoplexy within the adenoma resulting in either extraocular palsy or visual deterioration, altered sensorium, and signs of

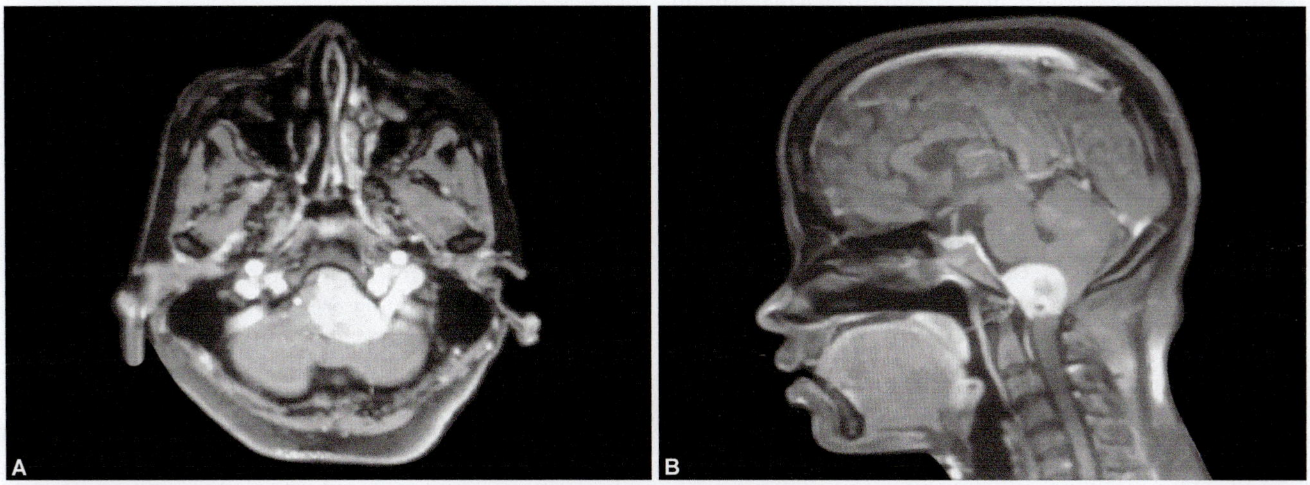

FIGS. 12A AND B: 48-year-old male with a foramen magnum meningioma—(A) MRI-axial contrast and (B) sagittal MRI contrast.

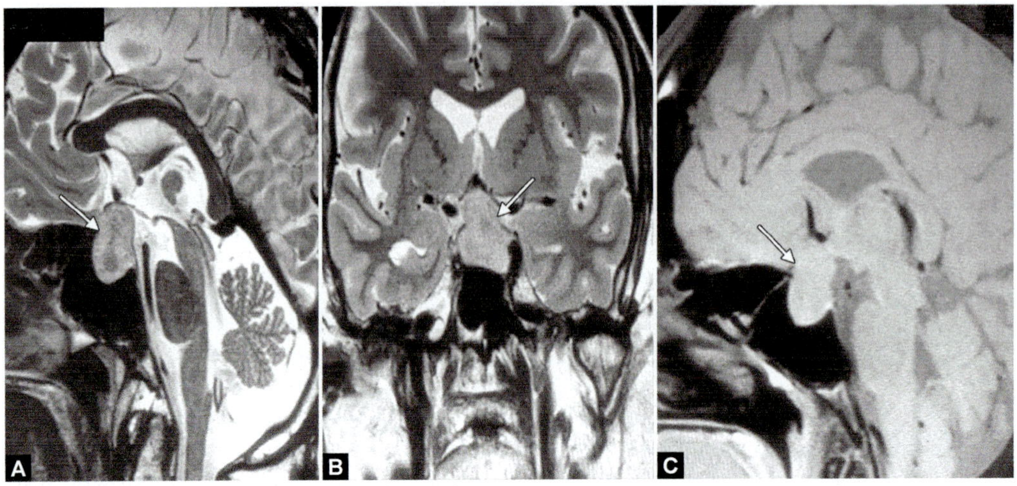

FIGS. 13A TO C: 56-year-old male presenting with hypopituitarism and bitemporal hemianopia MRI shows a nonfunctional pituitary macroadenoma—(A) sagittal T2 showing compression of chiasm, (B) coronal T2 shows the lateral extension of the tumor into the cavernous sinus, (C) noncontrast T1.

acute hypocortisolism. In this scenario, urgent surgical intervention may be indicated, however, this is performed after medical management of hypocortisolism and other metabolic derangements.

Epidermoids and Dermoids

Epidermoids are benign brain tumors that arise from ectopic epithelial cells rests that occur during closure of the neural tube. The capsule of the epidermoid cysts consists of stratified squamous keratinized epithelium. Epidermoids have a linear rate of growth resulting from gradual aggregation of desquamated epithelial cells and cholesterol. Malignant transformation to squamous cell carcinoma has been reported. Dermoids are similar to epidermoids, however, dermoids also contain dermal elements like hair, sebaceous, and sweat glands. Dermoids may arise from defects in gastrulation and disruption of neural tube closure. Surgical resection is the treatment of choice of these tumors, complete resection may not be possible due to attachment of the capsule to nerves, pial surface of the brain or blood vessels and the capsule can be spared in such cases. Complete tumor resection decreases the rates of chemical meningitis which is a complication of surgery for these tumors. Residual tumors can be observed with periodic MRI and symptomatic recurrences may be resected. There is no role for radiotherapy in the treatment of these tumors.

Vestibular Schwannoma

Schwannomas of the cerebellopontine angle present commonly with tinnitus, hearing loss, ataxia, and headache. They have also been known as acoustic neuromas. These tumors arise from the vestibular component of the vestibulocochlear nerve usually the inferior vestibular nerve, followed by the superior vestibular nerve in the frequency of origin **(Figs. 14A to D)**. The microscopic appearance of a vestibular schwannoma (VS) consists of two patterns: (1) Antoni A and (2) Antoni B. Antoni A areas contain spindle-shaped cells with rod-shaped nuclei and dense reticulin arranged with palisading of nuclei forming a Verocay body. Antoni B areas have stellate or spindled-shaped cells with small hyperchromatic nuclei, prominent cytoplasmic processes and loose myxoid stroma. Bilateral VSs may occur on NF-2 which is an autosomal dominant disease resulting from a mutation in the *NF-2* gene on chromosome 22. Small VS especially in elderly patients may be observed with serial imaging. Surgical resection is indicated when the VS has become large and causes symptoms related to cerebellar or brainstem compression. In patients who have hydrocephalus, successful surgical resection results in resolution of hydrocephalus. In cases where the patient has features of normal pressure hydrocephalus or when they are acutely symptomatic due to hydrocephalus with altered sensorium an emergent endoscopic third ventriculostomy (ETV) or ventriculoperitoneal (VP) shunt may performed and definitive tumor resection may be performed after symptoms of hydrocephalus have resolved. VSs which are smaller than 3 cm may also be treated with stereotactic radiosurgery.

Hemangioblastomas

Hemangioblastomas are WHO grade 1 tumors and occur almost exclusively in the CNS, with nearly 90% of these tumors seen in the brainstem, spinal cord, and the cerebellum. These tumors are sporadic in 60–75% of cases while in around 25–40% cases, occur as a part of the Von Hippel-Lindau (VHL) syndrome which is an autosomal dominant syndrome resulting from mutations in the VHL tumor suppressor gene on chromosome 3p25. VHL results in multiple CNS hemangioblastomas which involve the brain and the spinal cord, retinal angiomas, renal

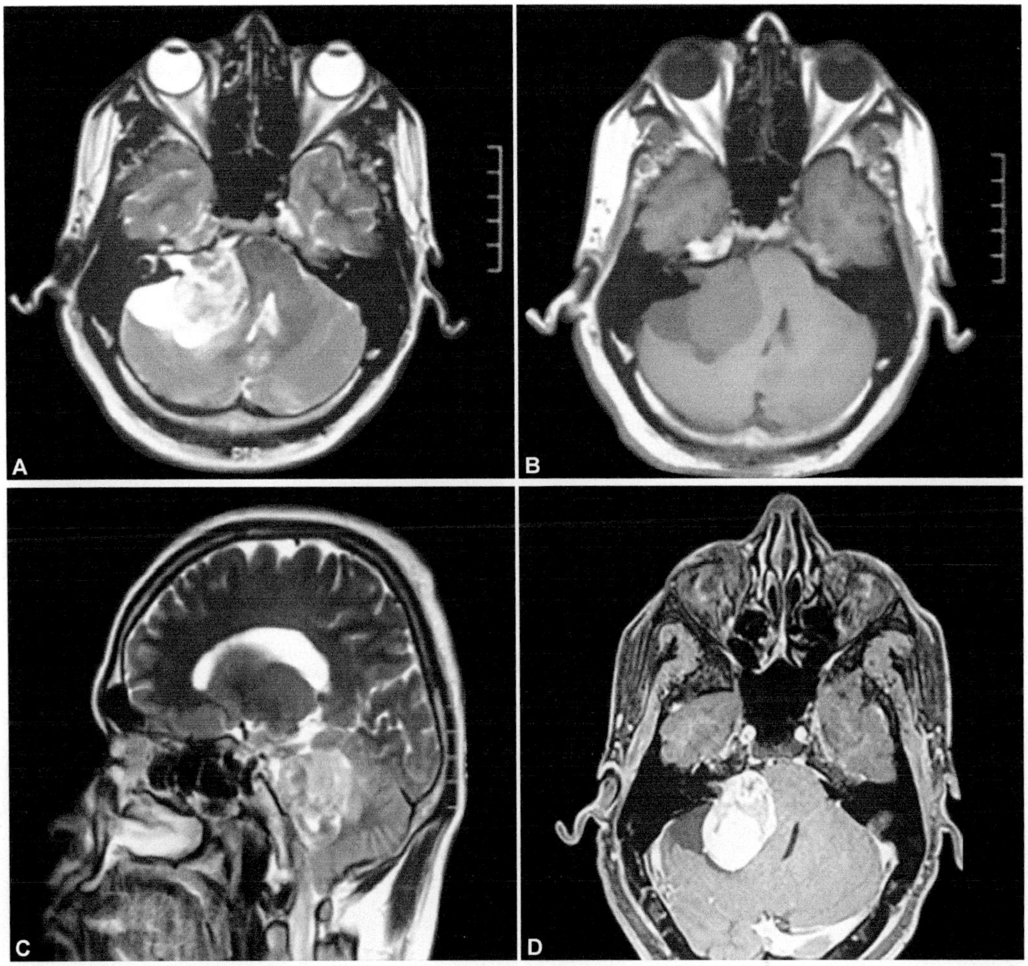

FIGS. 14A TO D: 56-year-old female presenting with right sided hearing loss and mild ataxia. MRI shows a right vestibular schwannoma—(A) T2 axial, (B) T1 axial, (C) T2 coronal, and (D) contrast axial.

cell carcinoma, pancreatic cysts, pheochromocytoma, epididymal cyst in males and broad ligament cyst in females, and endolymphatic sac tumors. Surgical resection is the treatment of choice of CNS hemangioblastomas. Tumor resections result in collapse of the cyst wall. Preoperative embolization of the tumor is needed in some cases to minimize intraoperative blood loss.

PINEAL REGION TUMORS

The pineal region may be the site of a variety of tumors of diverse histology. Pineal region tumors can be classified into four categories: (1) germ cell tumors, (2) pineal parenchymal cell tumors, (3) glial cell tumors, and (4) other miscellaneous tumors which include meningiomas, hemangioblastomas, epidermoid, choroid plexus papillomas, metastasis, lymphoma, etc. Pineal region tumors may initially present with clinical signs of obstructive hydrocephalus and upward gaze palsy. In this scenario, hydrocephalus is first treated by an ETV and a tumor biopsy when feasible or a VP shunt when an ETV is not possible. The cerebrospinal fluid (CSF) collected during the procedure can be sent for analysis of tumor markers like alpha-fetoprotein (AFP) or beta-human chorionic gonadotropin (β-HCG). The management of pineal region tumors is guided by the histology of the tumor. Germ cell tumors are subclassified by WHO as germinoma, yolk sac tumors, choriocarcinoma, embryonal carcinoma, and teratoma (mature or immature). Malignant germ cell tumors result in the appearance of AFP or β-HCG in the CSF or serum, CSF levels being more sensitive for tumor diagnosis than serum levels. AFP is secreted by cells of the fetal yolk sac and AFP levels are elevated in endodermal sinus tumors, embryonal cell carcinomas, and immature teratomas. β-HCG is produced by the cell of the fetal syncytiotrophoblast and is elevated in choriocarcinomas and occasionally embryonal cell carcinomas. Germinomas without spinal dissemination are treated with adjuvant radiotherapy along with chemotherapy and have 5-year survival rates exceeding 90%. Nongerminomatous germ cell tumors (NGGCT) are treated with chemo and radiotherapy except in cases of mature teratoma which requires surgical resection. In patients with NGGCT, residual tumors that do not completely regress following adjuvant chemo and radiotherapy may also be surgically resected.

Pineal parenchymal tumors, epidermoids, and dermoids are treated by surgical resection with good long-term results. In other pineal region, tumors tissue biopsy may also be obtained by a stereotactic biopsy or by a craniotomy.

Pediatric Brain Tumors

Diffuse intrinsic pontine gliomas (DIPG): Brainstem gliomas account for 10–20% primary brain tumors, of these 60–75% are DIPG. DIPG present with symptoms of cerebellar dysfunction, lower cranial nerve palsy, and long tract signs. Nearly 20% of these patients have obstructive hydrocephalus at the time of presentation. DIPG have a mutation in histone H3K27, this mutation is associated with a poor long-term prognosis. Due to its location within the brainstem, surgical resection is never feasible. Radiotherapy confers transient clinical improvement in the clinical course of the DIPG, without any improvement in overall survival. DIPG has a poor prognosis, with a median survival time of 10 months.

Medulloblastoma

Medulloblastoma is the most common malignant brain tumor in children **(Figs. 15 and 16)**. The WHO 2016 classification subdivided medulloblastomas into four genetically different subtypes with distinct clinical outcomes, these sub-types were: (1) wingless/integrated (WNT)-activated, (2) sonic hedgehog (SHH)-activated, (3) group 3, and (4) group 4 **(Table 4)**. Children with medulloblastoma present with complaints of headache, lethargy, and vomiting. Very young children and infants may manifest loss of appetite, weight loss, and failure to thrive. Obstructive hydrocephalus may also be seen with symptoms of increased intracranial pressure, including vomiting, a tense anterior fontanelle and upgaze palsy. Patients have clinical features of cerebellar vermian involvement like ataxia or cranial nerve palsies. Management of medulloblastoma involves surgery, radiation, and chemotherapy. Surgical resection of the tumor is the first line of treatment. Surgery yields tissue for biopsy and molecular analysis. Patients can be grouped into average risk or high-risk based on the

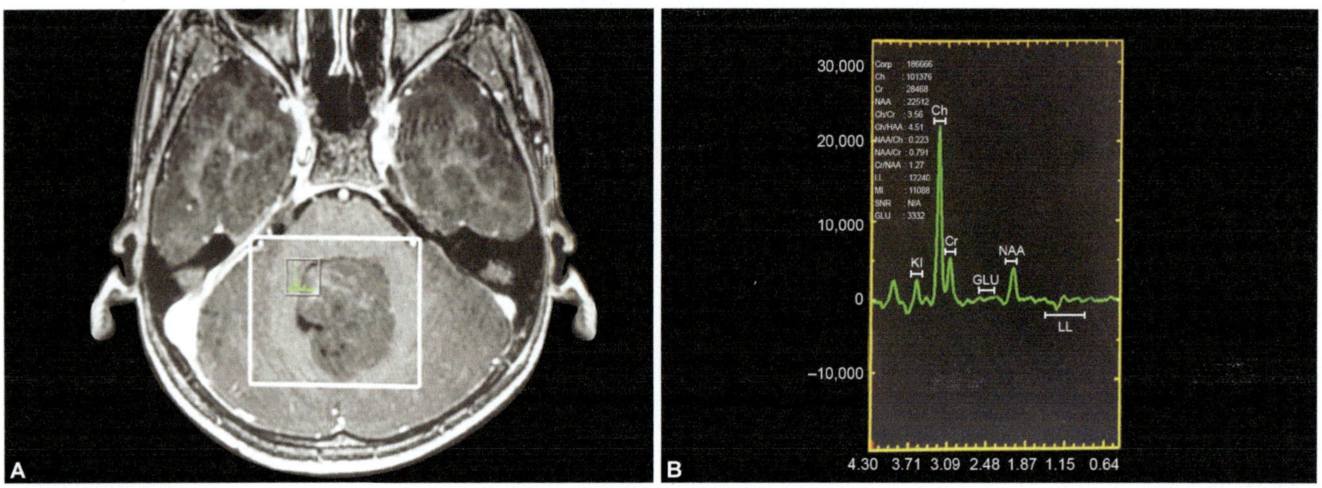

FIGS. 15A AND B: 4-year-old male medulloblastoma—(A) MRI axial (contrast) and (B) MR spectroscopy showing a choline peak.

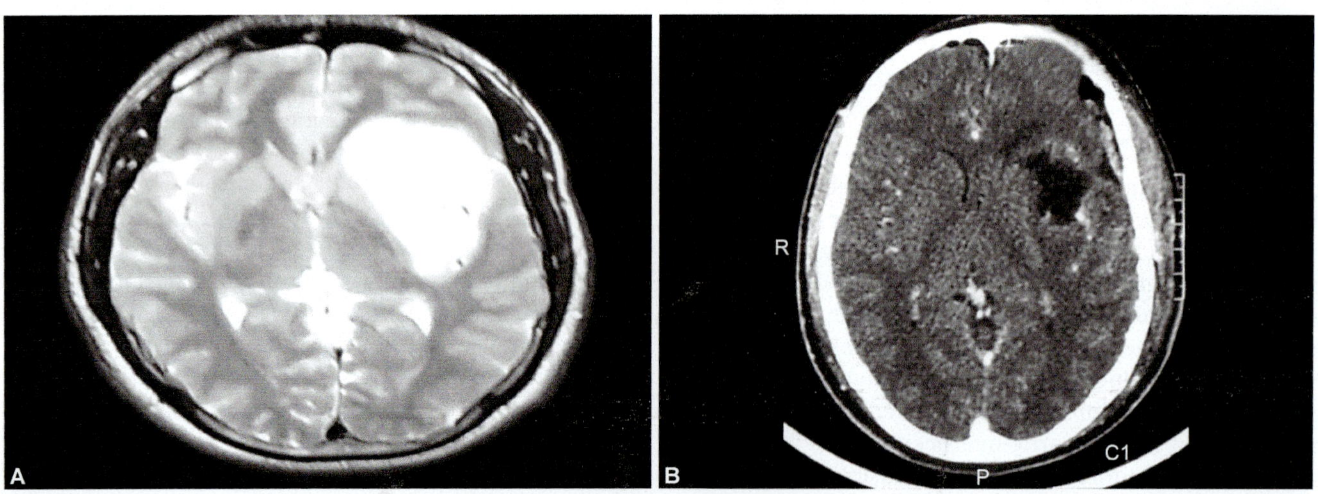

FIGS. 16A AND B: 25-year-old male with left insular glioma—(A) T2 MRI shows a hyperintense tumor involving the left insula—preoperative; (B) postoperative CT demonstrating tumor resection.

TABLE 4: Classification of medulloblastoma.

Type	Age	Site	Prognosis (5-year survival)
WNT group	Infants and children	Cerebellar peduncle/CPA cistern	Very good (100%)
SHH group	Infants and adults (bimodal distribution)	Lateral cerebellum	Good (75%)
Non-WNT/non-SHH/group 3	Infants and children	Midline vermis and 4th ventricle with CSF spread	Poor (40–60%)
Non-WNT/non-SHH/group 4	Children	Midline vermis and 4th ventricle	Intermediate (75%)

(CPA: cerebellopontine angle; CSF: cerebrospinal fluid; SHH: sonic hedgehog; WNT: wingless/integrated)

extent of resection, subtype, and dissemination into the subarachnoid space. In addition to the molecular subtype, the patient's age at diagnosis and the extent of CSF or extraneural metastasis determines the prognosis of the patient. Average risk patients include children >3 years without evidence of gross or microscopic metastatic disease at diagnosis and with <1.5 cm^2 of residual tumor. High-risk patients include those <3 years or with metastatic tumor in the subarachnoid space in the spine or the ventricles or extraneural spread or significant residual tumor (>1.5 cm^2) after surgery. Patient's may also require surgery for hydrocephalus, in which case, CSF diversion in the form of either an ETV or a VP shunt may be needed. Following surgery, patients are managed with adjuvant radiotherapy to the craniospinal axis and chemotherapy.

PROGNOSTIC FACTOR

Recently, discovered biomarkers that indicate improved survival in gliomas include O6-methylguanine-DNA methyltransferase (MGMT), IDH mutation, and a glioma cytosine-phosphate-guanine island methylator phenotype. Pilocytic astrocytoma (grade I) has the highest relative survival. Glioblastoma has the poorest overall survival, with only 0.05–4.7% of patients surviving 5 years past diagnosis. In general, gliomas with an oligodendroglial component have increased survival, as opposed to those with an astrocytic component **(Table 5)**.[12,13]

TABLE 5: Prognostic factors for glial tumors.

Glioma type	Positive prognostic factor	Negative prognostic factor
Low-grade glioma	Maximum safe resection	Subtotal resection
	Oligodendroglial lineage	Age >40
	Seizures at presentation	Astrocytic lineage
	IDH mutant status	Tumor diameter >6 cm
	1p19q codeletion	Tumor crossing midline
	TERT mutation	Neurological deficits at presentation
	ATRX loss	Presence of motor deficits
		Cognitive deficits
		Contrast enhancement
		Poor KPS
		IDH wild type
High-grade glioma	Maximum safe resection	Subtotal resection
	Age 40 years or below	Age >65
	KPS >70	KPS <60
	IDH mutant status	Astrocytic lineage
	MGMT methylation	Tumor >5 cm
	1p19q codeletion	Tumor crossing midline
		Thalamic/brainstem location
		Neurological deficits at presentation
		IDH wild type
		TERT mutation
		EGFR amplification with gain of chromosome 7, loss of chromosome 10

(ATRX: alpha-thalassemia/mental retardation syndrome X-linked; IDH: isocitrate dehydrogenase; KPS: Karnofsky performance score; MGMT: O6-methylguanine-DNA methyltransferase; TERT: telomerase reverse transcriptase)

Glial Tumors

Codeletion of 1p/19q

The combined deletion of 1p and 19q is the hallmark molecular signature of oligodendrogliomas. It leads to loss of entire chromosomal arms t(1;19)(q10;p10). A high proportion of oligodendrogliomas with 1p/19q loss demonstrated response to chemotherapy regimes such as PCV or single agents like temozolomide.[20] This also conferred better long term survival. In contrast, in patients with 1p/19q deleted tumors resection alone without any adjuvant chemotherapy or radiation does not confer a longer progression free survival.

IDH1 Mutation

Isocitrate dehydrogenase 1 mutations are present at high frequency in secondary glioblastomas that originate from prior lower-grade gliomas when compared to in primary glioblastomas (<1%). IDH1 mutations do not exist in certain other conditions cerebritis, cerebral infarction, viral infections, or radiation change and may be used differentiate these conditions during histopathological examination. These findings are of particular diagnostic value because they enable the distinction of reactive gliosis from low-grade diffuse astrocytoma, when biopsy samples are scanty.

Isocitrate dehydrogenase 1 and IDH2 mutations are associated with a favorable prognosis and an overall prolonged survival time independent of treatment. The survival of patients with IDH1 mutation in astrocytomas or oligodendrogliomas and glioblastoma is longer than IDH1 wild-type tumors.[22]

MGMT

MGMT is a DNA repair enzyme involved in DNA repair following damage from ionizing radiation and alkylating agents. A majority of glioblastomas have been found to express decreased levels of MGMT due to methylation of the promoter site, which makes these tumors more susceptible to alkylating agents used during chemotherapy. Glioblastoma with MGMT promoter hypermethylation also responds better to temozolomide, because they lack the ability to efficiently repair the damage introduced by alkylation. Hypermethylated MGMT promoters treated with temozolomide and radiation showed significantly increased survival times.[23]

Epidermal Growth Factor Receptor

The identification of epidermal growth factor receptor (EGFR) amplifications and overexpression, especially EGFRvIII, has been associated with poorer prognosis and in general is considered indicative of high-grade malignancy. The *EGFR* gene at 7p12 has been described as the most frequently amplified and overexpressed gene in approximately 60% of glioblastomas and has been associated with shorter survival times.[24]

Pituitary Adenomas

In the WHO 2017 classification of pituitary adenomas, certain subtypes of pituitary adenomas have been classified as high risk tumors which include (1) plurihormonal Pit-1-positive adenoma, (2) Crooke's cell adenoma, (3) silent corticotroph adenoma, (4) lactotroph adenoma in males, and (5) sparsely granulated somatotroph adenoma **(Box 1)**. High-risk pituitary adenomas have a higher rates of local invasion, tendency to recur, and a higher incidence of apoplexy compared with that in low-risk types.[25,26]

BOX 1 High-risk pituitary tumors (WHO 2017).

- Plurihormonal Pit-1–positive adenoma
- Crooke's cell adenoma
- Silent corticotroph adenoma
- Lactotroph adenoma in males
- Sparsely granulated somatotroph adenoma

Futuristics

Cancer immunotherapy is the stimulation of a patient's immune system to activate specific immune cells to attack cancer cells. Immunotherapy strategies currently studied in brain tumors include cancer vaccines, oncolytic virotherapeutics, monoclonal antibodies (checkpoint inhibitors), and adoptive T-cell therapies (CARTcell). Tumor-specific vaccines like rindopepimut target EGFRvIII and are currently being used in trial setting against glioblastoma.[27] Targeted therapy for glial tumor is based on targeted delivery directed to specific receptors or genes on the tumor with the aim to selectively eradicate it without damaging the normal brain **(Table 6)**. Gene therapy is the technique of introducing genetic material (DNA or RNA) into cells for altering the DNA expression of a cell, the most effective means of transferring DNA is by using viral-based vector like an adenovirus. This modality has been used for recurrent glioblastomas with limited response, but has not shown clinical benefit in the trial setting till date.

TABLE 6: Targeted therapy in glioblastoma.

EGFRvIII amplification	EGFR vaccine rindopepimut
KIT amplification	KIT inhibitor imatinib
PDGFRA amplification	PDGFR inhibitor dasatinib
PTEN deletion or mutation	AKT inhibitor or mTOR inhibitor voxtalisib
MDM2 amplification	MDM2 inhibitor AMG 232
TP53 wild-type	MDM2 inhibitor AMG 232
RB1 wild-type	CDK4/6 inhibitor ribociclib

CONCLUSION

The advent of genome sequencing and DNA methylome profiling has revolutionized prognostic predictions in brain tumor care. Nevertheless, survival statistics have not measured up to show a concurrent marked improvement. Molecular profiling and immunohistochemical markers are not easily available in several developing countries, limiting their widespread utilization. Imaging and surgical adjuncts of the current era, with newer adjuvant therapy modalities have improved surgical resection rates with better functional outcomes. The future stage is now set for personalized medicine in brain tumor treatment guided by broad general principles, yet individualized for each patient based on unique tumor-specific genetic signatures.

REFERENCES

1. Miller K, Ostrom Q, Kruchko C, Patil N, Tihan T, Cioffi G, et al. Brain and other central nervous system tumor statistics, 2021. CA Cancer J Clin. 2021;71(5):381-406.
2. Strong MJ, Garces J. Brain Tumours: Epidemiology and current trends in treatment. J Brain Tumours amp; Neurooncol. 2016;1:1.
3. Komori T. The 2021 WHO classification of tumours, 5th edition, central nervous system tumours: the 10 basic principles. Brain Tumour Pathol. 2022;39(2):47-50.
4. Bondy M, Scheurer M, Malmer B, Barnholtz-Sloan JS, Davis FG, Il'yasova D, et al. Brain tumour epidemiology: Consensus from the Brain Tumour Epidemiology Consortium. Cancer. 2008;113(S7): 1953-68.
5. Dasgupta A, Gupta T, Jalali R. Indian data on central nervous tumours: A summary of published work. South Asian J Cancer. 2016;5(3):147-53.
6. Sarkar C, Jain A, Sharma M, Suri V, Kale SS, Mahapatra AK, et al. Spectrum of pediatric brain tumours in India: A multi-institutional study. Neurol India. 2011;59(2):208-11.
7. Ostrom Q, Bauchet L, Davis F, Deltour I, Fisher JL, Langer CE, et al. The epidemiology of glioma in adults: a "state of the science" review. Neuro Oncol. 2014;16(7):896-913.
8. Jalali R, Datta D. Prospective analysis of incidence of central nervous tumors presenting in a tertiary cancer hospital from India. J Neurooncol. 2008;87(1):111-4.
9. Preul M. History of brain tumour surgery. Neurosurg Focus. 2005;18(4):1.
10. George C, Shreykumar P, Biren K, Darshan R, Easwer V. History of brain tumour surgery—A global and Indian perspective. Arch Med Health Sci. 2021;9(1):156.
11. Miller K, Ostrom Q, Kruchko C, Patil N, Tihan T, Cioffi G, et al. Brain and other central nervous system tumour statistics, 2021. CA Cancer J Clin. 2021;71(5):381-406.
12. Gould J. Breaking down the epidemiology of brain cancer. Nature. 2018;561(7724):S40-1.
13. Ullrich N. Neurocutaneous syndromes and brain tumours. J Child Neurol. 2016;31(12):1399-411.
14. Ostrom Q, Fahmideh M, Cote D, Muskens IS, Schraw JM, Scheurer ME, et al. Risk factors for childhood and adult primary brain tumours. Neuro Oncol. 2019;21(11):1357-75.
15. Alther B, Mylius V, Weller M, Gantenbein A. From first symptoms to diagnosis: Initial clinical presentation of primary brain tumours. Clin Transl Neurosci. 2020;4(2):2514183X2096836.
16. Thomas V, Choudhury J, Hussey M. Review of presenting symptoms and time to diagnosis of children with primary brain tumours. Arch Dis Child. 2011;96(Supplement 1):A85-A86.
17. Ozawa M, Brennan P, Zienius K, Kurian KM, Hollingworth W, Weller D, et al. Symptoms in primary care with time to diagnosis of brain tumours. Fam Pract. 2018;35(5):551-8.
18. Girardi F, Allemani C, Coleman M. Survival from brain tumours in children: A systematic review of geographical variation and time trends. SSRN Electronic Journal. 2019.
19. Louis DN, Perry A, Wesseling P, Brat DJ, Cree IA, Figarella-Branger D, et al. The 2021 WHO Classification of Tumours of the Central Nervous System: a summary. Neuro-Oncol. 2021;23(8): 1231-51.
20. Claus EB, Walsh KM, Wiencke JK, Molinaro AM, Wiemels JL, Schildkraut JM, et al. Survival and low-grade glioma: the emergence of genetic information. Neurosurg Focus. 2015;38(1):E6.
21. Nanda A, Bir SC, Maiti TK, Konar SK, Missios S, Guthikonda B. Relevance of Simpson grading system and recurrence-free survival after surgery for World Health Organization Grade I meningioma. J Neurosurg. 2017;126(1):201-11.
22. Olar A, Wani KM, Alfaro-Munoz KD, Heathcock LE, van Thuijl HF, Gilbert MR, et al. IDH mutation status and role of WHO grade and mitotic index in overall survival in grade II–III diffuse gliomas. Acta Neuropathol (Berl). 2015;129(4):585-96.
23. Riemenschneider MJ, Hegi ME, Reifenberger G. MGMT promoter methylation in malignant gliomas. Target Oncol. 2010;5(3): 161-5.
24. Saadeh FS, Mahfouz R, Assi HI. EGFR as a clinical marker in glioblastomas and other gliomas. Int J Biol Markers. 2018;33(1): 22-32.
25. Fountas A, Lavrentaki A, Subramanian A, Toulis KA, Nirantharakumar K, Karavitaki N. Recurrence in silent corticotroph adenomas after primary treatment: A systematic review and meta-analysis. J Clin Endocrinol Metab. 2019;104(4):1039-48.
26. Lloyd RV, Osamura RY, Klöppel G, Rosai J. WHO Classification of Tumours of Endocrine Organs, 4th edition. France: International Agency for Research on Cancer; 2017.
27. Fecci PE, Sampson JH. The current state of immunotherapy for gliomas: an eye toward the future: JNSPG 75th Anniversary Invited Review Article. J Neurosurg. 2019;131(3):657-66.

105

CHAPTER

Traumatic Brain Injury

Prahlad K Sethi, Nitin K Sethi

INTRODUCTION

The Centers for Disease Control and Prevention defines traumatic brain injury (TBI) as a disruption in the normal function of the brain caused by a bump, blow, or jolt to the head, or penetrating head injury.[1] TBIs can be broadly divided into closed (nonpenetrating) or open (penetrating). They can also be characterized as mild, moderate, or severe usually based on increasing structural damage visualized on either computed tomography (CT) or magnetic resonance imaging (MRI) of the brain. TBIs are one of the most common causes of acute and chronic neurological disability in both developed and developing countries. India has witnessed an explosive rate of industrialization, urbanization, and economic development in the last two decades. Urbanization has led to a rapid increase in motorized transport in cities and towns across India. India is soon expected to be among the top automotive markets in Asia. The current Indian road infrastructure is ill-equipped to handle this exponential increase in nonmotorized and motorized forms of transport. As a result, TBIs are increasing and have been rightfully referred to as the silent pandemic sweeping India. Traumatic brain injuries lead to adverse acute and chronic cognitive, neuropsychiatric, and functional outcomes. In this review, TBIs are analyzed concerning Indian context with special attention to those occurring in the context of road traffic accidents. Existing medical infrastructure to manage these TBIs is discussed and recommendations for improvement follow.

EPIDEMIOLOGY

Traumatic brain injury affects millions around the world on an annual basis. While incidence and prevalence rates are known in developed countries, data is scarce for developing countries in Asia and Africa.[2] It is generally acknowledged that there is an enormous unmet burden concerning management of these injuries in India.[3] Worldwide the two most common causes of TBIs are falls and motor vehicle accidents. In India, it is estimated that nearly 1.5–2 million persons are injured and 1 million die every year. Road traffic injuries are the leading cause (60%) of TBIs followed by falls (20–25%) and violence (10%).[3,4] The high burden of TBIs leads to significant morbidity and functional disability. Brain-injured persons frequently sustain polytrauma leading to significant rehabilitation needs which are challenging to meet in a resource-limited environment such as India.

Sports-related TBIs are likely common in India though incidence and prevalence numbers are lacking. Most of these injuries occur about combat sports such as boxing, mixed martial arts, wrestling, and popular contact sports such as football and rugby. The incidence of TBIs in sports such as cricket and field hockey, both played widely at school and college levels is largely unknown. Most of these injuries are of mild grade and are classified as concussions.[5] In the absence of validated biofluid (blood/CSF) and imaging biomarkers separating concussion as a distinct pathophysiological entity from mild TBI is not easy. This may lead to misconceptions and biases in the diagnostic process. Recent studies have also highlighted the risks of multiple head impact exposure in combat sports such as boxing and contact sports such as American Football. The burden of chronic neurological injuries such as chronic post-traumatic headache, post-traumatic dizziness, post-traumatic Parkinsonism, and chronic traumatic encephalopathy in these athletes is likely high but remains largely hidden coming to medical attention after the athlete has retired.[6]

Falls are another common cause of TBIs especially in the elderly. India's population is steadily graying due to rising life expectancy and falling birth rate. While the contribution of mechanical falls to the overall incidence of TBIs in the Indian population is unknown, it is likely substantial. Falls remain a leading cause of morbidity and mortality in the elderly.

The contribution of other miscellaneous causes such as nonmotor vehicle traffic accidents, and gunshot injuries whether in the civilian arena or the Indian armed forces involved in counter-terrorism operations is also unknown. The Indian army is the third largest army in the world. India is also got large numbers of paramilitary forces. Indian army is deployed in battlefields at the high attitude and adverse climate conditions where the incidence of head injuries and polytrauma is high. Paramilitary forces are constantly deployed in Naxalite areas. Unfortunately, there is a dearth of epidemiological studies from the Indian armed forces.

Traumatic brain injury can be graded into mild, moderate, and severe based on the duration of loss of consciousness, duration of post-traumatic amnesia, Glasgow Coma Scale (GCS) score, and degree of structural damage on imaging study of the brain either a CT of the head (CTH) or MRI of the brain.[7,8] While patients with moderate to the severe grade of TBI usually present to the attention of a physician or an acute care facility such as trauma centers in hospitals, the burden of mild TBI is likely very high and largely hidden. A significant number of patients with TBI experience cognitive and motor deficits acutely after the head impact exposure. In some of these patients, these deficits lead to long-term adverse cognitive, neuropsychiatric, and functional outcomes and poor quality of life.

PATHOLOGY AND PATHOPHYSIOLOGY

The pathophysiology of TBI has now been well elucidated in animal models and can be broadly divided into:

1. Primary injury, caused by biomechanical forces during the initial insult; and
2. Secondary injury, which refers to tissue and cellular damages which follows the primary insult.

Primary Brain Injury

The immediate impact of biomechanical forced brain can result in two types of primary injuries: (1) focal and (2) diffuse brain injuries. The coexistence of both types of injuries is common in patients who suffer moderate-to-severe TBI. Diffuse axonal injury (DAI) is common in moderate-to-severe TBI cases.[9,10] MRI is the modality of choice to identify DAI and the injury is frequently missed if only CTH is carried out following TBI. In both closed head and penetrating TBI there is focal brain damage with evidence of localized brain contusion at the site of the head impact exposure (coup). At the coup necrotic neuronal and glial cells cause further compression of blood supply. Extra-axial blood collection causes the occurrence of epidural and subdural hematoma (SDH) which may further compromise cerebral blood flow (CBF) by increasing intracranial pressure (ICP). As per the Monro-Kellie doctrine, the sum of volumes of the brain, CSF, and intracranial blood is constant. So, an increase in one should cause a decrease in one or both remaining two.

Monro–Kellie Doctrine

Cerebral perfusion pressure (CPP) = Mean arterial pressure (MAP) – ICP.

Secondary contusion may occur in tissues opposite to or surrounding the coup (contrecoup) due to secondary impact when the brain rebounds and strikes the inside of the skull. In contrast to focal injury, the main mechanism of diffuse brain injury is rapid deceleration and acceleration causing shearing and stretching injury of brain tissue. The biomechanical forces cause damage to neuronal axons, oligodendrocytes, and blood vasculature, leading to brain edema and ischemic injury. The release of mediators such as glutamate, lactate, H^+, K^+, Ca^{2+}, nitric oxide, arachidonic acid, free oxygen radicals, kinins, and histamine leads to vasogenic and cytotoxic edema.[11,12] Diffuse TBI pathologically is characterized by extensive axonal damage in subcortical and deep white matter tissue such as that of the brain stem and corpus callosum. Disruption of axonal cytoskeleton leads to impairment of axonal transport and conduction.[13] TBI because of explosive injury such as that which occurs in soldiers exposed to the improvised explosive device (IED) blast injuries displays the characteristics of a typical diffuse brain injury and is the result of shock waves as against inertial forces.

Secondary Brain Injury

Biochemical, cellular, and physiological events that occur during primary injury cause delayed and prolonged secondary brain injury. Processes of excitotoxicity, mitochondrial dysfunction, oxidative stress, lipid peroxidation, neuronal inflammation, axon degeneration and apoptotic cell death cause adverse cognitive, neurobehavioral, and functional outcomes which can last for months to years and at times are irreversible.[11-14] Many drugs and therapeutic strategies including targeted hypothermia are aimed at preventing and reversing secondary brain injury. Research in this important field is ongoing.

CLINICAL PRESENTATIONS, DIFFERENTIAL DIAGNOSIS, AND INVESTIGATIONS

Patients with concussive brain injury, the term often used synonymously with mild TBI, present with subjective symptoms such as headache, dizziness, lightheadedness, light sensitivity, sound sensitivity, nausea, impaired attention, impaired concentration, and feeling foggy and fuzzy. Objective signs are lacking though patients may display short-duration gross motor instability and incoordination immediately after the head impact exposure. Multimodal concussion assessment batteries are more sensitive than stand-alone measures of concussion. Structural imaging such as CTH and MRI brain is usually normal.

Electroencephalography if carried out is also normal. Symptoms are self-limited and complete recovery can be expected in most patients in about 2–4 weeks. Some patients experience prolonged postconcussive symptoms. In these patients, a formal neurocognitive evaluation demonstrates deficits in multiple cognitive and neuropsychiatric domains. Underlying anxiety disorder and depression at times leads to the persistence of symptoms in these otherwise young healthy adults who have experienced a mild grade of closed head injury.

Patients with moderate to severe TBI present with altered mental status and varying degrees of motor, sensory, and cerebellar deficits. The GCS score is <13 and may decline precipitously over a short period. CTH and MRI brain show an increasing level of structural brain damage. MRI techniques such as gradient echo and susceptibility weight imaging are more sensitive for identifying microhemorrhages and other stigmata of TBI. The role of diffusion tensor imaging (DTI) is still evolving in the identification and management of these patients. At present, these advanced imaging modalities are only carried out in research settings.

MANAGEMENT

Management of a patient with concussion/mTBI is usually supportive. Patients experience postconcussion symptoms and are usually advised a period of cognitive and physical rest till acute symptoms begin to abate. It is important not to cocoon these patients as this leads to the persistence of symptoms. After a few days of cognitive and physical rest, patients are instructed to begin a graded and gradual return to work and exercise. They should be further instructed to keep themselves well hydrated, avoid inversions, and alcohol till symptoms have resolved. The benefit of supplements such as magnesium oxide, vitamin B2, vitamin B12, and fish oil has not been systematically studied but these are routinely prescribed.

The first step in the management of a moderate to severe brain injured person involves a detailed neurological examination. This is accomplished in the hospital setting usually after the primary and secondary surveys have been completed by the trauma or emergency room teams. The duration of loss of consciousness, the duration and degree of post-traumatic amnesia, the initial GCS score, and the degree of structural damage on neuroimaging help to establish the severity of TBI and serve as a baseline against which future assessments are carried out. Assessment of the intubated patient with a much lower GCS score is more challenging. Checking for pupil reactivity, symmetry, as well as cough/gag, and corneal reflexes is important in these patients. Intubated patients are usually pharmacologically sedated and paralyzed with intravenous sedatives and neuromuscular blockers and these medications hinder the neurological assessment. It is important to remember that the contribution of these medications to the degree of cerebral dysfunction is generally unaccounted for in basic grading scales such as the GCS. Under these circumstances, the sedative/paralyzing medications used, the timing of their administration, their half-lives, and any other potential confounding factors to the neurological examination should be a factor when prognosticating about injury severity and outcome. If decisions are made based on one factor alone whether the initial neuroimaging or GCS score it may not be in the best interest of the patient.

Medical Interventions for TBI

Following a moderate-to-severe TBI, the patient should be evaluated and medically stabilized as soon as possible. As in other trauma patients, evaluating the airway, breathing, and circulation is the first step. Securing the airway, ensuring adequate oxygenation, and maintaining circulation help to prevent secondary brain injury and nontraumatic anoxic brain injury. These patients are best managed in dedicated neurological intensive care units where serial neurological assessments are carried out and expertise for intracranial pressure monitoring is available.

Role of Head Elevation

Raising the head of a TBI patient in a simple intervention that leads to a reduction in ICP both by displacement of CSF from the intracranial compartment as well as due to promotion of venous outflow.[15] While the mean carotid pressure is reduced by the head of the bed elevation, ICP is reduced, and CBF remains unaffected.

Role of Hyperventilation

Hyperventilation lowers ICP by reducing the intra-arterial carbon dioxide partial pressure ($PaCO_2$), which results in vasoconstriction.[16] This ultimately results in the reduction of cerebral blood volume. Prophylactic hyperventilation is generally not recommended in TBI patients. Currently, hyperventilation is used in the setting of severe TBI only for brief periods during acute neurological deterioration.[17]

Role of Anticonvulsants for Seizure Prophylaxis

Patients with moderate to severe TBI have a lower seizure threshold and increased propensity to seizures in the immediate aftermath of the head injury. Hence, many patients while in the hospital are started on an anticonvulsant drug regimen for seizure prophylaxis. Usually, a broad-spectrum anticonvulsant such as levetiracetam is preferred. Levetiracetam is an efficacious broad-spectrum anticonvulsant with a favorable side-effect profile and few drug-drug interactions. It can also be administered intravenously in the unconscious intubated patient. Post-traumatic seizures may be divided into immediate, early, and late based on when they occur after the head injury. Immediate post-traumatic seizures also at times referred to as impact seizures occur at the time of the head injury. The etiology of these seizures is thought to be the initial head impact exposure. Immediate post-traumatic seizures usually have a good prognosis and do not lead to post-traumatic epilepsy. As a result, these patients do not warrant long-term anticonvulsant drug therapy. Seizures occurring within 6 months of the head injury are labeled early post-traumatic seizures. These patients are usually treated with anticonvulsant drug therapy for varying periods. If they remain seizure free, a gradual and cautious taper of anticonvulsant should be attempted. An EEG study may help in characterization and prognostication before anticonvulsant wean is attempted. Seizures may occur as far as 5 years out after a head injury. These patients with late post-traumatic epilepsy usually need long-term anticonvulsant therapy.[18] In some, seizures are refractory warranting antiseizure medication polypharmacy.

Role of Hyperosmolar Therapy

Hyperosmolar therapy in the setting of a TBI can be administered in the form of a bolus or an infusion to reduce ICP. The immediate effects of mannitol are likely due to alterations in blood rheology.[19] As blood rheology improves and blood becomes less viscous, an increase in CBF occurs. The body's autoregulatory response to this is transient vasoconstriction, which ultimately limits the degree of CBF. Mannitol also does have osmotic diuretic properties, but this mechanism of decreasing ICPs is not thought to take place until after the primary effect.

Role of Surgical Intervention in the Management of Moderate and Severe TBI Craniotomy: For Evacuation of Extra-axial Hematoma

Surgical intervention in the form of craniotomy and hematoma evacuation is generally warranted when there is a significant mass effect from either an epidural hematoma (EDH) or SDH or a contusion and/or intracranial hematoma with a significant volume of blood. Usually in these cases, the mass effect is significant causing midline shift and herniation. The underlying brain injury associated with an EDH is usually quite minor, however, the rapidity of an EDH expansion makes this surgery a neurosurgical emergency and frequently lifesaving. The mainstay of treatment of a large EDH with mass effect is a generous craniotomy over the desired region, evacuation of the hematoma, and cauterization of the bleeding vessel, often the middle meningeal artery or its branches.[20]

Acute SDH is usually associated with a much more significant underlying brain injury. SDH is the most common cause of boxing (combat sports)-related neurological mortality **(Fig. 1)**. In these otherwise young healthy athletes, a decompressive hemicraniectomy is at times lifesaving but patients are left with significant neurological deficits.[21] SDH varies in age from acute to subacute, chronic, and mixed. After a few days, acute SDH generally enters a process of liquefaction, making them amenable to minimally invasive surgical evacuation through a burr hole. Limitation to this type of drainage is when there are multiple subdural septations and loculations, allowing chronic blood to be evacuated from only the pocket the burr hole is overlying. In the case, multiple burr holes or craniotomy is performed.[22,23]

SPECIAL FEATURES OF TBIs CONCERNING INDIAN CONTEXT

Massenburg *et al.*, have done an excellent work by reviewing quantitative research on TBI in India, pooling data from nearly 2,000 patients, over 27 years, across 14 states.[24] In India, the rapid urbanization, economic growth, and lifestyle changes have led to a tremendous increase in the incidence of TBI, so much so that it is rightfully referred to as a "silent epidemic" **(Figs. 2 and 3)**. It is challenging to obtain reliable

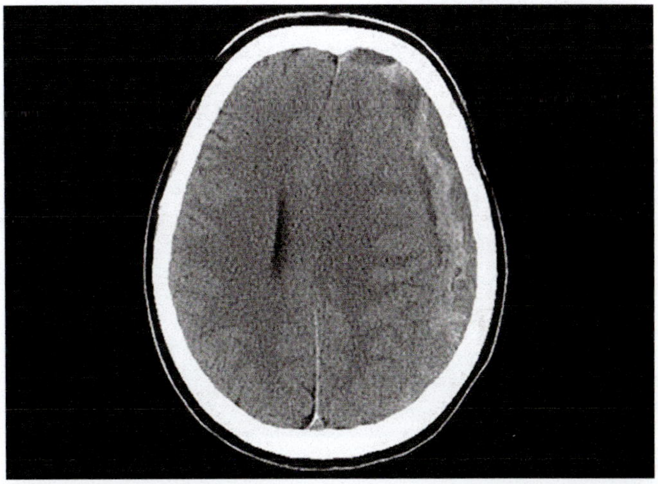

FIG. 1: Subdural hematoma is a common cause of traumatic brain injury (TBI) related mortality.

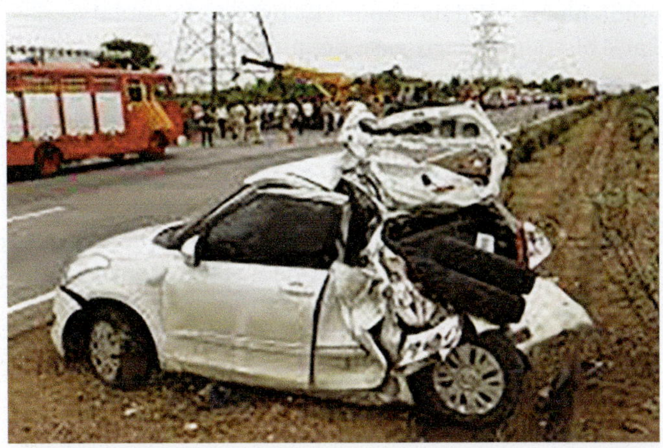

FIG. 2: Motor vehicle accidents have led to a tremendous increase in incidence of traumatic brain injury (TBI) in India, rightfully referred to as a "silent epidemic".

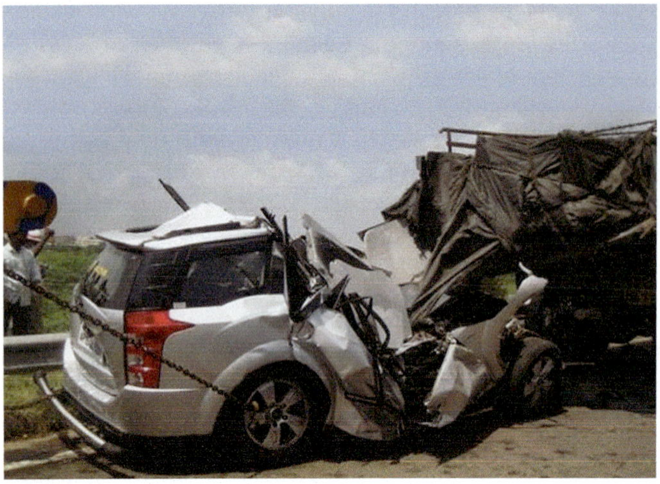

FIG. 3: Motor vehicle accidents are common on poorly maintained Indian roads.

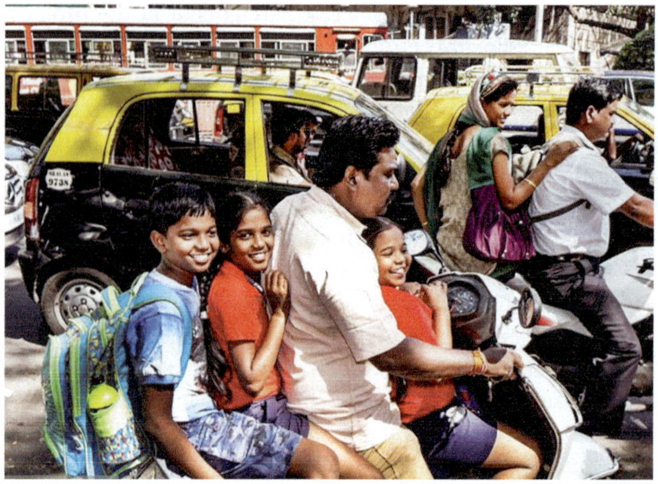

FIG. 5: In India drivers disobey traffic rules with impunity, drive without helmets, and do not wear seat belts and many on the road are minors without a valid driving.

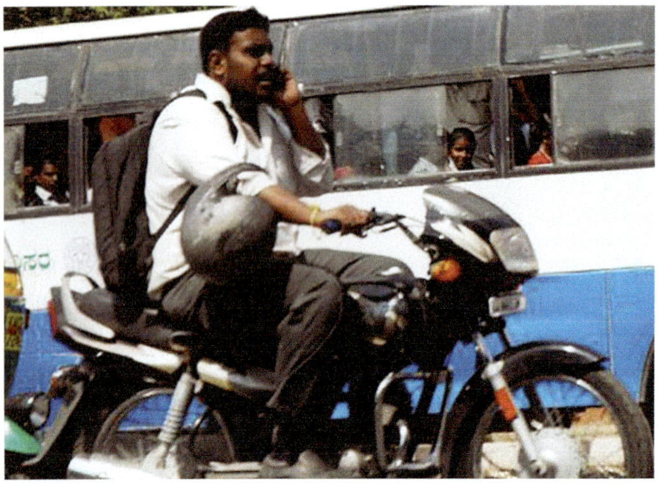

FIG. 4: People in India commonly ride motorcycles and scooters without helmets.

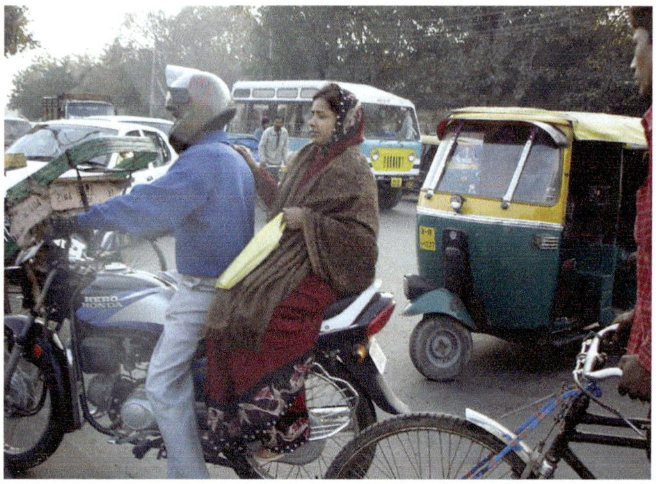

FIG. 6: Trucks, buses, cars, scooters, cyclists, and pedestrians jostle with each other on poorly maintained Indian roads leading to frequent accidents.

epidemiological data about TBI from India and Asia.[25-27] Lack of standardized case definition, lack of centralized reporting mechanisms from urban and rural hospitals, lack of population-based studies, absence of standardized survey protocols, and inadequate mortality statistics present some of the major obstacles.

Across India, rapid urbanization and industrialization have led to an exponential increase in motorized transport and along with-it accidents. India has the second-largest road network in the world, spanning a total of 5.89 million kilometers (km) but the quality and maintenance of this vast infrastructure are very poor. The traffic is heterogeneous and plies on narrow poorly maintained roadways. Roads in India are poorly illuminated at night, and frequently lack appropriate lanes and the median strip (central reservation) to separate opposing lanes of traffic. In many places, traffic signals and signs are either missing or broken. Drivers frequently lack knowledge of traffic rules and signs. People disobey traffic rules with impunity, drive without helmets, do not wear seat belts, and many on the road are minors without a valid driving license **(Figs. 4 and 5)**. Trucks, buses, cars, scooters, cyclists, and pedestrians jostle with each other leading to frequent accidents **(Fig. 6)**. India lacks a coordinated and integrated prehospital emergency healthcare system staffed by well-trained emergency medical services (EMS) responders.[28,29] India also lacks a coordinated and integrated hospital trauma system. Accident victims who need level I trauma center care and neurosurgical expertise are frequently taken to hospitals ill-equipped to handle their complex needs.

Nontraffic accident injuries such as falls among the elderly, domestic and nondomestic violence, and construction accidents are also likely very common in India

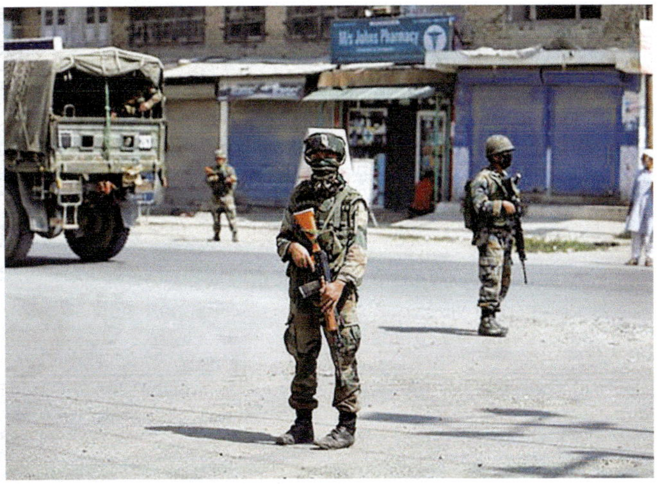

FIG. 7: The incidence of head trauma in the Indian army and paramilitary forces deployed in counter insurgency operations is unknown.

but their contribution to the total burden of TBI is largely unknown.

The Indian army with a reported strength of over 1.4 million active personnel is the world's second-largest military force. Indian armed forces are deployed in field areas and have been in battles with neighboring countries' armed forces. Surprisingly, very few studies are available on head trauma in the Indian army and paramilitary forces **(Fig. 7)**.

Brain injury rehabilitation centers in western countries offer comprehensive inpatient and outpatient programs offering occupational, physical, speech, and cognitive therapy. These services are provided by highly skilled staff including physiatrists, physical therapists, occupational therapists, speech and language therapists, neuropsychologists, pain medicine specialists, skilled nurses, and social workers. India currently lacks dedicated brain injury rehabilitation centers.

PREVENTION

Prevention is said to be better than cure. This is especially true when it comes to TBIs. Interventions designed to prevent TBI such as efficient first aid care, proper stabilization, and transfer of injured persons, referral to the appropriate trauma center based on triage and early transfer to definitive treatment centers will help save lives and reduce disabilities. It is important to remember that most deaths occur at the crash site or en route to hospitals. Emphasis should be placed on developing and upgrading road infrastructure, introduction, and enforcement of road safety laws and traffic education.

To prevent falls in the elderly, there should be an emphasis on early recognition and management of neurodegenerative disorders which predispose to falls. Mechanical falls are also common in this subgroup due to degenerative disorders which affect the hip and knees. Physical therapy is helpful in these patients. Most falls occur in the home at night when the patient is going to use the bathroom and can be prevented by fall-proofing the bedroom and bathroom.

To prevent TBIs in combat and contact sports such as boxing, wrestling, and football (soccer), emphasis should be placed on educating athletes and coaching staff on concussion recognition and management.

CONCLUSION

Traumatic brain injury is a leading cause of death and disability worldwide. There is likely a high burden of TBI in India too but is largely hidden. Prevention of TBI and proper management will save countless lives and prevent major disabilities. In India, we cannot ignore this silent pandemic anymore. Developing and maintaining a comprehensive TBI registry and developing national guidelines on triaging and management of these patients are the need of the hour. Time = brain not just in stroke but also in TBI!

REFERENCES

1. Centers for Disease Control and Prevention. (2019). Traumatic brain injury and concussion report. [online] Available from https://www.cdc.gov/traumaticbraininjury/pubs/index.html (Last accessed January, 2023).
2. Rutland-Brown W, Langlois JA, Thomas KE, Xi YL. Incidence of traumatic brain injury in the United States, 2003. J Head Trauma Rehabil. 2006;21:544-8.
3. Gururaj G. Epidemiology of traumatic brain injuries: Indian scenario. Neurol Res. 2002;24:24-8.
4. Pal R, Ghosh A, Kumar R, Galwankar S, Paul SK, Pal S, et al. Public health crisis of road traffic accidents in India: Risk factor assessment and recommendations on prevention on the behalf of the Academy of Family Physicians of India. J Family Med Prim Care. 2019;8:775-83.
5. Kelly JP, Rosenberg JH. Diagnosis and management of concussion in sports. Neurology. 1997;48:575-80.
6. McKee AC, Cantu RC, Nowinski CJ, Hedley-Whyte ET, Gavett BE, Budson AE, et al. Chronic traumatic encephalopathy in athletes: progressive tauopathy after repetitive head injury. J Neuropathol Exp Neurol. 2009;68:709-35.
7. Sternbach GL. The Glasgow coma scale. J Emerg Med. 2000;19: 67-71.
8. Besenski N. Traumatic injuries: imaging of head injuries. Eur Radiol. 2002;12:1237-52.
9. Skandsen T, Kvistad KA, Solheim O, Strand IH, Folvik M, Vik A. Prevalence and impact of diffuse axonal injury in patients with moderate and severe head injury: a cohort study of early magnetic resonance imaging findings and 1-year outcome. J Neurosurg. 2010;113:556-63.
10. Smith DH, Meaney DF, Shull WH. Diffuse axonal injury in head trauma. J Head Trauma Rehabil. 2003;18:307-16.

11. Schmidt OI, Infanger M, Heyde CE, Ertel W, Stahel P. The Role of Neuroinflammation in Traumatic Brain Injury. European Journal of Trauma. 2004;30:135-49.
12. Ray SK, Dixon CE, Banik NL. Molecular mechanisms in the pathogenesis of traumatic brain injury. Histol Histopathol. 2002;17:1137-52.
13. Maxwell WL, Domleo A, McColl G, Jafari SS, Graham DI. Post-acute alterations in the axonal cytoskeleton after traumatic axonal injury. J Neurotrauma. 2003;20:151-68.
14. Povlishock JT, Katz DI. Update of neuropathology and neurological recovery after traumatic brain injury. J Head Trauma Rehabil. 2005;20:76-94.
15. Feldman Z, Kanter MJ, Robertson CS, Contant CF, Hayes C, Sheinberg MA, et al. Effect of head elevation on intracranial pressure, cerebral perfusion pressure, and cerebral blood flow in head-injured patients. J Neurosurg. 1992;76:207-11.
16. Grubb RL Jr, Raichle ME, Eichling JO, Ter-Pogossian MM. The effects of changes in $PaCO_2$ on cerebral blood volume, blood flow, and vascular mean transit time. Stroke. 1974;5:630-9.
17. Darby JM, Yonas H, Marion DW, Latchaw RE. Local "inverse steal" induced by hyperventilation in head injury. Neurosurgery. 1988;23:84-8.
18. Torbic H, Forni AA, Anger KE, Degrado JR, Greenwood BC. Use of antiepileptics for seizure prophylaxis after traumatic brain injury. Am J Health Syst Pharm. 2013;70:759-66.
19. Burke AM, Quest DO, Chien S, Cerri C. The effects of mannitol on blood viscosity. J Neurosurg. 1981;55:550-3.
20. Bullock MR, Chesnut R, Ghajar J, Gordon D, Hartl R, Newell DW, et al; Surgical Management of Traumatic Brain Injury Author Group. Surgical management of acute epidural hematomas. Neurosurgery. 2006;58(3 Suppl):S7-15.
21. Sinha S, Raheja A, Garg M, Moorthy S, Agrawal D, Gupta DK, et al. Decompressive craniectomy in traumatic brain injury: A single-center, multivariate analysis of 1,236 patients at a tertiary care hospital in India. Neurol India. 2015;63:175-83.
22. Bullock MR, Chesnut R, Ghajar J, Gordon D, Hartl R, Newell DW, et al; Surgical Management of Traumatic Brain Injury Author Group. Surgical management of acute subdural hematomas. Neurosurgery. 2006;58(3 Suppl):S16-24.
23. Tanaka Y, Ohno K. Chronic subdural hematoma—an up-to-date concept. J Med Dent Sci. 2013;60:55-61.
24. Massenburg BB, Veetil DK, Raykar NP, Agrawal A, Roy N, Gerdin M. A systematic review of quantitative research on traumatic brain injury in India. Neurol India. 2017;65:305-15.
25. Kamalakannan SK, Gudlavalleti ASV, Murthy Gudlavalleti VS, Goenka S, Kuper H. Challenges in understanding the epidemiology of acquired brain injury in India. Ann Indian Acad Neurol. 2015;18:66-70.
26. Puvanachandra P, Hyder AA. The burden of traumatic brain injury in Asia: A call for research. Pak J Neurol Sci. 2009;4:27-32.
27. Agrawal A, Munivenkatappa A, Shukla DP, Menon GR, Alogolu R, Galwankar S, et al. Traumatic brain injury related research in India: An overview of published literature. Int J Crit Illn Inj Sci. 2016;6: 65-9.
28. Tripathi M, Tewari MK, Mukherjee KK, Mathuriya SN. Profile of patients with head injury among vehicular accidents: An experience from a tertiary care centre of India. Neurol India. 2014;62:610-7.
29. Burton A. A key traumatic brain injury initiative in India. Lancet Neurol. 2016;15:1011-2.

106

CHAPTER

Severe Acute Brain Injury

Prafulla Shembalkar, Roop Gursahani, Rajinder K Dhamija

INTRODUCTION

Neurocritical illnesses involve the brain, spinal cord, or neuromuscular system. Survival after these became a likely outcome only after the introduction of modern critical care. Lifesaving therapies (LSTs) such as ventilatory and inotropic support are essential in addition to specific treatment depending on the etiology. The largest subset is of patients who present in altered mental status due to serious acute brain injury and are in coma as defined below, either at admission or during their course in the hospital. In some of them, brain death (BD) criteria will be met and can be declared once irreversibility is confirmed. A proportion of them will remain persistently or even permanently incapacitated, and they are subsumed under the term chronic disorders of consciousness (C-DoC). Some features are common to all severe acquired brain injuries (SABIs). These illnesses often occur as acute events in previously functional individuals. Families are faced with the possibility of mortality rates of 40–60% or permanent disability of varying severity. Sometimes, these patients need salvage procedures such as thrombectomy, decompressive craniectomy (DC), and external ventricular drainage. LST can support or replace the functions of various organ systems for varying periods of time. However, eventual quality of life (QoL) largely depends on neurologic recovery, which can be prolonged and both emotionally and economically burdensome, for the family and perhaps for the patient, if she is aware. Hence, assessment of neurologic prognosis must be incorporated into this decision-making as early as possible. In the Indian situation, with limited resources, an ethical approach has to balance medical feasibility against practicality.[1] It is increasingly recognized that a palliative care (PC) approach can and should be incorporated early for optimal neurocritical care.[2] PC focuses on clear and compassionate communication in the face of uncertainty. Moreover, it also provides clinical and psychosocial support to the surviving family as they work through determining goals of care and planning either for withdrawal of LST or for a prolonged and uncertain future.

COMA

Definitions

Coma is a "state of unarousable unresponsiveness without evidence of awareness of self and environment."[3] Normal consciousness is the inverse of this: "the presence of a wakeful arousal state coupled with awareness and motivation to respond to internal or external events and stimuli."[4] Consciousness comprises content and arousal. Content refers to all cognitive and affective functions that need a functioning cerebral cortex, and it is the recovery of these that determines long-term outcomes of coma. The comatose state is thus a clinical determination that has to be made at the bedside, and a consensus clinical and operational definition is provided in **Box 1**. At the upper limits of this state is an individual that opens eyes to pain, utters incomprehensible or moaning sounds, and at best

BOX 1 Definition of coma.[4]

- No arousal, either spontaneous or stimulus-induced
- GCS of 8 (E2 M4 V2) or less
- No purposeful response to visual, vocal, or tactile/painful stimulus (withdrawal, posturing, or triple flexion may occur)
- No eye opening/closing or visual pursuit/fixation/saccades to command
- No intelligible speech or recognizable gesture
- Not due to paralytic agents or sedatives
- Not due to another neurologic (locked-in state, neuromuscular paralysis, akinetic mutism) or psychiatric disorder (catatonia, functional neurologic disorder)
- No cognitive motor dissociation on electrophysiologic testing or functional MRI (if testing is available)

(GCS: Glasgow coma scale; MRI: magnetic resonance imaging)

withdraws from pain. Brainstem functions may be variably impaired and are a crucial determinant of prognosis. The only physiologic equivalent is normal sleep where brainstem functions are intact. The definition above does not include duration, but one study included patients only if they had been in a coma as defined for 6 hours or more, possibly because reversible causes are unlikely to persist beyond that time after reaching medical attention. In coma survivors with brainstem recovery, the sleep-like state lasts 2–4 weeks. As the "forebrain shock" due to dysfunction of arousal systems wanes, sleep–wake cycles return and these patients then transition to one of the C-DoC states. The term coma is reserved for patients who are alive, which means that they have some evidence of brainstem function.

Etiology

Box 2 lists, in sequence, the 10 most common causes of SABI presenting in a coma as determined by consensus.[4] The frequency of individual causes will vary depending on geography and level of care (e.g., tertiary vs. primary and developed country vs. low- to middle-income country). The most frequent currently seem to be intracerebral hemorrhage, traumatic brain injury (TBI), and hypoxic-ischemic encephalopathy (HIE) following cardiopulmonary resuscitation (CPR) and return of spontaneous circulation.

Mechanisms and Course

Consciousness needs awareness, processing, integration, and responsiveness. It is maintained by complex networks that link central thalamic (anterior and posterior intralaminar nuclei) neurons with the cortex (thalamocortical) and with the striatum (thalamostriatal). Pathways connect the cortex, thalamus, and basal ganglia (cortico-striatopallidal-thalamic) and this is termed the anterior forebrain mesocircuit. The mesocircuit, together with the ascending reticular activating system (ARAS), maintains awareness. This circuit works with the frontoparietal circuit (discussed below) for the other components of consciousness. Coma is due to one of the following etiopathologies: (1) bilateral diffuse or multifocal hemispheric structural pathologies, (2) unilateral massive lesion/s with herniation, (3) metabolic/toxic encephalopathies, (4) status epilepticus, and (5) focal lesions involving the diencephalon and brainstem (bilateral thalamic with extension into the midbrain and/or rostral dorsolateral pontine tegmentum). The forebrain dysfunction of coma is possibly due to one or more of three possibly overlapping mechanisms:[5]

1. *Destruction of forebrain neurons*: If extensive, this is associated with BD or permanent vegetative state (VS), and the likelihood of recovery is negligible.
2. *Thalamocortical disconnection*: The widespread point-to-point connections of central thalamic neurons to the cortex make them particularly vulnerable to deafferentation and disconnection. This may occur, for example, with diffuse axonal injury in TBI, permitting late recovery as structural alterations compensate for the original damage.
3. The "mesocircuit hypothesis" postulates the third mechanism. Normally the globus pallidus, mainly interna (GPi) but possibly also externa (GPe), inhibits thalamocortical activity. Both GPi and GPe[6] are controlled by the medium spiny neurons (MSNs) of the striatum. Damage to these neurons (vulnerable to hypoxia) and/or cortico-thalamo-striatal damage and disconnection reduce this GABAergic input to the globus pallidus. The GPi and perhaps the GPe then actively inhibit the thalamus and reduce its excitatory glutamatergic output to the cortex. Electrophysiologically, withdrawal of this cortical excitatory activity in a coma, either by destruction or by active inhibition, produces "disfacilitation" and passive hyperpolarization followed by the appearance of very slow rhythms (<1 Hz) across the corticothalamic system.[7] This particular mechanism allows the possibility of pharmacologic manipulation or neuromodulation. Which mechanism dominates in a given patient is crucial to long-term prognosis.

Mechanisms of Recovery from Coma

Recovery begins with reactivation of the ascending activating network (AAN), also termed ARAS, which is relatively resilient to hypoxia and herniation. In TBI studied with magnetic resonance imaging (MRI) diffusion tensor imaging (DTI), restitution of brainstem–thalamic connectivity has been shown to correlate with the recovery of consciousness.[8] The central thalamus then presumably begins providing facilitatory input to the anterior forebrain mesocircuit. This is the stage of the VS. Transition to the minimally conscious state (MCS) is marked by reactivation of the frontoparietal subcircuits (also termed "intrinsic" networks). Of these the default mode network (DMN) subserves internal self-awareness while the executive control network is responsible for attention, especially to the environment. Restitution of cognition corresponds with the reappearance of intrinsic network (especially DMN) connectivity with "extrinsic" or "task-positive" networks, which are active in goal-directed functions. These are the visual, auditory, sensorimotor,

BOX 2 Etiologies of coma.[4]

- Traumatic brain injury
- Intracerebral hemorrhage
- Cardiac arrest/HIE
- Spontaneous subarachnoid hemorrhage
- Ischemic stroke
- Metabolic/toxic encephalopathy
- Epilepsy/status epilepticus
- Sepsis
- CNS infection
- Brain tumors

(CNS: central nervous system; HIE: hypoxic-ischemic encephalopathy) and salience networks that process sensory stimuli and are active in cognitive tasks. When these reactivate, clinically the patient transits from MCS to a confused state (see below). In patients with SABI, mesocircuit and intrinsic (frontoparietal) network function recovery can potentially occur within weeks while extrinsic network connectivity recovers over months. Early recovery probably corresponds with the resolution of edema and electrical dysfunction.

Prognosticating in the First Few Weeks

The initial decision-making is for the identification of BD and confirmation of irreversibility (see below). Of the remainder, many of these patients improve slowly over 3–12 months or plateau in a severely disabled state. Adequate rehabilitation can speed up, prolong, and elevate this trajectory. However, since the availability of rehabilitation is limited, there is an unfortunate triage of those judged least likely to benefit. The likelihood of self-fulfilling prophecy is an important concern and has been demonstrated especially in intracerebral hemorrhage.[9] Frontera et al.[2] estimate that in the USA, LST is withdrawn in up to 15% of these patients and this accounts for about 60% of the mortality in this category. Rizoli et al.,[10] studying prediction in coma [Glasgow coma scale (GCS) < 8 at admission and surviving >24 hours] due to TBI, found severe residual disability [Glasgow outcome scale-extended (GOSE) ≤4] in 43% at 6 months. This is best delineated by GOSE. A score of 4 (upper severe disability) means an individual who can look after herself at home for 8 hours but cannot manage longer (24 hours) or travel outside the home. A systematic literature review[11] of nontraumatic coma showed a mortality rate of 25–87% with moderate-to-severe residual disability in 5–25%. Bates (2001)[12] reviewed earlier literature on outcomes in a medical coma and identified four important clinical factors for prognostication: etiology, depth of coma, duration of coma, and clinical signs **(Table 1)**. These figures, although dated, are essentially clinical and hence are unlikely to become truly obsolete, but they should be used subject to caveats as discussed below. In HIE, since the brainstem is relatively resistant to hypoxia, diffuse hemispheric damage determines outcomes and can be largely identified by MRI diffusion-weighted imaging. Electrophysiology, especially evoked potentials, have also been used. Clinically the motor score is predictive of outcomes.[13] Ischemic stroke is easier to predict and recovers consciousness unless the crucial thalamic and brainstem structures are involved. Intracerebral and subarachnoid hemorrhage, especially the latter (because of vasospasm and seizures), can fluctuate in the first few weeks. The most challenging is TBI because injuries are both multifocal and heterogenous with hemorrhages of various sizes and diffuse axonal injury. Multiple models have been developed[14] mainly for identifying the poorest prognosis in the initial few days,[10] and the focus is on specificity rather than sensitivity. Overall prognostic determinations for all etiologies in the initial 2–3 weeks focus on identifying candidates for withdrawal of LST. Patients who are likely to do well transition out of coma and into C-DoC early. Covert consciousness (CC) (see below) is an important indicator of a likely better prognosis than expected.

TABLE 1: Indicative features and outcomes in medical/nontraumatic coma (after 6 hours of admission).[10]

Feature	Death, PVS, and severe disability (%)	Moderate disability or better (%)
Hypoxic-ischemic etiology	89	11
Cerebrovascular	93	7
At admission: Absent two of three: corneal, pupillary, oculovestibular	99	1
At admission: Brainstem reflexes present but motor responses absent or only abnormal extensor or flexor posturing	83	17
At 24 hours: Absent oculovestibular or pupillary responses	98	2
At 7 days: Still in coma (GCS ≤ 8)	94	6

(GCS: Glasgow coma scale; PVS: persistent vegetative state)

BRAIN DEATH

Pathogenesis

Any of the causes of SABI can trigger the final common pathway. The massive increase in intracranial pressure (ICP), in addition to manifesting as herniation, also reduces cerebral perfusion causing further secondary hypoxia. Eventually, cerebral circulatory arrest ensues due to ICP exceeding mean arterial pressure. Brain damage proceeds from anterior to posterior, and the last to be lost is the medullary function, with the onset of apnea.

Definitions

Death is both a medical diagnosis and a legal issue, and hence terminology matters. The World Brain Death Project[15] defines BD and death by neurologic criteria (DNC) as follows: "the complete and permanent loss of brain function as defined by an unresponsive coma with loss of capacity for consciousness, brainstem reflexes, and the ability to breathe independently, resulting from the permanent cessation of oxygenated circulation to the brain and/or devastating brain injury." Permanent means that function cannot be restored or resume spontaneously or through intervention. Since BD is the common term familiar to the lay public, they suggest retaining it but with a combined acronym, hence BD/DNC. However, the semantics of the words "complete" and "coma" in this definition are not consistent. This is because some jurisdictions use the term "whole BD" and/or "brainstem death." Whole (or complete) BD is not appropriate since some neuroendocrine hypothalamic functions (hypophysiotropic hormone secretion, osmoregulation, and responsiveness to anterior pituitary stimulation) persist in patients who otherwise meet BD/DNC criteria. Brainstem death refers to irreversible loss of brainstem reflexes with possible preservation of some cerebral and/or neuroendocrine function,[16] and this has led to some controversy. As mentioned above, the terms coma and BD/DNC should not be combined.

Diagnosis

The clinical determination of brainstem death (apnea and loss of brainstem reflexes) and the confirmation of etiopathogenesis (imaging evidence of primary SABI and/or cerebral circulatory arrest) are both necessary for the diagnosis of BD/DNC.[17] These have evolved from the AAN criteria for adults that were formulated in 1995 and updated in 2010.[18] There are no published reports of any recovery of neurologic function after BD/DNC diagnosis by these criteria, although individuals have been maintained on ventilators for prolonged periods.[19] Irreversibility is confirmed by the diagnosis of a condition that is sufficient to cause BD and an adequate waiting period that depends on the etiology. For instance, in HIE, waiting 24 hours is appropriate since imaging abnormalities may not emerge till 3–5 days. In adults, only a single examination (see **Table 2** for details) suffices with only a single positive apnea test, since irreversibility can be confirmed by adequately delaying the first test. A second test (in India) is required after a minimum of 6 hours if BD/DNC is for organ harvesting.[20] In children, two tests with a minimum gap of 24 hours are required, especially for neonates (gestation 37 weeks to 30 days postnatal). In some jurisdictions, this is shortened to 12 hours for children (up to 14 or 18 years of age). In patients who have been subjected to targeted temperature management or therapeutic hypothermia for anoxic insult, BD/DNC requires imaging confirmation of severe cerebral edema and then a waiting period of 24 hours after rewarming to 36°C. Sedative medication effects require a delay of five half-lives of the slowest metabolized drug. Other toxicologic

TABLE 2: Clinical examination to check for BD or DNC.

Test	Anatomical level	Procedure	Congruent responses	Cautions and exclusions
Consciousness and motor responses	Whole neuraxis	*Deep pressure*: TMJ condyles, supraorbital notch, sternum, all four extremities (proximal + distal) Nasal tickle with cotton-tipped stick	No grimace, facial movement, or limb movement	• Spinal reflex movements, especially with stimulation below neck, should not be confused for response • Ancillary testing required for severe facial injury, severe neuromuscular disorder, unclear interpretation of limb movement (spinal vs. cerebral)
Pupillary reflex	Upper brainstem	Shine bright light into each eye and assess pupillary diameter	• *No response*: Pupils fixed in mid- to-dilated position (4–6 mm) • Small/constricted pupils are not consistent with BD/DNC	• Use magnifying glass or pupillometer • Ancillary testing recommended if pupils cannot be seen
Corneal reflex	Upper and mid-brainstem	Touch cotton-tipped stick at external border of iris	No eyelid movement	*Ancillary testing*: If severe orbital or scleral edema
OCR and OVR	Mid-brainstem	*OCR*: Rotate head briskly to both sides *OVR*: Head elevated to 30°. Then instill 30–50 mL ice water over 1 minute, on either side with 5-minute interval between them	• No eye movements with either maneuver • In case of cervical spine injury or suspected spine fracture, check only OVR and if it is conclusive, no need for ancillary testing	Ancillary testing required if response is obliterated by skull fracture (base or petrous temporal) or restricted by orbital/scleral edema
Gag and cough reflexes	Lower brainstem	*Gag*: Stimulate posterior pharyngeal wall bilaterally with suction catheter *Cough*: Stimulate tracheo-bronchial wall at carina level with suction catheter	No gag or cough	Ancillary testing required with high cervical spine injury since cough may be lost due to phrenic paralysis
Apnea testing	Lower brainstem	Please see text		

(BD: brain death; DNC: death by neurologic criteria; OCR: oculocephalic reflexes; OVR: oculovestibular reflexes; TMJ: temporomandibular joint)

confounders that can mimic brainstem failure include snake envenomation, drug overdose (baclofen, tricyclic antidepressants, bupropion, barbiturates), alcohols (ethanol and ethylene glycol), and organophosphates.[21] Of these the longest durations reported were with ethylene glycol (over 2 months).

Apnea Testing

Medullary respiratory centers are very responsive to hypercarbia and acidosis but not so to hypoxia. For testing, ventilation is discontinued and partial pressure of carbon dioxide (pCO_2) levels are allowed to rise to see if respiratory efforts are triggered. This should only be performed after the following criteria are met:

- Identification of etiology and confirmation of irreversibility as above
- Absent brainstem reflexes (see **Table 2**), which clearly means that apnea testing is done last
- *Vasomotor stability*: If need be with fluid repletion and/or vasopressors/inotropes
- *Normothermia*: At least 36°C, if required with warming measures
- Preoxygenation with 100% O_2 for 10 minutes

Ideally, normocarbia (pCO_2 35–45 mm Hg), partial pressure of oxygen (pO_2) >200 mm Hg, and normal pH should be confirmed by arterial blood gas (ABG) testing before proceeding. The ventilator is then disconnected, and the oxygen supply (4–6 L/min) is maintained by insufflation through a catheter in the lower trachea for 10 minutes. Oxygen supply can also be maintained with continuous positive airway pressure (CPAP)/positive end-expiratory pressure (PEEP) settings on the ventilator. Testing must be aborted if (1) respiratory efforts are seen, (2) systolic blood pressure drops below 100 mm Hg, and (3) arterial oxygen saturation (SaO_2) drops below 85%. At the end of 10 minutes, an ABG sample is sent, the ventilator is reconnected, and the patient is hyperventilated for a short period. ABG should now show pCO_2 over 60 mm Hg or a rise of 20 mm Hg above the previous baseline for confirmation of loss of respiratory drive. If no respiratory effort is seen, a declaration of death and further procedures will follow local rules. The main risk is vasomotor collapse during testing.

Ancillary Testing

These are mandatorily required in some countries as part of BD/DNC diagnosis. Clinically, they are recommended under the following circumstances: (1) inability to complete apnea test (e.g., due to vasomotor instability), (2) facial injuries restricting brainstem reflex testing, (3) confounders such as hypothermia and toxic exposures, (4) severe spinal injury, and (5) uncertain interpretation of possible spinal movements (i.e., if the family is not willing to accept the diagnosis based on posturing). Ideally, these tests should confirm the cerebral circulatory arrest. Hence, the current reference gold standard is conventional four-vessel digital subtraction angiography, which shows no filling beyond the level where the internal carotid and vertebral arteries enter the skull, with patent external carotid circulation. Radionuclide studies [single photon emission computed tomography (CT)] are an acceptable and recommended alternative. Transcranial Doppler is also acceptable (not recommended) and requires expertise and adequate acoustic windows and must be repeated once after 30 minutes for confirmation. CT angiography and MR angiography are widely available but their validity is still uncertain and hence are not recommended yet. Electrophysiologic testing has a long history but is not recommended for BD/DNC determination unless mandated by local legal requirements. Electroencephalogram (EEG) (no detectable activity ≥ 2 μV) is confounded by the same issues that can confound apnea and clinical testing (sedation, hypothermia, etc.). Sensitivity and specificity are approximately 50–80%. Evoked potential testing (preferably multimodality) runs into the same problems and is perhaps better used to identify poor prognosis in individuals who are not brain dead. Clinical exams should always be completed to the fullest extent possible before performing any ancillary tests, even if these are legally required. If the ancillary test picks up blood flow or activity, then BD/DNC declaration has to be suspended. If the apnea and clinical testing continue to be consistent with BD, alternate end-of-life or PC may have to be considered.

Ethical and Other Controversies

The first controversy is philosophical. This is based on a point of view that if death is the cessation of the organism as a whole, BD/DNC is not adequate proof, since various components are still functional. Bernat,[22] in response, argues that the brain is responsible for the critical emergent functions of the human organism. Conceptually, biological entities follow a hierarchical organizational pattern. Lower-level components integrate to form a higher level of structure. Functions then emerge that would not be possible for the individual components at the lower level. The brain is responsible for the emergent functions of conscious awareness, circulatory control, and respiratory drive. As a practical answer, beyond about a week of BD, hormonal, autonomic, and immune functions begin to deteriorate, and maintaining these "individuals" becomes a complex exercise in critical care. The second major controversy is due to the somewhat loose concept in the American Uniform Determination of Death Act, which allows BD/DNC to be determined by acceptable medical standards.[23] Since these "standards" varied significantly from state to state and even between institutions, the inconsistencies led to misdiagnoses, especially in younger individuals with TBI. Cases emerged of individuals certified brain dead who were completely normal a year or so later! Lewis et al.[23] argue that the acceptable standard has to be the guidelines generated consensually by professional societies such as the AAN and these must be specified by law. The third major controversy relates to whether the process of diagnosing BD/DNC can begin without the consent of family or surrogates as proposed by Lewis et al. Apnea testing is a potentially lethal procedure. Given our current emphasis on patient autonomy and shared decision-making, the reasoning that "death gives no choice, hence no consent" has to be reexamined.[24] Notably, the World Brain Death Project supports "no consent required" but suggests that there needs to be legislative or regulatory sanction for doing away with this requirement and for withdrawal of somatic support after confirmation. The last controversy is about the religious rejection of BD/DNC. Since this obviously links to the rejection of cadaveric organ donation, all countries have worked on resolving this with religious authorities. No major world religion clearly opposes BD/DNC, but local communities and families do raise objections based on religious concerns.

Current legal status in India: The only legislation to deal with BD/DNC in India is the Human Organ Transplantation Act. This offers no guidance for BD when a transplant is not envisioned. The Aruna Shanbaug judgment mentioned this issue in passing and clearly stated that it was acceptable to withdraw.[25] Even earlier, statutory regulations under the Indian Medical Council Act had permitted withdrawal of supports using the same process as in the Transplantation of Human Organs and Tissues Act (THOTA). Currently, three state governments (Kerala, Karnataka, and Gujarat) have passed government resolutions that permit ventilator disconnection in BD. The Kerala order in fact clarifies that no consent is required for either BD/DNC determination or withdrawal of support. The only end-of-life judgment passed so far in India concerns a Delhi hospital that was penalized for holding a boy who was brain dead on the ventilator beyond medical necessity. Thus, Indian practitioners who proceed with the termination of LST after BD/DNC should have no concerns about adverse litigation. In a private healthcare system, the bigger issue is who will pay for ventilating a dead body. If insurance objects, the hospital may be left holding the bill. It is quite likely that in the near future, the central government will officially include BD/DNC in a uniform declaration of death regulation that is specific to India.

CHRONIC DISORDERS OF CONSCIOUSNESS

Evolving Nosology

Chronic DoC begins at or after 28 days post-injury as per the operational definition of the AAN guideline.[26] The lowest state above coma is the VS, termed persistent if stable for 1 month and permanent once further recovery is deemed unlikely (3 months nontraumatic and 12 months TBI). Because of the negative perceptions of "vegetative," it is now often termed an unresponsive wakefulness state (UWS). It consists of arousal without awareness and is marked by spontaneous eye opening as part of sleep-wake cycles, which are random and not controlled by circadian rhythms. There is no response to stimulation even though crying, laughing, and vocalization may occur spontaneously. The next level is the MCS minus (MCS–) in which awareness appears and inconsistent, minimal, but reproducible signs of voluntary response are seen. The earliest evidence is usually visual fixation or tracking and can be sought by the mirror test, as the subject looks at her own face. Localizing motor responses, avoidance of noxious stimuli, and object manipulation may all be seen. In MCS+, some language reappears and is marked by command following, yes-no responses, intelligible verbalization, and intentional communication.[27] Functional interactive communication and/or functional object use marks the next level, termed the confusional state or emergence from MCS (e-MCS). Locked-in syndrome (LIS) is often included in the differential diagnosis of C-DoC but is due to de-efferentation, with injury to the pyramidal tracts usually in the mid-pons leaving the patient conscious but aphonic and quadriplegic. The only mode of communication remaining in LIS is through partly preserved eye movements. In all C-DoC, evaluation for recovery of cognitive and motor functions must be performed systematically using the coma recovery scale-revised (CRS-R). Nonsystematic assessment using current bedside methods has a miscategorization rate of 30–40%. Typically, MCS is not identified and is mistaken for UWS/VS, and this distinction is very important for prognosis. The CRS-R needs training and about 30 minutes for administration per session. Because responses in MCS fluctuate widely, it must be repeated five (nontraumatic coma) or six (traumatic coma) times, over a period of 1–3 weeks[28] for confirming a negative response. For patients in e-MCS, the confusion assessment protocol (CAP)[29] tests for disorientation, cognitive impairment, psychosis, restlessness and fluctuations, or diurnal variations **(Table 3)**.

Covert Consciousness or Cognitive-motor Dissociation

The first report of this condition appeared in 2006[30] and was soon followed by others. This condition refers to approximately 15–20% of individuals with a clinical diagnosis of coma or UWS/VS or MCS–, in whom voluntary brain activity can be detected by functional MRI (fMRI) or EEG (together termed advanced imaging and electrophysiology-based techniques or AIE).[31] EEG techniques[32] utilize advanced computing and machine learning and include resting state alpha power and evoked potentials such as the N400. The most promising is combined transcranial magnetic stimulation (TMS) and EEG, utilizing the perturbation complexity index. Task-based AIE depends on subjects following a command by performing motor imagery ("imagine hitting a ball with a bat/racquet") or mental navigation ("imagine entering your home and walking around it"). External network activation is lateralized, and this can be identified by AIE. Some subjects were trained enough to answer yes-no to questions by choosing which task to perform. If command-following is identified in a patient who has no behavioral evidence of language

TABLE 3: Nosology of chronic disorders of consciousness.

Assessment	Findings	Clinical states			
Confusion assessment protocol (CAP)	Functional communication				Confusional state or e-MCS
Motor function with CRS-R*	Command following			MCS+	
	Purposeful movements		MCS–	MCS+	
CRS-R	Eye opening	Vegetative state (Unresponsive wakeful state)	MCS–		
	No response: Clinical or covert	True negative			
Covert cognition testing by AIE	Passive response	VS with covert cortical processing	Without command following		
Advanced imaging and EEG techniques	Active response		MCS with cognitive motor dissociation	With command following	

(CRS-R: coma recovery scale-revised; EE: Electroencephalogram; MCS: minimally conscious state)

function, this is termed cognitive-motor dissociation (CMD). These studies have a false-negative rate of up to 25% in normal volunteers. Hence, if no response is obtained, a passive response to language (affectively salient stimuli, e.g., loved one's voice) or music is tried with resting-state fMRI or electrophysiologic study. Passive responses in association cortex indicate covert cortical processing or CC. Patients in whom CMD is identified are considered to be in MCS+. Monti and Schnakers discuss the clinical relevance of AIE.[31] The first is the clear evidence of the prognostic significance of CMD (but not CC), in terms of functional recovery in both acute and chronic DoC. Claassen et al.[33] could identify brain activation in 16 of 104 patients in a single intensive care unit (ICU), a median of 4 days after the onset of coma. At 12 months, 7 of these 16 patients (as against 12 of the remaining 84) had attained a GOSE level of 4 or higher, denoting functional independence. This obviously allows clinicians to prioritize those in whom rehabilitation is most likely to provide benefit. Second, knowing about CC/CMD alters goals of care, especially end-of-life decisions (withholding or withdrawing LST) and pain management. Third, these patients would also be prime candidates for neuromodulation with brain-computer interfaces.

Prognosis after the Initial Few Weeks

Faugeras et al.[34] found that patients who were in UWS/VS at 3 months largely (97%) remained in the same state (GOSE < 4) over the following 6–12 months while those who had reached MCS had a significantly better outcome (47% GOSE ≥ 4). Noé et al.[35] reported on the neurobehavioral progress of 100 consecutive patients (40 traumatic and 60 nontraumatic) with UWS/VS admitted to inpatient multidisciplinary rehabilitation in a network of four hospitals in Valencia, Spain. With systematic weekly standardized assessments, these patients were followed till discharge, death, or emergence from MCS. Over the course of the study, 34 progressed to MCS, 12 emerged from MCS, and 10 died. These 12 patients who emerged were all younger (13–33 years of age) and 10 were due to trauma. In a parallel paper from the same group, Olaya et al.[36] found that the 1 year post-emergence, most patients were still severely dependent. Of the 12 patients, 2 required minimal-to-moderate assistance with activities of daily living, 3 were completely independent as regards to sphincter management, 1 was mobile with supervision, and 2 had died. But all required moderate-to-total assistance with executive, i.e., day-to-day functioning. Estraneo et al.[37] reported on a 5-year follow-up of 13 similar patients who had emerged from VS/UWS and had been discharged from inpatient rehabilitation. Two had succumbed to complications and 11 survived but none was completely independent on activities of daily living or in transfers. All had cognitive and behavioral issues but were able to communicate adequately with relatives and caregivers. In addition to these two systematic reports, there are multiple reports with similar outcomes. Of course, there are random reports of individuals who regain functional independence years after TBI but that seems to be too rare to be predictable. Mortality is significant:[37] over a 2-year period, over 42% in VS/UWS versus 16% in MCS. Predictors of mortality[38] included age > 51 years and comorbidities.

Management

Ideally, these patients should be managed in specialized inpatient multidisciplinary rehabilitation units. Essentials of management include (1) daily physiotherapy with passive range-of-motion exercises and placing into an upright/sitting position preferably with a tilt table, (2) control of agitation with beta blockers and neuroleptics (quetiapine, olanzapine, risperidone), (3) management of pain by monitoring for it and using simple analgesics, and (4) multisensory stimulation with massage, music, aromatherapy, etc. Trials with drugs that have been reported to improve consciousness are indicated. Amantadine[5] (200–400 mg/day for 4–6 weeks) has some evidence in TBI. Other neurostimulants with positive but limited evidence include methylphenidate, modafinil, levodopa, apomorphine, memantine, and citalopram. A single dose of 10 mg of zolpidem can be tried and repeated with systematic assessment using the CRS-R. In one study it produced >5-point improvement in the CRS-R in 5% of patients. Noninvasive brain stimulation with either transcranial direct current or magnetic devices is often used. Invasive neuromodulation with deep brain stimulation (DBS) has not shown many results. Medical complications are common in these patients[37,38] and include pressure sores, urinary infections, tracheostomy-related issues, upper gastrointestinal complications related to gastrostomy and hepatic dysfunction, in addition to age-related comorbidities. Paroxysmal sympathetic hyperactivity syndrome is uncommon but is marked by motor hyperactivity in addition to the sympathetic storm and can cause weight loss. Some patients will continue to have epileptic seizures.

ETHICAL DECISION-MAKING IN SEVERE ACUTE BRAIN INJURY AND DISORDERS OF CONSCIOUSNESS: THE INDIAN PERSPECTIVE

Decision points in the clinical trajectory of SABI are as follows:

- *Day 1-5*: Curative or salvage therapies provide variable benefit. In selected cases, dramatic results are seen but, in many others, expensive interventions may not justify the final outcome[39,40] and have been strongly criticized on ethical grounds. These include neurointervention (thrombectomy) and neurosurgery including DC.
- *Day 1-3*: BD/DNC: This is often obvious from the severity of the original insult. In some patients, it may be decided not to perform DC and try medical therapy instead for raised ICP. Here, brain herniation may evolve over a longer period.
- *Day 10–20*: Tracheostomy and gastrostomy versus palliative extubation. Wijdicks[41] terms this the "fork in the road" when families with our support must decide about forgoing LST and accepting PC versus embarking on a long and uncertain journey with a loved one in C-DoC. In India, specialized inpatient rehabilitation is not easily available, and much depends on the caregiver/s' commitment and capacity. Families contemplating withdrawal often ask about organ donation but that is possible only in countries with legislation supporting donation after cardiac death, as has been proposed for India.[42] See Ramchand[43] for a wonderfully evocative story of how this works.
- *Weeks to months*: As discussed above, at 2–4 weeks patients transition to a C-DoC. Earlier and higher trajectories raise hopes for a full recovery but by 3 months, final outcomes are largely predictable, especially in nontraumatic coma. In older patients, medical complications now determine the course. In a traumatic coma, especially in younger individuals, permanent VS/UWS can be accepted only after 12 months. This is a period of intense caregiver burden. If medical advances improve outcomes, this stage will also produce new challenges, eloquently explained by Fins.[44]
- *Months to years*: Families/surrogates may decide to withdraw care once it is certain that the condition has plateaued. In most countries, this decision has to go through the courts. Withdrawal of assisted nutrition and hydration produces death by dehydration and renal shut down over a period of 10–14 days.[45]

Family Meetings and Shared Decision-making

The initial contact just after admission tends to be fraught. Information may be limited, and it may be best to suggest a time-limited trial of maximal therapy for a period of 48–72 hours. This usually satisfies the requirements of ethics, economics, and common sense. It is recommended that the first full meeting be scheduled and held within 72 hours. Setting up and running this meeting is a core competence for anyone practicing neurointensive care.[46] It is important to make sure that all concerned surrogates are available and present. Ideally, a surrogate hierarchy is set by legislation but since we do not have that in India, we depend on the All India Institute of Medical Sciences (AIIMS), Delhi, end-of-life guidelines.[47] Decision-making in these situations is preference-based, as opposed to the evidence-based decision-making that we normally use. The order to be followed is:

1. *Patient's known wishes*: Ideally in the form of advance medical directives (AMDs) but if not available, then clearly expressed verbal wishes must be taken into account.
2. *Substituted judgment*: Ideally this should be a designated healthcare proxy (as part of the AMD) but if not specified, it must follow the surrogate hierarchy. It has to be clearly explained to the surrogates that this decision-making is not about their own wishes and that their role is to be the voice of the absent patient.
3. *Best interests decision-making*:[48] This is often the clinician's responsibility and should ideally be consensual and if this is not possible, it is best left to the judicial system. As clinicians, our responsibility is to share information appropriately (see Chapter 129: Breaking Bad News) on our prognostic estimates of neurologic outcome and future QoL. Surrogates' input consists of

their estimate of the patient's goals and values for an acceptable QoL. Shared decision-making then leads to setting of goals of care. When decision-making is difficult, a time-limited trial should be negotiated. This sets out a therapeutic plan, anticipated outcomes, and a time point at which a further meeting can be held, usually at 3–5 days. As clinicians, we need to be aware of our own biases,[49] which can be either positive or negative. If negative, we run the risk of self-fulfilling prophecies: withdrawal of LST converts possible mortality to certain death. For surrogates, the two major risks are of the focusing illusion (healthy people focus on what is lost, while devaluing those aspects of life that will continue) and the disability paradox (people with severe disabilities report better QoL than healthy people asked to imagine being in the same situation). This decision-making becomes especially complex in C-DoC,[1] because of ethical challenges in judging the benefits, harms, feasibility, and practicability of any course of action.

Forgoing LST: The Indian legal scenario: In 2011, a two-judge bench of the Supreme Court of India (SCI) first weighed in on the issue of withdrawal of LST and declared it legal in the Aruna Shanbaug case. Then in 2018, a five-judge Constitution Bench confirmed the constitutional validity of the right to die with dignity and of AMDs. Both judgements have been considered infructuous because of the impractical procedures that have been prescribed.[50] But prescribing procedures and penalties is the job of the state legislatures and/or Parliament, and that has not happened so far. So we are in an evolving situation, and the ethical practitioner must and can safely follow institutional or society guidelines.[47,51,52] Decisions to forgo LST should follow due process and must be consensual, transparent, and adequately documented.

CONCLUSION

Managing SABI requires a combination of scientific knowledge and clinical acumen with clarity about the ethical and legal frameworks. Every patient's and family's situation is unique. It is our responsibility to do right and to be seen to have done right. If not done well, it can leave the surviving family traumatized. Futile care that leaves them with debts and a death can have adversarial consequences. Our commitment to shared decision-making is necessary to support the surrogates through the process and minimize their sense of guilt if withdrawal is appropriate. If they wish to continue, we must respect their commitment and support them.

REFERENCES

1. Peterson A, Young MJ, Fins JJ. Ethics and the 2018 practice guideline on disorders of consciousness: a framework for responsible implementation. Neurology. 2022;98(17):712-8.
2. Frontera JA, Curtis JR, Nelson JE, Campbell M, Gabriel M, Mosenthal AC, et al. Integrating palliative care into the care of neurocritically ill patients: a report from the improving palliative care in the ICU Project Advisory Board and the Centre to Advance Palliative Care. Crit Care Med. 2015;43(9):1964-77.
3. Brogan ME, Provencio JJ. Spectrum of catastrophic brain injury: coma and related disorders of consciousness. J Crit Care. 2014;29(4):679-82.
4. Helbok R, Rass V, Beghi E, Bodien YG, Citerio G, Giacino JT, et al. Curing Coma Campaign and its contributing members. The Curing Coma Campaign International Survey on coma epidemiology, evaluation, and therapy (COME TOGETHER). Neurocrit Care. 2022;37(1):47-59.
5. Schiff ND. Recovery of consciousness after brain injury: a mesocircuit hypothesis. Trends Neurosci. 2010;33(1):1-9.
6. Zheng ZS, Monti MM. Cortical and thalamic connections of the human globus pallidus: implications for disorders of consciousness. Front Neuroanat. 2022;16:960439.
7. Edlow BL, Claassen J, Schiff ND, Greer DM. Recovery from disorders of consciousness: mechanisms, prognosis, and emerging therapies. Nat Rev Neurol. 2021;17(3):135-56.
8. Snider SB, Bodien YG, Frau-Pascual A, Bianciardi M, Foulkes AS, Edlow BL. Ascending arousal network connectivity during recovery from traumatic coma. Neuroimage Clin. 2020;28:102503.
9. Lun R, Yogendrakumar V, Ramsay T, Shamy M, Fahed R, Selim MH, et al. Predicting long-term outcomes in acute intracerebral hemorrhage using delayed prognostication scores. Stroke Vasc Neurol. 2021;6(4):536-41.
10. Rizoli S, Petersen A, Bulger E, Coimbra R, Kerby JD, Minei J, et al. ROC investigators. Early prediction of outcome after severe traumatic brain injury: a simple and practical model. BMC Emerg Med. 2016;16(1):32.
11. Horsting MW, Franken MD, Meulenbelt J, van Klei WA, de Lange DW. The etiology and outcome of nontraumatic coma in critical care: a systematic review. BMC Anesthesiol. 2015;15:65.
12. Bates D. The prognosis of medical coma. J Neurol Neurosurg Psychiatry. 2001;71(Suppl 1):i20-3.
13. Nolan JP, Soar J, Cariou A, Cronberg T, Moulaert VR, Deakin CD, et al. European Resuscitation Council; European Society of Intensive Care Medicine. European Resuscitation Council and European Society of Intensive Care Medicine 2015 guidelines for postresuscitation care. Intensive Care Med. 2015;41(12):2039-56.
14. Gao J, Zheng Z. Development of prognostic models for patients with traumatic brain injury: a systematic review. Int J Clin Exp Med. 2015;8(11):19881-5.
15. Greer DM, Shemie SD, Lewis A, Torrance S, Varelas P, Goldenberg FD, et al. Determination of brain death/death by neurologic criteria: the World Brain Death Project. JAMA. 2020;324(11):1078-97.
16. Machado C. Brain death diagnosis in primary posterior fossa lesions. Neurol India. 2022;70:670-5.
17. Greer DM. Determination of brain death. N Engl J Med. 2021;385(27):2554-61.
18. Wijdicks EF, Varelas PN, Gronseth GS, Greer DM. American Academy of Neurology. Evidence-based guideline update: determining brain death in adults: report of the Quality Standards Subcommittee of the American Academy of Neurology. Neurology. 2010;74(23):1911-8.
19. Shewmon DA. Chronic "brain death": meta-analysis and conceptual consequences. Neurology. 1998;51(6):1538-45.

20. Srivastava A, Mani A. Deceased organ donation and transplantation in India: promises and challenges. Neurol India. 2018;66(2):316-22.
21. Murphy L, Wolfer H, Hendrickson RG. Toxicologic confounders of brain death determination: a narrative review. Neurocrit Care. 2021;34(3):1072-89.
22. Bernat JL. Refinements in the organism as a whole rationale for brain death. Linacre Q. 2019;86(4):347-58.
23. Lewis A, Bonnie RJ, Pope TM. It's time to revise the Uniform Determination of Death Act. Ann Intern Med. 2020;172(2):143-4.
24. Muramoto O. Is informed consent required for the diagnosis of brain death regardless of consent for organ donation? J Med Ethics. 2021;47:e5.
25. Gursahani R. Life and death after Aruna Shanbaug. Ind J Med Ethics. 2011;8:68-9.
26. Giacino JT, Katz DI, Schiff ND, Whyte J, Ashman EJ, Ashwal S, et al. Practice guideline update recommendations summary: disorders of consciousness: report of the Guideline Development, Dissemination, and Implementation Subcommittee of the American Academy of Neurology; the American Congress of Rehabilitation Medicine; the National Institute on Disability, Independent Living, and Rehabilitation Research. Neurology. 2018;91(10):450-60.
27. Thibaut A, Bodien YG, Laureys S, Giacino JT. Minimally conscious state "plus": diagnostic criteria and relation to functional recovery. J Neurol. 2020;267(5):1245-54.
28. Yang H, Ye C, Liu X, Sun L, Wang A, Wang J, et al. Estimating the minimal number of repeated examinations for random responsiveness with the coma recovery scale-revised as an example. Front Integr Neurosci. 2021;15:685627.
29. Sherer M. (2004). Introduction to the Confusion Assessment Protocol. [online] Available from http://www.tbims.org/combi/cap. [Last accessed January, 2023].
30. Owen AM. The search for consciousness. Neuron. 2019;102(3): 526-8.
31. Monti MM, Schnakers C. Flowchart for implementing advanced imaging and electrophysiology in patients with disorders of consciousness: to fMRI or not to fMRI? Neurology. 2022;98(11):452-9.
32. Bai Y, Lin Y, Ziemann U. Managing disorders of consciousness: the role of electroencephalography. J Neurol. 2021;268(11):4033-65.
33. Claassen J, Doyle K, Matory A, Couch C, Burger KM, Velazquez A, et al. Detection of brain activation in unresponsive patients with acute brain injury. N Engl J Med. 2019;380(26):2497-505.
34. Faugeras F, Rohaut B, Valente M, Sitt J, Demeret S, Bolgert F, et al. Survival and consciousness recovery are better in the minimally conscious state than in the vegetative state. Brain Inj. 2018;32(1):72-7.
35. Noé E, Ferri J, Olaya J, Navarro MD, O'Valle M, Colomer C, et al. When, how, and to what extent are individuals with unresponsive wakefulness syndrome able to progress? Neurobehavioral progress. Brain Sci. 2021;11(1):126.
36. Olaya J, Noé E, Navarro MD, O'Valle M, Colomer C, Moliner B, et al. When, how, and to what extent are individuals with unresponsive wakefulness syndrome able to progress? Functional independence. Brain Sci. 2020;10(12):990.
37. Estraneo A, Magliacano A, Fiorenza S, Formisano R, Grippo A, Angelakis E, et al. Risk factors for 2-year mortality in patients with prolonged disorders of consciousness: an international multicenter study. Eur J Neurol. 2022;29(2):390-9.
38. Pagani M, Leonardi M, Covelli V, Giovannetti AM, Sattin D. Risk factors for mortality in 600 patients in vegetative and minimally conscious states. J Neurol. 2014;261(6):1144-52.
39. Estraneo A, Moretta P, Loreto V, Santoro L, Trojano L. Clinical and neuropsychological long-term outcomes after late recovery of responsiveness: a case series. Arch Phys Med Rehabil. 2014;95(4):711-6.
40. Lönnqvist PA. Medical research and the ethics of medical treatments: disability-free survival. Br J Anaesth. 2017;118(3): 286-8.
41. Wijdicks EFM. Predicting the outcome of a comatose patient at the bedside. Pract Neurol. 2020;20(1):26-33.
42. Seth AK, Mohanka R, Navin S, Gokhale AG, Sharma A, Kumar A, et al. Organ donation after circulatory determination of death in India: a joint position paper. Indian J Crit Care Med. 2022;26(4): 421-38.
43. Ramchand P. The gift. Lancet. 2019;394(10216):2283-4.
44. Fins JJ. The Jeremiah Metzger lecture: disorders of consciousness and the normative uncertainty of an emerging nosology. Trans Am Clin Climatol Assoc. 2020;131:235-69.
45. Turner-Stokes L. A matter of life and death: controversy at the interface between clinical and legal decision-making in prolonged disorders of consciousness. J Med Ethics. 2017;43(7):469-75.
46. Gao L, Zhao CW, Hwang DY. End-of-life care decision-making in stroke. Front Neurol. 2021;12:702833.
47. All India Institute of Medical Sciences. (2022). Guidelines for end-of-life care, AIIMS, New Delhi. [online] Available from https://www.aiims.edu/images/pdf/notice/irch-9-3-20.pdf. [Last accessed January, 2023].
48. British Medical Association. (2019). Best interests decision-making for adults who lack capacity: a toolkit for doctors working in England and Wales. [online] Available from https://www.bma.org.uk/media/1850/bma-best-interests-toolkit-2019.pdf. [Last accessed January, 2023].
49. Creutzfeldt CJ, Holloway RG. Treatment decisions for a future self: ethical obligations to guide truly informed choices. JAMA. 2020;323(2):115-6.
50. Bandewar SV, Chaudhuri L, Duggal L, Nagral S. The supreme court of India on euthanasia: too little, too late. Indian J Med Ethics. 2018;3(2):91-4.
51. Myatra SN, Salins N, Iyer S, Macaden SC, Divatia JV, Muckaden M, et al. End-of-life care policy: an integrated care plan for the dying: a joint position statement of the Indian Society of Critical Care Medicine (ISCCM) and the Indian Association of Palliative Care (IAPC). Indian J Crit Care Med. 2014;18(9):615-35.
52. Mani RK, Simha S, Gursahani R, Mehta D, Garg P, Mathur R. DNAR guidelines from ICMR: meeting a felt need. Indian J Med Ethics. 2020;V(4):1-5.

107

CHAPTER

Inborn Errors of Metabolism

Hansashree Padmanabha, Bidisha Banerjee, Nagaraj AR

INTRODUCTION

Inborn errors of metabolism (IEMs) are rare heterogenous group of inherited disorders that result from disruption of activity in the metabolic pathway leading to either deficiency or accumulation of a specific metabolite. The term was first coined by Sir Archibald Garrod in the early 20th Century to describe four metabolic conditions namely—"alkaptonuria, benign pentosuria, albinism, and cystinuria."[1] Since the discovery of phenylketonuria (PKU) in 1934 by Folling, numerous IEMs have been unraveled with >1,000 IEMs being described to date. It is a common misnomer that IEMs are only seen in neonates and children. IEMs can present at any age from conception to adulthood with protean clinical manifestations affecting any organ/system. IEMs left undiagnosed and untreated lead to significant morbidity and mortality. It is thus important for clinicians to recognize and diagnose IEMs early as many have treatment potential. In this context, the authors describe the clinical presentations, differentials, investigations, and available treatment options for various IEMs to increase awareness among clinicians.

EPIDEMIOLOGY

Though IEMs are individually rare, they are collectively common with a global birth prevalence of 50.9 per 100,000 live births being the highest in eastern Mediterranean regions.[2] However, in the earlier reports, a higher prevalence (1in 784 live births) has been reported in West Midlands, UK due to the effects of ethnicity and consanguinity.[3] More than a century since its initial description, still the exact prevalence of IEMs in India is not known. Available data is limited to anecdotal case reports, case series, and independent small-scale studies mainly because of the wide heterogeneity in the clinical manifestations, relative rarity, and lack of specialized laboratories for diagnostic testing. A noteworthy study from south India had identified metabolic disorders in 3.2% of 3,550 symptomatic children by screening through tandem mass spectrometry.[4] Studies from India suggest a higher prevalence of congenital hypothyroidism (CH), congenital adrenal hyperplasia (CAH), and glucose-6-phosphate dehydrogenase deficiency (G6PD). Overall, the prevalence of IEMs is estimated to be >1 per 1,000 live births worldwide, 1 in 2,497 live births in India and 1 in 1,000 newborns in Andhra Pradesh, India.[5]

PATHOPHYSIOLOGY

Inborn errors of metabolism primarily result from disruption of metabolic activity, which is a continuous process of tissue breakdown and regeneration. Enzymes, cofactors, and specific transport proteins are essential for the same. Mutations in the genes of any of these play an important role in the pathophysiology of inherited metabolic disorders by the following mechanisms either directly by: (1) accumulation of the toxic substrate proximal to the block (e.g., aminoacidopathies—PKU, organic acidemias—methylmalonic acidemia), (2) deficiency of the product of a specific reaction [e.g., thyroid hormone deficiency in CH, "metabolic steal" in case of glycogen storage disorders (GSDs), "metabolic sequestration" due to transport protein defects like in hyperammonemia-hyperornithinemia-homocitrullinemia (HHH) syndrome], (3) accumulation of a normally minor metabolite (e.g., psychosine in Krabbe disease), and indirectly by (4) activation of the secondary metabolic process (e.g., hyperammonemia and hyperglycinemia in patients with methylmalonic acidemia) **(Fig. 1)**.[1,6] Often, more than one mechanisms can contribute to the disease process (e.g., argininosuccinic aciduria—a urea cycle disorder, methylmalonic acidemia, and organic acidemia). Genetics also plays an important role in the pathophysiology as the disease phenotype varies among different affected individuals based on the type of mutation, the influence of other genes (gene-gene interactions), and the environment (gene-environment interactions). Most of the metabolic disorders follow the mendelian

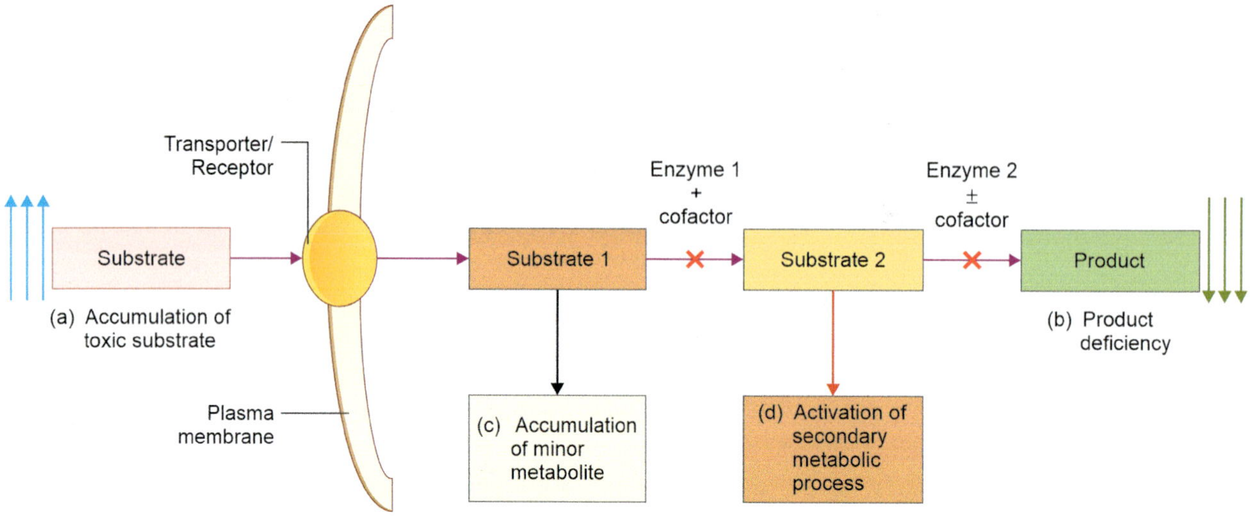

FIG. 1: *Pathogenic mechanisms in the inborn errors of metabolism*. The effect of enzyme/cofactor deficiency results in—(a) direct toxicity from the accumulation of the substrate, (b) deficiency of the product, (c) accumulation of minor metabolite, (d) activation of secondary metabolic process.

pattern of inheritance with the majority being inherited in an autosomal recessive manner as residual enzyme activity in heterozygote carriers is sufficient to prevent the development of disease. However, autosomal dominant, X-linked, and mitochondrial inheritance are also possible. Some of the X-linked recessive disorders are ornithine transcarbamylase deficiency, Lesch-Nyhan syndrome, Fabry disease, hunter syndrome, Menkes syndrome, and X-linked adrenoleukodystrophy (ALD). Autosomal dominant inherited metabolic disorders are cystinuria, glucose transport 1 deficiency, POLG1-related progressive external ophthalmoplegia, and porphobilinogen (PBG) deaminase deficiency. Mitochondrial diseases are of mendelian (nDNA) or maternal inheritance (mtDNA) and show phenotype variability based on mutant mitochondrial DNA.[1,6]

CLASSIFICATION

Traditionally, IEMs were classified in numerous ways based on the clinical manifestations, pathophysiology, or size of the molecules. These are broadly classified into two clinical categories. Category 1 consists of disorders affecting single organs (intestine, renal tubules, etc.) or systems (immune system, coagulation factors, etc.) where the manifestations are uniform and the diagnosis is easier. Category 2 are the disorders affecting a metabolic pathway or a single organ with a multitude of manifestations. Category 2 was subdivided into three distinct groups for diagnostic ease: (1) Group 1 includes disorders of intermediary metabolism affecting small molecules, (2) Group 2 includes disorders of energy metabolism, and (3) Group 3 includes disorders of complex molecules with each group having distinct clinical presentations and management as described in **Table 1**.[6]

Eventually, there was a hierarchical classification by the Society for the Study of Inborn Errors of Metabolism (SSIEM) in 2014 and a proposed nosology by Ferreira et al. in 2019.[7,8] With the evolution of time, a better understanding of the disease process, advancements in genetics, the concept of inclusivity, and option for continuous updation, there came in the International Classification of Inherited Metabolic Disorders (ICIMD) by the ICIMD advisory group in 2021. ICIMD included any disease or disorder with a defined genetic cause in which there are primary alterations in the metabolic pathway, irrespective of the detection of biochemical alterations in the presently available laboratory tests. ICIMD classified IEMs into 24 categories consisting of 124 groups with a total of 1,450 disorders.[9]

CLINICAL PRESENTATIONS

Clinical manifestations of metabolic disorders are heterogenous, often nonspecific, affecting any organ/system and can manifest at any age. The age of onset and the course often provide a clinical indication to the type of IEM. In general, small molecule disorders (intermediary metabolism and energy metabolism) present early as acute metabolic crisis associated with encephalopathy, with periods of relapse and remission, often severe and catastrophic, and a brisk response to treatment. While organelle disorders (complex molecules) manifest late as a chronic, slowly progressive disease, with characteristic examination and histopathological findings with poor response to medications. It is important to keep in mind that some organelle disorders can present with a metabolic crisis requiring emergency intervention. The common noteworthy clinical manifestations, which give clues to an underlying IEM, are briefly described here.

TABLE 1: Broad categorization of IEMs based on the pathophysiology.

Classification	Components		
Category 1	Disorders affecting single organ (intestine, renal tubules, etc.) or system (immune system, coagulation factors, etc.) where the manifestations are uniform and the diagnosis is easier		
Category 2	This category involves disorders affecting a metabolic pathway or a single organ with multitude of manifestations		
Group 1	Disorders of intermediary metabolism affecting small molecules	Characteristics	Subclassification
		• Presents early as acute metabolic crisis associated with encephalopathy, with periods of relapse and remission, often severe and catastrophic, and a brisk response to treatment • Attacks are precipitated by fever, intercurrent illness, catabolism, and food intake • *Diagnosis*—mainly by plasma and urine amino acids, organic acids, and chromatography • *Treatment*—reduce formation of toxic metabolites, enhance the excretion of toxic metabolites, specific cofactor therapy and supportive care	• Amino acid disorders • Organic acidemia • Urea cycle disorders • Metal disorders • Inborn errors of neurotransmitter synthesis • Inborn errors of neurotransmitter and brain amino acid synthesis
Group 2	*Disorders involving energy metabolism*	• Disorders that result from deficiency in energy production or utilization within the liver, cardiac, muscle, brain, or other tissues • Hypoglycemia, hepatomegaly, hyperlactatemia, developmental delay, myopathy, cardiomyopathy, and failure to thrive are common symptoms • Diagnosis relies on functional tests, enzymatic analysis, biopsies, and molecular analysis	• Congenital lactic acidemias • Mitochondrial respiratory chain disorders • Fatty acid oxidation disorders • Cytoplasmic energy disorders—disorders of glycolysis, glycogen metabolism and gluconeogenesis, and glucose transporter defect • Disorders of creatine metabolism • Pentose phosphate pathway defects
Group 3	*Disorders involving complex molecules*	• This group includes disorders that disturb the synthesis, remodeling, recycling, trafficking, and catabolism of complex molecules • Symptoms most often manifest late as chronic, slowly progressive disease, with characteristic examination and histopathological findings and are permanent • In general, symptoms are not precipitated by metabolic triggers (unrelated to food/ intercurrent illness)	• Lysosomal storage disorders • Peroxisomal disorders • Purine and pyrimidine disorders • Cholesterol and bile acid synthesis disorders • Intracellular triglycerides, phospholipids, and glycosphingolipids synthesis disorders

(IEM: inborn error of metabolism)

Neurological Manifestations

Neurological symptoms are the most common and well-known manifestations seen in the majority of metabolic disorders.[1,6] Apart from the extent of neurological involvement, it is important to look for association with any non-neurological manifestations. The six common neurological presentations of IEMs are described here.

Chronic Encephalopathy

Chronic encephalopathy with isolated neurological involvement: Based on whether gray matter (poliodystrophy) or white matter (leukodystrophy) of the nervous system is involved, psychomotor retardation (developmental delay, intellectual disability, or regression of milestones), seizures, blindness, extrapyramidal symptoms, and tone abnormalities are the most common clinical presentations. Progressive cognitive decline/dementia is a manifestation usually seen in adolescents/adults. The baseline developmental milestones and scholastic performance give clues to the cognitive status of the patients.

Though developmental delay or intellectual disability is an otherwise common manifestation with enormous causes, it becomes difficult to decide in whom to evaluate for IEM.

Routine screening for metabolic disorders in developmental delay has a diagnostic yield of 1%. It increases to 5% if there are specific clinical indications. This group is largely contributed by organelle (storage disorders) and mitochondrial disorders. But late-onset small molecule disorders can also present as developmental delay and cerebral palsy mimics. Some clinical pointers, which can alert the physician to the possibility of an underlying IEM, are that—(1) developmental delay tends to be global affecting all spheres of development, (2) in older children/adolescents with intellectual disability, verbal quotient is better than performance quotient, (3) behavioral issues including irritability, aggressiveness, hyperactivity-impulsivity, and self-mutilation are common, (4) usually the course is progressive with either arrest or regression of the developmental milestones in younger children and cognitive decline in adolescents/adults, and (5) the presence of objective neurological signs such as tone abnormalities, pyramidal, or extrapyramidal signs. One must always rule out causes for pseudoregression such as emotional deprivation, malnutrition, or infections before concluding as true neuroregression. In children with autism failure to thrive, seizures and hypotonia may suggest IEM as an underlying cause. In a child with a cerebral palsy-like presentation, absence of perinatal risk factors for brain injury, family history, the onset of motor symptoms after initial normal development, marked fluctuation of motor symptoms, clinical exacerbation in a catabolic state, and isolated generalized hypotonia or ataxia may suggest IEM.

Recurrent seizures by themselves, in absence of any metabolic abnormalities and normal neuroimaging, are an uncommon manifestation of IEM. However, one should think of a metabolic disorder if the seizures have an onset early in life, are drug-refractory, nonresponsive to usual anticonvulsant medications, and associated with other neurological signs such as dysmorphism, cognitive decline, or visual impairment. The semiology is often a mixture of focal seizures, erratic myoclonus of the face and extremities, or West syndrome. Some conditions, which can present with metabolic epilepsies, are enlisted in **Table 2**.

In the case of white matter involvement, the clinical presentation is dominated by motor difficulties in form of motor delay, recurrent falls, tone abnormalities like progressive spasticity or weakness, and incoordination. The presence of peripheral neuropathy detected either clinically or by electrophysiological examination is an important clue suggesting altered myelin lipid metabolism, e.g., Krabbe or metachromatic leukodystrophy (MLD). Hypotonia occurs in conditions like acid maltase deficiency, mitochondrial diseases, congenital disorders of glycosylation, and lysosomal storage diseases. Spasticity is a prominent feature of metabolic leukodystrophies. Spastic diplegia-like presentation can be seen in arginase deficiency, X-linked ALD, and HHH syndrome. White matter involvement is primarily a manifestation of complex molecule disorders and can still be a manifestation of late-onset small molecule disorders demanding evaluation for both. Some notable conditions are inherited leukodystrophies (Canavan's disease, Alexander's disease, X-ALD), late-onset GM2-gangliosidois, and mitochondrial respiratory chain defects.[10-12]

Chronic encephalopathy with neurological and additional systemic involvement: The pattern of non-neurological involvement gives an important etiological clue to the type of underlying metabolic defect. Most often, they are seen in organelle disorders and the symptoms overlap. Additional systemic involvement can be there either in the form of involvement of the liver, spleen, heart, muscle, or

TABLE 2: Classification of metabolic epilepsies based on the age group.

Early infantile onset	Late infantile to childhood onset	Childhood to adolescent onset
Urea cycle defects	Organic acidemias	Sialidosis type 1
Organic acidemias	GM2 gangliosidosis	Myoclonic epilepsy ragged-red fibers
Maple syrup urine disease	Biotin–thiamine responsive basal ganglia disease	Mitochondrial encephalomyopathy, lactic acidosis, and stroke-like episodes
Biotinidase deficiency	Mitochondrial respiratory chain defects	Niemann–Pick C type 3
Pyridoxine-dependent deficiency	Classical late infantile onset neuronal ceroid lipofuscinosis	Gaucher disease type 3
Pyridoxine phosphate-dependent epilepsy	Congenital disorders of glycosylation	Wilson disease
GLUT1 deficiency	Folate receptor deficiency	X-linked adrenoleukodystrophy
Molybdenum cofactor deficiency	Succinic semialdehyde dehydrogenase deficiency	
Mitochondrial disorders	GLUT1 deficiency	
Peroxisomal disorders		
Congenital disorders of glycosylation		
Pyruvate dehydrogenase deficiency		

(GLUT1: glucose transporter type 1)

skeletal system or they can manifest as dysmorphism in storage disorders. The four common clinical presentations suggesting hepatic involvement are the presence of jaundice, hypoglycemia, asymptomatic hepatomegaly, and hepatocellular dysfunction (coagulopathy with bleeding tendencies, cirrhosis, growth failure, myopathy, and neuropsychiatric disturbances). Etiology varies based on the age group with galactosemia, GSDs, tyrosinemia, fatty acid oxidation defects (FAODs), and Wilson disease are a few to mention.

Some notable inherited metabolic disorders associated with cardiomyopathy are Pompe disease, disorders of fatty acid metabolism, mitochondrial respiratory chain defects, and lysosomal storage disorders. In general, its associated noncardiac signs such as skeletal myopathy, hepatosplenomegaly, and a few cutaneous findings such as angiokeratomas and tuberous xanthomas point towards specific IEM. The symptom constellation of characteristic facies (dysmorphism), bone abnormalities (skeletal dysostosis and short stature), and organomegaly (hepatosplenomegaly and megalencephaly) with neurological involvement suggests an underlying storage syndrome. Dysmorphism is usually nonspecific, and becomes more pronounced with age. They generally tend to have coarse facies, i.e., prominent forehead, puffiness of eyelids, broad and depressed nasal bridge with thick upper lip, large tongue, and thickened gums. Mainly, lysosomal disorders (mucopolysaccharidosis, fucosidosis, and Gaucher disease), peroxisomal disorders (Zellweger syndrome), and mitochondrial disorders [pyruvate dehydrogenase (PDH) deficiency] are the metabolic disorders with significant dysmorphism.[10-12]

In addition to the above-mentioned clinical presentations, non-neurologic signs in chronic encephalopathy may provide clues to the diagnosis of specific IEMs. Eye signs, skin and hair changes, presence of dysmorphism, organomegaly, and skeletal changes require attention as enlisted in **Table 3**.[13] Overall, a comprehensive approach for

TABLE 3: Non-neurological signs suggesting IEMs.

Organ	Abnormality	Condition
Facies	Coarse	Mucopolysaccharidosis (MPS)
	Flat	Peroxisomal
	Cherubic	Menkes
	Dysmorphism	• *Zellweger syndrome*: High forehead, epicanthal fold, large anterior fontanelle, hypoplastic supraorbital ridges, epicanthal folds, deformed ear lobes with broad nasal bridge • *Mucopolysaccharidoses*: Coarse facies • *Smith–Lemli–Opitz disease*: Ptosis, cleft palate, syndactyly, and congenital heart disease with midline brain anomalies • *Congenital disorders of glycosylation*: Nonspecific facial dysmorphism
Hair	Alopecia	Biotinidase deficiency
	Pigmentary change (hypopigmentation)	PKU, Menkes disease
	Wooly, kinky hair	Menkes
	Brittle hair	Argininosuccinic aciduria and citrullinemia type I
Skin	Rash	Biotinidase deficiency, holocarboxylase deficiency (diaper area and perioral)
	Subcutaneous nodules	Farber
	Fat pads, focal lipoatrophy	Congenital disorders of glycosylation
	Persistent Mongolian spots	GM1 gangliosidosis, Hunter, Hurler, Mannosidosis, Neiman–Pick
	Angiokeratomas	Fabry's, fucosidosis, sialidosis II, MPS I
	Hyperpigmentation	X-ALD
	Blonde	PKU
	Ichthyosis	Refsum disease, tyrosinemia type II, Sjogren–Larsson syndrome
Abdomen	Hernia	MPS, GM1 gangliosidosis
	Hepatosplenomegaly	MPS, GM1 gangliosidosis, Gaucher
Cardiovascular	Cardiac dysfunction	MPS, Zellweger, Fabry (valve) Kearns Sayre (conduction defect) FAOD, mitochondrial, Friedrich, AVED, Pompe (cardiomyopathy)

Continued

Continued

Organ	Abnormality	Condition
Eye	Corneal opacities	MPS, ML
	Cataract	• Galactosemia • Wilson (+KF rings) • Zellweger's
	Cherry red spot	• GM1 gangliosidosis • Gaucher's • Tay–Sachs • Sandhoff's • Nieman–Pick's • Sialidosis
	Retinitis pigmentosa	• NCL • Zellweger's • Mitochondrial
	Optic atrophy	• MLD • Krabbe's • Canavan • NCL • GM2 gangliosidoses
	Ophthalmoplegia	• HSGP—Gaucher • VSGP—Nieman–Pick
Ears	Exaggerated startle	Tay–Sachs, Krabbe's
	Hearing impairment	• Sensorineural—MPS, mitochondrial, and peroxisomal disorders • Cortical—ALD
Skeletal abnormalities	• Dysostosis, joint laxity, and short stature • Osteoporosis • Pathological fractures	• MPS especially type IV • All IEMs, galactosemia, phenylketonuria, and homocystinuria • Wilson disease and Pompe disease

(ALD: adrenoleukodystrophy; FAOD: fatty acid oxidation defect; HSGP: horizontal supranuclear gaze palsy; IEM: inborn error of metabolism; MLD: metachromatic leukodystrophy; NCL: neuronal ceroid lipofuscinosis; PKU: phenylketonuria; VSGP: vertical supranuclear gaze palsy)

patients presenting with chronic encephalopathy is depicted in **Flowchart 1**.

Acute Encephalopathy

Acute encephalopathy irrespective of the cause is a medical emergency and a presenting feature of the majority of metabolic disorders which may potentially be dangerous if untreated. They usually present abruptly in a previously normal child and progress rapidly. In newborns, symptoms start after several days of feeding due to the accumulation of the toxic metabolite, which earlier were cleared by maternal circulation. In infants and children, the symptoms are precipitated by acute stressful conditions such as fasting, infections, surgery, etc. Symptoms are vast and age-based with neonates presenting with feeding problems, lethargy, coma, respiratory abnormalities, and seizures. Often missed if it starts as subtle behavioral abnormalities. Acute intermittent ataxia with periods of normalcy in-between is an important manifestation of acute encephalopathy in older children/adolescents. Acute encephalopathy is often reversible if recognized early and appropriate treatment is initiated. Delay in diagnosis results in chronic metabolic decompensation, progressive neurological injury, or death.

Urea cycle defects, organic acidemias, FAODs, and mitochondrial respiratory complex chain defects are the prototype IEMs manifesting as an acute encephalopathy. The diagnosis of acute encephalopathy can be done based on clinical phenotype and routine diagnostic tests [complete hemogram, arterial blood gas, liver function tests, renal function tests, serum electrolytes, ammonia, lactate, and cerebrospinal fluid (CSF) glucose]. Hypoglycemia, hyperammonemia, metabolic acidosis, leucine encephalopathy, and Reye-like syndrome are the common metabolic phenotypes to watch out for when a patient presents with acute encephalopathy. The evaluation of this is described in the investigation section below.

Stroke

Stroke and stroke-like lesions precipitated after metabolic decompensation suggest a possibility of IEM. The unique feature of metabolic strokes is they do not conform to vascular territories except in classic homocystinuria. In addition,

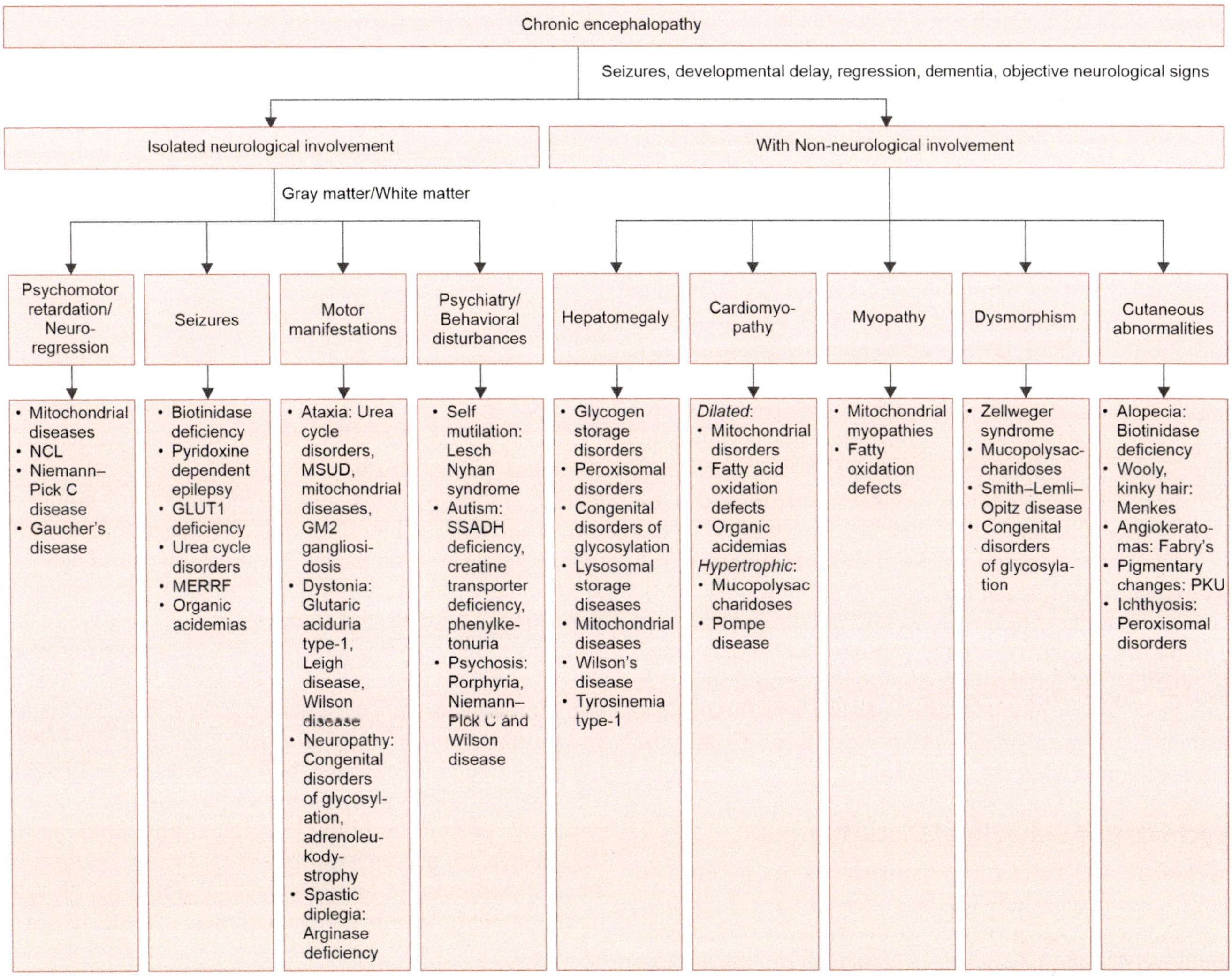

FLOWCHART 1: The comprehensive approach for patients presenting with chronic encephalopathy.

(GLUT1: glucose transporter type 1; MSUD: maple syrup urine disease; NCL: neuronal ceroid lipofuscinosis; PKU: phenylketonuria; SSADH: succinic semialdehyde dehydrogenase)

they may show hyperperfusion in the acute stage, unlike ischemic stroke. A metabolic cause of stroke is suspected when they present at a young age, have a family history, recurrent strokes, systemic symptoms like failure to thrive, developmental delays, acidosis, and migraine-like headache, seizures and visual symptoms. They can be seen in small, large, or complex molecule disorders—urea cycle disorders, organic aciduria, mitochondrial encephalomyopathy, lactic acidosis, and stroke-like episodes (MELAS), homocystinuria, and Fabry disease to name a few. Early diagnosis is essential as there are both acute and chronic medical interventions to prevent recurrent strokes and progressive neurological damage.

Myopathy

Myopathy in IEMs presents as either intermittent or progressive proximal muscle weakness, exercise intolerance with muscle cramps, and myoglobinuria or can be a manifestation of multisystemic disease. Pompe disease (GSD II) and GSD III are striking examples for progressive myopathy. McArdle disease and carnitine palmitoyltransferase II (CPT II) deficiency are the prototypes for muscle cramps and myoglobinuria. Mitochondrial electron transport chain (ETC) defects present with myopathy as a part of multisystemic involvement. While GSD may come as exercise-induced muscle cramps relieved by rest (second wind phenomena), FAODs may come with muscle weakness, fatigue, or pain after exertion or fasting and be relieved with carbohydrate ingestion.

Movement Disorders

Movement disorders are also common manifestation of metabolic disorders. In IEMs that cause diffuse CNS or selective basal ganglia involvement, 29% have movement disorder; while 22% of pediatric movement disorders are due to IEM.[14,15] Ataxia and dystonia are one of the most common presentations of IEM and can manifest at any age. Acute or subacute onset of more than one movement disorder type, progressive course, developmental delay, cognitive decline, and psychiatric symptoms are suspicious for an underlying IEM. Fever, fasting, and exercise may be triggers. In addition, diurnal fluctuation may be seen in neurotransmitter disorders. The most common disorders, which present with dystonia, are glutaric aciduria type I, Leigh disease, biotin-thiamine basal ganglia disease, and GM1 gangliosidosis. Methylmalonic and propionic acidemias present with the late-onset extrapyramidal disease. Ataxia in IEM can manifest as episodic ataxia, chronic progressive ataxia, and progressive myoclonic ataxia. Intermittent ataxias following a metabolic decompensation are common in urea cycle disorders, organic acidurias, maple syrup urine disease (MSUD) variants, and PDH deficiency. Progressive ataxias are seen in late-onset organelle disorders such as MLD, NPC, GM1, or GM2 gangliosidosis. Childhood-onset static ataxias are unlikely to be due to an IEM. Progressive and treatable ataxia may be seen in primary CoQ10 deficiency. Choreoathetosis and dystonia can suggest neurotransmitter disorders. Not to forget Wilson disease, which can have dystonia-parkinsonism phenotype with neuropsychiatric manifestation in adolescents/adults.

Psychiatry or Behavioral Disturbances

Psychiatric and behavioral disturbances are a common manifestation especially in those presenting with chronic encephalopathy. A few to name are the disruptive behavior in Sanfilippo disease, implacable irritability in Krabbe disease, episodes of acute irritability in hepatorenal tyrosinemia and acute psychiatric emergency in patients with porphyria manifesting as delirium, psychosis, and neurovisceral crisis. In late-onset disorders most often behavior or personality changes may be the first manifestation of the disease, e.g., X-linked ALD. Self-mutilation with behavioral disturbances and hyperuricemia points toward Lesch-Nyhan syndrome. Personality changes can also be seen in homocystinuria and Wilson disease. Language delay/abnormalities occur in succinic semialdehyde dehydrogenase deficiency, methionine adenosyl transferase deficiency, sepiapterin reductase deficiency, Niemann-Pick C, and neuronal ceroid lipofuscinoses (NCLs). An exaggerated startle response may be seen in GM2 gangliosidosis, sulfite oxidase deficiency, asparagine synthase deficiency, and hyperekplexia. Seizures can occur in all forms of IEM.

Autonomic Dysfunction

Some metabolic disorders such as Fabry disease, mitochondrial neurogastrointestinal encephalomyopathy (MNGIE), neurotransmitter disorders, mucopolysaccharidosis, and occipital horn syndrome can have autonomic symptoms as their presenting manifestation.

Vision/Hearing Abnormalities

Visual impairment can occur in IEM either due to degenerative changes in the retina or primary involvement of the optic nerve. Some examples are NCL; neuropathy, ataxia, and retinitis pigmentosa (NARP); ornithine aminotransferase (OAT) deficiency; congenital disorders of glycosylation; etc. Sensorineural hearing loss (SNHL) is a more common hearing abnormality in metabolic disorders than conductive hearing loss. The most common diseases, which were associated with SNHL, are adrenomyeloneuropathy, MELAS, biotinidase deficiency, mucopolysaccharidoses, peroxisomal disorders, and Smith-Lemli-Opitz syndrome.

Neonatal Presentations

Neonatal presentations are usually nonspecific (poor feeding, lethargy, drowsiness, hypotonia, and failure to thrive) and delay in identification invariably results in death or irreversible brain damage.[16] These are often misdiagnosed as neonatal sepsis. Some pointers, which suggest a metabolic disorder in neonates, are nonresponsiveness to the usual antibiotics, deterioration after a period of apparent normalcy due to accumulation of toxic metabolites, consanguinity and family history of unexplained sibling loss, fluctuating sensorium, presence of unexplained hypoglycemia, hyperammonemia, and metabolic acidosis on evaluation. The five pathognomonic presentations of IEMs in the neonatal period include: (1) acute encephalopathy, (2) seizures, (3) hepatic syndromes, (4) cardiac syndromes, and (5) nonimmune hydrops fetalis.[16] Some not to miss treatable IEMs in the neonatal period are MSUD, urea cycle enzyme defects, pyridoxine-dependent seizures/vitamin-responsive epileptic encephalopathies, and organic acidurias.

IEMs in Adults

Adult-onset IEMs are suspected typically if a patient presents with an unexplained and bizarre neurological or psychiatric manifestation in whom the usual etiologies have been excluded by appropriate tests. Adults/adolescents with IEM may have a residual enzymatic activity that allows slow accumulation of metabolic products over a long time and results in the disease at a later age. Some metabolic disorders commonly seen in adults are hemochromatosis, Gaucher disease type 1, X-linked adrenomyeloneuropathy, Wilson's disease, Fabry disease, porphyria, GM2 gangliosidosis, CPT II deficiency, homocystinuria, ornithine transcarbamylase deficiency, and 3-methylcrotonyl-CoA carboxylase deficiency. The clinical manifestations, which are suggestive of IEMs in adults, are described in **Box 1**.[17]

DIAGNOSIS OF IEMS

The diagnosis of metabolic disorders rests solely on a high index of clinical suspicion. A detailed clinical evaluation

BOX 1	Clinical features suggesting a metabolic disorder in adults.

- Fluctuating clinical symptoms or signs, especially when triggered by fever, stress, exercise, fasting, or postpartum
- Multisystemic/multiaxial involvement like neurological signs with systemic involvement or involvement of different parts of the nervous system such as leukoencephalopathy with polyneuropathy, cerebellum, and optic nerve
- Neurological features such as unexplained recurrent encephalopathy (urea cycle disorders), acute/subacute myelopathy (homocysteine remethylation defects), exercise-induced paroxysmal dyskinesia (GLUT1 deficiency), and diurnal fluctuating dystonias (dopa-responsive dystonia)
- Ophthalmological features such as cherry red spot (Tay–Sachs disease, sialidosis), supranuclear gaze palsy (Niemann–Pick C, Gaucher disease), bilateral optic neuropathy (energy metabolism defects like respiratory chain defects; pyruvate dehydrogenase defects, and *PLA2G6* mutation), cataract (cerebrotendinous xanthomatosis, Refsum disease, and Wilson's disease), and pigmentary retinopathy (neuropathy, ataxia, and retinitis pigmentosa; Kearns–Sayre syndrome; neuronal ceroid lipofuscinosis)
- Dermatological manifestations such as angiokeratomas (Fabry disease), tendon xanthomas (cerebrotendinous xanthomatosis), and ichthyosis (Sjogren–Larsson syndrome, Refsum disease)
- Other features such as gout, nephrolithiasis (purine disorders), splenomegaly (lysosomal diseases, Tangier disease), and cholestasis (Niemann–Pick C, hereditary spastic paraparesis type 5)

(GLUT1: glucose transporter type 1)

needs to be done considering the clinical presentations as described above. Additional points to be noted in history are the antecedent illness or the precipitating factors, a detailed developmental history with premorbid developmental status, and an elaborate antenatal, natal, and perinatal history (HELLP syndrome in mother may be due to FAOD in the fetus). It is a must to draw a three-generation pedigree while evaluating any patient with suspected IEM. History of consanguinity, sudden infant death syndrome, epilepsy, and siblings with other neurological disorders should be noted. The presence of unexplained sibling deaths strongly suggests a metabolic disorder. A comprehensive examination needs to be done in all the patients keeping in mind the points suggested in **Table 3** and **Figures 2A to E**. Unusual urinary odors may suggest an IEM as enlisted in **Table 4**. Always try to exclude the possibility of neuroinfections, toxins, and child abuse. Diagnosis is later confirmed by appropriate biochemical investigations, enzyme analysis, and genetic studies. One must always be aware that IEMs might not always manifest as classical presentations as described in textbooks.[18,19]

DIFFERENTIAL DIAGNOSIS

Diagnosis is often delayed or misdiagnosed probably because of one of the common sources of errors either—(1) usually mistaken with common acquired conditions such as infections, toxins, or nutritional deficiency, (2) overemphasizing the intercurrent illness which has triggered the metabolic decompensation or (3) due to genetic heterogeneity—similar phenotype caused by different mutations, e.g., mucopolysaccharidosis, NCL, etc.[1,6] Intoxication phenotype may be mimicked by sickness related to sepsis, hypoxic-ischemic encephalopathy, duct-dependent lesion in congenital heart disease, and drugs. Hence, we need to consider an IEM in any critically ill neonate especially if deterioration after an initial period of apparent good health following an uncomplicated pregnancy. In term infants who develop the symptoms of sepsis without risk factors or have unexplained neonatal or sudden infant deaths in siblings, parental consanguinity increases the likelihood of autosomal recessive IEM. Similarly, nonspecific presentation with developmental delays may be mimicked by acquired brain injury or other neurogenetic disorders. Behavioral disturbances as initial manifestations may be incorrectly diagnosed as primary nonorganic psychiatry disorders. Low vitamin B12, methylmalonic acidemia, and hyperhomocysteinemia may be underdiagnosed as a nutritional deficiency. The hepatic syndrome is often misdiagnosed as valproate toxicity.

INVESTIGATIONS

The goal of laboratory investigations is to classify inherited metabolic disorders, establish a proper diagnosis, and to determine the extent and severity of organ involvement. The routine laboratory tests include complete hemogram, liver function tests, renal function tests, serum electrolytes, random blood glucose, serum ammonia, plasma lactate, arterial blood gases with anion gap, urine, and blood ketones.[20,21] The measurement of serum ammonia is done by enzymatic autoanalyzer and it is still subject to significant errors because of poor venepuncture techniques, environmental contamination, and careless sample handling. The sample should be collected from a free-flowing vein directly into an anticoagulated tube, transported on ice to the laboratory and plasma separated and analysis to be done within 15 minutes. Normally, plasma ammonia concentrations will be slightly higher in newborn patients. Even while collecting the sample for plasma lactate, same procedure needs to be followed. The levels of plasma lactate will be more significant in arterial blood and CSF than in venous sample.[20,21] Plasma lactate levels will be elevated in delayed sampling testing and with the use of a tourniquet while collecting the sample. Pyruvate in the blood is unstable and its level will be lower than the lactate. The ratio of lactate to pyruvate is more significant than individual values, but it should be interpreted cautiously if plasma lactate levels were normal. **Table 5** summarizes the list of investigations to be done on an IEM-suspected patient.[1]

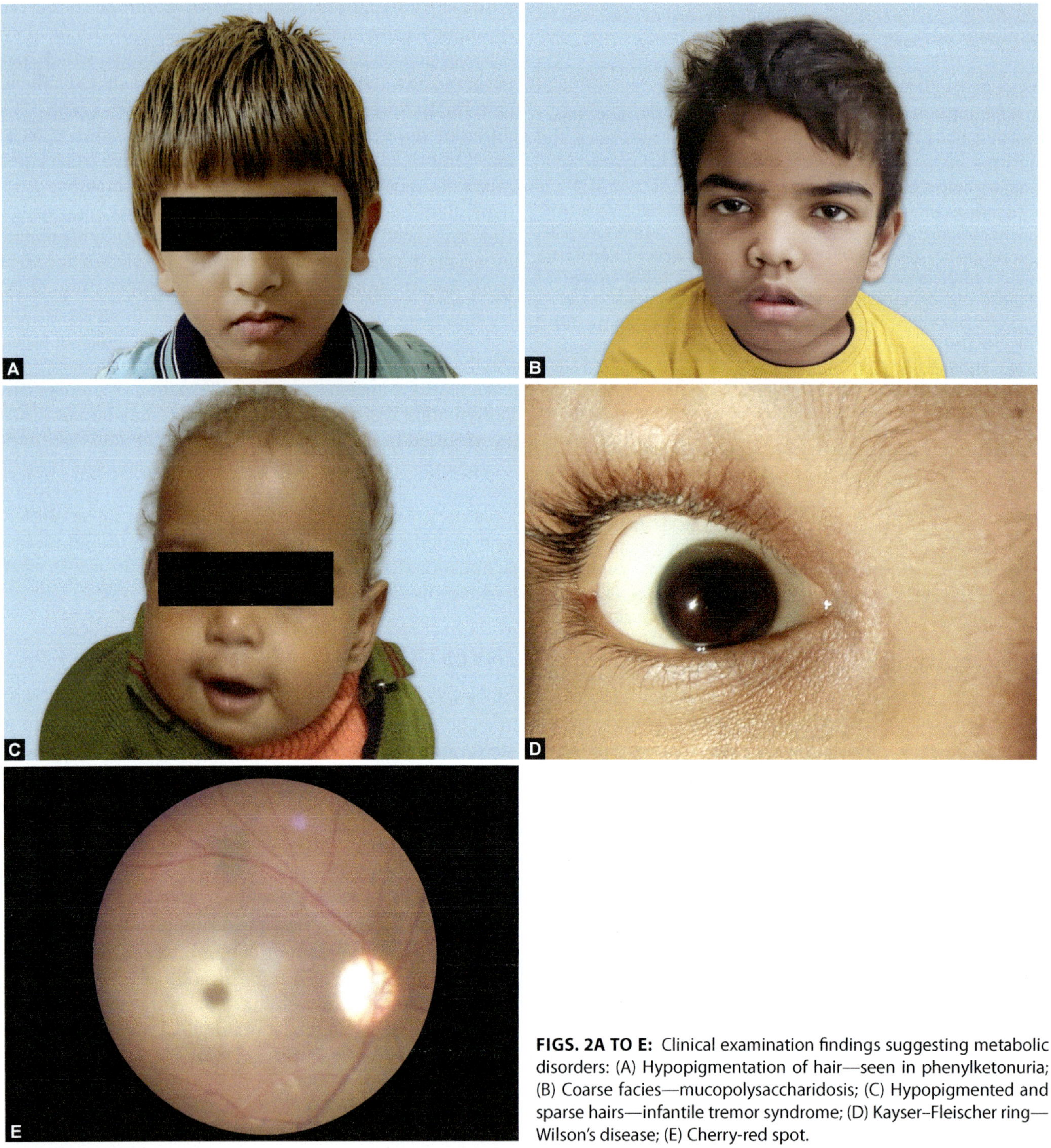

FIGS. 2A TO E: Clinical examination findings suggesting metabolic disorders: (A) Hypopigmentation of hair—seen in phenylketonuria; (B) Coarse facies—mucopolysaccharidosis; (C) Hypopigmented and sparse hairs—infantile tremor syndrome; (D) Kayser–Fleischer ring—Wilson's disease; (E) Cherry-red spot.

Blood Glucose

Hypoglycemia (<45 mg/dL in all age groups, <30–35 mg/dL in neonates, and <25 mg/dL in preterm infants) is defined as plasma concentration of glucose lower than the normal which is enough to cause clinical symptoms and signs resulting in impaired brain function. The plasma concentration of glucose levels will be normally lower in newborns before 48 hours as there is a transition from intrauterine to extrauterine life. Hypoglycemia commonly occurs in disorders of carbohydrate metabolism, FAODs, organic acidemias, and certain aminoacidopathies. The normal physiological response to hypoglycemia is increased mitochondrial fatty acid beta-oxidation and ketone body production. Urinary ketone measurement provides indirect evidence of hypoglycemia whether its due to inadequate production or overutilization of glucose. Absence of urinary ketones is a strong indicator of increased glucose utilization conditions such as hyperinsulinism and FAOD. Low-free fatty acid levels during hypoglycemia indicate abnormally elevated insulin levels. Hypoglycemia in postprandial state or short fasting hours (<4 hours) signifies glucose overutilization disorders like hyperinsulinism whereas intermediate fasting and long fasting hours suggest carbohydrate metabolism and fatty acid oxidation disorders.[21]

When hypoglycemia is associated with hepatomegaly, then deficiencies of glucose-6-phosphatase (GSD I), glycogen debrancher (GSD III) or glycogen synthase (GSD 0), and fructose 1,6-bisphosphatase (FBP) should be considered as the most probable diagnosis. Patients with GSD I disease typically show hypoglycemia, lactic acidosis, hyperuricemia, hypertriglyceridemia, and hypophosphatemia. The characteristic feature of this disease is hypoglycemia which will not respond to glucagon administration and there will be a significant increase in plasma lactate levels. An oral glucose test helps to differentiate GSD I from GSD III, in which there will be an increase in the level of lactate in GSD III, whereas its levels decrease in GSD I. The definitive diagnosis of these disorders requires the measurement of relevant enzymes. Hypoglycemia due to mitochondrial fatty acid oxidation disorders can be confirmed by demonstrating the presence of a high concentration of C6–C10 dicarboxylic acids and the characteristic acylcarnitines in plasma during acute decompensation. **Flowchart 2** depicts the approach to hypoglycemia.

TABLE 4: Classical urine odors in some inborn errors of metabolism.

Urine odor	Metabolic disorder
Mousy	Classical phenylketonuria
Sweaty feet	• Isovaleric acidemia • Multiple acyl-CoA dehydrogenase deficiency
Maple syrup urine disease	Maple syrup
Cabbage like/Rancid butter	Tyrosinemia type 1
Cat urine	3-methylcrotonyl CoA carboxylase deficiency

Blood Gas Analysis

Metabolic acidosis is one of the important manifestations of neurometabolic disorders.[10,20] In metabolic acidosis, there will be a disturbance in the acid-base balance due to loss of bicarbonate, reduced renal excretion, or increased production of acids. An increased anion gap is observed in metabolic disorders due to abnormal accumulation of lactic acid, ketoacids, and other organic acids. Metabolic acidosis with normal anion gap is seen in renal tubular acidosis or diarrhea. If acidosis is present then other parameters such as hypo-/hyperglycemia, hyperammonemia, ketosis, and lactate should be evaluated in conjunction. Organic acidemias present with metabolic acidosis and ketosis, whereas mitochondrial FAODs present with metabolic acidosis, and hypoglycemia without ketosis. However, postprandial paradoxical ketonuria may be seen in mitochondrial disorders.

TABLE 5: The list of investigations to be done in an IEM-suspected patient.

Small-molecule and organelle metabolism disorders	Small-molecule disorders	Disorders of organelle metabolism
Complete hemogram	Gas chromatography mass spectrometry (GCMS) of urine	Skeletal survey
Liver function tests	High-performance liquid chromatography (HPLC)	*Fasting lipid profile*: Low HDL in Gaucher disease and Niemann–Pick C disease
Renal function tests	Tandem mass spectrometry to look for plasma amino acids and acyl carnitine profile	Creatine kinase
Serum electrolytes	Urinary organic acid and urine orotic acid	Plasma very long-chain fatty acid (VLCFA) levels
Blood glucose	*Enzyme assays*: Biotinidase assay, GALT (galactose-1-phosphate uridyltransferase) assay, etc.	Purine–pyrimidine panel
Serum ammonia (*normal value*: 15–45 µ/dL)	CSF analysis	Skin, skeletal muscle, liver biopsy—histopathology and electron microscopy
Plasma lactate (*normal values*: 0.5–1.6 mmol/L)	Electroencephalogram	Molecular analysis
Arterial blood gas analysis	*Neuroimaging*: MRI brain with magnetic resonance spectroscopy	
Urine and blood ketones	Genetic analysis	
Urine routine: Color, odor, and dipstick examination		

(CSF: cerebrospinal fluid; MRI: magnetic resonance imaging)

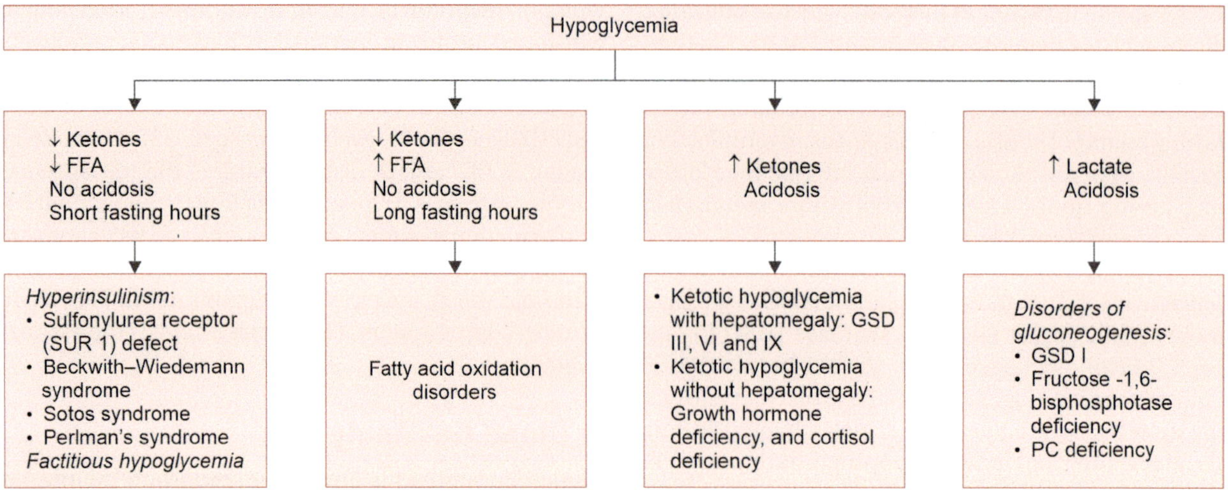

FLOWCHART 2: An algorithmic approach to differential diagnosis of hypoglycemia.
(FFA: free fatty acid; GSD: glycogen storage disorder; PC: pyruvate carboxylase)

Ammonia

Hyperammonemia is an important laboratory finding in neurometabolic disorders, which manifests as an acute encephalopathy. Normally, plasma ammonia levels range <45 mmol/L. Ammonia is a neurotoxic byproduct of amino acid (AA) metabolism which is normally excreted as urea through series of enzymatic steps. In urea cycle disorders, ammonia levels will be elevated up to 10–100 times of upper limit of normal. Hyperammonemia can also occur in nonmetabolic conditions such as a hepatic failure, valproate use especially in higher doses or concomitant use of topiramate/zonisamide, portocaval shunt, and glutamate dehydrogenase hyperactivity.

The inherited metabolic disorders, which present with hyperammonemia, are urea cycle defects, organic acidemias, congenital lactic acidosis, FAODs, dibasic AA defects, and hyperammonemias secondary to hepatic dysfunction (tyrosinemia type 1, galactosemia, α1 antitrypsin deficiency, and respiratory chain defects). In organic acidemias, the accumulated substrates or organic acid intermediates inhibit proximal urea cycle enzyme N-acetylglutamate synthase (NAGS), producing an overall decrease in the urea cycle-detoxifying efficacy. Whereas in mitochondrial fatty acid oxidation disorders, hyperammonemia results from the combined effects of substrate depletion and urea cycle inhibition by toxic acylcarnitine species. Acetyl-CoA is the end product of fatty acid beta oxidation, which is required for the production of N-acetyl glutamate that in turn allosterically activates the enzyme carbamoyl phosphate synthetase 1 (CPS1). Lysosomal storage diseases, mucopolysaccharidoses, and some peroxisomal disorders result in the accumulation of complex large molecules within the liver leading to hepatocellular damage and a decrease in urea cycle efficacy. An approach to hyperammonemia is shown in **Flowchart 3.**[10,20]

Plasma AA analysis is essential while evaluating patients with hyperammonemia to ascertain the type of urea cycle disorder. The concentration of citrulline is important in the interpretation of the results of the AA analysis. In argininosuccinate synthetase defect, there will be a marked elevation of the concentration of citrulline, resulting in citrullinemia. Very low citrulline levels suggest a defect in citrulline biosynthesis, which is the result of a deficiency of CPS 1, NAGS, and ornithine transcarbamylase. A normal citrulline concentration with elevated arginine levels occurs in arginase deficiency. Hyperinsulinemia-hyperammonemia syndrome is characterized by defective transport of ornithine into the mitochondria with markedly elevated plasma ornithine level, urinary orotic acid, and orotidine levels.

Lactate

The plasma levels of lactate and pyruvate depend upon their equilibrium between the cytoplasmic production from glycolysis and their consumption by different tissues. Abnormal accumulation of lactic acid causes metabolic acidosis. Blood lactate elevates in conditions with hypoxic insult, circulatory collapse, and failure of cellular respiration and these conditions should be ruled out prior considering the IEM. The inherited metabolic causes of lactic acidosis are mitochondrial electron transfer chain defect, pyruvate metabolism defects, glycogen storage diseases, organic acid metabolism, and defects of biotin metabolism. Ketosis associated with hyperlactacidemias is a nearly constant finding in inherited metabolic disorders except for fatty oxidation defects, glycogen storage disease type I, and pyruvate dehydrogenase deficiency. The plasma lactate/pyruvate ratio correlates with the NAD+/NADH ratio and indirectly reflects the cytosolic redox state.[10,20]

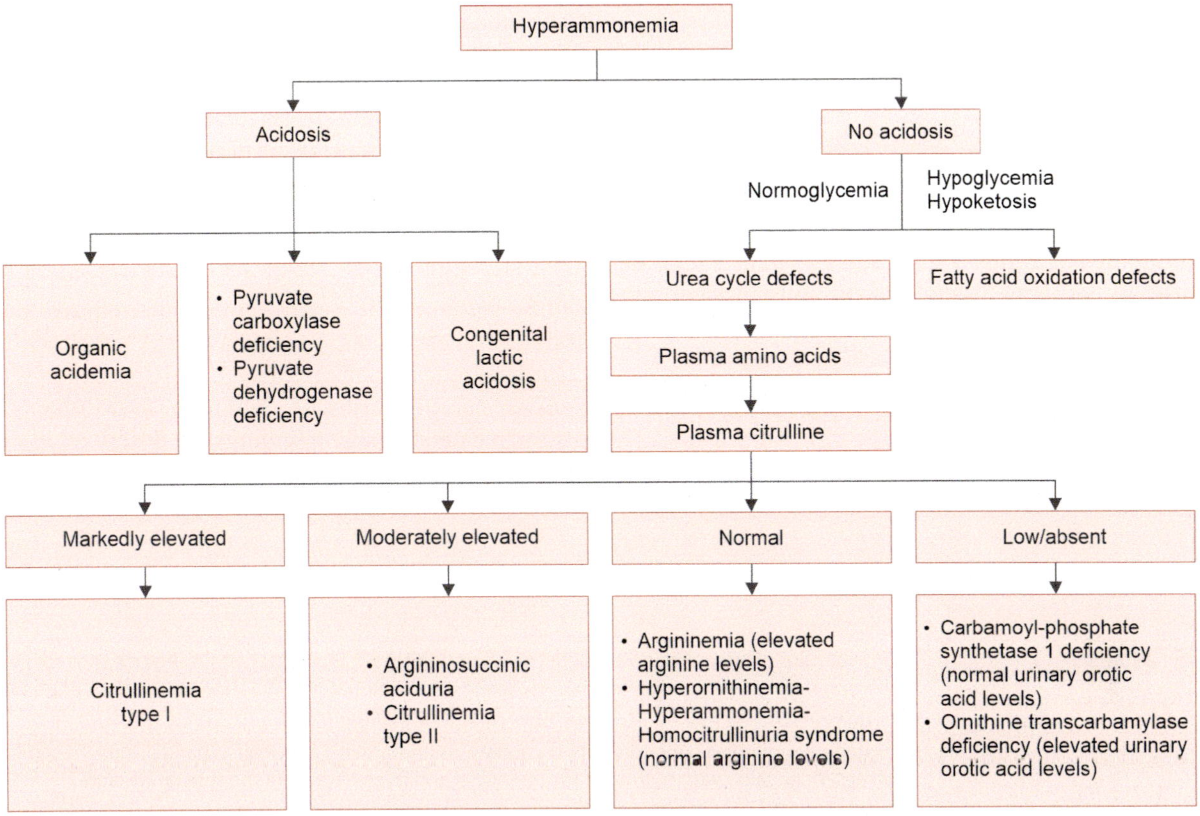

FLOWCHART 3: An algorithmic approach to differential diagnosis of hyperammonemia.

Ketones

Acetoacetic acid, 3-OH butyric acid, and acetone are the normal end products of mitochondrial fatty acid beta oxidation. Ketonuria without hypoglycemia or metabolic acidosis is found physiologically in late infancy, childhood, and adolescents. Fasting hypoglycemia or postprandial hyperglycemia with hyperlactatemia and severe ketonuria occurs in disorders of gluconeogenesis. Pure marked ketonuria in a fed or fasting state occurs in ketone body handling disorders such as succinyl-CoA transferase (SCOT) deficiency or beta-ketothiolase (BKT) deficiency. Hypoketotic hypoglycemia occurs in vomiting, generalized catabolic states, and mitochondrial FAODs.

Urine Routine Examination

Urine color and odor give diagnostic clue to the specific types of IEM. The urine color in some of IEM was as follows: green–blue in Hartnup disease, red in porphyria, dark black/brown in alkaptonuria, and orange/red in hypoxanthine-guanine phosphoribosyltransferase deficiency. Reducing substances in the urine are tested by using benedict or Fehling test. Ehrlich test is used to detect PBG and urobilinogen in the urine sample, and ferric chloride test is used to look for the presence of oxoacids.[18]

Plasma Amino Acids

Quantitative AA levels in plasma are used to confirm the urea cycle disorders and disorders of AA metabolism.[10,20] The quantitative AA analysis will be performed by high-performance liquid chromatography or tandem mass spectrometry to measure the levels of AAs. Mild elevation of AAs up to 5–10% is not considered as significant. The concentration of AAs depends on the metabolic state of an individual. Prolonged fasting will result in the elevation of branched-chain AAs, valine, leucine, and isoleucine, whereas in the postprandial state, the levels of essential AAs will be elevated. Increased AA levels in the urine without corresponding increase in plasma levels occur due to inherited or acquired renal transport defects.

Urine Organic Acids

Organic acids comprise key metabolites of all pathways of intermediary metabolism as well as exogenous compounds. Analysis of urinary organic acids is performed by gas chromatography or mass spectrometry. A qualitative analysis of these compounds is sufficient because pathogenic organic acids are not present in significant amounts in the urine.

Acylcarnitine Profile

Analysis of carnitine and glycine esters is an important part of investigation in FAODs and organic acidemias. The analysis of acylcarnitines will be performed by tandem mass spectrometry in a plasma sample or a filter-paper bloodspot. In carnitine transporter defect, plasma carnitine levels are severely reduced (<5% of the normal level) whereas in carnitine palmitoyl transferase-1 (CPT-I) deficiency, the total carnitine levels (150–200% of the normal level) are elevated. Nearly 25–50% of the total carnitine level will be reduced in all other defects of fatty acid beta oxidation.[10,20]

Neuroimaging

Neuroimaging plays an important role in the diagnosis and treatment monitoring in inherited metabolic disorders. Neuroimaging depends on the maturity of the brain at the time of insult, type/severity of pathway defect, amount of toxic byproduct accumulation, duration of injury, the timing of imaging during the disease course, and compensatory mechanisms. The pattern of brain involvement in some IEMs is characteristic such as in organic acidemias—involvement of deep gray matter, and white matter involvement in AA disorders, whereas in energy defect disorders, both deep gray and white matter involvement will be present. MR spectroscopy may help in detecting abnormal metabolites, e.g., lactate peak in mitochondrial disorders, leucine peak in MSUD, and absence of creatine peak in cerebral creatine deficiency syndromes.[19] Few distinctive neuroimaging findings are described in **Table 6** and depicted in **Figures 3A to H**.

TABLE 6: Neuroimaging features of common metabolic disorders.

Disease	MRI findings
Urea cycle disorders	Central pattern of edema involving peri-insular, peri-Rolandic and basal ganglia regions with sparing of thalamus (distinguish between hypoxic–ischemic encephalopathy). MRS shows glutamate/glutamine ratio peak between 2 and 2.5 ppm during times of hyperammonemia
Wilson's disease	• Bilateral symmetrical hyperintensity in caudate and putamen. Face of giant panda sign—hyperintensity of mesencephalon with sparing of the red nuclei and lateral aspect of the substantia nigra • Panda cub sign—seen within the pontine tegmentum: ○ *Eyes of panda*: Relative hypointensity of the central tegmental tract and medial longitudinal fasciculi ○ *Nose and mouth*: Hyperintensity of the aqueduct opening into the fourth ventricle ○ *Cheeks*: Superior cerebellar peduncles • *Bright claustrum sign*: T2W bilateral symmetrical hyperintensity arising from claustrum • *Double panda sign*: Face of giant panda sign + panda cub sign • *Trident sign*: Abnormal hyperintensity in the pons with characteristic hypointensity in the middle forming a star shape in T2-weighted axial images
Glutaric aciduria type 1	Basal ganglia hyperintensity, poor opercularization ("Bat wing appearance"), widened sylvian fissure, and subdural fluid collections
Mitochondrial diseases: (a) Leigh's disease	• *SURF1 mutation*: T2W hyperintensity in the brainstem, periaqueductal gray matter, medulla, midbrain, and occasionally basal ganglia involvement • *Other etiologies*: T2W hyperintensity involving caudate, putamen, globus pallidi, thalami, brainstem, and sometimes diffuse supratentorial white matter involvement • *MRS*: Lactate peak
(b) Mitochondrial myopathy, encephalopathy, lactic acidosis, and stroke-like episodes (MELAS)	Stroke-like lesions predominantly affecting the gray matter lesions not confined to vascular territory commonly involving parieto-occipital and parietotemporal region. MR angiography will be normal, while MRS shows lactate peak
(c) Kearns–Sayre syndrome and mitochondrial neurogastrointestinal encephalomyopathy (MNGIE)	Diffuse cerebral, cerebellar, and brainstem atrophy. T2W images show diffuse white matter signal abnormalities with basal ganglia calcification
Molybdenum cofactor deficiency (MCD) and sulfite oxidase deficiency (SOD)	Neuroimaging features are similar to hypoxic ischemic encephalopathy. Imaging reveals caudate head involvement (usually spared in HIE), thalamic sparing (often involved in HIE) and chronic lesions show necrotic/hemorrhagic basal ganglia lesions. MRS showed abnormal elevation of metabolites such as S-sulfocysteine (3.61 ppm), taurine (3.42 and 3.24 ppm), and cysteine (2.92 and 2.97 ppm)
GM2 gangliosidosis	T1 hyperintensity and T2 hypointensity in the thalamus
Biotin-responsive basal ganglia disease	Bilateral lesions in the caudate nuclei with complete or partial involvement of putamen and sparing of the globus pallidi
Succinic semialdehyde dehydrogenase deficiency	T2W hyperintensity in globus pallidus, subthalamic nucleus, and dentate nucleus

(HIE: hypoxic–ischemic encephalopathy; MRI: magnetic resonance imaging; MRS: magnetic resonance spectroscopy)

Very Long-chain Fatty Acids

The quantitative analysis of very long-chain fatty acid (VLCFA) is required for the diagnosis of peroxisomal disorders. Methods used to detect VLCFA and phytanic acid are isotype dilution gas chromatography/mass spectrometry. Increased levels of VLCFA are seen in Zellweger syndrome and X-linked ALD, whereas increased phytanic acid levels occur in Refsum disease.

Molecular Testing

With the advances in the technology, next-generation sequencing significantly improved the genetic diagnosis of IEMs. Many of recently identified IEMs do not have specific biochemical and enzymatic markers. So, the only way to identify them is through genetic testing. Molecular testing also plays a significant role in assessing eligibility for novel therapies.[22]

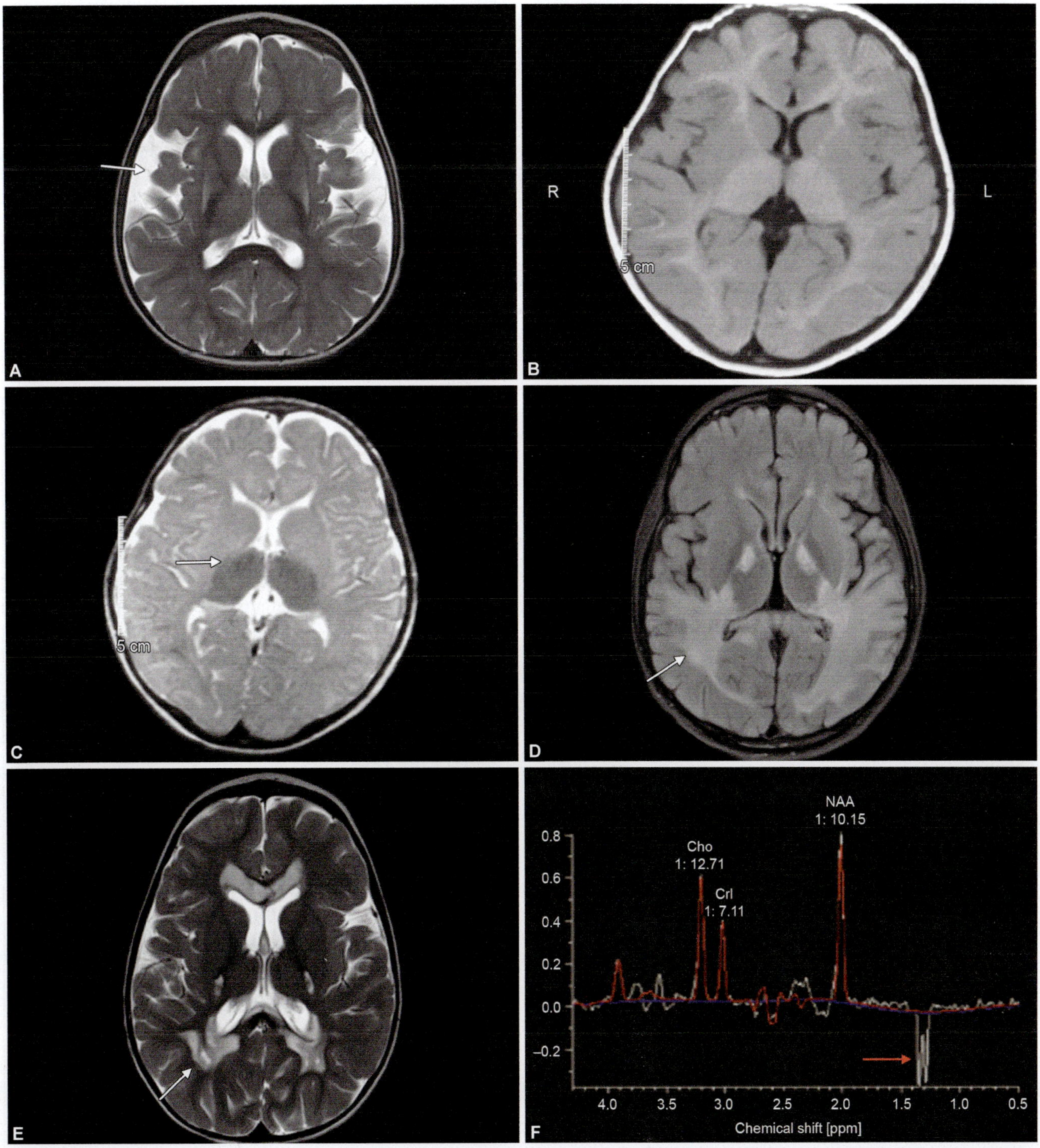

FIGS. 3A TO H: *Continued*

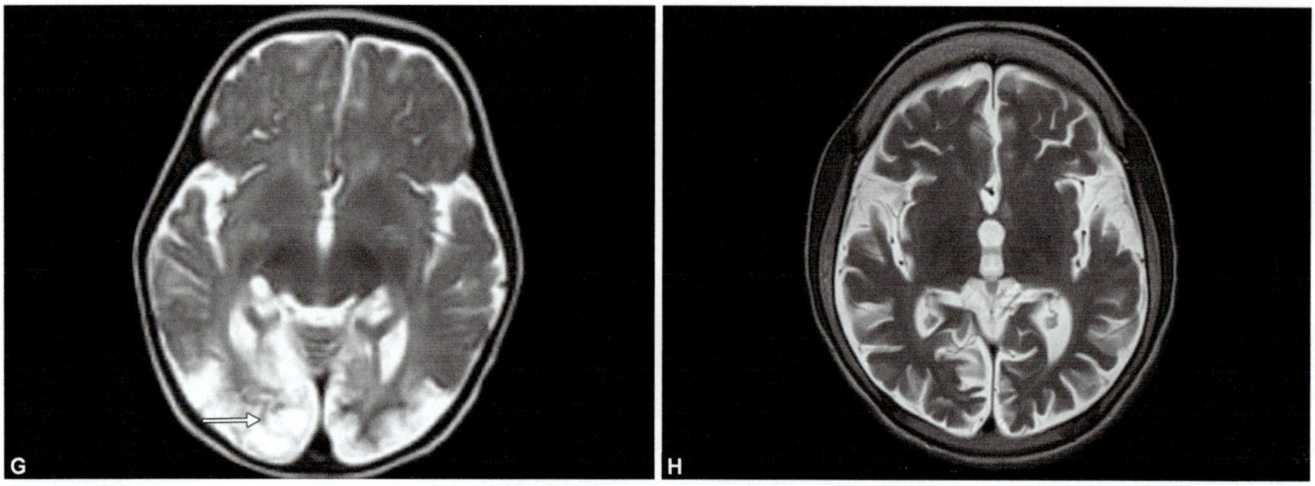

FIGS. 3A TO H: Neuroimaging findings suggesting inborn errors of metabolism: (A) Axial T2W image showing symmetrical widening of sylvian fissure (bat wing appearance) with hyperintensity in globus pallidum—glutaric aciduria type I; (B and C) Axial T1W iso to hyperintense and T2W hypointense symmetrical signal changes in bilateral thalami suggestive of GM1 gangliosidosis; (D) Posterior onset leukoencephalopathy seen in X-linked adrenoleukodystrophy; (E and F) Axial T2W image showing confluent symmetrical hyperintensity in parieto-occipital region predominantly involving periventricular white matter and corpus callosum. Few small cysts are noted within bilateral parietal lobe deep white matter. MRS showing raised NAA levels with inverted lactate peak at 1.33 ppm suggestive of mitochondrial respiratory complex chain defect; (G) Axial T2W images showing bilateral infarcts in a nonvascular territory in a child with MELAS; and (H) Diffuse cerebral atrophy seen in a patient with neuronal ceroid lipofuscinosis.

(MELAS: mitochondrial encephalomyopathy, lactic acidosis, and stroke-like episode; MRS: magnetic resonance spectroscopy; NAA: N-acetylaspartate)

Others[23-25]

- *Cardiac evaluation*: Echocardiography to be done in patients with long-chain fatty acid metabolism and mitochondrial disorder to rule out cardiomyopathy.
- Serum uric acid levels will be elevated in patients with glycogen storage disease and Lesch-Nyhan disease. It is decreased in patients with defects of purine metabolism or molybdenum cofactor deficiency.
- Skeletal surveys are used to detect dysostosis multiplex or cartilage stippling, which is seen in lysosomal storage diseases and peroxisomal biogenesis disorders.
- Urine sulfocysteine levels for sulfite oxidase and molybdenum cofactor deficiencies in patients with early onset seizures.
- Urinary glycosaminoglycans and urinary oligosaccharides to evaluate the cause of lysosomal storage disorders.
- Plasma and urine creatine and guanidinoacetate levels will be done to assess the abnormalities of creatine metabolism.
- Skin, skeletal muscle, or liver biopsy for enzyme assays, histopathology, or electron microscopy if these tissues are involved.
- Cerebrospinal fluid analysis for measurement of glucose, protein, lactate, pyruvate, pyruvate/lactate ratio, glycine, serine, alanine, organic acids, neurotransmitters, or other disease-specific metabolites.
- Metabolomic profiling is an emerging clinical diagnostic test that screens many small molecules in a single test. Metabolomic profiling combined with clinical exome sequencing is most effective in diagnosing the inherited metabolic disorders.

Metabolic Autopsy

In babies who are critically sick and in those children with suspected IEM but undiagnosed at the time of death, postmortem evaluation is essential to determine the cause of death. The establishment of diagnosis helps in prenatal counseling, reducing the recurrence risk, and early identification and management for treatable IEMs.[26] The following samples should be taken to enable a specific diagnosis within 1–2 hours after death.

- *Blood 5–10 mL*: Heparinized (for chromosomal) and EDTA (for DNA)
- *Newborn screening (NBS) card*: 4–6 blood spots (four to six) on filter paper
- *Urine*: Frozen at –20°C in plain sterile containers
- *CSF*: Store at –20°C
- *Punch skin biopsy*: Store at 4–8°C; do not freeze in normal saline
- *Liver, muscle, kidney, and heart biopsy*: As indicated
- Clinical photograph (in cases with dysmorphism)
- Infantogram (in cases with skeletal abnormalities)

TREATMENT

Herein, an overview of the general principles of treatment is provided. Small-molecule disorders, especially the intoxication phenotype, may require urgent and intensive medical treatment. This includes supportive treatment and specific measures as outlined below. However, family education about disease and adherence to long-term treatment and regular monitoring needs to be emphasized upfront to reduce neuromorbidity from repeated acute episodes. Limited specific treatment options are available for complex/storage disorders including enzyme replacement and bone marrow transplantation. In mitochondrial ETC disorders, coenzyme Q10 for primary deficiency, L-arginine and L-citrulline for MELAS, folinic acid for Kearns–Sayre syndrome and POLG-related disorders, L creatine for mitochondrial myopathy, and thiamine/ketogenic diet for PDH deficiency may constitute specific/precision therapies. In addition, mitochondrial cocktail consisting of B vitamins, antioxidants (vitamin E/alpha-lipoic acid with biotin), coenzyme Q, and N-acetylcysteine, if glutathione deficiency, has been recommended by Mitochondrial Medicine Society **(Table 7)**.[1,6] An overview is depicted in **Flowchart 4**.

Aims of acute treatment:
- *Reduce the formation of toxic metabolites*:
  - By decreasing substrate (stop feeds)
  - By providing adequate calories and preventing endogenous catabolism
- Enhance the excretion of toxic metabolites—hemodialysis, ammonia scavengers, and carnitine.
- Institute cofactor therapy for specific disease/empirically if a diagnosis is not established.
- *Supportive care*: Treatment of seizures (avoid valproate), maintaining euglycemia and normothermia, fluid, electrolyte and acid-base balance, treatment of infection, and mechanical ventilation if needed.

Management of hyperammonemia:
- *Discontinue feeds*: Adequate calories by intravenous glucose and lipids. Maintain glucose infusion rate (GIR) of 8–10 mg/kg/min. Intralipid 0.5 g/kg/day (up to 3 g/kg/day).

TABLE 7: Mitochondrial cocktail.

Drug	Dosage
CoQ10 as ubiquinone	• 2–8 mg/kg daily divided in two doses • 10–30 mg/kg daily divided in two doses
Riboflavin	50–400 mg/day
L-creatine	0.1 g/kg/day; maximum 10 g/day
L-arginine (in case of suspected MELAS only)	• *Acute*: 500 mg IV/kg/day for 1–3 days • *Maintenance*: 150–300 mg/kg orally or IV in 2–3 divided doses
L-carnitine	10–100 mg/kg/day IV or orally in 3 divided doses
Vitamin E	1–2 IU/kg/day
Vitamin C	5 mg/kg/day
Folinic acid	0.5–1.5 mg/kg/day
Alpha-lipoic acid	50–200 mg/day
Thiamine	100–200 mg/day
Biotin	5–10 mg/day

(MELAS: mitochondrial encephalomyopathy, lactic acidosis, and stroke-like episode)

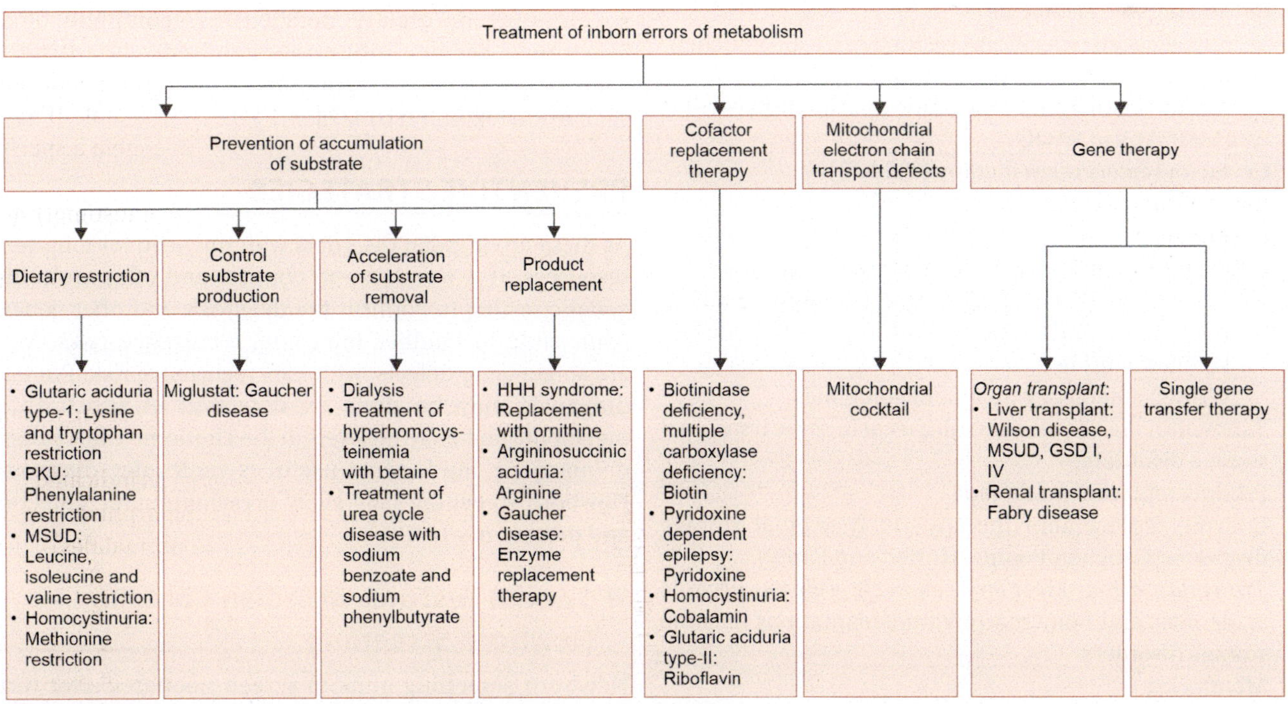

FLOWCHART 4: An overview to treatment of Inborn errors of metabolism.

(GSD: glycogen storage disorder; HHH: hyperammonemia–hyperornithinemia–homocitrullinemia; MSUD: maple syrup urine disease; PKU: phenylketonuria)

- *Alternate pathways for ammonia excretion*:
  - *Sodium benzoate*—loading dose 250 mg/kg then 250–400 mg/kg/day in four divided doses
  - *L-arginine*: 300 mg/kg/day in three divided doses
  - *L-carnitine (oral/IV)*: 100–200 mg/kg/day
- Dialysis for rapid removal of ammonia (if comatose or ammonia >500 µg/dL or rapidly rising); hemodialysis better than peritoneal dialysis. Exchange transfusion is not useful.
- *Supportive care*: Treatment of sepsis, seizures, and ventilation. Avoid valproate.
- After stabilization, gradually add protein 0.25 g/kg till 1.5 g/kg/day while monitoring clinical and laboratory parameters.

Therapeutic measures for organic acidemia:
- Discontinue oral intake temporarily.
- 10% glucose and intravenous lipids 1 g/kg/24 h. Add minimal amounts of protein and mixture of essential AAs (0.25 g/kg/24 h) during the first 24 hour of therapy. Add insulin to prevent catabolism.
- Bicarbonate/carnitine/sodium benzoate/arginine.
- Dialysis should be considered for severely acidotic neonates/infants and children with organic acidemias.
- Vitamins are often given in cocktails after samples for laboratory investigations are obtained for establishing diagnosis. These include biotin, pyridoxine, B12, riboflavin, thiamine, and folate.
- Metronidazole—to reduce organic acids by gut flora.

Long-term therapy:
- *Dietary management*:
  - General protein restriction in urea cycle disorders and organic acidemias
  - Specific diets/specific AA restrictions, e.g., branched-chain AAs in MSUD, phenylalanine in PKU
  - Avoid fasting/use medium-chain triglycerides (MCTs) oil in FAODs
- Co-factor replacement therapy **(Table 8)**
- *Crisis management protocols*:
  - *Intercurrent illness*: Sick day diet (adequate calories, reduced proteins), double the dose of carnitine
  - *Early recognition of danger signs*: Lethargy, vomiting, poor oral intake, fast breathing, and moderate ketones in urine
  - Written emergency treatment guidelines
- *Substrate reduction therapy*: Miglustat in some lysosomal storage disorders
- Product replacement therapy
- Enzyme replacement therapy—in lysosomal storage disorders (Gaucher, Pompe, Hurler, and Fabry)
- *Transplantation*: Liver in urea cycle defects, organic acidemias, and bone marrow transplantations in some storage disorders
- *Monitoring*
- Growth standard charts
- Developmental surveillance—early intervention

TABLE 8: Vitamins/cofactors used in treatment of IEMs.

Vitamin/cofactor	Disorder	Dose
Thiamine	MSUD	100–200 mg per day
Riboflavin	Glutaric aciduria-I and -II	100 mg/day
Biotin	Biotinidase/ holocarboxylase synthetase deficiency, PA, biotin–thiamine-responsive basal ganglia disease	10–40 mg/day
Vitamin B12 (hydroxocobalamin)	Methylmalonic acidemia, disorders of cobalamin metabolism	• 1–2 mg/day • 0.3 µg/kg/day IM
Carnitine	MSUD, propionic acidemia, and isovaleric acidemia	50–100 mg/kg/day
Arginine	MELAS	300–500 mg/kg/day
Pyridoxine	• Pyridoxine-dependent epilepsy • Homocystinuria	• 20–30 mg/kg/day • 100 mg/day
Folinic acid	Kearns–Sayre/POLG/ disorder of cobalamin metabolism	20–30 mg/kg/day
Betaine (trimethylglycine)	Hyperhomocysteinemia	200–300 mg/kg/day
Coenzyme Q	Primary CoQ deficiency, ETC defects	5–10 mg/kg/day
L-creatine	Mitochondrial myopathy	0.1 g/kg

(CoQ: coenzyme Q; MELAS: mitochondrial encephalomyopathy, lactic acidosis, and stroke-like episode; MSUD: maple syrup urine disease)

- Monitor for dietary deficiencies—complete blood count, serum albumin, calcium, quantitative plasma aminoacidogram [high-performance liquid chromatography (HPLC)]

PREVENTIVE STRATEGIES

As these are lifespan disorders with the need for long-term resources, it is necessary to counsel and offer molecular genetic testing to confirm the diagnosis and offer genetic counseling to families informing recurrence risks. Most are single-gene defects, with 25% recurrence risk. Prenatal diagnosis may be done by detection of substrate or metabolite and enzyme levels in the chorionic villus sample or amniotic fluid. Most useful is molecular diagnosis. Newborn screening may allow presymptomatic detection and prevent morbidity.

Special Features in Indian Context: Newborn Screening

Newborn screening aims to screen neonates after birth for metabolic disorders that can cause severe morbidity or mortality unless detected and treated early. It is a norm in the developed countries. In India, small studies from various centers across India, private hospitals, and laboratories, and few state-level NBS programs provide a glimpse into the challenges and the inroads made. In 2008, Indian Council of Medical Research (ICMR) launched a pilot multicenter NBS program to screen 100,000 newborns for CH and CAH in five metropolitan cities—Chennai, Delhi, Hyderabad, Kolkata, and Mumbai. State-level NBS programs of note are the Chandigarh Program initiated in 2007 which screened for CH, CAH, and G6PD; Kerala State and Goa state NBS Program (under PPP model). However, universal NBS as a National program is not yet initiated in India. Applying Wilson and Jungner's screening criteria (1996) for selecting disorders into NBS programs in India, the biggest challenges are—the cost/benefit and availability of diagnosis and treatment facilities. 40 of the 54 disorders recommended for newborn screening by the American College of Medical Genetics and Genomics (ACMG) expert committee are diagnosed by MS/MS. A few drops of blood from a heel prick are taken on a filter card paper and air-dried for a few hours before sending to the laboratory. The use of quaternary ammonium compounds should be avoided to clean skin as it may lead to a false diagnosis of malonic aciduria. Filter paper should be attached to a card that carries all the relevant clinical information. Samples are usually collected for NBS between 24 and 72 hours of age. Prematurity, type of feeding, parenteral nutrition, neonatal jaundice, and some drugs may affect metabolite levels. Collected samples should be sent to the laboratory within 24 hours. Delays or adverse transport conditions may result in false-negative results due to metabolite degradation. False positivity of <0.3% should be the aim for any laboratory performing NBS. Additional testing on the same initial blood spot confirms the results with increased specificity. In 2011, the national neonatology forum recommended CH, CAH, and G6PD as the screening panel to implement for NBS in India. It is probably feasible to universally screen for CH in India, because it is easy and inexpensive to treat, with excellent outcomes.[27-29]

CONCLUSION

Inherited metabolic disorders though individually rare are collectively common with a wide range of clinical manifestations across age groups. These are often missed/misdiagnosed if a high index of clinical suspicion is not present. Early and timely recognition of IEMs is essential for the initiation of appropriate treatment for a better outcome as many have treatment potential.

REFERENCES

1. Clarke JTR. A clinical guide to inherited metabolic diseases, 3rd edition. Cambridge, UK; Cambridge University Press; 2005.
2. Waters D, Adeloye D, Woolham D, Wastnedge E, Patel S, Rudan I. Global birth prevalence and mortality from inborn errors of metabolism: a systematic analysis of the evidence. J Glob Health. 2018;8(2):021102.
3. Sanderson S, Green A, Preece MA, Burton H. The incidence of inherited metabolic disorders in the West Midlands, UK. Arch Dis Child. 2006;91(11):896-9.
4. Nagaraja D, Mamatha SN, De T, Christopher R. Screening for inborn errors of metabolism using automated electrospray tandem mass spectrometry: study in high-risk Indian population. Clin Biochem. 2010;43(6):581-8.
5. Verma IC. Burden of genetic disorders in India. Indian J Pediatr. 2000;67(12):893-8. Erratum in: Indian J Pediatr. 2001;68(1):25.
6. Saudubray JM, Garcia-Cazorla À. Inborn Errors of Metabolism Overview: Pathophysiology, Manifestations, Evaluation, and Management. Pediatr Clin North Am. 2018;65(2):179-208.
7. Zschocke J. SSIEM Classification of Inborn Errors of Metabolism. In: Blau N, Duran M, Gibson K, Dionisi Vici C (Eds). Physician's Guide to the Diagnosis, Treatment, and Follow-up of Inherited Metabolic Diseases. Berlin, Heidelberg: Springer; 2014.
8. Ferreira CR, van Karnebeek CDM, Vockley J, Blau N. A proposed nosology of inborn errors of metabolism. Genet Med. 2019;21(1):102-6.
9. Ferreira CR, Rahman S, Keller M, Zschocke J; ICIMD Advisory Group. An international classification of inherited metabolic disorders (ICIMD). J Inherit Metab Dis. 2021;44(1):164-77.
10. Christopher R, Sankaran BP. An insight into the biochemistry of inborn errors of metabolism for a clinical neurologist. Ann Indian Acad Neurol. 2008;11(2):68-81.
11. Shevell M, Ashwal S, Donley D, Flint J, Gingold M, Hirtz D, et al.; Quality Standards Subcommittee of the American Academy of Neurology; Practice Committee of the Child Neurology Society. Practice parameter: evaluation of the child with global developmental delay: report of the Quality Standards Subcommittee of the American Academy of Neurology and The Practice Committee of the Child Neurology Society. Neurology. 2003;60(3):367-80.
12. Campistol J, Díez-Juan M, Callejón L, Fernandez-De Miguel A, Casado M, Garcia Cazorla A, et al. Inborn error metabolic screening in individuals with nonsyndromic autism spectrum disorders. Dev Med Child Neurol. 2016;58:842-7.
13. Garanto A, Ferreira CR, Boon CJF, van Karnebeek CDM, Blau N. Clinical and biochemical footprints of inherited metabolic disorders. VII. Ocular phenotypes. Mol Genet Metab. 2022;135(4):311-9.
14. Ferreira CR, Hoffmann GF, Blau N. Clinical and biochemical footprints of inherited metabolic diseases. I. Movement disorders. Mol Genet Metab. 2019;127(1):28-30.
15. Ortigoza-Escobar JD. A Proposed Diagnostic Algorithm for Inborn Errors of Metabolism Presenting with Movements Disorders. Front Neurol. 2020;11:582160.
16. Sharma S, Kumar P, Agarwal R, Kabra M, Deorari AK, Paul VK. Approach to inborn errors of metabolism presenting in the neonate. Indian J Pediatr. 2008;75(3):271-6.
17. Saudubray J, Baumgartner M, Walter J. Inborn Errors of Metabolism in Adults: A Diagnostic Approach to Neurological and Psychiatric Presentations. Inborn Metabolic Diseases. Diag Treat. 2016;32(6):72-6.
18. Ezgu F, Makowski GS. Inborn errors of metabolism. Adv Clin Chem. 2016;73:195-250.

19. Lai LM, Gropman AL, Whitehead MT. MR Neuroimaging in Pediatric Inborn Errors of Metabolism. Diagnostics (Basel). 2022;12(4):861.
20. Gurrero RB, Salazar D, Tanpaiboon P. Laboratory diagnostic approaches in metabolic disorders. Ann Transl Med. 2018;6(24):470.
21. Thornton PS, Stanley CA, De Leon DD, Harris D, Haymond MW, Hussain K, et al. Pediatric Endocrine Society. Recommendations from the Pediatric Endocrine Society for Evaluation and Management of Persistent Hypoglycemia in Neonates, Infants, and Children. J Pediatr. 2015;167(2):238-45.
22. Cleary MA, Green A. Developmental delay: when to suspect and how to investigate for an inborn error of metabolism. Arch Dis Child. 2005;90:1128.
23. van Karnebeek CDM, Wortmann SB, Tarailo-Graovac M, Langeveld M, Ferreira CR, van de Kamp JM, et al. The role of the clinician in the multi-omics era: are you ready? J Inherit Metab Dis. 2018;41(3): 571-82.
24. Chakrapani A, Cleary MA, Wraith JE. Detection of inborn errors of metabolism in the newborn. Arch Dis Child Fetal Neonatal Ed. 2001;84(3):F205-10.
25. Weiner DL. Metabolic emergencies. In: Fleisher GR, Ludwig S, Henretig FM (Eds). Textbook of Pediatric Emergency Medicine, 5th edition. Philadelphia: Lippincott, Williams and Wilkins; 2006. p. 1193.
26. Burton BK. Inborn errors of metabolism in infancy: a guide to diagnosis. Pediatrics. 1998;102(6):E69.
27. Mookken T. Universal implementation of newborn screening in India. Int J Neonatal Screen. 2020;6(2):24.
28. Verma IC, Bijarnia-Mahay S, Jhingan G, Verma J. Newborn screening: need of the hour in India. Indian J Pediatr. 2015;82(1):61-70.
29. Shibata N, Hasegawa Y, Yamada K, Kobayashi H, Purevsuren J, Yang Y, et al. Diversity in the incidence and spectrum of organic acidemias, fatty acid oxidation disorders, and amino acid disorders in Asian countries: Selective screening vs. expanded newborn screening. Mol Genet Metab Rep. 2018;16:5-10.

108

CHAPTER

Neuroepidemiology

Abhinay M Huchche, Nadir E Bharucha

INTRODUCTION

The year 2022 marks 2 years of the coronavirus disease 19 (COVID-19) pandemic, and has been a testament to the importance of epidemiological research studies in understanding disease behavior and also helping in devising advanced treatment and prevention measures. The face of neurology has changed over the last two decades in terms of advances in stroke treatment and other fields. Thus, we have moved forward from diagnosticians to therapists. As neurologists and neurology trainees, the topic of epidemiology seems quite mundane, but considering the dynamic evidence-based medicine, we ought to know the nitty-gritties of epidemiological studies in order to draw sensible inferences and apply them to clinical practice. The history of neuroepidemiology dates back >50 years. One of the seminal neuroepidemiological studies that have set a benchmark for the future concerned multiple sclerosis in US veterans in World War II.[1] It was a large study wherein almost 5,000 Veterans diagnosed with multiple sclerosis were compared with controls. These studies were supported by the US Veterans administration. It described the ethnic, geographic, and genetic predispositions to multiple sclerosis and is one of the first-class studies in multiple sclerosis. Other studies that set a benchmark for the future need a quick mention. The Kuru study in the geographical isolate of the Fore group of people which was linked to ritualistic cannibalism led to the discovery of the slow virus and set a reference for prion diseases such as human Creutzfeldt-Jakob disease (CJD).[2,3] The neurological damage caused by consumption of fish and the link to mercury was established by Douglas Mcalpine and Shukuro Araki in the 1950's.[4]

Epidemiology literally means study (logos) among (epi) people (demos). Neuroepidemiology is the study of neurologic diseases in a population including assessment of frequency, natural history, risk factors, and treatment. Knowledge of the disease burden is important for public health policy makers to enable allocation of resources and institute community measures and also to help practitioners in prevention, diagnosis, and treatment.

FREQUENTLY USED TERMS IN EPIDEMIOLOGY (CENTER FOR DISEASE CONTROL)

It is vital to know the definitions of terms used in epidemiological studies in order to understand the importance and authenticity of the study. These basics have been covered during our medical schooling, but as pure practicing clinicians, we usually lose touch and thus it's a good idea to keep brushing up our knowledge from time-to-time.

Neuroepidemiological studies are designed to answer a particular question (research question) pertaining to the neurological disorder.

The prerequisites for measuring the frequency of the disorder are:
- Study population of interest (sample)
- Event (case) and
- Time frame (per year)

Let us understand them in detail below.

Sampling

The types of sampling differ depending on how individuals are chosen from the source population.

Types of Sampling

There are four types of sampling:
1. *Cluster sampling*: Here, individuals from a particular cluster are selected randomly, e.g., school cluster and neurology clinic cluster.
2. *Stratified sampling*: Population is divided into strata based on age, gender, and ethnicity and then sampling is done randomly from each stratum.

3. *Multistage sampling*: An example can best explain this first-stage sampling—Hyderabad city, second-stage sampling—Rangareddy district, third-stage sampling—Paradise circle, and so on.
4. *Random sampling*: Each individual in the population has an equal chance of getting selected in the sample.

Sample Size

Another crucial step is deciding the number of individuals chosen for the study, i.e., sample size. Too small a sample size might undermine the strength of the differences found, whereas a large sample size needs a larger human resource and longer time for the study. It is essential to carefully consider the appropriate sample size depending on the parameters to be studied.

Terminology Related to Data Description

Mean, Median, and Mode

The midpoints in the data collected are represented by these terms. The term used depends on the type of data that is taken into consideration. Mean is basically an average of the sum of all values divided by the number of values. Median is used for data that is continuously distributed, thus it is the midpoint of all the values arranged in an ascending order, e.g., median age for the data collected. Mode is the value that appears most frequently in a given database.

Gaussian or Normal Distribution (Bell-shaped Curve)

Wherein the data is continuously distributed along a bell-shaped curve.

Standard Deviation

Variability that can be probable around the mean is standard deviation. Usually, applicable for Gaussian data. Two standard deviations usually cover about 95% of the variability around the mean.

Standard Error of the Mean

It tells us about the variability when comparing means from two different samples.

CLASSIFICATION OF NEUROEPIDEMIOLOGY

Epidemiological studies are broadly classified into:
- Observational and
- Experimental

Observational Studies

Descriptive Studies

An observational epidemiological study includes description of the neurological disease frequency, distribution, and severity in the defined population. Disease frequency is quantified by the incidence and prevalence rates. Age and gender-specific rates elaborate disease distribution in the population. Mortality and morbidity rates give us an idea of the disease severity. The definitions for the above-mentioned rates are given below:
- *Incidence rate*: Frequency of occurrence of new cases of a disease within a specified population over a given time interval at a particular place.
- *Prevalence rate*: Frequency of all current cases of a disease in a defined population at a particular time and place. If this number is identified over a time period, it is termed *period* prevalence; whereas if they were identified at a single point in time, it is called *point* prevalence.
- *Mortality rate*: Number of deaths due to a disease over a time frame divided by the population. One of the major hindrances when describing mortality from low- and-middle-income countries (LMIC) is the lack of death certificate data. Thus, we need to rely on verbal accounts for comparison across the globe (verbal autopsy).
- *Standardized mortality ratio (SMR)*: This is used when we compare mortality data across two different populations. The standardization is usually done by age and gender and thus in addition to the age-specific mortality data, we need to know the age and gender structure for the population.

Analytical Studies

Analytical studies look at the relationship between risk factors and disease and some studies in addition look at the frequency of occurrence of risk factors. For example, hypertension is not only an important risk factor for stroke but also, as untreated hypertension is common in the community, a significant burden of stroke may be attributed to hypertension. Analytical studies are further subdivided into case control and cohort studies.

Case Control Study

A "case" is a person with the neurological disease being studied, whereas a "control" is a healthy age and gender-matched person from the same population. The study design is a retrospective one wherein people with established neurological disease are compared with controls to study the risk factors associated with the disease. The case control study of stroke in Parsis from Bombay is an early example from India.[5] Here, Parsis from Mumbai (then Bombay) with completed strokes were identified by a prevalence survey and were compared with healthy age- and gender-matched Parsis selected randomly from the same population. This study reiterated that hypertension and diabetes are important risk factors for stroke. Thus, preventive lifestyle measures for diabetes and hypertension and regular adequate medical treatment for these conditions can help reduce stroke burden.

Cohort Study

A cohort is a group of people with a shared characteristic, e.g., people living in a particular district. The study design is usually prospective wherein people from the defined population are longitudinally followed up over a period of time, in order to study the neurological disease of interest. The Rotterdam study performed in the 1990's is an example of a prospective cohort study, where people aged 45 years and above living in the Ommoord district in the city of Rotterdam were followed up for neurological diseases such as stroke, Parkinson's disease (PD), and dementia.[6] Cohort studies are a precious source of information as they give us volumes of information about incidence, prevalence, and natural history of the neurological disease. They help understand risk factors for these diseases. The Framingham study of cardiovascular disease is one of the oldest cohort studies performed in the 20th century.[7] Framingham town population was chosen as there was very little migration and had a limited population, thus making it suitable for regular assessment. The age group selected for the study was between 30 and 62 years of age as people below this age group had a very low probability and people over 62 would have had established coronary disease. Thus, this age group was appropriate to study incidence of coronary artery disease in the population.

In these studies, we observe exposures and subsequent outcomes without a bias. Measures used in observational studies of the relation between the exposure (risk factor) and outcome (disease) are mentioned below:

- *Relative risk or risk ratio*: This measure indicates risk of developing neurological disease following exposure to a particular factor, e.g., when we divide the incidence of stroke in hypertensives by the incidence in normotensives, we ascertain relative risk of stroke due to hypertension. The definition of hypertension has changed over time. Now we have more stringent definitions of hypertension. Therefore, comparison of earlier with later studies needs to account for differences in definition. For calculating the relative risk, we need to know the incidence rate in people with and without the risk factor. If the incidence is not known, prospective studies in comparable groups with and without the factor can be compared to know the relative risk.
- *Odds ratio*: A retrospective case control comparison for the presence or history of a risk factor gives us the odds ratio which is shown in the **Table 1**.

TABLE 1: Details of how the odds ratio is calculated.

Hypertension	Stroke	Control	Total
Present	a	c	a + c
Absent	b	d	b + d

Note: Odds ratio = ad/bc

The product "ad" represents the correct calls made, whereas the product "bc" represents the errors wherein b is no hypertension in stroke and c is hypertension in controls.

- *Attributable risk*: The difference between the incidence of disease in the exposed and the incidence in the nonexposed is a measure of the contribution of the risk factor (attribution) to the disease being studied.

Descriptive epidemiological studies are a part of *classical epidemiology* and can help devise primary prevention strategies and help initiate screening programs for identifying and treating the concerned risk factors for neurological diseases. Clinical epidemiology deals with application of the principles of epidemiology for diagnosis and treatment of neurological disorders in an evidence-based fashion in order to increase safety and avoid unwarranted treatment. An accurate diagnosis is essential for initiating treatment and to predict outcome. In neurology, clinical diagnosis is supported by tests—imaging, serology, and electrophysiology. However, a clinician needs to be cautious before interpreting the test results and needs to take into consideration factors such as pretest probability of the disease and sensitivity and specificity of the test.

UTILITY OF DIAGNOSTIC TESTS[8,9]

Questions that can be used to evaluate the utility of a diagnostic test will be discussed in the following section:

- How reliably can the test be performed? The test should be accurate and precise for it to be applied in practice. Accuracy is the proportion of all results (positive and negative) that prove to be correct. A diagnostic test which produces the same result when repeated in the same individual/population is termed precise. Some diagnostic tests are highly influenced by the observer performing the test and the center where it is performed, e.g., neck Doppler for the carotid arteries to determine the amount of stenosis. Literature for these diagnostic tests is usually derived from tertiary care centers which have advanced machinery and expert people. Correlating these results with local results either at individual or population level does not seem practical.
- What population was tested? It is important that the test be performed in the population with and without the disease, each being represented in adequate numbers and sharing similarities in clinical features.
- Was a gold standard or reference standard used? A gold standard or reference standard test is the best measure we have to differentiate diseased individuals from the healthy population. The diagnostic test under evaluation should be compared with the reference standard to increase the value of the test.
- What was the cutoff used? The cutoff should be such that it balances the sensitivity and specificity of the test. Sensitivity and specificity are best understood from the **Table 2**.
- *Disease prevalence*: The baseline prevalence of the disease in the population determines the predictive value of a positive test. If the disease is uncommon, the predictive value of a positive test is very low.

TABLE 2: Incident table for the calculation of diagnostic test properties.

	Disease	No disease
Positive test	a	c
Negative test	b	d
Total	a + b	c + d

- Sensitivity of the test = a/a + b (i.e., proportion of diseased people testing positive)
- Specificity of the test = d/c + d (i.e., proportion of people without the test who tested negative)
- Positive predictive value = a/a + c (i.e., proportion testing positive actually having the disease)
- Negative predictive value = d/b + d (i.e., proportion testing negative and not having the disease)
- False positive rate = 1—specificity
- False negative rate = 1—sensitivity

- What's the cost effectiveness? Cost is an ever-changing game because of the dynamic market. Also, it varies based on the place, country, and institute where it is being performed, thus lacking uniformity. Severity of the disease also plays a role in deciding whether cost should be considered before ordering the test.

Experimental Epidemiology

After having understood the utility and evaluation of diagnostic tests, we need to move forward toward understanding the use of epidemiology to facilitate treatment. Here comes the most advanced part of neuroepidemiology also known as experimental epidemiology. Most of us can recall our school days in the science laboratory where we used to be excited to perform experiments with chemicals and our college days wherein, we were busy proving hypotheses in the physics laboratories. The basis of an experimental study is the formation of a hypothesis that a drug or procedure "X" helps a particular neurological disease "Y". The role of the experimental study is to prove the hypothesis by comparing the results (primary outcome) in the people receiving the therapy vis-à-vis, those not receiving therapy. Also, if there is a difference in the outcomes, we use statistical methods to determine if the difference is significant enough to recommend therapy. Thus, guidelines are framed based on the quality of evidence and strength of recommendation for therapy and the disease of interest.

Randomized Double Blind Placebo Controlled Trial

This is a study design wherein individuals are randomly selected and assigned to either a drug or procedure arm or a placebo agent or procedure. The investigator and the participant are both blinded as to what they are analyzing or receiving in terms of the therapy. These studies are less prone to bias and thus provide the best possible evidence. During the trial tenure, some patients may not be compliant with the treatment assigned. These people need to be included while analyzing the results. This kind of inclusion and analysis serves the purpose of randomization and also helps minimize bias and is termed *"intention to treat"* analysis. A drug that is effective but has unacceptable adverse effects will have a low compliance. If noncompliant participants are excluded from the analysis, it might give a false impression that the drug has a good scope for treatment which is not the true case. An "as-treated" analysis might be useful to study the adverse effects of the therapy.

SYSTEMATIC REVIEW AND META-ANALYSIS

Summary of all the available evidence for a particular research question forms a systematic review.[10] While framing evidence for a systematic review, studies which meet predefined standards are included. The rest are excluded. Meta-analysis is a statistical method wherein results obtained in different studies are combined onto a single graph and thus benefit or risk of therapy is ascertained in a more mathematical manner.[11] A single trial can never answer the research question with certainty. There are instances, where many trials refute the findings in the previously performed trials. In systematic reviews, by combining studies, the sample size increases and thus the confidence intervals are narrow compared with single randomized controlled trials.[12] These reviews are different from narrative review articles and textbook chapters, which are descriptive and more subjective. A systematic review goes through different stages and at each step, precautions are taken to avoid bias. Two studies addressing the same research question cannot be entirely similar resulting in heterogeneity. Studies differing in terms of eligibility criteria, intervention, or measures of outcome are not suitable for meta-analyses. These are clinically heterogeneous studies.[13] Studies with quantitative differences in outcomes, but similar in other aspects, are statistically heterogeneous. Statistical heterogeneity is addressed by tests like I2. The I2 index measures the variability amongst two studies in terms of effect size. It is graded as 25% (low), 50% (medium), and 75% (high); the higher the percentage, the higher the chances of true heterogeneity amongst studies. To summarize, systematic reviews and meta-analyses are simplified evidence guidelines for the practitioners.

BIAS IN STUDIES

Bias can change results of a study and point us away from the truth. It can arise at different stages of study design. A sample is a subset of individuals chosen from a larger population (source population) in order to answer the research question related to the neurological disorder. Sampling is a crucial step for a study to be valid, as the sample should aptly represent the source population *(external validity)* and inferences drawn for an individual in the sample should be applicable to the whole sample *(internal validity)*. Only then can the conclusions drawn be broadly applicable to the population at large. Bias is usually created due to the lack of internal validity.

Bias can be broadly classified into three types, i.e., *(1) selection bias, (2) information bias, and (3) confounding bias*. Selection bias arises when the study population is not representative of the target population. Selection bias is further subdivided into different types based on the stage at which the error is introduced. Selection bias is introduced at the time of sampling. For example, cases with disease for a longer duration are more likely to be included in the study, but are not representative of the case spectrum in the population. This bias is termed "length bias sampling error". Citation bias may be seen in systematic reviews where articles that are more frequently cited are easily found and included. Citation depends on the impact factor of the journal in which the article has been published. Information bias is introduced during data collection. A typical example that can be quoted is that of recall bias, which is seen in case control studies. As people already have the disease, they may better recall possible risk factors. Underreporting bias is a form of information bias seen with substance abuse such as alcohol and smoking. In addition, socially stigmatized conditions such as epilepsy may not be reported. Confounding bias occurs when the variable in exposed and nonexposed people affects outcome.[14]

NEUROEPIDEMIOLOGY GLOBAL PERSPECTIVE[15]

As nations and continents, we differ in terms of our culture, lifestyle, and geographical aspects. It is always interesting to know how these factors influence the cause and outcome of neurological diseases. The per capita income, which differs amongst nations and continents, also influences healthcare, prevention, treatment, and allocation of resources toward research. Comparison of burden of neurological disease at the national, regional, and global levels helps clinicians and policy makers in allocating resources for neurological disorders.

The Global Burden of Disease Study 2015 (GBD) was a comprehensive estimate for other disorders, but data was lacking for many neurological disorders such as stroke, cancer, and communicable diseases. The GBD 2015 neurological disorders collaborators group did a systematic analysis of all the epidemiological studies between 2013 and 2015. The inclusion of the missing neurological disorders in GBD 2015 made us realize that neurological disorders in general and stroke in particular top the list of global disability and rank second when considering global mortality estimates. The parameters used for describing the global burden were prevalence, disability-adjusted life years (DALY's), and deaths. This data was calculated across 195 countries and regions worldwide. The other highlights of the study were the comparison of trends over time and correlation with the sociodemographic index (SDI) (clubs per capita income, education, and fertility) across various regions.

Stroke (around 45%), migraine (around 15%), and Alzheimer's disease (along with other dementias around 10%) shared the first, second, and third positions, respectively in terms of DALY's. Stroke retained its position at the top, accounting for almost two-thirds of global neurological deaths, followed by dementia at the second spot (around one fifth). Communicable diseases ranked higher in regions such as South Asia and sub-Saharan Africa. Meningitis was the largest contributor in sub-Saharan Africa. Tetanus figures were the highest in Somalia and Sudan, whereas encephalitis topped the Indian charts. The figures for headache are in contrast to communicable diseases, with highest figures for high income countries and lowest in sub-Saharan Africa.

Population explosion and increase in the life expectancy over time has indirectly led to an alarming increase (almost 100%) in the number of DALY's, prevalence, and deaths for Alzheimer's disease and other dementias as compared with the data in 1990. The same is true for PD. Meningitis, encephalitis, and tetanus figures have decreased over time, probably because of the improvement in vaccination trends and the overall improvement in hygiene and health. The DALY's and death rates for combined neurological disorders decreased, compared with the 1990's. Thus, there has been a shift from communicable diseases to noncommunicable diseases at the global level.

Figures in accordance with respect to SDI suggest that DALY rates for neurological disorders are higher in regions with a low SDI. The steadily increasing number of people with neurological disorders cautions us to plan for the future. Access to neurological care has been a problem in resource poor countries with a disproportionate health sector to population ratio.

NEUROEPIDEMIOLOGY: INDIAN PERSPECTIVE

India is a nation with a diverse cultural background across parts of the country. Conducting research in India is not an easy task, taking into consideration shortage of trained manpower and funds and the diversity of language. After having understood the global estimates, it is essential to know the trends and figures from India in order to understand how we differ from other countries and also what we (as practitioners and Indian health policymakers) need to do in order to address local issues.

Neuroepidemiology in India has evolved over time from single disorder studies to community and population-based studies. World Health Organization (WHO) pilot studies to detect the burden of neurological disorders in Nigeria were replicated in India in the 1980's.[16] Using a validated questionnaire, trained social workers performed surveys to detect people with possible neurological disorders such as stroke, epilepsy, peripheral neuropathy, and PD. People identified on the basis of a screening procedure were later examined by neurologists and diseases confirmed or ruled out. In India, the neuroepidemiological studies in Parsis were very much a part of these initial studies. The Parsi population was relatively stable. In Bombay, many stayed in housing communities known as colonies thus facilitating the survey. Gourie-Devi et al. modified and expanded the questionnaire and performed a survey of neurological disorders in the Gowribidanur town.[17] These were some of the pioneering initial studies in India thus promoting research and grants from the Indian Council of Medical Research.

Studies conducted in resource poor countries had many deficiencies like small sample size and nonrepresentative samples differences in case definition. The Bangalore Urban Rural Neurological survey (BURN) addressed some of these deficiencies by developing questionnaires and training healthcare workers, thus forming a framework for future neuroepidemiological studies in India.[18]

Estimates of the prevalence of neurological disorders in India stems from a pool of studies which were door to door surveys conducted from West, South, North, and East India. These were conducted by Bharucha et al. from Bombay, Gourie-Devi et al. from Karnataka, Kapoor et al. from Delhi, Razdan et al. from Kashmir, Das et al. from Malda, and Saha et al. from South 24 parganas [19-23] The average crude prevalence rate of neurological disorders was 2,394 people per 100,000 population. In studies with both an urban and a rural component, prevalence rates were higher in rural areas. Epilepsy, headache, febrile seizures, and stroke accounted for almost 80% of the neurological disorders. There were people detected with postpolio sequelae and people with post-Japanese encephalitis sequelae. These kinds of community studies help us plan preventive, therapeutic, and rehabilitative strategies for neurological disorders in the Indian community.

EPILEPSY STUDIES FROM INDIA

As per the GBD, more than two-thirds of people with epilepsy live in resource poor countries. There were about 14 epilepsy surveys performed in India in between 1968 and 2008. The principal investigators for these population studies need to be acknowledged taking into consideration the methodological difficulties faced while conducting those studies a few decades back. Goel et al., Kokkat et al., Kapoor et al., and Koul et al. conducted studies among rural portions of Dehradun, Haryana, and Kashmir.[20,24-26] Bharucha et al. conducted a prevalence survey in the urban Parsis in Bombay, Das et al. studied epilepsy in the urban population of Kolkata.[22,27] There were many studies from South India. Mathai et al. (1968) and Rajshekhar et al. (2003) studied epilepsy in the combined urban and rural populations of Vellore, Tamil Nadu.[28,29] Mani et al. published his data from rural Yelandur in Karnataka, wherein there was a high prevalence of hot water epilepsy.[30] Radhakrishnan et al. published studies from Kerala whereas Gourie Devi et al. and Satishchandra et al. conducted studies in Gauribidanur and Bengaluru in Karnataka.[18,31] The questionnaires used were NIMHANS, WHO, and ICEBERG. The mean crude prevalence rate of 5.7 per 1,000 population was comparable to developed countries. Two studies (Goel et al. and Rajshekhar et al.) focused on neurocysticercosis and epilepsy, a special contributor to epilepsy in India and other developing countries.[24,29] The treatment gap varied amongst different studies, with the gap being as high as 75% owing to lack of awareness, myths, and misunderstandings about epilepsy and inadequate healthcare services.

STROKE AND PARKINSON'S DISEASE STUDIES FROM INDIA

As per the GBD, stroke contributed to the major burden of deaths and DALY's in India as well. The mortality in stroke study by Joshi et al. from Andhra Pradesh through verbal autopsy highlighted stroke as a major contributor to deaths in the community.[32] There are many hospital-based studies of stroke, but few population-based studies. The prevalence rates calculated from community studies had a wide range (52–472 per 100,000 population).[33-36] Abraham et al. conducted one of the earliest studies on stroke in India in the urban and rural population of Vellore.[37] However, this study considered only hemiplegic stroke with residual disability. Hence, prevalence rate was low. The highest prevalence rate was from the study in Parsis by Bharucha et al. (842.3 per 100,000 population). The age-adjusted ratio was 424/100,000, slightly lower than the world average at that time. Age-adjusted incidence rates were available from the Trivandrum and Mumbai stroke registries and were about 135 and 152 per 100,000 population, respectively.[38,39] Almost all the studies highlighted the importance of hypertension as a risk factor for stroke.

Parkinson's disease prevalence rates from the Indian studies by Gourie-devi et al., Razdan et al., and Saha et al. are in the range of 6–53 per 100,000 population.[18,21,23] The study by Bharucha in the Parsi community had a higher age-adjusted prevalence ratio of 328.3/100,000. Age-specific rates of neurodegenerative disorders such as Parkinson's and Alzheimer's diseases increase with age. Hence, the prevalence of these conditions is higher in aging populations such as the Parsis and is expected to increase in the whole community as it ages. WHO questionnaires to detect neurological disorders in the community were used for PD. Specific questionnaires to increase the sensitivity for PD would give more correct estimates of this steadily increasing disease. Mentioning all important studies performed in India is beyond the scope of this chapter. Readers should refer to the relevant chapter on a specific disease for more detailed information.

The number of neurology practitioners qualifying every year in India is increasing. More and more private hospitals offer neurology training programs. As the number of neurologists increases, neurology care is being taken further into rural areas. Neurology practitioners from different parts of the country further supplement rural healthcare of conditions such as epilepsy. They organize camps in rural areas conducted in collaboration with the State Government under the aegis of the National Rural Health Mission where medicines are provided free of cost. The Lifeline Express epilepsy clinics are another such effort to extend the reach of epilepsy care and research to remote villages from Uttar Pradesh, Madhya Pradesh, and West Bengal.[40]

Rural primary health centers (PHCs) need to be strengthened with more doctors and paramedical healthcare workers and availability of essential medicines, e.g., antiepileptic drugs. Training programs focusing on common neurological conditions would enable timely identification, management, and where necessary referral of patients by PHC doctors. Training programs in neurology for nurses and physicians would facilitate and improve stroke care even in remote areas. Also, access to rehabilitation services in remote areas is essential to improve neurologic outcomes.

CONCLUSION

Resource poor countries contribute most to the global burden of neurological disorders such as epilepsy. Ironically, the majority of epidemiological research globally takes place in resource rich countries. Conducting research in resource poor settings has its own challenges—methodological difficulties, lack of adequate funds, people not consenting to give details especially of conditions such as epilepsy where there is stigma, diverse often migrating populations, and inadequate remuneration and recognition of investigators. Many of the studies performed in these settings fail to appear in indexed international journals. Hence, valuable information is overlooked leading to publication bias. Systematic reviews and meta-analyses also overlook these studies.

Advances in technology, especially the widespread use of mobile phones, using short messaging services (SMS), devices enabling use of the internet and cloud computing and the e-Aadhaar system would further help data collection and communication between healthcare workers and the population. These services would also help to remain in touch with people who migrate for better work opportunities. Thus, a quantum leap in Indian healthcare services has been brought about by the technology as illustrated by the response to COVID.

Organizations such as the Indian Academy of Neurology (IAN) and the Neurological Society of India (NSI) constantly strive to promote research and provide a platform for neurologists to present their work in journals and interact with colleagues at annual conferences. There seems to be a lot of hope and light for future neurology in India, both in terms of care and research.

REFERENCES

1. Kurtzke JF, Beebe GW, Norman JE Jr. Epidemiology of multiple sclerosis in U.S. veterans: Race, sex, and geographic distribution. Neurology. 1979;29(9 Pt 1):1228-35.
2. Zigas V, Gajdusek DC. Kuru: Clinical study of a new syndrome resembling paralysis agitans in natives of the eastern Highlands of Australian New Guinea. Med J Aust. 1959;44:745-54.
3. Zigas V, Gajdusek DC. Kuru: Clinical, pathological and epidemiological study of a recently discovered acute progressive degenerative disease of the central nervous system reaching "epidemic" proportions among natives of the Eastern Highlands of New Guinea. Papua New Guinea Med J. 1959;3:1-31.
4. McAlpine D, Araki S. Minamata disease. An unusual neurological disorder caused by contaminated fish. Lancet. 1958;2:629-31.
5. Bharucha NE, Bharucha EP, Bharucha AE, Bhise AV, Schoenberg BS. Case-control study of completed ischemic stroke in the Parsis of Bombay: a population-based study. Neurology. 1988;38(3):490-2.
6. Hofman A, Breteler MB, Van Duijn C, Krestin GP, Pols HA, Stricker BHC, et al. The Rotterdam study: Objectives and design update. Euro J Epidemiol. 2007;22(11):819-29.
7. Mahmood SS, Levy D, Vasan RS, Wang TJ. The Framingham Heart Study and the epidemiology of cardiovascular disease: a historical perspective. Lancet. 2014;383(9921):999-1008.
8. Ewigman BG, Crane JP, Frigoletto FD, LeFevre ML, Bain RP, McNellis D; RADIUS Study Group. Effect of prenatal ultrasound screening on perinatal outcome. N Engl J Med. 1993;329(12):821-7.
9. Leitich H, Kaider A. Fetal fibronectin—how useful is it in the prediction of preterm birth? BJOG. 2003;110:66-70.
10. Chalmers I, Altman DG. Systematic reviews. London: BMJ Publishing; 1995.
11. Briere JB, Bowrin K, Taieb V, Millier A, Toumi M, Coleman C. Meta-analyses using real-world data to generate clinical and epidemiological evidence: a systematic literature review of existing recommendations. Curr Med Res Opin. 2018;34(12):2125-30.
12. Lau J, Ioannidis JP, Schmid CH. Quantitative synthesis in systematic reviews. Ann Int Med. 1997;127(9):820-6.
13. Higgins JP, Thompson SG, Deeks JJ, Altman DG. Measuring inconsistency in meta-analyses. BMJ. 2003;327:557.
14. Delgado-Rodriguez M, Llorca J. Bias. J Epidemiol Community Health. 2004;58(8):635-41.
15. Feigin VL, Abajobir AA, Abate KH, Abd-Allah F, Abdulle AM, Abera SF, et al. Global, regional, and national burden of neurological disorders during 1990–2015: a systematic analysis for the Global Burden of Disease Study 2015. Lancet Neurol. 2017;16(11):877-97.
16. Osuntokun BO, Schoenberg BS, Nottidge VA, Adeuja A, Kale O, Adeyefa A, et al. Research protocol for measuring the prevalence of neurologic disorders in developing countries. Neuroepidemiology. 1982;1(3):143-53.
17. Gourie-Devi M, Rao VN, Prakashi R. A protocol to detect neurological disorders in the community. Indian J Med Res. 1988;88:443-9.
18. Gourie-Devi M, Gururaj G, Satishchandra P, Subbakrishna DK. Prevalence of neurological disorders in Bangalore, India: a community-based study with a comparison between urban and rural areas. Neuroepidemiology. 2004;23(6):261-8.

19. Bharucha NE, Bharucha EP, Dastur HD, Schoenberg BS. Pilot survey of the prevalence of neurologic disorders in the Parsi community of Bombay. Am J Prev Med. 1987;3:293-9.
20. Kapoor SK, Banerjee AK. Prevalence of common neurological diseases in a rural community of India. Indian J Community Med. 1989;14(4):171.
21. Razdan S, Kaul RL, Motta A, Kaul S, Bhatt RK. Prevalence and pattern of major neurological disorders in rural Kashmir (India) in 1986. Neuroepidemiology. 1994;13(3):113-9.
22. Das SK, Sanyal K. Neuroepidemiology of major neurological disorders in rural Bengal. Neurol India. 1996;44:47-58.
23. Saha SP, Bhattacharya S, Das SK, Maity B, Roy T, Raut DK. Epidemiological study of neurological disorders in a rural population of Eastern India. J Indian Med Assoc. 2003;101:299-300,302-4.
24. Goel D, Dhanai JS, Agarwal A, Malhotra V, Saxena V. Neurocysticercosis and its impact on crude prevalence rate of epilepsy in an Indian community. Neurol India. 2011;59:37-40.
25. Kokkat AJ, Verma AK. Prevalence of seizures and paralysis in a rural community. J Indian Med Assoc. 1996;96:43-5.
26. Koul R, Razdan S, Motta A. Prevalence and pattern of epilepsy (Lath/Mirgi/Laran) in rural Kashmir, India. Epilepsia. 1988;29:116-22.
27. Bharucha NE, Bharucha EP, Bharucha AE, Bhise AV, Schoenberg BS. Prevalence of epilepsy in the Parsi community of Bombay. Epilepsia. 1988;29:111-5.
28. Mathai KV. Final report. Investigations into methods for rehabilitation of persons disabled by convulsive disorders. SRS Project No. 19-P-58113- F-0l. Vellore, Dept of Neurol Sci., CMC; 1971.
29. Rajshekhar V, Raghava MV, Prabhakaran V, Oommen A, Muliyil J. Active epilepsy as an index of burden of neurocysticercosis in Vellore district, India. Neurology. 2006;67:2135-9.
30. Mani KS, Rangan G, Srinivas HV, Kalyanasundaram S, Narendran S, Reddy AK. The Yelandur study: A community-based approach to epilepsy in rural South India—epidemiological aspects. Seizure. 1998;7:281-8.
31. Radhakrishnan K, Pandian JD, Santoshkumar T, Thomas SV, Deetha TD, Sarma PS, et al. Prevalence, knowledge, attitude and practice of epilepsy in Kerala, South India. Epilepsia. 2000;41:1027-35.
32. Joshi R, Cardona M, Iyengar S, Sukumar A, Raju CR, Raju KR, et al. Chronic diseases now a leading cause of death in rural India-mortality data from the Andhra Pradesh rural health initiative. Int J Epidemiol. 2006;35:1522-9.
33. Bansal BC, Dhamija RK. Epidemiology of stroke in Haryana (North India). In: Bansal BC, Agarwal AK (Eds). Recent concepts in stroke. New Delhi: Indian College of Physicians, Association of Physicians of India; 1999. Pp. 22-5.
34. Banerjee TK, Mukherjee CS, Sarkhel A. Stroke in the urban population of Calcutta—An epidemiological study. Neuroepidemiology. 2001;20:201-7.
35. Das SK, Banerjee TK, Biswas A, Roy T, Raut DK, Mukherjee CS, et al. A prospective community-based study of stroke in Kolkata, India. Stroke. 2007;38:906-10.
36. Razdan S, Kaul RL, Motta A, Kaul S. Cerebrovascular disease in rural Kashmir, India. Stroke. 1989;20:1691-3.
37. Abraham J, Rao PS, Inbaraj SG, Shetty G, Jose CJ. An epidemiological study of hemiplegia due to stroke in South India. Stroke. 1970;1:477-81.
38. Sridharan SE, Unnikrishnan JP, Sukumaran S, Sylaja PN, Nayak SD, Sarma PS, et al. Incidence, types, risk factors and outcome of stroke in a developing country: The Trivandrum stroke registry. Stroke. 2009;40:1212-8.
39. Dalal PM, Malik S, Bhattacharjee M, Trivedi ND, Vairale J, Bhat P, et al. Population-based stroke survey in Mumbai, India: Incidence and 28-day case fatality. Neuroepidemiology. 2008;31:254-61.
40. Singh M. Epilepsy care by rail. Ann Indian Acad Neurol. 2010;13(3):234.

109
CHAPTER

Functional Neurological Disorders

Sudhir Kothari, Rajesh Benny, Devashish Ruikar, Bhushan Mishal, Parthvi Ravat

INTRODUCTION

Functional neurological disorders (FNDs) are a significant and common reason for neurological symptoms that appear to be "medically unexplained," as there is no abnormal finding on tests or neuroimaging. These disorders are caused by an impairment of neurological function, without any observable underlying pathology. They are indeed located in the patient's mind, but this statement should not be dismissive. The suffering and disability are real, not fabricated, and they lead to significant disability and strain on financial and healthcare resources, and, if not handled sensitively, can damage the relationship between patients and doctors.[1]

Both the neurologist and the psychiatrist may find themselves struggling with these patients; the neurologist has difficulty in managing them while the psychiatrist has difficulty diagnosing them. As a result, these patients often feel unwelcome and neglected by both specialists. The approach to diagnosing and managing these disorders has improved and can now be more positive, like other neurological disorders.

The way forward involves a collaborative and multidisciplinary approach to managing these illnesses. Despite the label "FND," they are not solely a neurological disorder, and psychiatric components are important in management.[1,2]

HISTORICAL BACKGROUND[1]

Patients with neurological symptoms that are not explainable by medical means have been recognized across different cultures for over 4,000 years. At one time they were attributed to disease of the uterus (the Greek word hystera means uterus.) In the mid-twentieth century, particularly after Sigmund Freud, the focus shifted to the mind. An artificial divide was created between disorders of the brain and disorders of the mind, one the domain of neurologists and the other of psychiatrists.[3] The name conversion disorder implied that somehow psychological factors got "converted" into these physical symptoms. Patients did not like this name or the implied mechanism.

The criteria laid down by the Diagnostic and Statistical Manual of Mental Disorders or the DSM-IV, for making the diagnosis of conversion disorder, required neurologists to do three very uncomfortable and difficult tasks first ruling out any other diseases, second making sure the patient was not faking illness, and third finding some linked psychosocial stressors. These criteria led to several problems. The criterion to rule out other diseases promoted excessive and unnecessary investigations. The way the diagnosis was presented gave patients the feeling that its only basis was the inability to find another cause and so they would wonder whether another neurologist or a new or repeat test could find the missing diagnosis. This gave rise to "doctor shopping." Making sure the patient was not being deceptive or faking the illness was an uncomfortable and almost impossible task. The doctor had to try and trick the patient into "revealing the truth." Conversion disorder was the only disorder that required doctors to explicitly rule out fake illness. This led to patients rejecting the diagnosis, the doctor, and even the medical system.

Finally, probing for linked psychological factors often could feel insensitive and spoil the relationship with the patient. Neurologists could get misled either way, thinking the disorder to be functional just by finding some stressor or by not considering it as functional due to the apparent absence of any stressor. Psychological factors are recognized as important risk factors but are neither necessary nor sufficient for the diagnosis.[4] Their importance would come later during management.

To add insult to injury, almost immediately after making the diagnosis, neurologists would disassociate themselves from the patient and hand them over to psychiatrists.

The new DSM-V criteria **(Box 1)** have addressed all the above issues, and now it is given the more neutral

BOX 1 **Functional neurological disorders and the Diagnostic and Statistical Manual of Mental Disorders (DSM)-V.**

DSM-V criteria for conversion disorder (functional neurological symptom disorder):

- One or more symptoms of altered voluntary motor or sensory function
- Clinical findings provide evidence of incompatibility between the symptom and recognized neurological or medical conditions
- Symptom or deficit is not better explained by another medical or mental disorder
- Symptom or deficit causes clinically significant distress or impairment in social, occupational, or other important areas of functioning or warrants medical evaluation

and acceptable name of FND rather than conversion disorder and now neurologists are actively involved in the management.

The name itself emphasizes it is neurological rather than psychological.

It is no longer dependent on ruling out, but on finding "positive" or rule-in signs. It is no longer mandatory to rule out factitious disorders and malingering nor to demonstrate a linked psychological factor.

Now neurologists can make the diagnosis like they do for any other category of neurological illness, by finding certain "positive" signs. Patients also accept the diagnosis more readily due to the removal of the stigma, realizing the positive signs, and the comfort and confidence of the doctor in making the diagnosis. There is transparency and no longer any sense of being tricked. This has generated tremendous clinical interest and spurred research and is expected to improve management strategies and the uniformly poor prognosis.

ROLE OF NEUROLOGISTS IN FUNCTIONAL NEUROLOGICAL DISORDERS

A patient with FND has neurological symptoms and so presents to general medicine and neurology and not to psychiatrists. It is disconcerting for them to get abruptly handed over to psychiatrists for management, without understanding what and why. Neurologists have crucial responsibilities in the management of FND, apart from diagnosis. They are better placed than anyone else to diagnose and look for mimics and using the new diagnostic criteria, they can make the diagnosis much more confidently, without worrying about misdiagnosis and asking for unnecessary tests. They are also in a unique position to correct fundamental misconceptions about diagnosis and mechanisms, offer simple tips for rehabilitation, and facilitate further management by mental health professionals or physical therapists.

Their next important task is to properly convey the diagnosis and explain the rationale behind making it. It is important to reassure the patient that there is no dangerous disorder such as a stroke, multiple sclerosis (MS), or a tumor, but their focus should be on what it is rather than only on what it is not. Getting the patient and the family to understand and accept the diagnosis is crucial. Sometimes this itself can be enough to solve the problem, but at the least, it sets the stage for acceptance of physical therapy and psychological intervention. Neurologists should learn basic skills in psychological evaluation and handling, so they feel comfortable in this step. Rather than banish the patient to mental health professionals, the neurologist must remain connected, call for follow-up, detect any new neurological symptoms or signs, and ascertain improvement.

EPIDEMIOLOGY

Functional neurological disorder commonly affects adults between ages 35 and 50 years but can afflict even children and the elderly. Around 60–75% of patients are female.

Up to one-third of patients attending neurology clinics have unexplained symptoms. FND may account for 1 in 10 to 1 in 20 of all neurological presentations and is the second most common reason for new neurology consultations. Patients may present in various settings including emergency settings, stroke, and rehabilitation services.[1,5] Psychologic comorbidity is seen in up to 50%, with anxiety at around 40% and depression between 20 and 40%.[1]

Various risk factors have been described, predisposing, triggering, or perpetuating. Some predisposing factors are female sex and young age, emotional and personality disorders, and adverse childhood events. Though no longer mandatory for making the diagnosis, stressors may be precipitating factors as can injury, illness, and surgery, especially in sudden-onset cases. Perpetuating factors may be biologic, psychologic like abnormal illness beliefs, and social like secondary gain.[1]

Medical and neurological diseases are risk factors for developing FND. Though the diagnostic criterion requires that "the symptom or deficit is not better explained by another medical or mental (health) disorder," up to 1 in 10 cases of definite FND can have an underlying medical or neurological disorder. More than one in six persons with neurological disease may have superadded FND, for example, functional seizures in cases of epilepsy or disability in a person with MS.[5]

PATHOPHYSIOLOGY

The focus has shifted to brain dysfunction and so in a way, it has been sent back to neurologists.[1] We now know that our perceptions do not only depend on "what is out there" but to a great extent on what the brain predicts or expects. This may explain phenomena such as excessive suggestibility, and "tunnel vision" (because that is what the brain expects to "see").

It is now hypothesized that FND occurs due to imbalance, hypofunction, or over function in various brain networks, leading to various combinations of dysfunction in emotion processing, sense of agency, attention, interception, and predictive processing/inference.

These circuits and predictions can be affected by various factors, including genetics, early life events, and sociocultural beliefs.[6] Various neuroimaging studies, including positron emission tomography (PET) and functional magnetic resonance imaging (fMRI), have shown consistent abnormal activation patterns in various above brain networks and circuits, suggesting genuine brain dysfunction.[7]

- Altered sense of agency, whereby the person no longer feels in control of a movement, may be related to the temporoparietal junction (TPJ)-based circuit.
- Impaired or excessive emotional responses and heightened arousal may be explained by abnormalities in the salience and limbic circuits.[8]
- Abnormal attention may be attributed to the frontoparietal circuits.
- Abnormal interception may lead to an improper assessment of what is happening inside the body, causing abnormal predictions and self-regulatory actions.

DIAGNOSIS OF FUNCTIONAL NEUROLOGICAL DISORDER

Let us reiterate that now the DSM-V criteria have made diagnosis easier for neurologists by demonstrating typical positive signs and no longer just because it seems bizarre, unexplained, no other diagnosis is found, tests are abnormal, or there is some old or new psychosocial stressor.

A good history can alert you to the possibility, but only an examination can confirm the diagnosis. Appropriate targeted investigations have an important role. Adequate time is needed, probably at least 30 minutes for a new patient. Multiple somatic symptoms and disorders, such as chronic pain, fatigue, and memory symptoms, are common accompaniments and can raise suspicion of FND. In many patients, these symptoms determine the quality of life more than motor or sensory symptoms.[5]

History Taking in Functional Neurological Disorder: Some Guidelines

- Ask the patient to enumerate all their important symptoms without too much interruption. Ask specifically about motor and sensory symptoms, fatigue, pain, sleep, concentration, or memory issues.
- Ask them to describe a typical day to understand real disability and subtly uncover any anxiety or depression.
- Ascertain onset, duration and progress, any triggers.
- Abrupt onset, fluctuations of the motor symptom, comorbid pain, and fatigue predict functional movement disorders (FMDs).[9]
- Ask what they think might be wrong, how their experience has been with earlier doctors, and what they expect from you. Ask about earlier encounters with doctors and allow them to vent and explain what went wrong.
- Prior history of psychiatric illness should not be used to make a diagnosis, but to be kept in mind for management later.
- Do not ask questions about depression, anxiety, stress, or abuse too early. Explicitly exploring past traumatic life events may be considered an intrusion and cause distress. It should be done with sensitivity at a pace that is suitable to the patient, often best at follow-up visits.

The examination is the only way to make a diagnosis by finding positive signs. The neurological assessment is a very important part of the treatment, with opportunities for education, treatment, and rapport building at each step of history taking, examination, and finally when delivering the diagnosis and formulating a plan of action.

- As you examine, explain what you are doing and what you find to show transparency and inspire confidence.
- Thorough general and neurological examinations are needed to show the patient that symptoms are being taken seriously and alternative or underlying disorders are not missed.
- Diagnosis is now rule-in with various positive signs. Finding incongruency with the known pathophysiological disease needs specific expertise in neurological examination, particularly FND. One also tries to show inconsistency or unexplained fluctuations, either randomly with time or with distraction. Excessive demonstration of effort when trying to follow the examiner's instructions may also support the diagnosis.
- At the bedside, the clinical neurological examination will show how distraction is an important component of proving FND. For example, in this patient with a complaint of imbalance and dizziness, the Romberg test is positive initially **(Video 1)**. When he is distracted by asking him to do some other hand movement, even with his eyes closed, he stops losing balance and Romberg's test turns negative **(Video 2)**.
- Several signs have been described and validated, in the different types of FND, which we shall see subsequently.

Investigations[5]

- Certain routine blood tests and other investigations for common disorders are needed because of the diagnostic uncertainty and to look for comorbid neurological disease.
- It can be helpful to inform that the tests are expected to be normal or may show minor incidental abnormalities. They should not feel that the diagnosis is made after the test results are negative. Incidental abnormal findings may be found in one in six patients and should not detract from the diagnosis and lead to inappropriate treatment.

- Tests should be completed before starting therapy so that doubts do not linger.
- Investigations should be targeted and not overdone out of fear of missing a diagnosis.
- Diagnosis should not be based solely on negative investigations for other conditions.
- FND should not be ruled out, if the tests do show some incidental findings or even other disorders, such as epilepsy or MS.
- Certain tests are diagnostic such as video electroencephalogram (VEEG) for functional seizures or electrophysiology in FMDs.

Missing the Diagnosis

- Certain bizarre symptoms, such as gaits or movement disorders, need expertise. When suspected, the patient should be referred to a specialist to avoid errors.
- Neurologists often are afraid of overdiagnosis of FND, but it has been found that their diagnosis holds over time; misdiagnosis is less than 1-4% like any other cause of limb weakness.[10] On the other hand, missing FND and diagnosing it as some neurological disorder may harm by unnecessary, invasive, or dangerous treatment, apart from psychological and socioeconomic costs.[11]
- New symptoms in a known FND must be evaluated on their own merit, as FND can have relapses and remissions, as well as an unrelated new disorder.

Points to Keep in Mind to Prevent Missing the Diagnosis

- Patient can be old, male, look normal, or be intelligent.
- It can happen for the first time, without any history of functional symptoms.
- Stressors may not be present in one-third of patients.
- Injury or illness may trigger.
- Having an organic illness is a risk factor for FND.
- Rather than accepting another's diagnosis evaluate for yourself.
- Abnormal magnetic resonance imaging (MRI) or tests can be unrelated or incidental.
- Missing a diagnosis is harmful too, so do not worry only about overdiagnosing FND.

Avoiding Overdiagnosis

- Do not get carried away by obvious psychosocial factors but base diagnosis on positive signs. Psychosis or schizophrenics do not usually present with FND.
- Organic illness is more likely if the patient attributes the symptoms to stress or presents with a new-onset mood or behavioral change.
- Positive signs are needed for diagnosis, not just unusual or unexplained signs or normal tests and MRIs.
- Remember that "la belle indifference" is seen as often in organic diseases, and degenerative diseases might initially present with vague symptoms and no signs. **Video 3** shows an example of la belle indifference in a lady who is smiling even while describing her 6-month facial twitching.

How to Tell the Patient?

Unlike many other diagnoses in neurology, the diagnosis of FND must be conveyed carefully and sensitively because it is not well known and there has been a lot of stigma and wrong concepts, for example, not real, especially since not seen on any scan or test. Successful treatment needs the active acceptance and participation of the patient, and so breaking the diagnosis and explaining it properly is a crucial first step and opportunity in the treatment. The doctor must not hold a false brain-mind dichotomy, be aware that faking illness is rare, know how to make the diagnosis accurately by rule-in signs, not worry unduly about missing or liability and respect the symptoms, given enough time and be sensitive, and have basic training in handling psychological issues.

The doctor should anticipate that patients will often be skeptical, as they have often never heard of the disorder; may not like the diagnosis or the implications; may have had a traumatic experience with earlier doctors, being made fun of, blamed, or shamed or disrespected; may not realize how important psychological factors are; and may feel that the diagnosis is based on some psychological issue just because nothing else is found, or else they may be emotionally attached to the earlier diagnosis. One must remember that just getting a diagnosis finally is often a relief for the patient, and honest, transparent, and sincere communication helps. It is imperative to make sure that the family also understands that the symptoms and the illness are real, and do not harbor false brain-mind dichotomy and also educate them about FND. **Box 2** gives the steps in conveying the diagnosis.

TREATMENT

There are many treatment options, tailored to the specific patient and the symptom. For treatment to be successful, it must be rehabilitative, with the active cooperation and participation of the patient. Proper communication of the diagnosis and explanation sets the stage for all further management. Sometimes a good explanation and acceptance combined with simple lifestyle changes can suffice as treatment and bring about results like a simple cognitive behavioral therapy (CBT).

In the majority, further multidisciplinary treatment is required. Neurologists must remain in the picture, not let the patient feel abandoned, and make sure that the patient recovers and does not turn out to have another

BOX 2 Steps in conveying the diagnosis.

1. Take out time. Do not rush
2. Make sure that the patient feels listened to, and properly understood
3. Validate the symptoms, tell them that you know they are genuine and common
4. Use respectful language, and functional is preferred over older terms such as hysteria or psychogenic or "medically unexplained"
5. Believe and convey that you believe in the patient
6. Explain the diagnosis like any other neurological diagnosis
7. Give a clear and confident diagnosis not just "nothing wrong" or "good news, all the tests are normal"
8. Focus on what they have but do reassure about what they do not have
9. Tell them why you are making the diagnosis and explain the significance of the positive signs
10. Explain why magnetic resonance imaging (MRI) and tests are normal
11. Focus on what and not why
12. Emphasize the potential for improvement seen even during the examination
13. Use metaphors, for example, software hardware problem and overactive alternate pathways
14. Encourage and optimize functioning over excessive "rest"
15. Provide information, for example, handouts and websites
16. Explain the role of psychotherapy, physiotherapy, and drugs
17. Fix up follow-up visit and do not abandon them

disorder or develop another disorder on follow-up. They must take the primary responsibility for these patients like gastroenterologists take for their functional disorder patients, calling on members of a multidisciplinary team to help as and when needed.

Physical therapy can be a first-line treatment for patients with motor FND. It needs to be optimized and personalized. Important components of the physical therapy include education, creating a positive expectation of improvement, open and consistent communication between the multidisciplinary team and the patient, encouraging early weight bearing, avoiding the use of adaptive equipment where possible, psychological information, and paying attention to unhelpful thoughts and behaviors.

Psychological treatments, including psychoeducation, CBT, and hypnosis, have been used. The role of placebo is controversial. Transcutaneous magnetic stimulation or TMS can also been postulated to help, possibly by disrupting and altering various dysfunctional or over-functioning brain circuits. Sedation may have a role. Antidepressants such as selective serotonin reuptake inhibitors (SSRIs) and serotonin and norepinephrine reuptake inhibitors (SNRIs) do not help FND directly but are often used to manage frequent concurrent anxiety or depression. Inpatient therapy may be needed for selected patients.

PROGNOSIS

The prognosis has not been good till now, but hopefully, more awareness among doctors, patients, and society implementing new approaches to management is expected to improve the prognosis. It has been one of the most common causes of serious long-term neurological disability and on long-term follow-up, 80% of patients remained with symptoms and disability, poor quality of life, and working status.[10] The long duration of symptoms was the most distinct negative predictor. Early diagnosis and young age seem to predict good outcomes.[12]

We now briefly review some of the common subtypes of FND, including FMDs, functional gait disorders (FGDs), functional motor paralysis, functional seizures, functional coma, functional cognitive disorder (FCD), functional dizziness or persistent postural perceptual dizziness (PPPD), functional hearing loss, sensory loss, visual disorders, functional eye movement disorders, functional speech, and voice disorders.

FUNCTIONAL MOVEMENT DISORDERS

Functional movement disorders are a subset of FND, which present with a disorder of movement, such as tremor, dystonia, myoclonus, tics, or gait disorders not fitting the patterns of known movement disorders. FMDs can be considered when the onset is abrupt or there are unexplained fluctuations, comorbid pain, or fatigue.[13] Positive signs are based on variability, distractibility, inconsistency, incongruency, and suggestibility. Sometimes electrophysiologic testing, for example, tremor, can help in diagnosis. Management hinges on education with the help of positive signs, and multidisciplinary treatment particularly physical therapy and less on drugs. Proper communication of the diagnosis and psychoeducation followed by CBT or physical rehabilitation using motor retraining, adding visual feedback or biofeedback can help in a multidisciplinary approach.

Psychogenic Tremor[14]

Psychogenic tremor is the most common FMD, accounting for up to 50% of patients. It may be suspected if the tremor is sudden in onset; has unexplained remissions; is precipitated by some trauma; shows unusual combinations of rest, postural, and kinetic tremors; or shows variability in severity, frequency, direction, or location. Positive signs are changing frequency or direction, entrainment (on asking the person to tap the contralateral limb voluntarily, the frequency of the tremor adapts to that frequency), and "whack-a-mole" sign (suppressing the tremor causes it to shift to another site). This can be seen in **Video 4**, with a changing location of the tremor. **Video 5** shows attenuation of a tremor in the left hand when the patient is asked to do some task with the right hand.

Psychogenic Dystonia[15]

Psychogenic dystonia is the second most common FMD, with a prevalence up to 47%. It can be fixed, mobile, or paroxysmal. The suspicion is raised by sudden onset of fixed dystonia, early local pain, and history of peripheral trauma or if there are unexplained variations, fluctuations, remissions, and relapses. Pain is particularly common in fixed ones. Unilateral fixed dystonia is the most common pattern, with distal affection, the foot more often than the hand. Various positive signs have been described, depending on the area affected, such as isolated lower facial spasm or pulling of the lip, flexion of digits three-to-five with sparing of pincer function, and foot inversion with plantar and toe flexion. **Video 6** shows functional oromandibular dystonia induced by a suggestion by the physician with the help of a tuning fork.

Psychogenic Parkinsonism[16]

Psychogenic parkinsonism accounts for 3–5% of all FMDs and less than 1.5% of all cases of parkinsonism. It should be suspected when it begins suddenly, remains stable, and shows a poor response to dopaminergic therapy. Various positive signs are distractibility, entrainment of tremor, oppositional stiffness without cogwheel rigidity, and slow movements but no reduced amplitude, unlike bradykinesia. If the diagnosis remains in doubt, a TRODAT scan can be helpful.

Functional Jerky Movements or Myoclonus

This common disorder is typically acute and paroxysmal. Axial jerks are more likely than limb jerks in functional cases. Sometimes one can document distractibility, inconsistency, entrainment, or variability, but since the jerks are intermittent, this may not always be possible.

Facial Functional Movement Disorder[17]

Facial FMD is more common than previously thought, either unilateral or bilateral and affects the upper face, lower face, or both. Some "positive" signs based on inconsistency and incongruity are the lack of Babinski sign **(Figs. 1A to C)**, tonic contractions > 3 seconds, bilateral or alternating hemifacial spasm, isolated lower face spasm, or lower lip pulling (see isolated lower face pulling in **Video 7**).

Functional Gait Disorders[18]

Functional gait disorders are very common, seen either in isolation or along with other FMDs. Various components of gait may be affected, including equilibrium and locomotion. Patients may show difficulty in bearing weight despite not having any motor deficit when tested in bed. Other pointers are excessive slowness or effort when walking, intermittent buckling at the knees, lurching without falling, and magnet-like attraction to the adjacent walls. Accordingly, various patterns have been described such as hesitant or slow gait, astasia-abasia, knee buckling, wide-based gait, limping, bouncing, scissoring, and lower limb dystonia. Positive signs show inconsistent, incongruent, or variable patterns, such as the "huffing and puffing" sign (excessive demonstration of effort during gait out of proportion to clinical examination), dragging the leg like a stick, excessive slowness, extremely hesitant and cautious gait, noneconomic postures which demonstrate good balance or strength, sudden knee buckling, and ability to propel a chair with wheels unexpectedly well. **Video 8** shows an example of astasia-abasia, where the person complaining of imbalance shows exquisite balance, despite swaying wildly. **Video 9** shows a child with a magnetic gait, swaying toward the wall whether he walks away or toward it, thus swaying once to the right and once to the left. **Videos 10 and 11** show the patient walking as if dragging the weak leg like a stick. **Video 12** shows a jerky gait and stance with the movement changing when lying

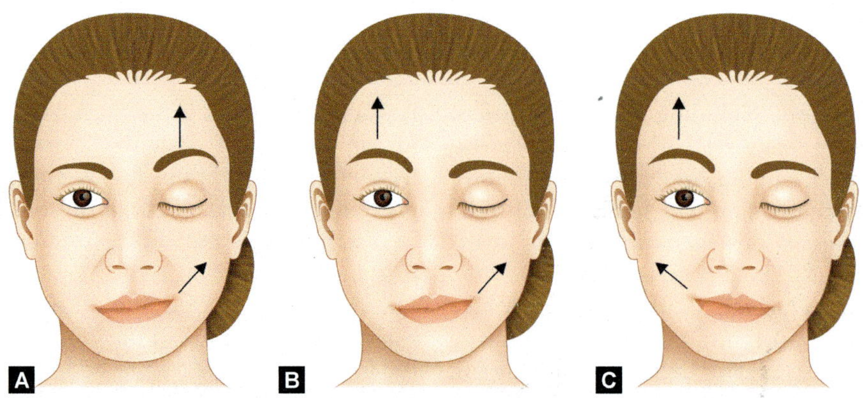

FIGS. 1A TO C: (A) True hemifacial spasm shows elevation of the frontalis on the same side as the orbicularis oculi (Babinski's "other" sign); (B and C) Functional movement disorder (FMD) may show the eyebrow rising contralateral to the closing eye.

in bed like whack-a-mole sign again. **Video 13** shows a peculiar gait, with noneconomic postures and good balance. **Video 14** shows a combined astasia-abasia with wild flinging and sudden giving way at the knee. **Video 15** shows a girl with unexplained sudden falls, but one can see her check out the area before falling and making sure she does not get injured.

Functional Limb Weakness

Functional movement disorder which presents with weakness of one or more limbs is one of the most common presentations of FND. The typical age of onset is between 30 and 40 years, and they are more common in women. The onset may be sudden or gradual, and it may involve one side of the body or less often a single limb or both lower limbs. It may be mild or severe, and the complaint may therefore be a heaviness in a limb, dropping objects from the hand, dragging or buckling of an affected leg. Functional weakness or inability to move facial muscles is extremely rare.[17] The affected limb almost always shows reduced sensation and may have pain. There may be some triggers such as an injury or surgery. One must look for an underlying neurological disorder, since they confer a high risk of FND, in general.[1]

The history may arouse suspicion, but the diagnosis must be made by positive motor signs such as distractibility, variability, inconsistencies, or unusual patterns of weakness, not consistent with known neurological disorders. Many such validated positive signs have been described. Most show high specificity (80–100%) but not all are sensitive.[13] These are listed below:

- *Discordance/inconsistency of limb weakness*: A movement cannot be done, but the same muscle can be used later in another movement. Movement is seen in the paralyzed limb, for example, when trying to wear clothes or being able to stand on tiptoes, but not able to flex the foot in bed **(Fig. 2)**.
- Expressions of disproportionate effort when attempting the movement.

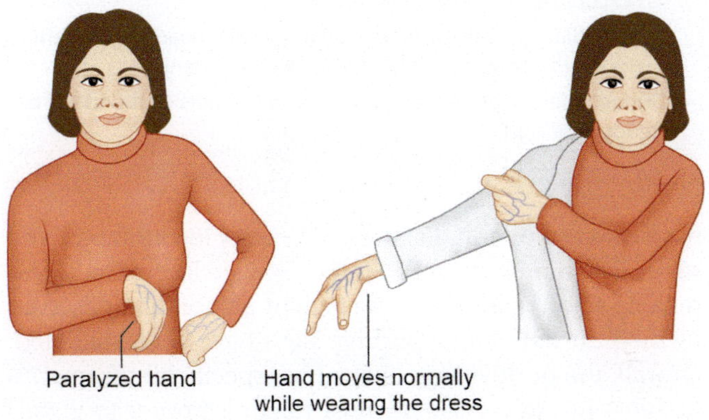

FIG. 2: The paralyzed upper limb might show movement when dressing, when attention is diverted.

- Global pattern of weakness in a limb with an equal affection of all muscle groups, unlike upper motor neuron weakness or weakness in the territory of a nerve
- *Give-way weakness*: The force exerted by the patient suddenly seems to give way with initial or intermittent good force.
- *Sternocleidomastoid test*: Rotation of the head is weak, typically to the affected side.
- *Tests for leg weakness*:
    - *Hoover's sign*: The hip extension is often weak in functional limb weakness when the person is asked to extend the hip in bed. But when one flexes a hip against resistance, the contralateral hip is involuntarily extended, so one can detect hip extension in the affected leg when asking the person to focus on flexing the other limb, while placing a hand below the affected limb to detect extension **(Fig. 3)**.
    - *Hip abductor sign*: It is like Hoover's sign, but here we look for abduction when the person is attempting contralateral hip abduction against resistance **(Fig. 4)**.

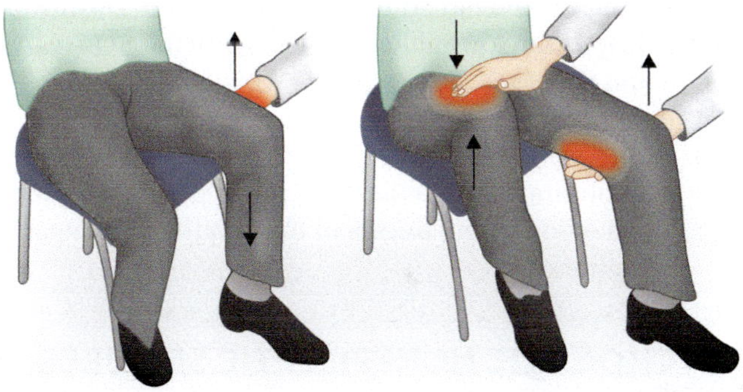

FIG. 3: Hoover's sign: Hip extension is weak when tested directly (left), but becomes normal when the patient is asked to do contralateral hip flexion against resistance (right).

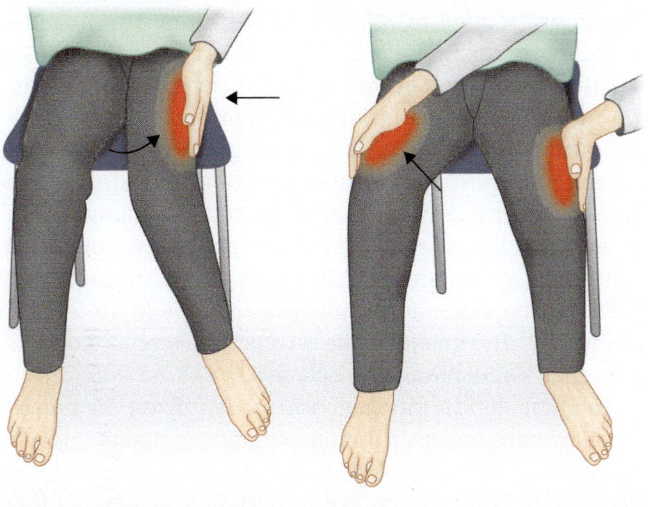

FIG. 4: Hip abductor sign: Left hip abduction is weak when tested directly (right), but seems normal when the person is asked to abduct the right hip against resistance (left).

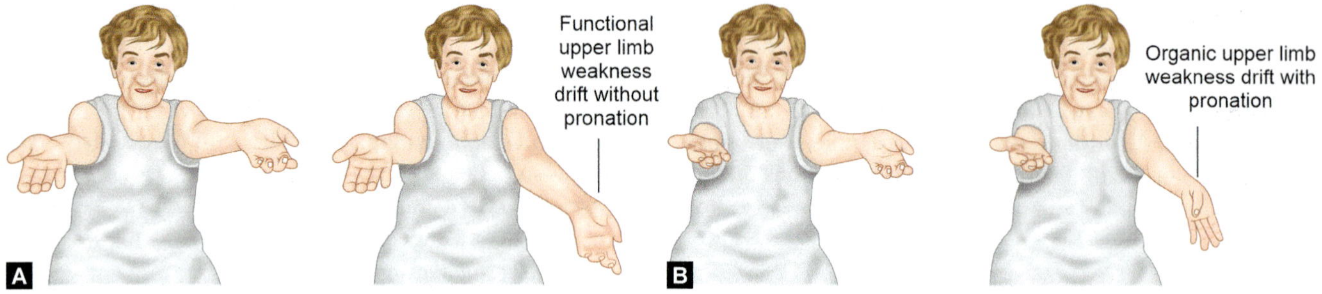

FIGS. 5A AND B: (A) Pronator drift in an outstretched weak left upper limb due to a stroke. Note how the hand pronates as it drifts down. (B) Drift without pronation in a case of functional left upper limb weakness.

- Dragging of monoplegic leg like a piece of wood without circumduction **(Videos 10 and 11)**.
- Sudden buckling of knee, often with each step **(Video 14)**.
- *Tests for upper limb weakness*:
  - Delayed, slow, or jerky descent when the clinician positions the outstretched arm in front of the patient and then releases it.
  - *Drift without pronation sign*: With eyes closed the arms are stretched out and palms face upward. Downward drift without pronation suggests functional **(Figs. 5A and B)**.
  - *Abductor finger sign in severe unilateral hand weakness*: Fifth finger in the weak hand shows involuntary abduction when the patient attempts abduction of the fingers of the healthy hand against resistance.

PSYCHOGENIC NONEPILEPTIC SEIZURES

Functional seizures are paroxysmal attacks that mimic a seizure (change in responsiveness, abnormal movement, and/or behavior). However, these events are not the result of abnormal electrical discharges in the brain and instead are related to psychological factors. Psychogenic nonepileptic seizure (PNES) has been reported in 5–15% of patients who are referred to outpatient epilepsy centers, and the number goes up to 25–40% of patients evaluated for intractable epilepsy. It is among the most frequent nonepileptic paroxysmal manifestations in adolescents but may occur at any age including children younger than 10 years and the elderly.[19] Like other FNDs, it occurs more commonly in females.[20,21] It needs to be stressed that PNES can be associated with true seizures in 10–20% of patients.[22,21] The quality of life is consistently reported to be lower than populations with epilepsy.[13]

The first step in the diagnosis is identifying the paroxysmal event as epileptic or nonepileptic. As it rarely occurs before the doctor, one must mainly rely on history, witness accounts, or home videos. It is important to remember that no single feature is pathognomonic for PNES, but multiple ones make it more likely. Like with many of the FNDs, this has become a rule-in diagnosis.[13] Urinary incontinence and self-injury can occur in PNES too. Tongue laceration is less reliable when reported by the patient, rather than observed by medical staff. Some positive signs have been validated. Overall, the positive signs have high specificities from 77% to 100% but lower sensitivities ranging from 9 to 96%.[13] These are listed below **(Box 3)**.

BOX 3 Validated positive signs for functional seizures.

General signs:
- Duration > 2 minutes
- Waxing and waning/fluctuating course

Clues that the patient has preserved awareness during attack:
- Able to recall the event later
- Able to repeat a phrase or name an object told during attack
- Others can alleviate or intensify the attack
- Eyes respond to environment and stimuli specificity
- Able to respond
- Generalized shaking without loss of consciousness
- *Motor behavior:*
  - Eyes are closed or resist attempted opening or eyelids flutter during the seizure
  - Asynchronous limb movements
  - Pelvis thrusting
  - Side-to-side head movements
  - Arching back
  - Rotation in bed
- *Accompanying behavior during the attack:*
  - Crying
  - Whispering
  - Stuttering
  - Hyperventilation throughout an attack
- *Postictal behavior:*
  - Irregular, rapid, and shallow breathing and not snoring
  - Immediate recovery
  - No confusion or disorientation
  - Immediately after the attack, blinks or brief head shaking after the event, looks around, and asks "what happened"
- During video electroencephalogram (VEEG) gets a stuffed toy or "teddy bear sign"

Video 16 shows a girl with functional seizures, showing closed eyes, resisting eye-opening, and also the abrupt termination of the attack with immediate recovery and no postictal confusion. **Video 17** shows suggestibility during the attack with asynchronous limb movements and responding during the attack. **Video 18** again shows the ability to induce attack by suggestion, asynchronous limb movement, arching back, and immediate recovery on suggestion.

On the other hand, some signs are suggestive of epilepsy. These are VEEG attack arising in sleep, epileptic cry, lateral tongue bite, bodily injury, and postictal Babinski sign within 5 minutes. Keeping both these aspects in mind, the International League Against Epilepsy (ILAE) has developed criteria for the diagnosis of PNES[23] which are as follows **(Table 1)**.

The only blood test that may be a useful adjunct is a raised prolactin level done within 10–20 minutes of the ictus suggesting a generalized tonic-clonic seizure (GTC). But it can be normal in focal seizures or if done late and therefore the practical value is reduced. Proper communication of the diagnosis is occasionally enough to ameliorate or stop the attacks. Everyone should be reassured that the events are not usually dangerous and do not need to be urgently taken to the emergency department.[22] A multidisciplinary approach with mental health professionals is the key. Many patients have early warning symptoms, at which time they should move or be moved to a safe place with minimal stimulation. The patient can be taught to calm themselves by deep breathing. Everyone else should be told to remain calm and allow the patient to calm themselves without distractions.[22] The next step is psychological counseling, in particular CBT. Drugs are not effective unless there are comorbid mood or anxiety disorders. The neurologist should remain actively involved and carefully withdraw antiseizure medications (ASMs) while monitoring the outcome and watching for any new symptoms or epileptic seizures.

TABLE 1: ILAE-proposed diagnostic levels of certainty for PNES.

Diagnostic level	History	Witnessed event	EEG
Possible	+	Patient/witness	Normal routine EEG
Probable	+	Clinician sees attack/ video	Normal routine EEG
Clinically established	+	Attack/video when not on EEG, seen by a clinician experienced in seizure semiology	Ictal EEG normal during the attack
Documented	+	Attack/video when on VEEG, seen by a clinician experienced in seizure semiology	Normal immediately before, during, or after ictus on ictal VEEG

(EEG: electroencephalogram; ILAE: International League Against Epilepsy; PNES: psychogenic nonepileptic seizure; VEEG: video electroencephalogram)

FUNCTIONAL COMA

Functional coma can be defined by some as an involuntary coma-like state that occurs in the absence of structural lesions or metabolic damage to the brain while showing evidence of normal waking brain activity during this state.[24,25] It is a relatively rare type of FND, representing less than 0.5% of coma. Males and females are equally affected. In some patients, the attack occurs after a trauma or after some surgery. There is usually some associated or underlying psychiatric disorder. Functional coma recovers usually between an hour and 4 days. It is distinct from catatonia and functional seizures. Catatonia may have characteristic motor signs, rarely recovers spontaneously, often has abnormal vital signs, and typically has underlying psychiatric or medical conditions. Functional seizures tend to repeat and are brief (less than 30 minutes) with a different semiology.[24]

Functional coma shows normal vital signs and normal pupillary and corneal reflexes. Patients may resist eye-opening, show spontaneous flickering, fluttering, or blinking of the eyelids or purposeful eye movements, uprolling of eyes on attempted eye-opening. Doll's eye examination is usually suppressed, while caloric testing shows normal oculovestibular reflex. Decerebrate or decorticate posturing is unusual. Applying noxious stimuli is not very reliable and doing it repeatedly is unethical. Positive signs demonstrate the inconsistency between an apparent comatose state and normal nervous system functioning, for example:

- *Eye gaze sign*: The patient's eyes are observed while turning him from one side to the other and eyes deviate down; when the patient is turned to the other side, the eyes deviate down to the other side.
- *Tightly shut eyelids*: The patient actively resists the examiner's attempts to open the closed eyelids and usually closes the eyelids rapidly as soon as they are released.
- *Bell's phenomenon*: During attempts to open the closed eyelid, the eyes roll up.
- *Harvey's sign*: The patient reacts to the adverse but harmless stimulus of a high-frequency tuning fork (440–1,024 Hz) applied to the mucosa of the nasal septum.
- *Hand drop test*: When the hand is lifted by the examiner and allowed to fall back, it does not fall limply on the face; either the hand falls on the side to prevent self-injury or more reliably, the rate of fall slows down.

It is essential that all structural and metabolic causes of coma need to be excluded, but it is important to consider and look for functional coma at an early stage to avoid unnecessary investigations and interventions. Investigations including laboratory tests, computed tomography (CT) scan, MRI brain, and electroencephalogram (EEG) should be normal, with certain exceptions. Supportive measures should be started until the inevitable recovery from the functional coma. There is no specific treatment, though sometimes it reverses with barbiturates or benzodiazepines.

FUNCTIONAL COGNITIVE DISORDER

Functional cognitive disorder is a subtype of FND, in which cognitive symptoms are present, associated with distress or disability, but caused by functional alterations rather than degenerative brain disease or another structural lesion.[26]

An increasing number of patients seek help for a self-experienced decline in cognitive capacity, but do not have any impairment when tested objectively. This condition is called SCD or subjective cognitive impairment.[27] It had been assumed that over time SCDs would develop measurable cognitive impairment and qualify to be called MCI or minimal cognitive impairment and later they would develop frank dementia. But, in fact, the majority stabilize and even improve **(Fig. 6)**.[26] FCD is believed to be the cause of many such SCD cases and may account for 12–56% of new referrals in memory clinics.[27,28] It is important to recognize these patients as they are at risk of harm due to drugs or wrong prediction of progressive worsening.[26]

The typical age at onset of FCD is midlife (overlapping with early onset dementia). It presents mainly with memory impairment, often with difficulty in attention and concentration, and usually does not affect functions such as praxis, language, or executive function.[28] The pointers toward the diagnosis of FCD are mentioned below **(Box 4)**.

It can be fallacious to diagnose based on the Ganser syndrome or the tendency to give "approximate answers" as these can be difficult to distinguish from wrong answers.[28] Diagnostic criteria emphasize inconsistency between observed and measured cognitive functions or show variation from time to time. What the patient reports seems out of proportion to what is reported at other times or what is evident during the interview. The inconsistency should be in the same cognitive domain, as inconsistency can be seen across different domains in various brain disorders, for example, selective deficits in visual comprehension or language in certain types of dementia.[28] Detailed neuropsychological testing can also demonstrate inconsistency, for example, delayed recall is better than the immediate.[28] The subjective cognitive difficulties seen in FCD are very similar to those seen in fibromyalgia, chronic fatigue syndrome, and other FNDs where they are described as "brain fog." Possibly pain, fatigue, and excessive inward attention lead to reduced external attention, impaired cognitive function, especially multitasking, and a feeling of undue effort in doing these tasks.[29]

FUNCTIONAL DIZZINESS OR PERSISTENT POSTURAL PERCEPTUAL DIZZINESS

Functional vestibular disorders are a subtype of FND, which present with dizziness. The main cause is a disorder termed PPPD. It is a positive diagnosis and not one of exclusion, given for unexplained chronic vestibular symptoms. The detailed criteria for diagnosis are given in **Box 5**.[30,31] This new term is now preferred over earlier names such as chronic subjective dizziness, phobic postural vertigo, visual vertigo, and space-motion discomfort. It may account for most chronically dizzy patients. It may comprise up to 15–20% of all patients presenting for evaluation of vestibular symptoms, ranking among the top three diagnoses with

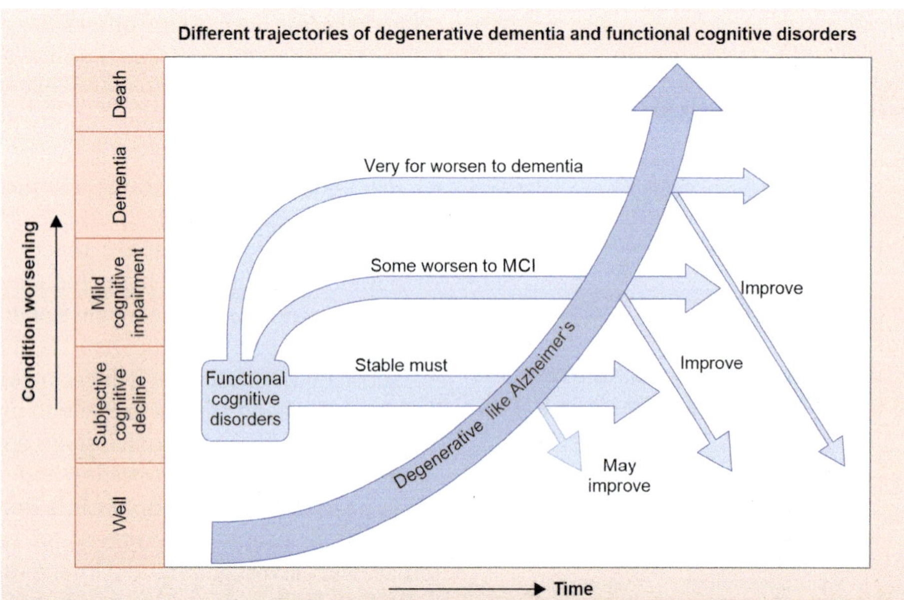

FIG. 6: Degenerative brain disease and functional cognitive disorder trajectories.

BOX 4 **Functional cognitive disorder (FCD) more likely than degenerative dementia.[26]**

Characteristics of the patient:
- Visits alone rather than with someone
- May bring along a written list of complaints
- Seems more aware and concerned than the accompanying person
- Gives even elaborate answers independently, remembers details
- Forgets recent as well as remote autobiographical memories
- Gives the exact date of onset

Characteristics of the cognitive impairment:
- Memory loss for specific periods or persons
- Cognitive impairment varies from time to time
- Cognitive impairment remains static or even improves over time

BOX 5 **Criteria for diagnosis laid down by the International Classification of Vestibular Disorders (ICVD). All five must be fulfilled.**

1. One or more symptoms of dizziness, unsteadiness, or nonspinning vertigo are present on most days for 3 months or more. They may last hours but may wax and wane
2. Persistent symptoms occur without specific provocation but are exacerbated by upright posture, active or passive motion, and exposure to moving visual stimuli or visual patterns
3. Disorder is precipitated by conditions that cause vertigo, unsteadiness, dizziness, or problems with balance including acute, episodic, or chronic vestibular syndromes, other neurologic or medical illnesses, or psychological distress
4. Symptoms cause significant distress or functional impairment
5. Symptoms are not better accounted for by another disease or disorder

benign paroxysmal positional vertigo (BPPV) and vestibular migraine. Like with other FNDs, the average age is around 40 years and females outnumber males.

It can arise de novo or often after a trigger that causes dizziness, or vertigo, or affect balance acutely, episodically, or even chronically. Some studies suggest up to 25% of BPPV; vertiginous migraine or panic disorder may have PPPD-like symptoms on follow-up.[31] The International Classification of Vestibular Disorders (ICVD) has laid down the criteria for the diagnosis which are listed below.

The mechanism seems to be changed in activity and connectivity in certain cortical networks dealing with balance and spatial orientation causing visual dependence by giving more weightage to visual input over vestibular and proprioceptive, leading to a stiffening of stance and gait. It is hypothesized that a trigger may set off these changes in a susceptible person **(Fig. 7)**.

Untreated, most continue to have symptoms, while with treatment, most do well. Treatment includes education, reassurance, CBT, vestibular rehabilitation, and sometimes a small dose of SSRI **(Fig. 7)**.[31]

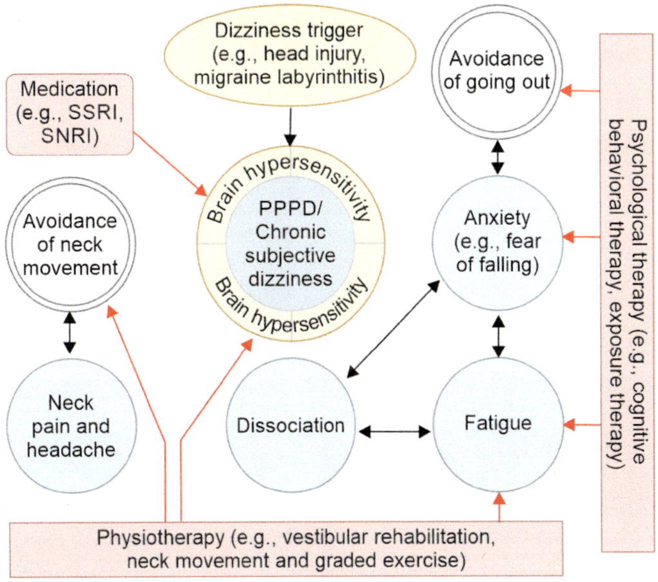

FIG. 7: Mechanism of functional dizziness.

(PPPD: persistent postural perceptual dizziness; SNRI: serotonin and norepinephrine reuptake inhibitor; SSRI: selective serotonin reuptake inhibitor)

FUNCTIONAL HEARING LOSS

The situation in which patients may behave as if they have a significant hearing loss, both in general communication and in pure-tone audiometry, is not borne out by specialized or objective testing. It tends to happen in teenagers, or individuals claiming compensation or trying to gain attention from family. When suspected, different strategies of audiometry may be helpful in confirming, for example, trying random stimuli, or stimuli at only low intensity, or at nonpredictable intervals. Objective testing of auditory brainstem responses are useful, as they are independent of patient cooperation.[1]

SENSORY LOSS

Functional sensory symptoms are those in which the patient experiences alteration or absence of normal sensation in the absence of neurologic disease. Up to one-third of patients of FND may have sensory symptoms, usually along with other symptoms.[1] Quite often patients notice the sensory impairment for the first time during the neurologic examination, possibly due to a suggestion by the physician. Sometimes it may follow an episode of functional coma or get superimposed on a neurological disorder like ulnar neuropathy.

Certain patterns of sensory loss are very suggestive of a functional disorder. The sensory loss is not anatomical and does not follow dermatomes or nerve territories **(Fig. 8)**.

The most common pattern is hemisensory, varying from a small area like the face to one side of the whole

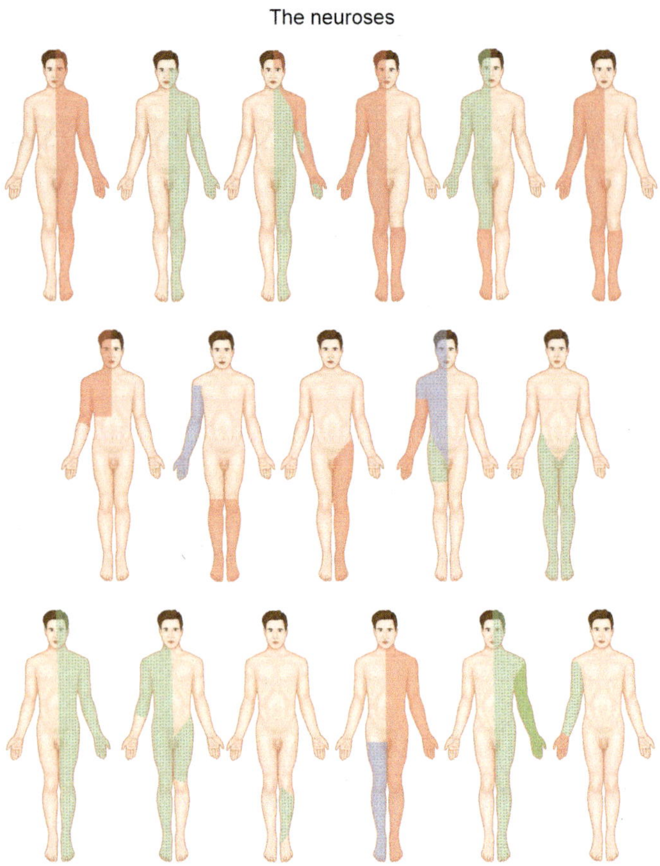

FIG. 8: Patterns of sensory loss that are suggestive of a functional disorder.

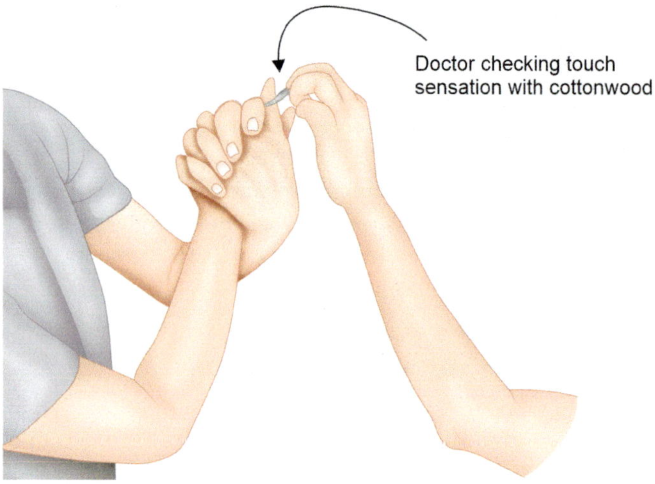

FIG. 9: Bowlus–Currier test.

body. Midline splitting of the sensory deficit is suggestive of functional sensory symptoms. More localized loss of sensations is also possible, like sock or glove sensory loss. Sensory loss may be patchy or irregular or restricted to joints or one foot or hand.

Positive signs hinge on showing internal inconsistency, variability or incongruence, or suggestibility, for example, midline splitting of sensation, midline splitting of vibration sense, nonanatomic sensory loss, inconsistent sensory loss, yes–no test, the Bowlus–Currier test **(Fig. 9)**, and sensory loss modified by suggestion. In general, the positive signs are not as reliable as those for functional limb weakness or FMD, because the sensory examination is very much subjective and prone to bias. They often do not need any specific treatment and improve if the other symptoms are treated, for example, weakness.[1]

FUNCTIONAL EYE MOVEMENT DISORDERS

There are several functional eye movement disorders. The most common one is convergence spasm but others such as convergence paralysis, gaze limitation, and voluntary nystagmus may be underreported.[1] They are infrequently the presenting symptom; it is more common to find them or elicit them in a patient coming for another functional neurologic disorder such as gait or movement disorder.[13] Patients with convergence spasm may present with intermittent blurring of vision or diplopia or squint, which corrects on temporary crinkling of the eye. If not seen initially, they can be "induced" by asking the patient to sustain an ocular contraction (>10 seconds). There may be tell-tale eyelid fluttering and effortful facial expressions during the examination. **Video 19** is a video of a girl coming for reduced vision but also showing convergence spasm.

Like with other motor types of FND, the diagnosis can often be clearly established by positive signs, such as fluctuations or inconsistency or reversibility with distraction or suggestion or by inducing other eye movements. In convergence spasm, on attempted abduction, one or both eyes may remain adducted with strong medial rectus contraction, mimicking unilateral or bilateral sixth nerve palsy. Miosis at the same time as convergence is the diagnostic sign. Sometimes the head impulse test, optokinetic nystagmus, or doll's eye maneuver can override the spasm and help in the diagnosis.

FUNCTIONAL BLINDNESS

Functional vision disorder (FVD) is the proposed new term for nonorganic visual loss and is defined as a decrease in visual acuity and/or visual field that does not have an anatomic or physiologic basis.[32] Like with other FNDs, FVD is now a rule-in diagnosis. Like with the other FNDs, around one-fourth to half of the cases have FVD superimposed onto some underlying cause of visual loss.

One still needs to look for other causes of visual loss, but now the diagnosis is a positive one and not just based on ruling out these other disorders. Some hints might be obtained right in the beginning as the patient walks in, with exaggerated movements or bumping into objects out of proportion to their visual loss, having sunglasses on inside the clinic. There may be subtle indicators of good vision, when they shake hands, have eye contact, write out forms, etc. The history may clarify onset and whether it affects one or both eyes, as well as associated symptoms. Diagnosis is essentially based on demonstrating that the person can see better than reported. This can be done by various simple tests in the clinic to show inconsistency, fluctuations, or incongruency with known diseases or laws of optics.

Monocular Vision Loss

One way is to see if vision with both eyes open is maintained, even when vision in the good eye is gradually hindered with the use of various lenses or prisms. Evaluating depth perception can help as it requires good vision in both eyes.

Binocular Vision Loss

Binocular vision loss is more common and more challenging to test. Patients with FVD may report the same visual acuity even when brought closer to the chart. The fingertip test and signature test, which depend on proprioception rather than can be used (see video and add a photo of signature of your patient, and illustration of mirror test). The mirror test looks at the patient's eye movements when a mirror is suddenly brought in front of the face and rotated. These tests are useful only in cases of severe loss. Eliciting nystagmus with an optokinetic drum, or stimulus, suggests a visual acuity of at least 20/200. **Video 20** shows preservation of both horizontal and vertical optokinetic nystagmus in a lady with blindness. The so-called "shock tests" using menace reflexes are no longer advised as the other tests are less objectionable.

Field testing, manually or automated, often shows concentric loss of peripheral vision, resulting in tunnel vision, for example, confrontation testing at 1 and 2 m. In a normal person the visual field should enlarge as the distance of testing increases, but in a person with functional blindness, it may remain the same and this is called "tunnel vision" **(Fig. 10)**.[32]

The mirror test is another objective way to prove functionality. The examiner turns a large mirror slowly back and forth in the horizontal direction, while the subject gazes at the reflected image. Both distant and near objects will appear to move with the same angular velocity, eliciting eye movements that the examiner can easily see. It is almost impossible for the subject with an intact vision to suppress the movements unless he/she can fix his/her gaze on some stationary object. Hence, the use of a large mirror fills the field of view as widely as possible. The examiner must take care to note the subject is not looking intently at some stationary object outside the margin of the reflected image **(Fig. 11)**.

Monocular blindness testing involves asking the patient to touch the tips of both his fingers with one eye at a time. While testing the affected eye, the patient might not be able to touch the tips of the fingers, which he/she will be able to do with the normal eye. **Video 21A** shows preserved ability to touch the tips to each other accurately when the bad eye is patched while the "seeing eye" is not patched. **Video 21B** shows an inability to touch the tips to each other accurately when the "seeing eye" is patched while the patient is unable to see with the left unpatched eye.

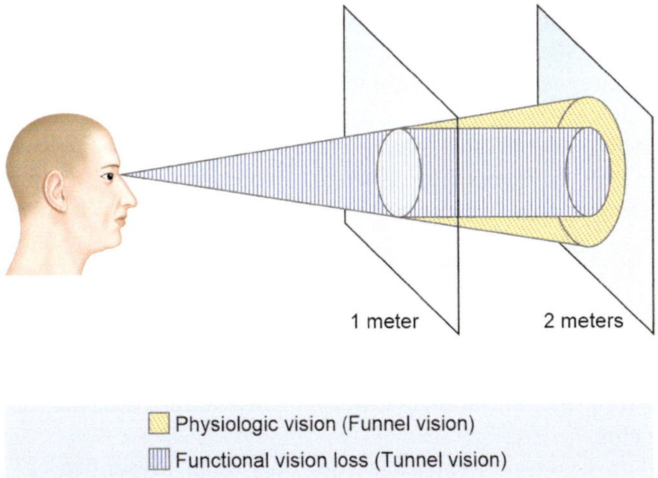

FIG. 10: Field testing.

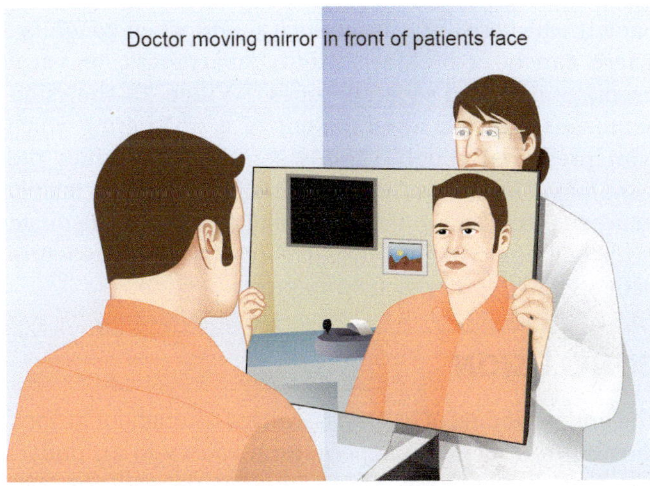

FIG. 11: Pursuit eye movements induced by moving a mirror side-to-side in front of a person with functional blindness.

Treatment

Eye movement disorders do not typically cause disability and may settle down with treatment of the presenting FND. One can treat convergence spasm symptomatically by atropine eye drops to cause temporary ciliary muscle paralysis along with reading glasses.[1]

FUNCTIONAL DISORDERS OF SPEECH AND VOICE

Functional speech and voice disorders (FSVDs) can affect any aspect of speech production but most often they present with dysphonia, stuttering, or prosodic abnormalities. They have been described in up to

25–50% of patients with FMDs. The speech patterns may demonstrate incongruity or inconsistency, distractibility, or suggestibility.[33] Functional stuttering (FS) may be differentiated from organic stuttering by the absence of dysarthria, aphasia, or apraxia of speech, excessive variability, excessive consistency, or struggle behavior while trying to speak. **Video 22** is a case of a patient with FS who then gets hyperventilation and jerking of whole body without impaired consciousness. Those with prosodic disturbances may start talking in a foreign accent or speaking like infants or children. Articulation distortions may show inconsistent lingual, jaw, or facial weakness on tasks unrelated to speech. Wrong-way deviation of the tongue in a hemiparesis may be a clue.

A functional voice disorder may often present to ear, nose, and throat (ENT) surgeons with a change in voice. There may be a sudden onset of aphonia or a whispering voice. As seen in this video of functional aphonia, the patient whispers but can produce sound when coughing. There can be a breathy falsetto, hoarseness, or vocal production of two separate tones.[34] **Video 23** shows an acute onset of the development of a whispering voice with preserved cough. Globus sensation describes the symptom of a painless "lump" or "ball" in the throat, mainly between meals and in the absence of dysphagia. Adequate investigations with the negative results could reassure patients and improve their symptoms.

CONCLUSION

The understanding of FNDs has evolved throughout history, moving from belief in supernatural causes to an understanding that they are related to networks and errors in the brain. These disorders cause significant disability and suffering, as well as a strain on resources. They have historically fallen between the jurisdiction of neurologists and psychiatrists. However, with the new criteria for diagnosis in the DSM-V, it is hoped that these disorders will be recognized as genuine neurological disorders. Neurologists must understand that these disorders are real, and not to be confused with feigned disorders. They should also be aware of the signs for making a confident diagnosis, and not do test after test to rule out nonexisting illnesses. They should also be aware of various pitfalls in over- and underdiagnosis, and learn the language of empathy and sensitivity in dealing with such patients, building rapport with the patient, and making sure the patient is with them in facing the disorder and not on the "other side." They should also know how teamwork with physiotherapists and mental health professionals can help in improving the erstwhile poor prognosis of such patients. The "dark ages" for patients with FND are over and the future looks bright for them.

VIDEO LEGENDS

Video 1: A boy with functional imbalance falls to either side when doing the Romberg test with his feet close and eyes closed.

Video 2: Now when the boy is asked to stand the same way with feet close, but instructed to focus on doing rapid alternating movements with the hands (dysdiadochokinesia), he no longer loses balance, even when his eyes are closed as in the earlier Romberg test. This shows the effect of distraction on the Romberg test.

Video 3: La belle indifference seen in a lady with focal "dystonic" movements of the left lower face.

Video 4: A man with functional tremor first affecting the whole hand. When the thumb is plugged into the ear, preventing it from moving, only the hand moves. When the thumb is removed, only the thumb moves. When the hands are placed on a pillow the hands tremble again, and finally when the feet are placed against each other they get the same tremor immediately. This is the whack-a-mole sign where movement (tremor) suppression of one body part is followed by immediate reemergence of movement (tremor) in another.

Video 5: An irregular tremor in the outstretched left hand, which slows down and almost stops when the person is asked to do tapping movements with the normal right thumb and finger.

Video 6: This video shows how suggestion using a tuning fork could induce the dystonia of the lips and jaw that the patient came for. On reminding, even her eyes close, like in her "spontaneous attacks." In the later part of the video, just pressing on the cheeks abruptly ends this dystonia.

Video 7: A lady showing functional hemifacial movements of the left face involving only the left lower face, with rhythmic movements unlike the irregular jerks of hemifacial spasm. The movements abruptly cease when she is asked to show her teeth. When she holds her hands outstretched, there emerges the tremor of the right hand on suggestion.

Video 8: A person with functional imbalance of gait demonstrates exquisite balance when doing tandem walking. The wild, flailing movements actually show excellent balance.

Video 9: A boy with functional ataxic gait suddenly veers and takes support of the wall, both when walking toward us and walking away from us and also when standing.

Video 10: A girl with functional hemiplegia dragging the right leg like a stick without circumduction, as would be expected in hemiplegic gait.

Video 11: A man with functional hemiplegia dragging the right leg very slowly like a stick without circumduction.

Video 12: This lady with shrug-like jerking of her shoulders while walking and standing later starts getting a tremor of her feet when she lies down in bed. This is also akin to whack-a-mole sign.

Video 13: A lady with a functional gait disorder shows her suddenly coming backward without losing balance, every time she takes a few steps ahead.

Video 14: A lady with a functional gait disorder shows wild swinging and swaying, as well as giving way at the knees without actually losing balance or falling.

Video 15: This girl with functional drop attacks shows how she walks quite normally, and then gets some sort of warning in her head and falls down without any injury.

Video 16: A girl with functional seizures shows a dystonic posture of the right hand, neck, face, and body as she holds her breath and keeps her eyes clenched tightly and resists opening. The attack stops suddenly when the doctor speaks to her, and she takes a breath again without any postictal confusion.

Video 17: This boy with functional seizure shows the gradual buildup of asynchronous limb and body movements. The video also demonstrates preserved consciousness as shown by him showing the tongue when asked to.

Video 18: A boy with a functional seizure, which is induced by suggestion with the use of a tuning fork. The attack shows typical asynchronous limb movements as well as arching of the back. It also shows how suggestion abruptly stops the attack, and there is no postictal confusion.

Video 19: A girl with functional loss of vision who also shows convergence spasm.

Video 20: Preserved optokinetic nystagmus in a lady who is functionally blind.

Videos 21A and B: (A) A lady able to touch her fingers to each other accurately when the "blind eye" is patched and she can see with the other one; (B) The same lady with functional blindness missing her fingers, when asked to touch both her index fingers to each other, when her seeing eye is patched. The ability to touch fingers to each other is not dependent on vision but on proprioception.

Video 22: Radio tactical shows a boy with functional voice order showing irregular stammering speech with hyperventilation and tremor of the body toward the end of the video.

Video 23: A person with an acute onset of whispering voice. He can make a sound when coughing though.

REFERENCES

1. Hallett M, Stone J, Carson AJ. Functional Neurologic Disorders, volume 139. Cambridge: Academic Press; 2016.
2. Burke MJ. "It's all in your head"—medicine's silent epidemic. JAMA Neurol. 2019;76(12):1417-8.
3. Sojka P, Paredes-Echeverri S, Perez DL. Are functional (psychogenic nonepileptic) seizures the sole expression of psychological processes? Curr Top Behav Neurosci. 2022;55:329-51.
4. Ludwig L, Pasman JA, Nicholson T, Aybek S, David AS, Tuck S, et al. Stressful life events and maltreatment in conversion (functional neurological) disorder: systematic review and meta analysis of case-control studies. Lancet Psychiatry. 2018;5(4):307-20.
5. Stone J, Burton C, Carson A. Recognizing and explaining functional neurological disorder. BMJ. 2020;371:m3745.
6. Drane DL, Fani N, Hallett M, Khalsa SS, Perez DL, Roberts NA. A framework for understanding the pathophysiology of functional neurological disorder. CNS Spectr. 2021;26(6):555-61.
7. Aybek S, Vuilleumier P. Imaging studies of functional neurologic disorders. Handb Clin Neurol. 2016;139:73-84.
8. LaFaver K, Maurer CW, Nicholson TR, Perez DL (Eds). Functional Movement Disorder. Cham: Springer International Publishing; 2022.
9. Lagrand T, Tuitert I, Klamer M, van der Meulen A, van der Palen J, Kramer G, et al. Functional or not functional; that's the question: can we predict the diagnosis functional movement disorder based on associated features? Eur J Neurol. 2021;28(1):33-9.
10. Gelauff JM, Carson A, Ludwig L, Tijssen MAJ, Stone J. The prognosis of functional limb weakness: a 14-year case-control study. Brain. 2019;142(7):2137-48.
11. Walzl D, Carson AJ, Stone J. The misdiagnosis of functional disorders as other neurological conditions. J Neurol. 2019;266(8):2018-26.
12. Gelauff J, Stone J. Prognosis of functional neurologic disorders. Handb Clin Neurol. 2016;139:523-41.
13. Aybek S, Perez DL. Diagnosis and management of functional neurological disorder. BMJ. 2022;376:o64.
14. Schwingenschuh P. Functional tremor. In: LaFaver K, Perez D (Eds). Current Clinical Neurology, 1st edition. Totowa: Humana Press Inc.; 2022. pp. 67-79.
15. Morgante F. Functional dystonia. In: LaFaver K, Perez D (Eds). Current Clinical Neurology, 1st edition. Totowa: Humana Press Inc.; 2022. pp. 81-91.
16. Akkaoui MA, Degos B, Garcin B. Functional parkinsonism. In: LaFaver K, Perez D (Eds). Current Clinical Neurology, 1st edition. Totowa: Humana Press Inc.; 2022. pp. 93-102.
17. Rohani M, Fasano A. Functional facial disorders. In: Kathrin L, Perez D (Eds). Current Clinical Neurology, 1st edition. Totowa: Humana Press Inc.; 2022. pp. 115-34.
18. Demartini B. Functional gait disorder. In: LaFaver K, Perez D (Eds). Current Clinical Neurology, 1st edition. Totowa: Humana Press Inc.; 2022. pp. 135-45.
19. Leibetseder A, Eisermann M, LaFrance WC, Nobili L, von Oertzen TJ. How to distinguish seizures from nonepileptic manifestations. Epileptic Disord. 2020;22(6):716-38.
20. Phakey N, Godara K, Garg D, Sharma S. Psychogenic nonepileptic seizures and psychosocial management: a narrative review. Ann Indian Acad Neurol. 2021;24(2):146-54.
21. Lopez MR, LaFrance WC. Treatment of psychogenic nonepileptic seizures. Curr Neurol Neurosci Rep. 2022;22(8):467-74.
22. Albert DV. Psychogenic nonepileptic seizures in children and adolescents. Semin Pediatr Neurol. 2022;41.100949.
23. Lafrance WC, Baker GA, Duncan R, Goldstein LH, Reuber M. Minimum requirements for the diagnosis of psychogenic nonepileptic seizures: a staged approach: a report from the International League Against Epilepsy Nonepileptic Seizures task force. Epilepsia. 2013;54(11):2005-18.
24. Ryznar E, Wilcox D. Functional coma: two case reports and a review of the literature. Psychosomatics. 2019;60(4):343-51.
25. Ludwig L, McWhirter L, Williams S, Derry C, Stone J. Functional coma. In: Hallett M, Stone J, Carson A (Eds). Handbook of Clinical Neurology. Amsterdam: Elsevier; 2016. pp. 313-27.
26. McWhirter L, Ritchie C, Stone J, Carson A. Functional cognitive disorders: a systematic review. Lancet Psychiatry. 2020;7(2):191-207.
27. Jessen F, Amariglio RE, Buckley RF, van der Flier WM, Han Y, Molinuevo JL, et al. The characterization of subjective cognitive decline. Lancet Neurol. 2020;19(3):271-8.
28. Ball HA, McWhirter L, Ballard C, Bhome R, Blackburn DJ, Edwards MJ, et al. Functional cognitive disorder: dementia's blind spot. Brain. 2020;143(10):2895-903.
29. Teodoro T, Edwards MJ, Isaacs JD. A unifying theory for cognitive abnormalities in functional neurological disorders, fibromyalgia, and chronic fatigue syndrome: systematic review. J Neurol Neurosurg Psychiatry. 2018;89(12):1308-19.
30. Staab JP, Eckhardt-Henn A, Horii A, Jacob R, Strupp M, Brandt T, et al. Diagnostic criteria for persistent postural-perceptual dizziness (PPPD): consensus document of the committee for the classification of vestibular disorders of the barany society. J Vestib Res. 2017;27(4):191-208.
31. Staab JP. Persistent postural-perceptual dizziness. Semin Neurol. 2020;40(1):130-7.
32. Raviskanthan S, Wendt S, Ugoh PM, Mortensen PW, Moss HE, Lee AG. Functional vision disorders in adults: a paradigm and nomenclature shift for ophthalmology. Surv Ophthalmol. 2022;67(1):8-18.
33. Duffy JR. Functional speech disorders: clinical manifestations, diagnosis, and management. Handb Clin Neurol. 2016;139:379-88.
34. Baker J. Functional voice disorders: clinical presentations and differential diagnosis. Handb Clin Neurol. 2016;139:389-405.

110

CHAPTER

Principles of Genetic Assessments in Neurological Disorders

Pragya Chaturvedi, Prachi Sahu, Rahul Khan, Gagandeep Singh, Anjana Munshi

INTRODUCTION

Neurological diseases are conditions affecting the central and peripheral nervous systems and are highly prevalent diseases across the globe, and hence, are also referred to as brain, behavioral, or cognitive disorders.[1] The Global Burden of Disease (GBD) 1990–2019 study demonstrated that tension-type headache, migraine, and dementias were the most prevalent disorders whereas migraine, dementias, and traumatic brain injuries were reported to be the most disabling neurological conditions, worldwide.[2] Among neurological diseases, dementia, Parkinson's disease, headache, epilepsy, and stroke are highly prevalent in India.[3] According to the International Classification of diseases 11th revision (ICD-11), neurological diseases are categorized into mental, behavioral, or neurodevelopmental disorders; sleep-wake disorders; and other diseases of the nervous system which are further classified into many subgroups. Disorders with prevalence of <1/2,000 in general populations referred to as rare diseases.[4] Some examples of rare neurological disorders include hemiplegic migraine, retinal vasculopathy with cerebral leukodystrophy (RVCL), mitochondrial encephalomyopathy with lactic acidosis and stroke-like episodes (MELAS) syndrome, headache with neurological deficits and cerebrospinal fluid (CSF) lymphocytosis (HaNDL), Sneddon's syndrome, Susac syndrome, and moyamoya angiopathy (MA).[5] Prenatal factors, lower socioeconomic status, older age, unhealthy diet, physical inactivity, hypertension, diabetes, heart disease, family history or genetics as well as environmental exposure pose a higher risk of developing neurological diseases.[6,7]

Proper investigation and diagnosis are important to treat these diseases effectively. Differential diagnosis strategies are used to distinguish the diseases with similar clinical symptoms. Many neurological diseases following Mendelian inheritance pattern are caused on account of mutations in various genes involved in the normal functioning of the spinal cord, brain, peripheral nerves, or even muscles.

In recent years, there has been rapid development in the field of neurogenetics and various genetic tests are being carried out to unravel the various neurological diseases rapidly. Genetic assessment also has the potential to carry out the pre- and postnatal diagnosis of the disease, especially in case of a family history. In addition to this the use of advanced genomic techniques, such as next-generation DNA sequencing is helping in the quick identification of various genes involved in inherited neurological diseases and opening new horizons for genetic testing.

These technologies also help to identify pharmacogenomic markers that help to identify the interindividual variations in drug response as well as adverse drug reaction. Pharmacogenomics is an emerging approach toward precision medicine helping clinicians to tailor the selection of drugs as well as those based on the patient's genomic architecture.

This chapter includes the various aspects of neurological diseases such as epidemiology, clinical presentations, investigation, diagnosis, differential diagnosis, pathology and pathophysiology, genetic assessment, management, and special features in the Indian context.

EPIDEMIOLOGY

Neurological diseases are mostly misinterpreted as their clinical manifestation is quite subtle. The influence of modifiable and nonmodifiable risk factors, clinical presentation, and the natural course of these diseases, all have a significant impact on the prevalence of various neurological diseases.[8] Although most neurological disorders are regarded as "complex," involving numerous genetic and environmental risk factors, their origin and causes are still poorly understood.[8] It has been estimated that one in two women and one in three men are prone to develop dementia, stroke, or Parkinson's disease at some point of their lives.[9]

According to the GBD study 2015, tension-type headache is the most prevalent neurological disorder globally with 1505.9 million cases [95% uncertainty interval (UI) 1337.3–1681.6)].[10] As per the GBD 2019, mental disorders are one of the top 10 leading neurological disorders across the world. The global prevalence of mental disorders has raised from 654.8 million (95% UI 603.6–708.1) to 970.1 (900.9–1044.4) from 1990 to 2019. In 2019, mental disorders were highly prevalent in Australasia, Tropical Latin America followed by high-income North America.[11] Nation-wise and worldwide prevalence, disability-adjusted life year (DALY), years of life lost (YLL), and years lived with disability (YLD), for mental disorders from 1990 to 2019 have been summarized in a report from GBD 2019.[11] For males age-standardized DALYs rate was reported to be 1426.5 (95% UI 1056.4–1869.5) per 100,000 population, whereas for females, it has been reported to be 1703.3 (1261.5–2237.8) across the globe. In 2019, the largest proportion of DALYs was reported for mental disorders followed by anxiety disorders and schizophrenia. Depressive disorders, anxiety disorders, and schizophrenia were ranked 2nd, 8th, and 20th among the top 25 leading cause YLDs in 2019.[11]

Global Burden of Disease, Injuries, and Risk Factor Study 2019, reported the DALYS, YLDs, and YLLs of three categories of neurological disorders in India, i.e., noncommunicable disorders, communicable disorders, and injuries. As per this largest comprehensive epidemiological research, i.e., GBD 2019, the prevalent cases of neurological disorders in India were highest for headache disorders, i.e., 488 million (95% UI 449–527) followed by epilepsy, Alzheimer's disease (AD) and other dementias, brain and central nervous system (CNS) cancer, Parkinson's disease, multiple sclerosis (MS), and motor neuron diseases. On the other hand, in the noncommunicable and communicable disorders category, the incident cases were highest for stroke, i.e., 1,291,200 (95% UI 1,150,700–1,453,000) followed by encephalitis, meningitis, and tetanus. Whereas incident cases in terms of injuries were 7,464,800 (95% UI 6,383,800–8,667,200) for traumatic brain injuries followed by spinal cord injuries.[12]

CLINICAL PRESENTATIONS

The term "clinical presentation" describes the typical signs or symptoms associated with a specific disease **(Figs. 1A and B)**. Clinical features of a disease include the age of onset, duration, and symptoms of the disease. The assessment and interpretation of clinical symptoms lead to diagnosis of the disease.

Neurodevelopmental Disorders

Characteristic features of the neurodevelopmental disorder include disruption in the process of brain development. Facial appearance of the patient is: a wide short nose with

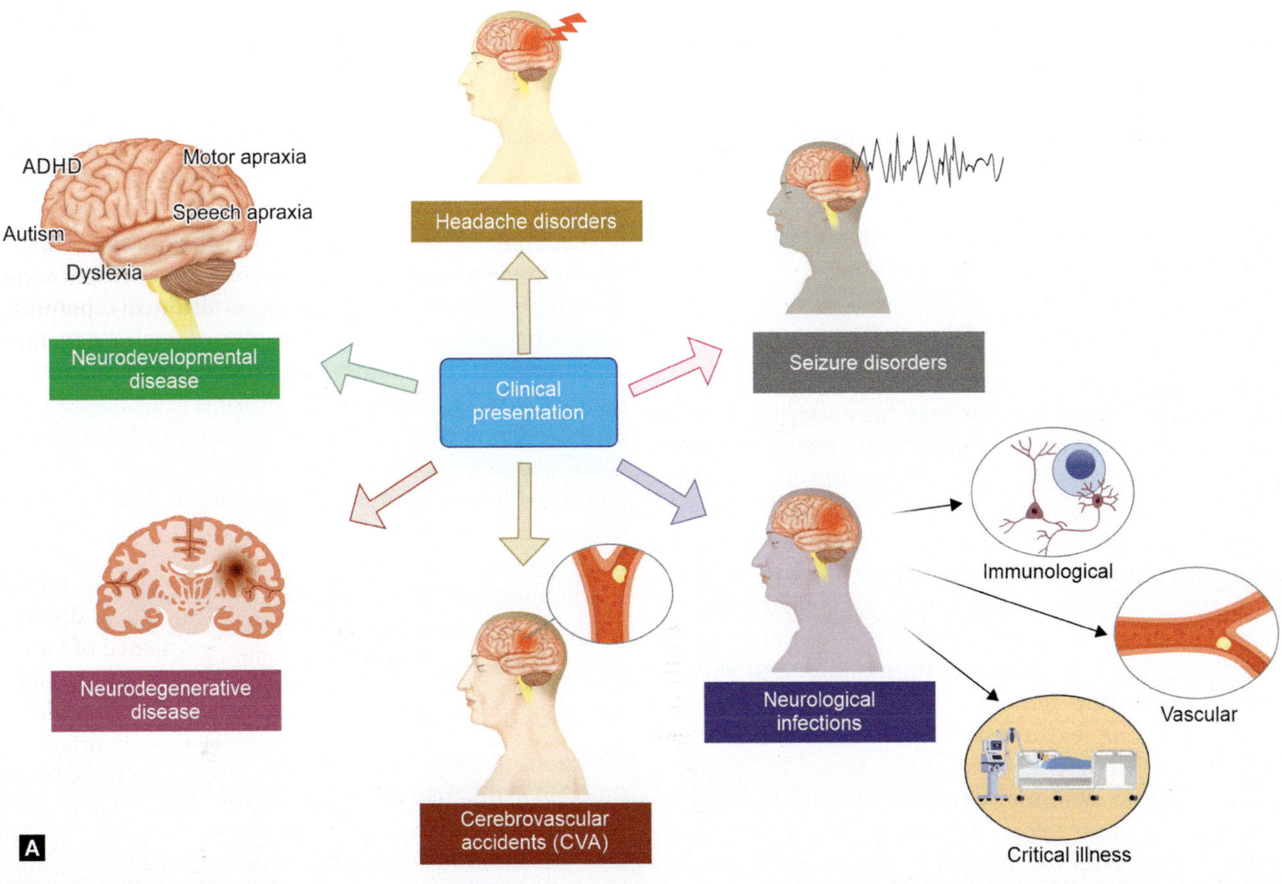

FIGS. 1A AND B: *Continued*

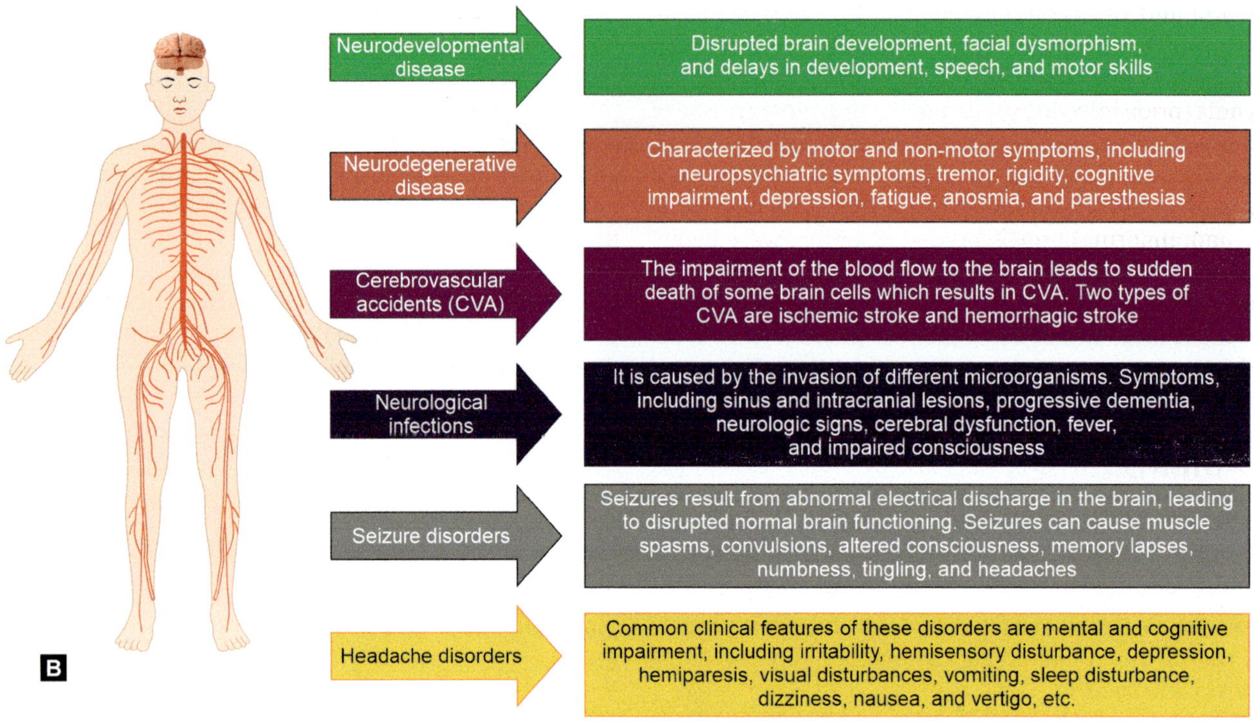

FIGS. 1A AND B: (A) Clinical presentation of neurological diseases; (B) Clinical characteristics of neurological disease.
Image courtesy: Created with BioRender.com.

full, upturned nasal tip, depressed nasal bridge, prominent forehead with a high anterior hairline, down slanted palpebral fissures, and prominent eyelashes. Development delay, speech delay, and motor delay are the significant features of the patients. Cerebral imaging usually shows cerebral abnormalities such as cortical dysplasia hippocampal hypoplasticity, perinatal hypoxic-ischemic encephalopathy, delayed myelination, hydrocephalus, and white matter lesions. In addition, patients might also have certain autistic, visual and gastrointestinal problems as well as abnormal behavioural and sleep-related features.[13]

Neurodegenerative Diseases

The degenerative condition is marked by several motor and nonmotor symptoms that may have varying degrees of neurological functional impairment. These disorders commonly affect specific subset of neurons and are also characterized by disappearance of neuronal cell bodies and glial proliferation. AD, frontotemporal lobe degeneration, Parkinson's disease, dementia, motor neuron disease, Huntington's disease, and multiple system atrophy are catcgorized in various groups based on their anatomical distribution, major molecular abnormalities, and clinical features.[14] Anterior temporal lobe or spinocerebellar degeneration or extrapyramidal is the anatomical distribution of neurodegenerative diseases.[14] In addition, neuropsychiatric symptoms, tremor, sialorrhea, rigidity, postural instability, decreased arm swing, hypomimia, dysarthria, bradykinesia, dysphagia, and shuffling gait are the motor symptoms associated with some of these disorders. While cognitive impairment, bradyphrenia, tip-of-the-tongue phenomenon, depression, apathy, anhedonia, fatigue, other behavioral and psychiatric problems, anosmia, ageusia, pain (shoulder and back), paresthesias, etc., are the nonmotor clinical features of neurodegenerative diseases.[15,16]

Cerebrovascular Accidents

Cerebrovascular accidents (CVAs) also refers to "brain attack" or stroke. The impairment of the blood flow to the brain leads to sudden death of some brain cells which results in CVA.[17] Out of the two types of CVA, ischemic stroke (IS) is caused by thrombi, emboli, or global hypoperfusion. In other words, when atherosclerotic plaque, thrombus, or embolus obstructs the arteries in cerebral circulation, it results in IS. Whereas another type, i.e., hemorrhagic stroke is caused by bleeding in the regions of brain due to bursting of blood vessels. Clinic features of CVA include sensory loss, aphasia sensory abnormalities, amaurosis fugax, motor neglect, speech disturbance, ipsilateral facial weakness, eye movement disturbance, hemisensory loss, sensory loss in contralateral leg, hemianopic visual loss and hemiparesis, contralateral gaze paresis, dysarthria, color blindness, memory disturbance, sensory loss, amnesia, and oculomotor palsy.[17-19]

Neurological Infections

Infectious diseases of the nervous system are caused by the invasion of different microorganisms. The infection can also be caused by fungus, parasite, prion diseases as well as brain abscess. Sinonasal and intracranial lesions, ventriculitis, or a solitary CNS granuloma (fungal infections); progressive dementia and neurologic signs such as visual problems, myoclonus, cerebral dysfunction, cerebellar ataxia, autonomic dysfunction, extrapyramidal symptoms, and insomnia (prion infection); increase in intracranial pressure, cerebritis, and abscess (bacterial infection); diurnal fever, impaired consciousness, brainstem dysfunction such as abnormal pupillary or corneal reflexed, a dysconjugate gaze, and abnormal breathing pattern (cerebral malaria); headache, swelling, redness, and fever are the characteristic features of neurological infection (common). In addition, certain infections might result in hydrocephalus, deafness, blindness, cognitive impairment, cerebral palsy along with permanent dysfunctioning of the nervous system.[20-23]

Seizure Disorders

Seizures result on account of abnormal electrical discharge in the brain leading to disruption of normal brain functioning. Seizures disorders are mainly grouped into epileptic, psychogenic, and nonepileptic seizures. Seizures can be caused due to many conditions, disorders, and other factors such as exposure to toxins, cerebral edema, CNS infection, brain malformations, genetic disorders, head trauma or injury, tumors growing in the brain, and stroke. The commonly reported clinical features of seizure disorders are muscle spasm, jerk or twitching in certain regions of body, intense stiffening of muscles or convulsions and altered consciousness, memory lapse, numbness, tingling in parts of body, pelvic thrusting, deep sleep, headache or hallucinations, depression and anxiety, etc.[24,25]

Headache Disorders

Head, neck, and facial pain disorders are come under the category of headache disorders. Common clinical features of these disorders are mental and cognitive impairment, including irritability, hemisensory disturbance, aphasia, ataxia, depression, hemiparesis, visual disturbances, focal neurologic events, vomiting, sleep disturbance, dizziness, nausea, diarrhea, lacrimation, and vertigo, etc.[26,27]

PATHOLOGY AND PATHOPHYSIOLOGY

Many factors contribute to the pathology or pathophysiology of a neurological disease. These can be genetic aberrations, upregulation, or downregulation of certain gene as well as altered levels of certain proteins or metabolites in the biological fluids or specific tissues.

Neurodevelopmental Disorders

Genetic aberrations along with the altered concentration of various molecules in biological fluids are found to be the most common pathophysiological alterations observed in most of the neurodevelopmental diseases.[28] Phenotypes of various neurodevelopmental diseases have been associated with the altered genes resulting in their aberrant expression.[28] For example, variations in phosphodiesterases (*PDE*) genes are found to be implicated in neurodevelopmental brain disorders.[29] Increased plasma level of endocannabinoids, anandamide (ANA) or N-arachidonoylethanolamine (AEA), sphingosine-1-phosphate (S1P d18:1), sphinganine-1-phosphate (S1P d18:0), and arachidonoylglycerol are found in attention deficit/hyperactivity disorder. Impairment of neural connectivity, synaptogenesis damage, and alteration in cerebral circuitry are the pathophysiological condition in autism spectrum disorders (ASDs).[30-32]

In case of schizophrenia, reduction of neuropil and layer-specific neurons in cortical regions are observed.[33-35] In addition, dysregulation of apoptosis in several cortical regions along with the progressive loss of cortical gray matter is also reported to be the neuropathologic features of schizophrenia.[33] Studies have also found the contribution of altered expression of the risk genes (DISC-1, neuregulin/ErbB4, dysbindin, Akt1, BDNF, and the NMDA receptor) in dysconnectivity observed in schizophrenia.[36]

Neurodegenerative Diseases

Abnormalities of structure and function as well as accumulation of neurotoxic proteins are the fundamental pathophysiological signatures of neurodegenerative disease.[37] Pathophysiology of these disorders varies as per the region affected. For example, when the disease affects cerebral cortex, cerebral white matter, and the basal ganglia or affects the brain homogenously then the associated pathophysiological features are poliodystrophies, leukodystrophies, corencephalopathies, and diffuse encephalopathies, respectively.[14] Accumulation of proteins in certain brain regions or spinal cord, release of cytokines, and increased neuroinflammation along with the microglial activation are some other pathophysiological mechanisms associated with various neurodegenerative disease.[38]

Cerebrovascular Accident

In CVA, there is a decrease in cerebral blood flow which triggers cellular metabolic processes and ultimately affects the cerebral function. Ischemia results in the deprivation of glucose and oxygen which cause acidosis along with depolarization of the cell membrane, and disturbances in intracellular calcium and sodium. Apoptosis and necrosis are the two mechanisms of cell death, occur on account of ischemia in which degradation of nucleus initiates a sequence of self-destruction and cellular architecture breakdown.[19]

Neurological Infections

Various pathogenic microorganisms causing infections are responsible for a variety of pathophysiology such as perivascular damage associated with intravascular sequestration of *Plasmodium*-infected red blood cells (RBCs) along with axonal injury, myelin loss, blood-brain barrier breakdown, and hemorrhagic punctate lesions in white matter areas (cerebral malaria); inflammation, intracranial complications, neuronal damage, and brain damage (bacterial CNS infection); neuronal cell death, synaptic degeneration, microglia and astrocyte activation, misfolding, aggregation, and spread of misfolded forms of prion protein (prion infection).[23,39,40] In case of meningitis, a high subarachnoid space inflammatory response results in cerebral edema, meningeal inflammation, and increased intracranial pressure.[41,42]

Seizure Disorders

Dysfunction at various levels such as cognitive-emotional information processing, volitional control, arousal tolerance, altered connections of brain regions associated with emotion processing, and unstable cognitive-emotional attention system (psychogenic nonepileptic seizure); and abnormal activation pattern of neurons, altered functioning of ion channels, and neurotransmitter receptors as well as changes in the levels of neurotransmitter and energy metabolism (acute symptomatic seizures).[43,44] Various physiologic imbalances such as cardiorespiratory instability, hypoxia, hypoglycemia, and hyperthermia are associated with prolonged convulsive status epilepticus.[45]

Headache Disorders

Underlying pathophysiological mechanisms of headaches (migraine) include spreading depression (SD).[46] SD is a wave of simultaneous depolarization associated with a transient depression of spontaneous electrical activity in certain regions of brain. It is known to activate another pathway, i.e., trigeminovascular nociceptive pathway which is responsible for cephalgia.[47] Intense transmembrane ionic, metabolite and neurotransmitter shifts, and cell swelling are found to be the SD-associated pathogenesis of headache.[46,48]

INVESTIGATION, DIAGNOSIS, AND DIFFERENTIAL DIAGNOSIS

Investigation of neurological diseases is also referred to as neuroinvestigation. With the increasing diversity of diseases, it is very important to distinguish among them. Differential diagnosis aids in differentiating between two or more diseases which share similar symptoms. This helps in the detection of therapeutic targets and in providing disease-specific treatment. Proper diagnosis also helps to monitor the disease progression. Based on the purpose and type of analysis, the diagnosis of the neurological disorders is carried out using various sophisticated and high throughput technologies. Diagnosis of the neurological diseases includes various approaches such as biochemical analysis, neuroimaging, neuropsychological assessment, and genetic testing **(Flowchart 1)**.

Neuroimaging a noninvasive method, carried out to study the structure and functioning of the nervous system.

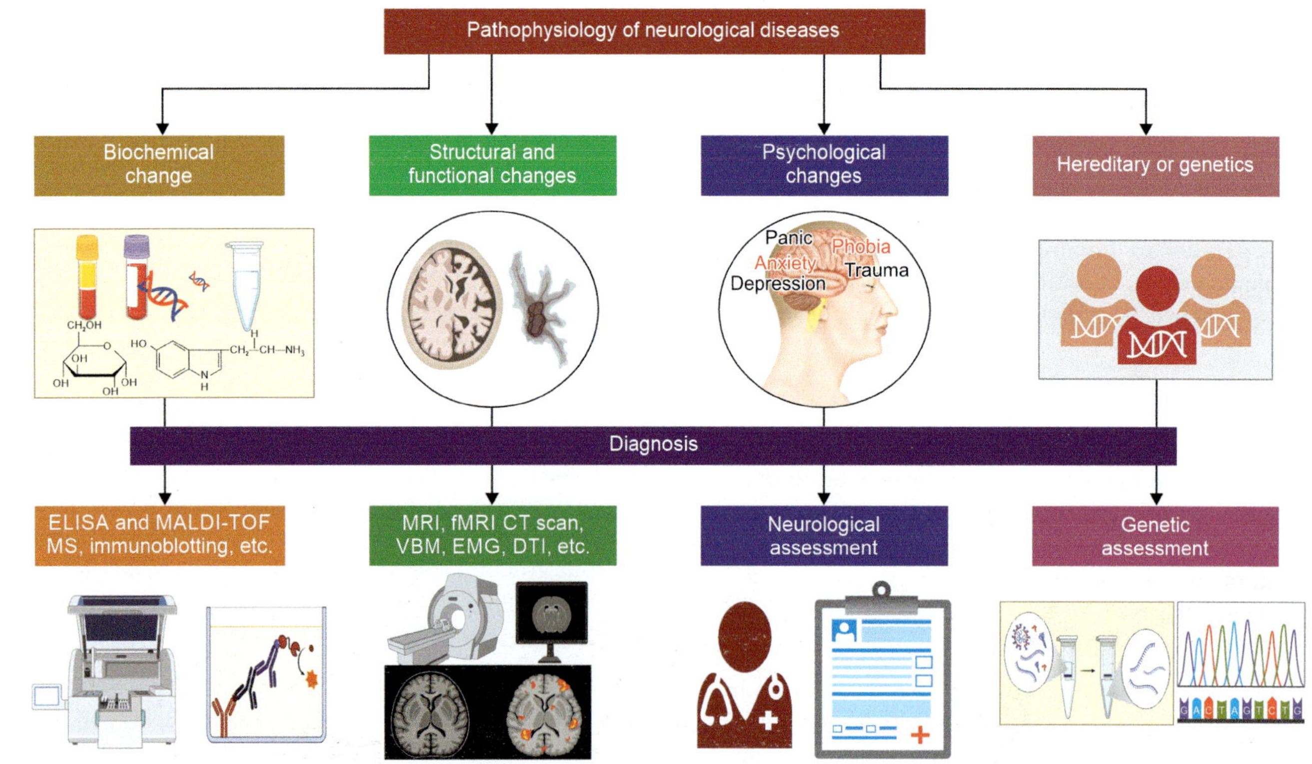

FLOWCHART 1: Different diagnostic methods available for neurological diseases based on their pathophysiology.

(CT: computed tomography; DTI: diffusion tensor imaging; ELISA: enzyme-linked immunosorbent assay; EMG: electromyography; fMRI: functional magnetic resonance imaging; MALDI-TOF: matrix-assisted laser desorption/ionization-time of flight; MS: multiple sclerosis)

Image courtesy: Created with BioRender.com.

It includes imaging of the nervous system and cerebral circulation, and study of the evoked potential and nerve conduction. Technologies used for neuroimaging (brain scans) are magnetic resonance imaging, functional magnetic resonance imaging (fMRI), magnetic resonance spectroscopy, computed tomography scan (CT-scan), single-photon emission CT (SPECT), voxel-based morphometry (VBM), electroencephalogram, magnetoencephalography (MEG), electromyography, and diffusion tensor imaging (DTI) and positron emission tomography (PET).[49]

Biochemical analysis is one of the conventional diagnostic approaches. It is the identification and measurement of the biomarkers in the biological samples such as CSF, whole blood, serum, saliva, and urine. Technologies used for this type of analysis are enzyme-linked immunosorbent assay (ELISA), immunoblotting, western blotting, immunohistochemistry, matrix-assisted laser desorption/ionization-time of flight (MALDI-TOF), Raman spectroscopy, mass spectrometry, etc. Biomarker detection has been moved from conventional laboratory settings to more portable, user-friendly equipment. With the evolving mobile technologies, researchers have developed optical detection-based portable medical devices for the comparable clinical measurement. These devices use three types of optical detection methods—(1) colorimetric, (2) chemiluminescent, and (3) fluorescent or phosphorescent. Based on the type of test, these biosensing methods are combined with chemical measurement accessories.[50]

Neuropsychological assessment is the evaluation of behavioral expression of brain dysfunction at clinical level. This is helpful in distinguishing between different neurological conditions.[51] Cognitive strength, relationship between the finding of the neuropsychological assessment, and the psychiatric condition of the individual are identified with this approach.[52]

Genetic Assessment: Many neurological diseases have a genetic component. Some neurological disorders are caused by single gene variations that interfere with the normal functioning of the nervous system and muscles such as neuropathies, myopathies, and ataxias.[53] Some neurological conditions run in families such as stroke, AD, Huntington's disease, Parkinson's disease, familial hemiplegic migraine, and epilepsy. Genetic tests have become a part of diagnostic process on account of high costs and lengthy procedures. It is mandatory especially in the single gene disorder showing a Mendelian pattern of inheritance. Even the multifactorial disorders are being subjected to genetic analysis to understand the role of significant genes involved in the disease development, progression, and drug response.

In addition to the demographic profile of the patient, pedigree analysis is also carried out to study the family history of a particular disorder and also understand the particular disorder.

Pedigree analysis helps to study family histories and inheritance of genes in humans. It is a chart that depicts a family tree, which maps out all relevant members of a family and exactly how they are related to one another as well as display the members of the family who are affected by a genetic trait. It can also use to predict the risk of developing a particular disorder in future generation by genetic counseling, genetic risk assessment, segregation analysis, and linkage analysis.[54]

GENETIC TESTING

The aim of the genetic testing is mainly based on the clinical state of the disease. It is usually to identify the carriers and to decide about the reproductive risk. Genetic testing can be carried out in a presymptomatic setting as well as in the symptomatic stage. A presymptomatic assessment (e.g., for the diagnosis of late-onset disorders such as Huntington's disease) can be done through screening programs, like in the neonatal and antenatal settings.[55] Genetic testing is usually recommended to the patients with proven family history of inherited neurological or neuromuscular diseases.

Based on the medical condition and the purpose of genetic test, these are classified into:

- Diagnostic testing (e.g., Fragile X syndrome in a boy with mental retardation)
- Presymptomatic testing
- Predictive testing (or predisposition genetic testing)
- Reproductive testing and pharmacogenetic testing (for individual-specific drug response, e.g., warfarin, carbamazepine, etc.)
- Newborns screening and identity testing (for paternity, zygosity, and forensic purposes)

Presymptomatic and Predictive Genetic Testing

Presymptomatic and predictive (or predisposition) types of genetic testing are the tests to identify a genetic mutation that results in a certain ailment before symptoms appear. Sometimes, the term presymptomatic, predictive, and susceptibility genetic testing are used interchangeably.[56,57] Presymptomatic genetic testing is generally carried out for those diseases for which positive result will surely lead to the disease development in life later on (in case of Huntington disease). On the other hand, predictive genetic testing refers to a wider spectrum of diseases where there is a higher possibility of developing a disease, without necessarily stating that there is any degree of certainty such as in case of hereditary cancers.[58] These types of test can be done for late-onset diseases includes Parkinson's disease, Tourette syndrome, AD, Huntington' disease, leukoencephalopathy amyotrophic lateral sclerosis (ALS), cerebral autosomal dominant arteriopathy with subcortical infarcts and, hereditary ataxia, neuromuscular disorders, and neurodevelopmental disorders such as Down syndrome and Rett syndrome.[56,59,60]

Reproductive Genetic Testing

Reproductive genetic testing reveals the likelihood that parents will pass on a genetic mutation to their offspring.

It also provides information about the genetic makeup of the in vitro fertilized embryos produced as well as about the fetus in utero. In this case, *Carrier testing* is done which ascertains whether a person has one altered gene copy for a specific recessive disorder (e.g., familial dysautonomia); *prenatal genetic testing*, i.e., genetic analysis of fetal cells obtained through amniocentesis and chorionic villus sampling; *preimplantation genetic testing* which involves genetic testing of in vitro fertilized eggs to determine which embryos should be implanted into a woman's womb (e.g., patients with a history of producing offspring with chromosomal abnormalities or with single gene disorders).[61]

Pharmacogenetic Testing

This type of testing helps in predicting the response of our body to specific medications based on the genetic profile. Pharmacogenetic testing aids in the diagnosis and treatment of multiple conditions.[62] It is the most promising clinical application of the genomic research. The use of pharmacogenetic indicators in clinical settings is expanding as more genetic variations linked to drug outcomes are identified and confirmed.[63] It also helps clinicians to predict the efficacy or toxicity of some drugs as the variations in activities of drug metabolizing enzymes depend on variations in DNA sequences **(Fig. 2)**.[64] These genetic variations result in varying drug responses such as poor metabolizer, extensive metabolizer, intermediate metabolizer, and ultrarapid metabolizers.[65,66] Personalized optimization of pharmacogenetics has a wide range of application in research and disease treatment. It has been explored in various diseases such as epilepsy, Parkinson's disease, psychoses, cerebral palsy, migraine, antipsychotic-induced movement disorders as well as in psychiatry.[67-80]

Methods Used for Genetic Testing

Genetic testing aims to find chromosomal aberrations and genomic alterations associated with various disorders using various cytogenetic and molecular techniques. Researchers also analyze the whole genome or exome (the protein coding part of the genome) in order to identify new or novel genes associated with neurological or any other diseases **(Flowchart 2)**. The identified and confirmed genes help in clinical testing in more focused way.

Methods or technologies such as karyotyping, fluorescent in situ hybridization (FISH), spectral karyotyping, and array comparative genomic hybridization (CGH) are used to analyze the chromosomal aberrations. The genomic alterations at candidate gene level or genome-wide association level are analyzed with the high throughput technologies like next-generation sequencing (NGS) of DNA or RNA **(Flowchart 2)**.

The other methods or techniques used for genetic testing include linkage analysis, genome-wide single nucleotide polymorphism (SNP) microarrays, target polymerase chain reaction (PCR), southern blot, multiplex ligation-dependent probe amplification (MLPA), and panel or pathway sequencing **(Flowchart 2)**.[81] Selection and platform of the test are guided by the clinical and demographic data of a patient such as phenotype, age, and family history as well as availability of specimen.[81]

Other than changes in genes, their expression analyses are also analyzed in different cell types that identify which genes are active or inactive or upregulated and downregulated in diseased condition. These tests study the gene expression which in turn affects protein levels. Functional analysis of the altered genetic variants or their expressions is also carried out at the level of animal

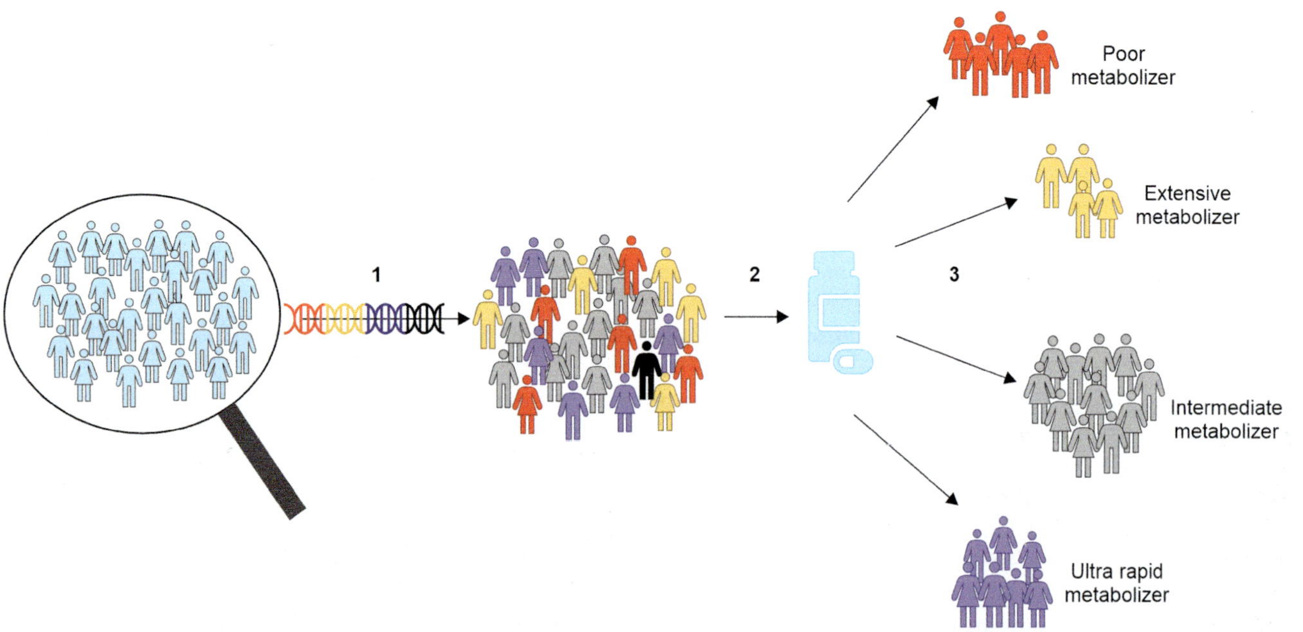

FIG. 2: Role of genetics in precision medicine—(1) Genetic screening of individuals; (2) same drug given to all the individuals; and (3) drug response based on the individual-specific genetic make-up.

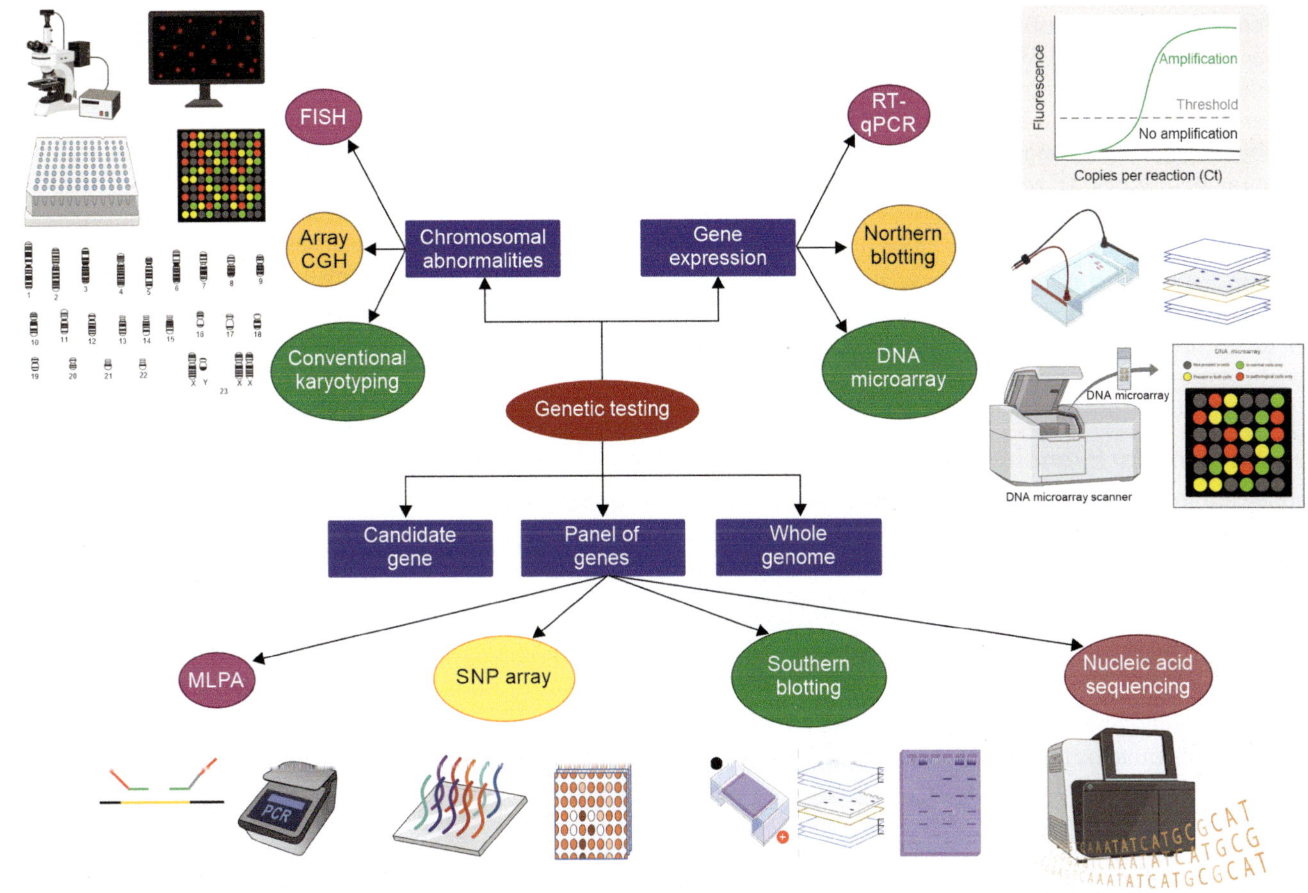

FLOWCHART 2: Various methods used to detect neurological diseases.

(CGH: comparative genomic hybridization; FISH: fluorescent in situ hybridization; MLPA: multiplex ligation-dependent probe amplification; PCR: polymerase chain reaction; SNP: single nucleotide polymorphism)

Image courtesy: Created with BioRender.com.

model to investigate and validate the pathophysiological mechanism of diseases at molecular level. Gene expression can be measured by either measuring the mRNA levels or by quantification of the proteins (product of gene expression). mRNA levels can be measured by northern blotting, reverse transcription followed by Quantitative PCR (RT-qPCR), RNA protection assay, serial analysis of gene expression (SAGE), DNA microarray, and RNA-sequencing **(Flowchart 2)**.

Typically, the gene product, which is often a protein, is quantified in order to measure the level of gene expression. Techniques for the quantification of proteins are western blotting and ELISA. These analyses are more helpful in exploring the rare neurological disease which in turn aids in proper diagnosis and management of these disease.

Linkage Analysis

Linkage refers to alleles being inherited together.[82] It is a classical genetic approach. Large pedigrees of multiple affected family members are used in linkage analysis. In this, functionality of genes is associated to their chromosomal locations by looking at cosegregation between genes and similarity in phenotypes between individuals sharing alleles at those marker loci. The phenomenon of recombination serves as the foundation for linkage analysis which takes place during meiosis via the exchange of DNA (crossing over) between two sister chromatids.[83] In a known pedigree, linkage studies analyze the transmission of both the disease phenotype and the marker alleles across two generations. These studies indicate whether the marker is linked to a causal locus.[82] A marker would be more likely to be coinherited with the trait locus if they are closely located due to low recombination rate than if it is located farther away.[83] DNA markers [such as variable number of tandem repeats (VNTRs), short tandem repeats (STRs), or SNPs] are used to map a region of interest or the complete genome in order to identify the linked regions.[82] The statistical significance of estimated recombination rate is evaluated using the log-likelihood (LOD) score. LOD scores required to be statistically significant is ≥ 3.[83]

Karyotyping

It is a cytogenetic technique used for the detection of structural and numerical chromosomal abnormalities.[84] Karyotyping is performed on specific body fluid or tissue which can be obtained in the following ways—phlebotomy, bone marrow aspiration, amniocentesis, and chorionic villus sampling. Chromosomal aberrations, such as copy number variations (CNV) which include microdeletion and microduplications, are significantly implicated in mental retardation and multiple malformations.[84,85] But these cannot be detected by conventional karyotyping and require high-resolution techniques. To resolve this, several new methods based on PCR, FISH and array techniques are developed for the early detection of microdeletion and microduplication.[86] Furthermore, chromosomal microarray analysis (CMA) has emerged as a first-line techniques in prenatal diagnosis for structural chromosomal abnormalities.[84,87] CGH chips and SNP chips are the two types of CMA which can detect CNVs up to 50–100 kb across the whole genome.[84,88]

Fluorescent in situ Hybridization

Fluorescent in situ hybridization is a molecular cytogenetic technique used for chromosome-wide detection and location of a specific DNA sequence. FISH helps in detection of chromosomal abnormalities. There are two components in FISH—(1) the DNA probe and (2) target DNA.[89] The location of a DNA sequence on a chromosome is identified based on its binding with fluorescently-labeled probe. In this, fluorescently-labeled probe binds to its complementary sequence and emits the fluorescence which can be observed under the microscope. Based on the application, various types of probes are used in FISH, e.g., locus specific, centromeric, and whole chromosome probes. FISH protocol has been diversified into a number of procedures in terms of improvement in resolution, sensitivity, and specificity along with the advancement in fluorescent microscopy, digital imaging, and increased availability of resources for genomic and bioinformatics data. These are ACM-FISH, armFISH, CARD-FISH, catfish, CB-FISH, CO-FISH, COBRA-FISH, COD-FISH, COMBO-FISH, Comet-FISH, Cryo-FISH, D-FISH, DBD-FISH, e-FISH, Fiber-FISH, Flow-FISH, Fusion-Signal FISH, Halo-FISH, Harlequin-FISH, Immuno-FISHLNA-FISH, M-FISH, Multilocus or ML-FISH, PCC-FISH, PNA-FISH, Q-FISH, QD-FISH, Rainbow-FISH, Raman-FISH, ReD-FISH, Reverse-FISH, RING-FISH, RNA-FISH, Rx-FISH, Split-signal FISH, T-FISH, 3-D FISH, and Zoo-FISH.[90]

Fluorescent in situ hybridization is widely used in detection of neurological diseases. It helps in the identification of gene expression in brain (CAT-FISH), the orientation of tandem repeats in centromeric region of brain (CO-FISH), copy number and protein amount quantification (COD-FISH), DNA damage (Comet-FISH), etc.[91] Out of these, CAT-FISH approach is used to examine the connection and interaction of neuronal populations which are associated with various behavioral or cognitive difficulties. This technique is employed to study and monitor the cellular distribution and the environment-specific gene expression of immediate early gene (IEG) Arc which is regulated by neural activity.[90]

Limitations of FISH include the difficulty in determining the probe to be used in case of the wide spectrum of developmental delay. A narrow range of the targets can be investigated reasonably due to the limited availability of materials.[86]

Array CGH

Array CGH analyzes quantitative increase or decrease of chromosomes by competitive DNA hybridization of patients and controls. Genomic imbalance, especially in pediatric neurologic diseases, can be identified using this method. Array CGH also has wider application in detecting chromosomal abnormalities such as deletions and duplication of certain regions of chromosome such as in case of mental retardation, developmental delay, dysmorphic face, atrial septal defect, hypotonia, lissencephaly, Kleefstra syndrome, Angelman syndrome, Prader–Willi syndrome, William–Beuren syndrome, Mowat–Wilson syndrome, Lennox–Gastaut syndrome, and epilepsy.[86]

Single Nucleotide Polymorphism Array

Combination of karyotype analysis and SNP array technology aids in detecting the fetuses with CNS abnormalities. The conditions which cannot be detected by CGH array such as regions of homozygosity, maternal cell contamination, and triploidy can be detected by SNP array. CNVs with different clinical significance can be detected with SNP array in case of CNS anomalies such as mental retardation, global developmental delay, ventriculomegaly and holoprosencephaly, choroid plexus cysts, posterior cranial fossa widened, abnormalities of the corpus callosum, abnormalities of septum pellucidum or CSP, cerebellar hypoplasia, arachnoid cyst, subependymal cyst, Blake's porch cyst, holoprosencephaly, and other CNS abnormalities which might be detected using this method.[84]

Multiplex Ligation-dependent Probe Amplification

Multiplex ligation-dependent probe amplification technique, based on multiplex PCR, can concurrently detect changes in DNA methylation, point mutations, and status of gene copy number.[92] Target sequence recognized by the MLPA probe is of only 50–100 nucleotides in length and hence aids in detection of small and heterozygous deletions. A smaller or higher relative amount of the probe amplification product is produced when the copy number of the MLPA probe-target sequence changes.[92] MLPA helps in the diagnosis of gliomas (malignant tumors in the CNS), neuroblastoma (*MYCN* gene and EGFR deletion variant III), subcortical band heterotopia (*DCX* gene deletion), Duchenne muscular dystrophy (DMD) and Becker muscular dystrophies (BMDs) (copy number of DMD exons or point mutations), idiopathic mental retardation (subtelomeric deletions), and phospholipase-associated neurodegeneration (novel intragenic *PLA2G6* gene mutations).[92-98]

Southern Blot

In this technique, DNA fragments are separated on a gel and then transferred straight to a second medium so that a hybridization assay can be performed. This technique is used to identify specific DNA sequences. Sothern blot is used in the combination with other techniques like PCR and has a wide application in the detection of specific DNA sequences. These techniques help in the diagnosis of spinocerebellar ataxia type 7 (CAG repeats in the *SCA7* gene), myotonic dystrophy (CTG trinucleotide expansion mutation), herpes simplex encephalitis, and multiple neurodegenerative syndromes (hexanucleotide repeat expansions).[99-102]

Real-time Quantitative PCR

Real-time PCR is the most commonly used accurate, sensitive, and fast technique to measure the gene expression. The process involves preparation phase, real-time PCR cycling, data analysis, and result interpretation.[103] Tissue-specific mRNA expression can also be measure using this technique. For example, in case of MS, cytokine mRNA expression was measured in CSF as well as peripheral blood mononuclear cells by Monteyne et al. (1997).[104] The technique has also helps to analyze the expression of inflammatory genes associated with ischemia reperfusion brain injury.[105] Furthermore, brain reference genes have also been assessed in neurodegenerative diseases using RT-qPCR.[106] Another wider application of this approach is to profile genome-wide expression of various genes in blood which helped in identifying biomarkers for Huntington's disease.[107]

Northern Blotting and DNA Microarray

Functional genomic studies of nervous system are quite difficult due to the complexity of nervous system. Northern blotting is one of the basic methods that aims to measure specific mRNAs. It is based on the fractionation and separation of RNA molecules as per their size, then their transfer on a blotting membrane followed by binding or hybridization of the probe to the complementary sequence of the target mRNA.[108]

Microarray has also emerged as a promising approach for identifying novel molecular markers in various neurological diseases.[109] In this, DNA and/or RNA hybridization is assessed in microminiaturized highly parallel formats.[110] In case of schizophrenia, the altered gene expression patterns have been identified using this method.[109] This method has also been applied to identify the gene expression in normal white matter (in MS); senile plaques and normal hippocampal CA1 neurons (in AD).[111,112]

Sanger Gene Sequencing, Whole-exome Sequencing, and Whole-genome Sequencing

The genetic heterogeneity of many neurological disorders makes it challenging to screen for disease-specific genes. Even when the condition is caused by mutations in well-known disease genes, specific diagnosis of many patients with genetic neurological disorders has not being done. New opportunities for diagnostic genetic testing have been created by recent technological advancements, especially high throughput DNA sequencing techniques, that help in quick identification of gene variants involved in various neurological disorders following Mendelian pattern of inheritance.

Comprehensive genomic testing of large panels of candidate genes or the entire genome is also possible by various sequencing technologies. Genome-wide association studies (GWAS) provide the data on genetic variation that is implicated in the pathogenesis of complex disorders without considering only the known candidate genes. New molecular pathways implicated in disease pathogenesis have come under focus on account of identification of rare disease-causing mutations.

Genome sequencing has been extremely helpful in identifying several disease-causing genes involved in the molecular pathogenesis of many disorders.[113] Sequencing technologies have improved a lot since they were discovered and have become time consuming and run at a reduced cost. These are classified into first generation (Sanger sequencing), second generation (pyrosequencing, sequencing by reversible terminator chemistry, and sequencing by ligation), third generation (single molecule fluorescent sequencing, single molecule real-time sequencing, semiconductor sequencing, and nanopore sequencing) and fourth-generation techniques which aim to analyze the genome directly in the cell.[114]

Sanger sequencing known as chain termination method is a first-generation DNA sequencing method. In 1970, Frederick Sanger and colleagues developed this method. This is ideal for medium to low throughput-targeted sequencing.[115] On comparison with other multiplex testing system, this approach is costly as it can analyze a gene-specific region or small subset of genes in individual Sanger sequencing reactions.[116] It provides a higher degree of accuracy, long read capabilities, and has wide range of applications. It helps in the validation of PCR results.[115] Recurrent single nucleotide mutations are frequently evaluated by Sanger sequencing in surgical neuropathology, have diagnostic, prognostic, and therapeutic implications as well. This has wider application in identifying mutations in case of oligodendrogliomas (IDH1 exon4), anaplastic astrocytomas (IDH2 exon 4), glioblastomas (*H3F3A* and *HIST1H3B*), pleomorphic xanthoastrocytoma (*BRAF* exon 15), extracerebellar pilocytic astrocytoma (*BRAF* exon 15), and anaplastic (malignant) meningioma (*TERT* promoter region), etc.[117]

Next-generation sequencing technologies allow the examination of genetic variability at a large scale and unprecedented resolution. NGS has wider applications in rapidly sequence whole genome or exome, deep sequences target regions, RNA sequencing to identify novel RNA variants, splice sites, or quantification of mRNAs for gene expression analysis. NGS can identify novel gene mutations underlying the phenotype in rare Mendelian diseases.[118] Detailed analysis, precise interpretation helps in the integration of the genomic data into the clinical diagnosis and management of the neurological diseases.[119]

These technologies have established as to how the genetic may provide information on disease phenotype, allowing testing of millions of known markers in a large number of individuals as well as the identification of extremely rare or novel mutations in smaller cohorts.[120] whole-genome sequencing (WGS) aids in the GWAS to provide the role of genetics from rare to common diseases. While the whole-exome sequencing (WES) allows the rapid and cost-effective identification of aberrant Mendelian genes associated with various neurological disorders.[120,121] To understand the effect of genetic variations results of the genotyping data can be integrated with the results of gene expression, proteomics, and metabolomics studies and understand the disease pathogenesis using a systems biology approach.

Whole-genome sequencing can help in faster diagnosis of neurological disorders such as Fragile X syndrome, Huntington's disease, neuropathic pain disorders, ALS and frontal lobe or frontotemporal dementia (FTD), Leber's hereditary optic neuropathy, and various neurodevelopmental disorders.[122]

Whole-exome sequencing has helped to identify *GM2A, SPG20, CYP27A1, NPC2, PNKP, WDR81, ADCK3, SBF1*, and *RYR1 genes significantly associated with GM2-gangliosidosis*, spastic paraplegia, cerebrotendinous xanthomatosis, Nieman-Pick disease, infantile-onset seizures, cerebellar ataxia, cerebellar atrophy, Charcot-Marie-Tooth disease, and minicore myopathy, respectively. *PNKP* gene has also been found to be implicated in progressive microcephaly and developmental delay.[118,123]

As far the GWAS are concerned the common disease-common variation hypothesis underlies this approach, which confers as to how the unknown gene mutation is associated with the development of common neurological diseases. Neurological diseases such as MS, ALS, AD as well as Parkinson's disease (PD) are amenable to GWAS approach.[118]

Genetic Counseling and Risk Assessment

Genetic counseling is a significant aspect of genetic testing since it is used to address the clinical and societal repercussions of Mendelian disorders. The primary objective of genetic counseling is to educate the individual or family members at the risk of developing a disease, management, and manifestation of the disease. The information about the relative risk, absolute risk, and lifetime risks are also conveyed to the respective individuals during genetic counseling. In order to cope up with the untreatable diseases, psychological and emotional support is also provided to the patient and their family members.[124]

Risk analysis is a critical aspect of genetic counseling and testing, and it is important to estimate the genetic risk as precisely as possible for individual and family decision-making. The accuracy of the determination of a person's genetic risk is improved by collecting all pertinent data from population surveys, pedigree analysis, and genetic testing.[124]

MANAGEMENT

The current treatment and management for neurological diseases include the use of various drugs along with physical or occupational therapy for rehabilitation.

In case of *neurodevelopmental diseases*, self-injurious behaviors are very common in children. Hence management plans include behavior therapies along with pharmacotherapy.[125] Higher prevalence of sleep disturbance is also associated with these diseases. In order to manage these problems, melatonin therapy is given to the patients.[126]

In *neurodegenerative diseases*, it is critical to prevent neuronal damage or death. As most of these diseases are late onset, certain therapies are given at initial stages in order to prevent or halt the progression of the diseases by either eliminating the primary stressor or by restoration of the neuronal function. Flavonoid-based therapies are among the therapies given in the early management of these diseases. These compounds are known to have neuroprotective as well as antioxidant properties.[127] In *neurological infections*, concentration of tumor necrosis factor in CSF is found to be reduced by the attenuation of inflammatory responses with adjunctive dexamethasone therapy.[41] Furthermore, with interfering the host-derived cytotoxin generation and restricting the release of toxic bacterial products are other approaches for adjunctive therapy.[128] Use of thrombolytics, β-blockers, statin therapy, and antiplatelet therapy treatment of cardiovascular risk factors (such as carotid stenosis), hypertension, diabetes mellitus, and dyslipidemia are used in the management of *CVA*.[129-131]

Current treatment and management strategies as well as prevention of these debilitating diseases are not effective in a broad spectrum. Hence, novel approaches are being explored to cure and manage these diseases by targeting the causative mechanisms at molecular level.

With the advancement in the field of molecular biology, various studies have shown that therapies such as stem cell therapy and gene therapy (CRISPR and siRNA) hold the potential to be the next-generation therapies for individuals suffering with neurological diseases. These strategies aim to cure diseases by tissue regeneration, gene editing, and gene silencing, respectively.[132] Among these, stem cells have the ability to modify into specific type of cells. They have the potential of self-renewal and differentiate into specialized adult cells. Stem cells have great potential for tissue regeneration; hence, they can be used for regenerating the damaged cells or tissues in case of these diseases especially in neurodegenerative diseases.[132] On the other hand, gene editing using CRISPR-Cas has emerged to be a promising approach in order to cure the diseases by the deletion of the aberrant gene or insertion of the corrected gene. In addition, gene silencing using siRNA silences the gene by inhibiting protein translation thereby silencing its expression.[133]

These strategies are currently being carried out in-vitro as well as in-vivo in various disease models of neuropathy. Some of these have reached the clinical trial stage.[134,135]

SPECIAL FEATURES IN THE INDIAN CONTEXT

Neurological diseases are quite prevalent in India. Diverse socioeconomic status, ethnicity, culture, genetics, and health system in India are the parameters responsible for considerable differences in the terms of prevalence of neurological diseases across different regions of the country.[12] Among various neurological diseases, stroke, headache, Parkinson's disease, epilepsy, and dementia are reported to contribute to high disease burden in India especially in the urban population.[1] DALY rate of various neurological diseases varies among different states of India. **Table 1** shows the Indian states with the highest DALY rate for different neurological diseases.

In North Indians, perinatal factors, lower socio-economic status, and consanguinity are the significant risk factors for the development of neurological diseases such as epilepsy, global developmental delay, and motor vision and hearing defects in children.[6] A study has reported that, long-term stay at high altitude as well as polycythemia are associated with higher risk of stroke in Indians.[136] The risk factors of Parkinson's diseases have been reported to be family history of Parkinson's disease, male gender, and past history of depression of up to 10-year duration.[137] In case of cerebral palsy, perinatal asphyxia and prematurity are considered to be the major risk factors.[138,139]

TABLE 1: Highest DALY rate of neurological diseases in Indian states as per the GBD, 2019.[12]

Neurological diseases	State
Stroke	West Bengal, Chhattisgarh, and Tripura
Headache	Goa, Tamil Nadu, and Himachal Pradesh
Epilepsy	Odisha, Karnataka, and Uttarakhand
Cerebral palsy	Himachal Pradesh, Kerala, and Arunachal Pradesh
Alzheimer's disease	Kerala, Goa, and Andhra Pradesh,
Parkinson's disease	Goa, Kerala, and Tamil Nadu
Brain and CNS cancer	Delhi, Karnataka, and Odisha
Multiple sclerosis	Punjab, Himachal Pradesh, and Uttarakhand
Motor neuron diseases	Goa, Uttarakhand, and Punjab

(CNS: central nervous system; DALY: disability-adjusted life-year; GBD: Global Burden of Disease)

CONCLUSION AND FUTURE PERSPECTIVE

Neurological diseases affect a large fraction of population worldwide. Among these diseases, headache and dementia are the most prevalent disorders across the globe. Dementia, Parkinson's disease, headache, epilepsy, and stroke are found to affect the Indian populations at the most. Since the burden of various neurological diseases affects a significant proportion of individuals across the globe, it becomes important to provide timely diagnosis for proper therapeutic interventions. It is a challenge to distinguish the diseases with overlapping symptoms. Therefore, the differential diagnostic approach is used for proper identification and diagnosis. Currently, various approaches such as neuroimaging, neuropsychological assessment, biochemical analysis, and genetic testing are being used to diagnose various neurological diseases.

Some of the single gene neurological diseases follow different Mendelian inheritance patterns whereas others are multifactorial in nature with genetic, epigenetic, and environmental contribution. Genetic testing, genetic counseling, and risk assessment are the components of genetic assessment which helps in detecting and avoiding the birth of individuals with neurological diseases.

Advances in molecular and technological research from DNA to behavioral levels are helping to delineate the pathophysiological mechanism implicated in the development of these disorders. However, future research in this direction should be based on the convergence of various approaches such as genomics, transcriptomics, and metabolomics or in other words it should be "systemic biology approach" to generate more knowledge about these debilitating diseases. Novel molecular therapeutic approaches such as CRISPR-Cas and siRNA, and use of stem cells hold lot of promise but it has to reach the reach the bedside yet.

REFERENCES

1. Gautam R, Sharma M. Prevalence and diagnosis of neurological disorders using different deep learning techniques: A meta-analysis. J Med Syst. 2020;44(2):1-24.
2. Raggi A, Monasta L, Beghi E, Caso V, Castelpietra G, Mondello S, et al., Incidence, prevalence and disability associated with neurological disorders in Italy between 1990 and 2019: An analysis based on the Global Burden of Disease Study 2019. J Neurol. 2022;269(4):2080-98.
3. Mehndiratta MM, Aggarwal V. Neurological disorders in India: past, present, and next steps. Lancet Glob Health. 2021;9(8):e1043-4.
4. Jiao Q, Sun H, Zhang H, Wang R, Li S, Sun D, et al. The combination of whole-exome sequencing and copy number variation sequencing enables the diagnosis of rare neurological disorders. Clin Genet. 2019;96(2):140-50.
5. Scelzo E, Kramer M, Sacco S, Proietti A, OrnelloR, Parati EA, et al. Migraine and rare neurological disorders. Neurol Sci. 2020;41(2):439-46.
6. Kumar R, Bhave A, Bhargava R, AgarwalKumar GG. Prevalence and risk factors for neurological disorders in children aged 6 months to 2 years in northern India. Dev Med Child Neurol. 2013;55(4):348-56.
7. Lyketsos CG, Kozauer N, Rabins PV. Psychiatric manifestations of neurologic disease: where are we headed? Dialogues in clinical neuroscience. 2007;9(2):111-24.
8. Dumurgier J, Tzourio C. Epidemiology of neurological diseases in older adults. Revue Neurologique. 2020;176(9):642-8.
9. Licher S, Darweesh SKL, Wolters FJ, Fani L, Heshmatollah A, Mutlu U, et al. Lifetime risk of common neurological diseases in the elderly population. J Neurol Neurosurg Psychiatry. 2019;90(2):148-56.

10. GBD 2015 Neurological Disorders Collaborator Group. Global, regional, and national burden of neurological disorders during 1990–2015: a systematic analysis for the Global Burden of Disease Study 2015. Lancet Neurol. 2017;16(11):877-97.
11. GBD 2019 Mental Disorders Collaborators. Global, regional, and national burden of 12 mental disorders in 204 countries and territories, 1990–2019: a systematic analysis for the Global Burden of Disease Study 2019. Lancet Psychiatry. 2022;9(2):137-50.
12. India State-Level Disease Burden Initiative Neurological Disorders Collaborators. The burden of neurological disorders across the states of India: the Global Burden of Disease Study 1990–2019. Lancet Glob Health, 2021;9(8):e1129-44.
13. Dijck AV, Silfhout ATV, Cappuyns E, van der Werf IM, Mancini GM, Tzschach A, et al. Clinical presentation of a complex neurodevelopmental disorder caused by mutations in ADNP. Biol Psychiatry. 2019;85(4):287-97.
14. Shang H, Zhao X, Zhang X. Neurodegenerative diseases in Pediatric Neuroimaging. Netherlands: Springer; 2022. pp. 211-4.
15. Jankovic J. Parkinson's disease: clinical features and diagnosis. J Neurol Neurosurg Psychiatry. 2008;79(4):368-76.
16. Hardiman O, Doherty CP. Neurodegenerative Disorders. Netherlands: Springer; 2011.
17. Crow EL. Cerebrovascular Accident in Pediatric Clinical Advisor. Netherlands: Elsevier; 2007. pp. 105-6.
18. Siddique MAN, Nur Z, Mahbub MS, Alam MB, Miah T. Clinical presentation and epidemiology of stroke: A study of 100 cases. J Med. 2009;10(2):86-9.
19. Beal CC. Gender and stroke symptoms: a review of the current literature. J Neurosci Nurs. 2010;42(2):80-7.
20. Glatzel, M, Stoeck K, Seeger H, Lührs T, Aguzzi A. Human prion diseases: Molecular and clinical aspects. Arch Neurol. 2005;62(4): 545-52.
21. Garvey G. Current concepts of bacterial infections of the central nervous system: bacterial meningitis and bacterial brain abscess. J Neurosurg. 1983;59(5):735-44.
22. Barichello T, Generoso JS, Milioli G, Elias SG, Teixeira AL. Pathophysiology of bacterial infection of the central nervous system and its putative role in the pathogenesis of behavioral changes. Braz J Psychiatry. 2013;35(1):81-7.
23. Schiess N, Villabona-Rueda A, Cottier KE, Huether K, Chipeta J, Stins MF. Pathophysiology and neurologic sequelae of cerebral malaria. Malaria J. 2020;19(1):1-12.
24. Abubakr A,Kablinger A, Caldito G. Psychogenic seizures: Clinical features and psychological analysis. Epilepsy Behav. 2003;4(3):241-5.
25. Camfield P, Camfield C. Epileptic syndromes in childhood: Clinical features, outcomes, and treatment. Epilepsia. 2002;43:27-32.
26. Saper JR. Headache disorders. Med Clin North Am. 1999;83(3): 663-90.
27. Murtaza M, Kisat M, Daniel H, Sonawalla AB. Classification and clinical features of headache disorders in Pakistan: a retrospective review of clinical data. PloS One. 2009;4(6):e5827.
28. Yamamoto T. Genomic Aberrations Associated with the Pathophysiological Mechanisms of Neurodevelopmental Disorders. Cells. 2021;10(9):2317.
29. Delhaye S, Bardoni B. Role of phosphodiesterases in the pathophysiology of neurodevelopmental disorders. Mol Psychiatry. 2021;26(9):4570-82.
30. Kosel M, Perroud N. Neurodevelopmental disorders: From pathophysiology to novel therapeutic approaches. Biomedicines 2022;10(3): 623.
31. Mosconi MW, Wang Z, Schmitt LM, Tsai P, Sweeney JA. The role of cerebellar circuitry alterations in the pathophysiology of autism spectrum disorders. Front Neurosci. 2015;9:296.
32. Yenkoyan K, Grigoryan A, Fereshetyan K, Yepremyan D Advances in understanding the pathophysiology of autism spectrum disorders. Behav Brain Res. 2017;31:92-101.
33. Jarskog LF, Glantz LA, Gilmore JH, Lieberman JA. Apoptotic mechanisms in the pathophysiology of schizophrenia. Prog Neuropsychopharmacol Biol Psychiatry. 2005;29(5):846-58.
34. Grace AA, Dysregulation of the dopamine system in the pathophysiology of schizophrenia and depression. Nat Rev Neurosci. 2016;17(8):524-32.
35. Meisenzahl E, Schmitt GJ, Scheuerecker J, Möller HJ. The role of dopamine for the pathophysiology of schizophrenia. Int Rev Psychiatry. 2007;19(4):337-45.
36. Balu DT, Coyle JT. Neuroplasticity signaling pathways linked to the pathophysiology of schizophrenia. Neurosci Biobehav Rev. 2011;35(3):848-70.
37. Bang S, Lee S, Choi N, Kim HN. Emerging brain-pathophysiology-mimetic platforms for studying neurodegenerative diseases: Brain organoids and brains-on-a-chip. Adv Healthc Mater. 2021;10(12):2002119.
38. Businaro R, Vauzour D, Sarris J, Münch G, Gyengesi E, Brogelli L, et al., Therapeutic opportunities for food supplements in neurodegenerative disease and depression. Front Nutr. 2021;8: 669846.
39. Sellner J, Täuber MG, Leib SL. Pathogenesis and pathophysiology of bacterial CNS infections. Handb Clin Neurol. 2010;96:1-16.
40. Kim TK, Lee I, Cho JH, Canine B, Keller A, Price ND, et al. Core transcriptional regulatory circuits in prion diseases. Mol Brain. 2020;13(1):1-14.
41. Tunkel AR, Scheld WM. Pathogenesis and pathophysiology of bacterial meningitis. Clin Microbiol Rev. 1993;6(2):118-36.
42. Quagliarello V, Scheld WM. Bacterial meningitis: pathogenesis, pathophysiology, and progress. N Engl J Med. 1992;327(12):864-72.
43. Baslet G. Psychogenic non-epileptic seizures: a model of their pathogenic mechanism. Seizure. 2011;20(1):1-13.
44. Vaughan CJ, Delanty N. (2002). Pathophysiology of acute symptomatic seizures. [online] Available from https://link.springer.com/chapter/10.1007/978-1-59259-094-0_2 [Last accessed May, 2023].
45. Fernández IS, Goodkin HP, Scott RC. Pathophysiology of convulsive status epilepticus. Seizure. 2019;68:16-21.
46. Chen SP, Ayata C. Spreading depression in primary and secondary headache disorders. Curr Pain Headache Rep. 2016;20(7):1-8.
47. May A, Cluster headache: Pathogenesis, diagnosis, and management. Lancet. 2005;366(9488):843-55.
48. Somjen GG. Mechanisms of spreading depression and hypoxic spreading depression-like depolarization. Physiolo Rev. 2001;81(3): 1065-96.
49. Bandettini PA. What's new in neuroimaging methods? Ann N Y Acad Sci. 2009;1156(1):260-93.
50. Pham ATT, Wallace A, Zhang X, Tohl D, Fu H, Chuah C, et al. Optical-based biosensors and their portable healthcare devices for detecting and monitoring biomarkers in body fluids. Diagnostics. 2021;11(7):1285.
51. Lezak MD, Howieson DB, Loring DW. Neuropsychological Assessment. USA: Oxford University Press; 2004.
52. Laatsch L. Neuropsychological assessment. Encyclopedia of Psychotherapy Editors-in-Chief. Elsevier Science (USA). 2002;(2)223-8.
53. Biskup S. Gasser T. Genetic testing in neurological diseases. J Neurol. 2012;259(6):1249-54.
54. Lange K, Elston R. Extensions to pedigree analysis. Hum Hered. 1975;25(2):95-105.
55. Holtzman NA. Promoting safe and effective genetic tests in the United States: work of the task force on genetic testing. Clin Chem. 1999;45(5):732-8.
56. Reyes S, Kurtz A, Hervé D, Tournier-Lasserve E, Chabriat H. Presymptomatic genetic testing in CADASIL. J Neurol. 2012; 259(10):2131-6.
57. Skirton H, Goldsmith L, Jackson L, Tibben A. Quality in genetic counselling for presymptomatic testing—clinical guidelines for practice across the range of genetic conditions. Eur J Hum Genet. 2013;21(3):256-60.
58. Godino L, Turchetti D, Jackson L, Hennessy C, Skirton H. Impact of presymptomatic genetic testing on young adults: a systematic review. Eur J Hum Genet. 2016;24(4):496-503.

59. Smith CO, Lipe HP, Bird TD. Impact of presymptomatic genetic testing for hereditary ataxia and neuromuscular disorders. Arch Neurol. 2004;61(6):875-80.
60. Wakabayashi T, Hidaka R, Fujimaki S, Asashima M, Kuwabara T. MicroRNAs and epigenetics in adult neurogenesis. Adv Genet. 2014;86:27-44.
61. Kalfoglou A, Suthers K, Scott J, Hudson K. (2004). Reproductive genetic testing: What America thinks. [online] Available from https://jscholarship.library.jhu.edu/handle/1774.2/976 [Last accessed May, 2023].
62. Kumuthini J, Zass L, Chimusa ER, Chaouch M, Masimiremwa C. (2018). Minimum Information Required for Pharmacogenomics Experiments. [online] Available from https://www.sciencedirect.com/science/article/abs/pii/B9780128094143000097?via%3Dihub [Last accessed may, 2023].
63. Haga SB, Burke W. Pharmacogenetic testing: Not as simple as it seems. Genet Med. 2008;10(6):391-5.
64. Ikediobi ON, Shin J, Nussubaum RL, Phillips KA, Walsh JM, Ladabaum U, Marshall D. Addressing the challenges of the clinical application of pharmacogenetic testing. Clin Pharmacol Ther. 2009;86(1):28-31.
65. Ma MK, Woo MH, Mcleod HL. Genetic basis of drug metabolism. Am J Health Sys Pharm. 2002. 59(21): p. 2061-2069.
66. Meyer UA. Pharmacogenetics and adverse drug reactions. Lancet. 2000;356(9242):1667-71.
67. Clarke W, McMillin G. Application of TDM, pharmacogenomics and biomarkers for neurological disease pharmacotherapy: focus on antiepileptic drugs. Per Med. 2006;3(2):139-49.
68. Nussbaum L, Hogea LM, Călina D, Andreescu N, Grădinaru R, Ştefănescu R, et al. Modern treatment approaches in psychoses. Pharmacogenetic, neuroimagistic and clinical implications. Farmacia. 2017;65(1):75-81.
69. Della-Morte D, Guadagni F, Palmirotta R, Testa G, Caso V, Paciaroni M, et al., Genetics of ischemic stroke, stroke-related risk factors, stroke precursors and treatments. Pharmacogenomics. 2012;13(5):595-613.
70. Ross S, Paré G. Pharmacogenetics of stroke. Stroke. 2018;49(10): 2541-8.
71. Kurzawski M, Białecka M, Droździk M, Pharmacogenetic considerations in the treatment of Parkinson's disease. Neurodegener Dis Manag. 2015;5(1):27-35.
72. Agúndez JA, García-Martín E, Alonso-Navarro H, Jiménez-Jiménez FJ. Anti-Parkinson's disease drugs and pharmacogenetic considerations. Expert Opin Drug Metabo Toxicol. 2013;9(7): 859-74.
73. Pienaar IS, Gartside SE, Sharma P, De Paola V, Gretenkord S, Withers D, et al. Pharmacogenetic stimulation of cholinergic pedunculopontine neurons reverses motor deficits in a rat model of Parkinson's disease. Mol Neurodegener. 2015;10(1):1-22.
74. Masellis, M, Collinson S, Freeman N, Tampakeras M, Levy J, Tchelet A, et al. Dopamine D2 receptor gene variants and response to rasagiline in early Parkinson's disease: A pharmacogenetic study. Brain. 2016;139(7):2050-62.
75. Stevenson RD. Use of segmental measures to estimate stature in children with cerebral palsy. Arch Pediatr and Adolesc Med. 1995;149(6):658-62.
76. Capi M, Gentile G, Lionetto L, Salerno G, Cipolla F, Curto M, et al. Pharmacogenetic considerations for migraine therapies. Expert Opin Drug Metabol Toxicol. 2018;14(11):1161-7.
77. Borro M, Guglielmetti M, Simmaco M, Martelletti P, Gentile G. The future of pharmacogenetics in the treatment of migraine. Pharmacogenomics. 2019;20(16):1159-73.
78. Jalonen M. Evaluation of pharmacogenomics and drug-drug interaction databases in migraine. Finland: Helsingin yliopisto; 2020.
79. Özdemir V, Basile VS, Masellis M, Kennedy JL. Pharmacogenetic assessment of antipsychotic-induced movement disorders: contribution of the dopamine D3 receptor and cytochrome P450 1A2 genes. J Biochem BiophysMethods. 2001;47(1-2):151-7.
80. de Leon J, Arranz MJ, Ruano G. Pharmacogenetic testing in psychiatry: a review of features and clinical realities. Clin Lab Med. 2008;28(4):599-617.
81. Katsanis SH, Katsanis N. Molecular genetic testing and the future of clinical genomics. Nat Rev Genet. 2013;14(6):415-26.
82. Korf BR, Liu N. Human Genome Project, Genomics, and Clinical Research. In: Gallin J, Ognibene F (Eds). Principles and Practice of Clinical Research. Nederland: Elsevier; 2012. pp. 707-25.
83. Lai D, Schwantes-An TH, Corbin TJ, White KE. Skeletal Genetics: From Gene Identification to Murine Models of Disease. In: Burr DB, Allen MR. Basic and Applied Bone Biology, 2nd edition. Nederland: Elsevier; 2019. pp. 159-85.
84. Xie X, Wu X, Su L, Cai M, Li Y, Huang H, et al. Application of single nucleotide polymorphism microarray in prenatal diagnosis of fetuses with central nervous system abnormalities. Int J Gen Med. 2021;14:4239-46.
85. Vissers LE, de Vries BB, Veltman JJ. Genomic microarrays in mental retardation: from copy number variation to gene, from research to diagnosis. J Med Genet. 2010;47(5):289-97.
86. Byeon JH, Shin E, Kim GH, Lee K, Hong YS, Lee JW, et al. Application of array-based comparative genomic hybridization to pediatric neurologic diseases. Yonsei Med J. 2014;55(1):30-6.
87. Charan P, Woodrow N, Walker SP, Ganesamoorthy D, McGillivray G, Palma-Dias R. High-resolution microarray in the assessment of fetal anomalies detected by ultrasound. Aust N Z J Obstet Gynaecol. 2014;54(1):46-52.
88. Liang JS, Shimojima K, Yamamoto T. Application of array-based comparative genome hybridization in children with developmental delay or mental retardation. Pediat Neonatol. 2008;49(6):213-7.
89. Bayani J. Squire JA. Fluorescence in situ Hybridization (FISH). Curr Protoc Cell Biol. 2004;23(1):Chapter 22:Unit 22.4.
90. Volpi EV, Bridger JM. FISH glossary: An overview of the fluorescence in situ hybridization technique. Biotechniques. 2008;45(4):385-409.
91. Ratan ZA, Zaman SB, Mehta V, Haidere MF, Runa NJ, Akter N. Application of fluorescence in situ hybridization (FISH) technique for the detection of genetic aberration in medical science. Cureus. 2017;9(6):e1325.
92. Hömig-Hölzel C, Savola S. Multiplex ligation-dependent probe amplification (MLPA) in tumor diagnostics and prognostics. Diagn Mol Pathol. 2012;21(4):189-206.
93. Jeuken J, Sijben A, Alenda C, Rijntjes J, Dekkers M, Boots-Sprenger S, et al. Robust detection of EGFR copy number changes and EGFR variant III: technical aspects and relevance for glioma diagnostics. Brain Pathol. 2009;19(4):661-71.
94. Jeuken J, Cornelissen S, Boots-Sprenger S, Gijsen S, Wesseling P. Multiplex ligation-dependent probe amplification: A diagnostic tool for simultaneous identification of different genetic markers in glial tumors. J Mol Diagn. 2006;8(4):433-43.
95. Mei D, Parrini E, Pasqualetti M, Tortorella G, Franzoni E, Giussani U, et al. Multiplex ligation-dependent probe amplification detects DCX gene deletions in band heterotopia. Neurology. 2007;68(6):446-50.
96. Schwartz M, Dunø M. Improved molecular diagnosis of dystrophin gene mutations using the multiplex ligation-dependent probe amplification method. Genetic Testing. 2004;8(4):361-7.
97. Rooms L, Reyniers E, van Luijk R, Scheers S, Wauters J, Ceulemans B, et al. Subtelomeric deletions detected in patients with idiopathic mental retardation using multiplex ligation-dependent probe amplification (MLPA). Hum Mutat. 2004;23(1):17-21.
98. Crompton D, Rehal PK, MacPherson L, Foster K, Lunt P, Hughes I, et al. Multiplex ligation-dependent probe amplification (MLPA) analysis is an effective tool for the detection of novel intragenic PLA2G6 mutations: implications for molecular diagnosis. Mol Genet Metabol. 2010100(2):207-12.
99. Hsieh, M, Lin SJ, Chen JF, Lin HM, Hsiao KM, Li SY, et al. Identification of the spinocerebellar ataxia type 7 mutation in Taiwan: application of PCR-based Southern blot. J Neurol. 2000;247(8):623-9.
100. Hsiao KM, Lin HM, Pan H, Li TC, Chen SS, Jou SB, et al. Application of FTA® sample collection and DNA purification system on the

determination of CTG trinucleotide repeat size by PCR-based southern blotting. J Clin Lab Anal. 1999;13(4):188-93.
101. Lakeman FD, Whitley RJ. Diagnosis of herpes simplex encephalitis: application of polymerase chain reaction to cerebrospinal fluid from brain-biopsied patients and correlation with disease. J Infect Dis. 1995;171(4):857-63.
102. Beck J, Poulter M, Hensman D, Rohrer JD, Mahoney CJ, Adamson G, et al. Large C9orf72 hexanucleotide repeat expansions are seen in multiple neurodegenerative syndromes and are more frequent than expected in the UK population. Am J Hum Genet. 2013;92(3):345-53.
103. Derveaux S, Vandesompele J, Hellemans J. How to do successful gene expression analysis using real-time PCR. Methods. 2010;50(4): 227-30.
104. Monteyne P, Laere VV, Marichal R, Sindic CJ. Cytokine mRNA expression in CSF and peripheral blood mononuclear cells in multiple sclerosis: detection by RT-PCR without in vitro stimulation. J Neuroimmunol. 1997;80(1-2):137-42.
105. Berti R, Williams AJ, Moffett JR, Hale SL, Velarde LC, Elliott PJ, et al., Quantitative real-time RT—PCR analysis of inflammatory gene expression associated with Ischemia—Reperfusion brain Injury. J Cereb Blood Flow Metab. 2002;22(9):1068-79.
106. Rydbirk R, Folke J, Winge K, Aznar S, Pakkenberg B, Brudek T. Assessment of brain reference genes for RT-qPCR studies in neurodegenerative diseases. Sci Rep. 2016;6(1):1-11.
107. Borovecki F, Lovrecic L, Zhou J, Jeong H, Then F, Rosas HD, et al. Genome-wide expression profiling of human blood reveals biomarkers for Huntington's disease. Proc Natl Acad Sci. 2005;102(31):11023-8.
108. Trayhurn P. Northern blotting. Proceed Nutr Soc. 1996;55(1B):583-9.
109. Mirnics K, Middleton FA, Lewis DA, Levitt P. Analysis of complex brain disorders with gene expression microarrays: schizophrenia as a disease of the synapse. Trends Neurosci. 2001;24(8):479-86.
110. Heller MJ. DNA microarray technology: devices, systems, and applications. Ann Rev Biomed Eng. 2002;4(1):129-53.
111. Whitney LW, Becker KG, Tresser NJ, Caballero-Ramos CI, Munson PJ, Prabhu VV, et al. Analysis of gene expression in multiple sclerosis lesions using cDNA microarrays. Ann Neurol.1999;46(3):425-8.
112. Ginsberg SD, Crino PB, Hemby SE, Weingarten JA, Lee VM, Eberwine JH, et al. Predominance of neuronal mRNAs in individual Alzheimer's disease senile plaques. Ann Neurol. 1999;45(2):174-81.
113. Straiton J, Free T, Sawyer A, Martin J. From Sanger sequencing to genome databases and beyond. Biotechniques. 2019;66(2):60-3.
114. Ari Ş, Arikan M. Next-generation sequencing: Advantages, disadvantages, and future. In: Hakeem KR, Tombuloğlu H, Tombuloğlu G (Eds). Plant omics: Trends and Applications. Switzerland: Springer; 2016. pp. 109-35.
115. Crossley BM, Bai J, Glaser A, Maes R, Porter E, Killian ML, et al. Guidelines for Sanger sequencing and molecular assay monitoring. J Vet Diagn Invest. 2020;32(6):767-75.
116. Gomes A, Korf B. Genetic Testing Techniques. In: Robin N, Farmer M. Pediatric Cancer Genetics, Netherlands: Elsevier; 2018.
117. Solomon DA. Integrating Molecular Diagnostics with Surgical Neuropathology. In: Perry A, Brat DJ. Practical Surgical Neuropathology: A Diagnostic Approach. Netherlands: Elsevier: 2018. pp. 71-89.
118. Jiang T, Tan MS, Tan L, Yu JT. Application of next-generation sequencing technologies in Neurology. Ann Transl Med. 2014;2(12):125.
119. Rexach J, Lee H, Martinez-Agosto JA, Németh AH, Fogel BL, et al. Clinical application of next-generation sequencing to the practice of neurology. Lancet Neurol. 2019;18(5):492-503.
120. Matos CM, Alonso I, Leão M. Diagnostic yield of next-generation sequencing applied to neurological disorders. J Clin Neurosci. 2019;67:14-8.
121. Bras J, Guerreiro R, Hardy J. Use of next-generation sequencing and other whole-genome strategies to dissect neurological disease. Nat Rev Neurosci. 2012;13(7):453-64.
122. Turro E, Astle WJ, Megy K, Gräf S, Greene D, Shamardina O, et al., Whole-genome sequencing of patients with rare diseases in a national health system. Nature. 2020;583(7814):96-102.
123. Alazami AM, Patel N, Shamseldin HE, Anazi S, Al-Dosari MS, Alzahrani F, et al. Accelerating novel candidate gene discovery in neurogenetic disorders via whole-exome sequencing of prescreened multiplex consanguineous families. Cell Rep. 2015;10(2):148-61.
124. Baptista PV. Principles in genetic risk assessment. Ther Clin Risk Manag. 2005;1(1):15-20.
125. Sabus A, Feinstein J, Romani P, Goldson E, Blackmer A. Management of self-injurious behaviors in children with neurodevelopmental disorders: A pharmacotherapy overview. Pharmacotherapy. 2019;39(6):645-64.
126. Abdelgadir IS, Gordon MA, Akobeng AK. Melatonin for the management of sleep problems in children with neurodevelopmental disorders: A systematic review and meta-analysis. Arch Dis Child. 2018;103(12):1155-62.
127. Solanki I, Parihar P, Mansuri ML, Parihar MS. Flavonoid-based therapies in the early management of neurodegenerative diseases. Adv Nutr. 2015;6(1):64-72.
128. Koedel U, Klein M, Pfister HW. New understandings on the pathophysiology of bacterial meningitis. Curr Opin Infect Dis. 2010;23(3):217-23.
129. Albertson M, Sharma J. Stroke: Current concepts. S D Med. 2014;67(11):455.
130. Farkhondeh T, Samarghandian S, Yazdi HS, Samini F. The protective effects of crocin in the management of neurodegenerative diseases: A review. Am J Neurodegener dis. 2018;7(1):1.
131. Musuka TD, Wilton SB, Traboulsi M, Hill MD. Diagnosis and management of acute ischemic stroke: speed is critical. CMAJ. 2015;187(12):887-93.
132. Biehl JK, Russell B. Introduction to stem cell therapy. J Cardiovasc Nurs 2009;24(2):98-103;quiz 104-5.
133. Gonçalves GAR, Paiva RDMA. Terapia gênica: avanços, desafios e perspectivas. Einstein (São Paulo). 2017;15:369-75.
134. Tsai ST, Lee CH, Lin SZ, Ding DC. Stem cell therapy in stroke. Vessel Plus, 2021. 5: p. 9.
135. Suda S, Nito C, Yokobori S, Sakamoto Y, Nakajima M, Sowa K, et al., Recent advances in cell-based therapies for ischemic stroke. Int J Mol Sci. 2020;21(18):6718.
136. Jha SK, Anand AC, Sharma V, Kumar N, Adya CM. Stroke at high altitude: Indian experience. High Alt Med Biol. 2002;3(1):21-7.
137. Behari M, Srivastava AK, Das RR, Pandey RM. Risk factors of Parkinson's disease in Indian patients. J Neurol Sci. 2001;190(1-2): 49-55.
138. Chauhan A, Singh M, Jaiswal N, Agarwal A, Sahu JK, Singh M. Prevalence of cerebral palsy in Indian children: a systematic review and meta-analysis. Indian J Pediatr. 2019;86(12):1124-30.
139. Singhi PD, Ray M, Suri G. Clinical spectrum of cerebral palsy in North India—an analysis of 1000 cases. J Trop Pediatr. 2002;48(3):162-6.

5

SECTION

Investigations

111

CHAPTER

Electroencephalography

Sita Jayalakshmi, Anuja Patil

INTRODUCTION

Electroencephalography (EEG) is one of the most crucial and indispensable investigations for the evaluation of epilepsy as well as many other neurological disorders. Despite the recent advances in the structural and functional imaging, EEG still stands the test of time by providing the dynamic real-time assessment of cerebral activity. The concept of EEG has evolved since times when cerebral imaging was not as readily available. The paroxysmal discharges as well as basic rhythm changes and patterns were correlated with many epileptic as well as nonepileptic neurological conditions. The vast data generated needs astute interpretation and clinical application. Reading EEG is an art, a legacy passed on over generations via books and clinicians. Although detailed discussion over every aspect of this topic might be out of scope for this chapter, an attempt has been made to present as much information in a concise and practical manner.

The concept that electrical activity generated by nerve cells may play a role in behavior was postulated as early as 18th century. An initial attempt by British Physician, Richard Caton (1842–1926), to record cerebral electrical activity was made using a galvanometer on rabbits. This paved way for clinical *"electroencephalogram" in Greek "electr" meaning electric, "encephalon" meaning enkephalos, and gram from graphein meaning to write.* By 1929, Hans Berger, originally an Austrian neuropsychiatrist, published his first report on human EEG[1] and became widely known as the father of EEG. He used a bipolar fronto-occipital recording along with a simultaneous electrocardiogram and time marker, much like the present-day EEG tracing. He described the basic EEG rhythms, and variability noted with sleep and eye closure. Most of his work gained popularity much later (1969), after the English translation of his German text notes.

GENERATION OF THE EEG ACTIVITY

The human central nervous system (CNS) constitutes mainly neurons, which function as transmitter of signals and glial elements, which are the supporting elements. The neurons are arranged in a laminar pattern and the glial elements are located in-between these neurons. Each neuron consists of a cell body, which contains a nucleus, and it has numerous small branches which subsequently ramify, known as the dendrites. These dendrites make contact with other neurons. Each neuron has a membrane potential, which is the difference in voltage between inside and outside of cell's membrane, normally around –70 millivolts (mV). This potential is usually due to concentration difference of various ions between the intracellular and extracellular compartments with sodium ions present extracellularly and potassium ions in the intracellular compartment. The influx and efflux of ions make the inside of neuron more positive (depolarized). When this depolarization reaches a critical threshold, an action potential is generated **(Figs. 1 and 2)**. The action potential is a brief, larger amplitude potential, which has the phenomenon of all or none. *Sink* is the site where extracellular space is relatively negative and positive ions rush into depolarize, while *source* is the site where extracellular space is relatively positive and current flows

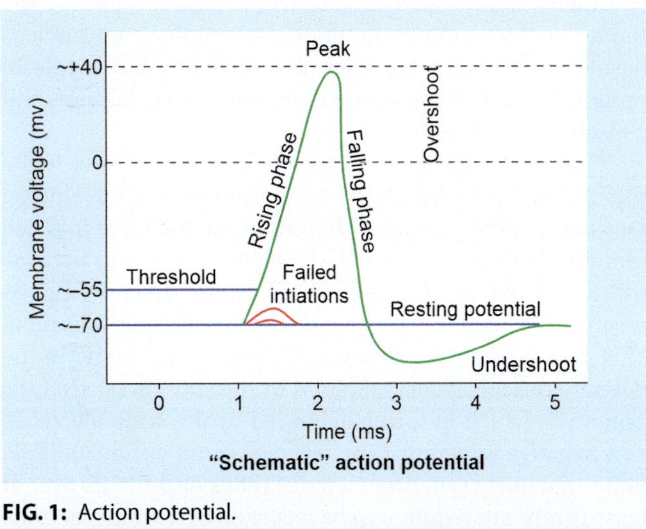

FIG. 1: Action potential.

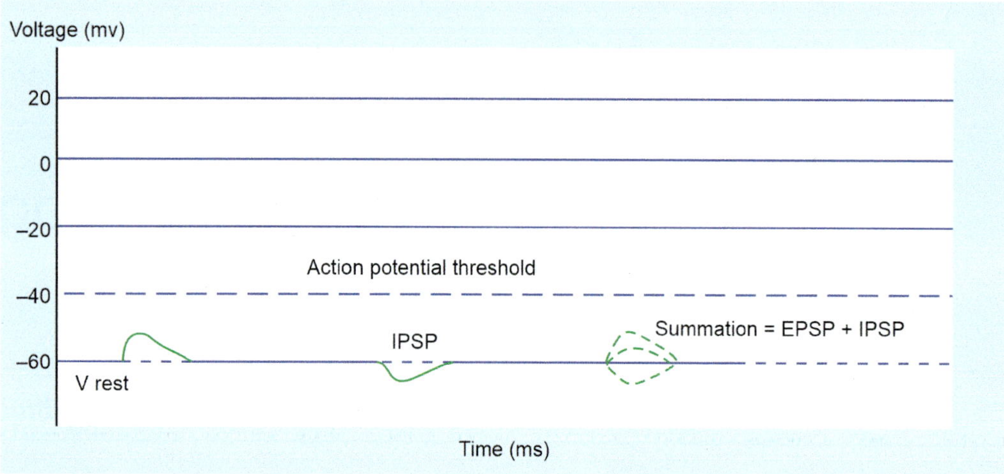

FIG. 2: Generation of EPSP and IPSP.
(EPSP: excitatory postsynaptic potential; IPSP: inhibitory postsynaptic potential)

out of the cell. The synapses that, in this way, excite nerve cells to discharge impulses are called excitatory synapses, and the depolarizing potentials that excitatory synapses produce in the postsynaptic membrane are called excitatory postsynaptic potentials (EPSPs). A second class of synapses that oppose excitation and tend to prevent the generation of impulses by excitatory synapses are called inhibitory synapses and the depolarizing potentials that inhibitory synapses produce in the postsynaptic membrane are called inhibitory postsynaptic potentials (IPSPs).

The conventional EEG is a spatial map recorded at the scalp surface, which records the synaptic activity of the cortex beneath **(Fig. 3)**. The EEG signals are generated due to summation of the excitatory and inhibitory potentials across the neurons. Human neocortex is a complex array of distinct layers and columns. Most of the cortical regions consist of six layers, with the pyramidal cells of Betz lying in layer 5. Each pyramidal cell's dendrites spanning over 3 mm form almost 10^{10} synapses constituting a macrocolumn driven by a unique thalamocortical input.[2] Other pathways including the dopaminergic projections form locus coeruleus, serotoninergic pathways from mesencephalic Raphe nucleus, and cholinergic projections from nucleus basalis of Meynert, although less specific, play a role in modulating the synaptic potentials as per sensory inputs and consciousness level.

The EPSPs generate negative EEG waveforms while the inhibitory potentials generate the positive waveforms. During an EPSP, positive charges enter the neuronal cell membrane thus causing the extracellular space to become more negatively charged, while more distant regions around the cell become relatively positively charged. This creates a dipole directed toward the positivity in the deeper cortical layers compared to the superficial synaptic potentials which in turn is recorded by the scalp electrode as a negative waveform. The reverse occurs during an IPSP. Simultaneously synchronized net IPSPs and EPSPs over at least 10 cm^2 are required to be recorded by a scalp electrode

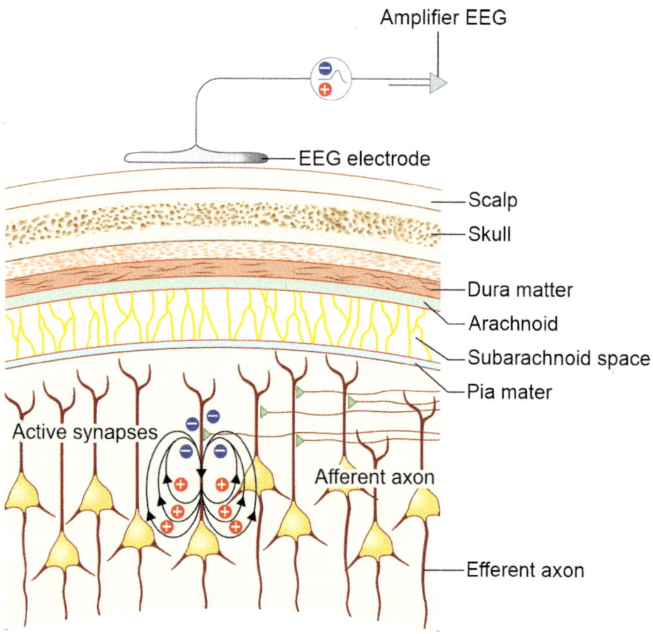

FIG. 3: EEG recording and relation to the neurons.
(EEG: electroencephalography)

as a specific discharge or pattern.[3] Summation of numerous small dipoles generates a current strong enough to be recorded at the surface. An electrode positioned directly over the excitatory cortical region will record a spike due to full force of the field generated, while the electrodes farther away will record lesser field causing smaller signals and those on opposite side of the cortical region will record inverted polarity though smaller signals. Also, the recording mainly oversees the superficial cortical surface as that along the deeper sulcal spaces carries the same dipole oriented in opposite directions due to the same cortical surface lining the sulci essentially cancelling out each other. The spatial orientation of the active neurons determines the generation of interictal and ictal discharges while the background activity will be generated by the underlying synaptic connections across all the neurons of layer IV and V. In view of the vast amount of information generated and high probability of artifacts due to intricacies in the recording, knowing the basic principles of recording an EEG should be known to interpret it correctly.

TECHNICAL ASPECTS OF EEG

The EEG recording involves measuring the potential difference between one surface electrode and either the next paired electrode or a reference electrode. The charges at the electrodes are passed through cables to high-impedance amplifier. The electrodes are about 10-mm sized cupped disks made of nonpolarized inert metals like silver chloride or gold to minimize the impedance for current flow. The electrode cups are filled with conducting paste rich in NaCl to maintain good contact between the electrode paste and skin, which generates electrode potential. Electrode impedance of >5,000Ω can cause noise artifacts while <100Ω means salt bridge causing short between surrounding electrodes.[4] Therefore, electrode impedance should be tested after applying the electrodes to the scalp, before and at the end of recording. Electrodes are applied as per standard arrays by International Federation of Clinical Neurophysiology (IFCN) called the international 10-20 system. Here, electrodes are placed successively at 10 or 20% of distance between landmark points of skull, such as nasion to inion, and left and right preauricular points **(Fig. 4)**. The standard names consist of first a letter abbreviation indicating the brain region and next a number

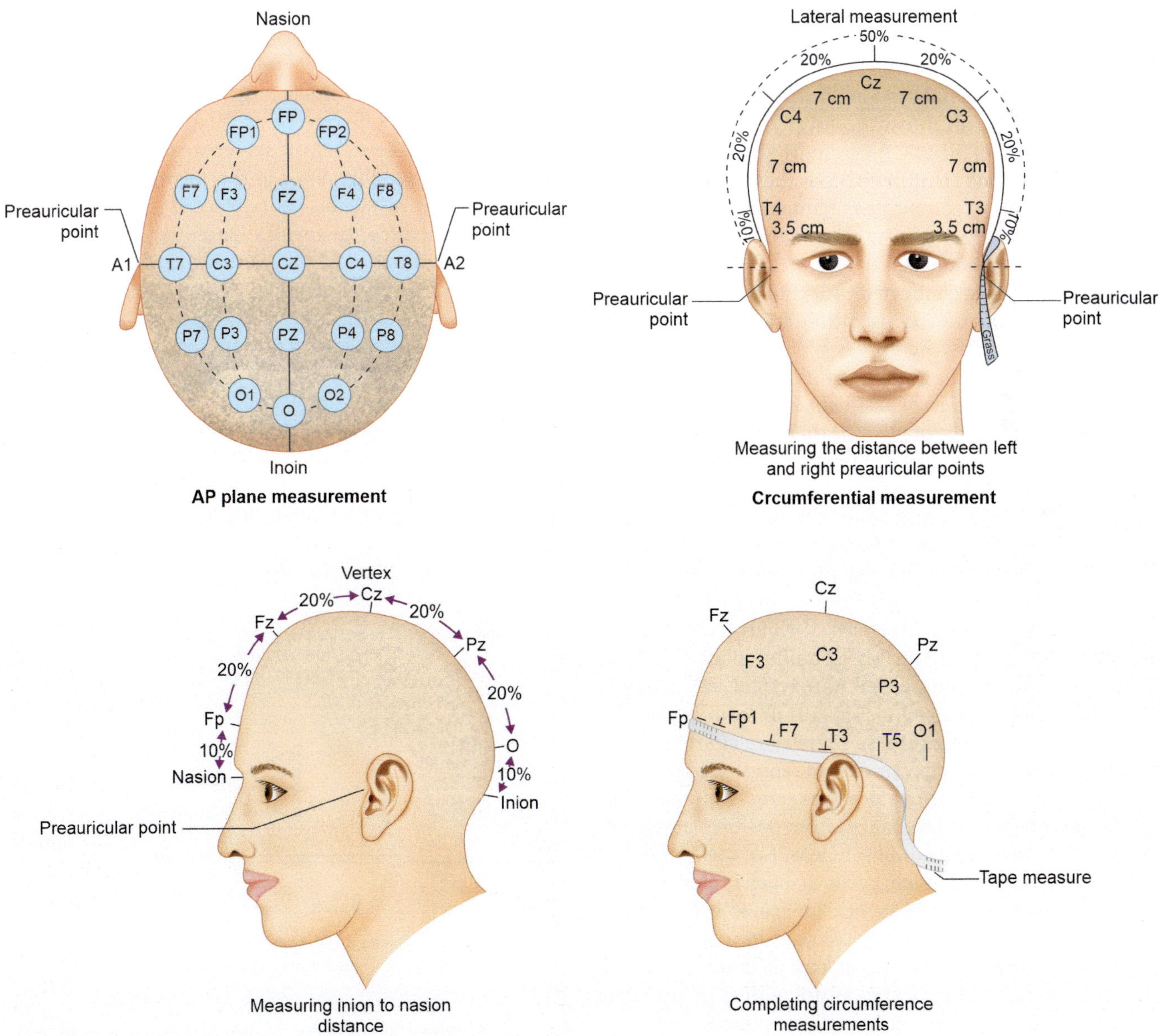

FIG. 4: International 10–20 system of electrode placement.

suggesting precise position at the location: Fp (frontopolar), F (frontal), C (central), P (parietal), O (occipital), and T (temporal). "Even" numbered electrodes indicate right side, "odd" numbers left side, while those at midline are denoted with letter "z". The nomenclature is not exclusive because clinically electrodes F7 and F8 record anterior temporal along with frontal region while P7 (T5) and P8 (T6) as per old 10-20 system record posterior temporal rather than parietal region. The standard IFCN array extends recording electrodes up to basal part of temporal lobe with T9 and T10. This has mostly supplanted need for sphenoidal electrodes used earlier to record inferior temporal regions.

Use of digital interpolation of the recorded electrode potentials can give localization details at points in-between the actual electrodes of the array. In addition to these, additional ground electrodes are connected to the jack box. The equipment in the EEG laboratory must be grounded to a common point, while the patient is connected with a separate "isolated" or "floating" ground electrode so that no ground loops are formed and current does not flow through the patient to the ground. One or more reference electrodes are also connected to the scalp. An ECG electrode forms an essential part of all EEG recordings giving information about likely cardiac rhythm changes due to or leading to ictal semiologies. In some cases, additional EMG channels may be required to monitor the correlation of movements or myoclonic jerks with ictal discharges.

Each electrode is connected with channels to amplifiers after a protection unit or isolation transformer, which ensures patient safety by one-way current transfer from patient's end toward the amplifiers and blocking the reverse. The potentials recorded at scalp surface are of very small amplitudes in the range of μVs. The differential amplifiers or grids magnify these potentials; the degree of amplification is called as *gain*. They also help in reducing the noise by subtracting out the components common to two inputs and only amplifying the difference in voltage between them. The analog signals are digitally converted into virtual signals. The sensitivity ranges from as low as 2-3 μV/mm (used to see low-amplitude signals as while reviewing brain death) to 100 μV/mm (for high-amplitude patterns like hypsarrhythmia or generalized paroxysmal fast activity). Conventionally, sensitivity of 7 (5-10) μV/mm is used for routine EEG recordings.[5] These signals are charted across the time windows during recording to represent a rhythm of voltage differences of various locations across the timeframe. The signals involve cyclic changes from positive to negative polarity. For accurate recording, at least two measurements need to be done for each cycle at each polarity. This represents the sampling frequency, for example, for a signal of 25 Hz, meaning 25 polarity changes in a second, one needs to measure the potentials at least 50 times per second (twice the number of cycles) so as not to miss or attenuate the signals. Thus, higher the sampling frequency, better is the resolution. For standard clinical EEG, the minimum sampling frequency should be 128 samples per second. Most of the modern EEG machines record at 256 Hz but may go up to as high as 2,000 Hz.[4]

Electroencephalogram amplifiers are designed to serve two main functions: differential discrimination and amplification. Discrimination is the ability of the amplifier to reveal differences in electrical potential between the amplifier inputs 1 and 2 while rejecting the potentials which are common to both. Signals from each electrode are led to a differential amplifier which subtracts one signal's voltage in relation to some reference electrode (which is usually the ground) from another signal, in relation to the same reference, and amplifies the difference. Signals common to both inputs of an amplifier are said to be in phase or common mode and are cancelled. Noise from a 50-Hz current line is an example of a signal likely to be in phase at all inputs and hence rejected. The ability of an amplifier to reject in-phase and amplify out of phase potentials is measured by *common-mode rejection ratio* (CMRR) of the amplifier. Good EEG amplifiers have a CMRR of at least 1,000. Analog machine has a CMRR 10,000 (80 dB). This means that an in-phase signal has to be 10,000 times larger than an out of phase signal in order for both to be recorded as the same size. The CMRR of digital EEG is >105 dB. It is important that reference electrode is reasonably close to the recording electrodes so that major noise signals get rejected by common mode (CMMR). While recording with differential amplifiers, the polarity convention for display is that negative waveforms cause an upward deflection and positive waveforms cause a downward deflection. If input 1 becomes more negative than the input 2, the signal deflects upward **(Fig. 5)** and if input 1 becomes more positive than input 2, then the signal deflects downward. This convention leads to the principle of *phase reversal* of the EEG signal. By this phenomenon, the negative potentials can be localized to an electrode demonstrating phase reversal between two channels sharing a common electrode. Such extracellular negativity occurs during

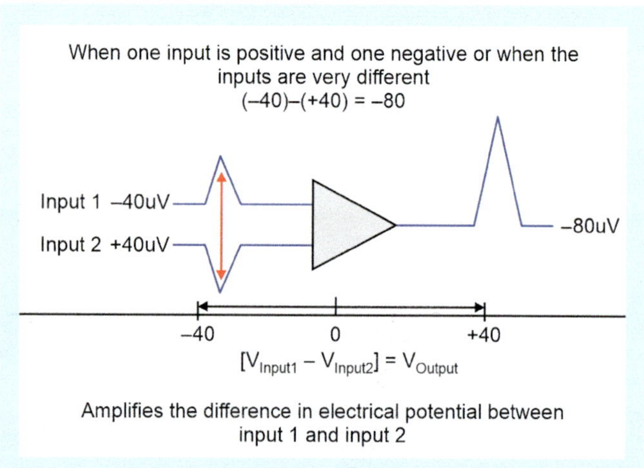

FIG. 5: Differential amplification in the EEG machine—amplifies the difference in the voltage at the two inputs (Input 1 – Input 2 = Output).

interictal spikes near an epileptic focus due to sudden influx of positive ions into the depolarizing neurons.

Apart from the synaptic potentials, the electrodes may record the noise, high-frequency signals from muscles, and surrounding electric structures. A high-frequency or low-pass filter attenuates signals of frequencies higher than the set value. Along with filtering out the high-frequency muscle artifacts from the scalp, this might at times attenuate high-frequency spikes in EEG as well. A low-frequency or high-pass filter attenuates the slower components like sweat artifacts, but may also attenuate slow frequency discharges or rhythms. Notch filters eliminate the electrical noise due to AC circuits during the recording. The recommended EEG settings are 0.5–1 Hz of high-pass filter, 70 Hz for low-pass filter and 50 Hz for the notch filter.[6]

Conventionally, negative potentials are shown as upward deflections while positive as downward. Usually, 10-second record is displayed on a routine computer screen. Each EEG channel display is similar to oscilloscope recording time on a horizontal axis from left to right while potential differences plotted vertically, where each second corresponds to 30 mm (30 mm/second). The paper speed (as per nomenclature for old analog EEG machines) can be adjusted during interpretation. Higher paper speed (60 or more mm per second) helps to better analyze rapidly propagating ictal discharges and to differentiate EMG artifacts from EEG fast activity. While slower paper speed (15 or less mm per second) helps in compressed visualization of periodic discharges or other EEG patterns. Slower paper speed helps in better visualization of periodic discharges (PDs).

The recordings derived thus from all the electrodes are compiled together and displayed in the form of montage (French for putting together or assembly similar to films compiled together from different video clips). Different montages need to be studied for proper interpretation of the recording **(Fig. 6)**. In a relatively circumscribed source with radial dipole oriented outward, the electrode overlying will show maximum peak negativity in referential montage while in bipolar montage, the overlying electrode will show peak negativity while the adjacent one will pick a positive

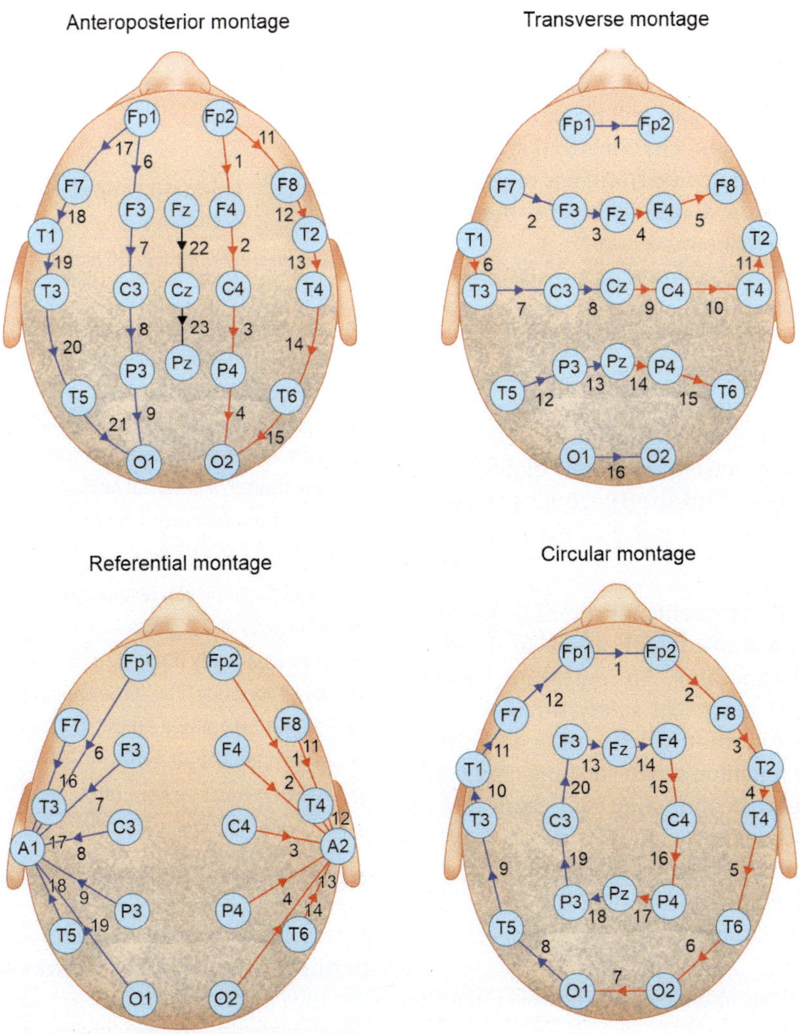

FIG. 6: The various types of montages.

signal subsequently showing a "negative phase reversal". With a more widespread source, two or more overlying electrodes will pick same potential, thereby the combined channel showing zero difference, isoelectric line, and phase reversal between channels before or after the isoelectric lines. In sources situated at either frontal or occipital poles, the peak negativity will be picked up by the end electrode of the chain, thus phase reversal is not seen rather only positive or negative deflection is noted in the end electrode (start or end of chain phenomenon). Tangentially oriented sources located in sulcus cause a positive and a negative pole on the scalp.

A bipolar montage can be in form of longitudinal, transverse, or circular arrangement. An identical potential in input 2 of one channel and input 1 of the next channel causes waveform deflections in opposite direction between these two channels. This reversal of phase is referred to as *instrumental phase reversal* because it only occurs by virtue of the arrangement of electrodes in successive channels and not because the polarity of the waveforms produced by the brain is reversed. The latter would be referred to as *true phase reversals*, which are quite uncommon. They are identified by the presence of a single-phase reversal in a reference montage or a double-phase reversal in a bipolar montage. Potentials that appear with greatest voltage in the last electrode in the chain of electrodes will produce waveform deflections in the chain of bipolar channels that are all in the same direction (i.e., no phase reversal) and it is referred to as *end of the chain phenomenon*. A circular bipolar montage is ideally used to study such a phenomenon.

Common electrode reference montages consist of a series of derivations in which same electrode is used in input 2 of each amplifier. Input 2 is ideally at a distance from the source of activity of interest so that it does not get intermixed with the activity occurring at the input 1 electrode. It is ideal for recording of high amplitude widely distributed activity. *Average reference montage* consists of a series of derivations in which potentials across all of the 10–20 electrodes are added together and placed in input 2 of every amplifier **(Table 1)**.

Electrical safety: Safety requirements for the EEG machines are more stringent than those which apply to domestic or industrial electrical apparatus. An important measure in defining standards of electrical safety for biomedical equipment is the leakage current which could pass through the patient's body if the machine's own earthing connection were disrupted. Both earth connection and earth leakage current of new apparatus must be checked on delivery and rechecked at regular intervals during routine maintenance. Extension cords should not be used with EEG machines. Use one common ground for all machines, for example, in the intensive care unit.

The optimum conditions and checklist for EEG recording are given in **Box 1**.

TABLE 1: Advantages and disadvantages of different EEG montages.

Montage	Advantages	Disadvantages
Bipolar	Effective in localizing the peak negative source, showing artifacts like eye movements, salt bridges	Poor detection of larger sources, distortion of actual waveforms, might miss strictly vertical (longitudinal or antero-posterior) or horizontal tangential (transverse) dipoles
Referential	Localization of greatest amplitude, visualizing positive potential of a dipole, comparison across all electrodes	Signals from the active reference electrode may contaminate the recordings
Common average	Precise representation of waveforms, visualization of diffuse abnormalities	Salt bridges between two adjacent electrodes may not be detected, erroneously show generalized discharges when several electrodes are active in one region
Laplacian (source derivation)	Shows electrode with highest potential, effective to read multifocal recording	Might miss more widespread slow waves

(EEG: electroencephalography)

BOX 1 Standard conditions and checklist for EEG recording.

Optimum conditions for EEG recording are:
- Quiet place
- Little machine vibrations
- The examination is best conducted in a shield room
- Low humidity
- Observation window should be there or monitoring camera to observe the patient's condition
- Low source of external noise
- Away from MRI room, X-ray, machines, artificial ventilator, syringe pump, cell phone etc.

Checklist for good EEG recording is:
- Sensitivity at 7 μV/mm
- High-frequency filter at 70 Hz
- Low-frequency filter/time constant at 1.6 Hz and 0.1 s
- Calibration voltage 50 μV
- Paper speed at 30 mm/s
- AC filters must be kept off

ACTIVATION PROCEDURES

Apart from passively recording the EEG, sometimes performing certain procedures to stimulate or reproduce the EEG discharges may be necessary. Routinely performed ones include mental alerting tasks, done early during

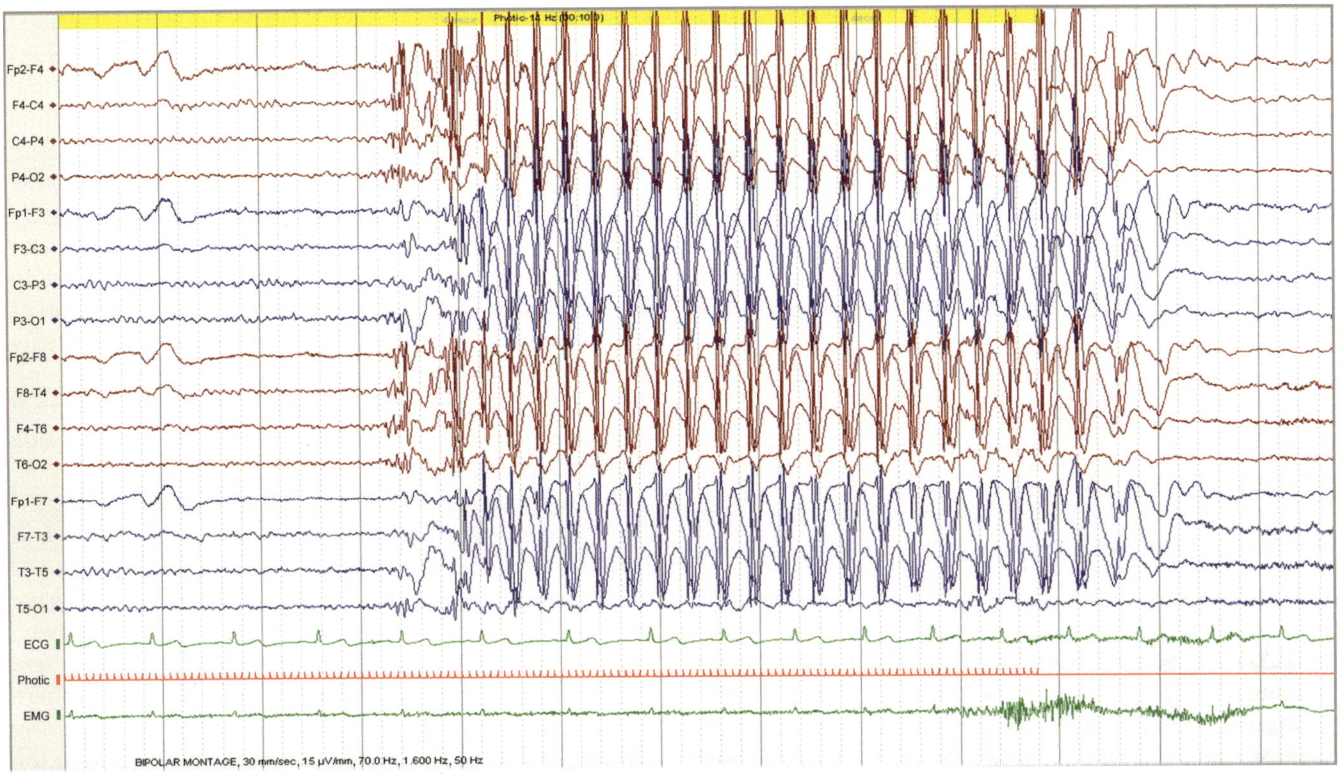

FIG. 7: Photoparoxysmal response in a case of idiopathic generalized epilepsy.

the recording, as the person undergoing the recording may fall asleep later. Calling out, testing response time, and mental arithmetic tests may attenuate posterior dominant rhythm and help to differentiate slow rhythms due to drowsiness (which will improve on alerting) versus pathological slowing. Hyperventilation may be performed for 3–5 minutes, following CO_2 washout resulting in cerebral vasoconstriction and, hence, slowing of the posterior dominant rhythm, which may be replaced by polymorphic theta range and later high-amplitude delta range activity termed as build-up or hyperventilation-induced high-amplitude rhythmic slowing (HIHARS). It may persist for a few seconds after the end of hyperventilation. Focal slowing and typical 3-Hz spike and wave activity of absence epilepsy may be induced during hyperventilation. This procedure is, however, contraindicated in people with history of obstructive airway disease, cardiac arrhythmias, sickle cell disease, moyamoya disease, subarachnoid haemorrhage, and pregnancy.

Sleep serves as an activation procedure especially in electrical status epilepticus (SE) of sleep, in which spike and slow-wave discharges occur in almost 85% of the slow-wave sleep period. In children with Rolandic epilepsy, centrotemporal spikes are prominent during sleep and could be absent during the awake record. Sleep may be induced using medications like melatonin or simply by sleep deprivation prior to scheduled EEG recording. Performing EEGs during the routine nap times in children helps to record routine sleep changes. Also after hyperventilation most candidates feel drowsy and sleep, so the procedure is usually performed towards end of the record.

Photic stimulation (PS) serves as an activation procedure especially in occipital epilepsies, juvenile myoclonic epilepsy (JME), and progressive myoclonic epilepsies. The "photic drive response" is time-locked potentials recorded at the occipital leads, similar in frequency to the rate of PS, and represents an occipital derivation of the P100 response evoked by visual stimulation (as in visual evoked potentials). Standard procedure includes stimulation across range of frequencies from 1 Hz to almost 30 Hz each lasting for 10 seconds. This works by reinforcing the thalamocortical networks thereby stimulating epileptiform activities termed photoparoxysmal response (PPR) seen particularly in idiopathic generalized epilepsies **(Fig. 7)**. PPR consists of spike or polyspike and wave discharges occurring in occipital leads at times generalized **(Table 2)**[7] and may outlast the

TABLE 2: Grades of photoparoxysmal response.

Grades of photoparoxysmal response (PPR)	Electroencephalography findings
Grade 1	Predominantly occipital spikes
Grade 2	Parieto-occipital spikes with biphasic slow waves
Grade 3	Parieto-occipital spikes spreading to frontal leads with biphasic slow waves
Grade 4	Generalized spike and polyspike wave discharges

PS and may evolve to a clinical seizure (photoconvulsive response). Progressive myoclonic epilepsies typically show PPR at relatively slow frequencies of PS (1-5 Hz) and may be responsive even at higher frequencies of PS.

Other procedures to activate the epileptiform discharges include repetitive eye opening and closure that can stimulate epileptiform discharges after closing eyes which may be self-limited (for a brief duration not entire period of eye closure) and are seen in most idiopathic generalized epilepsies (IGEs) especially in eyelid myoclonia with absences (EMA). Performing particular tasks known to trigger seizures like reading or sudden loud sounds in reflex epilepsies may be used as activation procedures.

INTERPRETATION

Analysis of EEG

An EEG record is described in terms of frequency, amplitude, location, symmetry, synchrony, reactivity, rhythmicity, morphology, background, and any abnormal activity. The four standard frequencies noted in routine EEG are: alpha (8-13 Hz) along occipital leads that disappears on eye opening, beta (14-30 Hz) along frontocentral leads, theta (4-7.5 Hz), and delta (01-3.5 Hz) **(Figs. 8 and 9)**. In case of focal lesions in one hemisphere, there may be failure of alpha activity attenuation on that side after eye opening, this is termed as *Bancaud's phenomenon.*

Amplitude may be described as an average across a run of EEG activity or as a range from minimum to maximum amplitude during the activity. Location may be described as a precise electrode location (focal) in case of specific EEG discharges, two or more contiguous electrodes (regional such as frontopolar, anterior temporal, etc.), lobar spanning across an entire lobe or hemispheric or diffuse. Asymmetry results from difference in frequencies of EEG activity among two hemispheres and can result from focal hemispheric abnormalities such as stroke, tumors, encephalitis, etc. Inherently, amplitude is slightly lower on the left due to higher skull thickness on left side and more prominent alpha activity over the nondominant cortex. Synchronicity is simultaneous occurrence of waveforms along both hemispheres. Severe hemispheric cortical or callosal anomalies may result in asynchrony, with epileptogenic side showing earlier occurrence of discharges.

Study of the normal EEG has dual purpose—to differentiate between normality and abnormality in clinical EEG and to enhance the understanding of the EEG as a phenomenon with important psychophysiological implications. In awake state, the EEG shows an alpha rhythm of 8-13 Hz activity, which is dominant in the posterior head regions and a beta rhythm at a frequency >13 Hz in the anterior areas. If there is a theta (4-7 Hz) or delta (<4 Hz) activity, it is seen during drowsiness and sleep, but it is abnormal if it occurs in the awake state.

Sleep EEG has less variations than awake EEG. It consists of slow waves, sleep spindles, positive occipital sharp transients (POSTs), vertex sharp waves, K complexes, medium-to-high-amplitude delta activity, and sawtooth waves. During stage 1 of nonrapid eye movement (NREM)

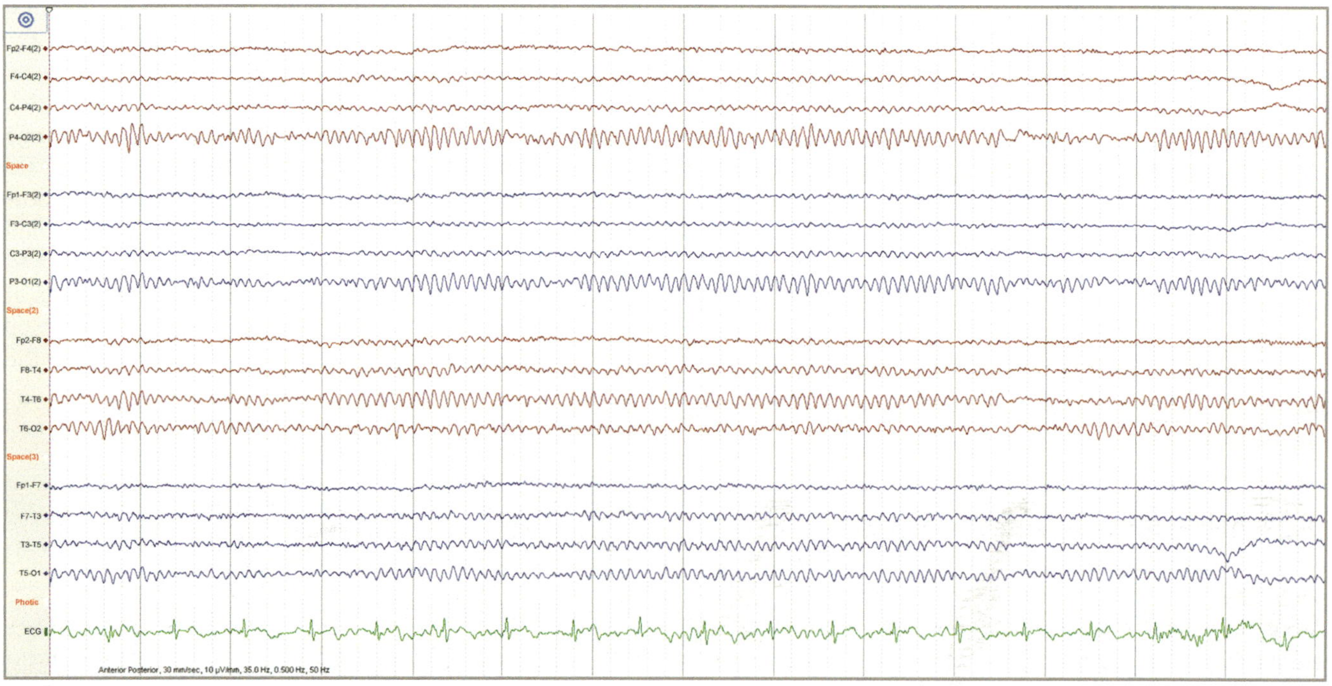

FIG. 8: Posterior dominant alpha rhythm during wakefulness.

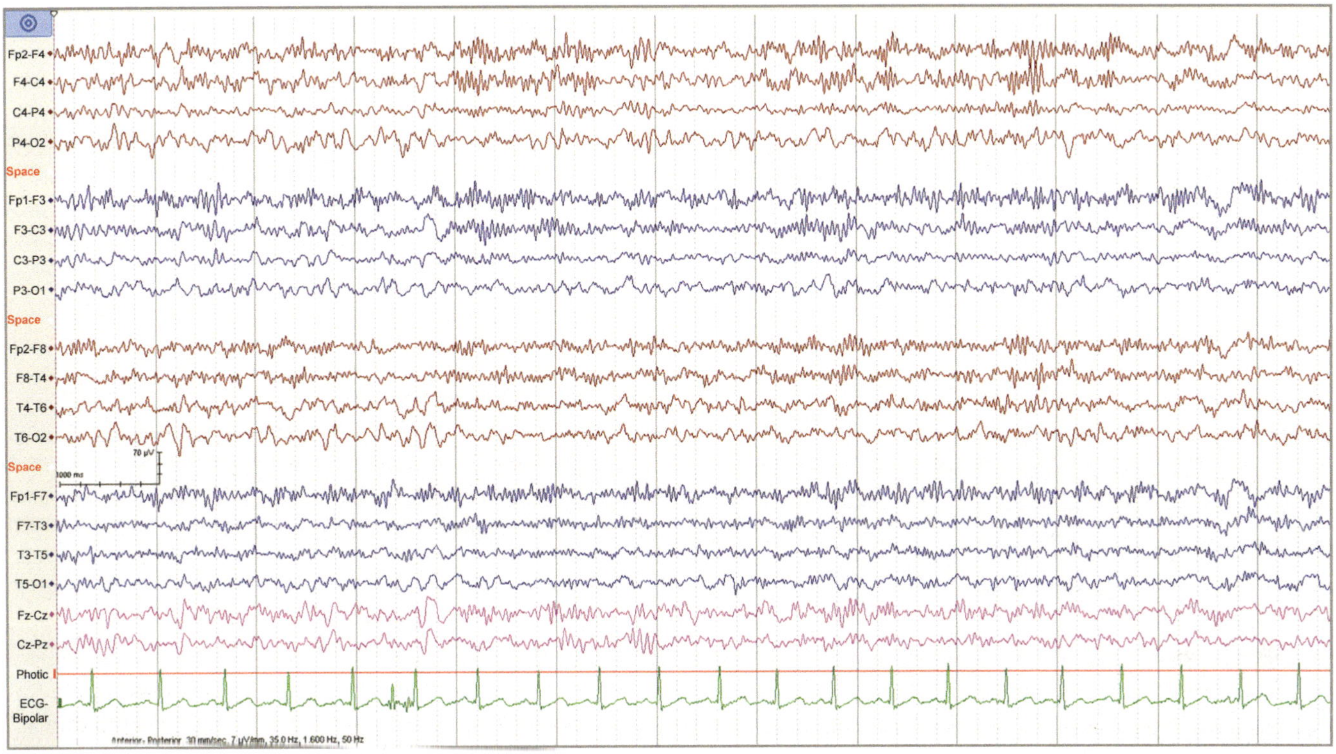

FIG. 9: Frontally dominant beta rhythm during wakefulness.

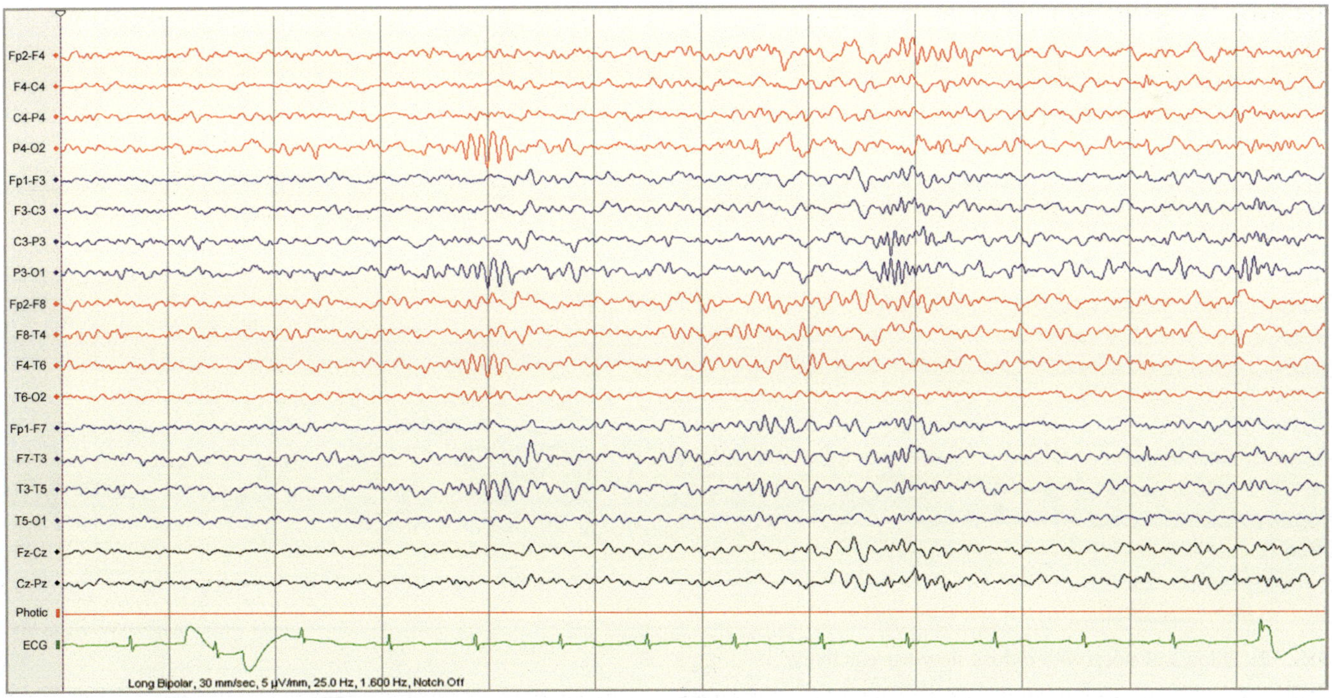

FIG. 10: Alpha dropout during stage 1 of sleep.

sleep, the EEG is characterized by low voltage, mixed frequency waves with highest amplitude in the 2–7 Hz range and vertex sharp waves may occur; their amplitude can reach 200 μV **(Fig. 10)**. Stage 1 is also scored when the epoch is characterized with alpha activity combined with mixed frequency waves and the amount of alpha activity comprises <50% of an epoch (recording of a fixed duration, usually taken as 30 seconds). Stage 2 of sleep is characterized by sleep spindles and K complexes, slow waves continue to be seen and are bilaterally synchronous, sleep spindles occur in 12–14-Hz frequency range **(Fig. 11)**. The duration of these patterns should be 0.5 seconds at minimum. If the

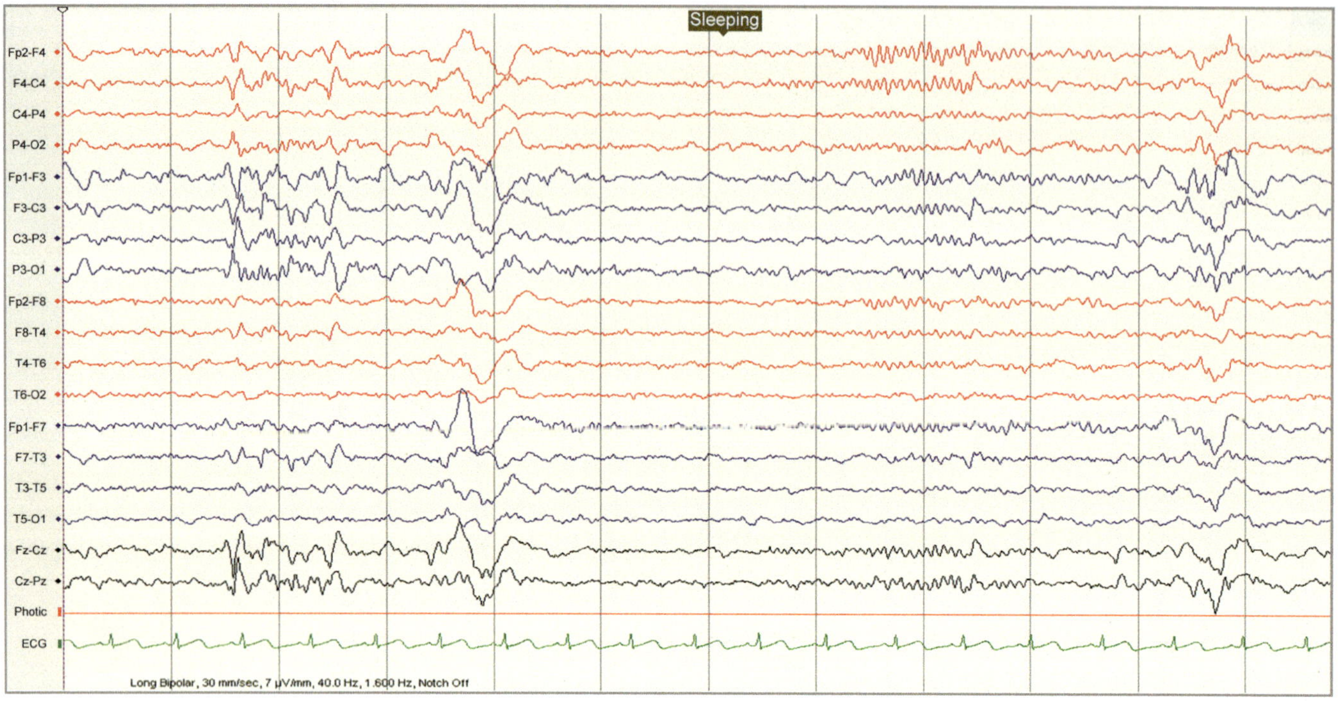

FIG. 11: Vertex sharp waves and sleep spindles during stage 2 of sleep.

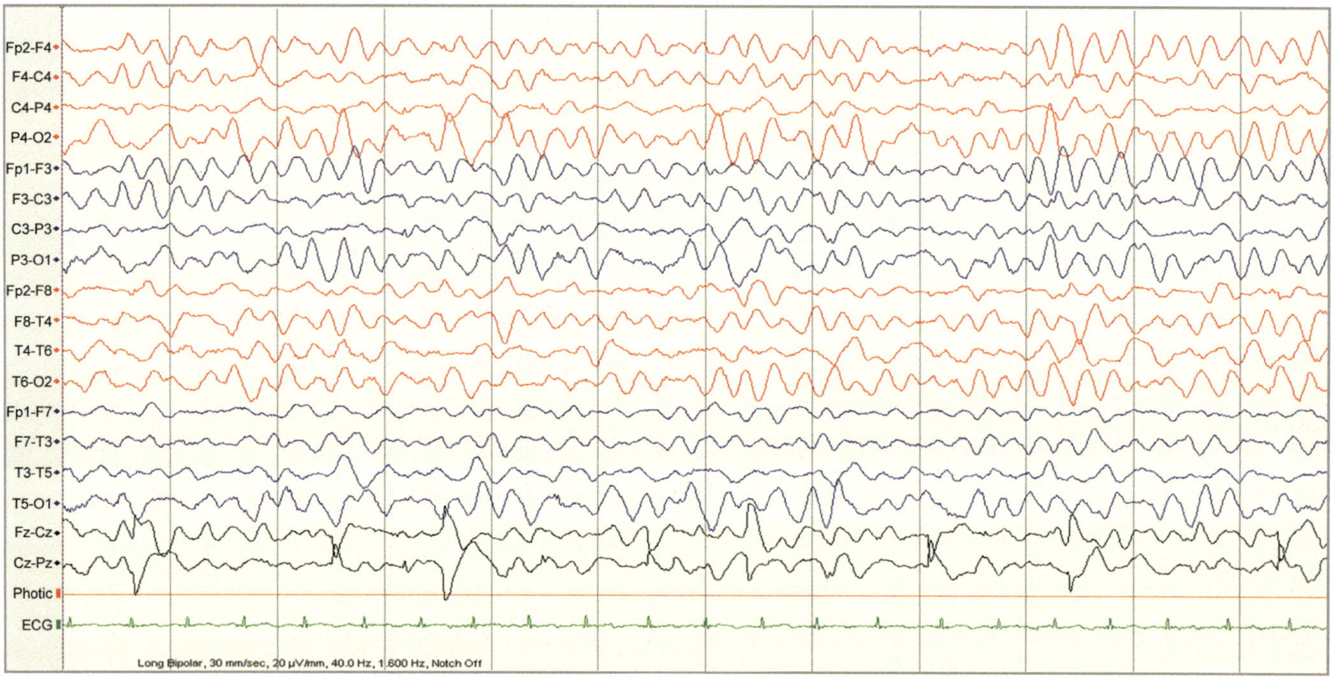

FIG. 12: Stage 3 of sleep with diffuse slow-wave activity.

time between two succeeding occurrences of sleep spindles or K complexes is <3 minutes, this interval is scored as stage 2, unless there are movement arousals or increased tonic activity. If the time interval is 3 minutes or more, it is scored as stage 1. In stage 3 of sleep, 20–50% of the epoch of EEG record should contain waves with 2 Hz or slower frequency and with the amplitudes above 75 μV in the sleep scoring system recorded in C3-A1 or C4-A2 **(Fig. 12)**. Sleep spindles and K complexes may occur during stage 3. Stage 4 has the same attributes as stage 3, but waves with 2 Hz and slower with the amplitudes >75 μV appear >50% of the epoch K-complexes blend with slow waves **(Fig. 13)**. During rapid eye movement (REM) sleep, the EEG shows low voltage, asynchronous and mixed frequency EEG with sawtooth wave pattern (brief runs of medium amplitude, sawtooth-shaped theta waves in central and frontal regions) is often present.

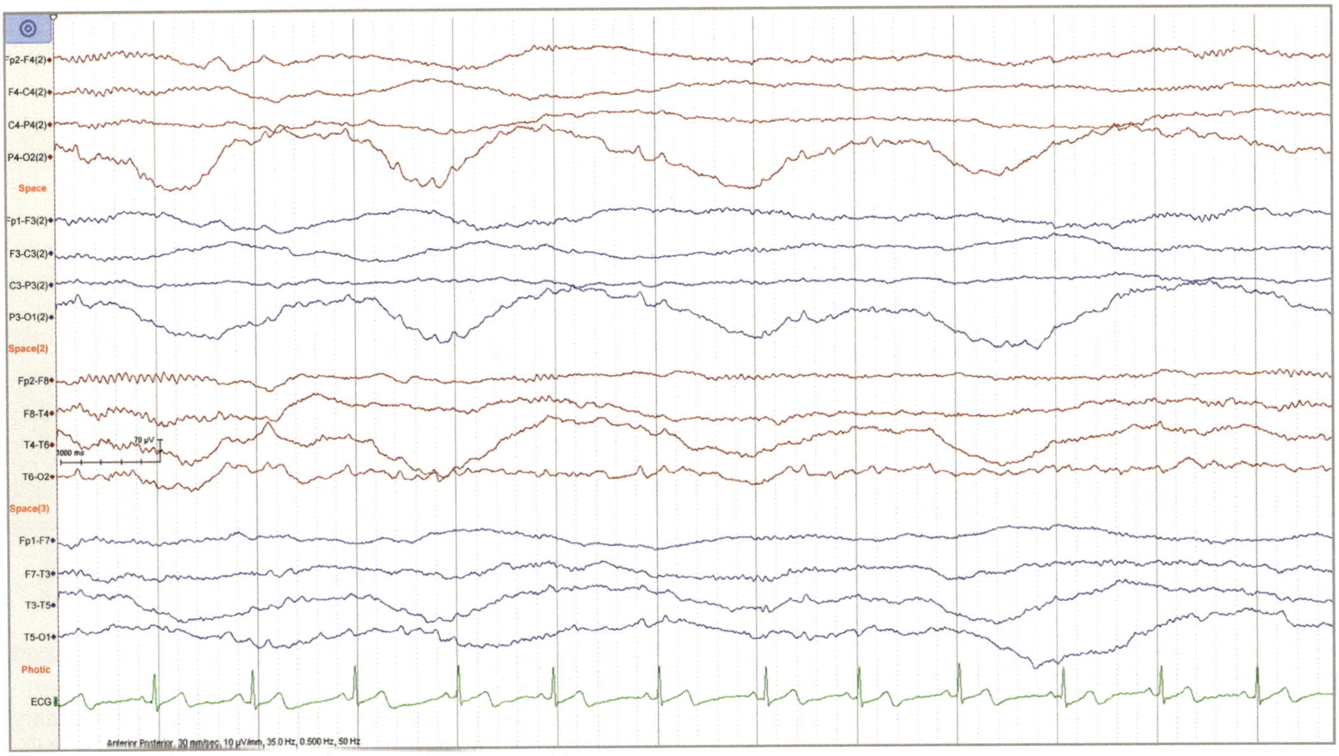

FIG. 13: Stage 4 of sleep.

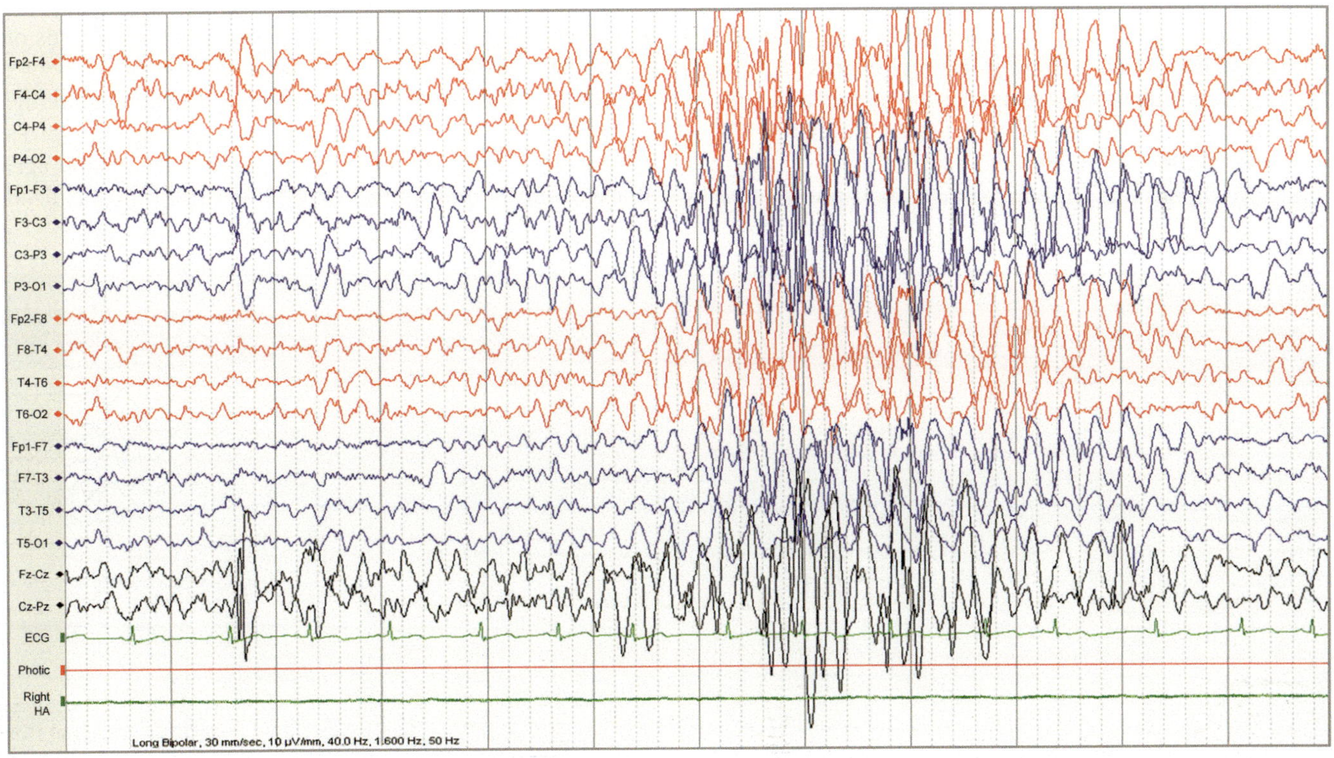

FIG. 14: Hypnagogic hypersynchrony in a 6-year-old child.

REM sleep is considered to be present if >50% of a 30-second epoch contains low-voltage EEG activity with prominent theta activity preceded by REMs and accompanied by reduced muscle tone on EMG.

Hypnagogic hypersynchrony is intermittent or sustained, moderate-to-high-amplitude sinusoidal, 3–5-Hz activity, for several seconds, occurring during the transition of awake to sleep in the frontal, central, and parietal regions **(Fig. 14)**.

It is a generalized, abrupt paroxysmal pattern, waxing and waning with a more gradual onset. It may have a notched appearance or a spike-like appearance due to a commingling of various waveforms. It usually appears at 3–5 months, is most prominent at the age of 2–5 years, and usually disappears by the age of 8–10 years.

EEG IN SPECIFIC EPILEPSY SYNDROMES

The yield of interictal epileptiform activity (IEA) is almost 51% when done within 24 hours of the first seizure.[8] It also depends upon the duration of EEG recording as routine 20-minute EEG can capture IEA in almost 37% of patients with established epilepsy while that recorded over 24 hours shows IEA in 89%.[9] Certain EEG findings are highly specific for seizures, including generalized 3-Hz spike and waves, localized anterior and midtemporal spikes, focal frontal spikes or pseudoperiodic or rhythmic epileptiform discharges.

Self-limited Epilepsy Syndromes of Childhood

Self-limited Epilepsy with Centrotemporal Spikes

This is a common childhood epilepsy syndrome and presents between 4 and 10 years of age, remits by 16–18 years of age, and is characterized by rare nocturnal events with facial twitching or interruption of speech or pharyngeal spasms occasionally followed by generalization.[10] Interictal EEG is characterized by normal for age background with frequent repetitive diphasic to triphasic sharp waves predominantly along central (C3 and C4) and midtemporal (T3 and T4) with a frontal positive dipole often unilateral or bilaterally synchronous. Occasionally, occipital or generalized discharges may also be seen. In almost 30% cases, these discharges are only seen in sleep.[11] The tangential dipole in self-limited epilepsy with centrotemporal spikes (SELECTS) is characterized by epileptiform spikes which arise at an angle that is parallel to the cortical surface, recording simultaneously both negativity from outer cortex and positivity from the deeper cortex. It produces anterior positivity and posterior negativity **(Fig. 15)**. It may produce a phase reversal in a referential montage and double-phase reversals in a bipolar montage. Persistence of spikes in wakefulness or bilaterally asynchronous discharges or associated language disturbances may be associated with risk of persistent seizures.

Self-limited Epilepsy with Occipital Paroxysms (Panayiotopoulos Syndrome)

This is benign focal epilepsy in early-to-mid-childhood (3–6 years of age) characterized by prolonged episodes with autonomic features such as vomiting, pallor, or rarely urinary incontinence. This may sometimes evolve into autonomic status lasting for several minutes to hours with preserved consciousness and can be associated with focal features like unilateral eye deviation. This may mislead evaluation for gastroenterological disorders or sometimes encephalitis or childhood migraine.

The EEG shows repetitive occipital spikes independently or synchronously in bilateral hemispheres **(Fig. 16)**. Spikes may occur in different regions and persist even in later age. Background is normal but may show diffuse or localized

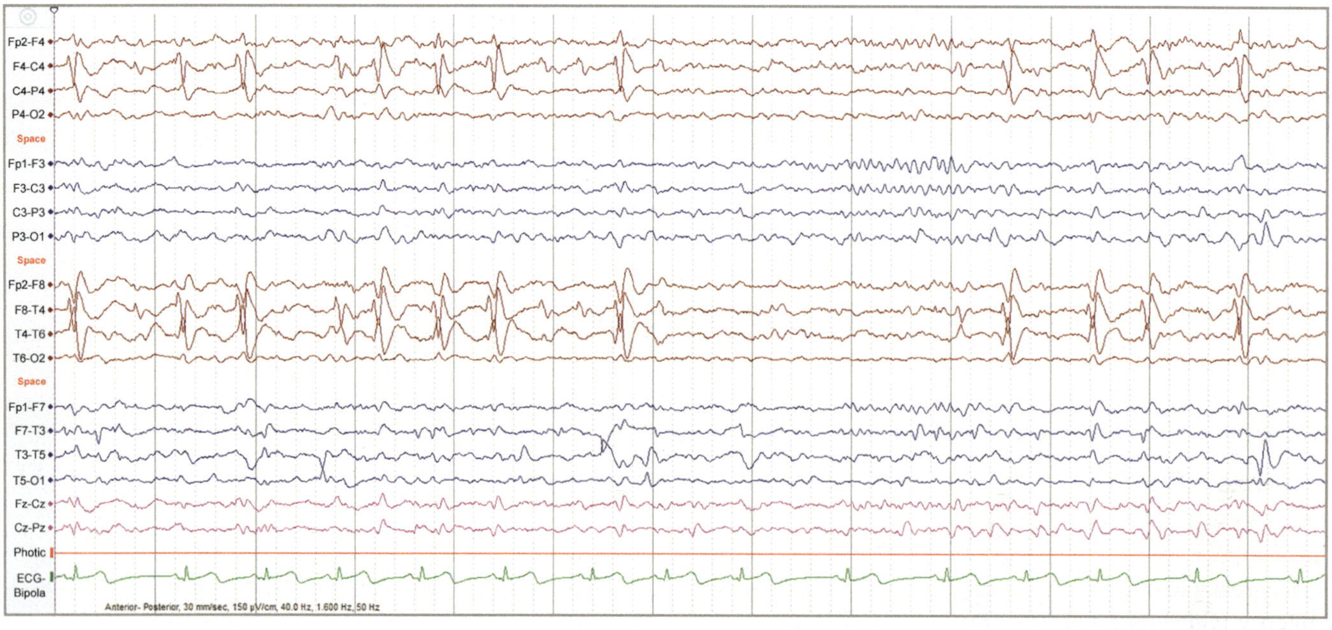

FIG. 15: EEG showing right frontocentral and temporal spikes in sleep in a child with benign Rolandic epilepsy, with frontal positivity and temporal negativity (tangential dipole).
(EEG: electroencephalography)

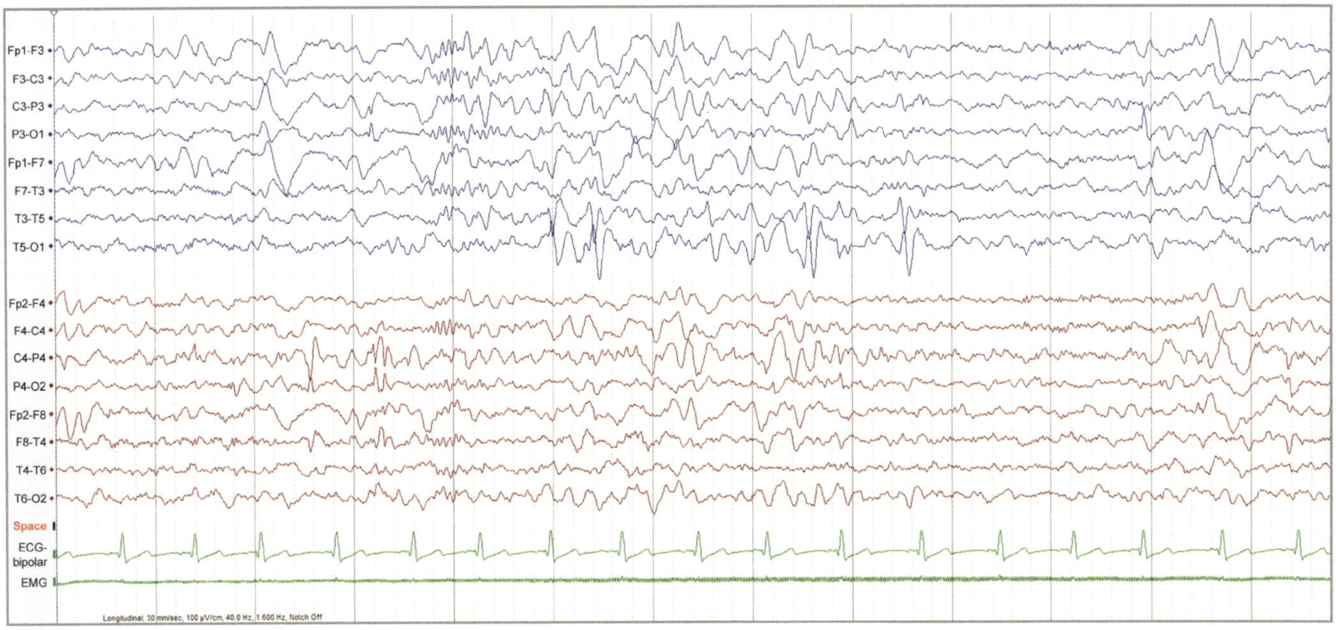

FIG. 16: Rhythmic left posterior temporal and occipital spikes in a child with early onset occipital epilepsy (Panayiotopoulos syndrome).

slow-wave discharges in some cases. Fixation-off sensitivity is rare. Ictal EEG although rarely captured often shows unilateral posterior or sometimes anterior or multifocal. Spikes may persist for years after clinical seizure remission.

Childhood Occipital Visual Epilepsy (COVE) or Occipital Epilepsy of Gastaut

This is an idiopathic occipital epilepsy of late childhood, occurring commonly around the age group of 3-15 years associated with prominent elementary visual hallucinations, eye deviation, blinking or ictal postictal blindness. EEG is characterized by occipital spikes, often more prominent during sleep. The EEG shows multifocal, high-amplitude epileptiform discharges with increased activation during drowsiness and sleep. Occipital discharges may be present and are suppressed with eye opening (fixation-off phenomenon) **(Fig. 17)**. Spikes usually subside with age along with seizure cessation. Ictal EEG correlates with seizure semiology. Fast spiking is associated with elementary visual hallucinations while slower spike activity occurs during complex visual hallucinations. Localized fast spike rhythm is associated with eye deviation while ictal blindness is associated with slow spike and wave activity.

Genetic Generalized Epilepsy Syndromes

Absence Epilepsy

Absence epilepsy is associated with brief 4-20-second seizures, occurring 10–100 times a day. Typically, it begins in 4–8-year-old children and constitutes childhood absence epilepsy (CAE) and generally remits by late adolescence. Juvenile absence epilepsy (JAE), however, begins by 9-13 years and has poor remission rate, about 44–55% persisting in late adulthood and frequently associated with early morning generalized tonic-clonic seizures or myoclonus.[10]

The interictal EEG shows most often normal background. Typical findings include symmetrical and synchronous diffuse single or biphasic sharp or spike wave discharges of 3–4.5-Hz frequency with abrupt start and cessation with frontal predominance, also termed as "egg and dart" discharges **(Fig. 18)**. Hyperventilation may increase the discharges in up to 30%, while these attenuate and become brief in sleep and in those on antiseizure medications (ASMs). Those with JAE show initial polyphasic spikes, at higher 4-6-Hz frequency with more irregular generalized discharges. Ictal events may be characterized with abrupt behavioral arrest with sometimes brief oral automatisms followed by abrupt cessation and resumption of prior activities.

Atypical absence seizures are characterized by inconspicuous start and cessation, more severe impairment of consciousness or tone. EEG shows slower spike wave of 1-2.5 Hz irregular discharges lasting for 4–10 seconds. These occur in symptomatic or cryptogenic epilepsies, Lennox-Gastaut syndrome, and epileptic encephalopathy with continuous spike wave during sleep and are associated with more severe learning disabilities, atonic or myoclonic seizures.

Juvenile Myoclonic Epilepsy

Juvenile myoclonic epilepsy is one of the most common epilepsy syndromes beginning by 12–15 years of age. Classical features include unilateral or bilateral myoclonic jerks with retained consciousness, often noted on awakening. About one-third have associated absence seizures and nearly 85% have generalized tonic-clonic seizures.

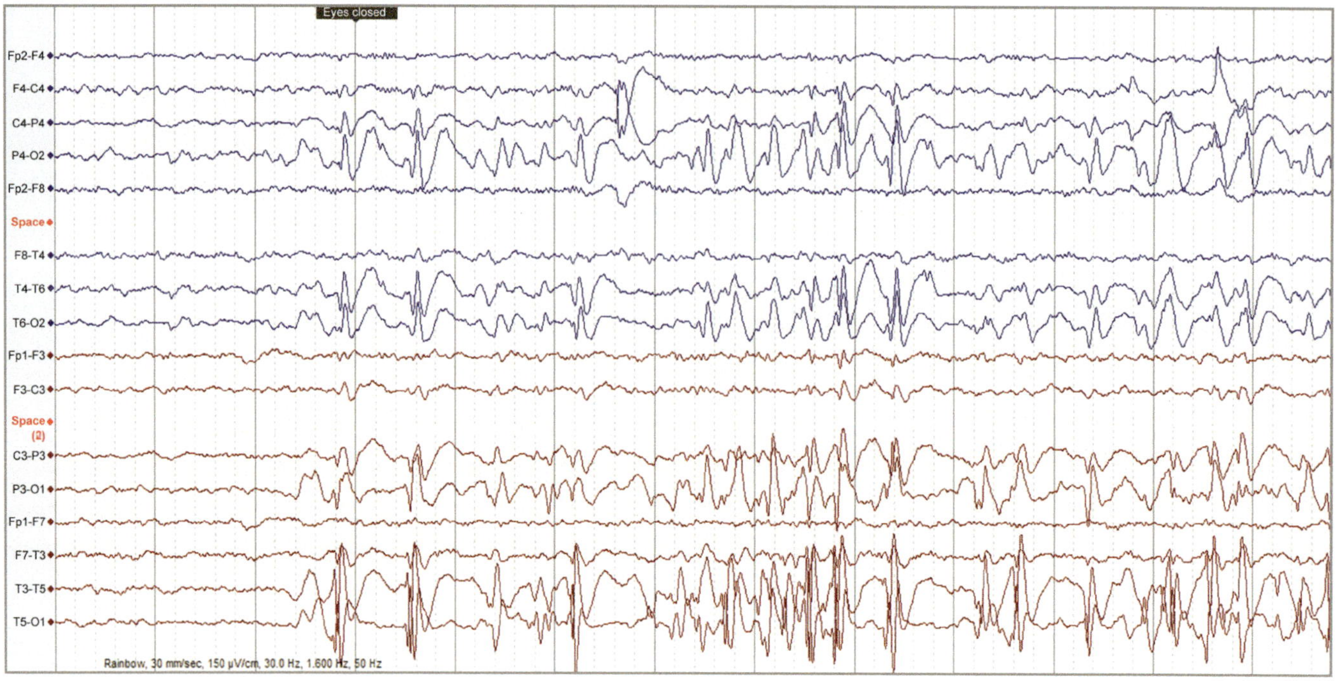

FIG. 17: Bilateral occipital spike discharges in a child with idiopathic childhood occipital epilepsy of Gastaut.

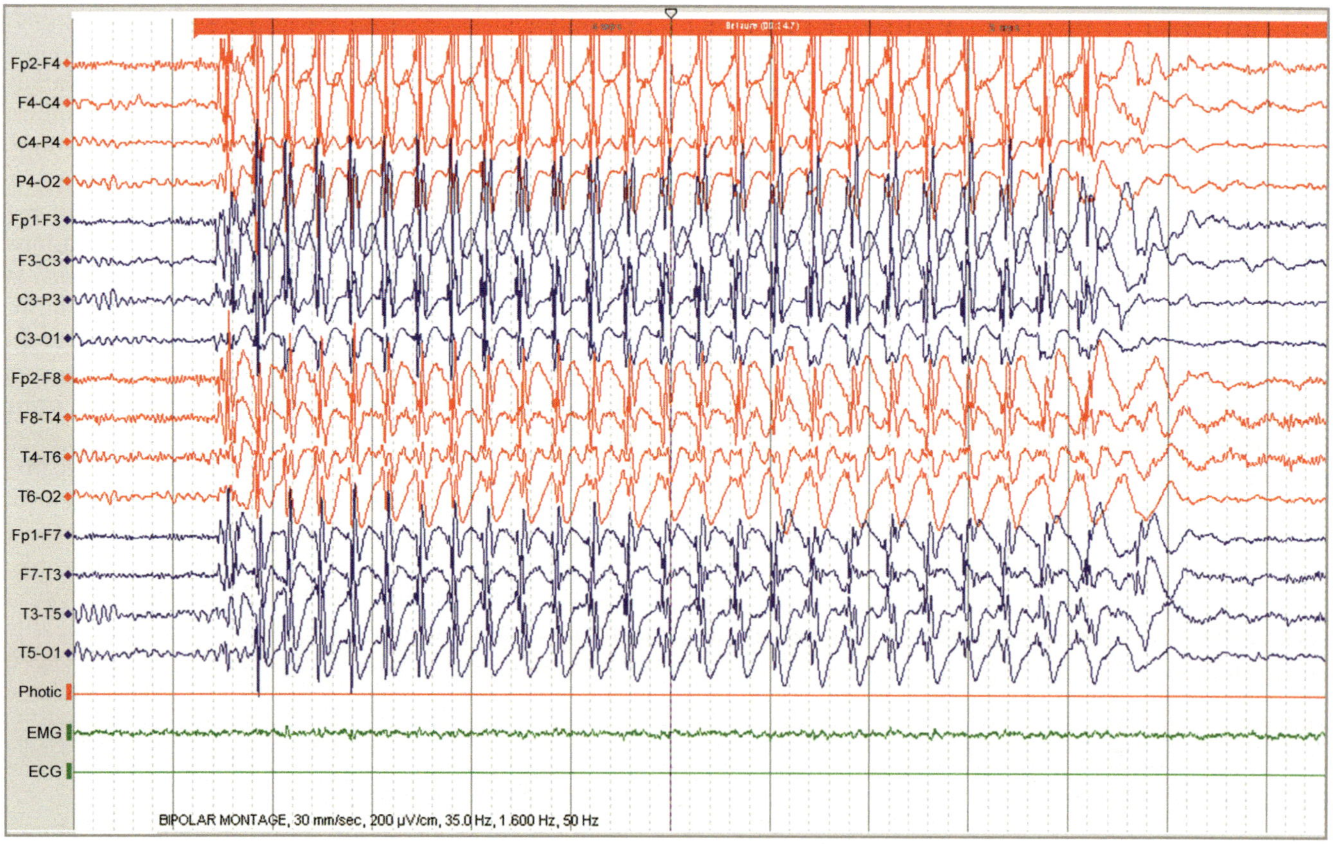

FIG. 18: EEG showing 3-Hz spike and wave discharge in a child during an absence seizure.
(EEG: electroencephalography)

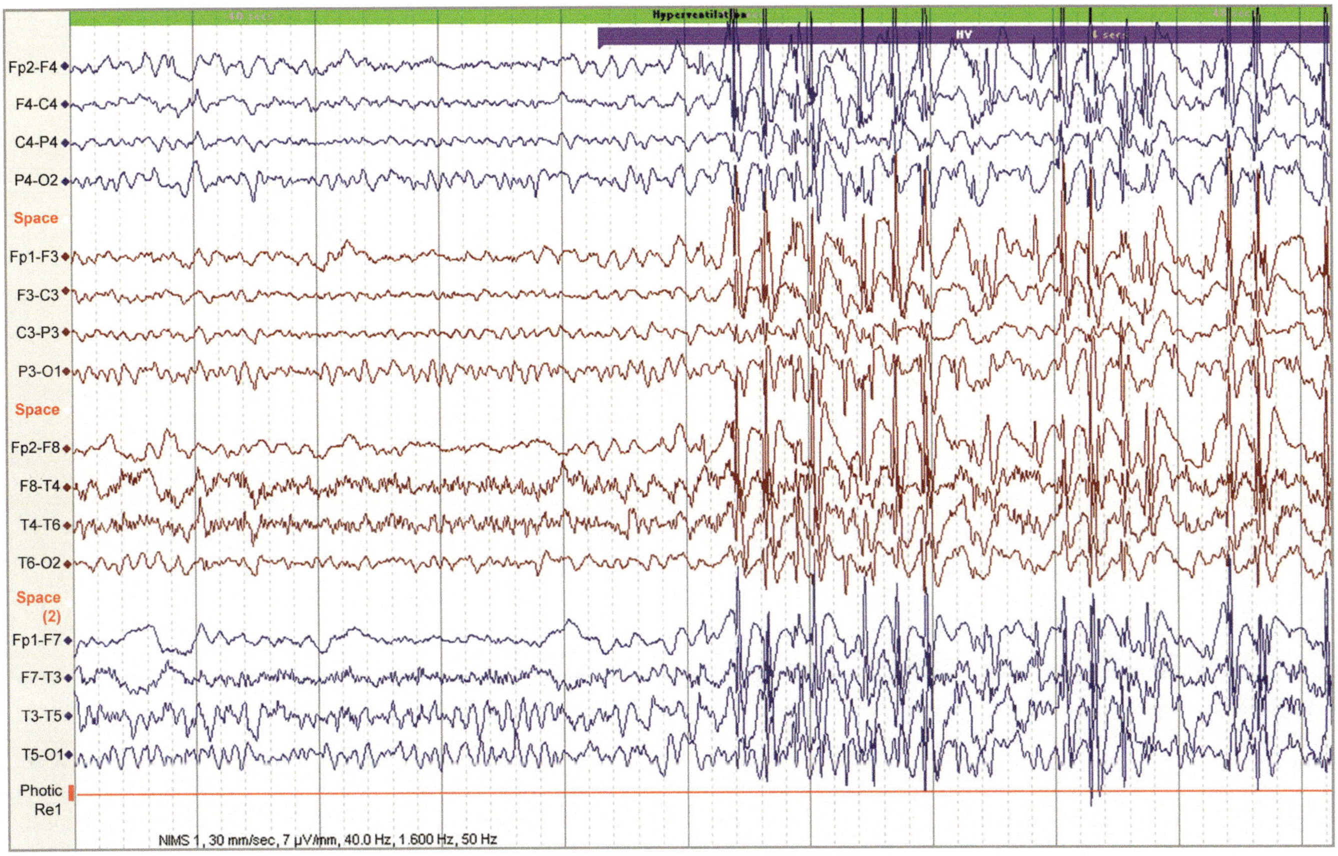

FIG. 19: Generalized 4–4.5-Hz SW/PSW discharges with fragmentation in a case of Juvenile myoclonic epilepsy.
(PSW: polyspike wave; SW: spike wave)

The interictal EEG in JME shows normal background with generalized polyspike wave discharges at faster frequencies of 3–6 Hz, with frontocentral predominance, brief, variable intradischarge frequency, fragmented than in typical absence epilepsy **(Fig. 19)**. The myoclonic jerks correlate with generalized burst of polyspikes lasting from 0.5 to 2 seconds. Arousal from sleep and hyperventilation potentiates this activity and has highest sensitivity to PS, i.e., 30–40% among all IGE syndromes.[10] The discharges may be attenuated with ASMs. Recorded seizures may show initial 3.5–5-Hz spike and wave activity evolving to fast 10–16-Hz polyspike discharges concomitant with the myoclonic jerks at times increasing in frequency leading to generalized seizure or resolving to a slower 2.5–5-Hz activity that outlasts the clinical jerks and then resumes background activity.

Epilepsy with Eyelid Myoclonia

Epilepsy with eyelid myoclonia (EEM) is a triad of eyelid myoclonia with and without absences, eye closure-induced seizures, and/or EEG paroxysms and photosensitivity. The age of onset is around 6–8 years and is twice more common in girls. Myoclonic jerks and generalized tonic–clonic seizures are the associated seizure types. The seizures are precipitated by eye closure more often than photosensitive stimuli. The EEG is characterized by EEG frequent high-amplitude, brief 3–6-Hz generalized spike and wave discharges with positive photoparoxysmal discharges. The discharges appear on eye closure within 0.5–2 seconds and are eliminated in darkness **(Fig. 20)**.

EEG in West Syndrome and Lennox–Gastaut Syndrome

West syndrome is a triad of infantile spasms, psychomotor delay, and grossly abnormal EEG characterized by hypsarrhythmia. The EEG typically shows hypsarrhythmia—irregular asymmetrical high, unstable voltage slow waves with irregular frequency, preceded by low-voltage EEG, suppression burst EEG, and multifocal spikes and sharps wave discharges **(Fig. 21)**. Spikes decrease and suppression burst pattern increases during sleep.

Lennox–Gastaut syndrome is a triad of severe generalized epilepsy, mental retardation, and an EEG pattern of slow spike wave (SSW) discharges. It is clinically characterized by high-seizure frequency with tonic, atonic, atypical absences, myoclonic, and generalized tonic–clonic seizures. Partial seizures also may be associated. SE is common. EEG shows bi- or triphasic surface negative sharp waves of 150–200-ms duration followed by high voltage (300–400 μV negative slow waves) **(Fig. 22)**. The SSW discharges are frequently bilateral, symmetrical, synchronous with high voltage

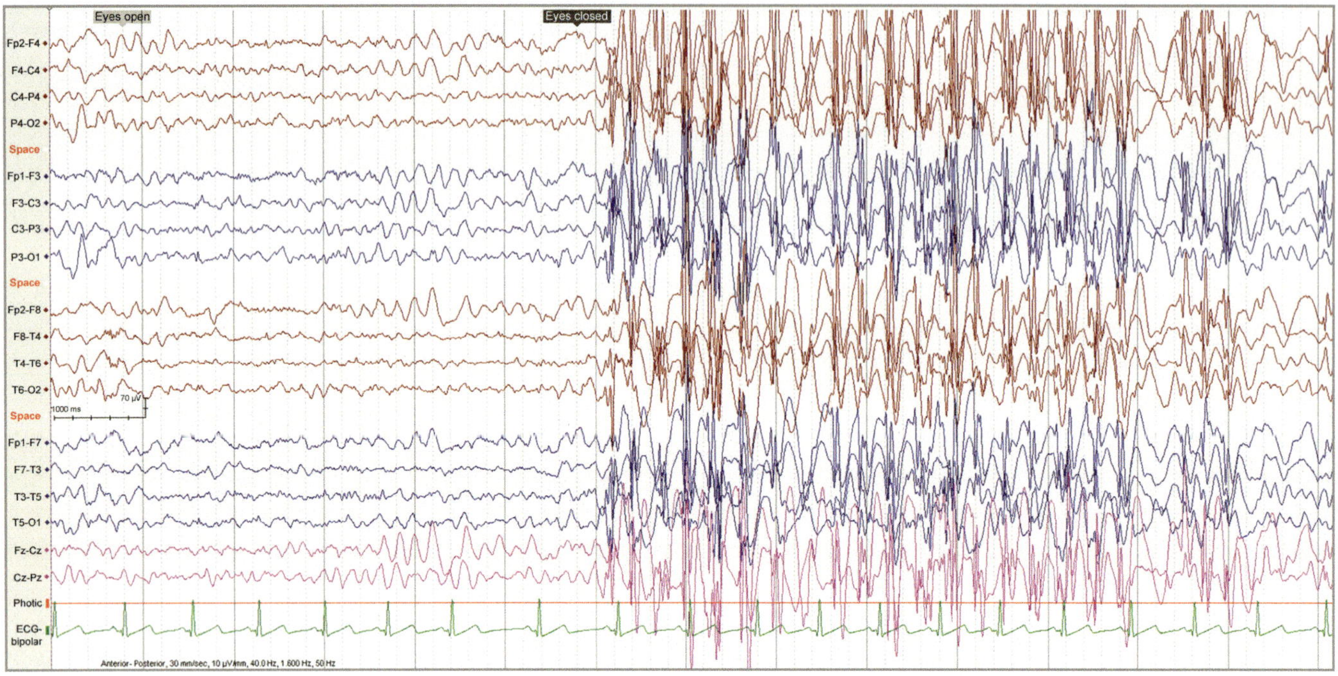

FIG. 20: High-amplitude generalized SW/PSW discharges on eye closure in a case of eyelid myoclonia with absences.
(PSW: polyspike wave; SW: spike wave)

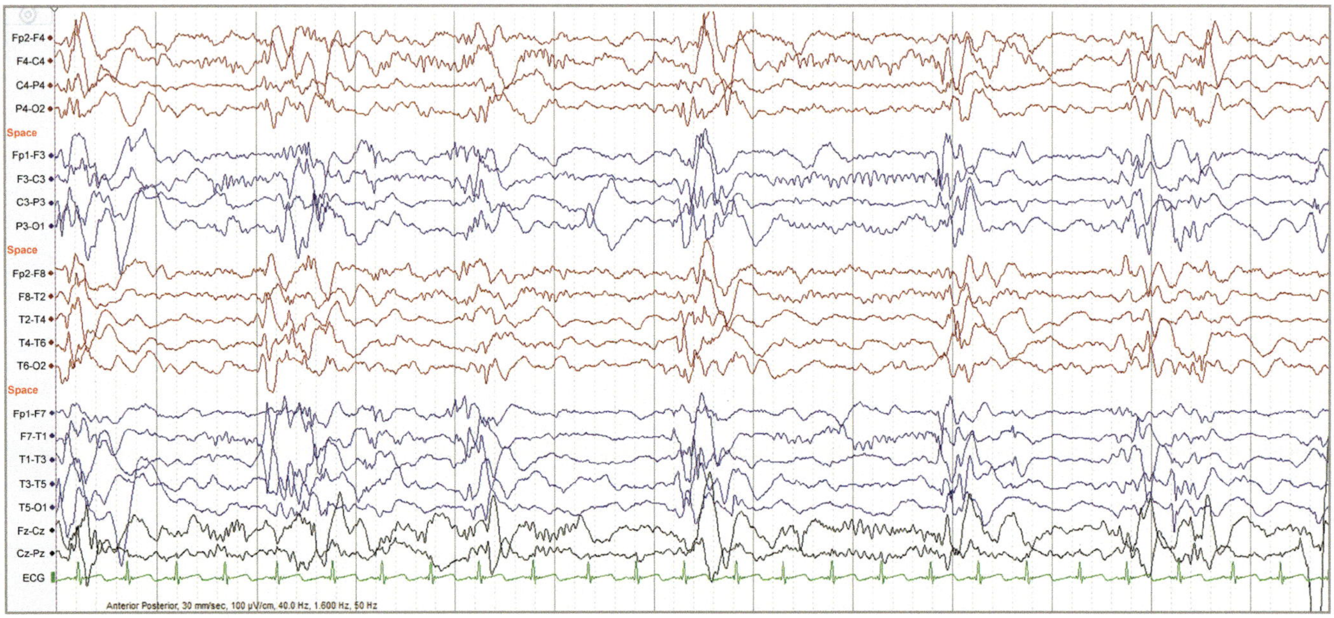

FIG. 21: High-amplitude slow-wave discharges with burst suppression in a case of West syndrome.

over frontocentral regions. They occur in bursts or runs. Hyperventilation and sleep enhance the SSW discharges. Persistent focal or lateralized asymmetries of SSW are common.

Focal Epilepsy Syndromes

Temporal Lobe Epilepsy

Temporal lobe epilepsy (TLE) is one of the well-characterized electroclinical epilepsy syndromes associated with greater detection of epileptiform discharges on routine scalp EEGs. However, EEG representation is based on the limited sampling of basolateral temporal neocortex.

Interictal EEG classically shows epileptiform discharges in the form of spikes, and sharp waves are seen on the anterior temporal region with phase reversals at T1/T2, F7/F8, and T3/T4 in 67% of the patients with mesial TLE and in approximately 30% of patients with neocortical TLE[12] **(Fig. 23)**. Consistent midtemporal and posterior temporal (T5/T6) or widespread temporally distributed epileptiform

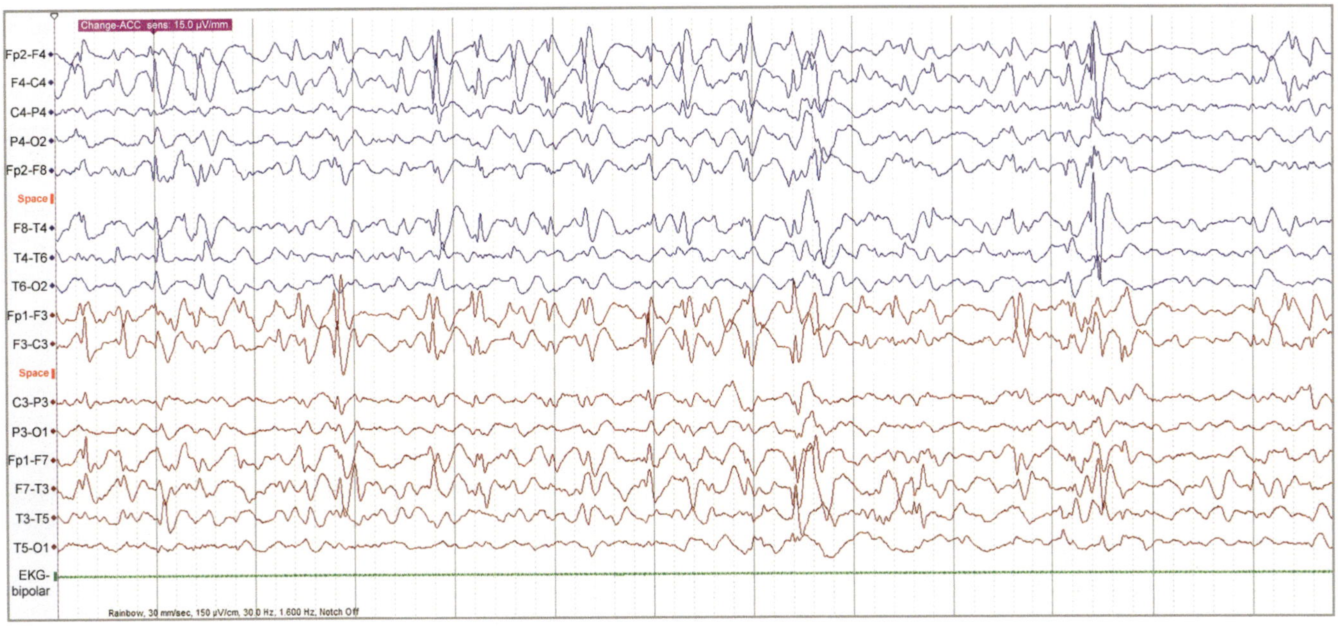

FIG. 22: Slow spike-wave discharges in a child with Lennox–Gastaut syndrome.

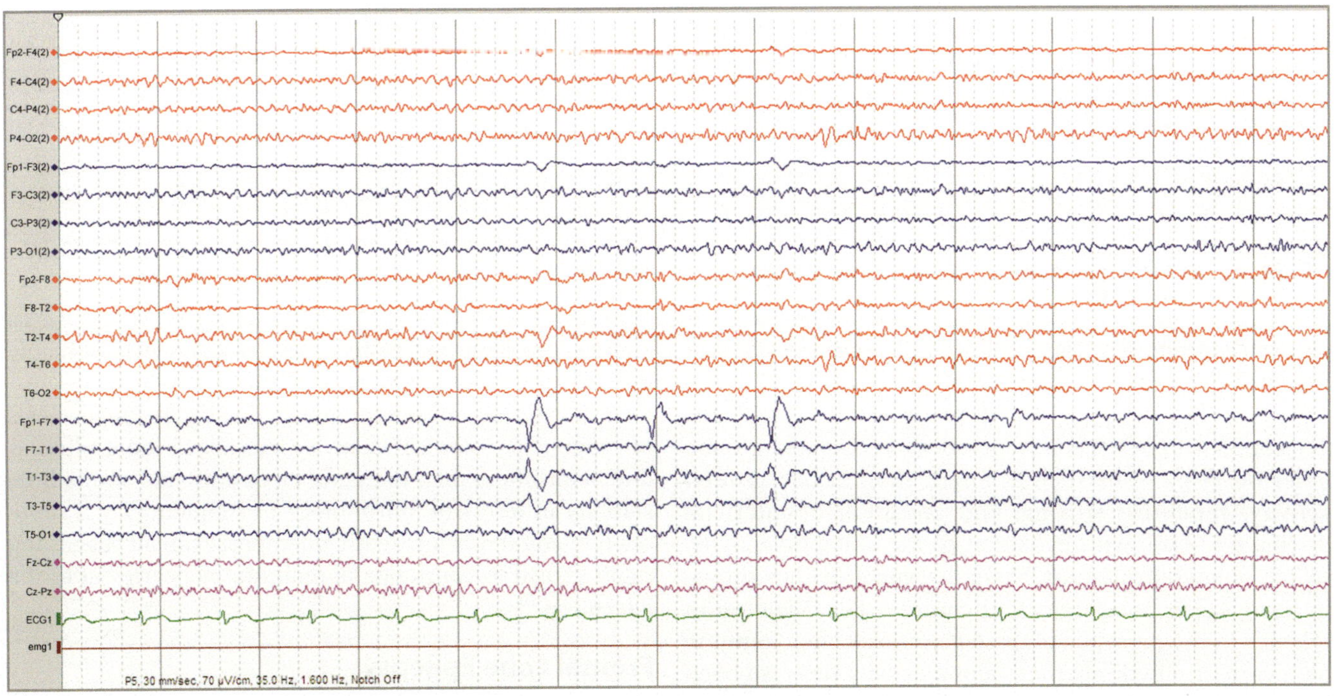

FIG. 23: Left anterior and mid-temporal spikes in a case of temporal lobe epilepsy.

discharges probably indicate a temporal neocortical focus. Focal delta slowing on the temporal region is seen in 30–90% of patients of TLE. Temporal intermittent rhythmic delta activity (TIRDA) is considered to be very specific (specificity—80%) for mesial TLE due to hippocampal sclerosis **(Fig. 24)** and temporal intermittent polymorphic delta activity (TIPDA) is common in temporal neocortical epilepsy and in TLE due to low-grade neoplastic lesions.[13] Bitemporal interictal epileptiform discharges (IEDs) may be seen in up to 30% of the patients with TLE and they may also have better postsurgical outcome provided they have unilateral ictal onset (40–56% seizure free) when compared to only 12% of patients who became seizure free with bitemporal ictal onset.[14] Bisynchronous spike-wave complexes are correlated with higher incidence of generalized seizures when compared to patients with focal spikes.

The most common pattern noted at ictal onset in mesial temporal lobe epilepsies associated with hippocampal sclerosis consists of rhythmic 5–9-Hz EEG activity of

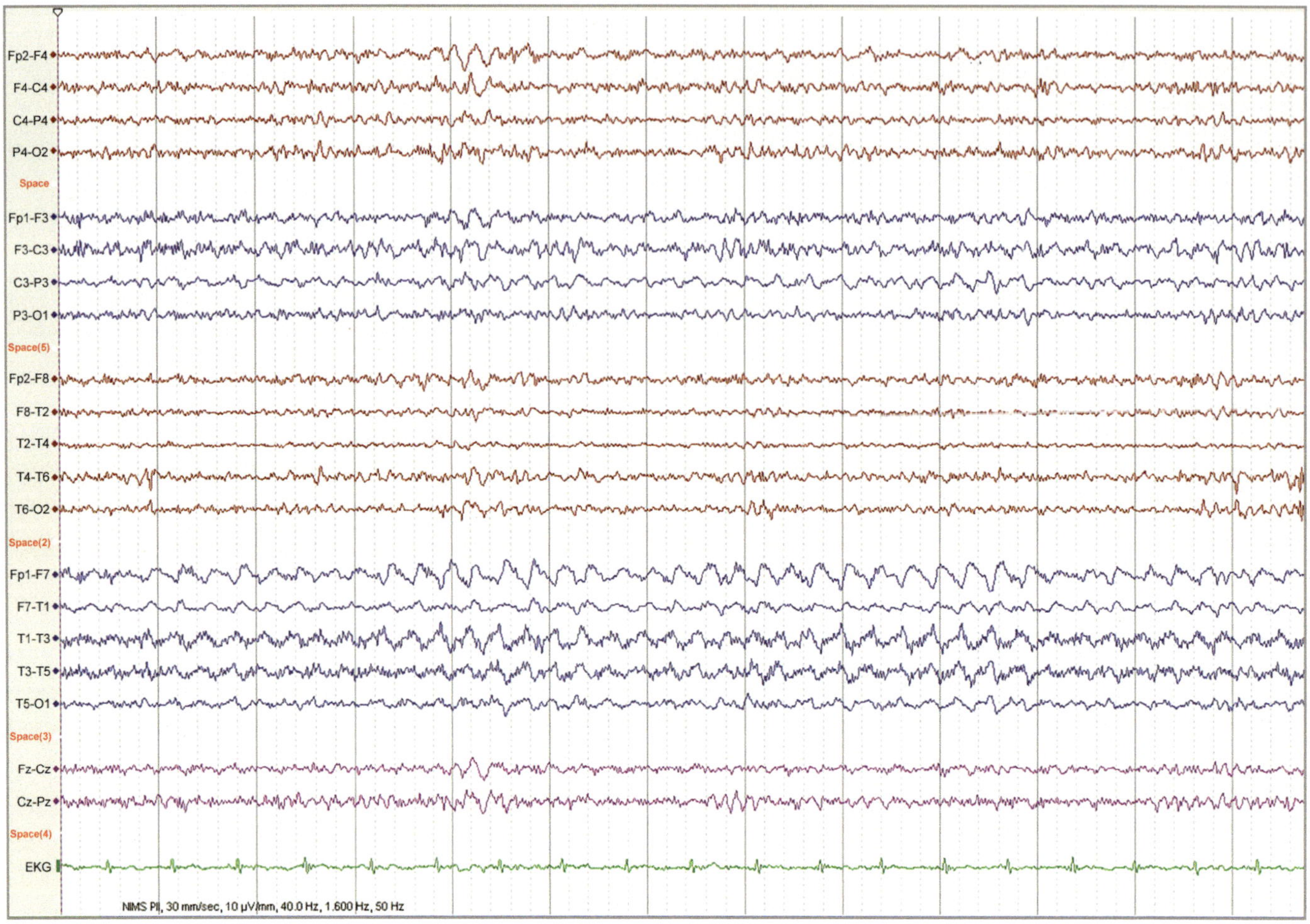

FIG. 24: Left temporal intermittent rhythmic delta activity in a case of temporal lobe epilepsy with left hippocampal sclerosis.

uniform morphology that persisted at least 5 seconds and localized principally to temporal electrodes **(Fig. 25)**. This pattern at onset (initial 3 seconds of the ictal EEG) has been associated with better seizure freedom as compared to the other onset patterns such as attenuation of background activity, repetitive spiking, and cessation of interictal discharges. Also, with evolution of the epileptic activity, switch of lateralization or bilateral asynchrony has shown to have worse postsurgical outcome as lateralization of seizures in the presence of these patterns is often found to be incorrect. Rhythmic theta/alpha activity has also been found to be the common late significant pattern (appears after 3 seconds following the patterns at onset and lasts for at least next 10 seconds). The sequential propagation of ictal activity has been shown more commonly first to ipsilateral frontal lobe, then contralateral frontal lobe, and lastly to contralateral temporal lobe. Although such sequential propagation is considered to be a better prognostic factor in terms of postsurgical outcome, the exact relevance is not yet established using scalp EEG analysis alone. Finally, termination of the ictal activity ipsilateral to the onset has been shown to have good surgical outcome.[15] Whenever present, low voltage fast activity with or without subsequent common evolving ictal patterns has been shown to be highly localizing for epileptogenic zone (EZ).

Typical neocortical temporal ictal onset rhythm consists of irregular 2–5-Hz EEG activity lateralized more often to one hemisphere than temporal electrodes and shows little stability in terms of morphology or frequency. It is more often bilateral or shows early bitemporal spread suggesting rapid spread to contralateral temporal neocortex after the ictal onset.[16]

Frontal Lobe Epilepsy

Next to temporal lobe epilepsies, frontal lobe epilepsy (FLE) is the most common etiology for focal epilepsies occurring in about 20–30% cases.[17] Often, the clinical features of frontal lobe seizures are so varied, subtle, or complex that the possible localization or lateralization becomes confusing. The semiologic features or EEG patterns may be varied and are often misdiagnosed as parasomnias or psychogenic episodes. Frontal lobe seizures are often brief with rapid recovery of awareness compared to temporal lobe seizures. EEG features are often noncontributory due to associated movement artifacts due to hypermotor nature of the seizures.

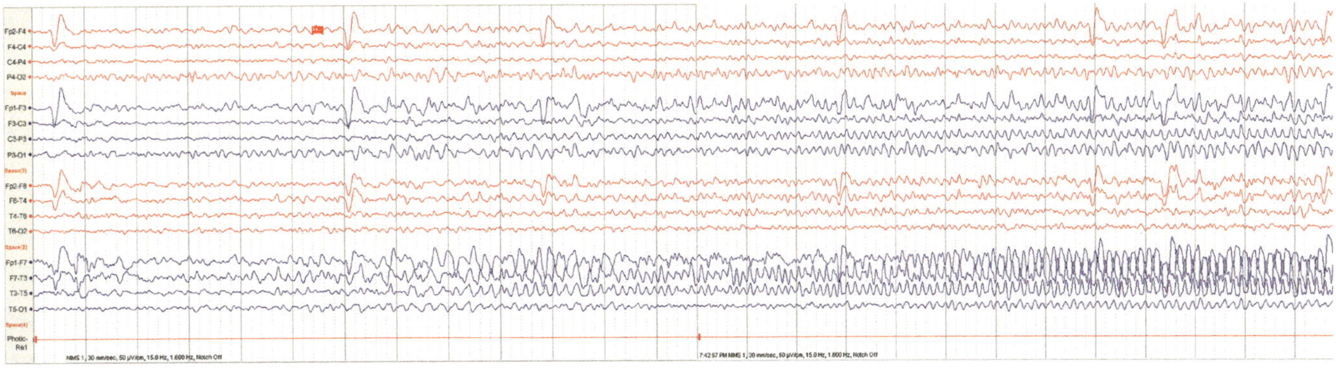

FIG. 25: Ictal EEG showing left anterior temporal 5–6-Hz rhythmic theta activity evolving in amplitude and frequency in a case of temporal lobe epilepsy with left hippocampal sclerosis.

(EEG: electroencephalography)

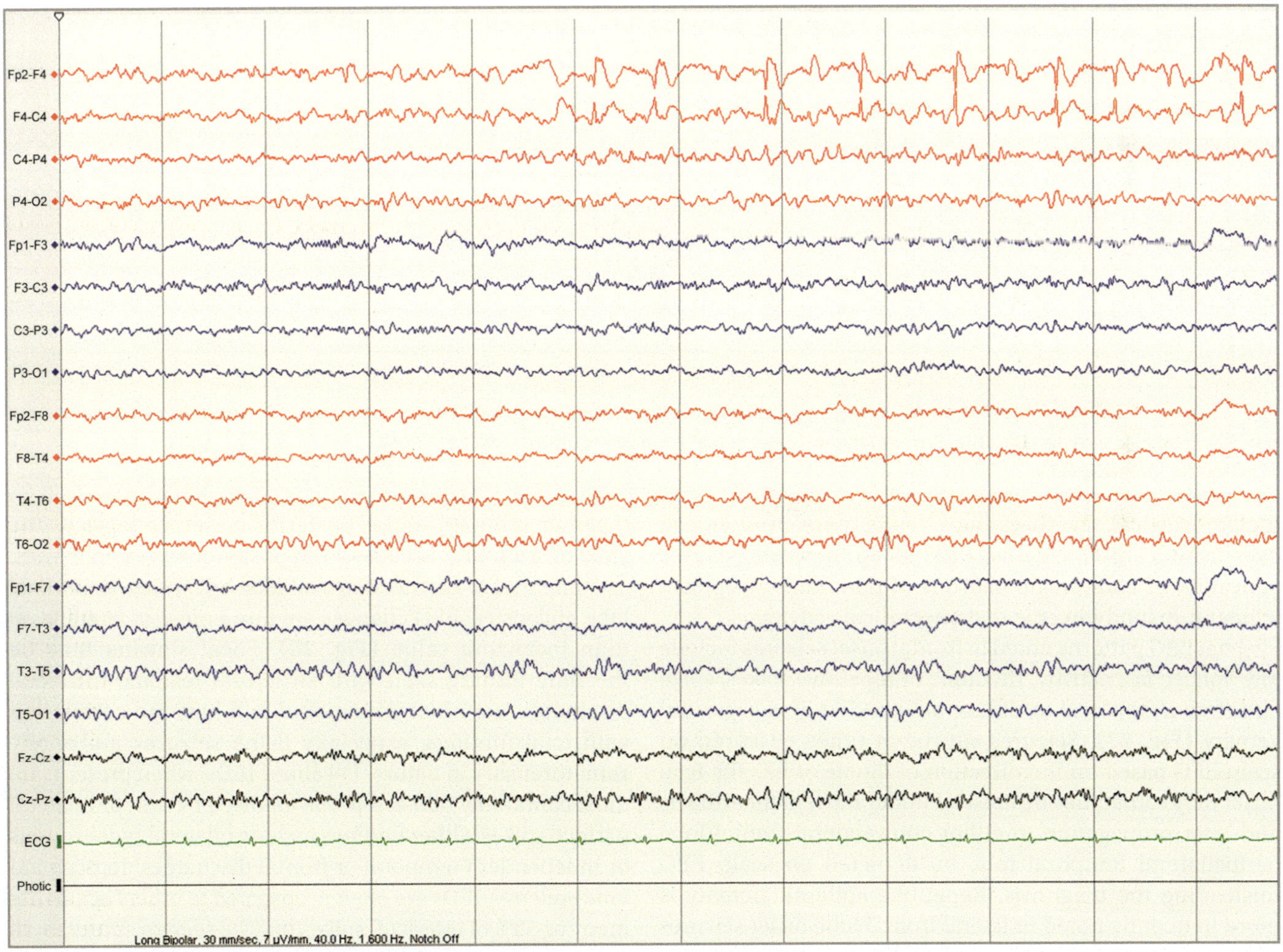

FIG. 26: Right frontal spikes in a case of frontal lobe epilepsy.

A third of patients with FLE may not have any IEDs in scalp EEG as large cortical areas such as orbitofrontal cortex, medial frontal cortex, and cingulate gyrus are inaccessible during scalp EEG recordings. The interictal discharges may present as focal, regional unilateral or multifocal, lateralized hemispheric or bifrontal symmetric, and asymmetric or generalized discharges **(Fig. 26)**. Parasagittal lesions causing bilateral or generalized slow-wave discharges due to *secondary bilateral synchrony* were shown by Tukel and Jasper in 1952.[18] Also, focal slow waves or rhythmic midline theta rhythm although not epileptiform may help in lateralization. IEDs and seizures are both accentuated in NREM sleep due to facilitation of phasic activity (including K complexes and sleep spindles) leading to synchronized

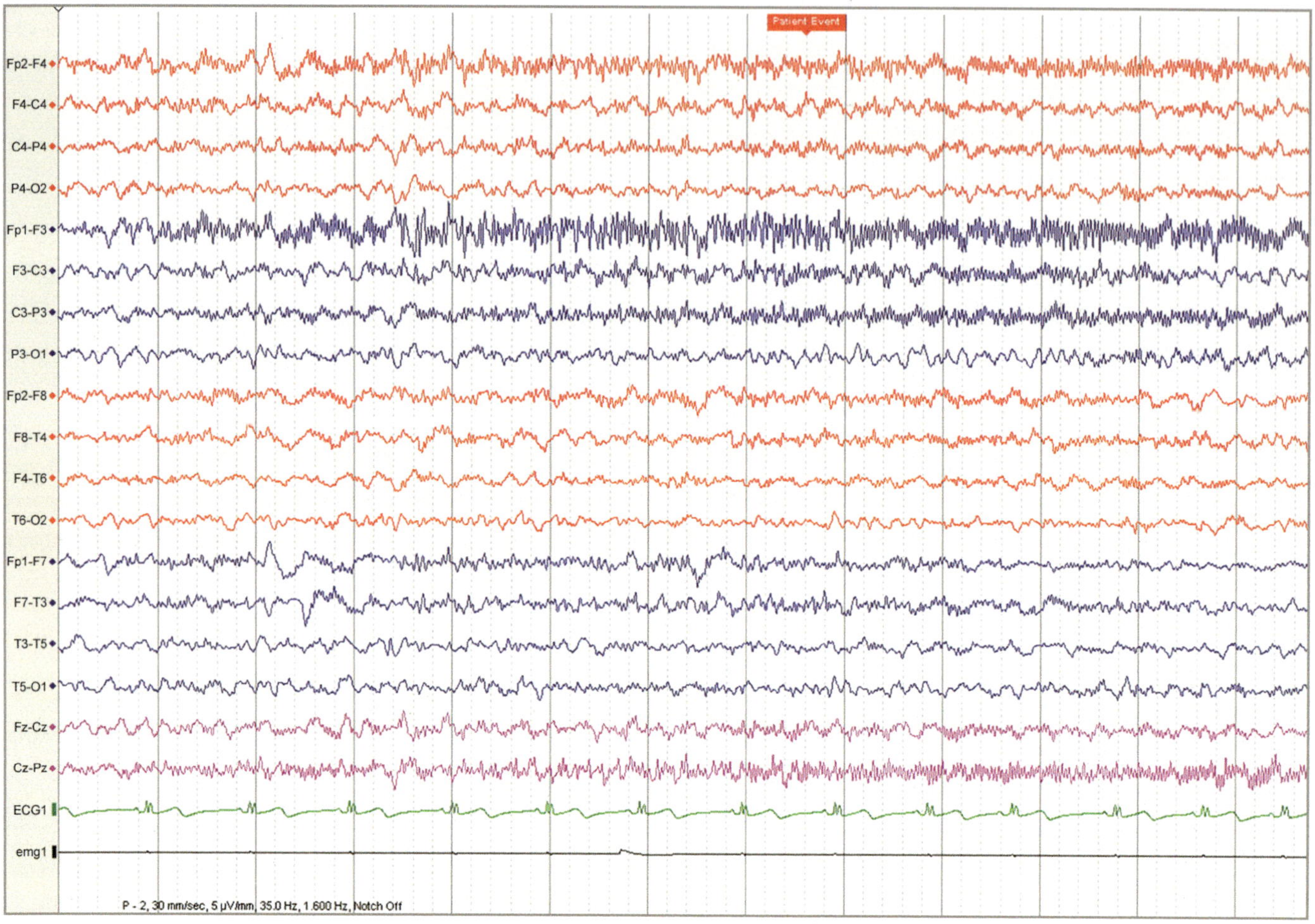

FIG. 27: Ictal EEG showing bifrontal low-voltage fast beta activity in a case of frontal lobe epilepsy.
(EEG: electroencephalography)

thalamocortical reverberating circuits more pronounced over frontocentral regions. REM sleep, however, causes activation of cholinergic neurons of pontomesencephalic tegmentum inhibiting the thalamocortical activity.

Ictal EEG patterns noted in frontal onset seizures include low-voltage fast activity, rhythmic or repetitive spikes, spike and slow wave, focal or diffuse attenuation of background activity **(Fig. 27)**. Seizures can be at times obscured on scalp EEG based on the direction of dipole of EZ. The ictal onset may sometimes be masked under movement artifacts and later propagation to either contralateral frontal lobe or ipsilateral temporal lobe be depicted on scalp EEG misleading the diagnosis. Repetitive epileptic activity is more frequently noted in lateral frontal lobe onset seizures while generalized ictal patterns with less than 2:1 amplitude difference over both hemispheres correlated with mesial frontal lobe onset seizures.[19] Postictal persistent spikes or prolonged suppression of background activity, sleep-enhanced activity, and use of different EEG montages especially circular may help in localization of the EZ in FLE.

Posterior Cortex Epilepsy

Seizures originating from occipital lobes, parietal lobes, posterior temporal regions, or combination of these are together grouped under posterior cortex epilepsies. The yield of scalp EEG is far lesser in posterior cortex epilepsies, as compared to classic temporal lobe epilepsies. In parietal lobe epilepsies, EEG changes are more often of lateralizing than localizing value **(Fig. 28)**. Focal slowing may be the only finding seen with structural lesions. Interictal discharges are often widespread and have no correlation with ictal findings, especially if the seizures are purely somatosensory in nature. Localized IEDs, when present, are most commonly mid-temporal, followed by uni- or bilateral parietal spikes. Other findings include bilateral synchronous or independent temporal or frontal discharges. In occipital lobe epilepsy, IEDs are often propagated to other regions. As many as 50% of interictal spikes may be seen over temporal, and sometimes noted even on frontal or central regions in an occipital lobe epilepsy. Isolated occipital discharges in confirmed occipital lobe epilepsy are seen in only 10–20% of cases.[20] Interictal spikes in occipital epilepsy are most often seen over the posterior temporal region, which often spread to the anterior temporal region. It has been postulated that spread usually occurs to the parietal and frontal electrodes, if the irritative zone is in the supracalcarine cortex, and in the ipsilateral temporal lobe if the focus is in the infracalcarine cortex. Frequently, bilateral occipital discharges may be

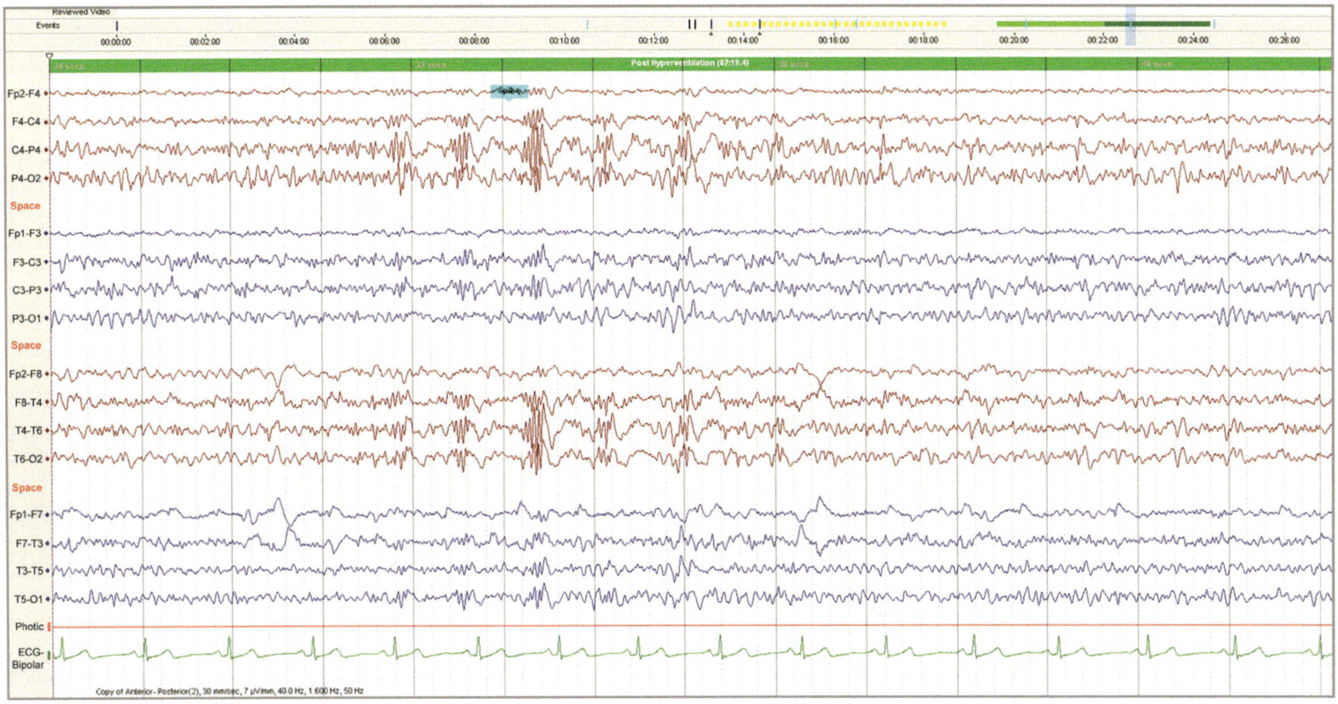

FIG. 28: Right posterior hemispheric focal polyspikes in a case of right parietal focal cortical dysplasia.

seen due to spread via the corpus callosum **(Fig. 29)**; here, the relatively lower voltage on the side of secondary spread is the clue.

The EEG information in posterior cortex epilepsy is limited because epileptiform discharges from basal and mesial occipital regions are not recorded from the scalp. The occipital lobe, because of its rich connectivity to the contralateral side through the splenium and to the frontal and temporal regions through the longitudinal fasciculi and inaccessibility of the mesial and basal regions for the scalp electrodes, the ictal onset is often nonlocalizing and nonlateralizing. The orientation of dipoles over the mesial occipital regions can result in false lateralization because the left mesial occipital dipoles may be facing the right occipital scalp electrode and vice-versa. There were very few points to differentiate between mesial and lateral occipital lobe ictal EEG pattern. Regional seizure patterns occur in 36% of lateral occipital lobe epilepsy and almost never in mesial occipital lobe epilepsy.[21] Parietal lobe epilepsy is a great masquerader and has the highest false lateralizing and localizing patterns predominantly due to its very rich connectivity with the rest of the brain. Ictal EEG patterns with parietal lobe epilepsy become visible on scalp after propagation to temporal or frontal lobe giving a wrong localization or spread to the contralateral lobe giving a wrong lateralization. False localization or lateralization in parietal lobe epilepsy is described in about 16%. Postictal EEG may have some localizing value when focal slowing or spike activation occurs.[22]

EEG in Critical Care Unit

Critical care patients often need prolonged EEG monitoring. It may help to rule out nonconvulsive seizures (NCS) or SE, characterization of various paroxysmal movements, prognostication of their neurological recovery postcardiac arrest or hypoxia, detection of complications like infarction in cases with subarachnoid hemorrhage or vascular intervention, and at times to certify brain death. Continuous EEG (cEEG) monitoring has shown NCS in 48% and nonconvulsive status epilepticus (NCSE) in 14% of critical care patients.[23] Monitoring with cEEG helps not only to detect seizure, but also to assess efficacy of antiepileptic and anesthetic treatment during SE with suppression of the epileptiform patterns.

Periodic Discharges

These occur as sharp/wave complexes of variable 50–300 μV amplitudes that recur at stereotypic time intervals. Lateralized periodic discharges (LPDs) or generalized periodic discharges (GPDs) are associated with worse outcome postcardiac arrest. These are also suggestive of SE but can be seen in other nonepileptic conditions such as acute infarcts, posterior reversible encephalopathy syndrome (PRES), *Herpes* encephalitis, autoimmune encephalitis, mitochondrial encephalopathies, and Creutzfeldt-Jakob disease (CJD). In *Herpes* encephalitis, EEG shows pseudoperiodic focal large-amplitude complexes, repeat at regular intervals, expressed maximally at involved temporal

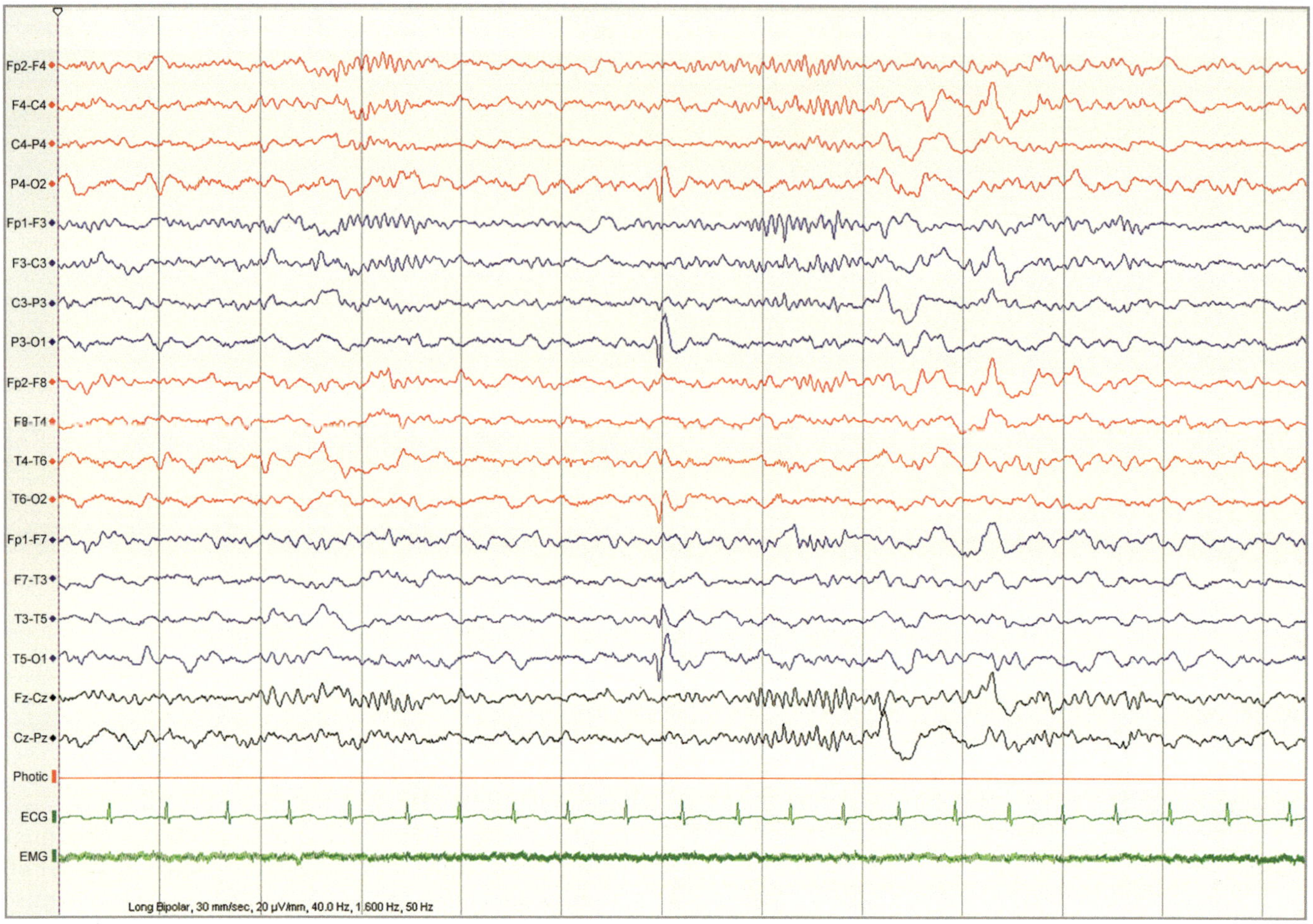

FIG. 29: EEG showing bilateral occipital spikes in a case of right occipital lobe epilepsy.
(EEG: electroencephalography)

lobe as single or group of waves, prominent of subtle, sharp, sawtooth, or delta waves, at 1–5 (2–3)-second interval. The periodic discharges can be unilateral or bilateral and may be synchronous or independent **(Fig. 30)**. The EEG in CJD shows generalized periodic discharges (GPDs) during stage 2 of the disease. They are characterized by periodic, bilaterally synchronous bi-/triphasic, 200–500-ms duration, and 300-μv sharp waves which occur at a frequency of 1 per second **(Fig. 31)**. LPDs may be predictive of seizure risk as <1-Hz discharges are associated with up to 40% risk of seizures while ≥2-Hz suggest 66% risk. LPDs plus suggest complex morphology with a prolonged ictal appearing after discharge along with fast activity (LPD + F), superimposed rhythmic activity (LPD + R), or both (LPD + FR). When occurring at faster rate, these are highly associated with clinical seizures.

Periodic complexes in slow virus disease like subacute sclerosing panencephalitis (SSPE) are highly characteristic and known as Radermecker complexes. They are bilateral, symmetrical, synchronous, stereotyped, and consist of 2–3 delta waves di-/tri-/polyphasic with an amplitude of 200–500 μv. The periodic discharges repeat at regular intervals of 4–10 seconds with a 1:1 relationship of jerks to EEG complexes **(Fig. 32)**.

Triphasic Waves

Triphasic waves (TWs) are characterized by high-amplitude (200–300 μV), bilaterally symmetrical and synchronous, positive sharp component preceded by short duration, small-amplitude negative component and followed by a long-duration negative slow wave, with fronto-occipital lag of 25–140 milliseconds **(Fig. 33)**. They may be monophasic, diphasic, or quadriphasic. The maximum amplitude is over fronto-central region. They may occur as isolated paroxysms or repeat at 2–4-Hz pseudoparoxysmal patterns. They are typically seen in hepatic encephalopathy but may also occur in uremic encephalopathy, anoxia, hyperosmolar state, and metabolic disturbances such as hypoglycemia, hyponatremia, hypercalcemia, and hyperthyroidism.

Extreme Delta Brush Activity

Rhythmic 1–3-Hz delta activity with superimposed 20–30-Hz beta rhythm riding on each delta wave resembling the pattern of delta brush in neonatal EEG is consistently noted in N-methyl-D-aspartate (NMDA) encephalitis patients independent of antibody status, clinical seizures, choreoathetotic movements, depth of anesthesia, or prognosis **(Fig. 34)**.

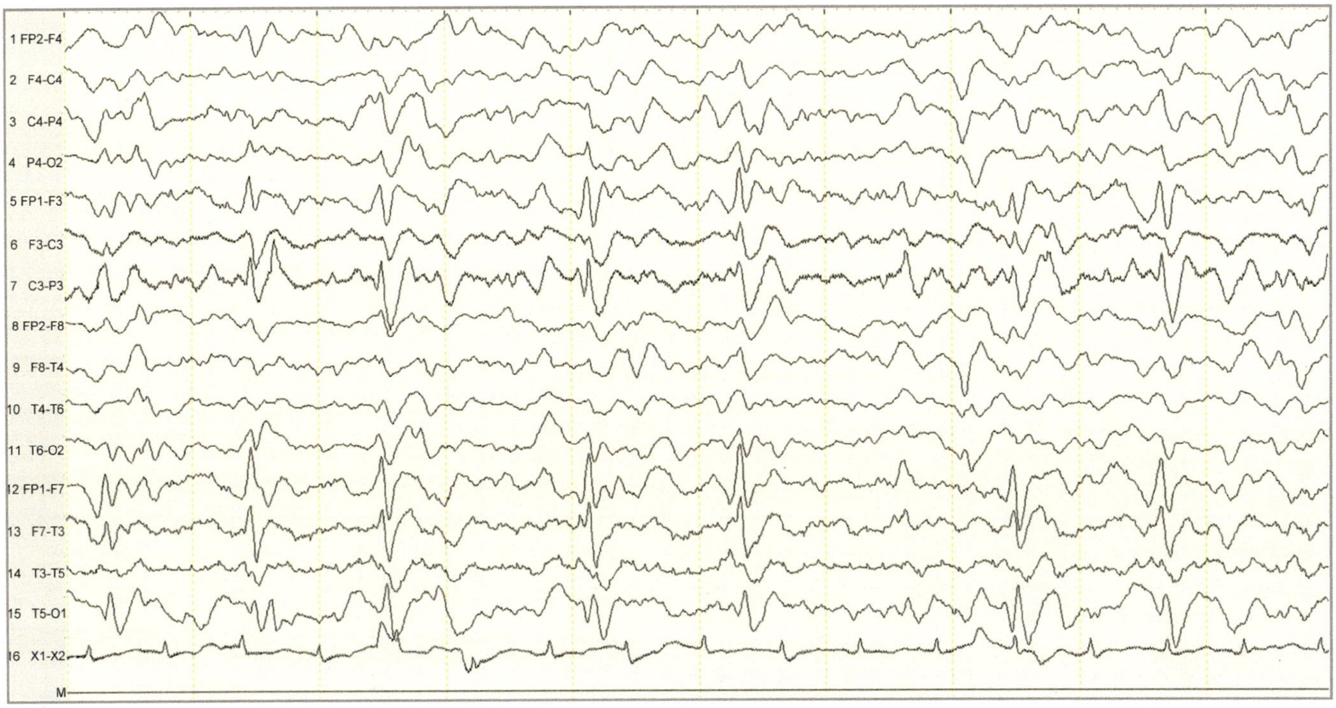

FIG. 30: Periodic lateralized discharges (left) in a case of herpes simplex viral encephalitis.

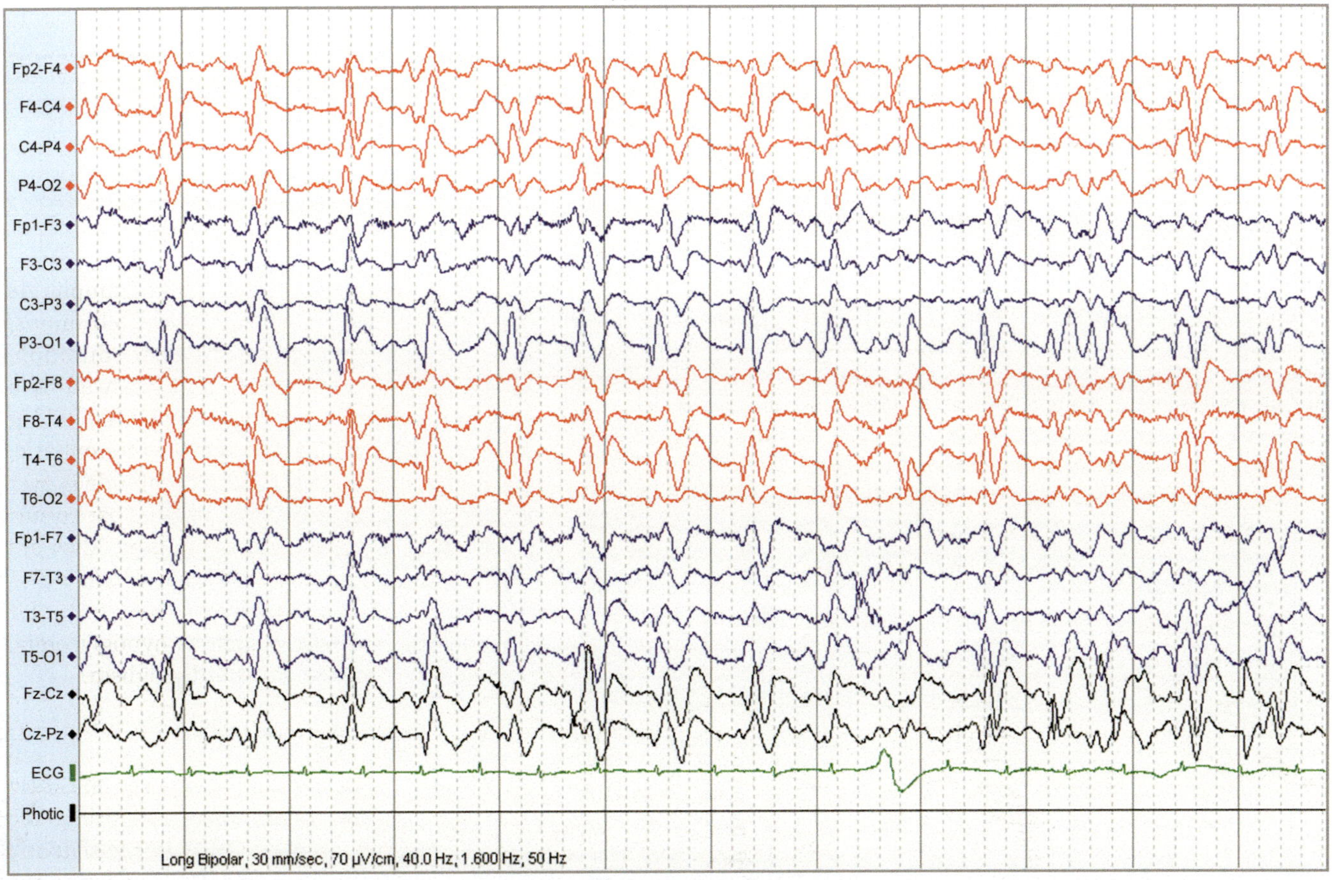

FIG. 31: Generalized 1/second periodic discharges in a case of Creutzfeldt–Jakob disease.

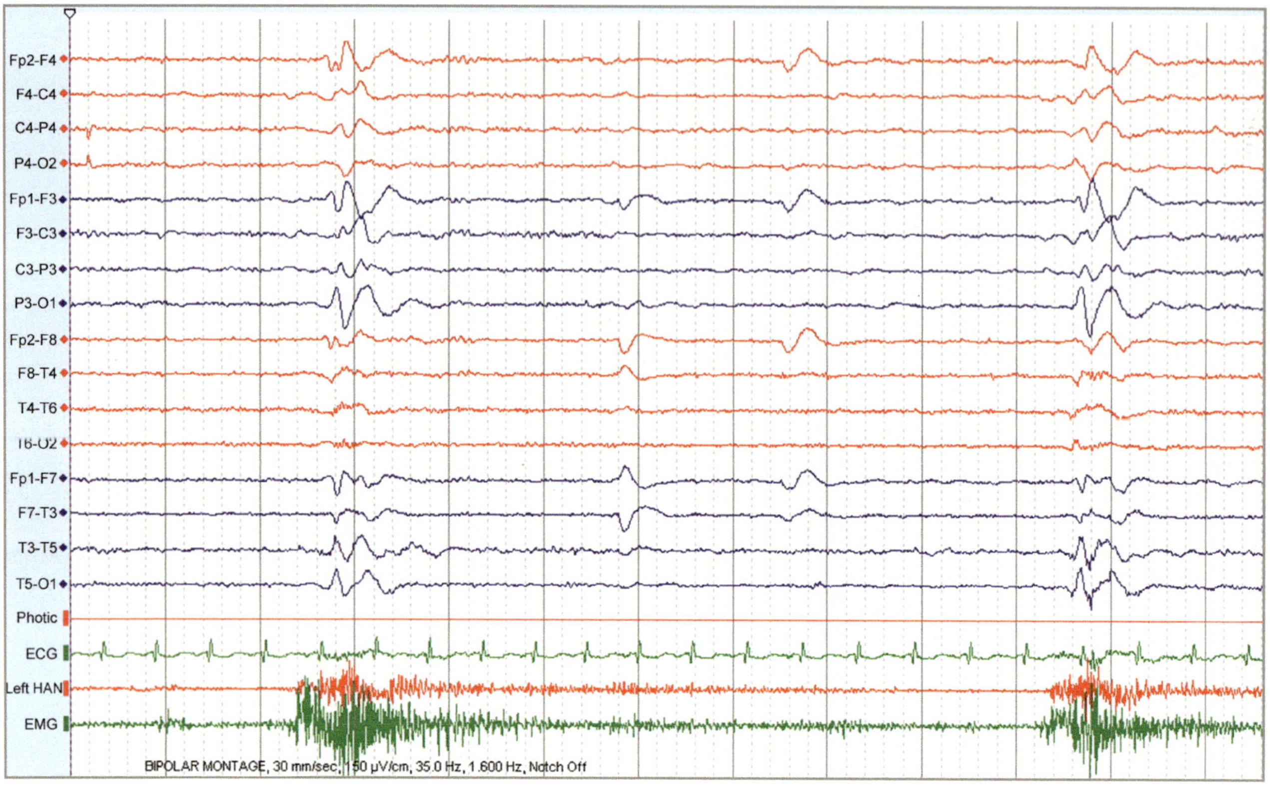

FIG. 32: EEG showing high-amplitude sharp and slow-wave generalized periodic discharges in a case of SSPE.
(EEG: electroencephalography; SSPE: subacute sclerosing panencephalitis)

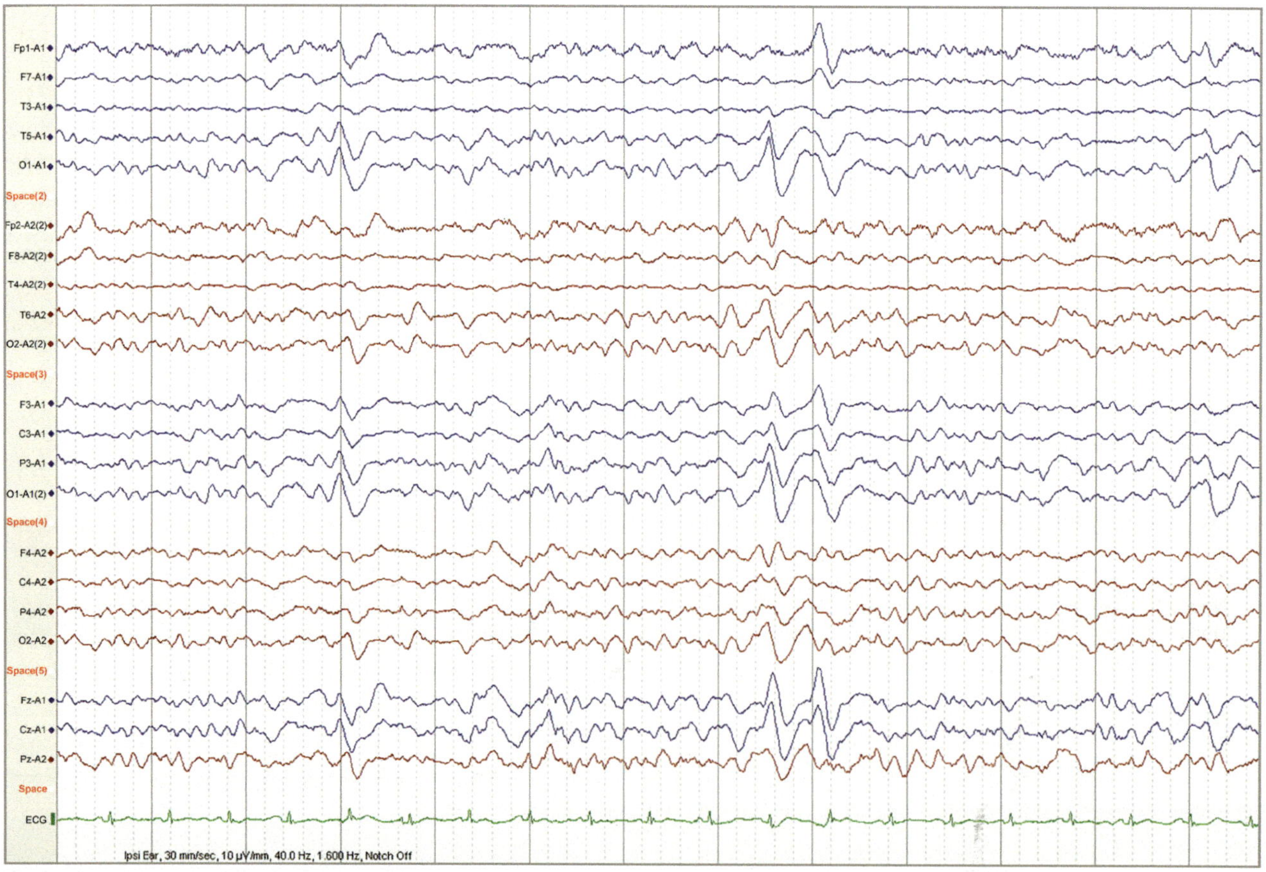

FIG. 33: Triphasic waves in a case of uremic encephalopathy.

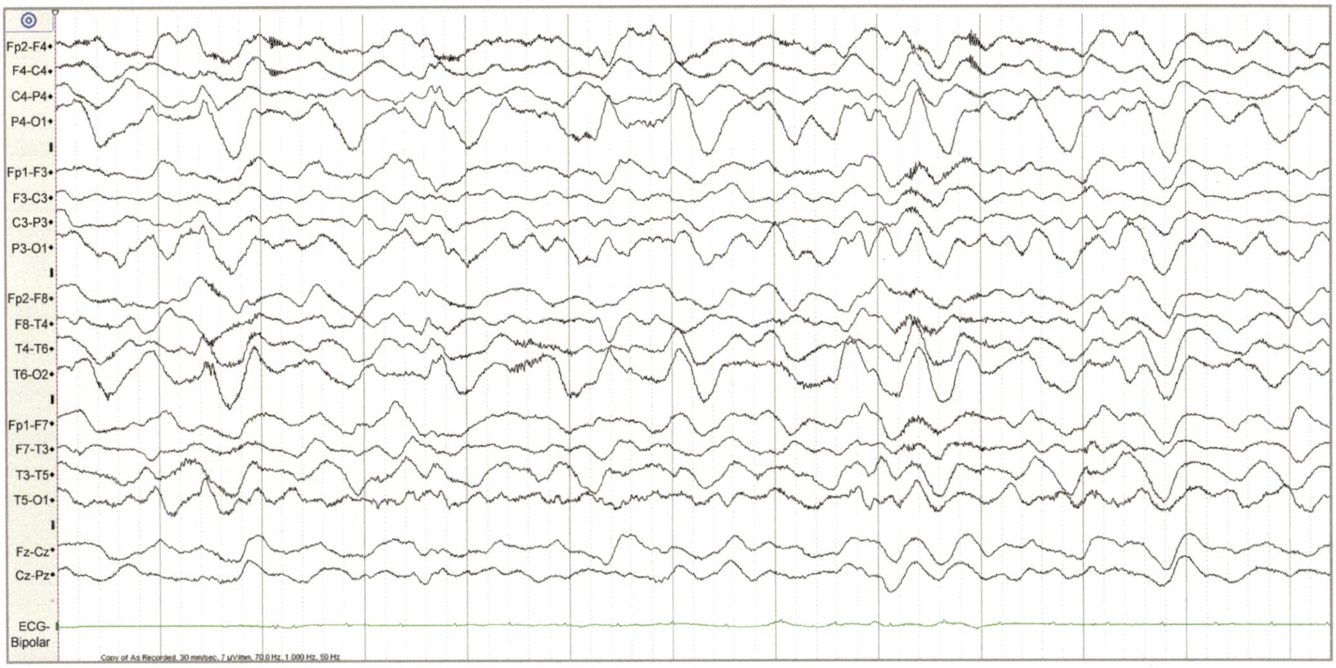

FIG. 34: Diffuse slowing with delta brush pattern in a case of NMDAR encephalitis.
(NMDAR: N-methyl-D-aspartate receptor)

LIMITATIONS

Electroencephalography represents only a summated form of synaptic potentials in superficial cortical layers. In order to be seen on routine EEG, large area of cortex has to be synchronously activated. Anatomical connections and pathways of propagation need to be considered while interpreting the evolving EEG activity else may lead to false localization of the EZ. Meticulous recording and dedicated infrastructure are a prerequisite to avoid generation of artifacts that can mask important EEG findings or cause misinterpretations. Reading EEGs is a patient and clinically oriented task and needs correlation with other imaging features.

CONCLUSION

Electroencephalography is an essential tool in the evaluation of epilepsies, encephalopathies, and in the intensive care unit, especially in the management of SE. EEG should be interpreted carefully with the clinical context in the background. The EEG recordings must be technically sound, and the interpretation should be performed by an experienced neurologist to avoid over-reporting.

REFERENCES

1. Britton JW, Frey LC, Hopp JL, Korb P, Koubeissi MZ, Lievens WE, et al. Introduction. In: St. Louis EK, Frey LC (Eds). Electroencephalography (EEG): An Introductory Text and Atlas of Normal and Abnormal Findings in Adults, Children, and Infants [Internet]. Chicago: American Epilepsy Society; 2016. [online] Available from https://www.ncbi.nlm.nih.gov/books/NBK390346. [Last accessed March, 2023]
2. Nunez P. Quantitative states of neocortex. In: Nunez P (Ed). Neocortical Dynamics and Human EEG Rhythms. New York: Oxford University Press; 1995. pp. 26-8.
3. Tao JX, Ray A, Hawes-Ebersole S, Ebersole JS. Intracranial EEG substrates of scalp EEG interictal spikes. Epilepsia. 2005;46(5):669-76.
4. Beniczky S, Schomer DL. Electroencephalography: basic biophysical and technological aspects important for clinical applications. Epileptic Disord. 2020;22(6):697-15.
5. Deuschl G, Eisen A. Recommendations for the practice of clinical neurophysiology: Guidelines of the International Federation of Clinical Neurophysiology, 2nd edition. Electroenceph Clin Neurophysiol. 1999;52:1-304.

6. Nayak DS, Sajeesh P. Technical standards for digital electroencephalogram recording in epilepsy practice. Ann Indian Acad Neurol. 2007;10:121-7.
7. Waltz S, Christen HJ, Doose H. The different patterns of the PPR--a genetic study. Electroencephalogr Clin Neurophysiol. 1992;83:138-45.
8. King MA, Newton MR, Jackson GD, Fitt GJ, Mitchell LA, Silvapulle MJ, et al. Epileptology of the first seizure presentation: A clinical, electroencephalographic, and MRI study of 300 consecutive patients. Lancet. 1998;352:1007-11.
9. Narayanan JT, Labar DR, Schaul N. Latency to first spike in the EEG of epilepsy patients. Seizure. 2008;17(1):34-41.
10. Panayiotopolus CP. A Clinical Guide to Epileptic Syndromes and their Treatment, 2nd edition. London: Springer; 2010.
11. Beydoun A, Garafalo EA, Drury I. Generalized spike waves, multiple loci and clinical course in children with EEG features of BECTS. Epilepsia. 1992;33:1091-6.
12. Pfänder M, Arnold S, Henkel A, Weil S, Werhahn KJ, Eisensehr I, et al. Clinical features and EEG findings differentiating mesial from neocortical temporal lobe epilepsy. Epileptic Disord Int Epilepsy J Videotape. 2002;4(3):189-95.
13. Brigo F. Intermittent rhythmic delta activity patterns. Epilepsy Behav EB. 2011;20(2):254-6.
14. Hufnagel A, Elger CE, Pels H, Zentner J, Wolf HK, Schramm J, et al. Prognostic significance of ictal and interictal epileptiform activity in temporal lobe epilepsy. Epilepsia. 1994;35(6):1146-53.
15. Sirin NG, Gurses C, Bebek N, Dirican A, Baykan B, Gokyigit A. A quadruple examination of ictal EEG patterns in mesial temporal lobe epilepsy with hippocampal sclerosis: onset, propagation, later significant pattern, and termination. J Clin Neurophysiol. 2013;30(4):329-38.
16. O'Brien TJ1, Kilpatrick C, Murrie V, Vogrin S, Morris K, Cook MJ. Temporal lobe epilepsy caused by mesial temporal sclerosis and temporal neocortical lesions. A clinical and electroencephalographic study of 46 pathologically proven cases. Brain. 1996;119 (Pt 6): 2133-41.
17. García-López B, Sueiras-Gil M, Gómez-Menéndez AI, Vázquez-Sánchez F, Lloria-Gil MC, González-Bernal JJ, et al. Morphological description of frontal EEG interictal and ictal discharges in an adult cohort of 175 patients. J Clin Med. 2021;10(6):1219.
18. Tukel K, Jasper H. The electroencephalogram in parasagittal lesions. Electroencephalogr Clin Neurophysiol. 1952;4:481-94.
19. Foldvary N, Klem G, Hammel J, Bingaman W, Najm I, Lüders H. The localizing value of ictal EEG in focal epilepsy. Neurology. 2001;57:2022-8.
20. Williamson P, Thadani V, Darcey T, Spencer D, Spencer S, Mattson R. Occipital lobe epilepsy: Clinical characteristics, seizure spread patterns, and results of surgery. Ann Neurol. 1992;31(1):3-13.
21. Blume WT, Wiebe S, Tapsell LM. Occipital epilepsy: lateral versus mesial. Brain. 2005;128(Pt 5):1209-25.
22. Kurian M, Seeck M, Wohlrab G, Korff C. Parieto-Occipital Epilepsies: Surgical Versus Non-Surgical Conditions. Epileptologie. 2010;27: 133-42.
23. DeLorenzo RJ, Waterhouse EJ, Towne AR, Boggs JG, Ko D, DeLorenzo GA, et al. Persistent nonconvulsive status epilepticus after the control of convulsive status epilepticus. Epilepsia. 1998;39(8): 833-40.

112
CHAPTER

Electroneuromyography

Khushnuma Mansukhani, Alika Sharma, Lajita Balakrishnan

INTRODUCTION

Modern electrodiagnosis owes its origin to experiments conducted by Galvani in the 18th century and a very comprehensive review is available in the book titled "Some Aspects of History of Neurosciences".[1]

Electrophysiology or electrodiagnosis in neurology, more aptly called electroneuromyography[2] (ENMG), consists of nerve conduction studies (NCSs), electromyography (EMG), and evoked potential (EP) studies. It is an often used but poorly understood tool for diagnosis of neuromuscular diseases. In India, it is often given a stepchild treatment, relegating it to unsupervised untrained technicians.

In India, the clinical neurologist faces a mammoth task. In 2012, there were only 1,100 neurologists for a population of 1.2 billion people.[3,4] With this kind of workload, performing lengthy electrodiagnostic studies may not be feasible for all clinical neurologists. Here comes the need for developing dedicated centers with trained physicians to perform these tests.

The practicing neurologist should, however, be critical of the work done and makes it a habit to analyze the report presented to him. It would be a good practice point to refer patients only to laboratories, which follow scientific protocols.

A good report should be lucid with numerical data, its interpretation, and traces. Traces form an important part of the report because the quality of the recording can be judged. Temperature measurements and corrections if necessary should be mentioned.

This article briefly outlines the ENMG tests and their utility for the management of neuromuscular disorders. Most importantly these tests should not be overused for "ruling out" diseases rather than "confirming" them.

NERVE CONDUCTION STUDY

Nerve conduction is a noninvasive method of studying the sensory, motor, and autonomic nerves. Special tests include H reflex and F wave recordings, repetitive nerve stimulation (RNS), the blink reflex study and short and long exercise tests (SET and LET) for channelopathies. Percutaneous (surface) stimulation of the nerve is the most commonly used technique. In special situations, the nerve can also be stimulated using needle electrodes, e.g., spinal root stimulation. Surface electrodes placed over the nerve or muscle record the responses, needle electrodes too can be used to record these responses, this is especially useful in a severely wasted muscle where the depth of the muscle being studied is difficult to assess.[5] To record the sensory nerve action potential (SNAP), the stimulating and recording electrodes are placed over the same nerve to be studied whereas in motor NCS the motor nerve is stimulated at two or more points along its course and the potential is recorded over the muscle supplied by the nerve. Standard acquisition and recording parameters have to be followed as those used when collecting the reference data.

The parameters measured are the distal latency, amplitude, and the velocity. In addition for motor conductions, the duration of the response, the percentage of area/amplitude drop or relative increase in the duration of the response between the sites of stimulation is also calculated.

Sensory Nerve Conduction Study

Sensory nerve conduction is performed by stimulating a nerve and recording the potential, called the SNAP **(Fig. 1)** at another site over the same nerve. They are thus true nerve action potentials as the potential is recorded over the same nerve being stimulated.[6] When the stimulating potential is travelling in the direction of the natural conduction pathway it is termed orthodromic potential and when it is directed in the opposite direction it is termed the antidromic potential. The latencies and velocities by both methods are comparable but their amplitudes differ.[7] The amplitudes obtained by antidromic techniques are larger as the digital nerves lie nearer to the surface making it easier to record. Also, they are easily obtained; hence, it is not necessary to average out the responses. However, the antidromic responses are sometimes difficult to mark as the amplitude may be obscured by the muscle potentials from the surrounding muscle. The cell body of the sensory nerves lies in the dorsal root ganglion. Hence, any lesion at or distal to the dorsal root ganglion abolishes the sensory potential. This is very helpful in localizing the site of lesion. In radiculopathies, dorsal root compression occurs within the spinal canal proximal to the dorsal root ganglion. The preganglionic sensory fibers are injured but the peripheral sensory axons remain intact. The SNAPs are therefore, normal in root compressions,[8] but there will be clinical sensory involvement. A general assessment of the sensory potentials requires the lower limb as well as upper limb study. One of the earliest markers of a length-dependent peripheral neuropathy is a low sural SNAP. The absence of the most distal sensory potentials in the feet, e.g., medial plantar SNAP or the dorsal sural study also gives clue to the presence of underlying peripheral neuropathy.[9] The length-dependent peripheral neuropathies follow the Wallerian degeneration whereby the lower limb SNAP amplitudes fall much before the upper limb amplitudes. A phenomenon seen in patients with acute inflammatory demyelinating peripheral neuropathy is absent/low median and ulnar SNAPs with normal sural SNAP amplitude signifying a nonlength-dependent peripheral nerve involvement.[10]

Motor Nerve Conduction Study

To record the motor nerve action potential, the recording electrode is placed over the belly of the muscle and the reference electrode is placed distally over the tendon of the same muscle. The amplitude of the compound muscle action potential (CMAP) **(Fig. 2)** is determined by the number of functioning motor units and muscle fibers. Any axon loss process at the nerve, plexus, root, or anterior horn cell level can decrease the CMAP amplitude. Similarly, if the number of muscle fibers is reduced as in severe myopathy the amplitude of the response is reduced. A multifocal demyelinating lesion is considered if there is temporal dispersion or conduction block. Temporal dispersion means a >30% in the duration of the response to proximal stimulation. Similarly, a conduction block implies a drop in area/amplitude of the response on proximal stimulation by 20% over a short segment or 50% over a longer segment, with minimal increase in the duration.[11,12]

Late Responses

Conventional NCSs assess the distal segments of the nerve. As the pathway of H reflex and F waves involves the most proximal segments, it is used for assessing the most proximal nerve roots.

H Reflex (Fig. 3)

It is a monosynaptic reflex mediated by the fast conducting Ia afferent fibers and after synapsing in the spinal cord the alpha motor neurons supply efferents to the muscle. It is analogous to the clinically elicited ankle jerk; but it is not mediated via the muscle spindles. Hence, it is possible to get an H reflex in the absence of an ankle jerk, but the reverse does not hold true. In infants, this reflex can be elicited in all muscles; however, as central nervous system (CNS) maturation occurs this reflex is restricted to only a few

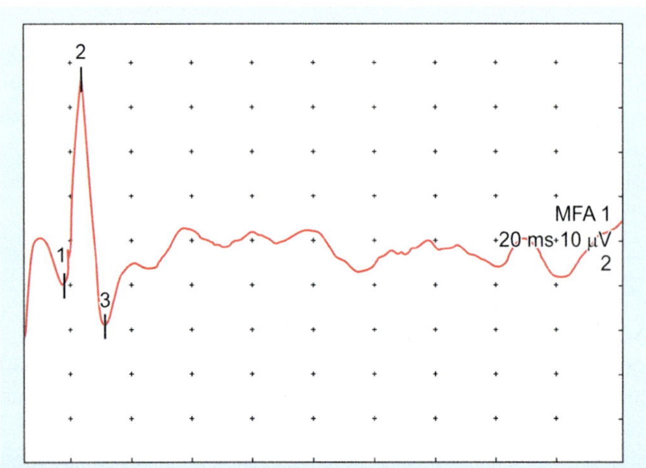

FIG. 1: Normal sensory nerve action potential (SNAP).

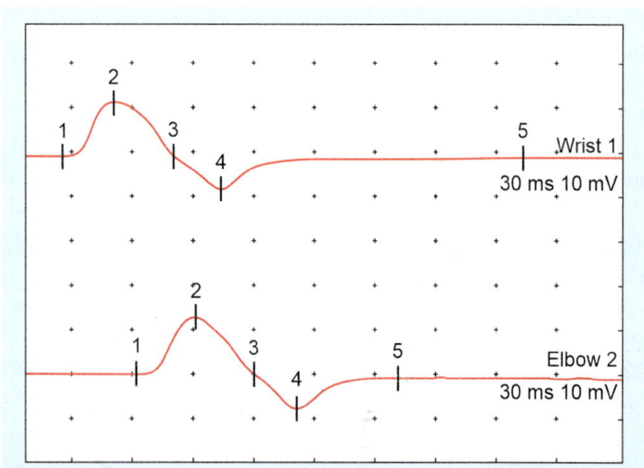

FIG. 2: Normal compound muscle action potential (CMAP).

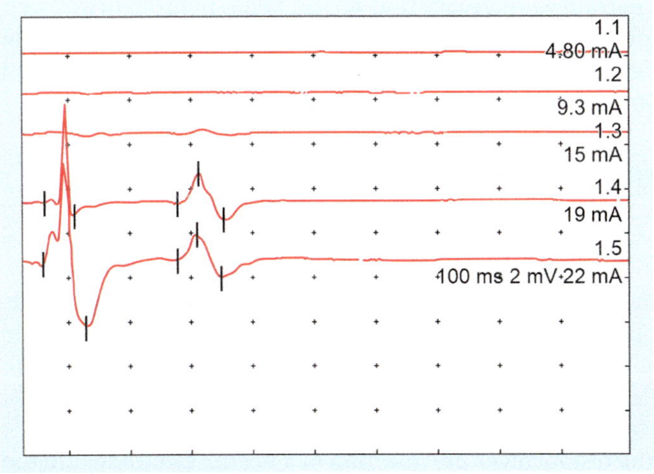

FIG. 3: Normal H reflex.

muscles. In adults, H reflex can be recorded from the tibial innervated gastrocnemius-soleus muscle or the median innervated flexor carpi radialis muscles in the upper limbs.

The absence of H reflex is an early marker of polyradiculopathy, e.g., acute inflammatory demyelinating polyradiculopathy (AIDP) with a sensitivity of 95%.[13] The amplitudes could also be attenuated as part of a generalized process like a diabetic or uremic neuropathy. An asymmetric low amplitude H reflex could suggest a S1 radiculopathy, a lumbosacral plexopathy, tibial, or a sciatic neuropathy. The difference in latencies between the two sides of 1.5 ms is considered to be significant. The maximum peak-peak amplitude of the H reflex can also be compared with the maximum peak-peak amplitude of the M response. This H/M amplitude ratio is found to be increased in upper motor neuron lesions. Similarly, the presence of H reflex in the small muscles of the feet where it is not present normally is an indicator of a central lesion. This has been attributed to the lack of inhibition of the higher centers on the alpha motor neurons.

F Wave (Fig. 4)

It has been so named as it was first recorded from the intrinsic foot muscles. The presence of F waves in deafferented experimental animals suggested that it arose from the motor nerve fibers. When a mixed nerve is stimulated some of the impulses travel antidromically and activates the alpha motor neurons. The parameters measured include the minimum latency, chronodispersion, persistence, and the F estimate. The difference in latencies of the F waves is due to the different firing rates of the alpha motor neurons. The F estimate is used to differentiate between proximal and distal slowing. If the F latency is more than the F estimate then the slowing is predominantly proximal. This is very helpful in early demyelinating lesions. Absence or prolonged latency of F waves has been considered a specific finding for proximal demyelination in AIDP.[8]

Repetitive Nerve Stimulation Test (Fig. 5)

It was first described by Harvey and Masland in 1941. It involves using low-frequency stimulation (<5 Hz) of the nerve and observing the decrementing responses. The basic principle is to stimulate the nerve at a level sufficient enough to overcome the safety factor and unmask the neuromuscular junction (NMJ) disorder. Normally, the amount of acetylcholine released with each nerve impulse is more than the amount required to elicit an endplate potential. This safety factor ensures that each nerve impulse results in an action potential and a muscle contraction.

In normal subjects, the endplate potential manages to cross the threshold level and always elicit an action potential. The amplitude of the response, however, gradually decreases but every stimulus still manages to elicit a muscle contraction.

In postsynaptic NMJ disorders there are less available receptors and some of the endplate potentials do not reach the threshold level to fire an action potential. Repetitive

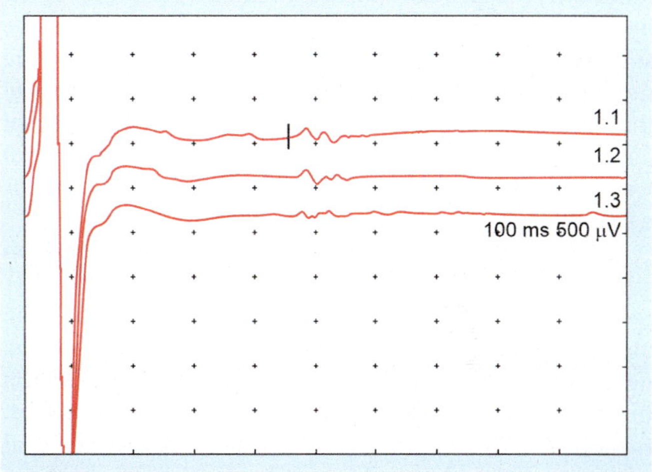

FIG. 4: Normal F waves.

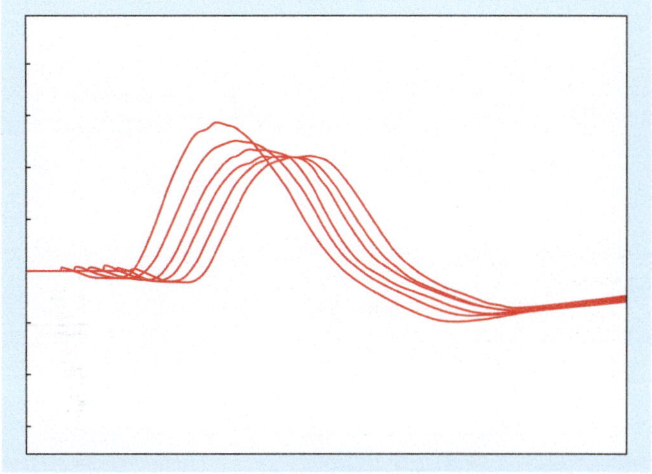

FIG. 5: Repetitive nerve stimulation (RNS) test showing a decrement.

stimulation precipitates this and a decrement is observed. In presynaptic neuromuscular disorders, the availability of acetylcholine is the basic problem and RNS unmasks this also as a decrement. The decrement is considered to be significant if the amplitude drops by 10% between the first and third or fourth responses.[14] Besides decrement, facilitation to 10-second exercise and postexercise fatigue should also be measured. In presynaptic neuromuscular disorders, a short exercise causes a >100% facilitation of the CMAP amplitude.

Blink Reflex (Fig. 6)

The blink reflex is useful for evaluating disorders affecting the fifth, seventh cranial nerves, and the brainstem. It is elicited by electrical stimulation of the supraorbital nerve. Surface electrodes placed over the orbicularis oculi record the responses. The afferent pathway is mediated by the trigeminal nerve and the efferent via the facial nerve. The reflex response consists of an early ipsilateral R1 and a later bilateral R2. The R1 response is an oligosynaptic pontine reflex whereas the R2 response is mediated via interneurons in the pons and medulla. Unlike direct facial nerve stimulation which assesses only the distal segments of the nerve, the blink reflex can study the proximal segments of the facial nerve. An abnormal blink reflex in the presence of a normal facial motor study indicates a lesion at a proximal level between the stylomastoid foramen and the facial motor nerve nucleus.

In facial nerve disorders, R2 response is abnormal on stimulation of the affected as well as the normal side. R1 response is abnormal only on the side of the lesion. The absence of blink reflex is a sign of poor prognosis in facial neuropathies. Involvement of the trigeminal nerve affects the ipsilateral R1 and R2 and the contralateral R2 responses. In addition to diagnosing an acute or subacute facial neuropathy, the blink reflex can also be used to check for

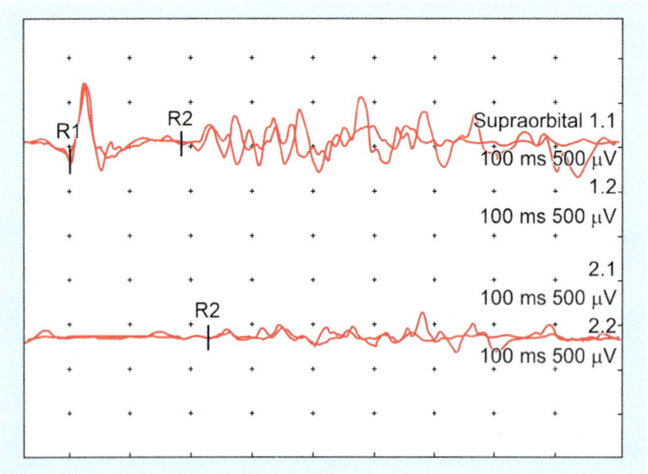

FIG. 6: Normal blink reflex.

aberrant reinnervation in an old facial neuropathy as well for observing synkinesis in hemifacial spasm.[15,16] Since the development of excellent imaging techniques for intracranial studies, the utility of this test had reduced.

NEEDLE ELECTROMYOGRAPHY

Mastering the technique and analysis of needle electromyographic examination (NEE) has a longer learning curve than NCS and being semiquantitative, analysis depends on the experience of the electromyographer.[17] Multiple software programs are now available to help quantify the findings and make teaching and learning an easier process. However, do remember the maxim "garbage in garbage out". The test involves the insertion of a needle electrode into the muscle and assessing electrical activity of the muscle at rest, during needle movement and with mild and full voluntary contraction.

The prerequisites for performing a needle electrode examination are:
- Sound knowledge of anatomy and physiology of nerves and muscles
- Good referral note or history and examination of the patient
- Preparing the patient for the test
- Skilled examiner
- Protocol based approach

Technique

Monopolar or concentric needles are used. Single fiber electrodes for jitter analysis are now replaced by small pore concentric needle electrodes. The selection of muscles is based on customized electrodiagnostic protocols, which take into consideration findings on clinical examination and NCS. Explaining the procedure and reassuring the patient often ensures good compliance.

Once the needle electrode is inserted, three types of activities should be observed:
1. *Insertional activity*: Associated with needle movement
2. *Spontaneous activity*: Activity noted at rest
3. *Voluntary activity*: Associated with muscle contraction/activation

Insertional Activity

It occurs in short bursts associated with needle movement. It is a normal finding if the duration is <300 ms.[18] It helps to identify that the needle is in the muscle and not in adipose tissue. Increased insertional activity, i.e., >300 ms, indicates unstable muscle membrane. This can be seen with acute neurogenic/myopathic disorders as a sign of early denervation and also in myotonic disorders (myotonic discharges).

Spontaneous Activity

The only normal spontaneous waveforms are endplate noise and endplate spikes observed in the end plate region. Various types of spontaneous activity have been classified based on source generators along the neuroanatomic axis and on morphology and firing characteristics **(Table 1)**.[14,18]

The spontaneous activity also helps in determining the temporal profile of the disorder, e.g., large amplitude fibrillation potentials indicate recent involvement and complex repetitive discharges indicate chronic disease process.

Voluntary Activity

It is the electrical activity noted with mild voluntary muscle contraction and consists of motor unit potentials (MUP). A motor unit is the basic unit of the peripheral nervous system. It is defined as an individual motor neuron, its axon and the associated NMJ and muscle fibers. The MUP represents the sum total of the action potentials of individual muscle fibers innervated by a single anterior horn cell within the pickup territory of the recording needle electrode. MUPs are assessed based on morphology, stability, and firing patterns.

- *Morphology*: The morphology of a normal MUP is usually biphasic or triphasic. It is best assessed at mild levels of contraction as increasing contraction leads to the recruitment of many motor units superimposed on each other.
- *Amplitude*: Normal MUPs vary in amplitude from 100 µV to 2 mV.[18] It is measured from peak-to-peak of the main spike of the potential. Important factors associated with increased amplitude include:
    - Proximity of the needle electrode to the motor unit
    - Increased number of muscle fibers in a motor unit
    - Muscle fiber hypertrophy
    - Synchronized firing of muscle fibers
- *Duration*: Measured from the initial deflection from the baseline to the final return to the baseline. It best reflects the number of fibers within a motor unit. Normal duration is between 5 and 15 ms.[18] Duration of a normal MUP indicates the synchrony of firing of motor units. Long duration MUPs indicate reinnervation following lower motor neuropathies. Short duration MUPs usually indicate loss of muscle fibers (myopathies).
- *Phases*: Phase of an MUP constitutes the part that deflects from and returns to the baseline. The number of phases is calculated as the number of baseline crossings of the MUP plus one. An increase in phases, i.e., polyphasics, is a nonspecific abnormality that indicates nonsynchronous firing of motor units. A 25% increase in polyphasics could be a normal finding in large proximal muscles.[19]
- *Stability*: Normal MUPs are identical in morphology and fire synchronously. Variation refers to a change in amplitude/duration of the potential when the contraction is maintained at a constant level without movement of the needle. NMJ disorders and neurogenic disorders causing reinnervation lead to instability of MUPs with moment-to-moment variation of waveform configuration.
- *Firing pattern*: A normal MUP fires semirhythmically. As the muscle begins to contract, only few motor units are activated and more motor units fire with increased force of contraction. Firing pattern is assessed in terms of activation of MUPs and recruitment. Activation refers to the firing rate and represents a central process. Recruitment is the ability to add motor units as the firing rate increases. Recruitment frequency is the

TABLE 1: Various types of spontaneous activity.

Potential	Source generator	Sound	Firing rate	Stability	Firing pattern
Endplate noise	Miniature endplate potentials	Sea shell	20–40 Hz		Irregular
Endplate spike	Muscle fiber initiated by terminal axonal twig	Sputtering fat on a frying pan	5–50 Hz		Irregular
Fibrillation **(Fig. 7A)**	Muscle fiber	Rain on a tin roof	0.5–10 Hz	Stable	Regular
Positive sharp wave	Muscle fiber	Dull pops/rain on a tin roof	0.5–10 Hz	Stable	Regular
Myotonic discharges **(Fig. 7C)**	Muscle fiber	Revving engine	20–150 Hz	Waxing and waning	Waxing waning
Complex repetitive discharges (CRD) **(Fig. 7D)**	Multiple muscle fibers	Machine	5–100 Hz	Perfectly regular	Usually stable
Fasciculation **(Fig. 7B)**	Motor unit	Corn popping	0.1–10Hz		Irregular
Myokymia	Motor unit	Marching soldiers	1–5 Hz interburst, 5–60 Hz intraburst		Bursting
Cramp	Motor unit		20–150 Hz		Interference pattern/ several individual units
Neuromyotonia	Motor unit	Pinging	150–250 Hz	Decrementing	Waning

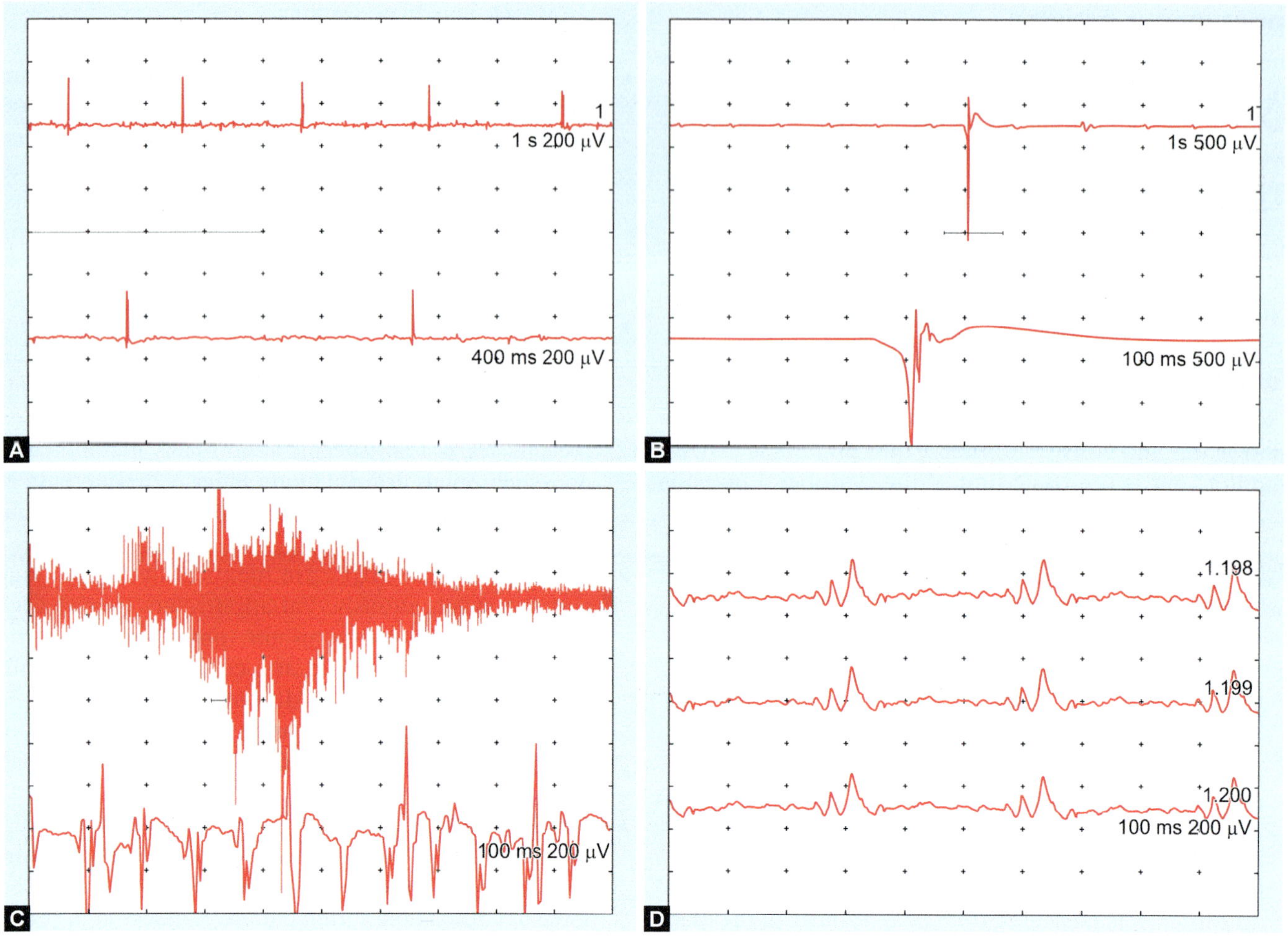

FIGS. 7A TO D: Spontaneous activity on needle electromyography: (A) Fibrillation potentials; (B) fasciculation potentials; (C) myotonic discharges; and (D) complex repetitive discharges.

firing frequency just before an additional motor unit is recruited with an increased force of contraction. Normal recruitment frequency ranges from 8 to 15 Hz.[19] The morphology and dimensions of a motor unit action potential (MUAP) vary with physiological factors such as patient age, temperature of the muscle, site of recording within muscle, size of the muscle, distance of motor unit from the recording electrode, and type of needle electrode.

ABNORMAL MOTOR UNIT ACTIVITY

Lower motor neuron disorders cause abnormalities in MUAP morphology as well as recruitment and the patterns of these abnormalities help in classification, localization, severity, and prognosis of the disorder. The various patterns could be:

- *Neuropathic*: Axonal/Demyelinating
- Myopathic
- NMJ transmission defect
- Acute/Chronic/End stage disorder

Neuropathic Abnormalities (Fig. 8A)

These include abnormal MUAP morphology due to axon loss—usually seen with peripheral nerve injuries, root/plexus lesions, and anterior horn cell disorders. The pattern of abnormalities varies with the time since onset of disease/injury. After acute but partial axon loss, Wallerian degeneration takes time and fibrillations may not be detected immediately—what is recorded on needle EMG is reduced recruitment due to loss of axons. To compensate for this, the rate of firing of motor units increases and hence the earliest finding is reduced recruitment of "normal looking" motor units with a fast firing rate. A fast firing rate is also noted when there is a conduction block in the motor fibers, however, these muscles have normal amplitudes on distal motor nerve testing (NCS) and do not develop fibrillations if there is a pure conduction block.[14]

What follows with time in partial axon loss lesions is collateral sprouting of axons which causes nonsynchronous firing of motor units leading to satellite and polyphasic MUPs indicating reinnervation. In complete acute axon degeneration (with physical continuity maintained), regeneration is seen with regrowth and when the axon reaches the target muscle. This is always delayed as the nerve grows at an approximate rate of an inch a month. Nascent, unstable, polyphasic MUPs which are small in amplitude are the first signs of reinnervation **(Fig. 8B)**. These then become large in amplitude and duration as time progresses and long duration, high-amplitude triphasic MUPs indicate a chronic process. In conditions that cause chronic ongoing denervation and reinnervation, a combination of findings is seen.

"Myopathic" Abnormalities

These are seen due to muscle fiber loss or dysfunction. Because of fewer numbers of muscle fibers per motor unit, the MUPs are of shorter duration and amplitude **(Fig. 8C)**. Also due to less synchronous firing of the remaining muscle fibers, there is an increase in polyphasic MUPs. Because of fewer numbers of muscle fibers in each motor unit, activation cannot generate as much force of contraction as a normal muscle. Hence for a small amount of contraction, a greater number of motor units need to be recruited leading to early recruitment and a full interference pattern. This early recruitment is a hallmark of myopathies.[20] Also with chronic myopathies, with an increase in loss of muscle fibers, the interference is reduced; however, the recruitment remains early. In some myopathies such as inclusion body myopathies and with very chronic myopathies, some large amplitude MUPs may be seen.

Neuromuscular Junction Disorders

Motor unit potential morphology usually remains normal in mild NMJ disorders. With the increase in severity, there is blocking of some muscle fibers in the motor unit leading to a change in morphology from potential to potential leading to unstable MUPs. With greater and more persistent block, the MUP becomes small, short, and polyphasic, similar to a myopathic MUAP.

Single Fiber EMG

This is a specialized electromyographic recording technique to assess neuromuscular transmission by recording individual muscle fiber action potentials. It requires specialized needle electrodes and software program for recording. Low-frequency filter is increased to 500 Hz to avoid recording from distant muscle fibers.[14] In voluntary

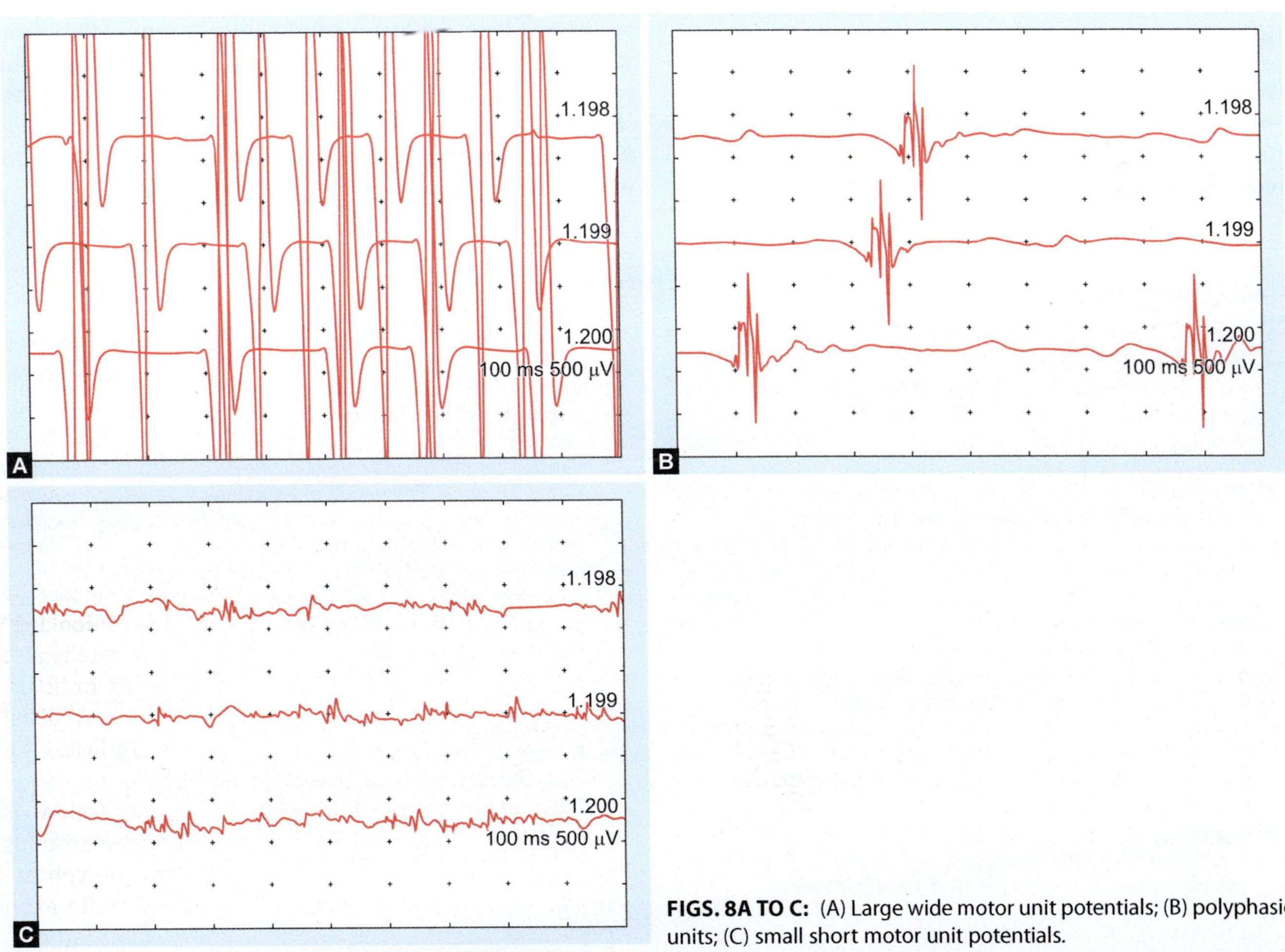

FIGS. 8A TO C: (A) Large wide motor unit potentials; (B) polyphasic units; (C) small short motor unit potentials.

activated single fiber EMG (SFEMG), the needle is inserted in the muscle and the patient is asked to voluntarily activate the muscle very minimally and steadily. The needle is focused on a "pair" of potentials from adjacent single muscle fibers from the same motor unit. The time interval between the two potentials is measured from discharge to discharge. The variation in the time interval from discharge to discharge reflects variation in neuromuscular transmission and is termed "Jitter". When the safety factor is reduced, some endplate potentials take longer to reach the threshold, muscle fiber action potential generation is delayed, and jitter increases. With more severe NMJ disorders, individual muscle fibers fail to discharge intermittently and produce "blocking" on SFEMG. Blocking correlates with clinical weakness. At least 20 different potential pairs are assessed from different areas of each muscle.[20] Results are reported as the mean/median jitter for all the pairs tested and pairs with impulse blocking. SFEMG is abnormal when >10% of fiber pairs exhibit increased jitter or the mean/median jitter is above the value specified for that muscle. Since the single fiber needle electrode is not disposable the same technique is now performed using the facial concentric needle electrode. The filter settings and techniques are well standardized and it is called "jitter analysis using facial concentric needle electrode" or "apparent SFEMG".

PROVOCATIVE TESTS

Over the last few years, provocative studies have been used for differentiating the various channelopathies using the effect of exercise and cooling on the CMAP. Exercise and cold affect the conduction of the NMJ and the excitability of the abnormal muscle membrane. Provocative tests were designed to objectively document these effects and use them for diagnosis in the electrodiagnostic (EDX) laboratory.[21]

Short Exercise Test

A 10-second exercise is given to the rested muscle and the CMAP is recorded immediately after stopping the exercise. In presynaptic neuromuscular transmission defects, facilitation (>60–100%) is noted. If three runs of SETs are given to a rested muscle the patterns observed after each run of exercise helps to differentiate autosomal dominant myotonia congenita, recessive myotonia congenita, and paramyotonia congenita.[22] Running the SET on the cooled muscle (SET with cooling) further helps in the differential diagnosis if the SET is not conclusive.[23]

Long Exercise Test

This involves testing the CMAP amplitude after exercising the muscle for 5 minutes. It is useful in the diagnosis of hypo/hyperkalemic periodic paralysis.[22]

CONCLUSION

Electroneuromyography when well performed and correlated with the history and clinical examination gives a wealth of information regarding the function of the nervous tissue being examined. It is up to the clinician to recommend this test with a good referral note stating his impression and the information he requires from the examining physician.

REFERENCES

1. Kumar JD. Some aspects of history of neurosciences. East Zone Neuro CME. 2003;177-229.
2. Katirji B. The clinical electromyography examination: an overview. Neurolo Clin N Am. 2002;20:291-303.
3. Khadilkar SV. Neurology: the scenario in India. J Assoc Physicians India. 2012;60:42-4.
4. Khadilkar SV, Wagh S. Practice patterns of neurology in India: Fewer hands, more work. Neurol India. 2007;55(1):27-3.
5. Mallik A, Weir AI. Nerve conduction studies: essentials and Pitfalls in practice. J Neurol Neurosurg Psychiatry. 2005;76 (Suppl 2):ii23-31.
6. Cohn TG, Wertch JJ, Pasupuleti DV, Loftsgarden JD, Schenk VA. Nerve conduction studies: Orthodromic vs antidromic latencies. Arch Phys Med Rehabil. 1990;71(8):579-82.
7. Shin OJ. Clinical electromyography: Nerve conduction studies. Philadelphia: Lippincott Williams & Wilkins; 2003. pp. 316-7.
8. Mondelli M, Aretini A, Arrigucci U, Ginanneschi F, Greco G, Sicurelli F. Sensory nerve action potential amplitude is rarely reduced in lumbosacral radiculopathy due to herniated disc. Clin Neurophysiol. 2013;124(2):405-9.
9. Papanas N, Trypsians G, Maltezos E. The sural sensory/radial motor amplitude ratio for the diagnosis of peripheral neuropathy in type 2 diabetic patients. Hipppokratika. 2010;14 (3):198-202.
10. Gordon PH, Wilbourn AJ. Early electrodiagnostic findings in Guillain-Barré syndrome. Arch Neurol. 2001;58(6):913-7.
11. Weber F Conduction block and abnormal temporal dispersion—diagnostic criteria. Electromyogr Clin Neurophysiol. 1997;37(5): 305-9.
12. Van den Bergh PY, Hadden RD, Bouche P, Cornblath DR, Hahn A, Illa I, et al; European Federation of Neurological Societies, Peripheral Nerve Society. European Federation of Neurological Societies/Peripheral Nerve Society guideline on management of chronic inflammatory demyelinating polyradiculoneuropathy: report of a joint task force of the European Federation of Neurological Societies and the Peripheral Nerve Society—first revision. Eur J Neurol. 2010;17(3):356-63.
13. Al-Shekhlee A, Hachwi RN, Preston DC, Katirji B. New criteria for early electrodiagnosis of acute inflammatory demyelinating polyneuropathy. Muscle Nerve. 2005;32(1):66-72.
14. Preston D, Shapiro BE. Electromyography and Neuromuscular disorders: Clinical–Electrophysiologic Correlations, 3rd edition. Baltimore: Williams and Wilkins; 2013.
15. Aminoff MJ. Electrodiagnosis in clinical neurology, 6th edition. Philadelphia: Elsevier Health Sciences; 2012.

16. Kimura J. Electrodiagnosis in Diseases of Nerve and Muscle: Principles and Practice, 3rd edition. New York: Oxford University Press; 2001.
17. Daube JR, Rubin DI. Needle electromyography. Muscle Nerve. 2009;39(2):244-70.
18. Katirji B. Neurologic Clinics: Clinical electromyography, Vol 20, Issue 2. Philadelphia: WB Saunders Company; 2002.
19. Katirji B. Electromyography in clinical practice: A case study approach, 2nd edition. Ohio: Elsevier Publication; 2007. pp. 35.
20. Ruben DI. Clinical Electromyography: An Issue of Neurologic Clinics, Vol 30. Philadelphia: Elsevier Publication; 2012. pp. 634.
21. Sanders DB, Arimura K, Cui LY, Ertaş M, Farrugia ME, Gilchrist J, et al. Guidelines for single fiber EMG. Clin Neurophysiol. 2019;130(8): 1417-39.
22. Fournier E, Arzel M, Sternberg D, Vicart S, Laforet P, Eymard B, et al. Electromyography guides toward subgroups of mutations in muscle channelopathies. Ann Neurol. 2004;56(5):650-61.
23. Gawel M, Szmidt-Salkowska E, Lusakowska A, Nojszewska M, Sulek A, Krysa W, et al. Value of short exercise and short exercise with cooling tests in the diagnosis of myotonic dystrophies (DM1 AND DM2). Muscle Nerve. 2014;49:277-83.

113

CHAPTER

Evoked Potentials

Karkal Ravishankar Naik, Aralikatte Onkarappa Saroja

INTRODUCTION

Evoked potentials (EPs) are the electrical responses from within the central nervous system to external stimulus. Majority of the EPs recorded from scalp and peripheral electrodes represent near-field potentials. Far-field potentials originating in deeper subcortical and brainstem structures are recorded using referential montages. Generators of these centrally-conducting volley of action potentials and synaptic potentials correlate with anatomical data, clinicopathological states, and neuroradiologic data. Recording during surgical procedures have provided confirmation of neural source generators of the EPs.

These potentials generally range from 0.01 to 10 μV and are much smaller than the simultaneously recorded electroencephalogram (EEG) from which they have to be extracted. Apart from the photic drive response from luminance-induced occipital responses in EEG, other EPs are not discernible in the raw EEG. Dawson described the use of signal averaging for extracting the somatosensory-EPs from the raw EEG in 1954. Introduction of signal processing and averaging paralleled by improvements in digital computations has made the EP extraction from EEG and other biological signals a simpler task. The responses to stimulations (signal) are time-locked to the stimulus and occur with each stimulus. The random electrical activities from nervous system (noise) are not time-locked to the stimulus. Averaging of multiple stimulus epochs removes the random noise leaving only the signal of interest which is time-locked. Signal-to-noise ratio (SNR) is proportional to the square root of the number of stimulus epochs. Increasing the number of stimulus epochs, therefore, increases the clarity of the signal by increasing the SNR **(Fig. 1)**. Averaging >1,000 epochs is needed for eliciting the small-amplitude (<0.5 μV) auditory evoked potentials (AEPs) whereas the larger-amplitude visual evoked potentials (VEPs) can be recorded with <100 stimulations. The stimulation should be continued till the EP waveform is robust and at least two trials should be averaged to demonstrate consistency.

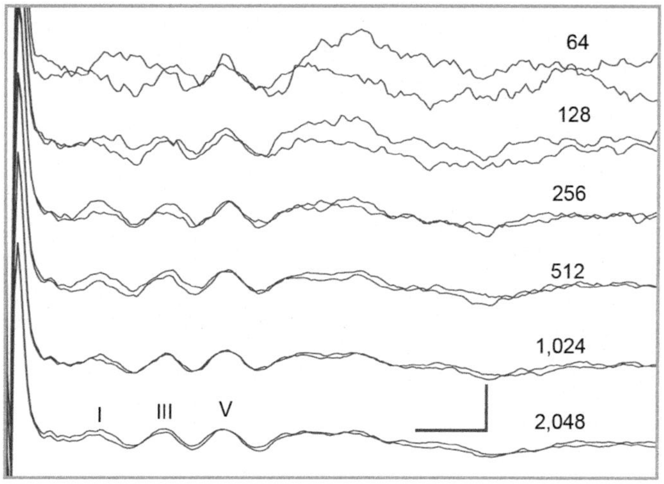

FIG. 1: The use of averaging to reduce noise in evoked potential recording with number of stimulus epochs ranging from 64 to 2,048; with increasing number of stimulations, the evoked potential waveform becomes well delineated due to progressive elimination of noise. Calibration 2 msec, 0.5 μV.

Laboratories performing EPs should obtain their normative data using guideline-based recording and use recommended parameters and nomenclature of the waveforms. It is recommended to use 2.5–3 standard deviations above the mean for latencies and intervals; and 2.5–3 standard deviations below the mean amplitude to avoid labeling a normal observation as abnormal.[1,2] It is customary to display the potentials with negativity upward in clinical neurophysiology laboratories. However, most ophthalmic and audiology electrophysiologists display positive activity above the baseline.

Auditory evoked potentials, VEPs, and somatosensory evoked potentials (SSEPs) are the routinely recorded EPs in clinical neurophysiology practice. Other EPs including electroretinograms (ERGs), vestibular evoked myogenic potentials (VEMPs) and event-related cognitive evoked potentials are evaluated less frequently. Intraoperative monitoring (IOM) of nervous system using EPs monitoring in special situations has contributed to better surgical outcome. Despite the advances in magnetic resonance imaging (MRI), including diffusion tensor imaging and functional imaging, EPs have important role in the diagnosis and monitoring of neurological disorders.

VISUAL EVOKED POTENTIALS

Visual evoked potentials are the averaged potentials from EEG recorded over the scalp overlying the visual cortex in response to visual stimuli. Adrian and Mathews demonstrated occipital EEG response to strobe flash in 1934. Visual stimuli used to record VEPs have evolved through stroboscopic flash, light-emitting diodes (LEDs), pattern onset–offset, and pattern reversal/shift to multifocal stimulation protocols. VEP is a complex response with many overlapping responses from the visual pathway. Primary visual cortex is located in the medial occipital lobe. Foveal visual field is in the calcarine fissure away from the occipital pole. Due to interindividual variations in visual-cortical representation, surface-recorded P100 amplitude varies between the midline and lateral electrodes. Generally, the surface-recorded VEP from hemifield stimulations have higher amplitude in the ipsilateral lateral occipital and posterior-temporal electrodes. Generators of the VEP components have major contributions from V1 and V4 areas. Multichannel recording, dipole modeling, and functional MRI with connectivity studies have provided insights into the surface distribution of the VEP signals. P100 can be recorded from the primary visual cortex and the dorsal extrastriate cortex in middle occipital gyrus.[3,4]

Visual Evoked Potential Methodology

Stroboscopic and LED flash stimulations excite the whole retina and produce luminance-induced visual response. It is less sensitive in detecting the visual pathway pathologies due to wide variation in latency and morphology even in normal individuals. Checkerboard pattern with equal number of black and white checks is the preferred stimulus for the clinical VEP recording. It produces consistent VEPs and is consistently abnormal in persons with visual pathway disorders. The black and white squares alternate without overall alteration change in luminance of the stimulus field and preferentially stimulate the central visual field. Central retina containing the macula and fovea is the major contributor of the retinal ganglion cell output to the optic nerve. Cortical representation of fovea accounts up to half of the primary occipital cortex.[5]

Small check size (<20 minutes) with small stimulus field size (≤4°) stimulates the central foveal and parafoveal visual field (*central field stimulation*). Patient attention and cooperation are very important with central field stimulation as the VEP can be easily degraded due to defocusing. For recording the clinical pattern reversal VEPs (PRVEPs), larger field size (>15°) along with larger check size (30–60 minutes) is utilized with viewing distance of at least 70 cm from the visual stimulator. Visual angle of the individual pattern and the display should be constant for all the examinations to avoid viewing angle-induced changes in latency and amplitude variations. The aspect ratio of the pattern display screen should not exceed 4:3. *Full-field stimulation* indicates that there are equal numbers of squares or bars of the pattern on both sides of the central fixation point. In the *hemifield stimulation*, pattern is displayed in either right or left hemifields with other hemifield kept blank.[6-9] The visual angle subtended at the viewing distance from the screen and pattern can be calculated using following formula:

$$Visual\ angle = tan^{-1}\ (check\ or\ screen\ width/distance\ from\ screen) \times 60$$

Brightness of the screen and the contrast between the black and white checks should be maintained constant for all the examinations to avoid brightness- and contrast-induced latency and amplitude changes. Stimulation using horizontal or vertical black-and-white bar or sinusoidal grating pattern can be utilized for obtaining the VEPs. Despite the identical spatial resolution of checkerboard and grating pattern, VEP latencies, amplitudes, and wave morphology from these patterns can be different **(Fig. 2)**.

Surface electrodes are placed after cleaning the skin with electrode impedance maintained <5 kOhms. Queen Square or 10–20 system of electrode placement can be used. With Queen Square system, midline occipital (MO) electrode is placed 5 cm above inion, mid-parietal (MP) is 5 cm above MO, and midfrontal (MF) electrode is placed 12 cm from nasion. The lateral occipital electrodes [right occipital (RO), left occipital (LO)] are placed 5 cm laterally on either side of MO. Lateral temporal electrodes [left temporal (LT), right temporal

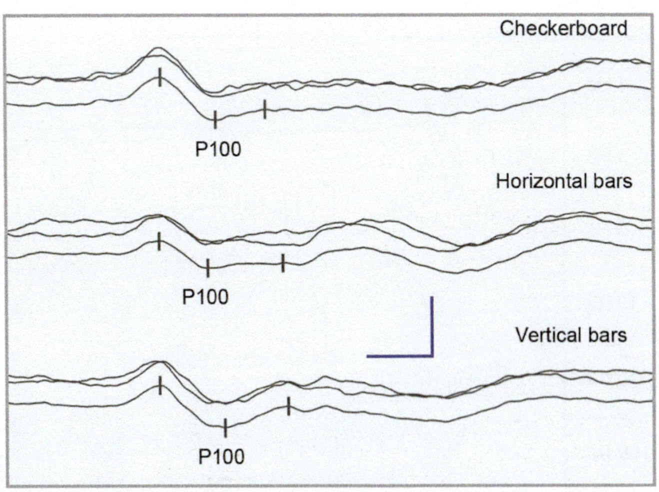

FIG. 2: Pattern visual evoked potentials (VEPs) elicited using 0.5 degree (30') reversed at 1.5 Hz displayed in a screen subtending 20° × 15° angle; top traces shows the VEP recorded using black-and-white checkerboard pattern, middle traces with horizontal bar pattern, and the bottom traces with vertical bar pattern. Latencies are increased with vertical bars and amplitude reduced with horizontal bars. Sensitivity 5 µV/division, sweep 30 ms/division.

(RT)] are placed 5 cm anterior to lateral occipital electrodes. The 10–20 system utilizes Oz, O1, O2, Pz, and Fz electrode placements.[7]

Low-frequency filter is set at 1 Hz and high frequency at 100 Hz with sweep duration of 300–500 ms. Full-field monocular stimulation for each eye is performed with covering of the opposite eye with opaque patch. Pattern reversals should be kept <4 Hz for the clinical transient VEPs as higher stimulation rates produce sinusoidal steady-state VEP **(Fig. 3)**. Two averages of 100–200 stimulus epochs are generally sufficient to record consistent VEP waveforms. If the responses are small, number of stimulations needs to be increased and more than two trials are needed.

P100, the major and consistent component of PRVEP, has a positive occipital and parietal electrical field. MF to ear derivation reveals concurrent N100 with similar latency but opposite polarity. Utilization of active MO and parietal electrodes referenced to MF electrodes increases the P100 amplitude due to concurrent opposite polarity potentials **(Fig. 4)**. The 2006 American Clinical Neurophysiology Society (ACNS) guidelines recommend the following montage for the full-field PRVEP:[7]

Channel 1: LO—MF

Channel 2: MO—MF

Channel 3: RO—MF

Channel 4: MF—Ai (ear/mastoid)

American Clinical Neurophysiology Society recommends an alternative montage with inion, MO, MP, and MF electrodes referenced to linked ear reference if the P100 amplitudes are small or absent. Few authors advocate simultaneous recording of pattern electroretinograms (PERGs) along with PRVEP. Conjunctival gold foil and Dawson, Trick, and Litzkow (DTL) electrodes are recommended for recording PERGs of consistent morphology and amplitudes. PERG amplitudes with subcanthal surface electrodes are small and require more number of stimulations to obtain consistent response.[10] Simultaneous PERG recording helps in identifying the retinal contributions to VEP and in the interpretation of VEP responses **(Fig. 5)**.

Major components of the VEP (N70, P100, and N145) are identified in the averaged response. Among these, P100 is the most consistent and least variable peak. The latencies are measured from the onset of the sweep to individual

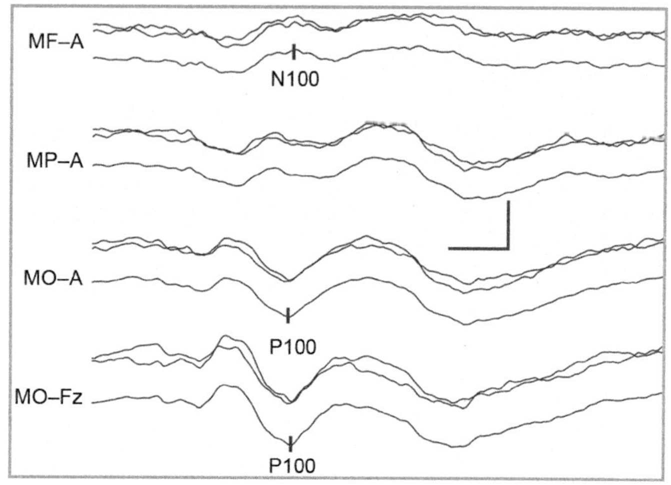

FIG. 4: Visual evoked potential (VEP) recorded from midfrontal (MF), mid-parietal (MP), and midoccipital (MO) electrodes using ear reference (A) shows higher P100 amplitude occipital than parietal recording. MF recording shows positive potential (N100) and MO recording reveals negative potential (P100). MO–MF derivation shows higher P100 amplitude due to interaction of simultaneous occipital negative with frontal positive activity. Sweep 30 ms/division, sensitivity 5 μV/division.

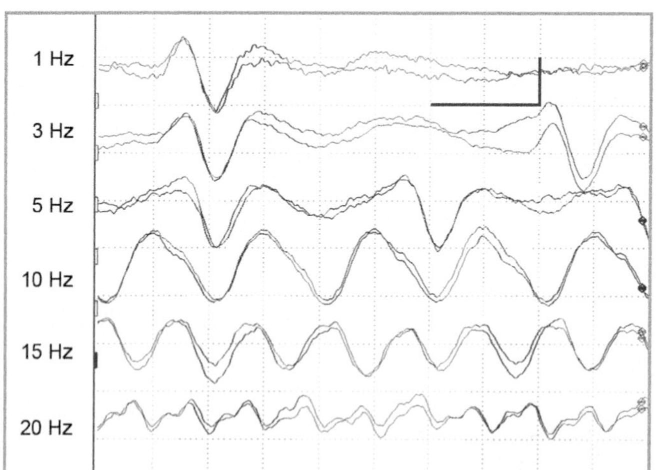

FIG. 3: The pattern reversal visual evoked potential (VEP) with increasing stimulation rates; with lower stimulation rates, individual VEP waves are identifiable. At stimulation rates above 5 Hz, steady-state VEP is seen with responses becoming sinusoidal. There is progressive reduction of amplitudes with increasing stimulation rates. Calibration 100 msec, 5 μV.

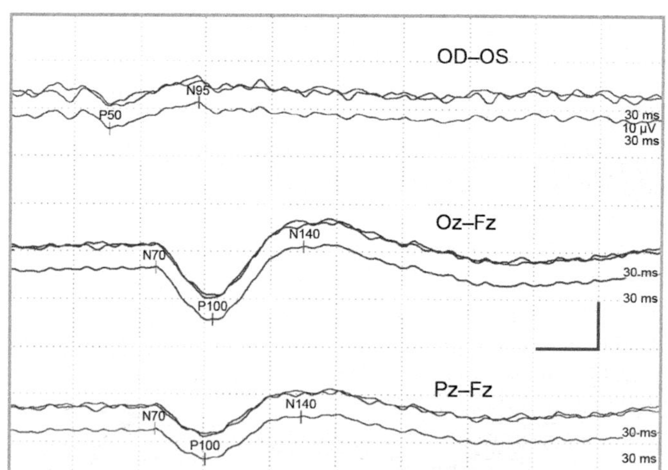

FIG. 5: Pattern reversal visual evoked potential and electroretinograms (ERGs) from normal subject; pattern electroretinogram was recorded with subcanthal surface electrode and the visual evoked potentials with Oz–Fz and Pz–Fz derivations. Pattern ERG amplitude (P50–N95) was 2.1 μV, P100 amplitude at Oz 6.5 μV, and at Pz 4.2 μV. P100 latency is 93 ms. Sensitivity 5 μV/division, sweep 30 ms/division.

peaks. Peak-to-peak amplitude of P100 is measured from N70 to P100 peak and N145 amplitude from P100 to N145 peak. Intertrial P100 latency difference should be <2.5 ms, and the amplitude difference <15%.[6,7,11] If the P100 amplitude is higher in the lateral occipital than the midline derivations, hemifield stimulation should be carried out.[7] The VEP waveform duration measured from N70 to N145 peaks becomes abnormal in pathological states, especially demyelinating disorders.

The measured P100 latency and amplitude on both sides are compared with age-specific normative data for absolute latency and amplitude values to identify abnormality in each eye. P100 latencies are markedly increased at birth and gradually reduce during infancy and early childhood to reach adult values.[12] In addition, interocular P100 latency difference and amplitude ratio in midline derivation are calculated. Interhemispheric P100 amplitude ratio in lateral occipital derivations is also calculated. The latency and amplitude abnormalities should be attributed to neurological dysfunction only after reasonable exclusion of abnormalities of refractive media and retina.[6,7] Prolongation of absolute P100 latencies or interocular P100 difference exceeding 2.5 or 3 standard deviations above the mean for the age-matched control population is considered abnormal. Absent VEP in multiple trials using midline and lateral derivations with sweep duration up to 500 ms, abnormally low P100 absolute amplitude, or abnormally high interocular P100 amplitude ratio are the amplitude criteria to consider VEP as abnormal.

Abnormal interhemispheric amplitude ratio can be caused by chiasmatic or postchiasmatic lesions. Hemifield stimulation is more sensitive than full-field stimulation in the evaluation of chiasmal and postchiasmal lesions. The pattern is displayed in one half of the screen with visual angle over 16° and pattern size about 50 minutes. Minimum of five channel recordings consisting of MO lateral occipital (RO, LO) and temporal (RT, LT) referenced to MF electrode is required. If additional channels are available, MP and ERG channels can be recorded. Other equipment settings including filters, sampling, epoch length, stimulation remain identical to full-field stimulation.[7]

Hemifield stimulation usually results in higher amplitudes of N70, P100, and N145 in the ipsilateral occipital and temporal electrodes due to orientation of the visual cortex. P100 latencies and amplitudes with each hemifield stimulation are measured. Measured parameters include interocular hemifield latency difference for left and right hemifields; latency difference between right and left hemifield stimulation in the each eye; amplitude difference for each hemifield and amplitude ratio for hemifields in each eye. Abnormalities detected in monocular hemifield or full-field stimulation suggest prechiasmatic and chiasmatic pathology. Binocular hemifield P100 amplitude reduction or latency prolongation suggests retrochiasmatic pathology.

Flash visual evoked potentials (FVEPs) are used in patients with markedly reduced visual acuity due to refractive error or opaque media, very young or uncooperative or sedated patients. FVEP is less sensitive than PRVEP in detecting abnormalities in the visual pathway. Stimulation can be carried out using LED goggles or Ganzfeld stimulator. Mydriasis is used to ensure adequate retinal stimulation. Monocular stimulation is carried out at 1 Hz. Recording montage consists of LO, MO, and RO electrodes referenced to Fz. In addition, ERG is recorded to look for retinal contribution to the abnormal FVEP **(Fig. 6)**. FVEP peaks are labeled sequentially in Roman numerals (I–VI) or according to polarity (N1, P1, N2, P2, N3, and P3). Increased latencies and/or reduced amplitudes in comparison to the normative data or the normal eye are documented. Presence of intact FVEP suggests that occipital cortex has received some visual input. Absent FVEP with normally elicited flash ERG suggests visual pathway pathology central to photoreceptors and bipolar cells whereas absent FVEP and flash ERG is due to retinal pathology.

Multifocal Visual Evoked Potential

Traditional full-field PRVEP evaluates the central retina and visual pathway. Patients with large scotomas may have reduced P100 amplitudes and patients with small scotomas in periphery generally have normal VEPs. Multifocal visual field stimulation expands the stimulated field beyond the central 40° and divides the stimulated visual field to radially oriented black-and-white dartboard patterns. Stimulation is performed with pseudorandom (*m-sequence*) protocol.[5] Multifocal VEPs (mfVEPs) from each individual focal stimulations are averaged and displayed radially as per the stimulated field.[13] Amplitude and latencies of individual mfVEPs from each side are measured and compared with opposite eye. The fovea does not produce response due to central fixation inhibition. Side-to-side comparison of

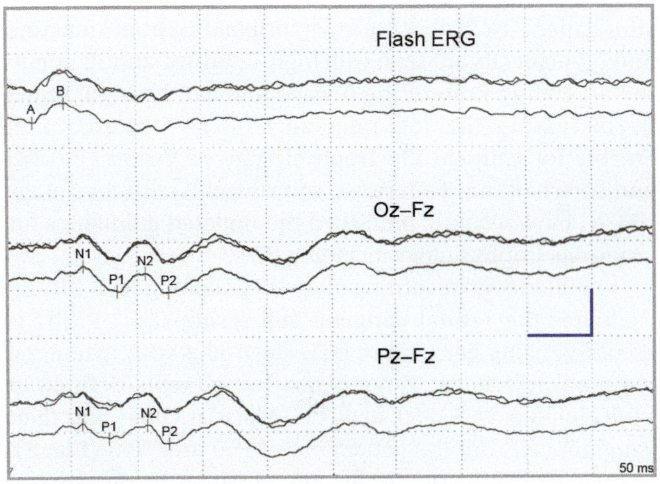

FIG. 6: Light-emitting diode (LED) flash visual evoked potential and electroretinograms (ERGs) from normal subject; LED ERG (displayed positivity upward) was recorded with subcanthal surface electrode and the visual evoked potentials (VEPs) with Oz–Fz and Pz–Fz derivations. Flash ERG amplitude was 22 μV with normal latencies and amplitude of VEP. Sensitivity 50 μV/division for ERG and 10 μV/division for VEP; sweep 50 ms/division.

amplitude and latencies for each stimulation field is checked. Latency prolongation or reduction/obliteration of waveform in focal visual field corresponds with localized lesions from retina to visual cortex. Studies on mfVEP in patients with multiple sclerosis (MS) and optic neuritis were more frequently abnormal compared with full-field stimulation.[14,15]

ELECTRORETINOGRAM

Electroretinogram was one of the first neural potentials to be recorded in 19th century. Electrical responses from different retinal elements contribute to generation of ERG. Full-field stimulation flash stimulus is performed under scotopic and photopic adaptation states with mydriasis. Ganzfeld stimulator is preferred for recording full-field flash ERG as it can deliver calibrated flashes of precise duration, brightness, and wavelength (color). Filters are used with Ganzfeld stimulator to deliver colored flashes for advanced ERG protocols.

Electroretinogram elicited by flash stimulus consists of early electronegative *a-wave* from the photoreceptors (rods and cones), electropositive *b-wave* from inner layers ON bipolar cells, Muller cells, horizontal and amacrine cells; and *c-wave* from pigment epithelium.[16] Early receptor potential from the outer photoreceptors segment representing density of visual pigments occurs in first 2 ms after stimulation is not discernible in the clinical ERG. For clinical flash ERG, only the a- and b-waves are evaluated in the scotopic and photopic states. The pupils are dilated to ensure adequate retinal stimulation. Corneal contact lens or conjunctival (gold foil or DTL) electrodes are used as active electrodes. Ipsilateral temporal reference and forehead ground electrodes are used. Scotopic rod function is evaluated initially during dark-adapted state using increasing intensity of the flash stimulus. Cone function is tested during light-adapted state using single flashes and 30 Hz steady-state stimulation. Oscillatory potentials originating from amacrine and bipolar cells are seen with high-intensity stimulation in the ascending limb of the b-wave and can be highlighted by increasing the low-frequency filter.[16] International Society for Clinical Electrophysiology of Vision (ISCEV) and International Federation of Clinical Neurophysiology (IFCN) have recently published the updated guidelines for visual electrophysiology including ERG.[8,11]

Simultaneous recording of the PERG along with PRVEP evaluates the retinal ganglion cell responses.[10] PERG is recorded using gold foil or DTL electrodes with ipsilateral temporal reference. Three major components defined in PERG include N35, P50, and N95. Macular cones and their ganglion cells are the generators of P50 and N95 **(Fig. 5)**. Transient PERG amplitudes are sensitive to the central retinal abnormalities and are reduced in retinal pathologies.

Pattern electroretinogram can be recorded with low frequency (transient PERG) and high frequency (steady state PERG) stimulation. Normal PERG in the presence of reduced amplitude of PRVEP points to retroretinal pathology beyond the retinal ganglion cells.[9] Calculated retinocortical time (RCT) measured between the PERG P50 and PRVEP P100 signifies the conduction interval from ganglion cell layer to visual cortex. RCT is prolonged in retroretinal demyelinating lesions including optic nerves, chiasm, and postchiasmatic visual pathway.

Multifocal ERG (mfERG) measures the cone function by stimulating the central 40°–50° of retina with radially oriented black and white hexagons centered around the macula. The pattern is scaled with smallest hexagon in the center and bigger hexagons in periphery corresponding to radially reducing retinal visual acuity. Corneal or conjunctival electrodes are mandatory for recording the mfERG as these potentials are very small. Stimulation is performed similar to mfVEP using pseudorandom (m-sequence) stimulation.[16] mfERG signals are mathematically stratified according to the spatial response to the stimulation sector. They consist of early negative N1 (cones and bipolar cells) and P1 (cone bipolar cells) components. mfERG represents function of the photoreceptors and bipolar cells whereas the PERG represents the function of ganglion cells. The signals are displayed as individual waves representing the retinal stimulation area. Graphic transformation as hexagons of different heights, color coded for the amplitude can simplify the demonstration of focal retinal dysfunction.[16] mfERG can demonstrate retinal pathologies including macular degeneration, enlargement of blind spot, focal retinal abnormalities, etc.

Clinical Utility of Visual Evoked Potential and Electroretinogram

Full-field PRVEPs are affected by ocular diseases including refractive errors, cataract, refractive media opacities, and retinal diseases which degrade retinal image projection. These ocular diseases reduce the P100 amplitude with mild increase of latency. P100 amplitude is also reduced by retinal diseases including macular degeneration, cone dystrophies, diabetic retinopathy, retinitis pigmentosa, etc.[17]

Optic nerve involvement in isolated optic neuritis, MS, neuromyelitis optica (NMO) spectrum, and myelin oligodendrocyte glycoprotein (MOG) disorder typically increase the P100 latency.[5,14,17-20] VEP is usually absent in patients with acute severe demyelination resulting in marked reduction of visual acuity. In milder cases P100 latency is prolonged, usually >35 ms with relative amplitude preservation. During recovery phase of optic neuritis, the absent VEPs reappear, and the reduced amplitudes recover over months. Despite clinical recovery of optic neuritis, P100 latency prolongation persists for years in adults. In children with optic neuritis, the latencies may normalize after years.[21] When recordable, PERG P50 and N95 latencies are normal with reduced N95 amplitude due to its origin from retinal ganglion cells. RCT prolongation between PERG P50 and VEP P100 may persist. In severe optic neuritis with atrophy, the flash ERG amplitudes are also reduced. PRVEP is almost always abnormal among patients with definite MS, especially those with clinical optic nerve involvement.[17] In patients with

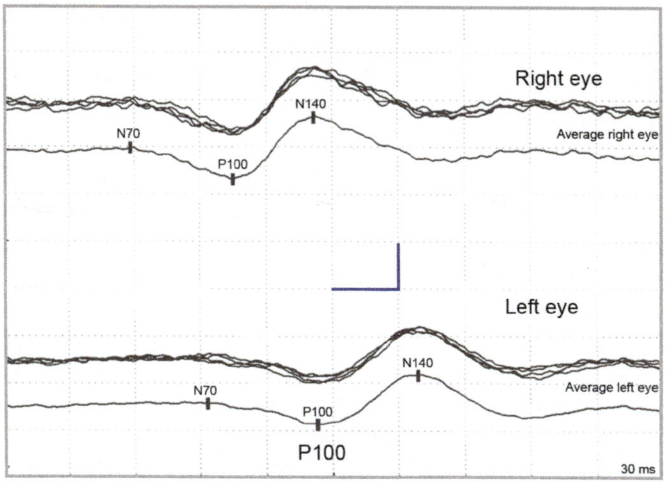

FIG. 7: Pattern reversal visual evoked potential (VEP) in a 45-year-old patient presenting with acute longitudinally extensive myelopathy and past history of clinically recovered left monocular impaired vision 6 months earlier. Serum aquaporin-4 antibodies were positive. VEP reveals persistent prolongation of P100 latency with left eye stimulation (141 ms) with increased interocular latency difference (38 ms) and normal P100 amplitude. Sweep 30 ms/division, sensitivity 10 µV/division.

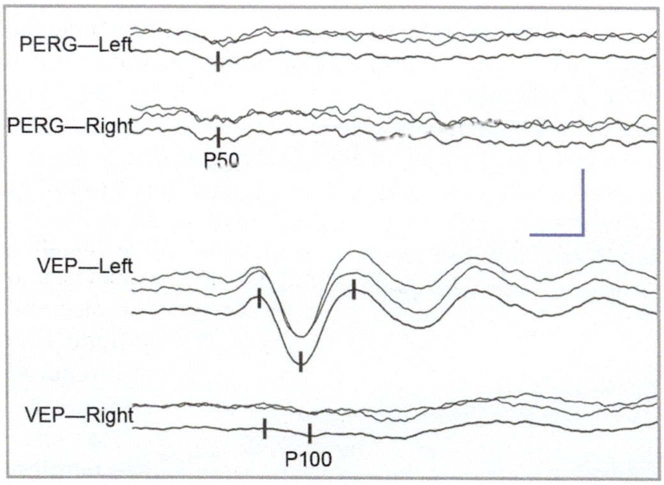

FIG. 8: Middle-aged lady with progressive right monocular blindness of 2 months. Examination revealed primary optic atrophy on right side with 6/36 vision and papilledema on right side. Visual evoked potential (VEP) from left eye stimulation is normal and VEP from right eye stimulation is poorly defined with reduced P100 amplitude (right eye 1.1 µV, left eye 10.4 µV) with mild increase in latency (103.2 ms vs. 95.7 ms). Concurrent surface recorded pattern electroretinogram (PERG) from both eyes show equal latency and amplitudes suggesting unilateral retroretinal pathology in right eye. Sweep 30 ms/division and sensitivity 10 µV/division.

possible MS, NMO, and MOG disorders, VEP abnormalities are seen in up to 50% **(Fig. 7)**. VEP in patients with ischemic optic neuropathy may be absent or show markedly reduced P100 amplitude. P100 prolongation is usually <10 ms in ischemic optic neuropathy.[22] With progressive extrinsic compression of optic nerve due to meningioma, pituitary tumors, craniopharyngioma, etc., the P100 amplitude progressively reduces with marginal increase in latencies **(Fig. 8)**. VEPs are abnormal in peripheral demyelinating diseases.[23] P100 amplitude is reduced in neurodegenerative disorders, and reduction in Alzheimer's disease reflects retinal cells loss.[24]

AUDITORY EVOKED POTENTIALS

Auditory evoked potentials are the scalp-recorded auditory pathway potentials produced in response to acoustic stimulation.[25] AEP is also termed as brainstem auditory evoked response (BAER), brainstem auditory evoked potentials (BAEPs), brainstem evoked response-auditory (BERA), auditory brainstem response (ABR), etc. AEP is the apt terminology as the recorded responses include potentials from auditory nerve, brainstem, thalamus, and cortical projections.[26]

Evoked responses occurring within 10 ms from stimulus onset are termed as short latency, those occurring between 10 and 50 ms are medium latency, and the responses beyond 50 ms are the long-latency AEPs. The short latency AEPs consist of surface recorded volley of potentials from auditory nerve to auditory cortex. These responses are highly consistent, reproducible, and can be recorded with relative ease despite their small amplitude. The short-latency AEPs are not affected by attention, concentration, and level of consciousness including anesthesia whereas the long-latency AEPs are markedly affected by these factors.[25,27]

Majority of the short-latency AEP components consist of far-field auditory pathway potentials and minor changes in the recording electrode position do not alter the recorded magnitude and polarity of these far-field responses. Auditory nerve responses originate near the recording electrode at ear lobe and are best recorded with electrode placed over the ipsilateral earlobe or mastoid. Electrocochleogram (ECochG) is the AEP with shortest latency and requires special external auditory canal electrodes.[28] ECochG is recorded predominantly in the audiological evaluations rather than in clinical neurophysiology laboratories.

Methodology

Short-latency AEPs are recorded by brief, monoaural, monophasic, acoustic stimulus delivered using calibrated headphone. Broadband acoustic click stimulus consists of frequencies encompassing low and high frequencies with dominance of higher frequencies. Shielded headphones are preferred as they produce lower stimulus artifact. The click stimulus should be loud enough to elicit the AEP without causing discomfort and sound-induced auditory damage.[28,29]

The acoustic click and tone stimulus intensities are measured in the logarithmic decibel (dB) scale. The absolute intensity is stated as sound pressure level (SPL). The average of the click intensity perceived by group of normal individuals is the normal hearing level (nHL). The hearing threshold is identified with gradual intensity adjustments with steps not exceeding 5 dB. Typically, the stimulus intensity 60–70 dB above the threshold level is used to record AEP. Monophasic 0.1 ms duration broadband clicks are presented monoaurally using over-the-ear headphones. The click stimulus is generated by square wave electrical impulses of positive or negative polarity which move the headphone diaphragm toward the tympanum (*condensation click*) or away from the tympanum (*rarefaction click*).[28,29] AEPs produced by rarefaction and condensation clicks differ marginally in latencies, morphology, and measured intervals among normal individuals **(Fig. 9)**. However, in pathological states, the latencies and intervals may differ markedly between the AEPs recorded with rarefaction and condensation clicks.[28] It is essential to have independent normative data for both types of stimulations. Masking white noise consisting of admixture of frequencies in human audible range is delivered to contralateral ear to prevent its stimulation by bone-conducted stimulation.[26,28,29]

Active electrode is placed over the ear lobes (Ai and Ac), reference electrode over the vertex (Cz), and ground electrode is placed over Fz with impedance maintained <5 kOhms. Simultaneous two-channel recording with Ai–Cz and Ac–Cz derivations is helpful as the fused waves IV and V with ipsilateral recording are generally separate with contralateral recordings **(Fig. 10)**. In neonates, children or persons with deformed/undeveloped pinna, the active electrode should be placed over the mastoid. However, the electromyographic artifacts from retroauricular and nuchal muscles are larger and wave I amplitude is smaller at mastoids.

Signals are filtered at 2–3 kHz high-frequency filter and 100 Hz low-frequency filter. Increasing the low frequency filter >100 Hz can make the peak separation easier at the cost of reduction of AEP amplitudes. In neonates and young children, low frequency filter should be reduced to 50 Hz. Data sampling at 25 kHz or higher avoids aliasing and provides undistorted AEP responses.[29] Acquisition length of 10 ms is used for adults and children older than 2 years. Sweep duration of 20 ms is used in neonates, infants and in patients with prolonged latencies.

Input sensitivity is kept at 5–10 μV and may be modified according to ongoing EEG activity. Due to the very small amplitudes of the AEP, averaging of two reproducible trials of >1,000 stimulus epochs is essential. When the waveforms are poorly defined, several averages of 2,000 stimuli may be needed. Intertrial peak latency differences should be <0.1–0.2 ms.[26,28] Stimulus repetition rate should be between 7 and 10 Hz. Use of lower stimulation rate increases the examination time and higher stimulation rate makes the initial AEP components less distinct. Recording during sleep and relaxed state reduces myogenic artifacts which degrade the AEP signal.

The AEPs represent the near- and far-field responses from the auditory pathway to acoustic stimuli. The recorded AEP is the end result of interplay of the potentials recorded between the "active" and "reference" electrodes placed over the head. It is worth noting that no electrode over the head is truly "inactive". The differential amplifier records the potential differences between the electrodes rather than the absolute voltages. Noncephalic reference electrodes reveal the true potential polarity of AEP components **(Fig. 11)**. Due to higher amount of artifacts and low SNR, noncephalic montages are not utilized for clinical AEP. The peaks are named using Roman numerals, beginning from I to VII for the successive electronegative peaks in the Ai–Cz derivation and from II to VII in the Ac–Cz derivation. The succeeding positive trough/peak is named with suffix of asterix or N (I*, IN).

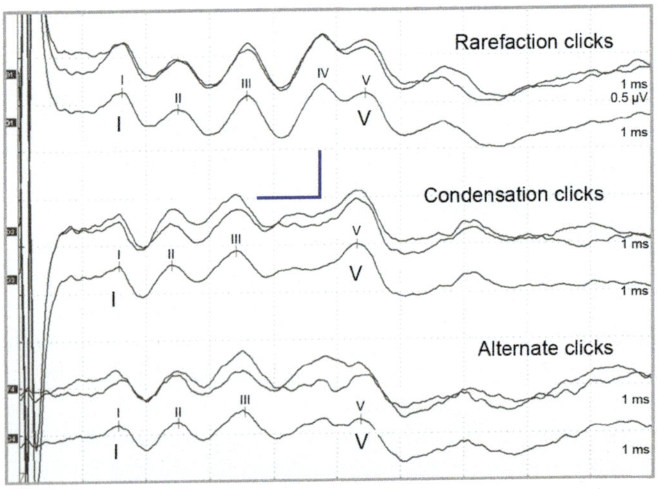

FIG. 9: Showing auditory evoked potentials recorded using rarefaction, condensation, and alternate clicks at 60 dB above the hearing threshold. Auditory evoked potential (AEP) elicited with rarefaction reveals all the waveforms with slightly longer latencies than condensation clicks. Wave IV was not elicitable with condensation clicks. The stimulus artifact preceding the wave I with rarefaction and condensation clicks are cancelled out with alternate clicks. Sweep 1 ms/division, sensitivity 0.5 μV/division.

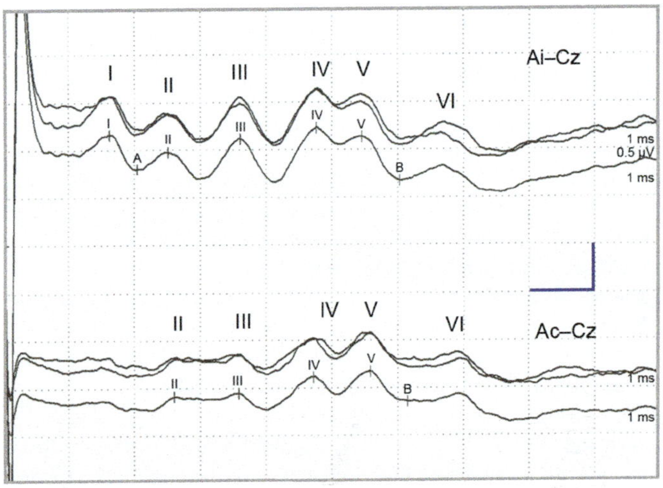

FIG. 10: Auditory evoked potential (AEP) recorded with rarefaction clicks at 60 dB above threshold with active electrodes at ipsilateral and contralateral ear lobes. Waves II–VI are seen on both sides whereas wave I is seen only in Ai–Cz derivation. Wave II and III are smaller with Ac–Cz recording and wave IV and V are seen separately on both sides. Sweep 1 ms, sensitivity 0.5 μV/division.

Wave I arises from the distal auditory nerve close to the cochlea and contributes to the N1 of the ECochG. Wave I arises from cochlear nerve and can be recorded in acoustic schwannoma, nerve transection, and brainstem death. It has surface negativity around the ipsilateral ear and mastoid. It is the first wave to occur after 1.4 ms from stimulus onset and is electronegative in Ai–Cz derivation.[28] In the Ac–Cz derivation, wave I is not commonly seen, though it may be rarely seen in some patients due to its dipole variations.[29] With high click intensities, relatively large amplitude cochlear microphonics appear and mask wave I. Digital average of trials with rarefaction and condensation clicks reveals the wave I by phase cancellation of cochlear microphonics. Averaging of alternating rarefaction and condensation clicks also reduces the cochlear microphonics artifact. Averaging of the alternating rarefaction and condensation clicks is very helpful in patients with elevated hearing threshold whose waves I and II are usually lost in the cochlear microphonics with monophasic stimulation **(Fig. 12)**.

Wave II originates from the central proximal parts of the auditory nerve. Intracranial recordings have demonstrated its origin from the nerve.[30] It can persist in patients with brain and brainstem death. It is the second negative peak in the Ai–Cz derivation. It may not be clearly seen in some people in the ipsilateral recording and may be seen with Ac–Cz derivation. Clinicopathological correlations confirm the pontine tegmentum and superior olivary nucleus origin of wave III. Intracranial recordings documented the caudal pons as the generator of wave III. It is seen as electronegative wave in Ai–Cz and Ac–Cz derivations. Wave III amplitude is generally larger in ipsilateral than contralateral recording.

Wave V occurs 5.5 ms after the stimulus and is broader and with generally higher amplitude than the preceding four peaks. There is large variation in the interaction between wave IV and V. The wave V can be seen as separate independent wave or completely fused with wave IV or seen as a separate peak in the ascending or descending limb of wave IV.[31] Recording from the contralateral ear with Ac–Cz derivation usually separates wave IV and V. The wave IV originates in lateral lemniscus and wave V from the inferior colliculus.[32] Wave IV originates predominantly from the contralateral lateral lemniscus. Wave V is absent in vascular midbrain lesions and lesions of lateral lemniscus.[33] Wave VI arises from medial geniculate body and VII from auditory cortex. Waves VI and VII are not routinely evaluated in clinical AEP recordings due to large variations in latency, amplitudes, and occurrence.

The peak latencies of the waves I to V are measured from the sweep onset. When the wave IV and V are combined into a single peak, it is termed as IV–V peak. The absolute latencies are compared with age-specific normative data. Interpeak latency intervals I–III, III–V, and I–V are measured from the peak latencies. The interpeak interval I–III denotes the time taken for the signal to travel from the auditory nerve to the auditory nucleus, interval III–V denotes the time taken from the auditory nucleus to the inferior colliculus. The amplitudes of wave I and wave V are measured from their peaks to the succeeding troughs.

For AEP recording in young children and comatose individuals, wave V threshold is identified by clicks delivered at higher stimulation rates as wave V persists at rates up to 70 Hz. Stimulation is started at 100 dB peak equivalent SPL delivered between 40 and 70 Hz. The click intensity

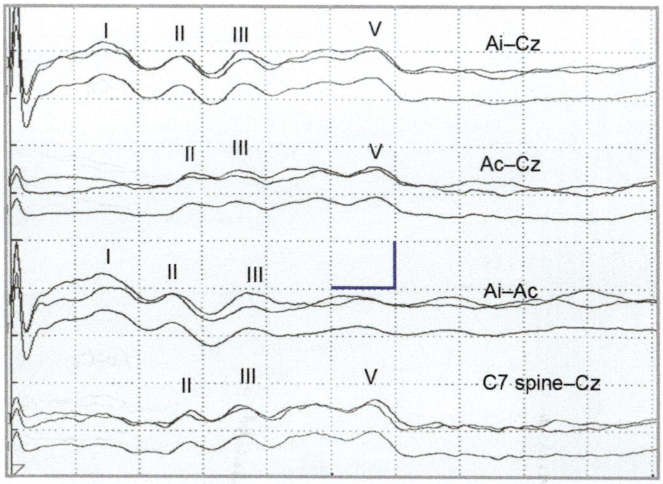

FIG. 11: Auditory evoked potentials (AEPs) recorded using Ai–Cz, Ac–Cz, Ai–Ac, and C7spine–Cz montages. Wave I is well seen with derivation using active electrode at ipsilateral ear (Ai–Cz, Ai–Ac). Wave IV better demonstrated in Ac–Cz than in Ai–Cz derivation. Noncephalic montage C7spine–Cz shows the far-field vertex positive AEP peaks from II to V; sweep 1 ms/division, sensitivity 0.5 μV/division.

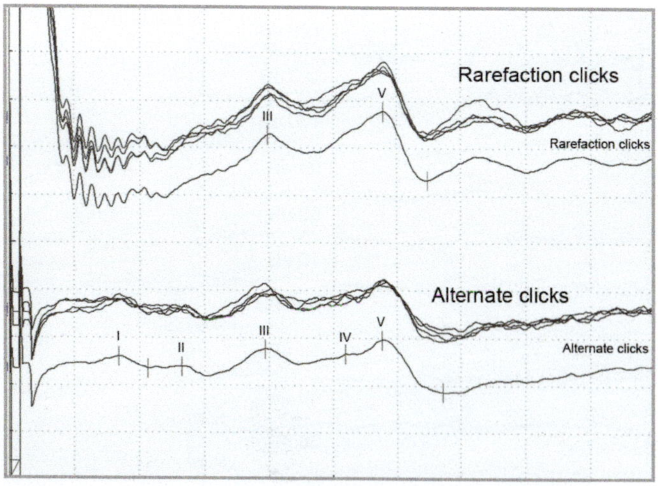

FIG. 12: Large amplitude cochlear microphonics with rarefaction clicks are shown in a patient with increased hearing threshold (100 dB). Wave I is obscured by the cochlear microphonics and only wave III and V are visualized. Averaging the alternating rarefaction and condensation clicks has removed the cochlear microphonics and waves I and II are discernible.

is reduced in 10 dB steps till wave V disappears to obtain wave V threshold **(Fig. 13)**. Stimulus intensity 60 dB above the wave V threshold is utilized for recording the AEP. If wave V is not recordable at 100 dB, intensity is increased in 10 dB steps to look for wave V.[26,28] The broadband click stimulus consists of admixture of different frequencies, predominantly >2 kHz and stimulates the proximal part of the cochlea. Low-frequency hearing loss may be missed in AEP recorded using click stimuli. Short tone pips at different frequencies are utilized to assess the hearing threshold at different frequencies.[34] The AEP testing can be performed in awake, asleep, and comatose patients by sequential stimulation at reducing intensities **(Fig. 14)**.

Due to the incomplete myelination and relative immaturity of the auditory pathway, the impulse conduction is slow in premature babies, neonates, and children up to 2 years. This results in prolongation of latencies and interpeak intervals which gradually approach adult levels by 2 years.[33] Interpeak interval I–V decreases at about 0.44 ms per weak over 26–40 weeks of gestation.[28] Data obtained from AEPs should be compared with age-specific normative data. Marginally shorter latencies in women has been attributed to temperature and skull volume. Hypothermia increases the latencies and intervals.

Clinical Applications of Auditory Evoked Potential

Auditory evoked potential abnormalities are divided into "central pattern" where I–V interpeak interval (central transmission time) is prolonged with normal wave I latency and "peripheral pattern" when all the waves including wave I are delayed. AEP in severe hearing impairment may have increased intervals due to submaximal stimulation as the click intensity cannot be increased beyond 130 dB. Auditory neuropathies due to genetically determined diseases including Friedreich's ataxia and Charcot-Marie-Tooth disease cause progressive decline of the AEP amplitudes culminating in complete absence with increasing duration of the illness.[35] Abnormalities of AEP in patients with MS is less frequent than VEP abnormalities. Among 202 patients with MS, 32% had prolonged I–V interval and in almost half of them the prolongation was monoaural.[36] AEP abnormalities are more frequent when the brainstem is involved (>50%) in contrast to those without brainstem involvement.

Auditory evoked potential was one of the investigations for evaluation of acoustic schwannomas till the widespread availability of MRI. AEP in patients with acoustic schwannoma reveal increased interpeak interval I–III and I–V using conventional methodology. AEP abnormalities are more frequent when the tumor is >1cm and can be normal when the lesion is small. Stacked AEP assessing response to specific frequencies was reported to be sensitive than conventional AEP with sensitivity of 95% and specificity of 85%.[37] Other posterior fossa tumors cause increased intervals when they distort the brainstem. In Meniere's disease, latencies of wave V can be increased, especially in acute severe episodes. Patients with posterior circulation infarction and transient ischemic attacks with brainstem involvement have abnormal AEPs.[38] Newborn and neonatal hearing assessment with threshold evaluation is useful in early identification and management of hearing impairment.

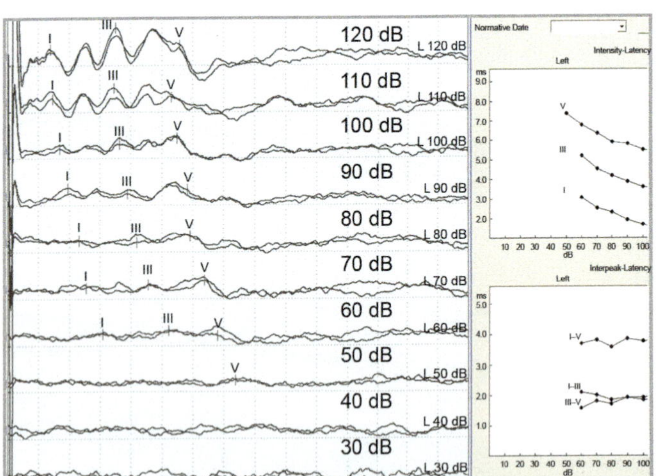

FIG. 13: The use of auditory click stimulus delivered at 44 Hz starting at 120 dB and reducing at 10 dB steps; with serial reduction of the click intensity, there is progressive prolongation of the auditory evoked potential (AEP) latencies. Wave V is the last wave to disappear at 50 dB intensity (wave V threshold). Intensity–latency curve is seen on right showing maintained interpeak intervals with different stimulus intensities.

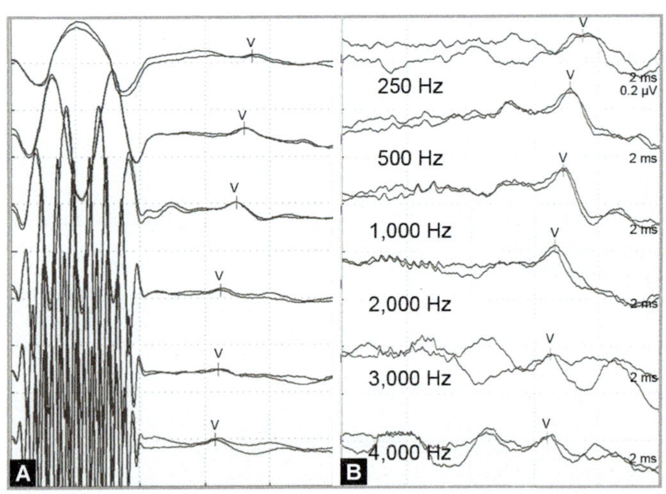

FIGS. 14A AND B: Use of tone pips to record auditory evoked potential (AEP); increasing stimulus frequencies from 250 Hz to 4 kHz are used. Due to longer duration of the tone stimulus, only wave V can be recorded, and earlier waves are difficult to record. Rarefaction stimulus was used in the traces in (A) Averaging of alternating rarefaction and condensation tone bursts in (B) removed the tone burst stimulus artifacts with better delineation of wave V.

SOMATOSENSORY EVOKED POTENTIALS

Somatosensory evoked potentials are time-locked obligatory potentials recorded along the peripheral and central sensory pathway from the nerve to sensory cortex in response to peripheral stimulation. Impulses from peripheral electrical stimulation of the mixed or pure sensory nerve travel in the lemniscal pathway. Conventional SSEP examination requires peripheral electrical stimulation of large diameter sensory axons. Mixed nerve or pure sensory nerve electrical stimulation is used to record the SSEPs. Mixed nerve stimulation preferentially excites the proprioceptive sensory fibers and in addition the afferents from tendons, joints, and muscles. The spinothalamic pathway SSEP recording requires peripheral selective small-fiber stimulation of nociceptive pain or temperature receptors.[39,40]

The large-fiber impulses conducting at 40–80 m/s enter the spinal cord through the posterior spinal roots. Structural and functional integrity of the whole sensory neuron including dorsal root ganglion cells, peripheral and central axon is essential for transmission of impulses to the spinal cord. These axons continue as cuneate and gracile tracts which synapse at their nuclei in medulla oblongata. The second order neurons cross over in medulla oblongata and ascend up in the medial lemniscus through medulla oblongata, pons, and midbrain to terminate on the ventral posterolateral (VPL) nucleus of the thalamus. Third order thalamic neuron projections terminate on the primary sensory cortex. Brodmann's area 3b and area 1 receive mechanoreceptor inputs and area 2 receives proprioceptive inputs.[39]

Somatosensory Evoked Potential Methodology

SSEP is recorded by monophasic peripheral electrical stimulation of mixed or pure sensory nerve using constant current stimulus of 0.2 ms. Cathode is placed proximally to avoid anodal block. Stimulus intensity of two to three times the sensory threshold is used for pure sensory nerves. Intensity sufficient to elicit visible consistent muscle twitch is used for mixed nerves. Use of higher intensities do not elicit higher amplitude SSEPs and are unnecessary. Ground electrode is placed between the stimulating and the recording electrodes. Stimulator impedance <5 kOhms ensures consistent stimulation at lower intensities and reduces patient discomfort.

The input data should be sampled at 10 kHz or higher to obtain precise latencies and waveform delineation. High frequency filter is set at 1,000–3,000 Hz. Low-frequency filter is set at 20 Hz which makes the peak identification and delineation easier for clinical studies. The filter setting for the normative data and the patient testing should be unchanged as the variations of filter settings alter the latencies, morphology, and amplitudes.[39,41,42] Patient relaxation is essential to reduce myogenic artifacts to improve SNR in the referential recording. Automatic artifact rejection helps to remove the electrocardiogram artifacts. SSEP examinations are performed on median, ulnar, posterior tibial, and fibular nerves out of which median and posterior tibial nerves are routinely tested nerves. At least four simultaneous channels are needed to document the peripheral and central nervous system responses. Additional channels may be used for characterization of specific responses.

Median Nerve Somatosensory Evoked Potential

The median nerve is stimulated with cathode at wrist 2 cm proximal to distal palmar crease and the anode is placed distally. Surface electrodes are placed at Erb's point (bilateral), C5spine, bilateral centroparietal scalp (CPi and CPc) and MF (Fz) locations. These electrodes help in recording the potentials from brachial plexus (N9 or EP), cervical spinal cord (N13), cervicomedullary junction (N14), sensory cortex (N20), and the far-field potentials (N11, P14). There are minor differences between the recommendations from ACNS[41] and IFCN.[39] Additional electrodes and montages can be used to obtain additional information. It is essential to maintain the same montage and settings through all studies.

The obligatory responses to be identified in the median nerve SSEP are N9 (EP), N13, P14, N18, and N20. Summated orthodromic sensory action potentials from C6 and C7 root elements are stimulated with median nerve stimulation and are recorded at Erb's point as triphasic N9 peak. Minor contributions from the muscle afferents and proprioceptive fibers also contribute to N9. Presence of N9 in the upper limb SSEP confirms adequacy of stimulation. N13 is the stationary peak generated in cervical spinal cord by the sensory inputs from the posterior C6 and C7 rootlets at dorsal root entry zone and the cuneate fascicle. It is recorded with active electrode at C5 spine referenced to anterior cervical (AC) or Fz electrode **(Fig. 15)**. C5S-AC derivation usually has higher

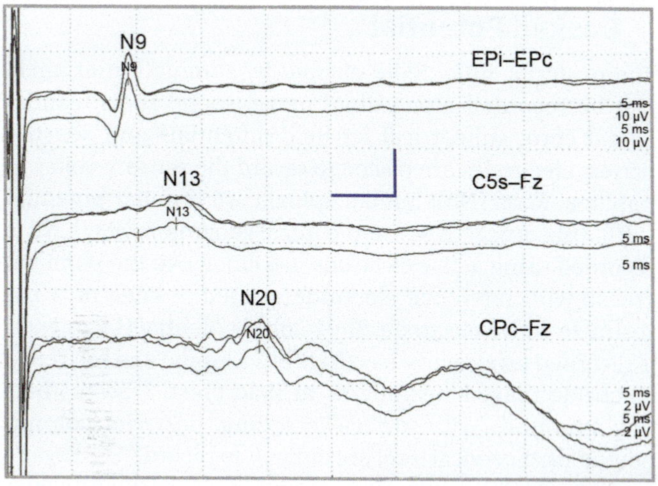

FIG. 15: The normal right median somatosensory evoked potentials recorded from Erb's point, cervical spine, and contralateral centro-parietal scalp; sweep speed 5 ms/division, sensitivity 10 μV/division for Erb's point and C5 spine; 2 μV/division for scalp recording.

amplitude due to the simultaneous anterior positivity at AC. In addition, C5S–AC is devoid of far-field potentials (N11, N14/P14). C5S–Fz records multiple far-field potentials (N11, N13, N14/P14) which can cause difficulty in identification of the peak.[39,40,41]

P14 arises from cuneate nucleus and caudal medial lemniscus. It has widespread scalp distribution and is recorded with combination of scalp and noncephalic derivation (Fz—contralateral Erb's point). Subcortical potentials arising from thalamic VPL nucleus and postsynaptic upper brainstem tracts result in P18 which is recorded as far-field potential using Fz–EPc or CPc–EPc. Sensory input to the hand area in the primary sensory cortex generates the N20 which is best demonstrated by the bipolar CPc–Fz derivation which phases out the far-field deep potentials.

The peak latencies of N9, N13, P14, and N20 are measured in appropriate channels. Interpeak intervals N9–N13 denote the transit time from brachial plexus to spinal cord, N9–N14 the transit time from brachial plexus to cuneate nucleus, P14–N20 measures conduction time from cuneate nucleus to sensory cortex.[39,41] Absence of any of the obligatory waveforms (N9, N13, N20) is considered abnormal in the presence of adequate stimulation. Absent scalp potentials could be due to cortical lesion or anywhere from median nerve to brachial plexus to cortical generators. In the presence of normal N9 and N20, absence of N13 or P14 may not be considered abnormal as it could be technical problem rather than true absence. Impulse conduction in central sensory pathways is better represented by interpeak intervals (N9–N13, N13/P14–N20, etc.) rather than the absolute peak latencies which are greatly affected by height and limb length. The initial components of upper limb SSEP (N9, N13, P14) are not affected by arousal state whereas N20 amplitude is reduced by deep sedation and anesthesia.

Posterior Tibial Somatosensory Evoked Potential

The posterior tibial SSEP elicited by stimulation at ankle can be recorded along tibial nerve, sacral roots, caudal spinal cord, subcortical far-field potentials and sensory cortex. Electrodes are placed to record the sensory volley at popliteal fossa (N8), lumbar spinal cord [lumbar potential (LP)], subcortical (N34), and cortical generators (P37). N8 is recorded using active electrode 4–6 cm above the popliteal crease with reference electrode at medial knee or 3 cm rostral to active electrode. The lumbar potential (LP or N22) is recorded using active electrode at T12 spine and reference electrode placed rostrally or at iliac crest. Due to their tiny amplitude with surface recording, posterior column potentials at cervical level are difficult to record.[39,40,41]

N30 and P31 are the far-field potentials representing the supraspinal and subcortical activity recorded with scalp–noncephalic derivation. N34 represents the postsynaptic activity from multiple generators in the brainstem and is preceded by small positive wave P31. P31 and N34 are considered analogous to P14 and N18 elicited with median nerve SSEP. These are recorded with C5spine–Fz or C5spine–CPi derivation. Sensory impulses from the posterior tibial stimulation terminate in medial parietal lobe and generate P37 and is usually recorded using CPz–Fz derivation. However, amplitude of P37 may be higher ipsilateral scalp with CPi–Fz or CPi–CPc derivation depending on P37 dipole. Using these three derivations simultaneously helps in recording its true surface amplitude (**Fig. 16**).[39] Four channels are needed to demonstrate posterior tibial SSEP. If only four channels are available, subcortical potential channel may be sacrificed. Five channel recordings help to record the nerve, caudal spinal cord, subcortical, and scalp SSEPs:

1. Popliteal fossa: N8
2. T12 spine–reference: LP (N22)
3. Fz–C5 spine: P31, N34
4. CPz–FPz: P37
5. CPi–FPz: P37

Stimulation is performed with patient in supine position after electrode placement. The nerve is stimulated at ankle with 0.2 ms duration monophasic stimulus with intensity enough to produce consistent visible small twitching of foot muscles. Stimulation at frequencies >2 Hz attenuates the P37 amplitude. Ground electrode is placed between the stimulator and popliteal electrode. Sweep duration of 100 ms is usually adequate and data is sampled at >10 kHz. Demonstration of the popliteal N8 suggests adequate stimulation of posterior tibial nerve. N8 may be absent in very obese patients or those with edema.

Peak latencies of N8, LP, P31 and P37 are measured and compared with normative data with due consideration for the height. Interpotential interval LP–P31 indicates impulse conduction from caudal spinal cord to cervicomedullary

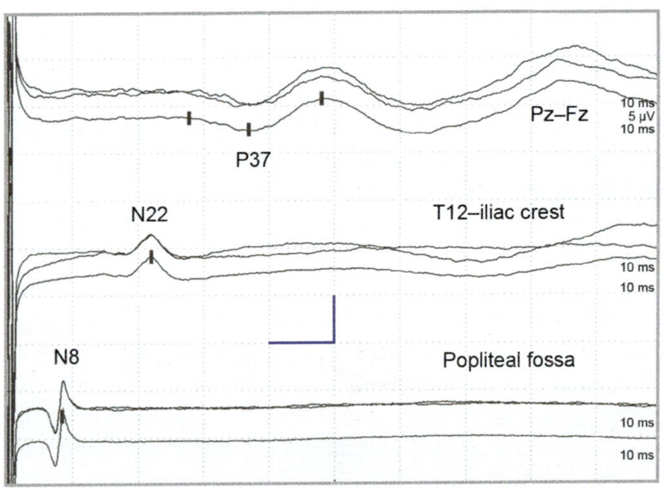

FIG. 16: The posterior tibial somatosensory evoked potentials recorded from popliteal fossa (N8), 12th thoracic spine (N22/lumbar potential) and midline parietal area (P37); sweep speed 10 ms/division, sensitivity 5 µV/division.

junction; P31–P37 represents conduction from cervicomedullary junction to sensory cortex. Absence of any of the obligatory waveform is considered abnormal, provided the stimulation and recording are technically adequate. N34 may be absent due to its small amplitude and low SNR in the noncephalic derivation.

Spinothalamic Somatosensory Evoked Potential

Stimulation of the nociceptive receptors preferentially stimulates A-delta and C fibers whose central impulses travel in the spinothalamic pathway. The proximal sensory axons reach the spinal cord through posterior roots and synapse at spinal cord. Second order neurons cross to opposite side to spinothalamic tract which ascends through spinal cord and brainstem to synapse on third order neurons in the thalamic ventral caudal (Vc) and ventromedial (VM) nuclei. Thalamic neurons project to dorsal insula, frontal operculum, and mid-cingulum in addition to the primary sensory cortex.[39] Pain-related evoked potentials (PREPs) evaluate the small-diameter sensory fibers and the spinothalamic system. PREPs can be elicited by laser, contact heat, intraepidermal electrical stimulation, pinprick and chemosensory stimulation. Due to small axonal diameter and the central processing, the cerebral PREPs latencies have long latency. In contrast to the oligosynaptic lemniscal pathway SSEPs, the PREPs are considered to be similar to polysynaptic event-related potentials (ERPs).[43]

Laser EPs elicited by cutaneous stimulation with CO_2 or solid-state laser generators produce vertex maximum positive polarity potential P2 preceded by negative potential N1 at temporal region. P2 results from simultaneous activity from multiple sources including middle part of cingulate gyrus, insula, and frontal operculum. Activity in upper bank of Sylvian fissure comprising secondary somatosensory area SII and posterior insula generates N1.[44,45] Latency of the P2 is proportional to the stimulation site, being shortest with facial stimulation and longest with foot stimulation.[39] PREPs are recorded from at least one midline site (Cz) and bilateral temporal sites (T3 and T4) referenced to ear. Additional midline sites (Pz and Fz) are useful and help to differentiate between the event-related P3 component. PREPs elicited by contact heat produce EPs of similar morphology with slightly longer latencies.[39,43] Subepidermal electrical stimulation SSEPs are technically simpler and require less complex stimulation equipment.[43]

Clinical Utility of Somatosensory Evoked Potential

Somatosensory evoked potentials may still be recordable due to central amplification in peripheral neuropathies with absent sensory nerve action potentials (SNAPs). Abnormal PREPs in patients with painful small-fiber neuropathies provide evidence for small-fiber involvement.[46] Utility of dermatomal SSEPs in radiculopathies is limited due to overlap of territories except when digital stimulation is used for evaluation of C6, C7, and C8 root lesions. Clinical and electromyographic evaluations are probably superior to SSEPs in evaluation of radiculopathies. SSEPs in inflammatory myelopathies due to MS, neuromyelitis optica spectrum disorder (NMOSD) and MOG antibody-associated disease (MOGAD) reveal normal peripheral potentials with delay or absence of spinal cord potentials (N13, N22) and cortical potentials (N20, P37). Calculated central conduction time between N13–N20 and N22–P37 are prolonged when the sensory tracts are involved. Patients without sensory or motor spinal cord involvement are less likely to have abnormal SSEPs. However, these findings are nonspecific as similar findings can occur in subacute combined degeneration, vitamin E deficiency, copper deficiency, hereditary spastic paraparesis, and spinocerebellar degenerations.[39,40] Therefore, the abnormal SSEPs in myelopathies need careful correlation with clinical, radiological, biochemical, and genetic data.

Traumatic brachial plexus lesions with spinal root avulsion without involvement of plexus have persevered SNAPs with reduced or absent evoked motor responses. Root involvement can be ascertained using SSEP which demonstrates normal Erb's point N9 with delayed and/reduced N13 and N20 depending on the completeness of the root lesion **(Fig. 17)**. Patients with cervical spondylotic myelopathy with neurological deficits usually have abnormal N13 potential.[47] SSEPs have been used for evaluation and electrophysiological follow-up of patients with spinal cord injuries. SSEPs in patients with spinal

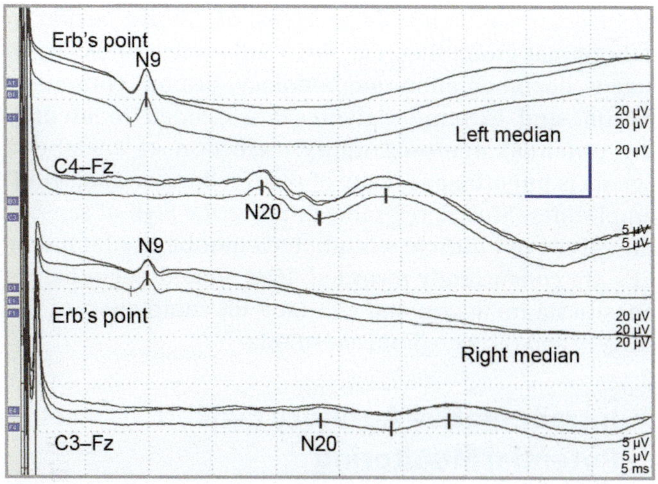

FIG. 17: Median nerve somatosensory evoked potential (SSEP) in a patient with longstanding right brachial plexus trauma with minimal recovery. Motor responses were markedly reduced and sensory nerve potentials normal in right upper limb. SSEP with left median nerve stimulation is normal. Right median SSEP reveals normal N9 with reduced amplitude and prolongation of N20 suggesting lesion at root level. Sweep speed 5 ms/division; sensitivity 20 µV/division for Erb's point and 5 µV/division for cortical potentials.

cord injury may be normal, attenuated, or show prolonged latencies.[48] In patients with traumatic brain injury, normal SSEPs predict good outcome and absent cortical potentials predict poor long-term outcome.[49]

Lesions involving compact spinothalamic projections (spinal cord, brainstem, thalamus, and internal capsule) result in reduced amplitude or abolition of P2. Patients with dissociated sensory loss from intramedullary spinal cord lesions including syringomyelia have intact lemniscal SSEP and abnormal PREP. Patients with nonorganic sensory loss have intact lemniscal and spinothalamic SSEPs. Peripheral responses equivalent to popliteal and brachial plexus and subcortical far-field potentials are difficult to demonstrate in PREPs.[43]

INTRAOPERATIVE EVOKED POTENTIALS MONITORING

Neurosurgical interventions on the spinal cord, brainstem, cranial nerves, and supratentorial compartment can be complicated by perioperative neurological deficits resulting from mechanical trauma, traction, or vascular manipulations. As clinical evaluations to assess the neurological status cannot be performed during anesthesia, intraoperative monitoring (IOM) of sensory and motor tracts is used to assess the integrity of these tracts. IOM is a useful tool to identify the impending and potential tissue damage which can result in postoperative neurological deficits. Depending on the site of surgery monitoring of visual, auditory, somatosensory lemniscal, and pyramidal tracts can be performed.

Recording the EPs in the operation theater is technically challenging due to multiple sources of artifacts including electrocautery, multiple sources of 50 Hz artifacts, suboptimal grounding, etc. Strict adherence to electrical safety, documentation, methodology, prompt communication, and extreme vigilance are needed to identify the potential neuronal injury. Selection of anesthetic agents is important as many of them reduce or abolish EP amplitudes. Muscle relaxants improve the SNR of sensory EPs. However, muscle relaxation cannot be used if motor EPs are concurrently recorded. IOM should begin before anesthesia induction and continue till completion of the surgery and recovery from anesthesia.

Intraoperative Auditory Evoked Potential Monitoring

Mechanical trauma, traction, or vascular manipulation during posterior cranial fossa surgeries may result in postoperative deficits due to brainstem or auditory nerve damage. Intraoperative AEP monitoring can detect potential damage and help the surgeon avoid permanent structural damage.

Monophasic broadband 100 μs clicks are delivered monoaurally using in-ear speakers or noncompressible tubal inserts. Bilateral sequential stimulation is required for side-to-side comparison. White noise at 60 dB SPL is delivered to contralateral ear to prevent bone-conducted crossover stimulation. Stimulus intensity of 60–70 dB above auditory threshold is used. Interleaved stimulation with alternating bilateral stimulation provides simultaneous independent averaging of AEP from both sides. However, masking of the unstimulated ear is not possible with interleaved stimulation. Alternating polarity clicks are utilized to reduce the stimulus artifact. Although optimal recording of AEP requires stimulation at 7–12 Hz, stimulation can be performed at rates up to 30 Hz to obtain rapid averaging and early feedback. Low frequency filter of 100–150 Hz and high frequency filter of 3 kHz is utilized with analysis time of 15 ms. Recording of AEP is performed using Ai–Cz and Ac–Cz derivation. Near-field recording of high-amplitude auditory nerve action potential (ANAP) can be done after surgical exposure which provides high SNR.

Absolute latencies of waves I and V; and I–V interpeak latency intervals are measured and monitored before and during surgery. Wave V latency, amplitude, and morphology are monitored. The baseline latencies and amplitudes are compared with sequential change with the patient serving as his/her own control. Surgeon should be immediately alerted when wave V prolongation exceeds 1 ms or amplitude is reduced by >50%. Reduction of body temperature or local cooling due to irrigation during surgery also increases the latencies.

Auditory evoked IOM is performed in surgery on cerebellopontine angle tumors and for other lesions in posterior fossa.[50] Compression, thermal injury, ischemia, traction, etc. are the common causes of surgically-induced auditory pathway damage which can be detected by AEP changes. Their recognition can prevent irreversible deficits. Sudden loss of all waves can occur from occlusion of internal auditory artery or severe injury to auditory nerve. Prolonged and low-amplitude wave I with proportional change in wave III and V without increase in I–V interval occurs from distal auditory nerve injury. Central injuries including caudal brainstem or proximal basilar artery cause delayed wave III and V with normal wave I. More rostral lesions in midbrain cause isolated abnormalities of wave V.

Intraoperative Visual Evoked Potential Monitoring

There is increased risk of visual impairment from injury to visual pathway during neurosurgical intervention for pituitary tumors, craniopharyngioma, sphenoidal meningioma, and other tumors in the close vicinity of anterior visual pathway. Intraoperative VEP monitoring during these surgeries can improve the postoperative outcome. Despite the early use of IOM using VEP in 1973, its utilization for monitoring was delayed till development of high intensity LED stimulators of small size which made the visual stimulation easier. Intraoperative VEP monitoring is performed with monocular stimulation using a small array of LED stimulators applied over the closed eyelids. Interleaved bilateral stimulation is used to reduce the time needed to record the VEP from both sides. Stimulation is delivered at 1–2 Hz with intensity of 10,000–20,000 lux with duration of 10–20 ms. Signals are recorded from Oz, O1, and O2 and referenced to linked ears (A1 + A2) using bandpass filter at 5–500 Hz.[51]

In patients with underlying visual impairment, it is difficult to record consistent VEP during IOM.[52] Progressive reduction of body temperature during surgery increases VEP latencies and at 25°–27°C, waveforms completely disappear.[53] Hypoxia and hypotension should be avoided as they can attenuate VEP amplitudes. Therapeutic levels of propofol and fentanyl do not reduce the VEP amplitude. However, ketamine, nitrous oxide, and fluorinated inhalational agents markedly reduce or abolish the VEP waveforms. Amplitude reduction >50% from baseline or latency prolongation should alarm the neurophysiologist and the neurosurgeon about early impairment of impulse conduction. Latency prolongation >8.65 ms was associated with postoperative visual deterioration.[54] Recent systematic review concluded amplitude reduction to be a strong predictor of postoperative visual deterioration.[55]

Intraoperative Somatosensory Evoked Potential Monitoring

Somatosensory lemniscal pathway monitoring can be performed for surgery on spinal cord lesions, posterior fossa, spinal deformities, carotid artery, and descending aorta. It has been also used for identification of the central sulcus.[56] Potentials recorded from proximal peripheral nerve, spinal cord, and sensory cortex have relatively high SNR and require fewer number of stimulations. Hence, multichannel recording from these sites is preferred for IOM. Far-field subcortical potentials having low SNR requiring >1,000 stimuli for elicitation are generally not recorded during IOM. The scalp recording location has to be optimized preoperatively in order to record cortical SSEP with high SNR for monitoring. In addition, rare presence of non-discussant lemniscal pathway projecting to ipsilateral sensory cortex needs to be identified preoperatively.[56]

Median nerve stimulation at wrist for SSEP IOM is used for monitoring the lemniscal pathway above C6, and ulnar nerve for monitoring lesions above C8 levels. Compound nerve action potential is recorded at elbow instead of Erb's point as it has high SNR at elbow. Preferred scalp montage for the decussant pathway is CPc–CPz (alternatively CPc–CPi/CPc–Fz) and for the nondecussant pathway is CPi–CPz (alternately CPi–CPc/CPi–Fz). For monitoring of pathway above lumbosacral level, posterior tibial nerve is stimulated at ankle with recording of the scalp potentials from CPz–CPc derivation in divergent pathway and CPz–CPi for nondivergent pathway.[57] Other derivations may be used if needed as per the preoperative SSEP optimization studies. Recording epoch length for median nerve is 50 ms and 100 ms for posterior tibial nerve, sampled >10 kHz. Signals are band-pass filtered at 30–300 Hz for scalp potentials and 0.2–1,000 Hz for the peripheral cubital or popliteal potentials.[56] SSEP amplitudes can be reduced or abolished by surgically-induced changes or be due to peripheral confounding factors including hypothermia, hypotension, anesthesia, and peripheral conduction failure due to compression.

Identification of the central sulcus and the precentral motor area is important in surgery on lesions in the peri-Rolandic area wherein the anatomy may be distorted due to the pathological states. Referential derivations using subdural electrode grids reveal reversal of polarity from N20 in postcentral gyrus to P20 in the precentral gyrus and help in planning the surgery.[58] Cortical ischemia during carotid endarterectomy, arteriovenous malformation interventions, and aneurysmal clipping reduces or abolishes the N20 response which resolves after restoration of perfusion.[59] During posterior fossa surgeries, integrity of the lemniscal pathway by median nerve SSEPs is preferred over posterior tibial due to higher SNR of the median nerve SSEPs. Motor deficits due to brainstem ischemia or injury can occur in the presence of normal SSEPs as the lemniscal pathway comprises only <20% of brainstem area.[60] Spinal deformity correction and abdominal aorta surgeries carry high risk of perioperative paraplegia and require simultaneous monitoring of SSEPs and motor EPs as only one of the modalities may be inadequate. Important surgical step of identification of posterior spinal cord midline in intramedullary lesions is helped by recording dorsal column volleys elicited by using transverse array of electrodes or by dorsal column stimulation.[61,62]

VESTIBULAR EVOKED MYOGENIC POTENTIALS

Short-latency muscle responses to vestibular stimulation using acoustic, vibration, or mechanical stimulation resulting from otolith organs activation are called the VEMPs. The response from the sternocleidomastoid is termed the cervical VEMP (cVEMP) and from the inferior oblique as ocular VEMP (oVEMP). These occur without contribution from semicircular canals. The VEMPs can be recorded using dedicated systems or with minor modifications of the AEP protocols in standard EP systems.[63]

The cVEMP is recorded from sternocleidomastoid muscle with surface belly-tendon recording. The response is part of the ipsilateral vestibulo-collic reflex consisting of P13 and N23. It can be elicited by acoustic stimuli (broadband click or pure tone pips) which preferentially stimulate the saccule. Impulses from saccule are carried to vestibular nucleus by inferior vestibular nerve. Fibers from vestibular nucleus descend to ipsilateral spinal accessory nerve nucleus and inhibit the tonically contracting sternocleidomastoid. oVEMPs with two peaks (N10 and P15) are recorded from tonically contracting contralateral inferior oblique muscle and represent activation of vestibulo-ocular reflex pathway.[63-65] Afferent fibers from the utricle traverse through the superior vestibular nerve and ascend in the medial longitudinal fasciculus and terminate on the contralateral oculomotor nucleus. cVEMP occurs due to inhibition of sternocleidomastoid and oVEMP due to stimulation of orbicularis oculi.

Cervical VEMPs are recorded with surface electrodes over bilateral sternocleidomastoid and oVEMP from surface electrodes below both eyes. Signals are filtered with 1–5 Hz low frequency and 200–1,000 Hz high-frequency filters. Subject is asked to tonically contract the sternocleido-mastoid by partially lifting and rotating the head for cVEMP and look upward for oVEMP recording. The stimulus is delivered monoaurally with click duration of 0.1 ms and intensity above 100 dB peak equivalent SPL. Tone stimulus of 500 or 1,000 Hz lasting <6 ms elicit bigger cVEMP than the click stimuli. Acoustic stimuli elicit smaller amplitude oVEMPs whereas vibration stimulus elicit larger amplitude responses. Preferred stimulus rate is about 5 Hz and higher stimulation rates reduce the cVEMP amplitudes. Sweep duration of 100 ms with 20 ms prestimulus epoch is used for both cVEMP and oVEMP to assess the prestimulus averaged electromyographic response. Two trials of 200 stimuli are averaged and the responses are measured. The random electromyographic signals average out and the time-locked VEMP are averaged.[63,65]

As cVEMP and oVEMP evaluate the function of saccule and utricle respectively, they are useful in the evaluation of disorders of balance and vertigo. In acute vestibular syndromes including acute vestibular neuronitis, either or both of cVEMP or oVEMP can be abnormal depending on involvement of superior or inferior vestibular nerves. Patients with episodic vertigo who have minor VEMP changes are likely to be having secondary positional vertigo.[66] VEMPs in Meniere's disease has predominant involvement of saccule and reveal higher occurrence of abnormalities with air-conducted stimulations. In the presence of third window syndrome with superior canal dehiscence, hearing is reduced with vestibular hypersensitivity evidenced by unusually large oVEMP and cVEMP amplitudes. Patients with acoustic schwannoma have reduced ipsilateral VEMPs and patients with posterior circulation infarctions have impaired VEMPs when the brainstem is involved.

EVENT-RELATED POTENTIALS

The obligatory stimulus-related potentials elicited by auditory, somatosensory, and visual stimuli do not require patient's attention and active response from the subject and can be recorded even during sleep and anesthesia. The endogenous ERPs require selective attentive perception and processing of the stimulus. ERPs provide noninvasive data on information and cognitive processing and are extracted from the scalp EEG by signal averaging. They have been utilized for evaluating the severity of the central nervous system disorders including cognitive, behavioral, and structural abnormalities affecting the information processing. Among the several ERPs P300, P400, and mismatch negativity (MMN) are more consistently recorded across the patient populations.

P300

Large, broad, positive component typically occurring at or beyond 300 ms after task-relevant rare stimulus termed P300 (P3) was reported by Sutton in 1965. It is the most studied ERP. It is elicited by using the oddball paradigm wherein the commonly occurring nontarget stimulus and randomly occurring perceptibly differing rare target stimulus (oddball) are utilized. Amplitude of the P300 increases with patient's attention. Subject must mentally count or press the response switch to each deviant (oddball) stimulus. Averages arising from the common and the deviant stimuli are averaged separately to demonstrate ERPs.

The amplitude of the P300 increases with decreasing occurrence of the deviant stimuli. P300 has its neural generators in hippocampus, superior temporal sulcus, ventrolateral cortex, and intraparietal sulcus. The P3a component occurs earlier with frontocentral distribution arising from initial attention reallocation due to detection of stimulus attribute changes. The larger amplitude P3b resulting from responded target stimuli has posterior parietal distribution and is related to voluntary stimulus categorization.[67,68]

P300 can be elicited using auditory, visual, or somatosensory stimulations using oddball paradigm. Auditory P300 is the most frequently evaluated ERP using stimulation with tones, environmental sounds or spoken words. The IFCN recommends tonal stimulation of 500 Hz and 1,000 Hz with 50–150 ms duration at 70 dB SPL intensity presented at 0.5–1 Hz with rare stimulus probability of 10–20%. For the visual P300 colors, shapes, words, or pictures can be utilized. Fz, Cz, and Pz serve as active electrodes referenced to earlobe to record P300. Simultaneous recording of eye movements is recommended to exclude artifactual distortion of the ERP. Signals epoch duration up to 1 second filtered at 0.01–0.1 Hz low frequency and 100 Hz high frequency filter are averaged separately for the target and nontarget stimuli.[69]

P300 has been studied in diverse neuropsychiatric disorders including dementia, schizophrenia, affective disorders, traumatic brain injury, developmental disorders, etc. Latencies of P300 are increased with amplitude reduction in Alzheimer's disease.[70] P300 amplitudes are reduced in patients with schizophrenia and unaffected family members. Patients with schizophrenia and psychosis-risk syndrome have reduced P300 amplitudes in comparison with controls.[71] Patients with bipolar affective disorders have more consistent deviations of latency and amplitudes compared to those with unipolar disorders.[72] Patients with alcohol dependence have reduced P300 amplitude which partially reverses with abstinence.[73]

Mismatch Negativity

Mismatch negativity is considered to reflect automatic process that can differentiate between incoming stimulus and sensory memory trace of preceding stimuli.[69] It is elicited by presentation of series of nondeviant stimuli interspersed with deviant (mismatch) stimuli which differ by intensity, duration, or frequency. Deviant stimulus probability is maintained <0.2 (20%) and is presented with interstimulus interval of 0.5–1 second. MMN is a small frontocentral surface negative potential of 0.5–5 μV occurring at 100–250 ms after the stimulus with simultaneous positive polarity at mastoid area. It is generated from bilateral auditory cortices irrespective of patient's attention. It is recorded by active electrodes at Fz, Cz, C3, C4, and mastoid with reference placed over nose. Responses are sampled at 200 Hz or higher and bandpass filtered at 0.1–30 Hz. MMN can be recorded in awake, inattentive, asleep, or unconscious patients as conscious discrimination between the common and deviant stimuli is not required.

Mismatch negativity has been studied in patients with schizophrenia, affective disorders, aphasia, cognitive decline, and coma.[69] MMN predicted the better outcome in coma due to traumatic brain injuries.[74,75] The amplitude of MMN is reduced in patients with dementia and in patients with aphasia.[76,77] Patients with schizophrenia and bipolar affective disorder have reduced P300 amplitude which correlated with reduced cortical thickness.[78]

CONCLUSION

Evoked potentials are noninvasive diagnostic modalities used for evaluation of disorders of the special and general sensory pathways. These help in assessment of demyelinating, degenerative, various structural and functional disorders involving the sensory pathways. Despite several advances in the structural and functional imaging of the nervous system, EPs have specific role in the neurological evaluation and monitoring. Optimal utilization of intraoperative monitoring is an additional tool for detection of potential harm to neuroaxis and to improve surgical outcome.

REFERENCES

1. Oken BS. Statistics for evoked potentials. In: Chiappa KH (Ed). Evoked Potentials in Clinical Medicine, 3rd edition. Philadelphia: Lippincott-Raven Publishers; 1997. pp. 565-77.
2. Davis CQ. Hamilton R. Reference ranges for clinical electrophysiology of vision. Doc Ophthal. 2021;143:155-70.
3. Slotnik SD, Klein SA, Carney T, Sutter E, Dastmalchi S. Using multi-stimulus VEP source localization to obtain a retinotopic map of human primary visual cortex. Clin Neurophysiol. 1999;110:1793-800.
4. Di Russo F, Martinez A, Sereno MI, Pitzalis S, Hillyard S. Cortical sources of the early components of the visual evoked potential. Hum Brain Mapp. 2001;15:95-111.
5. Creel DJ. Visually evoked potentials. Handb Clin Neurol. 2019;160:501-22.
6. Chiappa KH. Pattern-shift visual evoked potentials: Methodology. In: Chiappa KH (Ed). Evoked Potentials in Clinical Medicine, 3rd edition. Philadelphia: Lippincott Raven Publishers; 1997. pp. 31-94.
7. American Clinical Neurophysiology Society. Guideline 9B: Guidelines on visual evoked potentials. J Clin Neurophysiol. 2006;23:138-56.
8. Holder GE, Celesia GG, Miyake Y, Tobimatsu S, Weleber RG; International Federation of Clinical Neurophysiology. International Federation of Clinical Neurophysiology: Recommendations for visual system testing. Clin Neurophysiol. 2010;121:1393-409.
9. Odom JV, Bach M, Brigell M, Holder GE, McCulloch DL, Mizota A, et al; International Society for Clinical Electrophysiology of Vision. ISCEV standard for clinical visual evoked potentials: (2016 update). Doc Ophthalmol. 2016;133:1-9.
10. Tan CT, King PJ, Chiappa KH. Pattern ERG: Effects of reference electrode site, stimulus mode and check size. Electroencephalogr Clin Neurophysiol. 1989;74:11-18.
11. Robson AG, Nilsson J, Li S, Jalali S, Fulton AB, Tormene AP, et al. ISCEV guide to visual electrodiagnostic procedures. Doc Ophthalmol. 2018;136:1-26.
12. Lenassi E, Likar K, Stirn-Kranjc B, Brecelj J. VEP maturation and visual acuity in infants and preschool children. Doc Ophthalmol. 2008;117(2):111-20.
13. Klistormer A, Fraser C, Garrick R, Graham S, Arvind H. Correlation between full-field and multifocal VEPs in optic neuritis. Doc Ophthalmol. 2008;116:19-27.
14. Laron M, Cheng H, Zhang B, Schiffman JS, Tang RA, Frishman LJ. Comparison of multifocal visual evoked potential, standard automated perimetry and optical coherence tomography in assessing visual pathway in multiple sclerosis patients. Mult Scler. 2010;16(4):412-26.
15. Zafeiropoulos P, Katsanos A, Kitsos G, Stefaniotou M, Asproudis I. The contribution of multifocal visual evoked potentials in patients with optic neuritis and multiple sclerosis: a review. Doc Ophthalmol. 2021;142:283-92.
16. Creel DJ. Electroretinograms. Handb Clin Neurol. 2019;160:481-93.
17. Chiappa KH, Hill RA. Pattern-Shift visual evoked potentials: interpretation. In: Chiappa KH (Ed). Evoked Potentials in Clinical Medicine, 3rd edition. Philadelphia: Lippincott-Raven Publishers; 1997. pp. 95-130.
18. Leocani L, Guerrieri S, Comi G. Visual evoked potentials as a biomarker in multiple sclerosis and associated optic neuritis. J Neuroophthalmol. 2018;38:350-7.
19. Barton JL, Garber JY, Klistomer A, Barnett MH. The electrophysiological assessment of visual function in multiple sclerosis. Clin Neurophysiol Pract. 2019;4:90-6.
20. Guerrieri S, Comi G, Leocani L. Optical coherence tomography and visual evoked potentials as prognostic and monitoring tools in progressive multiple sclerosis. Front Neurosci. 2021;15:692599.
21. Tekavcic-Pompe M, Stirn-Krajnc B, Brecelj J. Optic neuritis in children—clinical and electrophysiological follow-up. Doc Ophthalmol. 2003;107:261-70.

22. Parisi V, Galllinaro G, Ziccardi L, Coppola G. Electrophysiological assessment of visual function in patients with non-arteritic ischaemic optic neuropathy. Eur J Neurol. 2008;15:839-45.
23. Stojkovic T, de Seze J, Hurtevent JF, Arndt C, Beaume A, Hache JC, et al. Visual evoked potentials study in chronic idiopathic inflammatory demyelinating polyneuropathy. Clin Neurophysiol. 2000;111:2285-91.
24. Krasodomska K, Lubiński W, Potemkowski A, Honczarenko K. Pattern electroretinogram (PERG) and pattern visual evoked potential (PVEP) in the early stages of Alzheimer's disease. Doc Ophthalmol. 2010;121:111-21.
25. Eggermont JJ. Auditory brainstem response. Handb Clin Neurol. 2019;160:451-64.
26. American Clinical Neurophysiology Society. Guideline 9C: Guidelines on short-latency auditory evoked potentials. J Clin Neurophysiol. 2006;23:157-67.
27. Legatt AD. Electrophysiology of cranial nerve testing: Auditory nerve. J Clin Neurophysiol. 2018;35:25-38.
28. Chiappa KH. Brain stem auditory evoked potentials: methodology. In: Chiappa KH (Ed). Evoked Potentials in Clinical Medicine, 3rd edition. Philadelphia: Lippincott Raven Publishers; 1997. pp. 157-98.
29. Legatt AD. Brainstem auditory evoked potentials: methodology, interpretation and clinical application. In: Aminoff MJ (Ed). Amionoff's Electrodiagnosis in Clinical Neurology. New Delhi: Elsevier; 2012. pp. 519-52.
30. Hashimoto I, Ishiyama Y, Yoshimoto T, Nemoto S. Brain-stem auditory-evoked potentials directly recorded from human brain-stem and thalamus. Brain. 1981;104:841-59.
31. Chiappa KH, Gladstone KJ, Young RR. Brain stem auditory evoked responses: studies of waveform variations in 50 normal human subjects. Arch Neurol. 1979;36:81-7.
32. Cho TH, Fischer C, Nighoghossian N, Hermier M, Sindou M, Mauguière F. Auditory and electrophysiological patterns of a unilateral lesion of the lateral lemniscus. Audiol Neurootol. 2005;10:153-8.
33. Ponton CW, Moore JK, Eggermont JJ. Auditory brain stem response generation by parallel pathways: differential maturation of axonal conduction time and synaptic transmission. Ear Hear. 1996;17: 402-10.
34. Gorga M, Johnson TA, Kaminski JR, Beauchaine KL, Garner CA, Neely ST. Using a combination of click- and tone burst-evoked auditory brain stem response measurements to estimate pure-tone thresholds. Ear Hear. 2006;27:60-74.
35. Rance G, Starr A. Pathophysiological mechanisms and functional hearing consequences of auditory neuropathy. Brain. 2015;138: 3141-158.
36. Chiappa KH, Harrison JL, Brooks EB, Young RR. Brainstem auditory evoked responses in 200 patients with multiple sclerosis. Ann Neurol. 1980;7:135-43.
37. Don M, Kwong B, Tanaka C. Interaural stacked auditory brainstem response measures for detecting small unilateral acoustic tumors. Audiol Neurootol. 2012;17:54-68.
38. Zhang XJ, Zhang LJ, Zhu J, He M, Wang Z, Wang J, et al. Clinical value of brainstem auditory evoked potential in the diagnosis of vertebrobasilar ischemia. Integr Med Int. 2015;1:199-204.
39. Cruccu G, Aminoff MJ, Curio G, Guerit JM, Kakigi R, Mauguiere F, et al. Recommendations for the clinical use of somatosensory-evoked potentials. Clin Neurophysiol. 2008;119:1705-19.
40. Muzyka IM, Estephan B. Somatosensory evoked potentials. Handb Clin Neurol. 2019;160:523-40.
41. American Clinical Neurophysiology Society. Guideline 9D: Guidelines on short-latency somatosensory evoked potentials. J Clin Neurophysiol. 2006;23:168-79.
42. Chiappa KH. Short-latency somatosensory evoked potentials: methodology. In: Chiappa KH (Ed). Evoked Potentials in Clinical Medicine, 3rd edition. Philadelphia: Lippincott Raven Publishers; 1997. pp. 283-340.
43. Verdugo RJ, Matamala JM, Inui K, Kakigi R, Valls-Solé J, Hansson P, et al. Review of techniques useful for the assessment of sensory small fiber neuropathies: Report from an IFCN expert group. Clin Neurophysiol. 2022;136:13-38.
44. Frot M, Magnin A, Mauguière F, Garcia-Larrea L. Human SII and posterior insula differently encode thermal laser stimuli. Cereb Cortex. 2007;17:610-20.
45. Kakigi R, Inui K, Tamura Y. Electrophysiological studies on human pain perception. Clin Neurophysiol. 2005;116:743-63.
46. Obermann M, Katsarava Z, Esser S, Sommer C, He L, Selter L, et al. Correlation of epidermal nerve fiber density with pain-related evoked potentials in HIV neuropathy. Pain. 2008;138:79-86.
47. Nardone R, Höller Y, Brigo F, Frey VN, Lochner P, Leis S, et al. The contribution of neurophysiology in the diagnosis and management of cervical spondylotic myelopathy: a review. Spinal Cord. 2016;54:756-66.
48. Curt A, Ellaway PH. Clinical neurophysiology in the prognosis and monitoring of traumatic spinal cord injury. Handb Clin Neurol. 2012;109:63-75.
49. Carter BG, Butt W. Review of the use of somatosensory evoked potentials in the prediction of outcome after severe brain injury. Crit Care Med. 2001;29:178-86.
50. Yingling CD, Gardi JN. Intraoperative monitoring of facial and cochlear nerves during acoustic neuroma surgery. Otolaryngol Clin North Am. 1992;25:413-48.
51. Hayashi H, Kawaguchi M. Intraoperative monitoring of flash visual evoked potential under general anesthesia. Korean J Anesthesiol. 2017;70:127-35.
52. Kodama K, Goto T, Sato A, Sakai K, Tanaka Y, Hongo K. Standard and limitation of intraoperative monitoring of the visual evoked potentials. Acta Neurochir (Wien). 2010;152:643-8.
53. Russ W, King D, Loesevitz A, Hempelmann G. Effect of hypothermia on visual evoked potentials (VEP) in humans. Anesthesiology. 1984;61:207-10.
54. Tao X, Yang X, Fan X, You H, Jin Y, Liu J, et al. Predication of post-operative visual deterioration using visual-evoked potential latency in extended endoscopic endonasal resection of craniopharyngiomas. Front Neurol. 2021;21:753902.
55. Jashek-Ahmed F, Cabrilo I, Bal J, Sanders B, Grieve J, Dorward NL, et al. Intraoperative monitoring of visual evoked potentials in patients undergoing transsphenoidal surgery for pituitary adenoma: a systematic review. BMC Neurol. 2021;21:287.
56. MacDonald DB, Dong C, Quatrale R, Sala F, Skinner S, Soto F, et al. Recommendations of the International Society of Intraoperative Neurophysiology for intraoperative somatosensory evoked potentials. Clin Neurophysiol. 2019;130:161-79.
57. MacDonald DB, Al Zayed Z, Al Saddigi A. Four-limb muscle motor evoked potential and optimized somatosensory evoked potential monitoring with decussation assessment: results in 206 thoracolumbar spine surgeries. Eur Spine J. 2007;16 (Suppl 2): S171-87.
58. Simon MV. Intraoperative neurophysiologic sensorimotor mapping and monitoring in supratentorial surgery. J Clin Neurophysiol. 2013;30:571-90.
59. Nwachuku EL, Balzer JR, Yabes JG, Habeych ME, Crammond DJ, Thirumala PD. Diagnostic value of somatosensory evoked potential changes during carotid endarterectomy: a systematic review and meta-analysis. JAMA Neurol. 2015;72:73-80.
60. Kodama K, Javadi M, Seifert V, Szelényi A. Conjunct SEP and MEP monitoring in resection of infratentorial lesions: lessons learned in a cohort of 210 patients. J Neurosurg. 2014;121:1453-61.
61. Mehta AI, Mohrhaus CA, Hussain AM, Karikari IO, Hughes B, Hodges T, et al. Dorsal column mapping for intramedullary spinal cord tumor resection decreases dorsal column dysfunction. J Spinal Disord Tech. 2012;25:205-9.

62. Nair D, Kumaraswamay VM, Braver D, Kilbride RD, Borges LF, Simon MV. Dorsal column mapping via phase reversal method: the refined technique and clinical applications. Neurosurgery. 2014;74:437-46.
63. Rosengren SM, Welgampola MS, Colebatch JG. Vestibular evoked myogenic potentials: past, present and future. Clin Neurophysiol. 2010;121:636-51.
64. Papathanasiou ES, Murofushi T, Akin FW, Colebatch JG. International guidelines for the clinical application of cervical vestibular evoked myogenic potentials: An expert consensus report. Clin Neurophysiol. 2014;125:658-66.
65. Rosengren SM, Colebatch JG, Young AS, Govender S, Welgampola MS. Vestibular evoked myogenic potentials in practice: methods, pitfalls and clinical applications. Clin Neurophysiol Pract. 2019;4:47-68.
66. Kim E, Oh S, Kim JS, Yang TH, Yang SY. Persistent otolith dysfunction even after successful repositioning in benign paroxysmal positional vertigo. J Neurol Sci. 2015;358:287-93.
67. Polich J. Updating P300: an integrative theory of P3a and P3b. Clin Neurophysiol. 2007;118:2128-48.
68. Wronka E, Kaiser J, Coenen AML. Neural generators of the auditory evoked potential components P3a and P3b. Acta Neurobiol Exp (Wars). 2012;72(1):51-64.
69. Duncan CC, Barry RJ, Connolly JF, Fischer C, Michie PT, Näätänen R, et al. Event-related potentials in clinical research: guidelines for eliciting, recording, and quantifying mismatch negativity, P300, and N400. Clin Neurophysiol. 2009;120:1883-908.
70. Hedges D, Janis R, Mickelson S, Keith C, Bennett D, Brown BL. P300 Amplitude in Alzheimer's Disease: A Meta-analysis and Meta-regression. Clin EEG Neurosci. 2016;47(1):48-55.
71. Hamilton HK, Woods SW, Roach BJ, Llerena K, McGlashan TH, Srihari VH, et al. Auditory and visual oddball stimulus processing deficits in schizophrenia and the psychosis risk syndrome: forecasting psychosis risk with P300. Schizophr Bull. 2019;45:1068-80.
72. Wada M, Kurose S, Miyazaki T, Nakajima S, Masuda F, Mimura Y, et al. The P300 event-related potential in bipolar disorder: a systematic review and meta-analysis. J Affect Disord. 2019;256:234-49.
73. Liu X, Zhou H, Jiang C, Xue Y, Zhou Z, Wang J. Cognitive control deficits in alcohol dependence are a trait- and state-dependent biomarker: An ERP study. Front Psychiatry. 2020;11:606891.
74. Fischer C, Morlet D, Bouchet P, Luaute J, Jourdan C, Salord F. Mismatch negativity and late auditory evoked potentials in comatose patients. Clin Neurophysiol. 1999;110(9):1601-10.
75. Zhou L, Wang J, Wu Y, Liu ZY, Yu Y, Liu JF, et al. Clinical significance of mismatch negativity in predicting the awakening of comatose patients after severe brain injury. J Neurophysiol. 2021;126:1 40-7.
76. Horvath A, Szucs A, Csukly G, Sakovics A, Stefanics G, Kamondi A. EEG and ERP biomarkers of Alzheimer's disease: a critical review. Front Biosci (Landmark Ed). 2018;23:183-220.
77. Lucchese G, Pulvermüller F, Stahl B, Dreyer FR, Mohr B. Therapy-induced neuroplasticity of language in chronic post stroke aphasia: a mismatch negativity study of (A)grammatical and meaningful/less mini-constructions. Front Hum Neurosci. 2017; 10:669.
78. Kim S, Jeon H, Jang K, Kim YW, Im CH, Lee SH. Mismatch negativity and cortical thickness in patients with schizophrenia and bipolar disorder. Schizophr Bull. 2019;45(2):425-35.

114

CHAPTER

Intraoperative Neurophysiological Monitoring

K Srinivasa Babu

INTRODUCTION

Intraoperative neurophysiological monitoring (IOM) has become an important adjunct tool in recent years. Various techniques are developed to identify and monitor neural structures that are at risk during the course of surgery. The objectives of IOM are to prevent any new neurological impairment during the course of surgery, to give reassurance to the surgeon to continue with the surgery so that a more radical excision/correction can be accomplished, and to modify surgical strategy if any changes occur in the recordings. IOM can be used to monitor the integrity of sensory pathways, and motor pathways, localize epileptic foci, and also to identify neural structures.

EQUIPMENT AND OPERATION THEATER

One must remember that an operation theater is a hostile environment for electrophysiological recordings. There are several electrical types of equipment such as cautery (monopolar and bipolar), electrocardiogram (ECG), ventilators, transformers, mains supply, etc., that will generate an electrical field and can interfere with the IOM recordings. With the advent of digital technology, it has been feasible to do averaging the signals and improve signals to noise ratio. Besides this, digital technology improved recording techniques while suppressing unwanted signals. An IOM machine looks and operates very much similar to what is in a diagnostic laboratory. However, it also differs in some ways. Since the operating area is a sterile environment, the IOM machine must be away from the sterile zone. Very often it will be required to do multimodality monitoring. Taking these facts into consideration, one must look for some of the following features in an IOM machine[1]—(1) a good common mode rejection; (2) amplifiers capable of withstanding cautery machines (diagnostic laboratory machines amplifiers are not built for this purpose); (3) cable length to be 6 or 8 meters long so that the IOM machine can be kept away from the sterile zone; (4) it must have at least 16 Channels for recording; (5) it must be capable of doing multimodality stimulation and recording; (6) IOM machine should be able to deliver monophasic and biphasic electrical stimulation; (7) the recording screen should indicate both voltage and current delivered at the same time, to ensure that the designated current/voltage is delivered; and (8) current IOM machines can deliver multipulse transcranial electrical stimulation (TES). However, it must have the capability to vary the frequency, pulse width, and the number of pulses. When delivering multisquare pulse stimulation, each square pulse must be of similar morphology for effective delivery of stimuli. The IOM machine should have good ground connectivity. Too much ground connectivity (from different machines in the operating room) can cause "ground loops", which can result in current flowing through the patient because of differential voltages **(Fig. 1)**. It will be helpful to consult the institutional bioengineering department to sort out some of these factors.

ANESTHESIA

Anesthesiologist plays a crucial role in IOM. To obtain consistent and reliable responses, anesthetic agents must be titrated in such a way as to get physiological homeostasis. The choice of anesthetic agents and depth of anesthesia has a direct impact on recordings. Since one needs consistent and reliable responses, any changes in recordings are attributed to risk/injury to neural tissue, it is important to maintain uniform physiological status (e.g., blood pressure). The IOM team needs to discuss their requirement the previous day with the anesthetist. The IOM team should bring to the attention of the anesthetists their areas of interest to place stimulating and recording electrodes (e.g., stimulating electrodes at the wrist/ankle, etc.) for monitoring.

Sensory evoked potentials (SEPs) in general are compatible with most anesthetic regimens that are currently used. However, a high concentration of volatile anesthetic agents can affect cortical SEPs. In contrast to this, motor evoked potentials (MEPs) require the cooperation of both

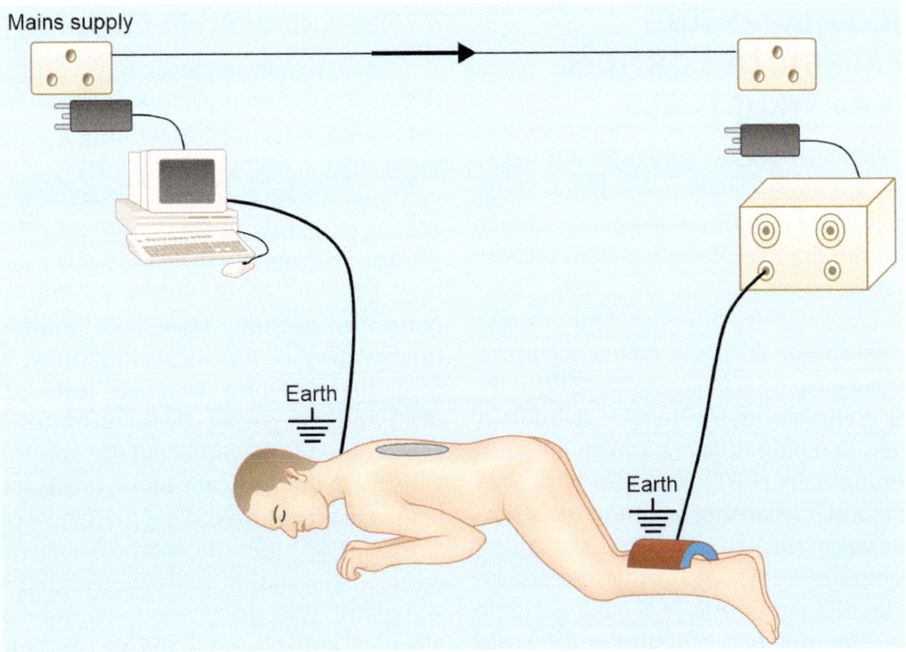

FIG. 1: Schematic diagram: Connecting multiple ground electrodes from different electrical equipment can sometime result in current flowing through the patient because of difference in voltages between each ground connection.

anesthetist and the surgeon. After induction, it is important to place "a bite block" between the molars and make sure that the tongue and cheek are clear of the teeth. When one is recording compound muscle action potentials (CMAP) for cases such as spinal cord surgery, where TES is used, it is important to control the use of muscle relaxants. The initial induction dose of anesthetics may take around 45 minutes to wear off and eliciting MEP responses during that period may not be possible. Some centers use a low level of muscle relaxants,[2] while others have avoided the total use of muscle relaxants.[3] In general, inhalational anesthesia has a significant effect on evoked potentials as compared to intravenous anaesthesia.[4-6] Intravenous agents such as propofol **(Fig. 2)** and remifentanil are short-acting and they enable the anesthetist to depend less on muscle relaxants.[7] The bispectral index (BIS) monitoring is recommended in cases that last >4 hours. Awake craniotomy procedure is considered in patients where intra-axial tumors are present close to functional areas, particularly near Broca or Wernicke or dominant angular gyrus. Intraoperatively, our practice is to give the block to the nerves of the scalp with a mixture of bupivacaine and lignocaine along with epinephrine.[7] It is also necessary to infiltrate the dura at the site of the incision. To keep the patient comfortable during craniotomy a low dose of propofol infusion is also administered. Combined use of local anesthetics and other drugs such as propofol, dexmedetomidine, and fentanyl have also been used. Dexmedetomidine has been suggested as an alternative due to its analgesic and sedative properties.[8,9]

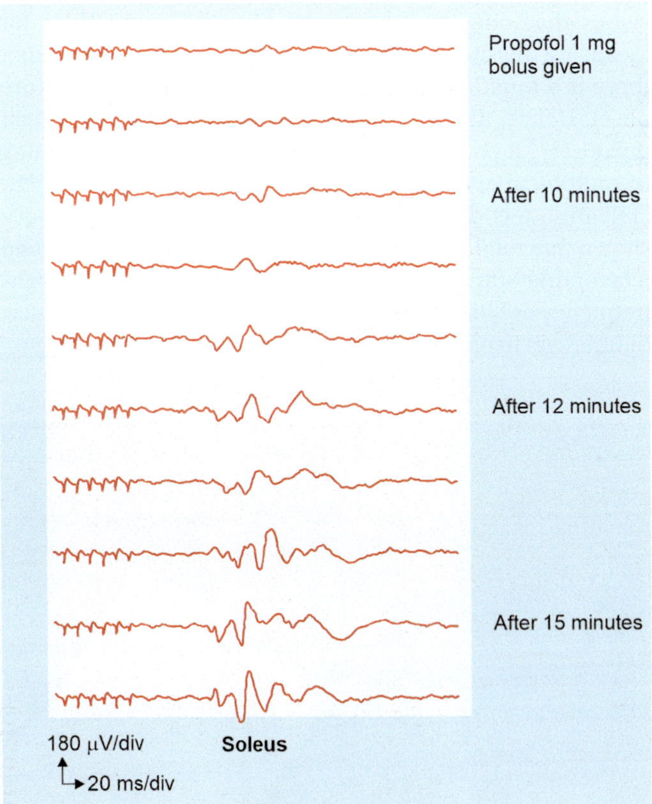

FIG. 2: Effect of propofol bolus on mMEPs. A 1 mg of bolus can completely attenuate mMEPs and it can take at least 10–12 minutes to wear off. IOM team must be aware and correlate anesthesia effect on electrophysiological recordings.

ELECTROCORTICOGRAPHY AND FUNCTIONAL MAPPING OF CORTICAL AND SUBCORTICAL STRUCTURES

Intraoperative electrocorticography (ECoG) has been used for mapping and monitoring electrical activity. These are used not only to localize functional areas but also in epilepsy surgery.[10] This requires the placement of electrodes directly over the exposed cortex (or over the dura). These electrodes come in different shapes and sizes and can also be custom-made. Depending on the requirement and space availability, one can use strip or grid electrodes **(Figs. 3A and B)**. Currently, for epilepsy surgery, there is technology available for functional mapping imaging known as fMRI, positron emission tomography (PET), and also improved intracranial and extracranial recording techniques such as magnetic encephalography (MEG), subdural electrodes, and chronic depth electrodes recording. In epilepsy surgery, the objective is to localize epileptic foci and irritable zones. ECoG has the same rhythms as found in the scalp recordings. The difference is 10 times bigger amplitudes and faster frequencies. However, one may not encounter spontaneous electrographic seizures intraoperatively. One has to rely on interictal epileptiform discharge (IED) to localize the site of epileptogenicity. There are several issues that one must be aware of while using IEDs for localizing the site for epileptogenicity. It is not absolute that there is a functional relationship between IED and seizure onset. Hence, the utility of IED has been a subject of much debate.[11,12] It could be much more complex and misleading in multifocal epilepsy. When patients have very few IEDs, activation techniques have been used. Some studies have shown that total resection of epileptiform abnormalities had a favorable outcome. Zijlmans et al.[13] suggested that high-frequency oscillations (80–500 Hz) can be considered as new biomarkers in epilepsy.

Functional Brain Mapping

Very often in epilepsy surgery, cortical mapping is also done to localize functional areas. Electrical stimulation of the cortex has been used to identify sensorimotor or language areas of the dominant hemisphere. Due to individual variations in the functional areas and the presence of lesions that can distort normal anatomy, intraoperative identification of functional areas based on anatomical landmarks may lead to postoperative morbidity. Currently, intraoperative magnetic resonance imaging (MRI), computed tomography (CT), ultrasonography, and navigators are available. Imaging language tasks preoperatively using fMRI and comparing it with electrical cortical stimulation, showed that fMRI predicted the absence of eloquent areas. However, the indications of fMRI activity in noncritical language areas lowered the predictive value of a critical area site by 51%.[14] Identification of eloquent areas using direct cortical stimulation remains the gold standard. However, using fMRI information and neuronavigation may speed up electrical cortical stimulation procedures and help tailor the size of craniotomy.[15]

Intraoperatively, functional mapping of the cortex can be done under light general anesthesia or in awake craniotomy surgeries. Awake craniotomy offers a more reliable and cost-effective method for maintaining neural integrity while excising tumors that are located within or proximal to eloquent areas. It also offers the advantage of continuous clinical monitoring of the awake patient for early detection of deficits in language, motor, or sensory domains. This instant availability of information to the surgeon will enable them to do a more safe and radical excision.

It has not been possible to obtain Class 1 evidence or data from a prospective randomized clinical trial, to prove that radical excision of low or high-grade gliomas is superior to a partial excision with radiation therapy. There are, however, several retrospective studies that have shown

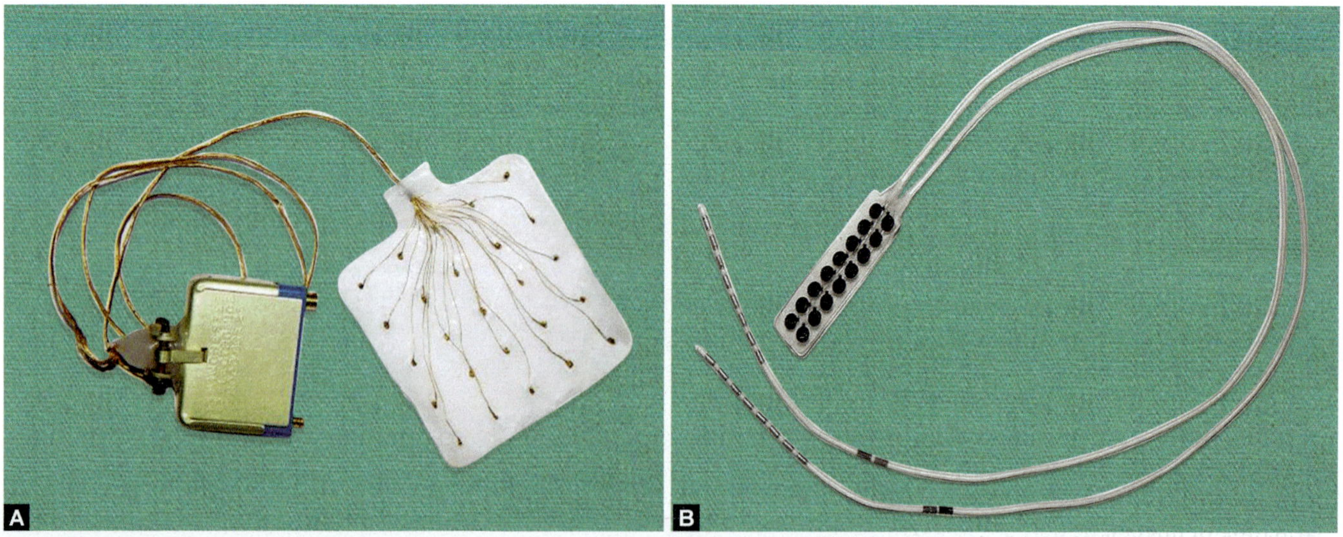

FIGS. 3A AND B: Electrocarticographic electrodes—(A) An array of 20 electrodes; and (B) Strip of 16 electrodes arranged in two rows. These strip electrodes can be used for recording and also for stimulating the cortex.

benefits in terms of longer recurrence-free survival in those patients undergoing more radical surgery for low and high-grade gliomas.[16] Quinones-Hinojosa et al.[17] described sulcal landmarks in the inferior frontal gyrus on a sagittal MR that closely correspond with speech arrest produced by intraoperative cortical stimulation. A preoperative study of the spatial relationship between these areas and the tumor would enable the surgeon to carry out a detailed plan of the surgery including the decision on whether intraoperative cortical stimulation would be required under awake conditions.

Awake surgeries have been done on children of 11 years of age.[18] However, not all patients are suitable for awake craniotomy surgeries. Some centers consider all patients with supratentorial intra-axial mass lesions and exclude those uncooperative due to aphasia, severe language barrier, mental retardation, emotional instability, and decreased level of consciousness.

Preoperative Patient Preparation

Patients are usually admitted a few days before the surgery so that the surgeons, the neuropsychologists, and the anesthesiologists can explain the entire procedure to them. Most patients accept the idea calmly when explained the advantages of awake surgery to locate and monitor motor and language areas thus preventing damage to these structures. The language in which the patient is most comfortable is chosen and the neuropsychologist gives the patient a battery of tests related to naming objects from a picture book. The patient needs to say out aloud, "This is a carrot" or "This is a house" upon being shown the appropriate picture. They are instructed to follow all commands, especially those related to the motor or sensory testing. Depending on the location of the lesion, the patient would be made familiar with the tasks that they are expected to do during surgery.[19] These would include repetitive voluntary movements of the contralateral limbs, such as finger and foot tapping. They have to report any abnormal sensations or feel an aura of a seizure. Preoperatively, it is important to establish the patient's ability to perform various tasks (baseline) so that intraoperative changes can be noticed.

Bipolar stimulating electrodes are ideal for cortical mapping in awake surgeries. Strip electrodes (recording) are placed over the cortex close to the stimulating area. This is to detect after discharge while stimulating. Detection of after discharge during stimulation would require a reduction of stimulus strength to avoid intraoperative seizures. Typically we start with 1 mAmp and increase in steps of 1 mAmp until responses are obtained (maximum 6 mAmp). Stimulation is done systematically in a grid fashion at a 5 mm distance between each stimulus point. Contralateral motor movements of upper and lower limbs are observed on stimulation of the motor cortex. A positive response area is marked with a sterile numbered ticket. One would notice twitching of fingers, flexion of the wrist, elbow, or shoulder, and flexion of toes and ankle on stimulation of the motor cortex. When stimulating supplementary motor areas, there will be a more complex multijoint movement (wrist, elbow, and shoulder movement). Paresthesia is noticed on stimulation of the primary sensory cortex. Stimulation of language areas results in speech arrest during the naming of visually presented images or during numerical counting tasks. Near the angular gyrus area, one needs to test the ability of a patient to calculate and to name colors before and during stimulation. Patients are asked to continuously perform motor tasks, such as opening and closing the fingers, raising the arm, finger tapping, and foot tapping. While operating on the dominant frontal and temporal opercula and insula, language assessment tasks are performed. One must observe for both positive and negative clinical correlation during stimulation.[20] For example, stimulation of supplementary motor areas can result in disruption of fine motor movements. While stimulating, the patient is asked to perform a continuous motor task. When a positive or negative phenomenon is observed, the test is repeated to validate the results. Whenever, the slightest weakness is noticed or a delay in obeying commands, resection, and retraction is stopped in that zone. Attention is shifted to other areas for tumor resection while clinically monitoring the patient. After a few minutes patient is retested where weakness was noted until improvement is noted.

We have not encountered problems at surgery due to raised intracranial pressure. This is likely to be a result of our exclusion criteria because we preferred to operate the higher grade gliomas with altered sensorium (due to extensive edema and midline shift) under general anesthesia. However, some workers have operated on large high-grade neoplasms, and have used mannitol, corticosteroids, rapid intratumoral decompression, and early decompression of cysts if present. None of our patients required conversion to general anesthesia. None have had generalized seizures but this could be treated with intravenous phenytoin or midazolam infusions. In our study on 67 consecutive patients, nine patients had persistent mild neurological deficits at the time of discharge,[21] and weakness persisted in four patients. Intraoperative focal seizures occurred in three patients and were controlled with ice-cold saline irrigation of the cortex. Another two patients who had no intraoperative seizures had postoperative seizures and progressed to status epilepticus. One patient recovered while the other succumbed due to status epilepticus and intractable brain swelling. Our experience showed that awake surgery enabled the surgeon to safely remove the tumor, while preventing any neurological deficit till that point in time, allowing the surgeon for maximal tumor resection.

Cortical Mapping under General Anesthesia

Not all patients are suitable for awake surgeries as mentioned in the above section. In awake surgeries, intraoperative seizures can cause complications such as airway control and postictal refractory effects. In such cases, functional areas can be localized using somatosensory evoked potentials (SSEPs) and direct cortical stimulation under general anaesthesia.[22]

Central Sulcus Localization using SSEPs

Central sulcus can be localized using SSEPs. Intraoperative SSEPs are relatively easy to obtain and are less affected by anesthetic agents and responses are not affected by muscle relaxants.[23] The stimulation and recording settings are similar to what is used in the diagnostic laboratory **(Table 1)**. Median nerve is stimulated at the wrist, contralateral to the side of surgery. Grid electrodes (2–64) are placed over the exposed cortex (can also be placed epidurally) with a referential electrode placed anteriorly (Fpz). When the contralateral median nerve is stimulated, if the electrodes are over the hand sensory and motor areas, then responses are elicited at around 20 ms. There will be both negative and positive responses at around 20 ms, indicating a reversal of phase **(Fig. 4)**. The channel showing the highest negative response at around 20 ms is considered as a sensory gyrus and the anterior and adjacent gyrus is considered as motor gyrus. Between these two gyri will be the central sulcus. Babu and Chandy[24] showed that even in patients with mild sensorimotor deficits, it is possible to obtain a phase reversal. While no phase reversal could be obtained in patients with gross sensory and motor deficits. The other possible reasons for failure to obtain a phase reversal could be the presence of a tumor that desynchronizes afferent volley along the thalamocortical pathways, mass effect distorting spatiotemporal projection, recording site not being appropriate for recording hand area potentials in the postcentral gyrus.[25]

TABLE 1: Central sulcus mapping.

Stimulation site	Contralateral median nerve at wrist
Rate of stimulation	4.1 Hz
Pulse width	200 μs
Stimulus intensity	25 mA
Average count	100 sweeps
Time base for recording	50 ms
Filters band width	10–1,000 Hz
Recording electrodes placement	• Strip electrodes placed over the dura/cortex • Reference electrode Fpz

Cortical Stimulation

There are different techniques available to elicit motor responses under light general anesthesia **(Table 2)**. One can use monopolar or bipolar stimulators. The stimulus can be monophasic or biphasic (anodal stimulation is more effective in cortical stimulation) **(Fig. 5)**. Pulse width could vary from 200 to 2,000 μs. The conventional stimulus frequency is 60/50 Hz. Taniguchi[26] used anodal rectangular pulses at a higher rate of stimuli to deliver a lesser amount of current for eliciting cortical responses. The optimal frequency for stimulation to elicit a large response was 500 Hz. Szelenyi et al.[27] used 1–2 ms stimulus duration for mapping the primary motor cortex and 2–4 ms for the secondary motor cortex. Studies have suggested that a charge density of 40 μC/cm^2/phase is the threshold limit to prevent damage to the neural tissue.[28]

Intraoperative Monitoring of Cortical and Subcortical Structures

Gliomas in general are infiltrative in nature, hence not possible to do a radical resection while preserving eloquent structures. The surgeon aims to achieve an "oncofunctional balance" during resection.[29] SSEPs can be used to monitor

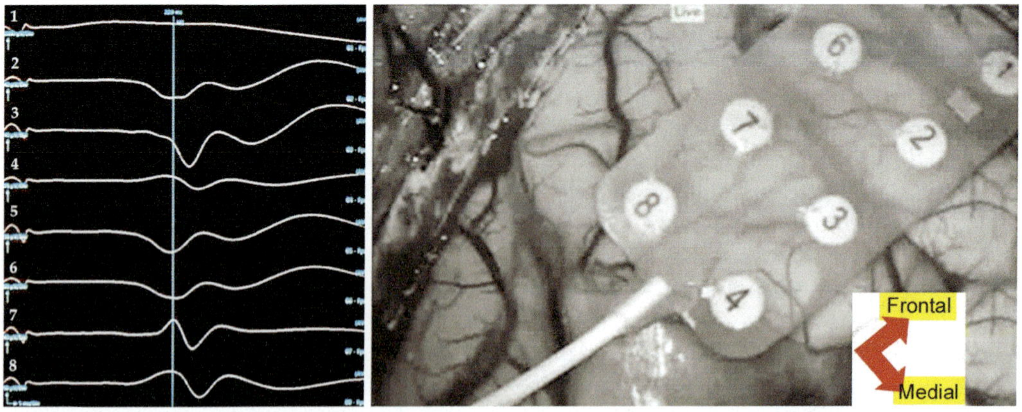

FIG. 4: Central sulcus localization: Intraoperative image of a grid of 8 electrodes placed over the cortex across the sulcus in anteroposterior manner is shown on the right side of the panel. On the left side of the panel is the response to stimulation of the contralateral median nerve at the wrist. Channels 3, 4, 7, and 8 showing negative responses (upward deflection). Channels 2, 5, and 6 showing a positive responses (downward deflection). Channel 7 shows maximum negative response at around 20 ms (N20), while Channel 6 (anteriorly placed to electrode 7) showing a positive response (P20) across the sulcus with inverse polarity. Channel 7 electrode where N20 response is obtained is the sensory gyrus and the anterior and adjacent gyrus (in this case Channel 6) is the motor gyrus. In between these two gyri is the central sulcus.

TABLE 2: Cortical stimulation and monitoring.

	Monopolar (penfield method)	Bipolar (awake)	Monopolar (localization and monitoring under general anesthesia)
Frequency of stimulation	50/60 Hz	4.7 Hz	300–500 Hz
Duration	200–300 µs	• 1–2 ms (motor cortex) • 2–4 ms (secondary motor cortex)	200–300 µs
Train of stimuli	Trigger	Trigger	2–5 pulses
Intensity	3–25 mA	1–7 mA	3–25 mA

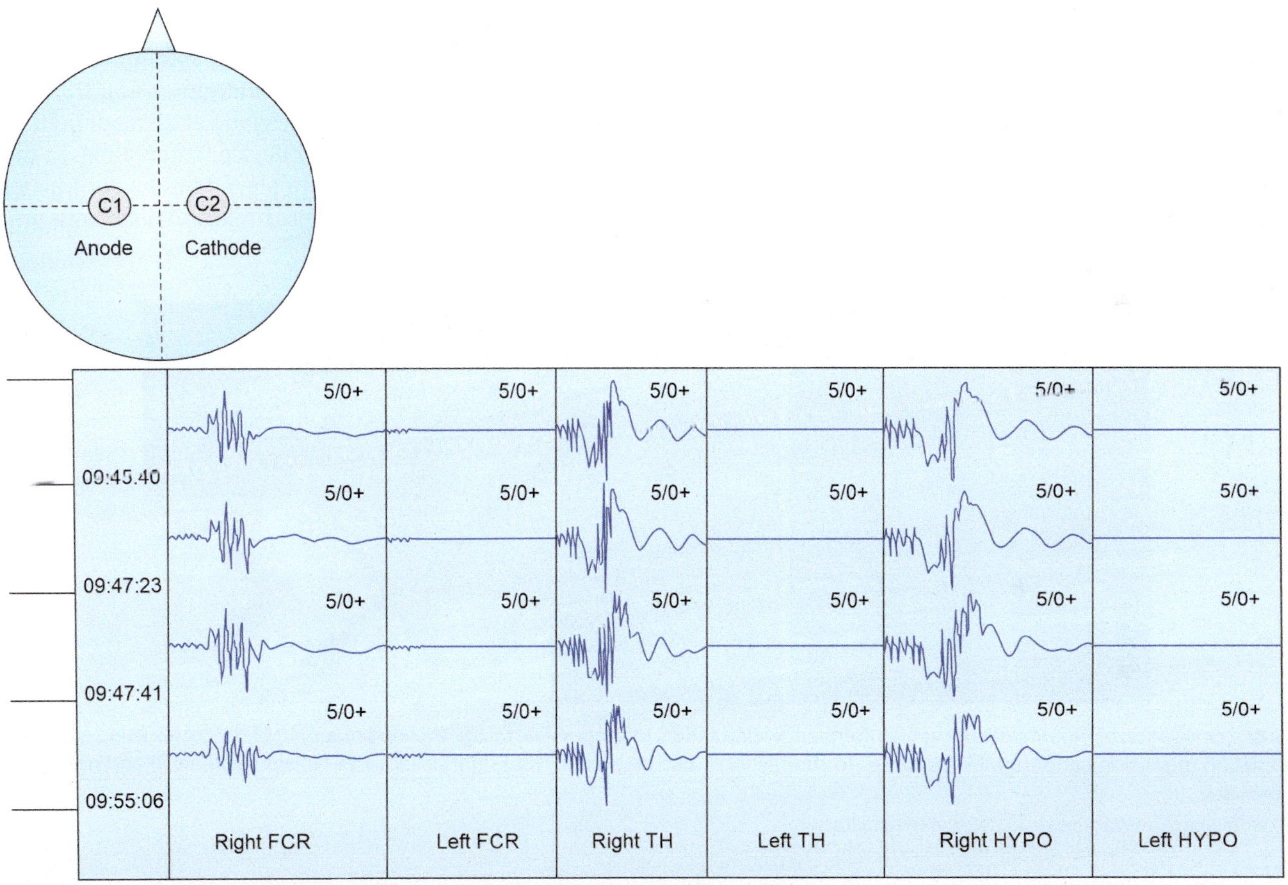

FIG. 5: Cortical response to anodal stimulation. When a monophasic stimulation is given with C1 as anode and C2 as cathode, largely mMEP responses are seen only contralateral to anode electrode. In this case, mMEP responses are seen only on the right side limb.
(FCR: flexor carpi radialis; HYPO: hypothenar muscles; TH: thenar)

sensory pathways but not motor pathways. TES again is not suitable for these surgeries as the activation of the descending motor pathways could be much deeper than the superficial surgical areas and could potentially bypass the injury site. Conventionally 60 Hz frequency of stimulation is used for cortical mapping **(Table 2)**. However, prolonged use of this frequency (1–6 s) often generates seizure activity. When high-frequency stimulation or multipulse was applied as first described by Taniguchi et al.[26] there was significantly less incidence of seizure generation. They showed that the total charge per train was < 8 µC, as compared to 600–5,000 µC/train for the Penfield 60 Hz technique. Unlike 60/50 Hz stimulation, high-frequency stimulation does not elicit visible movements so needle electrodes are needed to be placed in muscle groups (CMAPs) for identification of respective motor areas **(Table 3)**. After completion of cortical mapping **(Fig. 6)**, one can place a strip of electrodes (2–8 contacts at 1 cm apart) over the identified motor area and continuously monitor the corticospinal tract while excising the tumor in the vicinity **(Fig. 7)**. Each electrode in the strip can be used as a stimulating anodal electrode referenced to a distant cathodal electrode. Since, it is direct cortical stimulation very often responses can be obtained around 17mA **(Table 3)**. Since no averaging is

TABLE 3: Cortical stimulation under general anesthesia (triggered stimulation).

Stimulator anodal stimulation	Hand held monopolar stimulator (pedicle probe having a ball tip)
Rate of stimulation	4.1 Hz
Number of pulses	3 pulses
Interstimulus interval (ISI)	3 ms
Pulse width	300–500 µs
Stimulation strength	1–20 mA
Time base for recording	80 ms
Filters band width	10–1,000 Hz
Target muscles	• *Face*: Frontalis, orbicularis oris • *Upper limbs*: Thenar, hypothenar, and flexor carpi radialis • *Lower limbs*: Tibialis anterior, extensor digitorum brevis, and abductor hallucis

required and stimulus strength is at a near-threshold value, a repeated stimulus train can be delivered at 0.1 Hz. This practically allows real-time monitoring of the corticospinal tracts. A drop in amplitude of >30–40% is considered to be significant.[30]

To map and monitor subcortical structures handheld probe is used intermittently (monopolar or bipolar). Using high-frequency stimulation one can estimate the distance of corticospinal tracts from the margins of the resection cavity. Studies have suggested that the distance between the margins of the resection cavity to the corticospinal tract is proportional to the current required (1 mA/mm) to elicit CMAPs.[31] That is, if one can elicit CMAP responses with 1 mA of current, then the corticospinal tract is about 1 mm away from the resection margin. Using this high-frequency stimulation method Raabe et al.[32] adopted it to an electrically isolated suction device (stimulator). In these cases, recording electrodes are placed on the contralateral side muscles of the face, and proximal and distal muscles of

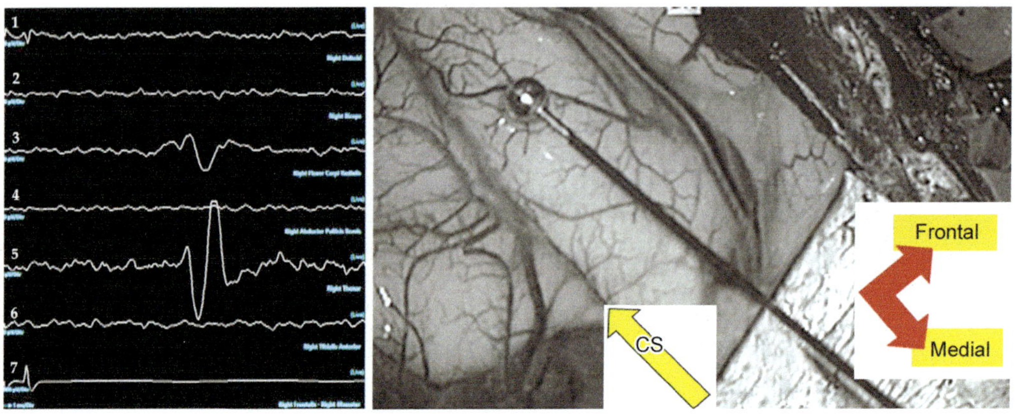

FIG. 6: Localization of motor areas using high-frequency stimulation. Intraoperative image showing mapping of the cortex using monopolar stimulation (right side panel). mMEP responses to stimulation could be elicited from right flexor carpi radialis (Channel 3) and right thenar (5) muscles.

(CS: central sulcus; mMEP: muscle motor evoked potentials)

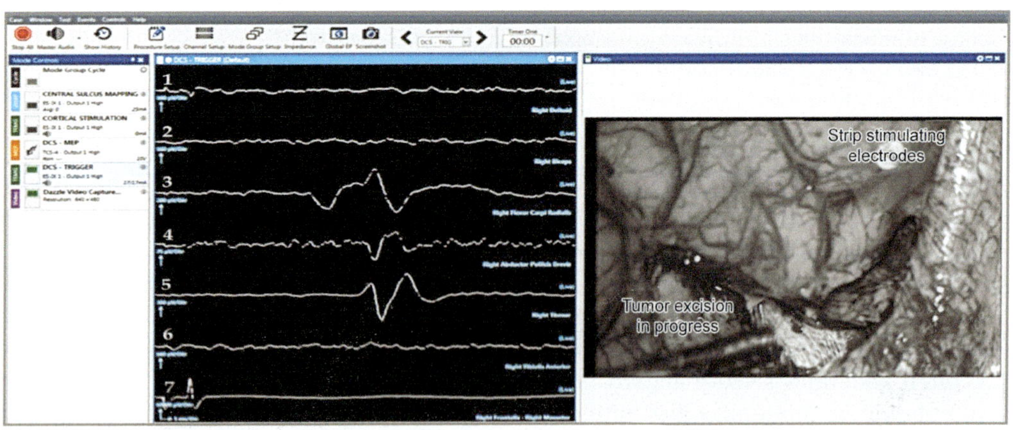

FIG. 7: Dynamic monitoring: Right side panel shows, strip electrodes placed over the identified motor area and stimulus delivered continuously while tumor is being excised. CMAP responses are elicited from right flexor carpi radialis (Channel 3), right abductor pollicis brevis (Channel 4) and right thenar muscle (Channel 5).

(CMAP: compound muscle action potentials)

the upper and lower limbs **(Table 4)**. Since the suction device also acts as a monopolar stimulator, it enables the surgeon to do continuous dynamic mapping of the corticospinal tracts **(Fig. 8)**. In this method, initially one can use a starting current of about 20 mA. While excising the tumor, if responses are elicited at 20 mA, it would suggest that the corticospinal tracts are 20 mm away from the operating margin. At that juncture, the stimulus current is reduced till no responses are elicited. This process of reducing stimulus strength continues as per the surgeon's intraoperative assessment. Usually, excision is stopped at about 3 mA of current. Seidel et al.[33] suggested that a response to stimulation at 1 mA or less can have postoperative deficits. Hence, they suggest stopping resection at 2 mA of current.

TABLE 4: Dynamic subcortical stimulation (triggered stimulation).

Stimulator Cathodal stimulation	Hand held monopolar suction stimulator
Rate of stimulation	4.1 Hz
Pulse width	50–75 μs
Number of pulses	3–5 pulses
Inter stimulus interval (ISI)	2–3 ms
Pulse width	500 μs
Stimulation strength	3–20 mA
Time base for recording	80 ms
Filters band width	10–1,000 Hz
Target muscles	• *Face*: Frontalis, orbicularis oris, and tongue • *Upper limbs*: Thenar, hypothenar, and flexor carpi radialis • *Lower limbs*: Tibialis anterior, extensor digitorum brevis, and abductor hallucis

CEREBRAL ISCHEMIA

Surgeries that involve vascular procedures leading to potential cerebral ischemia need to be considered for IOM. The common electrophysiological monitoring techniques that are employed are EEGs, SSEPs, and more recently MEPs. The cerebral blood flow (CBF) value is around 50 mL/100 g/min. Neuronal dysfunction can occur if the CBF falls below 22 mL/100 g/min. And this can be noticed by a drop in EEG amplitude and or EEG slowing. A drop in EEG amplitude of >30% and changes in EEG that last >30 seconds are considered to be significant.[34] The first changes in SSEPs can occur at a CBF of 18 mL/100 g/min. SSEPs disappear at CBF of 15 mL/100 g/min. In these cases, the pathway to be monitored must be at risk, e.g., in middle cerebral artery aneurysm, the hand area is monitored (contra lateral median nerve stimulation), in anterior communicating artery aneurysm the leg area is monitored (posterior tibial nerve stimulation) and in posterior communicating artery aneurysm, both hand and leg areas are monitored. In these cases, SSEPs can be used to give us an estimate of a "deadline" for correcting the blood flow back to above 18 mL before the brain spends too much time below this level. Very often surgeon applies temporary clips onto the parent vessel. The current norm is that if the SSEPs amplitudes drop by 50% then the temporary clips are removed or retractors are readjusted. After the removal of temporary clips, the surgeon waits for the responses to recover and then reapplies the temporary clips if necessary **(Fig. 9)**. MEPs

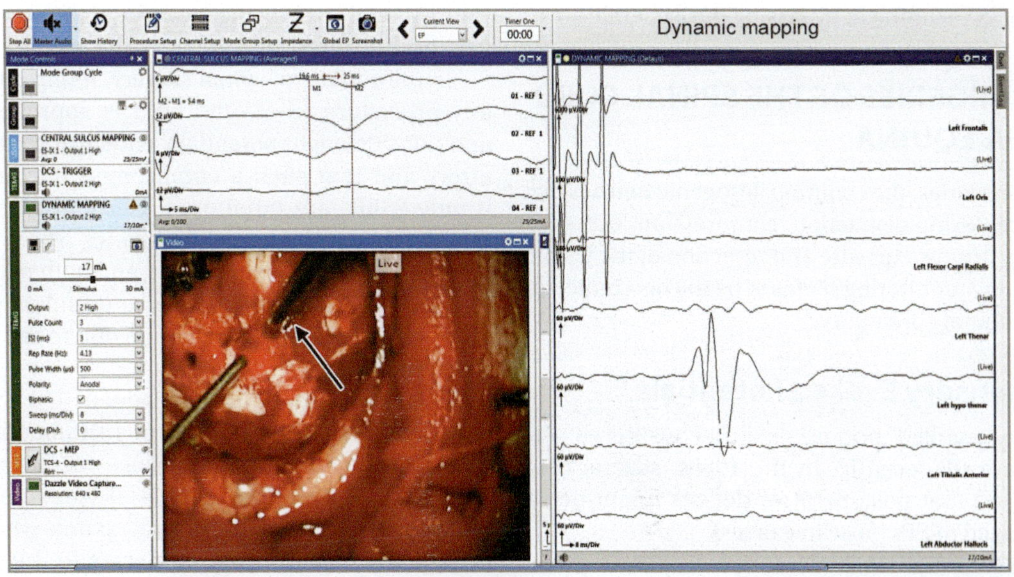

FIG. 8: Dynamic mapping: Intraoperative image showing subcortical lesion resection in progress using suction monopolar stimulator (arrow). A current strength of 17 mAmps elicited responses from the left hypothenar muscle, suggesting that the functional track is about 17 mm away from the margin of the tumor (arrow).

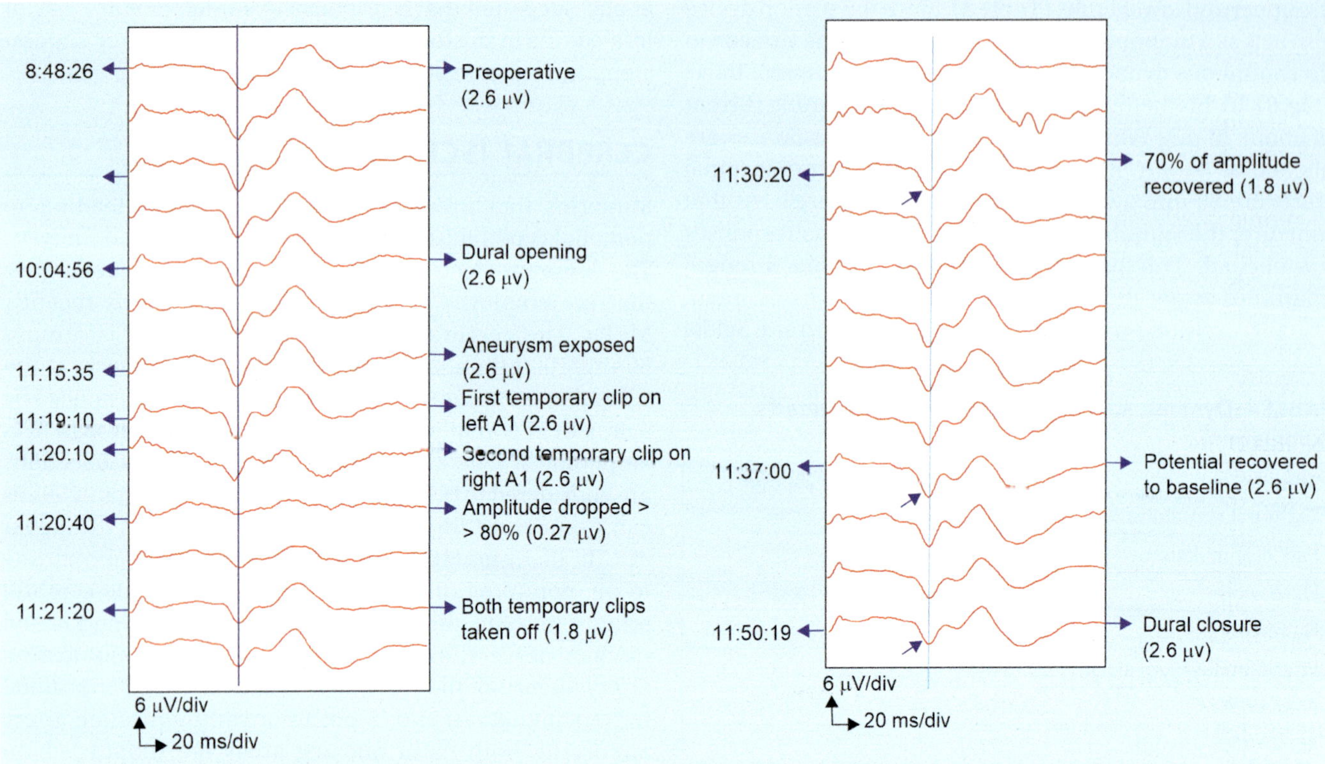

FIG. 9: Serial somatosensory evoked potential responses to right posterior tibial nerve stimulation in anterior communicating artery aneurysm surgery. Application of temporary clips to left and right A1 vessel, resulted in bilateral drop in amplitude (left tibial nerve responses not shown) by >50%. Immediate removal of temporary clips resulted in recovery after 10 minutes.

have also been used in these cases to improve the outcome. They are considered to give an early warning than SSEPs and are found to be useful in coiling procedures. A drop in muscle MEPs (mMEPs) amplitude of >50% is considered as significant. While using MEPs, one must be aware of the jerking movement during stimulation and activating deeper descending tracks resulting in bypassing the ischemic area.

IOM FOR SURGERIES OF THE SPINAL CORD AND CAUDA EQUINA

In spinal cord surgeries, the common iatrogenic injuries that can happen are during distraction, compression, excessive cord retraction, during exposure and resection of the lesion, etc. Multimodality monitoring seems to be the best indicator for impending spinal cord injury.[35]

Somatosensory Evoked Potentials

Somatosensory evoked potentials are considered the standard of care till recently. In the 1980s, several case reports indicated that postoperative deficits might occur despite unchanged SSEPs (false negatives).

In patients undergoing neurosurgical operations on the spine, several factors impact the importance of spinal cord monitoring and the methods available for use. These include preexisting myelopathy, possibly associated with impaired cord perfusion, the variety of surgical approaches and instruments that may be employed, and the effects of direct cord manipulation. Preexisting myelopathy was found to be the most significant risk factor associated with SSEP deterioration, the others being the level of surgery (more rostral levels being the riskier), the number of cervical vertebrae involved, and the use of instrumentation.

In the context of spinal surgery, it might be argued that any procedure where the cord is approached from the anterior side might potentially endanger the anterior spinal artery and that such a compromise may go undetected if only SSEPs are monitored. Currently, it is considered that SSEPs can be used in surgeries where external cord compression could cause injury and both pathways can get affected **(Table 5)**. They are also useful where successful MEP monitoring cannot be done due to the clinical status of the patient.

It is also widely acknowledged that SSEPs may be abolished during resection of intramedullary tumors, recovering again during closure or in the immediate postoperative period.[36] This is presumably due to neurapraxia of dorsal column axons when a midline myelotomy is performed for access to the tumor. Under these circumstances, MEP monitoring is considered essential by some surgeons.

Motor Evoked Potentials Monitoring

Different centers have used different techniques to monitor the spinal cord. Some centers have directly stimulated the spinal cord from the epidural space or outside the vertebral column. Their responses are recorded epidurally from a different level or recording CMAPs from leg muscles or recording mixed nerve potentials in the leg (electrodes over the tibial nerve at the popliteal fossa). The other popular method is to use TES to the cortex and record the responses from epidural space (D-wave) or the peripheral muscles as CMAP **(Fig. 10)**. With single electrical shocks of high intensity, descending volleys can be recorded from the dorsal epidural space.[37] These consist of one or more waves, the first D-wave being due to direct stimulation of pyramidal cells and the more variable—waves due to stimulation of cortical interneurons **(Table 6)**. D-wave is less affected by anesthetic agents and the duration of the recording is shorter, hence it is more feasible for continuous monitoring. The amplitude of the D-wave is large at the cervical level; it diminishes markedly at lower levels of the cord and may therefore require averaging. Since the fiber density decreases craniocaudally, D-waves are not recordable in the lumbosacral region (D-wave recording is limited to T10–T11). In situations where D-waves can be recorded, they are found to be more reliable than mMEPs and in intramedullary tumor surgeries; a 50% drop in D-wave amplitude can indicate postoperative deficit.[30]

To record mMEP responses to TES, it is necessary to deliver multiple (3–9) pulses with interpulse intervals of 2–4 ms[30] **(Figs. 11A to E)**. The square-wave pulse duration of 50–75 µs with stimulus strength ranging between 200 and 400 V, is usually sufficient **(Table 7)**.

A major disadvantage of MEP monitoring using CMAPs is the marked and widespread jerking of paraspinal muscles which often accompanies multipulse TES. This is often sufficiently "visible" that the surgeon must pause the operation to record MEPs. Tongue biting is a recognized complication that must be guarded against by using a bite block. However, the delivery of the pulse at electrodes close to the midline (C1 and C2 scalp locations, near-optimal for lower limb activation) reduces the tendency for paraspinal muscles to contract.

One limitation of CMAPs to multipulse TES is that the waveform varies quite markedly from one stimulus to the next, making it difficult to derive firm criteria for the degree of amplitude reduction deemed to be "significant". Some

TABLE 5: Somatosensory evoked potentials.

Stimulation site	Median nerve at the wrist, posterior tibial nerve at the ankle
Rate of stimulation	4.1 Hz
Pulse width	200 µs
Stimulus intensity	10–25 mA
Average count	100–200 sweeps
Time base for recording	50–100 ms
Filters band width	10–1,000 Hz
Recording electrodes placement	• C3'/C4'—Fpz (for median nerve stimulation) • Cz/Cz'—Fpz (for tibial nerve stimulation)

TABLE 6: Transcranial electrical stimulation for recording D-wave.

Stimulation site Anodal stimulation	C1–C2/Cz'–Fz
Rate of stimulation	0.7 Hz
Pulse width	50–75 µs
Number of pulses	3–5 pulses
Interstimulus interval (ISI)	2 ms (500 Hz)–4 ms (250 Hz)
Stimulation strength	100–400 volts
Time base for recording	100 ms
Average	1
Filters band width	10–1,000 Hz
Target	Spinal epidural electrodes with two or three contact points are placed cranially and caudally to the lesion

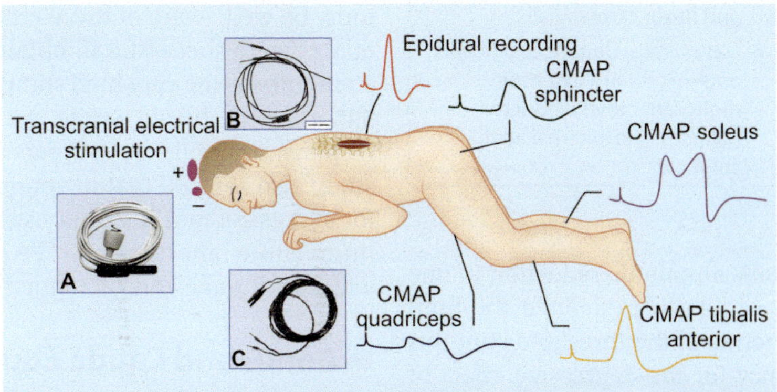

FIG. 10: Schematic diagram showing placement of TES electrodes on the scalp and responses that can be recorded from the epidural space (D-wave) and different peripheral muscles (CMAP/mMEPs) in the limbs. A—cork screw stimulating electrode, B—epidural electrode, inset showing recording electrode tip with two metal rings. C—subdermal needle electrode for recording mMEPs.

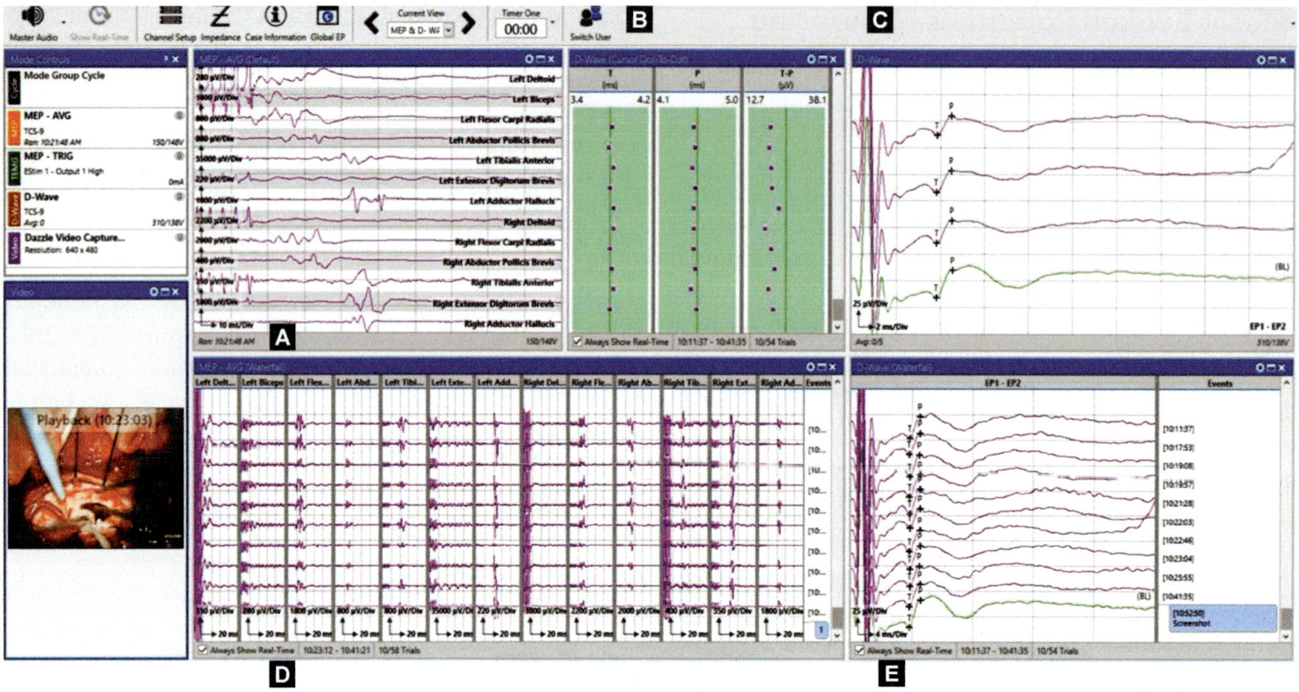

FIGS. 11A TO E: A typical screen shot of IOM recordings. Patient undergoing surgery for intramedullary hemangioblastoma. (A) mMEP responses from left and right upper and lower limb muscles. (B) D-wave latency and amplitude tracking during course of surgery. (C) D-wave recordings. (D) mMEP recordings during the course of surgery. (E) D-wave recordings during the course of surgery.

TABLE 7: Transcranial electrical stimulation for spinal cord monitoring.

Stimulation site Anodal stimulation	C1–C2/Cz′–Fz
Rate of stimulation	0.7 Hz
Pulse width	50–75 µs
Number of pulses	3–7 pulses
Interstimulus interval (ISI)	2 ms (500 Hz)–3 ms (300 Hz)
Stimulation strength	150–400 volts
Time base for recording	100 ms (10 ms/div)
Average	1–5 sweep
Filters band width	10–1,000 Hz
Target muscles	• *Upper limbs*: Thenar, hypothenar, and flexor carpi radialis • *Lower limbs*: Quadriceps, tibialis anterior, soleus, extensor digitorum brevis, abductor halluces, and external anal sphincter

authors used a criterion of 80% amplitude reduction in one of the monitored muscles, while others defined the limit of acceptable variability in terms of the threshold stimulus voltage.[38] There is a tendency for the depressive effect of anesthetic agents gradually to increase during the course of the operation.[39] A study into factors that could predict the feasibility of monitoring mMEPs in patients undergoing spinal cord tumor surgery showed that successful CMAP responses are significantly higher in patients with better functional grades and higher motor power. Patients with Nurick grades 0–3 and muscle power 3 [Medical Research Council (MRC)] and above have a better chance of obtaining mMEPs.[40] Failure to get baseline MEP responses in thoracic lesions may lead to the patient having postoperative deficits.[41] Hence, it is important to record mMEPS in as many muscles as possible. Our study on the influence on tumor location and other factors on predictive value showed that patients who had intraoperative mMEP changes undergoing surgery for thoracic segment intramedullary tumors, with >12 months of symptoms and age older than 21 years are likely to have postoperative deficits.[42] The warning criteria vary from one center to other and the monitoring team must be well aware of these criteria while using MEPs.[43] Yi et al.[44] were successful in obtaining mMEPs in children of <3 months using very high stimulating voltage (900 V; mean 596 ± 154V). In our study, we could successfully obtain responses in children <2 years (mean voltage 285 V). This study also showed that in young children, ideal anesthesia for successful mMEPs responses can be obtained with total intravenous anesthesia (TIVA) and balanced anesthesia with sevoflurane and ketamine.[45]

Conus and Cauda Equina Lesions

Patients can have significant postoperative morbidity due to intraoperative damage to neural elements during conus and cauda equina lesions surgery and can result in motor, sensory, bowel, bladder, and sexual dysfunctions. Conus and cauda equina lesions mainly include neoplasms and spinal dysraphism states that are frequently presented in children. Tethered cord cases in an adult often present with bladder dysfunction. Ischemia is the main pathophysiology in these cases[46] and there is an improvement when the cord is untethered.[47] During untethering and excision of tumors, continuous monitoring of neural structures (motor, sensory, or reflex circuits) can help in preventing damage due to traction, compression, or coagulation.

Monitoring in these cases has been classified into (1) mapping techniques and (2) monitoring techniques.[48]

Bulbocavernosus Reflex

There are several studies regarding the use of EMG of the external anal sphincter (EAS) to study bulbocavernosus reflex (BCR) in disorders of micturition, defecation, and sexual function. Deletes et al.[49] studied continuous monitoring of BCR by recording muscle action potentials from the EAS after stimulation of the dorsal penile or clitoral nerve by surface electrodes (on the dorsum of the penis in males, cathode on the clitoris, and anode on labia in females) **(Table 8)**.

Free Run Electromyography Monitoring

Free run electromyography (EMG) activity involves recording spontaneous EMG activity from muscles. This can be used in these surgeries to detect lower motor neuron damage, indicated by abnormal bursts or trains of motor unit potentials. Even though they have a high degree of specificity to injury, they have low specificity.[50] Romstock et al.[51] showed neurotonic discharges called A-waves as postoperative facial nerve dysfunction indicator in patients undergoing cerebellopontine angle surgery. In conus and cauda equina cases, irritation of sensory fibers causes periodic EMG activity. While irritation of motor fibers causes spontaneous EMG activity. Stretching or traction on the roots can cause irregular high-frequency activity with high amplitudes.[52]

Triggered Electromyography—Motor Mapping

Individual spinal root mapping and recording CMAPs can be done from lower limb segmental muscles.

Compound muscle action potential responses can be recorded by direct stimulation of the spinal roots using brief electric stimuli **(Table 9)**. One can use monopolar or bipolar concentric handheld stimulators. There is some concern while using a monopolar stimulator those responses could be from other nonspecific muscle groups due to the spread of current. This can be avoided by using a bipolar concentric stimulator; however, one must make sure that there is no excessive fluid present at the stimulation site. This is to make sure that the current is delivered to the nerve and does not get shunted. This technique helps during dissection at the neural placode, to identify nerve roots in the lipomas, distinguishing filum from the nerve roots. We have used this technique not only to identify nerve roots but also to verify if the filum has any functional nerves, if it is found to have any functional nerves then that filum is left tethered.[53,54] Initial current settings are set at 0.2 mA while identifying the roots. Before deciding to cut the filum the current is increased to 2 mA. Despite this high current, if there is no response, then the filum is severed.

For monitoring the bladder and bowel functions, sphincter pressures were recorded. Stimulation of the cauda equina was used for vesical pressure measurement to monitor detrusor function.[55] This method requires a high frequency of stimulation and the response of the sphincter was slow. Pang et al.[56] used monitoring the anal sphincter by recording anal squeeze pressure through a fluid-filled polyethylene balloon placed in the anal canal.

Pedicle Screw Placement

In scoliosis surgery, the insertion of screws can be a "blind" technique. The incidence of pedicle screw misplacement is as high as 40% due to pedicle wall breach. In these cases, triggered EMG can be very useful. Cathodal monopolar stimulation can be used by stimulating either the drilled hole or the screw. The frequency of stimulation is 4.1 Hz with

TABLE 8: Bulbocavernosus reflex (BCR).

Stimulation site	Males: Dorsum of penis Female: Cathode on the clitoris, anode on labia
Rate of stimulation	0.7 Hz
Number of pulses	3–5 pulses
Interstimulus interval	2 ms (500 Hz)–4 ms (250 Hz)
Pulse width	300–500 µs
Stimulus intensity	10–40 mA
Average count	1–10 sweeps
Time base for recording	80 ms
Filters band width	10–1,000 Hz
Recording site	External anal sphincter

TABLE 9: Direct nerve stimulation for tethered cord surgery (triggered stimulation).

Stimulator	Hand held concentric bipolar stimulator Cathodal stimulation when monopolar stimulator is used
Rate of stimulation	4.1 Hz
Pulse width	50–100 µs
Stimulus strength	0.1–2 mA
Time base for recording	50 ms
Filter band width	10–1,000 Hz
Target muscles	Quadriceps, tibialis anterior, soleus, extensor digitorum brevis, abductor halluces, and external anal sphincter

a pulse duration of 300 μs is used. CMAPs can be recorded from the lower extremity muscles. If no responses can be elicited at 20 mAmps then there is no breach. If no responses at 10 mAmps then probably there is no breach. Each center should develop their standards as multiple factors can affect the stimulus threshold. These could be pedicles to be of different thicknesses at different spinal levels, chronic nerve injury as in radiculopathy can have higher stimulus thresholds to elicit CMAP responses. Too much of relaxants or shunting of current can lead to false negatives. Wherever current shunting is suspected, it is better to use voltage stimulation than current stimulation.

Sensory Mapping

Sensory mapping can be performed by intraoperative stimulation of the dorsal roots and recording the muscle action potentials, similar to H-reflex. Sensory roots can only be identified by recording SSEPs using epidural or cranial electrodes.

Somatosensory Evoked Potentials

Somatosensory evoked potentials can be used to establish the functional integrity of the sensory pathways using epidural or scalp electrodes after stimulation of the tibial or pudendal nerve. Loss of SSEPs suggests an injury to the sensory pathways. Shinomiya et al.[55] and Kothbauer et al.[57] have used monitoring of SSEPs above the level of laminectomy (epidural, cervical spine, and scalp) to monitor the lower limb sensory pathway.

Motor Evoked Potential

The functional status of corticospinal tracts can only be monitored using MEPs. D-waves cannot be recorded in these conus cases. Similar to spinal cord monitoring, MEPs can be recorded from the lower limb. Hoving et al.[58] showed improved clinical outcomes in these cases when multimodality monitoring was done. Since untethering shows improvement in functional status, we proved it by using MEPs. In our study, 50% of the patients showed improvement in intraoperative MEPs after untethering of the cord. Pain is the most common improvement and to a lesser extent in bladder improvement.[54]

MONITORING OF CRANIAL NERVES AND BRAINSTEM

Whenever surgery requires an approach to the skull base or brainstem that can potentially put nuclei or nerves, or tracts at risk, the IOM of those structures could be useful.[59,60] Operating on the brainstem is considered a challenge and most surgeons will be reluctant to operate in this area and an injury can lead often to a deep coma. Depending on the requirement, multimodality monitoring can be used such as SEP, MEPs, and free and triggered EMGs. IOM could include corticospinal tract, corticobulbar tract (MEPs); cranial nerves 3rd, 4th, 6th, 7th, 10th, 11th, and 12th (EMGs); 8th [brainstem auditory evoked responses (BAER)].

In midbrain and skull base surgery (3rd and 4th); in pontine tumor (5th and 6th) resection, microvascular decompression (5th and 7th), and vestibular schwannomas (5th and 7th); pons, vestibular schwannomas, intracanalicular tumor resection, microvascular decompression, and skull base (8th); surgeries of the medulla, foramen magnum pathology, and skull base (9th); surgeries with the medulla, skull base, thyroid surgery, and fourth ventricle tumors (10th, 11th, and 12th) are considered to be monitored.

Intrinsic or extrinsic brainstem lesions can distort normal anatomy and identification of brainstem motor nuclei can be helpful. Identification of the 5th cranial nerve from other cranial nerves (7th and 8th) structures during microvascular decompression in trigeminal neuralgia cases could be helpful. Similarly, if the 9th and 10th complex can be differentiated from the 7th and 8th cranial nerve complex, it could help the surgeon. This identification can also help the surgeon to make an informed incision into the brainstem **(Figs. 12A to C)** Monitoring can also help in preventing excessive retraction of these structures that are out of the surgeon's sight during resection. To get focal responses, it is important to use small amounts of currents, to prevent adjacent structures from getting activated **(Table 10)**.

An increase in free-running EMG activity during dissection would indicate excessive retraction or pull on the tumor nerve. A silent EMG would predict normal neurological function. Prolonged EMG activity can indicate a severe and permanent neurological deficit postoperatively. Any increase in stimulus threshold could also indicate damage to those structures. However, there is no clear-cut correlation between these injury responses to postoperative outcomes.[60]

The 7th cranial nerve is the most extensively monitored nerve, particularly in vestibular schwannomas. They have proven to be useful in the identification of facial nerve during microsurgical resection of the vestibular schwannomas. Intraoperative functional integrity of the facial nerve at the end of surgery is a good indicator of long-term postoperative function.[61] As mentioned in the above subsubsection (IOM of cortical and subcortical structures), stimulus strength can be used in these surgeries to estimate the distance between the surgical plane and the facial nerve **(Fig. 13)**. This technique can also be used for mapping the course of the nerve during intracapsular decompression of the tumor **(Fig. 14)**.

Corticobulbar Motor Evoked Potentials

In brainstem lesions, corticospinal tracts can be monitored using TES and recording from the upper and lower limb muscles as described above. Stimulating corkscrew electrodes are placed at C1/C2 montage (international 10/20 EEG system) to monitor hand and leg corticospinal tracts. The same technique can be employed for monitoring

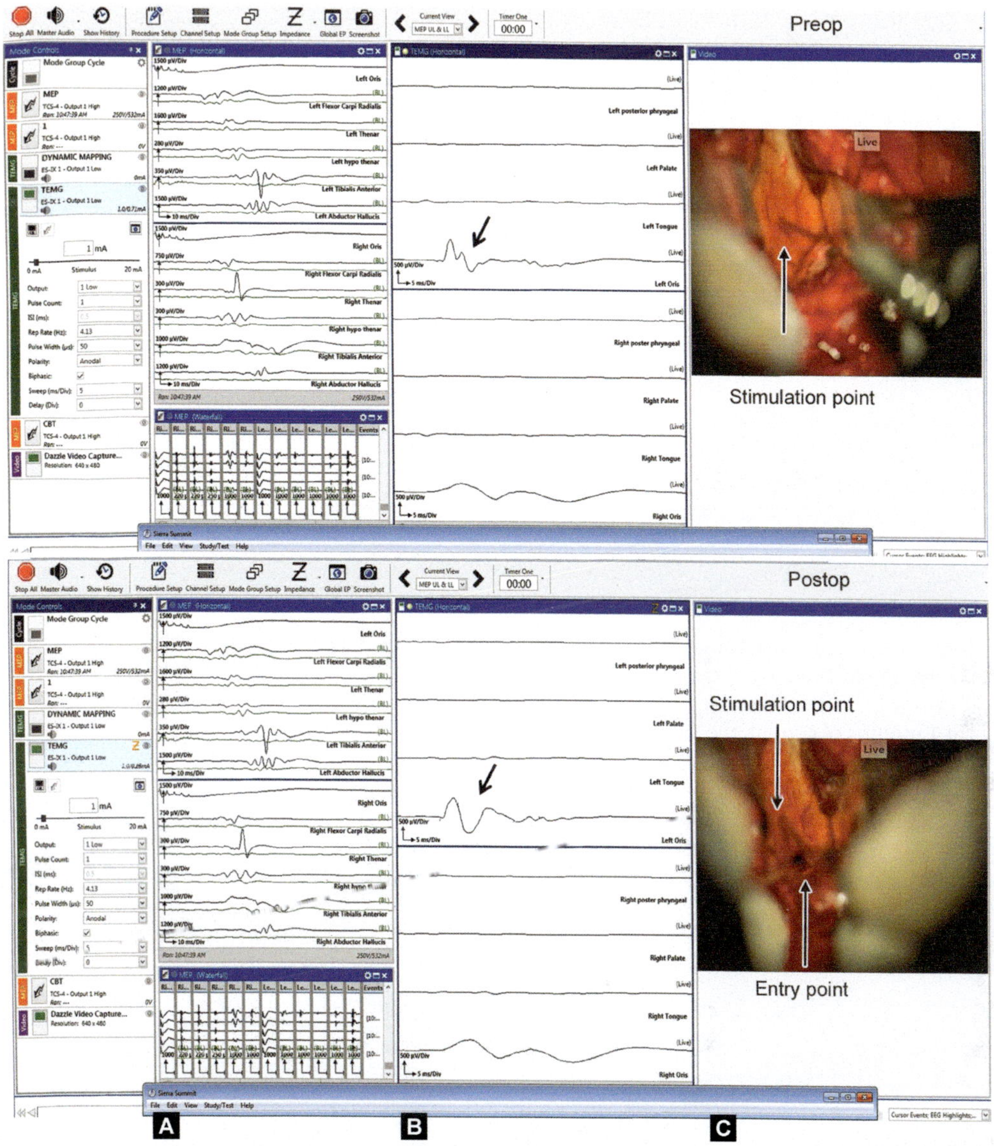

FIGS. 12A TO C: Brainstem monitoring; multimodality monitoring. (A) mMEP recordings. (B) Triggered EMG. Response elicited from left oris (arrow). (C) Preoperatively (top panel) motor nuclei were identified (arrow) before making an incision into the brainstem. Postoperatively (lower panel) responses could be elicited from the same muscle for the same stimulus strength. Bipolar concentric electric stimulation at 1 mAmps, pulse width 50 μs.

TABLE 10: Direct stimulation for cranial nerves and brainstem nuclei (triggered stimulation).

Stimulator	Hand held concentric bipolar stimulator
Rate of stimulation	4.1 Hz
Pulse width	50–100 μs
Stimulus strength	0.1–3 mA
Time base for recording	50 ms
Filter band width	10–1,000 Hz
Target muscles	• Extraocular muscles • Frontalis, orbicularis oris/oculi. posterior pharyngeal wall, and soft palate bilaterally • Vocal cords, sternocleidomastoid bilaterally • Tongue bilaterally

corticobulbar tracts, by placing stimulating electrodes more laterally C3 or C4 as nodes and a midline reference near Cz which acts as a cathode **(Table 11)**. The responses can be recorded from facial, pharyngeal, and tongue muscles. The disadvantage of using lateral stimulating electrodes is the spread of the current and activating the peripheral cranial nerve.[60] One must note that MEPs may not activate all the motor neurons, hence may result in inaccurate postoperative prediction.[62]

Brainstem Auditory Evoked Potentials

Brainstem auditory evoked responses are short-latency sensory potentials generated in the brainstem in response to auditory stimuli. Intraoperative BAER is used for the preservation of hearing and monitoring of brainstem function

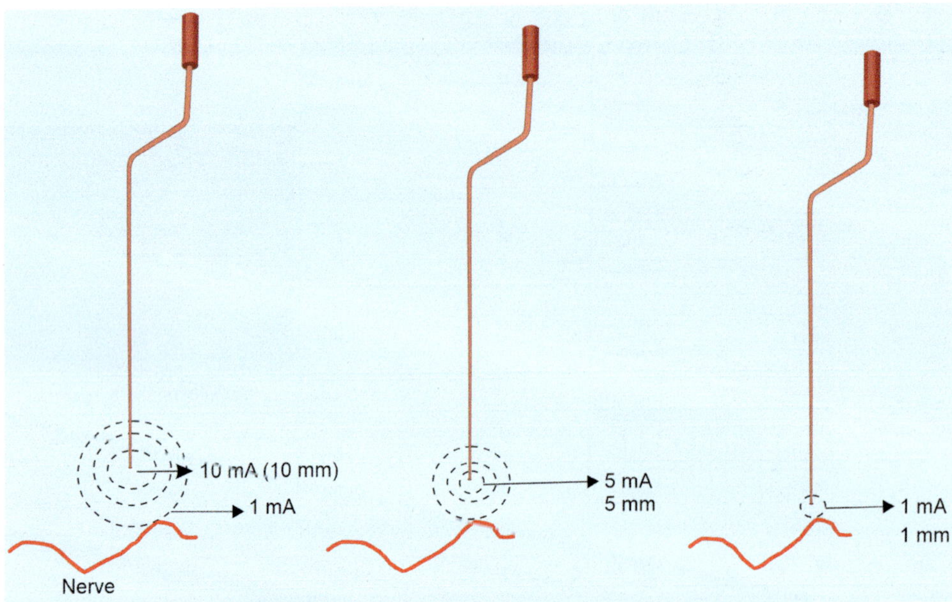

FIG. 13: Schematic diagram showing dynamic mapping using stimulus strength to know the distance between the tumor dissection margin to the underlying nerve. When high current is used stimuli can reach deeper structures to identify its presence (10 mAmps). As the surgery progresses, responses can be elicited with lesser current (5 mAmps) suggesting underlying nerve is 5 mm away from the tumor margin. At eliciting responses at 1 mAmps of current, the surgeon could be very close to functional nerve.

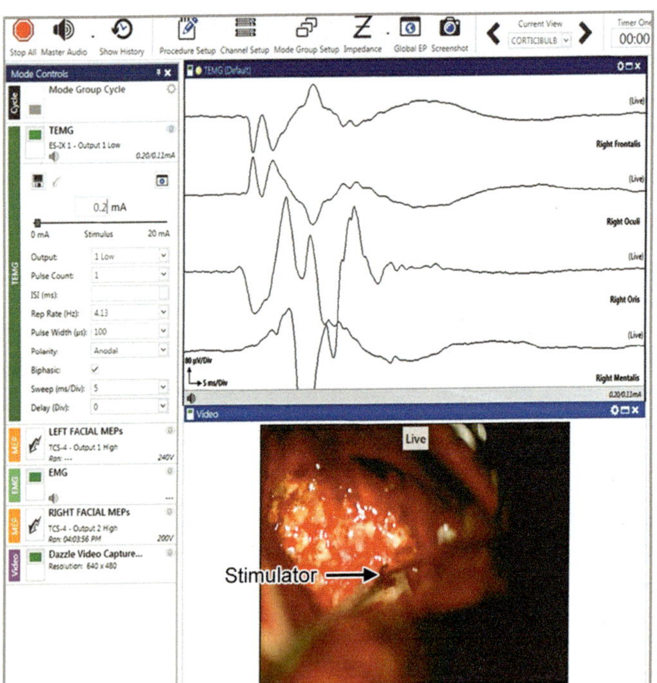

FIG. 14: Intraoperative recordings of a patient undergoing surgery for vestibular schwannomas. To identify facial nerve, recording needle electrodes are placed in frontalis, oculi, oris, and mentalis muscles. Surgeon used concentric bipolar stimulator during intracapsular decompression, to know the location and map the course of the nerve by stimulating inside the tumor capsule. In this case, the surgeon could elicit response at 0.2 mAmps at the stimulation point, suggesting that stimulating probe probably touching the facial nerve at that location. Pulse width 100 µs, biphasic stimulation. Current strength 0.1–5 mAmps.

TABLE 11: Transcranial stimulation for corticobulbar tract monitoring.

Stimulation site **Anodal stimulation**	**C1–C2; C3–C4 as anode with Cz reference**
Rate of stimulation	0.7 Hz
Pulse width	50–75 µs
Number of pulses	3–5 pulses
Interstimulus interval (ISI)	2 ms (500 Hz)–4 ms (250 Hz)
Stimulation strength	100–400 volts
Double train stimulation	Yes
Second stimulus	At 90 ms
Number of pulse	1
Time base for recording	150 ms
Average	1–5 sweeps
Filters band width	10–1,000 Hz
Target muscles	Facial, pharyngeal, and tongue muscles

during posterior fossa surgery. The BAER is recorded from an electrode placed at the vertex, with reference electrodes placed over the mastoid. The electrode on the mastoid hampers cleaning and draping for a retromastoid surgery, instead earlobe can also provide a satisfactory recording. A ground electrode was placed on the forehead. The stimulus is delivered through an insert earphone with an alternating click between 80 and 100 dB, and masking white noise at half this intensity is delivered to the other ear. Since the duration of the recording is only 10 ms (timebase) stimulus can be given at a higher rate and 2,000 stimuli are averaged. The response to stimulation is seen as seven waves, I through VII have been described. The amplitude and latency of waves I through V are commonly used in IOM. Measurement of the interpeak latencies I–III and III–V are considered important. Prolongation of I–V interpeak latency by >1 ms probably indicates hearing impairment or other neurological deficit.[63]

Brainstem auditory evoked response changes during surgery could indicate direct damage, reversible, or permanent, to the eighth nerve or brainstem up to the midbrain. Damage to the inner ear during drilling, or internal auditory artery ischemia affects all components of the BAER including wave I. The trauma of the intracranial portion of the eighth nerve will cause impairment or loss of all components of the BAER except for wave I. Mechanical, thermal, or ischemic damage to the brainstem in the region of the superior olivary complex can lead to attenuation or loss of wave III and subsequent components.

Hearing Preservation during Microvascular Decompression

In trigeminal neuralgia cases, microvascular decompression is performed. During cerebellum retraction, the nerve can be stretched **(Fig. 15)**. Changes in wave V latency and I–III interpeak latency prolongations are considered as warnings to adjust retractor position. In decompression of the facial nerve for hemifacial spasms cases, an increase in latency by >0.4 ms is significant, and >1 ms is critical.[64]

Hearing Preservation during Vestibular Schwannoma Excision

Prolongation of interpeak I–III latency should indicate that the cochlear nerve was being damaged while attempting to peel the tumor off it. For intraoperative prognostication, BAER is very sensitive but not very specific. Direct stimulation of the eighth nerve was found to be superior to BAER,[65] and electrocochleography was a useful supplementary tool.[66]

Preservation of Brainstem Function

Hahn and Latchaw[67] reported two patients dying after a bilateral loss of BAER during posterior fossa vascular malformations surgery. Raudzens and Shetter[68] described a patient who developed severe brainstem dysfunction after the loss of contralateral BAER. Intraoperative BAER in patients on cardiopulmonary bypass has been reported to be useful and in predicting cognitive problems.

SUCCESSFUL IOM PROGRAM

An IOM team comprises the monitoring team, surgeon, and anesthesiologist. The in-charge neurophysiologist must have training and exposure with an in-depth understanding of the evoked potentials, EEGs, and EMGs. They also should have worked in the operation theater. Studies have suggested that experience matters the most in interpreting any changes during surgery, they must be able to discriminate artifacts and reduce them and be able to do different monitoring

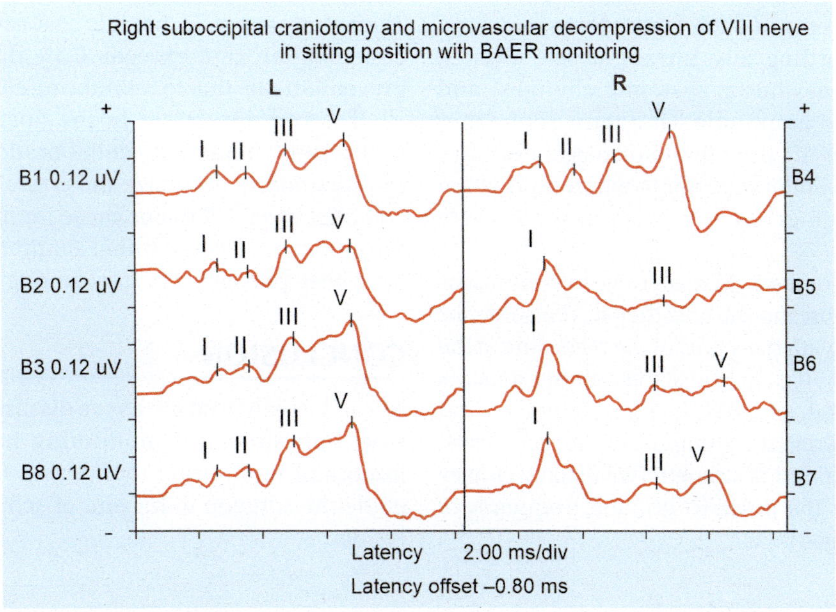

FIG. 15: Brainstem auditory evoked response (BAER) recordings: Intraoperative recordings of a patient undergoing microvascular decompression of VIII nerve on the right side. BAER responses are recorded from left (L) and right (right) side. During retraction, wave III and V peaks on the right side dropped. But the responses on left side were intact, suggesting no damage to brainstem. By the end of surgery wave III and V showed signs of recovery.

modalities and be aware of safety issues.[69] In accordance with the practice guidelines for the supervising IOM team, they have three distinct components, they are technology, interpretive, and interventional.[70]

It is important to have standard operating procedures. The day before the surgery the IOM team must know the clinical status of the patient and the modalities that would require monitoring. The IOM team must communicate to the anesthetist regarding their requirements such as placement of stimulating and recording electrodes, type of monitoring they will be conducting and optimum anesthetic conditions that are expected.

On the day of surgery in the operation theater, each person has their own space and time while preparing the patient for surgery. The IOM team must be familiar with these procedures so that each person will be able to operate smoothly. The IOM team must inform the anesthetist and the surgeon before approaching the patient. It is practice, to show the surgeon the date of sterilization before opening any sterile pack. Once sterile drapes are placed over the patient, it may not be possible to approach the patient. Hence, it is important to have backup electrodes, in case some electrodes pick up more noise or have poor contacts.

It is important to record baseline responses (latency and amplitude where applicable), this will be usually after 40 minutes of induction and usage of monopolar cautery would have been stopped. In our earlier IOM machines we noticed, the cautery ground electrode interfering with recordings and would require its disconnection after its use. Responses can be taken as baseline till opening of the dura (to adjust due to any anesthetic or systemic changes). The IOM team must be familiar with the surgical procedure and must enter comments at each stage. They also must enter comments regarding any intraoperative events, change in depth of anesthesia, systemic changes, and changes in latency and amplitude. One must remember that the IOM recordings are used for medicolegal purposes and it is important to enter comments where and when necessary. These recordings have a time stamp for this very purpose.

It is also important for the IOM team to be in continuous dialogue with the surgeon and the anesthetist. The surgeons are to be made familiar with the status of the recording at the beginning of the surgery, e.g., in MEPs, the number muscles that could be recorded, etc. While stimulating neural structures, before delivering the stimulus, the surgeon must be made aware of the stimulus strength (we usually convey current strength used. The pulse width, and frequency of stimulation is not changed).

When there is a change in the recordings, it could be due to surgical manipulation, ischemia, temperature changes (temporal dispersion), increase in the depth of anesthesia leading to systemic changes. At that juncture, it is important to repeat the recording at least three times and make sure that it is not due to any technical reasons. If it is not due to a technical reason, then the anesthetist should be approached to know if any bolus has been administered or an increase in the depth of anesthesia or a drop in temperature. If none of these are the factors, then it is important to inform the surgeon. Each center has developed different warning criteria in this regard. For example in scoliosis surgery when a unilateral or bilateral loss of >65% of MEP amplitudes for at least three trials, if it is related to any maneuver, then it needs to reverse. The blood pressure is raised to 90 mm Hg to promote spinal cord perfusion. If the MEPs do not recover in 10 minutes then a bolus of 30 mg/kg of methylprednisolone is administered.[71] Kothbauer[72] group have suggested that in spine neurosurgical cases, when there is loss of mMEPs, with >50% loss in D-wave could lead to transient postoperative weakness. On the other hand, if both mMEPs and D-wave are lost, could lead to permanent postoperative weakness. Currently more evidence is pointing to multimodality monitoring[73] being superior to single modality monitoring. Hence, the IOM team must have a clear idea of these various issues that influence recordings and the clinical outcome of the patient. Due to the clinical status of the patient or due to any technical reason, if the quality of the recording is poor or is not reproducible, it is very important to convey to the surgeon that recordings are not reliable.[74] Spinal cord surgery is involved in most medicolegal issues. Ney and Goes[75] studied the cost-effectiveness of spinal cord IOM. Their study suggests that it is cost-saving if the neurological complication rate exceeds 0.3% due to surgery and the prevention rate due to monitoring alert is >14.2%.

It is very important in the operation theater to have optimized interaction, collaboration, and awareness of the situation to minimize the errors to avoid postoperative complications.[76] A major cause for medical errors has been attributed to dysfunctional communication[77] and could have been prevented by trust among colleagues.

CONCLUSION

As can be seen from the above discussion, the intraoperative electrophysiological monitoring has evolved and is an important monitoring tool during surgical procedures, to guide the surgeon in his aim of achieving optimal surgical results.

REFERENCES

1. Rajshekhar V, Babu KS. Instrumentation for Intraoperative Monitoring. Textbooks of Operative Neurosurgery, Volume 2. New Delhi: BI Publications Pvt Ltd; 2005. pp. 125.
2. Pelosi L, Stevenson M, Hobbs GJ, Jardine A, Webb JK. Intraoperative motor evoked potentials to transcranial electrical stimulation during two anaesthetic regimens. Clin Neurophysiol. 2001;112(6):1076-87.
3. Jones SJ, Harrison R, Koh KF, Mendoza N, Crockard HA. Motor evoked potential monitoring during spinal surgery: responses of distal limb muscles to transcranial cortical stimulation with pulse trains. Electroencephalogr Clin Neurophysiol. 1996;100(5):375-83.
4. Lo YL, Dan YF, Tan YE, Nurjannah S, Tan SB, Tan CT, et al. Intraoperative motor-evoked potential monitoring in scoliosis surgery: comparison of desflurane/nitrous oxide with propofol total intravenous anesthetic regimens. Journal of neurosurgical anesthesiology. 2006;18(3):211-4.
5. Devadoss U, Babu S, Cherian VT. Quantifying the effect of isoflurane and nitrous oxide on somatosensory-evoked potentials. Indian J Anaesth. 2010;54(1):40.
6. Velayutham P, Cherian VT, Rajshekhar V, Babu KS. The effects of propofol and isoflurane on intraoperative motor evoked potentials during spinal cord tumour removal surgery–a prospective randomised trial. Indian J Anaesth. 2019;63:92-9.
7. Babu KS, Korula G. Intraoperative localization of eloquent areas during tumour surgery. In: Singh VP, Nair M (Eds). Progress in Clinical Neurosciences, Volume 27. India: Neurological Society of India publications; 2012. pp: 159-69.
8. Bekker AY, Kaufman B, Samir H, Doyle W. The use of dexmedetomidine infusion for awake craniotomy. Anesth Analg. 2001;92(5):1251-3.
9. Manikandan S. Dexmedetomidine: Its fascination, fad, and facts in neuroanaesthesia practice! J Neuroanaesthesiol Crit Care. 2014;1(03):163-5.
10. Daniel RT, Babu KS, Jacob R, Villemure JG. Posterior quadrantic resection and disconnection. In: Cataltepe O (Ed). Pediatric Epilepsy Surgery, Preoperative Assessment and Surgical Treatment. India: Thieme; 2010. pp. 196-204.
11. Bernier GP, Richer F, Giard N, Blume WT, Jones DC, Pathak P, et al. We believe the surgical treatment of epilepsy requires a multidisciplinary approach, and thus the additional information gathered by ECoG recordings may have a significant role in its success. Intraoperative Neurophysiology: A Comprehensive Guide to Monitoring and Mapping. 2009;10(4):127.
12. Kuruvilla A, Flink R. Intraoperative electrocorticography in epilepsy surgery: useful or not? Seizure. 2003;12(8):577-84.
13. Zijlmans M, Worrell GA, Dümpelmann M, Stieglitz T, Barborica A, Heers M, et al. How to record high-frequency oscillations in epilepsy: a practical guideline. Epilepsia. 2017;58(8):1305-15.
14. Rutten GJ, Ramsey NF, Van Rijen PC, Noordmans HJ, Van Veelen CW. Development of a functional magnetic resonance imaging protocol for intraoperative localization of critical temporoparietal language areas. Ann Neurol. 2002;51(3):350-60.
15. Picht T, Krieg SM, Sollmann N, Rösler J, Niraula B, Neuvonen T, et al. A comparison of language mapping by preoperative navigated transcranial magnetic stimulation and direct cortical stimulation during awake surgery. Neurosurgery. 2013;72(5):808-19.
16. Keles GE, Lamborn KR, Berger MS. Low-grade hemispheric gliomas in adults: a critical review of extent of resection as a factor influencing outcome. J Neurosurg. 2001;95(5):735-45.
17. Quiñones-Hinojosa A, Ojemann SG, Sanai N, Dillon WP, Berger MS. Preoperative correlation of intraoperative cortical mapping with magnetic resonance imaging landmarks to predict localization of the Broca area. J Neurosurg. 2003;99(2):311-8.
18. Berger MS. The impact of technical adjuncts in the surgical management of cerebral hemispheric low-grade gliomas of childhood. J Neurooncol. 1996;28(2):129-55.
19. Coello AF, Moritz-Gasser S, Martino J, Martinoni M, Matsuda R, Duffau H. Selection of intraoperative tasks for awake mapping based on relationships between tumor location and functional networks: A review. J Neurosurg. 2013;119(6):1380-94.
20. Rech F, Duffau H, Pinelli C, Masson A, Roublot P, Billy-Jacques A, et al. Intraoperative identification of the negative motor network during awake surgery to prevent deficit following brain resection in premotor regions. Neurochirurgie. 2017;63(3):235-42.
21. Chacko AG, Thomas SG, Babu KS, Daniel RT, Chacko G, Prabhu K, et al. Awake craniotomy and electrophysiological mapping for eloquent area tumours. Clin Neurol Neurosurg. 2013;115(3):329-34.
22. Thomas SG, Chacko AG, Thomas MM, Babu KS, Russell PS, Daniel RT. Outcomes of disconnective surgery in intractable pediatric hemispheric and subhemispheric epilepsy. Int J Pediatr. 2012;2012:527891.
23. Broughton R, Rasmussen T, Branch C. Scalp and direct cortical recordings of somatosensory evoked potentials in man (circa 1967). Can J Psychol. 1981;35(2):136.
24. Babu KS, Chandy MJ. Reliability of somatosensory evoked potentials in intraoperative localization of the central sulcus in patients with perirolandic mass lesions. Br J Neurosurg. 1997;11(5):411-7.
25. Romstöck J, Fahlbusch R, Ganslandt O, Nimsky C, Strauss C. Localisation of the sensorimotor cortex during surgery for brain tumours: feasibility and waveform patterns of somatosensory evoked potentials. J Neurol Neurosurg Psychiatry. 2002;72(2):221-9.
26. Taniguchi M, Cedzich C, Taniguchi M, Cedzich C, Schramm J. Modification of cortical stimulation for motor evoked potentials under general anesthesia: technical description. Neurosurgery. 1993;32(2):219-26.
27. Szelényi A, Bello L, Duffau H, Fava E, Feigl GC, Galanda M, et al. Intraoperative electrical stimulation in awake craniotomy: methodological aspects of current practice. Neurosurg Focus. 2010;28(2):E7.
28. Agnew WF, McCreery DB. Considerations for safety in the use of extracranial stimulation for motor evoked potentials. Neurosurgery. 1987;20(1):143-7.
29. Duffau H, Moritz-Gasser S, Gatignol P. Functional outcome after language mapping for insular World Health Organization Grade II gliomas in the dominant hemisphere: experience with 24 patients. Neurosurg Focus. 2009;27(2):E7.
30. Macdonald DB, Skinner S, Shils J, Yingling C. Intraoperative motor evoked potential monitoring–a position statement by the American Society of Neurophysiological Monitoring. Clin Neurophysiol. 2013;124(12):2291-316.
31. Prabhu SS, Gasco J, Tummala S, Weinberg JS, Rao G. Intraoperative magnetic resonance imaging–guided tractography with integrated monopolar subcortical functional mapping for resection of brain tumors. J Neurosurg. 2011;114(3):719-26.
32. Raabe A, Beck J, Schucht P, Seidel K. Continuous dynamic mapping of the corticospinal tract during surgery of motor eloquent brain tumors: evaluation of a new method. J Neurosurg. 2014;120(5):1015-24.
33. Seidel K, Beck J, Stieglitz L, Schucht P, Raabe A. The warning-sign hierarchy between quantitative subcortical motor mapping and continuous motor evoked potential monitoring during resection of supratentorial brain tumors. J Neurosurg. 2013;118(2):287-96.
34. Florence G, Guerit JM, Gueguen B. Electroencephalography (EEG) and somatosensory evoked potentials (SEP) to prevent cerebral

ischaemia in the operating room. Neurophysiol Clin. 2004;34(1): 17-32.
35. Fehlings MG, Brodke DS, Norvell DC, Dettori JR. The evidence for intraoperative neurophysiological monitoring in spine surgery: does it make a difference?. Spine. 2010;35(9S):S37-46.
36. Morota N, Deletis V, Constantini S, Kofler M, Cohen H, Epstein FJ. The role of motor evoked potentials during surgery for intramedullary spinal cord tumors. Neurosurgery. 1997;41(6): 1327-36.
37. Kothbauer KF, Deletis V, Epstein FJ. Motor-evoked potential monitoring for intramedullary spinal cord tumor surgery: correlation of clinical and neurophysiological data in a series of 100 consecutive procedures. Neurosurg Focus. 1998;4(5):E3.
38. MacDonald DB. Intraoperative motor evoked potential monitoring: overview and update. J Clin Monit Comput. 2006;20(5):347-77.
39. MacDonald DB, Al Zayed Z, Khoudeir I, Stigsby B. Monitoring scoliosis surgery with combined multiple pulse transcranial electric motor and cortical somatosensory-evoked potentials from the lower and upper extremities. Spine. 2003;28(2):194-203.
40. Rajshekhar V, Velayutham P, Joseph M, Babu KS. Factors predicting the feasibility of monitoring lower-limb muscle motor evoked potentials in patients undergoing excision of spinal cord tumors. J Neurosurg Spine. 2011;14(6):748-53.
41. Kim JS, Jang MJ, Hyun SJ, Kim KJ, Jahng TA, Kim HJ, et al. Failure to generate baseline muscle motor evoked potentials during spine surgery: risk factors and association with the postoperative outcomes. Clin Neurophysiol. 2018;129(11):2276-83.
42. Velayutham P, Rajshekhar V, Chacko AG, Babu SK. Influence of tumor location and other variables on predictive value of intraoperative myogenic motor-evoked potentials in spinal cord tumor surgery. World Neurosurg. 2016;92:264-72.
43. MacDonald DB. Motor evoked potential warning criteria. J Clin Neurophysiol. 2017;34(1):1-3.
44. Yi YG, Kim K, Shin HI, Bang MS, Kim HS, Choi J, et al. Feasibility of intraoperative monitoring of motor evoked potentials obtained through transcranial electrical stimulation in infants younger than 3 months. J Neurosurg Pediatr. 2019;23(6):758-66.
45. Nair BR, Ramamani M, Singh G, Babu KS, Rajshekhar V. Feasibility and diagnostic accuracy of intra-operative monitoring of motor evoked potentials in children <2 years of age undergoing tethered cord surgery: results in 100 children. Childs Nerv Syst 2021;37(7):2289-98.
46. Yamada S, Won DJ, Yamada SM. Pathophysiology of tethered cord syndrome: correlation with symptomatology. Neurosurg focus. 2004;16(2):1-5.
47. Schneider SJ, Rosenthal AD, Greenberg BM, Danto J. A preliminary report on the use of laser-Doppler flowmetry during tethered spinal cord release. Neurosurg. 1993;32(2):214-8.
48. Kothbauer KF, Novak K. Intraoperative monitoring for tethered cord surgery: An update. Neurosurgical focus. 2004;16(2):E8.
49. Deletis V, Vodusek DB. Intraoperative recording of the bulbocavernosus reflex. Neurosurg. 1997;40(1):88-93.
50. Paradiso G, Lee GY, Sarjeant R, Hoang L, Massicotte EM, Fehlings MG. Multimodality intraoperative neurophysiologic monitoring findings during surgery for adult tethered cord syndrome: analysis of a series of 44 patients with long-term follow-up. Spine. 2006;31(18):2095-102.
51. Romstöck J, Strauss C, Fahlbusch R. Continuous electromyography monitoring of motor cranial nerves during cerebellopontine angle surgery. J Neurosurg. 2000;93(4):586-93.
52. Coumans JC, Simon MV, Cooper JS, Winograd JM. Peripheral nerve surgery. In: Simon MV (Ed). Intraoperative neurophysiology, a comprehensive guide to monitoring and mapping. New York: Springer; 2010. pp. 267-98.
53. Gaddam SS, Santhi V, Babu S, Chacko G, Baddukonda RA, Rajshekhar V. Gross and microscopic study of the filum terminale: does the filum contain functional neural elements? J Neurosurg Pediatr. 2012;9(1):86-92.
54. Pratheesh R, Babu KS, Rajshekhar V. Improvement in intraoperative transcranial electrical motor-evoked potentials in tethered cord surgery: An analysis of 45 cases. Acta neurochirurgica. 2014;156(4):723-31.
55. Shinomiya K, Fuchioka M, Matsuoka T, Okamoto A, Yoshida H, Mutoh N, et al. Intraoperative monitoring for tethered spinal cord syndrome. Spine. 1991;16(11):1290-4.
56. Pang D, Casey K. Use of an anal sphincter pressure monitor during operations on the sacral spinal cord and nerve roots. Neurosurgery. 1983;13(5):562-8.
57. Kothbauer K, Schmid UD, Seiler RW, Eisner W. Intraoperative motor and sensory monitoring of the cauda equina. Neurosurgery. 1994;34(4):702-7.
58. Hoving EW, Haitsma E, Oude Ophuis C, Journée HL. The value of intraoperative neurophysiological monitoring in tethered cord surgery. Childs Nerv Syst. 2011;27(9):1445-52.
59. Deletis V, Fernández-Conejero I. Intraoperative monitoring and mapping of the functional integrity of the brainstem. J Clin Neurol. 2016;12(3):262-73.
60. Sala F, Manganotti P, Tramontano V, Bricolo A, Gerosa M. Monitoring of motor pathways during brain stem surgery: what we have achieved and what we still miss?. Neurophysiol Clin. 2007;37(6):399-406.
61. Turel MK, Babu KS, Singh G, Chacko AG. The utility of facial nerve amplitude and latency ratios in predicting postoperative facial nerve function after vestibular schwannoma surgery. Neurol India. 2014;62(2):178.
62. Dong CC, MacDonald DB, Akagami R, Westerberg B, AlKhani A, Kanaan I, et al. Intraoperative facial motor evoked potential monitoring with transcranial electrical stimulation during skull base surgery. Clin Neurophysiol. 2005;116(3):588-96.
63. Campbell KC, Abbas PJ. The effect of stimulus repetition rate on the auditory brainstem response in tumor and nontumor patients. J Speech Hear Res. 1987;30(4):494-502.
64. Polo G, Fischer C, Sindou MP, Marneffe V. Brainstem auditory evoked potential monitoring during microvascular decompression for hemifacial spasm: intraoperative brainstem auditory evoked potential changes and warning values to prevent hearing loss—prospective study in a consecutive series of 84 patients. Neurosurgery. 2004;54(1):97-106.
65. Danner C, Mastrodimos B, Cueva RA. A comparison of direct eighth nerve monitoring and auditory brainstem response in hearing preservation surgery for vestibular schwannoma. Otol Neurotol. 2004;25(5):826-32.
66. Schlake HP, Milewski C, Goldbrunner RH, Kindgen A, Riemann R, Helms J, et al. Combined intra-operative monitoring of hearing by means of auditory brainstem responses (ABR) and transtympanic electrocochleography (ECochG) during surgery of intra-and extrameatal acoustic neurinomas. Acta neurochirurgica. 2001 Oct;143(10):985-96.
67. Hahn JF, Latchaw JP. Evoked potentials in the operating room. Neurosurgery. 1984;31(CN_suppl_1):389-403.
68. Raudzens PA, Shetter AG. Intraoperative monitoring of brain-stem auditory evoked potentials. J Neurosurg. 1982;57(3):341-8.
69. MacDonald DB, Deletis V. Safety issues during surgical monitoring. Handb Clin Neurophysiol. 2008;8:882-98.
70. Skinner SA, Cohen BA, Morledge DE, McAuliffe JJ, Hastings JD, Yingling CD, et al. Practice guidelines for the supervising professional: intraoperative neurophysiological monitoring. J Clin Monit Comput. 2014;28(2):103-11.

71. Schwartz DM, Auerbach JD, Dormans JP, Flynn J, Drummond DS, Bowe JA, et al. Neurophysiological detection of impending spinal cord injury during scoliosis surgery. JBJS. 2007;89(11):2440-9.
72. Kothbauer KF. The interpretation of muscle motor evoked potentials for spinal cord monitoring. J Clin Neurophysiol. 2017;34(1):32-7.
73. Ito Z, Matsuyama Y, Ando M, Kawabata S, Kanchiku T, Kida K, et al. What is the best multimodality combination for intraoperative spinal cord monitoring of motor function? A multicenter study by the Monitoring Committee of the Japanese Society for Spine Surgery and Related Research. Glob Spine J. 2016;6(3):234-41.
74. Nuwer MR. Billing, Ethical, and Legal Issues. In: Husain A (Ed). A Practical Approach to Neurophysiologic Intraoperative Monitoring. India: Demos Medical Publishing; 2008. pp. 67.
75. Ney JP, van der Goes DN. Comparative effectiveness analyses of intraoperative neurophysiological monitoring in spinal surgery. J Clin Neurophysiol. 2014;31(2):112-7.
76. Skinner S, Holdefer R, McAuliffe JJ, Sala F. Medical error avoidance in intraoperative neurophysiological monitoring: the communication imperative. J Clin Neurophysiol. 2017;34(6):477-83.
77. Leonard M, Graham S, Bonacum D. The human factor: the critical importance of effective teamwork and communication in providing safe care. BMJ Quality Safety. 2004;13(suppl 1):i85-90.

115
CHAPTER

Computed Tomography and Magnetic Resonance Imaging

Paramjeet Singh, Vikas Bhatia

INTRODUCTION

Neuroimaging plays a crucial role in diagnosing and managing various neurological diseases. Cross-sectional imaging [computed tomography and magnetic resonance imaging (CT and MRI)] has revolutionized the understanding of pathologies by enabling their direct visualization in greater detail. It was the landmark work of Alan Cormark and Godfrey Hounsfield in the development of CT. They were awarded the Nobel Prize for Medicine in 1979.[1] The First CT scanners were installed in 1973. Since then, there has been a tremendous advancement in CT technology to the current state-of-the-art multislice CT scanners.[2] The concept of nuclear magnetic resonance has been known for many decades. Later studies revealed that normal and pathological tissues could be differentiated based on the different relaxation times of the various tissues. The first MR scanner was installed in 1980. Paul C Lauterbur, PhD, and Sir Peter Mansfield were awarded the Nobel Prize in 2003 in Medicine for their significant contribution to the development of MRI. Marked hardware and technology improvements have made MRI the major workhorse of neurological diagnosis and management.[3]

In this chapter, we will briefly discuss CT and MRI technology as applicable to neurological disorders.

COMPUTED TOMOGRAPHY IMAGING

Over the last few decades, CT has seen tremendous growth in hardware and software technologies. Current generation CT scans provide state-of-the-art imaging with isotropic volumetric data, submillimetric thickness, high spatial and temporal resolution, and short acquisition time.[4] CT is one of the most valuable imaging modalities in neuroimaging, particularly in stroke and trauma patients. The significant advantages of CT are summarized in **Table 1**.

Advancements in CT technology are summarized in **Table 2**.

Computed Tomography-based Modalities for Neuroimaging

The most common CT-based modalities with varied clinical applications are noncontrast CT (NCCT) for the head and spine, CT angiography (CTA), and CT perfusion (CTP). CT myelography and CT cisternography have limited roles currently.

Noncontrast Computed Tomography

Noncontrast CT is the initial neuroimaging modality in acute stroke, emergency, and trauma settings due to widespread and round-the-clock availability. It is essential to demonstrate ischemic stroke **(Fig. 1)**, hemorrhage **(Fig. 2)** and hydrocephalus **(Fig. 3)** in acute settings, which have important management implications.

The Hounsfield scale represents the tissue density on CT with water showing zero Hounsfield units (HU). The low-density tissues are assigned darker shades, and the high-density tissues are given brighter shades **(Fig. 4)**. **Table 3** shows the HU value for various tissues.

Due to the limited ability of the human eye to perceive all the gray shades, instead of displaying a full range of

TABLE 1: Advantages and disadvantages of computed tomography.

Advantages	Disadvantages
Widespread availability	Radiation exposure
Noninvasive	Use of iodinated contrast media when indicated
Fast acquisition (helpful in unstable and pediatric patients)	Low sensitivity for posterior fossa pathologies
High spatial and temporal resolution	Streak artifacts
Very high sensitivity to detect calcification and hemorrhage	
No contraindication to metallic implants	

TABLE 2: Advancements in computed tomography technology.

Advancement	Structure/principle	Clinical application
Multidetector CT	• It consists of multiple rows of detectors • Multiple slices per rotation are acquired (2–320) • High gantry speed results in faster imaging with a larger volume • Provides excellent multiplanar reformations (MPRs) and 3D reconstructions	• Whole brain perfusion imaging • CT angiography with excellent temporal resolution useful in stroke, stenosis or other vascular pathologies
Dual-energy computed Tomography (CT)	• It helps in differentiating tissues • Based on the principle that different materials show different (absorption) of energy at various kVp settings • Different vendors use different technologies, such as using an assembly of two X-ray tubes and detectors, Or single X-ray tube with fast kV-switching systems or dual-layer detection technology	• Better atherosclerotic plaque and tumor characterization • Reduction in the metal artifact • Improved CT angiography images due to effective bone removal
Cone beam CT	Utilizes a conical beam of X-ray with a cone-shaped area detector to image the entire region of interest in a single rotation	Mainly used in dental imaging; Also useful for imaging temporal bone imaging, paranasal sinus imaging and imaging implanted devices
Portable CT	• Portable CT is a system that can be moved from one place to another in a hospital • Higher cost and radiation concerns to the public and staff are an issue with these portable scanners	Useful for imaging in the ICU and perioperative setting
Advanced image reconstruction techniques	Iterative reconstruction methods to reduce noise and streak artifacts	• Improved image quality • Dose reduction

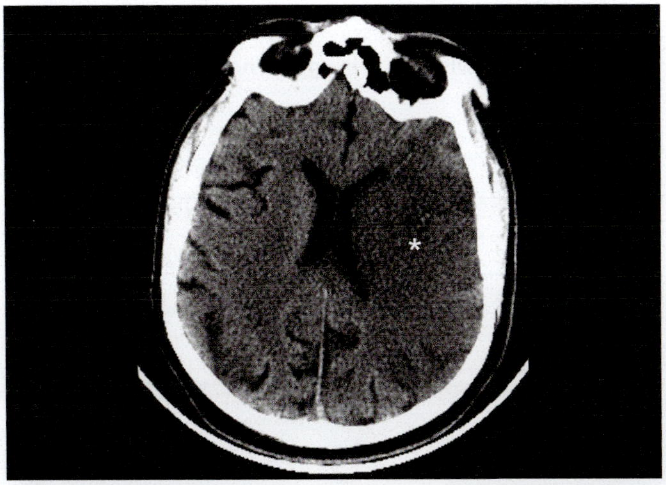

FIG. 1: Axial NCCT head of a patient shows hypoattenuation (star) involving left MCA territory s/o acute ischemic infarct.
(MCA: middle cerebral artery; NCCT: noncontrast computed tomography)

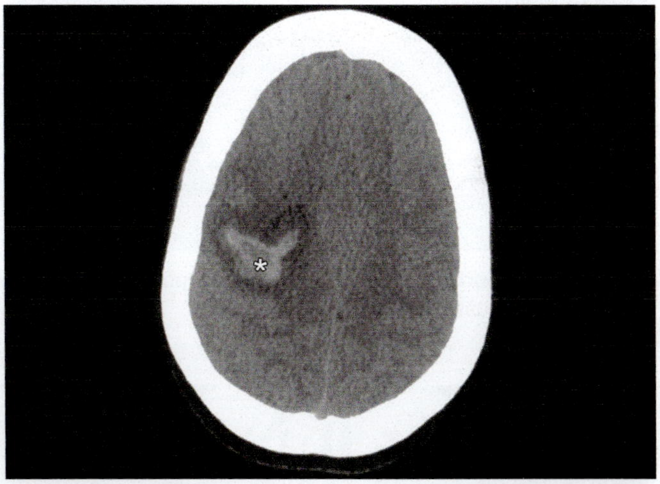

FIG. 2: Axial noncontrast computed tomography (NCCT) head shows hyperdense hematoma (star) in right frontal lobe with mild surrounding edema.

density values, only a narrow portion of the entire density range is displayed for the tissues of interest, known as windowing.

Before interpreting, it is of paramount importance to select the appropriate window width (WW) and window level (WL) as they can significantly alter the appearance of the CT image. A wide window setting is used for demonstration of the subdural lesion and a narrow window setting for stroke.

Various window settings for neuro-CT are shown in **Table 4**.

Computed Tomography Angiography

Computed tomography angiography provides excellent visualization of the extracranial and intracranial vessels. Multidetector CT (MDCT) with high spatial and temporal resolution allows rapid acquisition of high-quality data

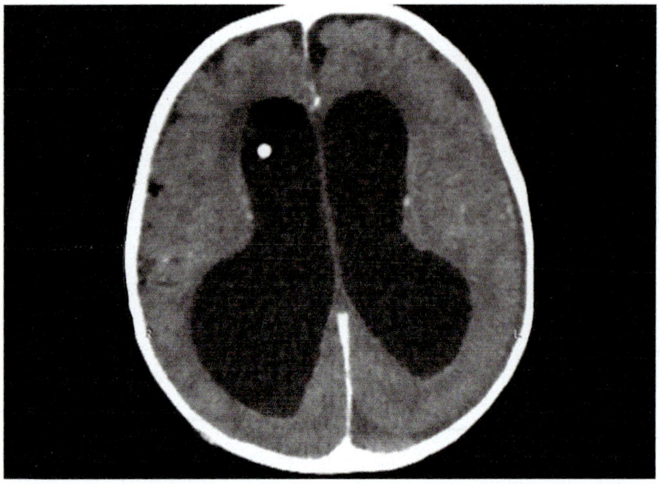

FIG. 3: Axial noncontrast computed tomography (NCCT) images showing dilated lateral ventricles suggestive of hydrocephalus.

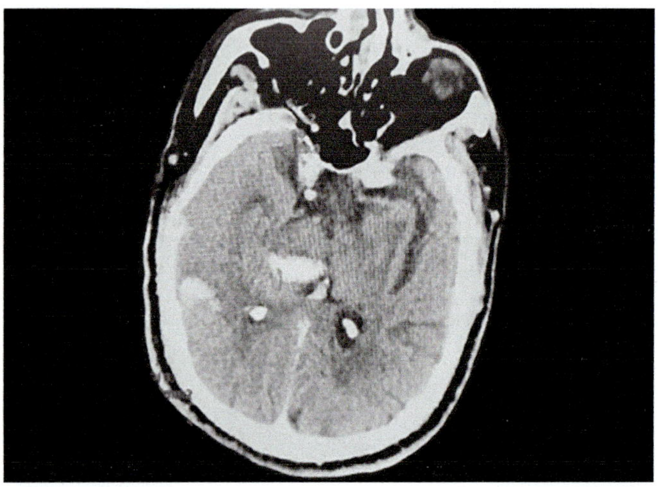

FIG. 4: Axial noncontrast computed tomography (NCCT) head showing CT attenuation values of various tissues.

for 2D and 3D reconstruction of vascular anatomy. For acquisition, the contrast is injected via a power injector at a rate (of 2–4 mL/s). Various methods such as bolus tracking, test bolus method, or an arbitrary delay (15–20 seconds) are used for optimal opacification.[5]

Different postprocessing techniques can be employed for additional information, such as maximum intensity projection (MIP), surface-shaded display (SSD), and volume-rendering techniques, which are mainly very useful in neuroimaging **(Figs. 5A and B)**.

The advantages of CTA are excellent anatomical and pathological detail of vessels, rapid acquisition, better

TABLE 3: Hounsfield units (HU) value for various tissues.

>1,000	Bone, metal
100–600	Iodinated contrast
30–500	Punctate calcifications
60–100	Hemorrhage
35–40	Gray matter
25–30	White matter
20–40	Soft tissue
0	Water
–30 to –80	Fat
–1000	Air

TABLE 4: Various window settings for neurocomputed tomography.

Brain	W: 80 L: 40
Subdural	W: 130–300 L: 50–100
Stroke	W: 8 L: 32 or W: 40 L: 40
Temporal bones	W: 2,800 L: 600 or W: 4,000 L: 700
Soft tissues	W: 350–400 L: 20–60

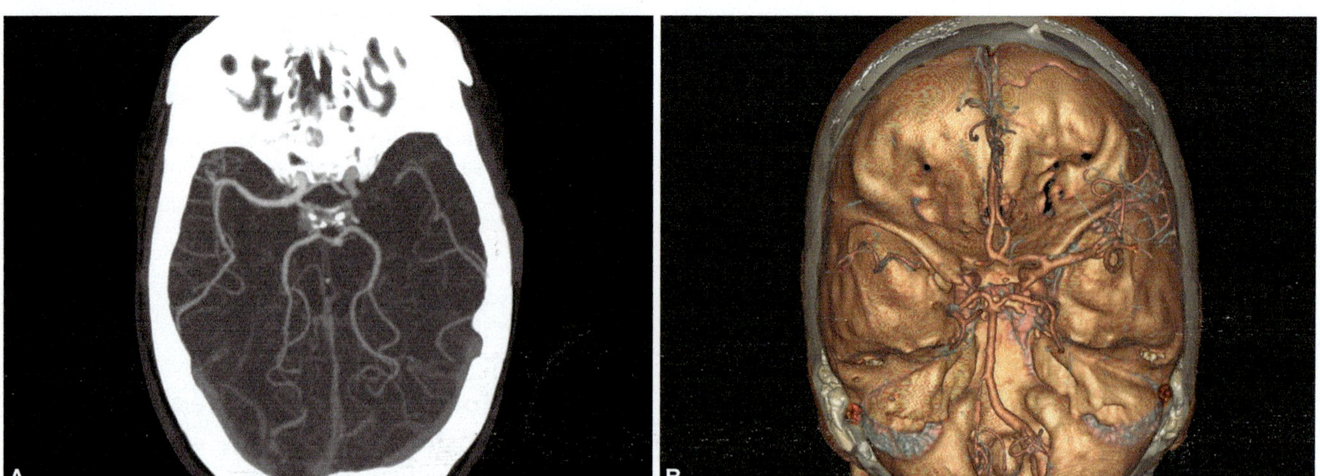

FIGS. 5A AND B: A 55-year-old female with acute onset of right hemiparesis. (A) Coronal MIP; and (B) VR images show nonopacification of left MCA.
(MCA: middle cerebral artery; MIP: maximum intensity projection; VR: virtual reality)

visualization of bony anatomical details, better visualization of calcification, and the ability to be used in patients with metallic implants. Drawbacks include the use of ionizing radiation and contrast requirements.

Major clinical use is seen in stroke assessment **(Figs. 5A and B)**, carotid stenosis **(Fig. 6)** and dissections, diagnosis and characterization of intracranial aneurysms **(Figs. 7A and B)**, and arteriovenous malformations. It is also used for surgical planning to assess tumor vascularity and preoperative assessment of vessel proximity.[6]

Computed Tomography Perfusion

It is a CT-based technique which is based on the principle of temporal changes in attenuation of brain tissue after administration of iodinated contrast medium. Indirectly, it reflects tissue vascularity and vascular physiology.

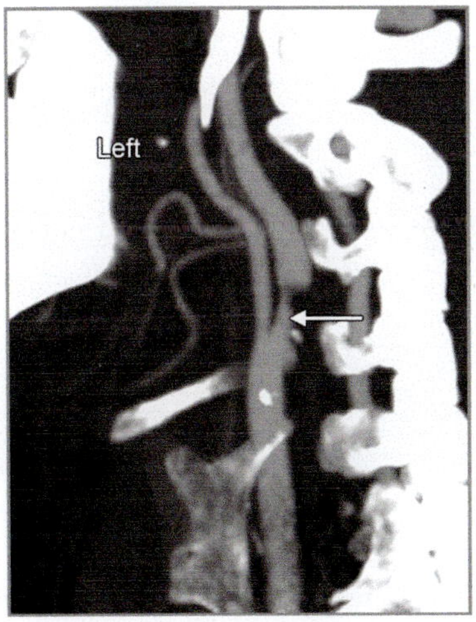

FIG. 6: CT angiography oblique MIP image shows 70–80% stenosis at the origin of left ICA.

(CT: computed tomography; ICA: internal carotid artery; MIP: maximum intensity projection)

Following an intravenous iodinated contrast injection, there is an initial phase of enhancement (40–60 seconds) mainly because of the contrast distribution within the intravascular space. Enhancement in the initial phase depends on tissue blood flow and volume. This is followed by the second phase, with the passage of contrast from the intravascular to the extravascular compartment occurring across the capillary basement membrane, followed by contrast distribution between the two compartments. Enhancements in this phase depend mainly on tissue permeability.[7,8]

To assess the perfusion data, the acquisition is acquired in rapid succession during these two phases after contrast injection, and the temporal changes in tissue attenuation are recorded. This data is then processed by complex mathematical algorithms such as deconvolution or compartmental analysis for quantitative information. Tissue-specific parameters from perfusion are cerebral blood volume (CBV), cerebral blood flow (CBF), mean transit time (MTT), and time-to-maximum (Tmax).

Primary clinical application is seen in acute stroke imaging **(Fig. 8)** to differentiate the ischemic core from the penumbra. Other clinical applications are seen in head trauma, intraparenchymal hemorrhage, vasospasm, and neoplasms. CTP is more useful in the emergency setting than MR perfusion due to its widespread availability, faster acquisition time, and low cost.[9]

Computed Tomography Venography

Computed tomography venography (CTV) is an excellent method for delineating the cerebral venous system. Rapid acquisition time and widespread availability make it an ideal imaging technique, particularly in the emergency setting. For CTV, the acquisition is made after 40 seconds of contrast injection. It has comparative diagnostic accuracy to MRI and demonstrates thrombosis as a filling defect **(Fig. 9)**.

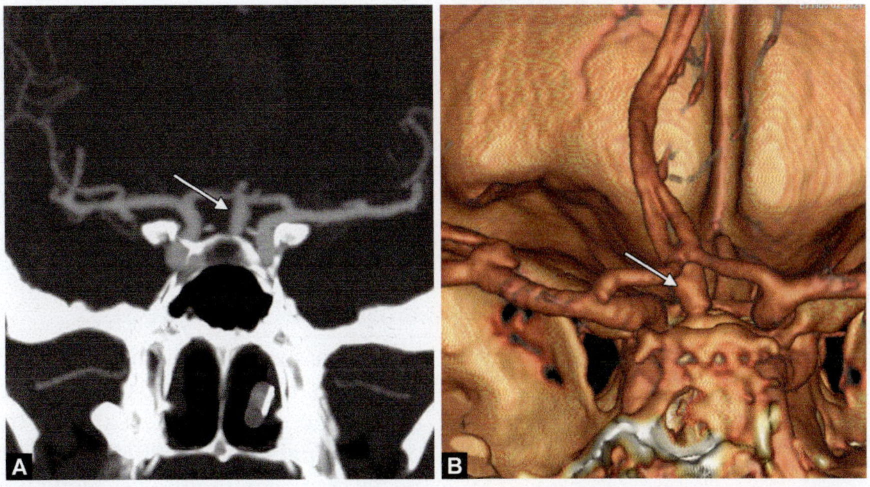

FIGS. 7A AND B: (A) Coronal MIP and (B) VR image showing narrow neck Acom aneurysm.

(MIP: maximum intensity projection; VR: virtual reality)

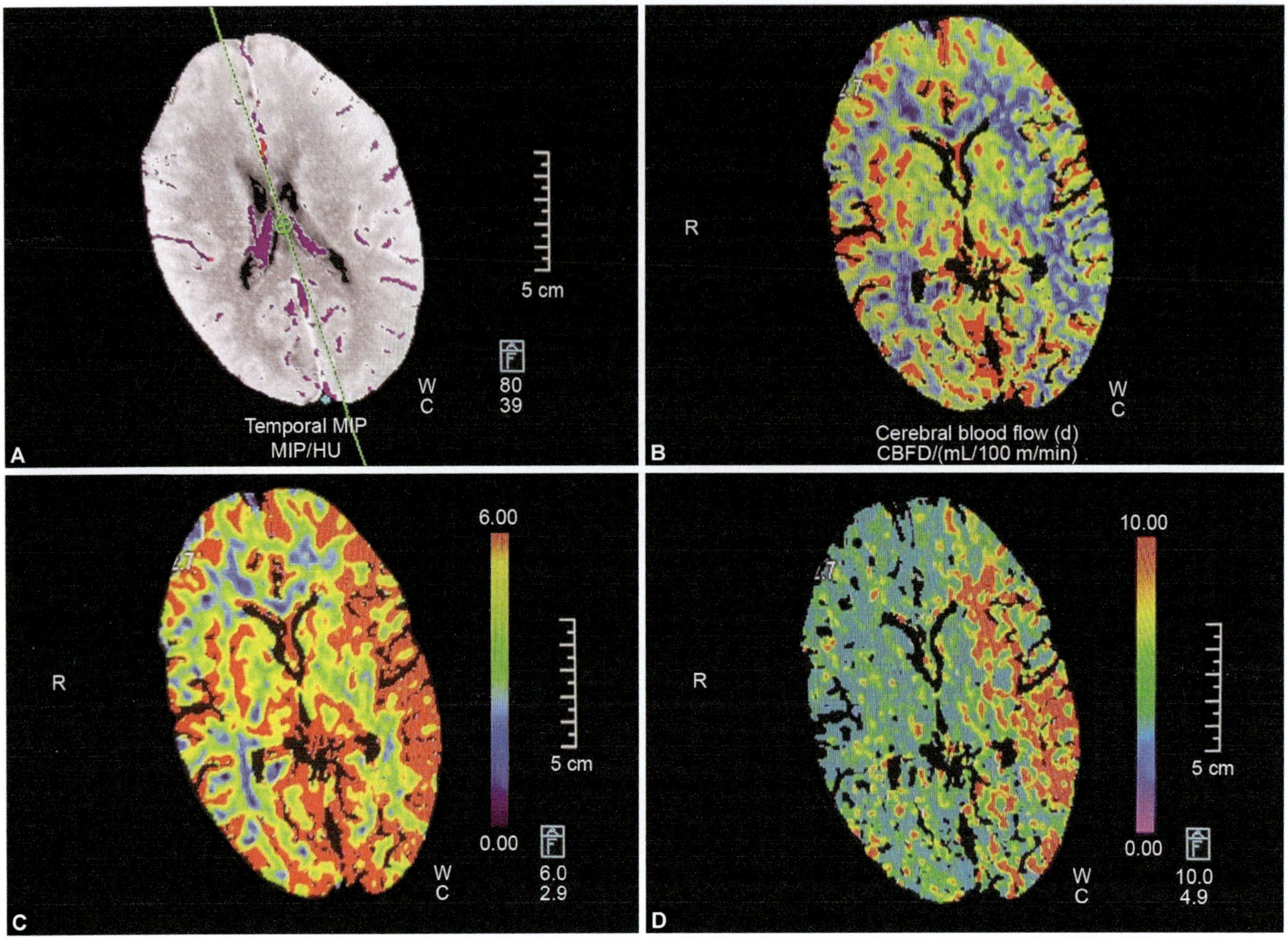

FIGS. 8A TO D: CT perfusion images in a patient with left MCA stroke shows reduced CBF, normal CBV and increased MTT suggestive of salvageable penumbra.

(CT: computed tomography; CBF: cerebral blood flow; CBV: cerebral blood volume; MCA: middle cerebral artery; MTT: mean transit time; VR: virtual reality)

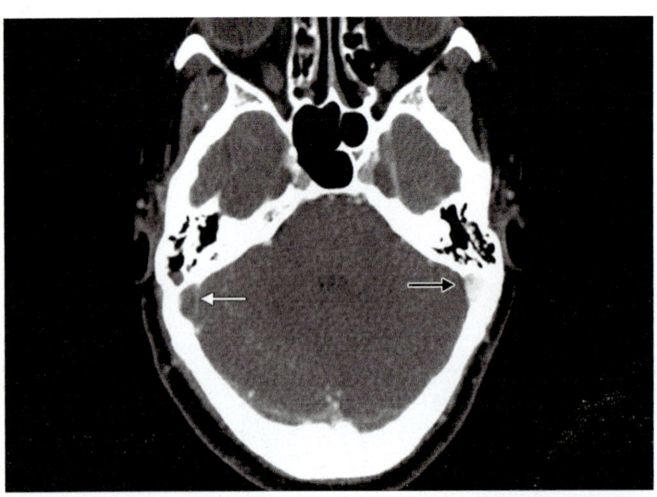

FIG. 9: Axial computed tomography (CT) venography images showing non opacification of right sigmoid sinus suggestive of thrombus (white arrow). Note made of normal left side sigmoid sinus (black arrow).

MAGNETIC RESONANCE IMAGING IN NEUROIMAGING

Magnetic resonance imaging is the workhorse of neuroimaging worldwide. It provides excellent anatomical details, better characterization of different pathologies and is devoid of radiation hazards. 1.5T and 3T MRIs are routinely used in clinical scenarios.

Limitations of MRI include prolonged acquisition time, limited availability compared to CT, issues in patients with metallic implants, and claustrophobia in few patients.

MRI Pulse Sequences

When an external magnetic field B0 is applied to the hydrogen nuclei in tissue, they start processing at a resonance frequency (Larmor frequency) which is proportional to the magnetic field strength. The hydrogen nuclei also align themselves along the axis of the magnetic field (z-axis), generating a net magnetic vector. At this stage, an external radiofrequency (RF) pulse is applied, which flips the net magnetization vector to a certain angle (flip angle) into the transverse plane (x/y axis). Free induction decay (FID) is generated when protons precess at the same frequency and direction. Due to magnetic field in homogeneities, this FID is rapidly lost due to the dephasing of protons. MR pulse sequences are employed to rephase these protons and generate a signal called echo. This can be done by a 180-degree refocusing pulse (spin echo sequences) or the use of gradients (gradient echo sequences) **(Tables 5 and 6).**[10]

TABLE 5: An overview of various spin echo pulse sequences used in MR neuroimaging.

Technique	Sequence name	Weighing	Features	Application
Spin echo	SE	T1, T2, PD	• High resolution • Less magnetic susceptibility artifacts • Prolonged acquisition time	Replaced by TSE sequences
Fast spin echo	• RARE • TSE • FSE	T1, T2, PD	• Fast sequences compared to SE • Less magnetic susceptibility artifacts	High-resolution Brain imaging
3D FSE	• CUBE VISTA • SPACE	• T1 • T2 • PD • FLAIR	3D isotropic resolution images	• Brain and inner ear imaging • MR neurography
Single shot FSE	HASTE	T2W	Faster acquisition	Fetal imaging
• Inversion recovery sequences	• TIRM • IR TSE • TURBO IR • FLAIR • STIR	• T1W • T2W • T1W and T2W	Fast and high resolution	• Epilepsy imaging • CSF suppression for white matter pathologies • Fat suppression for spine and orbital imaging

(FSE: fast spin echo; HASTE: half-Fourier acquisition single-shot turbo spin-echo; IR: inversion recovery; MR: magnetic resonance; PD: proton-density; RARE: rapid acquisition with relaxation enhanced; SPACE: sampling perfection with application-optimized contrasts by using different flip angle evolutions; STIR: short tau inversion recovery; T1W: T1 weighted; TIRM: turbo inversion recovery magnitude; TSE: turbo spin echo; VISTA: volume isotropic turbo spin-echo acquisition)

TABLE 6: An overview of various gradient echo pulse sequences used in MR neuroimaging.

Technique	Sequence name	Weighing	Features	Application
2D spoiled gradient (GRE)	• FLASH • T1-FFE • SPGR	T1W	Fast imaging	MR angiography
Ultrafast GRE	TURBO FLASH	T1W	Very fast imaging	Contrast tracking
Multiple GRE	• MERGE • MEDIC • M-FFE	T2*W	High contrast resolution	Spine imaging
3D ultrafast GRE	MP-RAGE	T1W	High-resolution 3D sequence	T1W cerebral imaging
Echo planar imaging	EPI	T2*W	Ultrafast acquisition	• Diffusion imaging • Perfusion imaging • Functional imaging
Preexcitation steady state refocused sequences	• PSIF • SSFP	T2W	High T2W weighting	• CSF flow studies • Inner ear imaging
Combined fully refocused steady-state sequences with and without phase change	• CISS • FIESTA-C	T2W	High-resolution imaging	• Inner ear • Cranial nerve imaging

(CISS: constructive interference in steady state; CSF: cerebrospinal fluid; EPI: echo-planar imaging; FFE: fast field echo; FIESTA-C: fast imaging employing steady-state acquisition cycled phases; FLASH: fast low angle shot; MR: magnetic resonance; MEDIC: multiple echo data image combination; M-FFE: merged fast field echo; MERGE: multiple echo recombined gradient echo; MP-RAGE: magnetization prepared rapid gradient echo imaging; SPGR: spoiled gradient recalled acquisition in the steady state; SSFP: steady state free precession; T1W: T1 weighted)

Magnetic Resonance Angiography

Magnetic resonance angiography (MRA) is a technique for noninvasive visualization of the cranial and extracranial vessels. These can be acquired after gadolinium contrast administration, known as contrast-enhanced MRA (CE-MRA). One advantage of MRA over CT is that angiographic images can also be acquired without contrast administration, such as time of flight (TOF) and phase contrast (PC) MRA.[11,12]

Time of flight MRA is based on the basic principle of application of repetitive RF pulses with short repetition time (TR) to the area of interest to suppress the signal from stationary tissues and get signal only from the inflowing blood. TOF imaging can be 2D or 3D or a combination such as MOTSA (multiple overlapping thin-slab acquisitions). TOF MRA is routinely used in day-to-day MR acquisition and provides important anatomical information about the vessels **(Fig. 10)**. Drawbacks include saturation and turbulence-related side effects, which may affect the signal in TOF MRA.

Phase-contrast MRA (PC-MRA) is another MR angiographic technique which is based on measurement in the area of interest by applying two equally flow-sensitized measurements in opposite directions to each other. By subtracting both measurements, any contribution from the stationary tissues not having motion or flow is removed. Although not used in routine practice, it provides crucial information regarding flow direction, velocity, and pressure.

Contrast-enhanced -MRA technique utilizes gadolinium-based contrast agent that results in T1 shortening and hence a brighter signal compared to the rest of the tissues. The acquisition can be made in a 2D or 3D manner. Use of ultrafast 3D gradient-recalled echo (GRE) sequences and parallel imaging results in faster acquisition of the angiographic data with isotropic resolution. Advantages over TOF MRA are fewer saturation artifacts, better coverage in all directions and time-resolved acquisition for understanding the angioarchitecture.[11,12]

Advanced MRI Techniques

Diffusion-weighted Imaging

Water molecules in biological tissue are not unrestricted and random but depend on the compartmentalized structure of the tissue consisting of intracellular, extracellular, and intravascular spaces. The diffusion of water molecules depends upon the interaction between the cell membrane structures and pathological processes. Thus, tissues containing high cellular density, intact cellular membranes, and the complex macromolecular system can show restricted diffusion as seen in cerebral abscesses, certain high cellularities neoplasms such as lymphoma and cytotoxic edema such as infarct and demyelination.[13]

Diffusion-weighted (DW) imaging is based on the application of spin echo-planar imaging (EPI) imaging. Two equal dephasing and rephasing gradients are applied to either side of an 180° refocusing pulse to track the movement of protons for restricted diffusion. A parameter 'b' value determines the distribution weighing along with a tissue-specific diffusivity factor called the "apparent diffusion coefficient" (ADC). Mean diffusivity trace images (DW) are used in daily practice. Almost all signals received are from diffusion-restricted molecules at the highest b value. A good diffusion weighting is achieved with a 'b value' of 1,000 s/mm. Tissues having restricted diffusion, such as high-grade brain tumors and acute brain infarct, will appear bright on DWI trace images and dark on ADC maps.

Clinical applications include encephalitis **(Figs. 11A and B)**, abscesses **(Fig. 12)**, acute ischemic stroke **(Fig. 13)**,

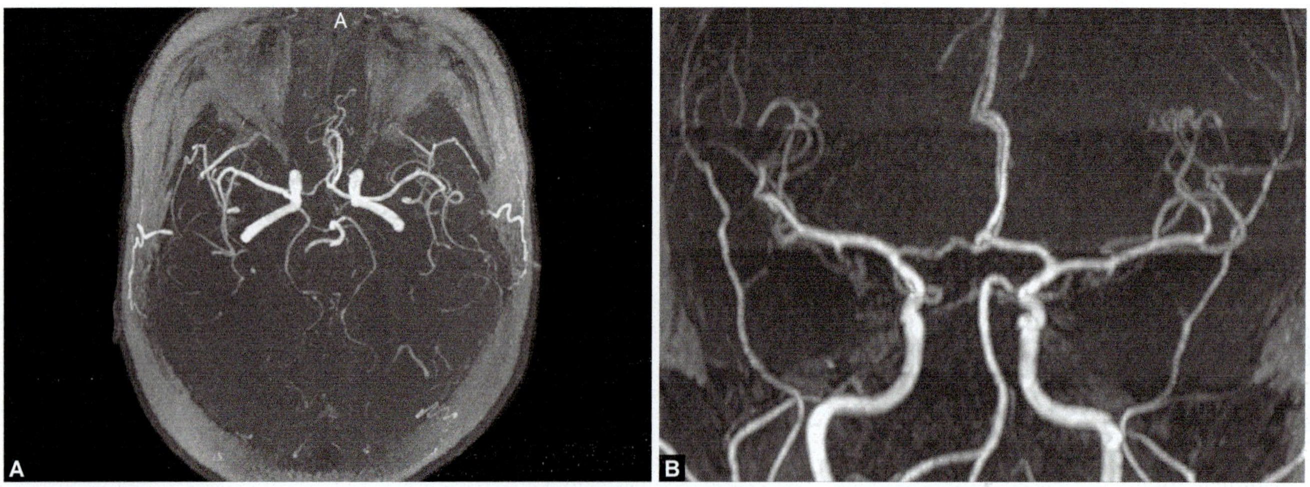

FIGS. 10A AND B: TOF MRA showing excellent depiction of intracranial vessels.
(MRA: magnetic resonance angiography; TOF: time of flight)

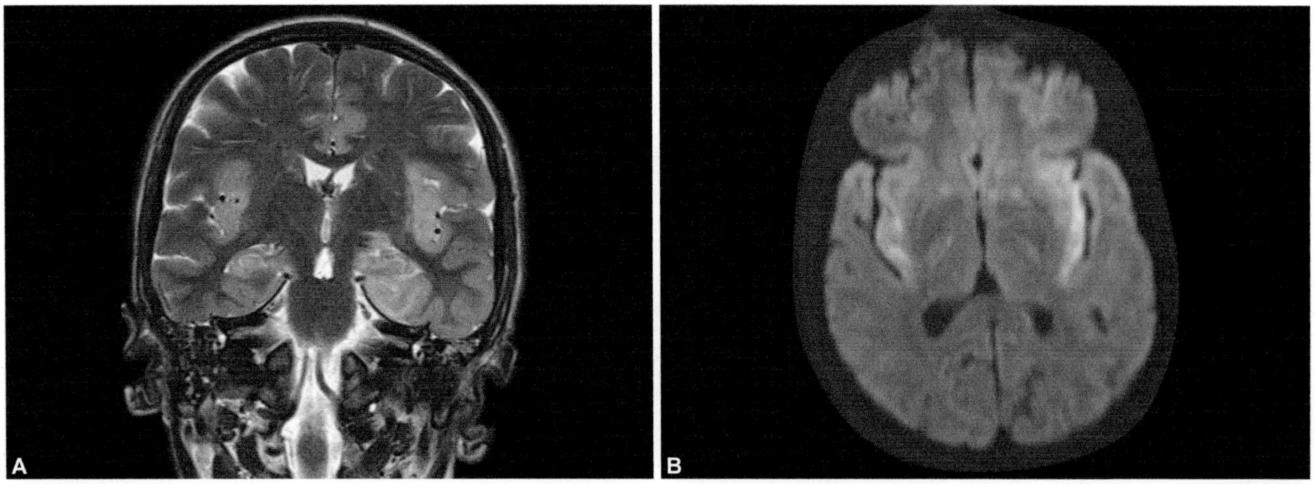

FIGS. 11A AND B: Coronal T2W MRI (A) shows asymmetric hyperintensity in bilateral temporal lobes and insular cortex; (B) DW images show diffusion restriction in these areas s/o herpes encephalitis.
(DW: diffusion-weighted; MRI: magnetic resonance imaging)

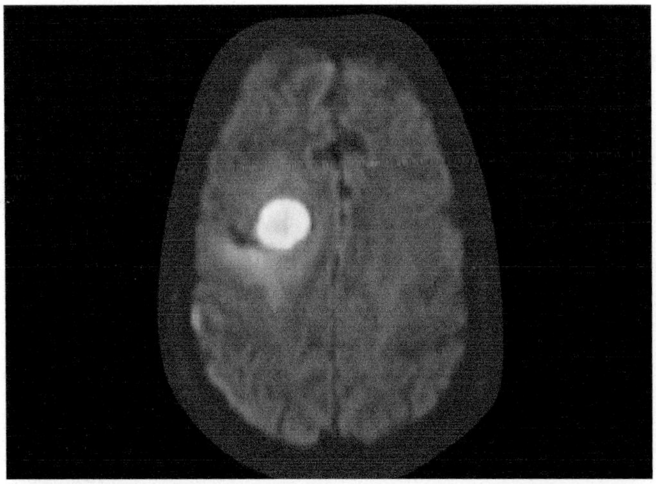

FIG. 12: Diffusion-weighted (DW) image shows central diffusion restriction in a case of pyogenic abscess.

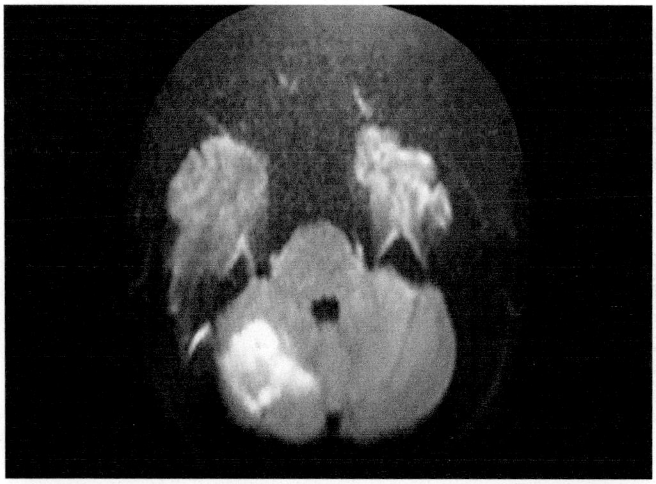

FIG. 13: Diffusion-weighted (DW) image showing restricted diffusion in right cerebellar hemisphere suggestive of acute ischemic infarct.

demyelination, characterization of neoplasms, diffuse axonal injury, and many more. DW has become the standard imaging sequence in all MRI examinations of the CNS.[13]

Diffusion Tensor Imaging

It is an advanced MR technique that employs complex mathematical models of diffusion tensors to delineate the anisotropy of water diffusion in multiple directions. Measurement of tensor data is usually done in six or more directions. Principle application is seen in imaging of the white matter. Due to its myelin sheath and macromolecular walls, water molecules in an axon move along the fiber axis, known as anisotropy.

Clinical applications are seen in stroke, demyelination, trauma, or any other disease-causing white matter structural disruption. It is also used to differentiate between tumor infiltration versus displacement of the white matter tracts. Fiber tracking is also used in developmental and psychiatric disorders.[14]

Susceptibility-weighted Imaging

Susceptibility-weighted imaging (SWI) is a velocity-compensated 3D GRE sequence consisting of contrast generation using magnitude and phase information. It exploits the magnetic inhomogeneity of the tissue, which results in signal distortion of the tissues showing high susceptibility. This results in signal loss as the protons become out of phase compared to surrounding tissues.

Clinical application is seen in traumatic brain injury, microbleed detection **(Figs. 14 and 15)**, coagulopathy, vascular malformation, neoplasms, calcified lesions, and neurodegenerative disorders with iron deposition **(Fig. 16)**. The signal of calcification and hemorrhage depends on the type of MR system whether left-handed or right-handed.[15,16]

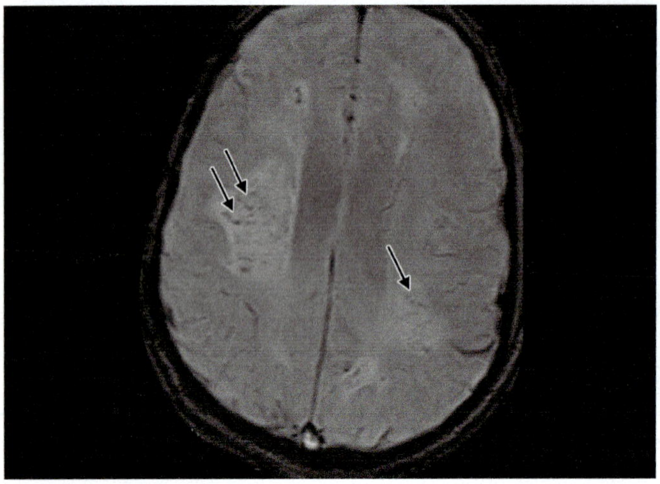

FIG. 14: Susceptibility-weighted (SW) image in a patient of vasculitis shows multiple microhemorrhages (arrows).

Perfusion-weighted Imaging

Perfusion-weighted imaging (PWI) provides necessary clinical quantitative and qualitative measures of blood flow and hemodynamic blood indices such as CBV, blood velocities, and blood transit times. MRI-based perfusion methods include dynamic susceptibility contrast (DSC), dynamic contrast enhancement (DCE), arterial spin labeling (ASL), and intravoxel incoherent motion (IVIM). Out of these, ASL and IVIM are noncontrast-based techniques **(Table 7)**.

Clinical applications of PWI: Major clinical applications are in stroke and tumor imaging **(Figs. 17A and B)**. MR perfusion can be used to differentiate the ischemic core and penumbra. The ischemic core is characterized by reduced relative CBV (rCBV), relative CBF (rCBF), and elevated MTT and TTP due to lack of signal drop after contrast arrival,

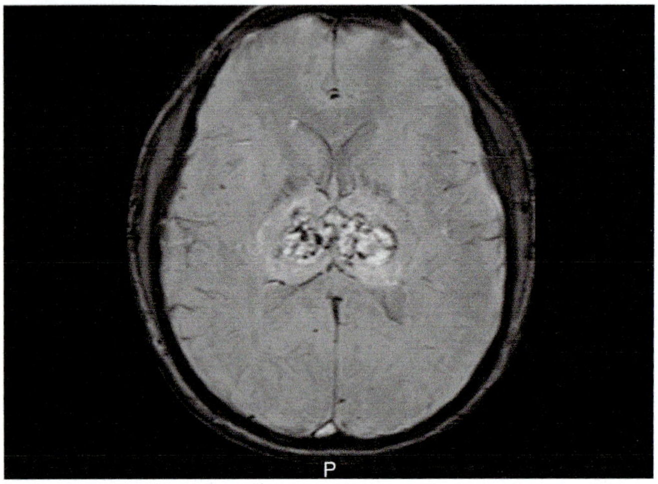

FIG. 15: Susceptibility-weighted (SW) image in a dengue. Patient shows bilateral thalamic hemorrhage.

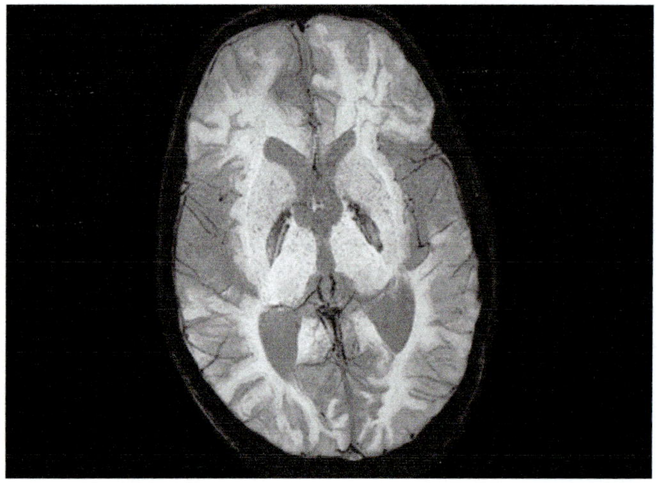

FIG. 16: Susceptibility-weighted (SW) image in a patient with neurodegeneration with brain iron accumulation (NBIA) shows brain atrophy with susceptibility changes in bilateral basal ganglia.

TABLE 7: Different PWI MR techniques.

	Imaging type	Acquisition	Sequences	Principle
DSC	T2/T2*W	2D/3D dynamic	2D single shot GRE EPI	The signal reduction during the passage of injected paramagnetic contrast agents, T2*W effects are measured
DCE	T1W	2D/3D dynamic	3D GRE	Dynamic acquisition of T1-weighted MR images resonance images are done before, during and after bolus injection of a contrast agent. By applying the physical principles of tracer-kinetic modeling, the generated data can be studied in terms of physiological tissue characteristics
ASL	Short TE/long TR sequence	2D/3D single time-point	single shot GRE EPI	Brain perfusion is measured by spin labeling of arterial water by tagging with alternating frequency. Two methods of ASL perfusion mainly used are pulsed ASL (PASL) and pseudocontinuous ASL (PCASL)

(ASL: arterial spin labeling; DCE: dynamic contrast enhancement; DSC: dynamic susceptibility contrast; EPI: echo-planar imaging; GRE: gradient-recalled echo; MR: magnetic resonance; PWI: perfusion-weighted imaging; TE: echo time)

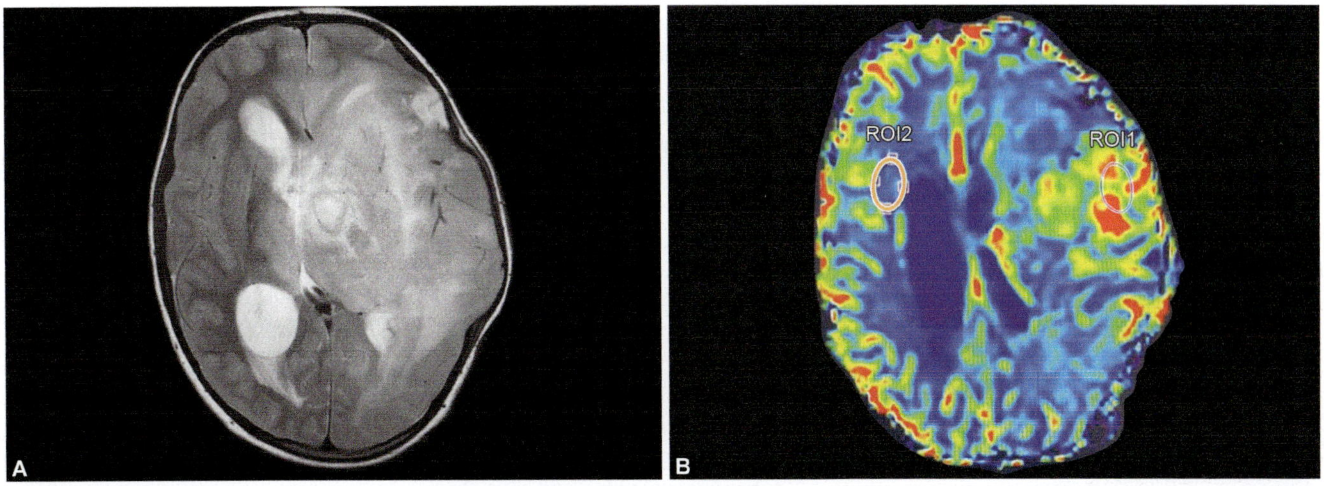

FIGS. 17A AND B: Follow-up imaging in a patient with postoperative high-grade glioma. Axial T2W (A) images shows heterogeneous mass in left frontotemporal region with mass effect; (B) Relative cerebral blood flow (CBF) perfusion maps show increase values suggestive of recurrence.

whilst the ischemic penumbra is characterized by reduced rCBF, elevated MTT, and TTP and normal or slightly elevated rCBV. The penumbra can also be identified as the areas of PWI and DWI mismatch, reflecting the presence of potentially salvageable tissue at risk.

In tumor imaging, perfusion can provide information regarding angiogenesis and grading of tumors which correlates well with rCBV. It can also help in differentiating tumor recurrence from radiation necrosis. It can also guide regarding the site for appropriate biopsy of the tumor. Another role is determining atypical infections and tumefactive demyelination which can mimic neoplasms. ASL perfusion is used in diagnostic utility for dementia, epilepsy, psychiatric disorders, and trauma. ASL can give perfusion information in patients with contraindication to gadolinium contrast.[16,17]

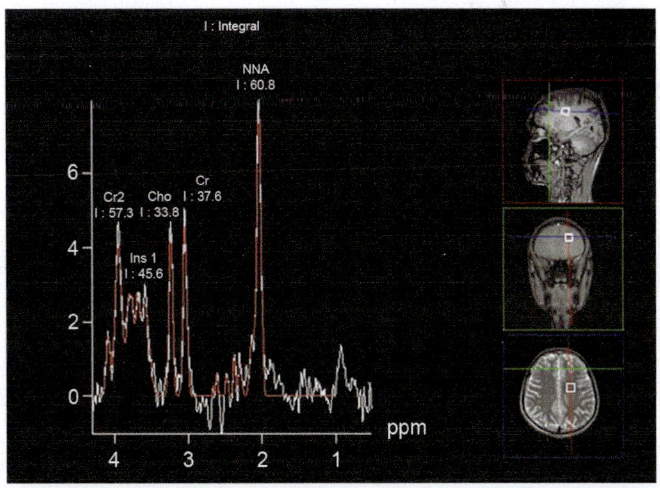

FIG. 18: A Normal spectroscopic display based on chemical shift of various metabolites.

Magnetic Resonance Spectroscopy

Magnetic resonance spectroscopy (MRS) is a technique employed to identify and localize various metabolites using spectral information from nuclei such as protons (1H) and phosphorus (31P) from a particular voxel. It is based on the principle of chemical shift. The spin frequency of each nucleus depends on the external magnetic field (B0) and local microenvironment. Because of the interaction of the electric shells of the nuclei with the surrounding molecule, each nucleus experiences a different magnetic field depending upon the shielding. This difference causes a change of spin frequency known as chemical shift. This information is utilized in MRS to express metabolite frequency in parts per million (ppm) displayed on the x-axis while the peak amplitude is shown on the y-axis **(Fig. 18)**.

Magnetic resonance spectroscopy can be acquired at short echo time (TE) (30), intermediate TE (135), and long TE (270), depending upon the pathology and expected metabolite to be detected. Some metabolites, such as lipids, are only seen at short TE, while glycine is seen at long TE. In addition, the lactate peak shows an inversion at intermediate TE, differentiating it from the lipid peak **(Table 8)**.

Magnetic resonance spectroscopy can be single-voxel spectroscopy (SVS) or multivoxel spectroscopy (MVS). A comparison between the two is shown in **Table 9**. Although there are indications for the use of each technique, more often, these are complementary to each other. For most cases, a combination of SVS at short TE and MVS at intermediate TE is appropriate.

TABLE 8: Various metabolites detected on magnetic resonance (MR) spectroscopy.

Metabolite	Peak resonance	Characteristic	Clinical significance
Creatine (Cr) and phosphocreatine (PCr)	3.0 and 3.9 singlet	Marker of brain metabolism	Decreased in hypoxic/ischemic injury, neoplasm, and trauma
Choline (Cho)	3.2 singlet	Required for membrane synthesis	• Decreased in hepatic encephalopathy, stroke, and SIADH • Increased in neoplasms, ischemic injury, demyelination, infections, and neonates
N-acetyl aspartate (NAA)	2.0 singlet	Indicative of normal neuronal function	• Decreased in hypoxia, ischemic injury, demyelination, neoplasms, trauma, and neurodegenerative disorder • Increased in Canavan's disease, PMD, normal developing infant brain
Lactate (Lac)	1.3 doublet inverted at TE 144 ms	Product of anaerobic metabolic activity	Increased in hypoxic/ischemic insult, hemorrhage, infections and neoplasms
Lipid	0.9–1.3	Indicates pathological process due to liberation of membrane lipids	Increased in necrotic neoplasm, lymphoma, tuberculoma, and brain abscess
Amino acids	0.9 doublet/triplet inverted at TE 144 ms	Necessary for protein synthesis	Increased in branched-chain ketonuria, MSUD, brain abscess
Succinate	2.4 single	Abscesses with anaerobic metabolism	Succinate >acetate indicative of parasitic abscesses
Acetate	1.9 singlet	Abscesses with anaerobic metabolism	Acetate >succinate indicative of pyogenic
Trehalose	3.6–3.8	Disaccharide	Fungal infections

(PMD: Pelizaeus–Merzbacher disease; SIADH: syndrome of inappropriate antidiuretic hormone secretion; TE: echo time)

TABLE 9: Difference between single-voxel spectroscopy (SVS) and multivoxel spectroscopy (MVS).

Technique	SVS	MVS
Voxel size (cm^3)	(4–20) large	(1–4) small
Scan time	Less	More
Lipid and water suppression	Good	poor
Processing	Simple	Time-consuming
Indications to use	• Single focal lesion or diffuse disease • Single query, e.g., abscess vs. tumor complementary to MRSI (e.g., different TE in SVS) • Areas close to the skull	• Multiple or heterogeneous lesions diffuse disease • Comparative assessment of brain regions required

(MRSI: magnetic resonance spectroscopic imaging; TE: echo-time)

Clinical Applications of Magnetic Resonance Spectroscopy [18,19]

- *Tumors*:
  - *Grading of tumors*: High choline peak with lipid and lactate in high-grade tumors **(Figs. 19A to C)**
  - *Differentiation between isocitrate dehydrogenase (IDH) mutant and wild-type astrocytomas* by showing 2-hydroxyglutarate (2-HG) peak resonating at 2.25 ppm in IDH-mutant astrocytoma
  - Alanine peak at 1.5 ppm in meningioma
  - Differentiation between metastasis and primary tumor with no abnormal spectroscopy findings in surrounding edema of metastasis
  - Planning of surgical biopsy from the lesion by demonstrating metabolite maps
  - The distinction between radiation necrosis and recurrence
- *Infections*:
  - Diagnosis of brain abscesses
  - Differentiation between pyogenic and tubercular abscesses **(Figs. 20A to D)**
  - Differentiate between NCC versus tuberculoma
- Pediatric disorders, e.g., Canavan disease, mitochondrial disorders, etc.
- Demyelinating diseases (active vs. chronic)
- Neurodegenerative disorders and dementia
- Epilepsy imaging
- Trauma
- Psychiatric disorders

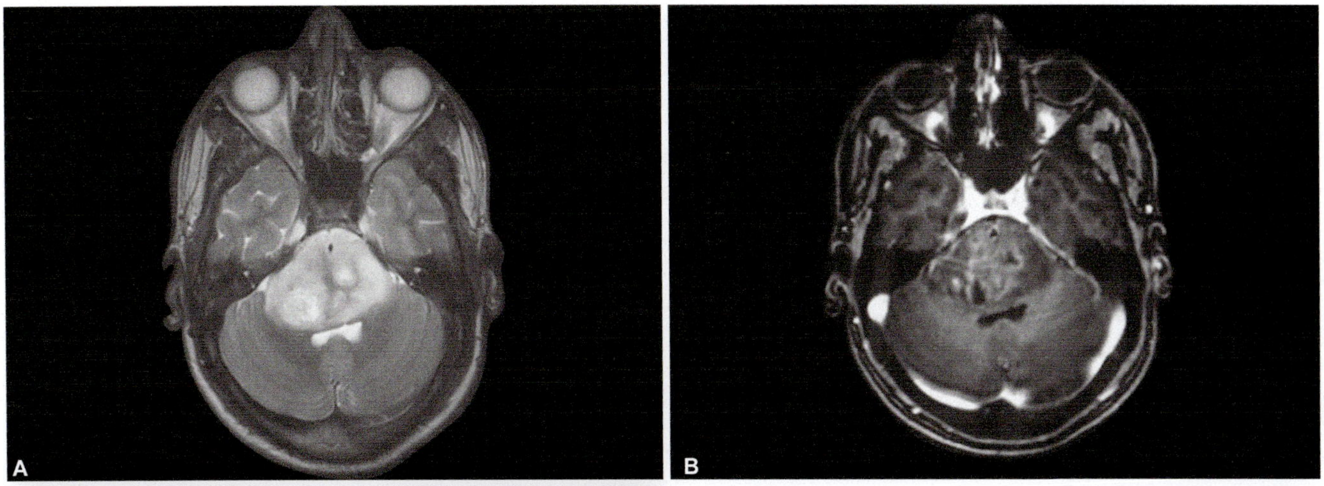

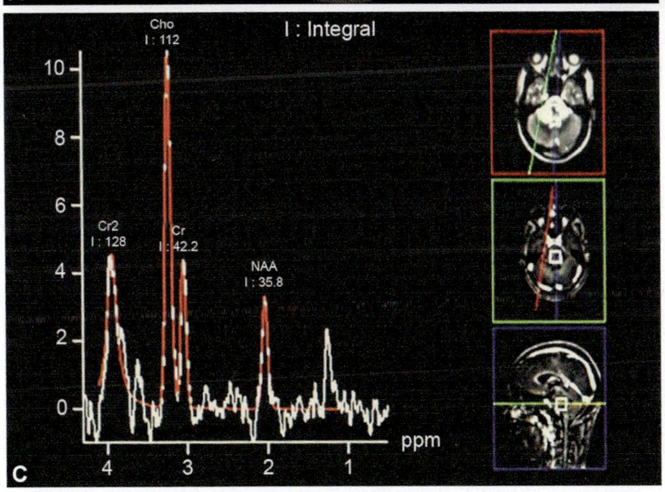

FIGS. 19A TO C: (A) Axial T2W images showing hyperintense expansile lesion in the pons region with encasement of the basilar artery; (B) Postcontrast axial images showing heterogeneous enhancement with necrotic areas; (C) Spectroscopy shows markedly raised choline peak with reduced N-acetyl aspartate (NAA) and presence of lactate peak suggestive of high-grade glioma.

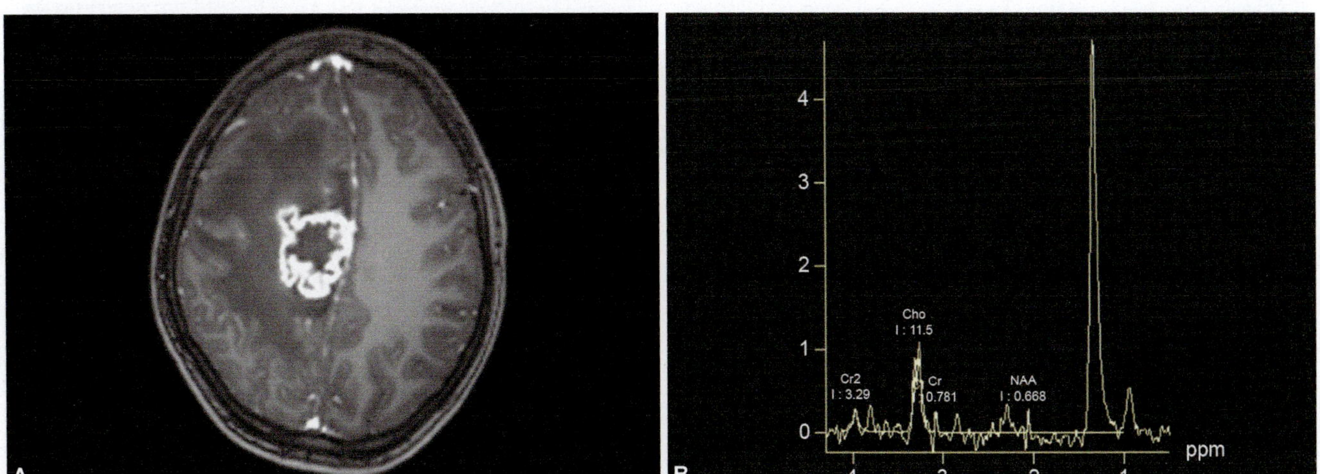

FIGS. 20A TO D: *Continued*

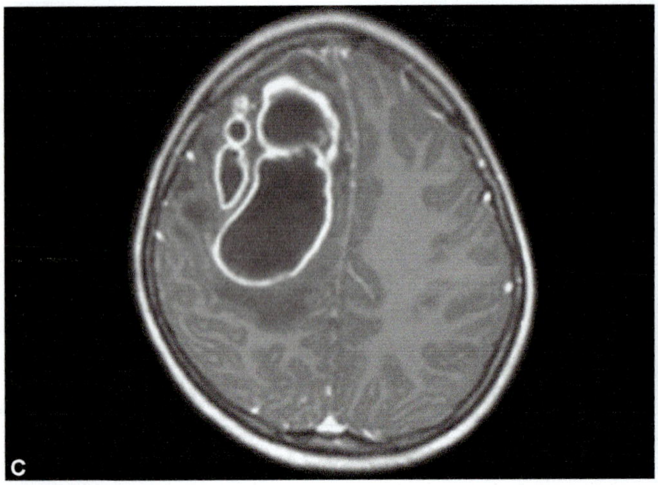

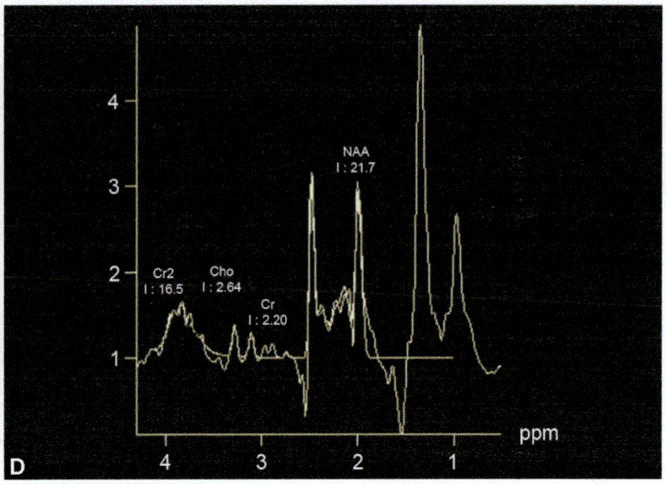

FIGS. 20A TO D: (A and B) Presence of ring enhancing lesion with magnetic resonance spectroscopy (MRS) showing prominent lipid peak suggestive of tubercular abscess; (C and D) Multiple ring enhancing lesions with MRS showing lipid/lactate and amino acid peaks suggestive of pyogenic abscess.

CONCLUSION

Computed tomography and MRI play an essential role in diagnosing and managing neurological disorders. It is crucial to have comprehensive knowledge of various primary and advanced techniques for the optimal imaging of the pathologies. These modalities should be judiciously used, keeping in mind the radiation hazards, contrast-related risks, and cost concerns to the patient.

REFERENCES

1. Bhattacharyya KB. Godfrey Newbold Hounsfield (1919-2004): The man who revolutionized neuroimaging. Ann Indian Acad Neurol. 2016;19(4):448-50.
2. Stockburger WT. CT imaging, then and now: a 30-year review of the economics of computed tomography. Radiol Manage. 2004;26(6):20-2.
3. Collins J. The history of MRI. Semin Roentgenol. 2008;43(4):259-60.
4. Ginat DT, Gupta R. Advances in computed tomography imaging technology. Annu Rev Biomed Eng. 2014;16:431-53.
5. Enterline DS, Kapoor G. A practical approach to CT angiography of the neck and brain. Tech Vasc Interv Radiol. 2006;9(4):192-204.
6. Madhuripan N, Atar OD, Zheng R, Tenenbaum M. Computed Tomography Angiography in Head and Neck Emergencies. Semin Ultrasound CT MR. 2017;38(4):345-56.
7. Miles KA. Brain perfusion: Computed tomography applications. Neuroradiology. 2004;46 (Suppl 2):s194-200.
8. Cianfoni A, Colosimo C, Basile M, Wintermark M, Bonomo L. Brain perfusion CT: principles, technique and clinical applications. Radiol Med. 2007;112(8):1225-43.
9. Krishnan P, Murphy A, Aviv RI. CT-based Techniques for Brain Perfusion. Top Magn Reson Imaging. 2017;26(3):113-9.
10. Jackson EF, Ginsberg LE, Schomer DF, Leeds NE. A review of MRI pulse sequences and techniques in neuroimaging. Surg Neurol. 1997;47(2):185-99.
11. Essig M, Nikolaou K, Meaney JF. Magnetic resonance angiography of the head and neck vessels. Eur Radiol. 2007;17 (Suppl 2):B30-7.
12. Hartung MP, Grist TM, François CJ. Magnetic resonance angiography: current status and future directions. J Cardiovasc Magn Reson. 20119;13(1):19.
13. Dmytriw AA, Sawlani V, Shankar J. Diffusion-weighted imaging of the brain: Beyond stroke. Can Assoc Radiol J. 2017;68(2):131-46.
14. Tournier JD. Diffusion MRI in the brain—theory and concepts. Prog Nucl Magn Reson Spectrosc. 2019;112-113:1-16.
15. Robinson RJ, Bhuta S. Susceptibility-weighted imaging of the brain: current utility and potential applications. J Neuroimaging. 2011;21(4):e189-204.
16. Cha S. Perfusion MR imaging: basic principles and clinical applications. Magn Reson Imaging Clin N Am. 2003;11(3):403-13.
17. Lanzman B, Heit JJ. Advanced MRI measures of cerebral perfusion and their clinical applications. Top Magn Reson Imaging. 2017;26(2):83-90.
18. Zhu H, Barker PB. MR spectroscopy and spectroscopic imaging of the brain. Methods Mol Biol. 2011;711:203-26.
19. Gupta RK, Jobanputra KJ, Yadav A. MR spectroscopy in brain infections. Neuroimaging Clin N Am. 2013;23(3):475-98.

116
CHAPTER

Vascular Imaging

Riddhi Patel, Narayan Deshmukh, Rakesh Singh

INTRODUCTION

Vascular disorders of brain and spine are commonly encountered in clinical practice. These often present as neurological emergencies. It is important to choose imaging modality wisely from available armamentarium.

Vascular imaging of brain and spinal cord gives information regarding angiographic architecture, which helps in better understanding of pathophysiology and better treatment modalities. Present chapter aims to impart basic information about vascular imaging and compare various modalities in vascular disorders.

COMPUTED TOMOGRAPHIC ANGIOGRAPHY

Computed tomographic angiography (CTA) is a noninvasive, relatively rapid method for evaluating head and neck vasculature. CTA offers advantage over magnetic resonance angiography (MRA) in presence of metallic implants like cardiac, orthopedic, and neuroimplants like stent and flow diverter (FD) where MRA is not possible or stent artifact shows (in FD and stent).

Technique

Helical computed tomography (CT) scanner acquires images from neck to vertex of the head within few minutes. CT parameters use a slice (collimated) thickness of 1–3 mm with a pitch of 1–2. A volume of contrast requires 100–150 mL to be injected at a rate of 2–3 mL/s. Image acquisition uses detection of bolus arrival and subsequent triggering of data acquisition. Techniques such as thin-slab maximum intensity projection (MIP), three-dimensional (3D) volume rendering, and multiplanar reformatting help in making 2D and 3D images. 4D CTA by 320 detectors is dynamic scanning with high-spatial and temporal resolution.

Clinical Applications

Acute Ischemic Stroke

Indication for vascular imaging in acute ischemic stroke (AIS) is to look for large-vessel occlusion. CT scan demonstrates bleed better, ischemic infarcts may appear prominently after 6 hours. Patients who are candidates for mechanical thrombectomy should undergo CT angiography to rule out proximal large vessel [internal cerebral artery, M1 segment of middle cerebral artery (MCA), and basilar artery] occlusion. **Figure 1** shows MCA hyperdense sign which is seen in acute stroke similar to basilar hyperdense sign.

Computed tomographic angiography is an alternative to MRA for AIS patients by rapid imaging and early treatment implications. The rapid imaging time has resulted in a significant escalation in the use of this modality during acute strokes. CTA source images (CTA-SIs) provide enhancement in the brain vasculature, which shows an

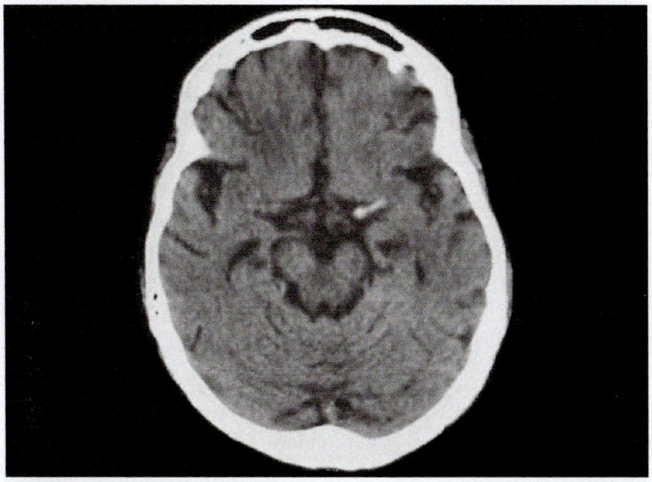

FIG. 1: CT scan showing left MCA hyperdense sign in case of acute infarct.

(CT: computed tomography; MCA: middle cerebral artery)

ischemic region with poor collaterals and there is no need for a second bolus injection for CT perfusion. The sensitivity of CTA-SI and diffusion-weighted images (DWIs) when directly compared has shown equal in detecting ischemia, but DWI is better for posterior fossa and smaller infarcts.

The 10-point Clot Burden Score (CBS) helps in determining prognosis in acute stroke by predicting final infarct size, functional outcome, and hematoma risk.[1] The Alberta Stroke Program Early CT Score (ASPECTS) is a 10-point score used in patients with MCA stroke.[2] A similar semiquantitative scoring system for patients presenting with acute basilar artery occlusion is termed the posterior circulation-ASPECTS. Various trials of acute stroke had different inclusion criteria such as various trial for mechanical thrombectomy in acute ischemic stroke used CTA for diagnosing large vessel occlusion (LVO) and perfusion imaging to identify infarct core, mismatch volume and penumbra.

The 4D-CTA (whole-brain dynamic time-resolved CTA) provides hemodynamic information on leptomeningeal collateral status as well as the extent of any retrograde flow.[3] Leptomeningeal collaterals and cross-flow from other vessels are important prognostic markers for outcome of AIS and success of mechanical thrombectomy. Multiphase CT angiography (mCTA) is an imaging technique that helps in the identification of patients who will be benefited from mechanical thrombectomy by evaluating the degree and extent of pial arterial filling in the whole brain in a time-resolved manner. mCTA is superior to single-phase CTA due to possibility to prognosticate, better inter-rater reliability, and identification of distal vessel occlusion ("delayed vessel sign").

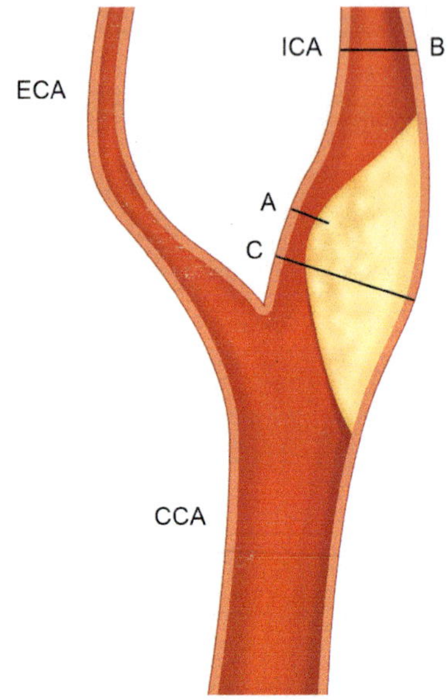

FIG. 2: Methods of measuring the degree of internal carotid artery (*ICA*) stenosis at contrast angiography. European Carotid Surgery Trial (*ECST*) method compares residual lumen (A) with original luminal diameter (C). North American Symptomatic Carotid Endarterectomy Trial (*NASCET*) method compares A with the distal internal carotid artery B.

(ECA: external carotid artery; CCA: common carotid artery)

Intra- and Extracranial Circulation

Atherosclerotic stenosis of extracranial vessels occurs commonly at origin of major vessels. The atherosclerotic plaque composition varies. Presence of calcified plaque can confound the degree of stenosis estimation by various modalities. Intracranial stenosis can cause reduced flow in vessel proximal to stenosis and, hence, may lead to inaccurate estimation of stenosis severity. CTA is primarily used to assess the severity of stenosis and to plan intervention. CTA is better than transcranial Doppler (TCD) in detecting intracranial stenosis due to high false-negative rate in later ones.[4] For extracranial diseases, CTA complements digital subtraction angiography (DSA) and alternative to MRA. Severity of carotid stenosis can be graded by North American Symptomatic Carotid Endarterectomy Trial (NASCET) or European Carotid Surgery Trial (ECST) (after ECST) criteria **(Fig. 2)**. Distal intracranial occlusion may appear as occlusion in proximal segment due to sluggish flow.

In dissections of the cervicocephalic arteries, there is narrowed eccentric arterial lumen in the presence of a thickened vessel wall, with occasional detection of a dissecting aneurysm. Dissections may be associated with narrowing of vessel with or without thrombus in the lumen.

Other steno-occlusive vascular disorders like fibromuscular dysplasia (FMD) may be detected unknown sensitivity and specificity. CTA may become difficult to detect skull base dissection because of artifacts.

Aneurysm

Aneurysms can present as unruptured, detected on incidental imaging, with subarachnoid hemorrhage (SAH), or with compression effects. CT and CTA is often performed as initial imaging modality to know the aneurysm characteristics, presence of bleed, or extent of mass effect. Aneurysm characteristics such as site, size, shape, dome-to-neck ratio, presence of mural thrombi, branch at the neck, and relation with skull may be well appreciated on CTA. The incorporation of 3D volume-rendered images provides better anatomy characteristics of an aneurysm which helps in guiding treatment options. Distal aneurysms are difficult to detect on CTA.

Postoperative aneurysm follow-up by CTA is a cost-effective, noninvasive alternative to DSA; however, DSA remains the gold standard. CTA had limited accuracy for small aneurysms (<3 mm)[5] with high false positivity (anterior communicating artery or basilar artery bifurcation) and false negativity [cavernous segment internal carotid artery (ICA) and MCA regions]. CTA is a good alternative to TCD to diagnose vasospasm.

CTA has diagnostic limitations in detecting small aneurysms, in postoperative assessment of residual neck of aneurysm, luminal patency of parent artery, specially due to coil and stent artifacts.

Intracerebral hemorrhage (ICH): CT is gold standard for ICH. It can diagnose various pathologies simultaneously. Acute ICH patients are at increased risk for hematoma expansion. Spot sign described as tiny foci which is enhancing within hematoma with or without clear contrast extravasation predicts the hematoma expansion.[7]

Cerebral Venous Sinus Thrombosis

Computed tomography scan is best imaging modality for detecting acute parenchymal hemorrhage, which can accompany venous sinus thrombosis. Spiral CT with acquisition is a single-section system which has limited spatial and temporal resolution. Multidetector CTA (MDCTA) may be equivalent to MR venography (MRV) in visualizing cerebral sinuses, but may have limited role in cavernous sinus, deep cerebral veins, and cortical venous thrombosis. The MDCTA has the advantage of visualizing arterial and venous phase simultaneously after single injection and shorter acquisition time. False-negative result can occur with subacute thrombus which may show enhancement after contrast administration and no filling defect. MDCTA with noncontrast CT helps in detecting presence of a spontaneously hyperattenuated clot to avoid dilemma with enhanced sinus known as cord sign [seen in 25–56% of acute cerebral venous thrombosis (CVT) cases].[8] Computed tomography venography (CTV) is helpful in visualizing filling defect (empty delta sign) in sinus in case of suspected CVT. Empty delta sign is a triangular area of contrast enhancement that surrounds a hypoattenuating area.

Vascular Malformations

Common indications for CTA include arteriovenous malformation (AVM), cavernoma, arteriovenous (AV) fistulas, etc. Vascular malformations present with hemorrhage at atypical sites (other than pons, basal ganglia, thalamus, and cerebellum) or typical sites in normotensive patients. Imaging is required to define nature of malformation, its exact site, extent, characteristics of feeding artery, presence of nidus, draining vein, presence of dysplastic vessels, or aneurysms. CTA has sensitivities of 96% and 87% for unruptured and ruptured AVMs, respectively. 4D CTA evaluates angioarchitecture and draining veins. For large AVMs (>3 cm), sensitivity is approximately 100%. CTA has limitations in evaluating arterial feeders, nidus, and draining veins. The sensitivity is 88% in diagnosing associated aneurysms.[9] CTA has limited utility in diagnosis of dural arteriovenous fistula (DAVF). The Spetzler–Martin (SM) grade is commonly used for cerebral AVMs[10] in which AVM is classified as 1–5 **(Table 1)**. This scale mainly assesses the risk of post surgical morbidity, and not the risk of hemorrhage.

TABLE 1: Spetzler–Martin grading scale for AVM.

Variable	Spetzler–Martin grading scale	
	Definition	**Points**
AVM size	<3 cm	1
	3–6 cm	2
	>6 cm	3
Deep venous drainage	No	0
	Yes	1
Eloquence	No	0
	Yes	1

(AVM: arteriovenous malformation)

Computed tomography has limited role in cavernoma due to low specificity as can mimic low-grade glioma, hemorrhage, and granuloma. However, it is useful in case of proven cavernoma to look for bleeding.

Limitations

CT imaging in patients with metallic implants such as clips, coils, and stents is safe (shown in **Figs. 3A to C**), but may lead to artifacts (more with cobalt than titanium). It can be reduced by adjusting gantry and taking thin sections (depends on operator). The degree of artificial lumen narrowing is inversely proportional to stent diameter. CT scan is contraindicated in pregnancy due to high risk of radiation exposure.

Due to the risk of contrast-induced nephropathy (CIN), it is mandatory to check serum creatinine levels before imaging. Precautions are required in patients who have a creatinine level >1.5 g/dL or an estimated glomerular filtration rate (GFR) <60 mL/min/1.73 m^2. Patients with chronic kidney disease (CKD) who are on dialysis should undergo hemodialysis as early as possible after the CTA to decrease the contrast exposure.[11]

MAGNETIC RESONANCE ANGIOGRAPHY

Magnetic resonance angiography (MRA) is a noninvasive imaging technique of vascular imaging without risk of radiation exposure.

Technique

Noncontrast-enhanced *MRA* is performed by time-of-flight (TOF) angiography, phase contrast (PC) angiography, and 3D electrocardiograph-triggered half-Fourier fast spin echo. Usually, these techniques are time-consuming as compared with contrast-enhanced (CE) MRA.

The TOF is the most commonly used noncontrast enhancement MRA technique. With TOF, both arteries

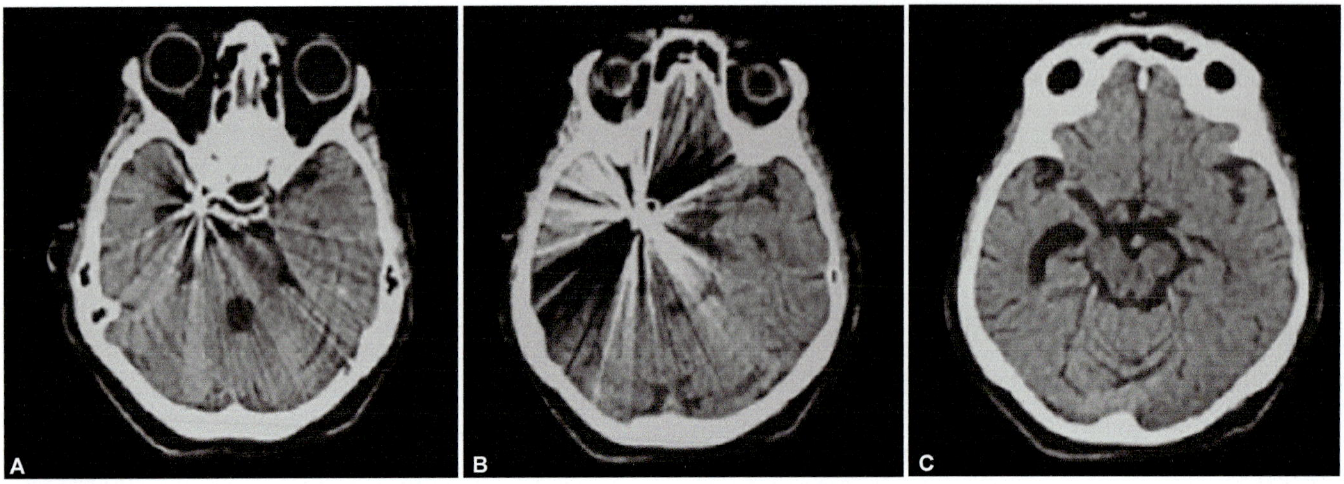

FIGS. 3A TO C: CT brain plain showing artifacts related to coils.
(CT: computed tomography)

and veins are seen with high-spatial resolution but provide no details regarding directional or flow velocity quantity. TOF image acquisition is due to effect of unsaturated spins inflowing into a region of saturated stationary spins. TOF has superior spatial resolution and decreased scan time as compared to phase contrast image acquisition. 3D TOF is preferred for the evaluation of intracranial arterial vasculature because of its higher spatial resolution, whereas 2D TOF is better for the evaluation of extracranial circulation because of its sensitivity to slower-flowing blood.

New TOF-based techniques, such as the hybrid of opposite contrast (HOP) MRA or the simultaneous TOF susceptibility-weighted imaging (SWI), are hoping to provide wide applications. PC is based on the phase shift acquired by spins moving along a magnetic field gradient which can be used to visualize and quantify arterial and venous blood flow as well as cerebrospinal fluid flow (helps in the understanding of normal physiology and for accessing altered hemodynamics). 4D flow MRI based on PC sequence promises to expand the range of applications of PC-MRA imaging. **Figure 4** is showing the normal intra- and extracranial circulation.

Contrast-enhanced MRA is a technique that involves 3D spoiled gradient echo (GE) sequences, with the administration of gadolinium-based contrast agents allowing shorter image acquisition time by perfect bolus time and fast image acquisition. The scan time after the bolus infusion of a gadolinium contrast agent (0.1–0.2 mmol/kg) per 3D volume is 5–10 minutes, and data is acquired in the first 10–15 minutes.

The MR cerebral venography can be contrast-enhanced or noncontrast sequences to assess the patency of the dural venous sinuses and cerebral veins.

The availability of MRI scanners with 3.0T or even higher field strengths (up to 7T) in selected centers may provide higher signal-to-noise ratios and parallel imaging.[12] 7T TOF-MRA provides better visualization of the large vessels

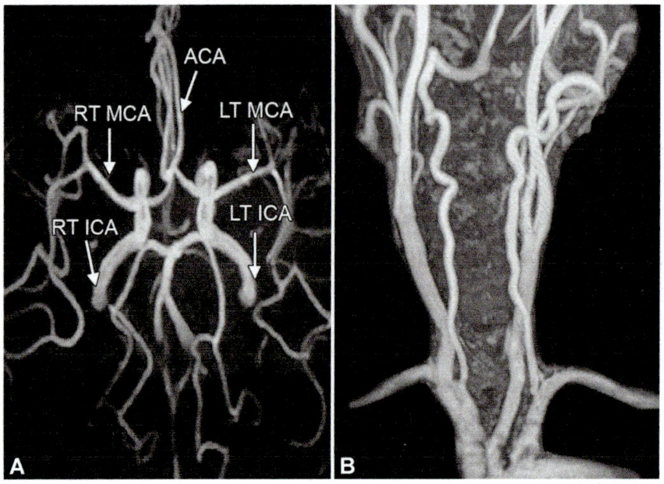

FIGS. 4A AND B: MRA showing normal intra- and extracranial vessels.
(ACA: anterior cerebral artery; ICA: internal carotid artery; MCA: middle cerebral artery; MRA: magnetic resonance angiography)

of the circle of Willis with significantly more first- and second-order branches and recognizes diminutive vessels in hypertensive patients.

Recently, 4D MRA (time-resolved or dynamic CE-MRA) is a vascular imaging method under investigation that uses novel processing techniques to achieve sub-second (60 times faster) temporal resolution while maintaining high-spatial resolution, 3T allows better characterization of various vascular lesions.[13]

Clinical Applications

Acute Ischemic Stroke

Magnetic resonance angiography offers better parenchymal visualization and delineates infarct site and size earliest with DWI sequencing. The CE-MRA may be better for localizing vessel occlusion, collateral vessels, and extracranial vessels.[14]

MRI and MRA of the brain are helpful in prognostication and in guiding treatment. TOF-MRA, rather than CE-MRA, is more commonly used for patients with an acute stroke which has higher sensitivity (81%) and specificity (95%), respectively.[15] A dynamic MRA method for AIS is being researched which showed a fast and reliable method of detecting cerebral hemodynamics and collateral circulation guide in thrombectomy patients. Currently, researchers are going to optimize rapid combined MRI and MRA stroke protocols with a shorter acquisition time. MRA takes slightly longer time than CTA. It can overestimate the degree of extracranial stenosis. Flow-related artifacts can miss precise localization in distal ICA occlusion. Large-vessel occlusion (LVO) detection is a major aspect in treatment of stroke vascular imaging.

Intracranial and Extracranial Circulation

The TOF 3D CE-MRA is better compared to 2D and 3D TOF-MRA for carotid arterial stenosis. Critical stenosis and plaque characteristics (e.g., ulcerated plaque and plaque hemorrhage) in case of arterial occlusions are easily identified by MRA. TOF-MRA MIP images show intravascular flow gaps in high-grade stenosis, which can be dealt with CE-MRA which has sensitivity and specificity values equivalent to CTA in determining the severity of stenosis.[16] **Figures 5 and 6** are showing the intracranial and extracranial stenosis, respectively. **Figure 7** shows intraluminal thrombus in MRA. MRA may overestimate the degree of stenosis. Intraluminal clot may be missed. Highly calcified plaque overestimates stenosis. Intracranial critical stenosis may dampen flow-related signal proximal

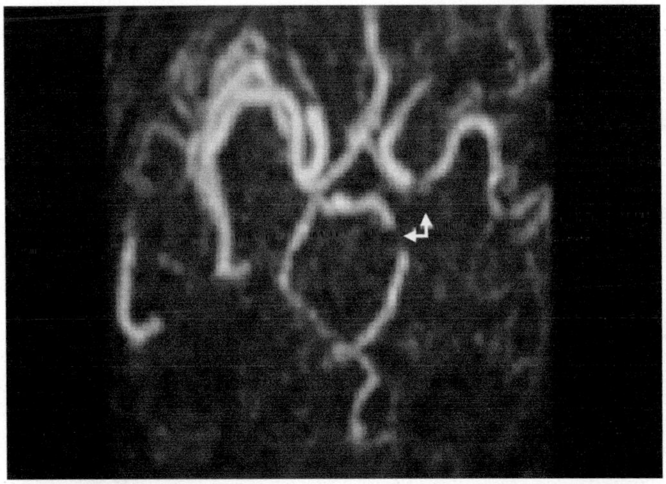

FIG. 5: MRA suggestive of intracranial vessel stenosis in MCA and PCA (shown by white arrow).

(MCA: middle cerebral artery; MRA: magnetic resonance angiography; PCA: posterior cerebral artery)

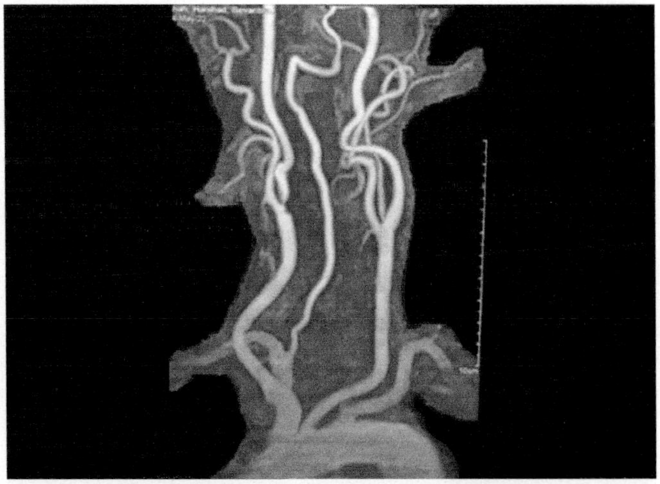

FIG. 6: MRA showing right ICA origin severe stenosis.

(MRA: magnetic resonance angiography; ICA: internal carotid artery)

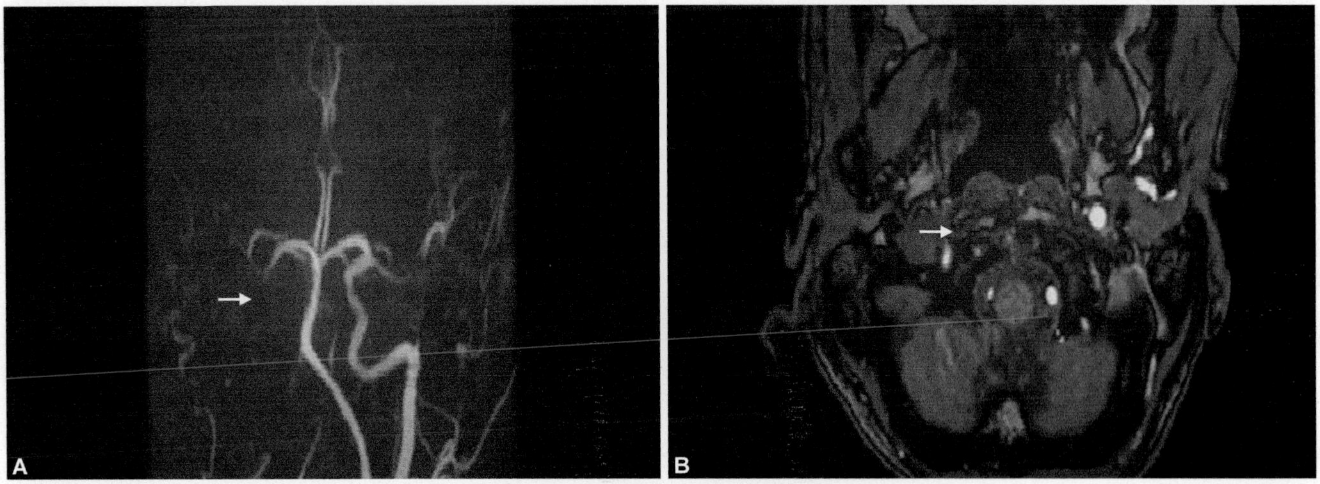

FIGS. 7A AND B: MRA showing absent right ICA flow and axial section showing thrombus in the vessel.

(MRA: magnetic resonance angiography; ICA: internal carotid artery)

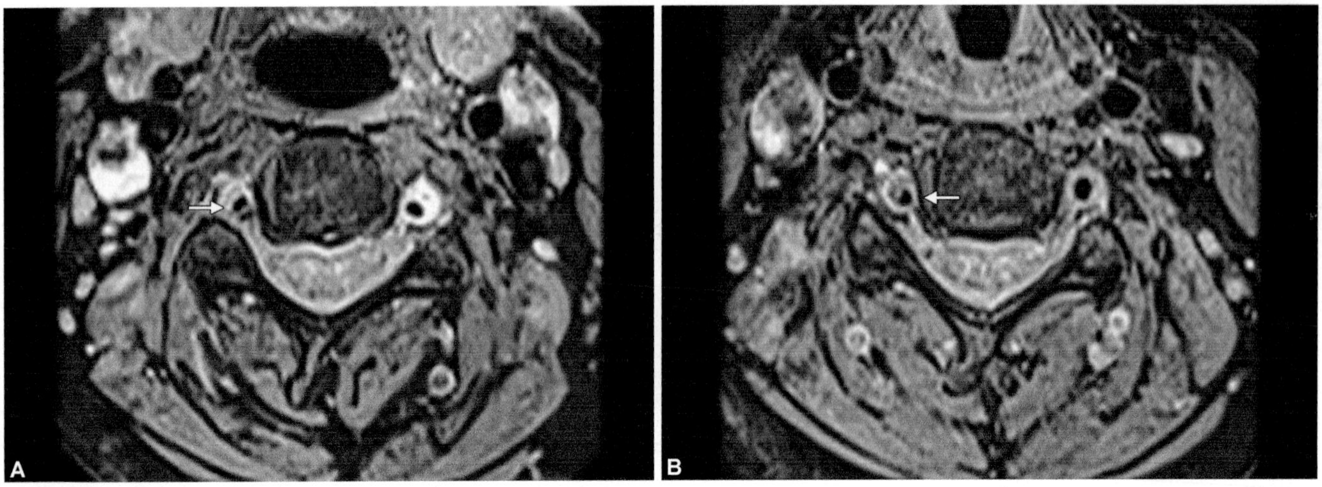

FIGS. 8A AND B: Dissection.

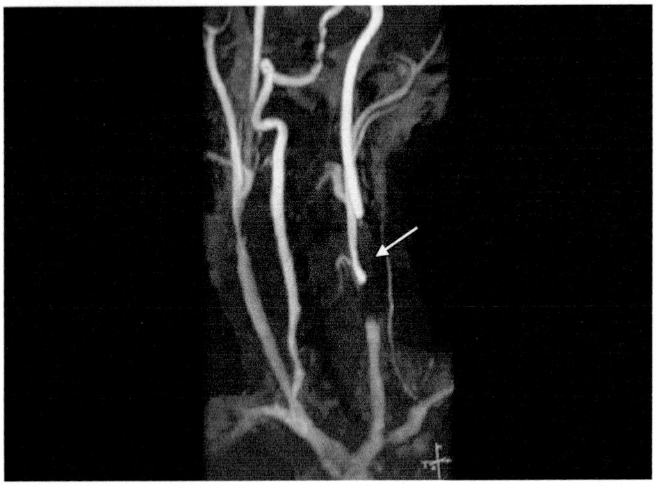

FIG. 9: MRA showing stent artifact (shown by white arrow).
(MRA: magnetic resonance angiography)

to stenosis and it may be visualized as long-segment stenosis. Benefits of parenchymal visualization, especially fluid-attenuated inversion recovery (FLAIR) images, are advantages of MRA.

In carotid or vertebral artery dissection, patient's fat-saturation sequences with CE-MRA help in characterizing intramural hematoma, clots, associated aneurysm, and features of the residual lumen[17] (as shown in **Figs. 8A and B**). T1-weighted images in addition to the above help in subacute hyperintense thrombus to eliminate the high-signal intensity from perivascular adipose tissue. Serial MRA scans may be performed during follow-up to see vascular recanalization and morphology of dissecting aneurysm at the site of hematoma.

After carotid stenting, MRA assessment of vascular stenosis shows turbulence and susceptibility artifacts due to metals **(Fig. 9)**. FMD detection by MRA remains unclear.[18]

Aneurysm T2*

Noninvasive imaging evaluation includes a review of T1- and T2-weighted (fast) spin-echo images, source images, MIP images, and T2*-weighted GE for the aneurysm detection. 3D TOF-MRA is evaluated for aneurysm detection, but the disadvantages are long scanning time and sometimes difficulty to distinguish between patent lumen, high-grade stenosis, and occlusion. False-positive (infundibulum and loops) and false-negative aneurysms are more commonly noted at the skull base and MCA.[19] For patients with SAH, 3T TOF-MRA with 3D volume is better for detecting aneurysms. Certain characteristics of an aneurysm such as sac shape, aneurysm neck detection, and visualization of branches originating at the sac or neck are better seen with CE-MRA than TOF-MRA.[20] TOF-MRA has low sensitivity for the detection of intracranial aneurysms <3 mm. Artifacts from coil embolization are less in 3T MRA compared to 1.5T MRA.[21] TOF-MRA is better for the localization of coil mass (as it is not related to contrast bolus accuracy). 4D MRA may help in follow-up for aneurysm re-canalization, and coil mass. Intra-aneurysmal flow disruption devices and FD are associated with more artifacts than coils.

Magnetic resonance angiography is important for parenchymal disease, presence of infarction, compression by aneurysm. However, MRA is less sensitive and specific compared to CTA.

Vascular Malformations

Routine MRA methods (2D and 3D TOF-MRA and PC-MRA) are an alternative option to DSA for evaluation of all components of AVM—feeding arteries, nidus, and draining veins **(Figs. 10A to C)**. For the patient who received any kind of treatment using surgery, embolization, or radiosurgery, 4D MRA is a noninvasive method for demonstrating the residual AVM, but as of now, the problems are low-spatial resolution and vessel superposition.[22]

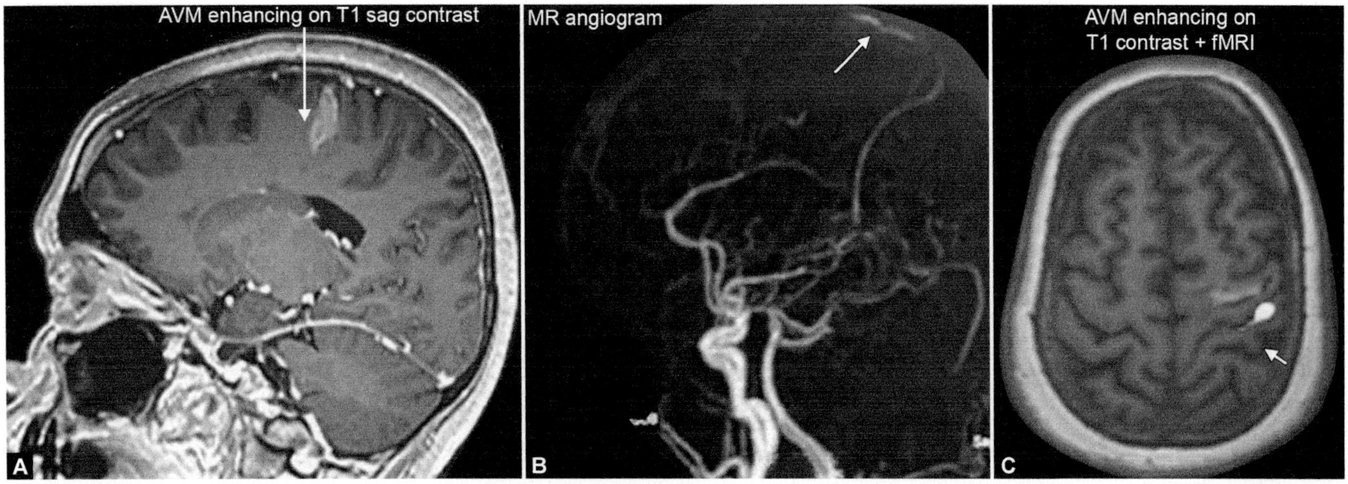

FIGS. 10A TO C: Interval imaging after 6 weeks is done to identify the eloquent cortex for open surgery. T1 postcontrast sagittal view showing sickle-shaped enhancement surrounding the AVM in precentral sulcus region white arrow (A). MR angiogram showing prominent early filling vein in sagittal section; white arrow (B). fMRI showed right hand and leg area very close to sulcal AVM (C).

(AVM: arteriovenous malformation; fMRI: functional magnetic resonance imaging)

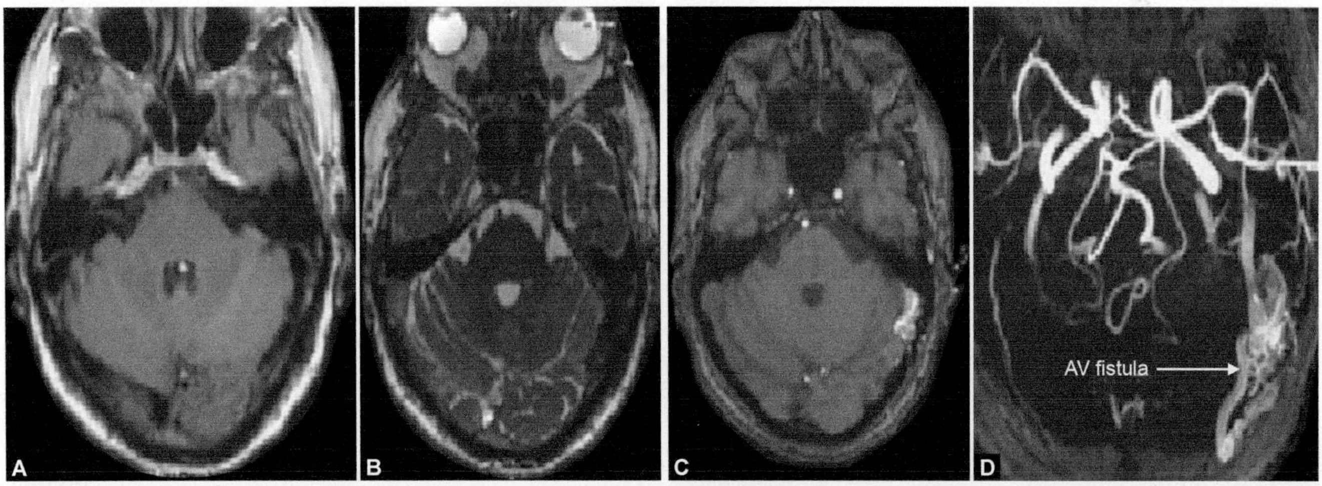

FIGS. 11A TO D: MRI in patients of left transverse sinus DAVF in patient with long-standing tinnitus—T1 (A) and T2 (B) hypointense structure on the left occipital region suggestive of dilated venous end of the fistula is enhancing following contrast injection (C). MRA showing complete fistula with arterial supply and venous drainage (D).

(DAVF: dural arteriovenous fistula; MRA: magnetic resonance angiography)

In Dural arterio-venous fistulas (DAVFs), arterial feeders not visible on spin-echo MRA are sometimes detected on 3D TOF-MRA.[23] Few sinuses such as transverse and sigmoid sinus occlusion and dilated cortical veins are better seen by MRA than spin-echo imaging but none is closer to DSA. **Figures 11A to D** are showing DAVF with fistulous component. The findings of cavernous sinus fistulas should be interpreted cautiously because of the lack of specificity. Cerebral cavernous venous malformations, usually known as cavernous hemangiomas or cavernomas, have characteristic appearance on the MRI as shown in **Figures 12A to E**.

Venous Disorders

MR venography with or without contrast is most commonly done for venous sinus thrombosis. It gives good additional information about parenchymal involvement. Contrast venography may help in distinguishing between hypoplastic sinus and complete/partial thrombosed sinus. Follow-up imaging in persistently symptomatic patients may show a developing arteriovenous fistula (AVF). Venography may help in diagnosing transverse sinus stenosis causing idiopathic intracranial hypertension (IIH) (to look for thrombus or stenosis; **Figs. 13A to C**).

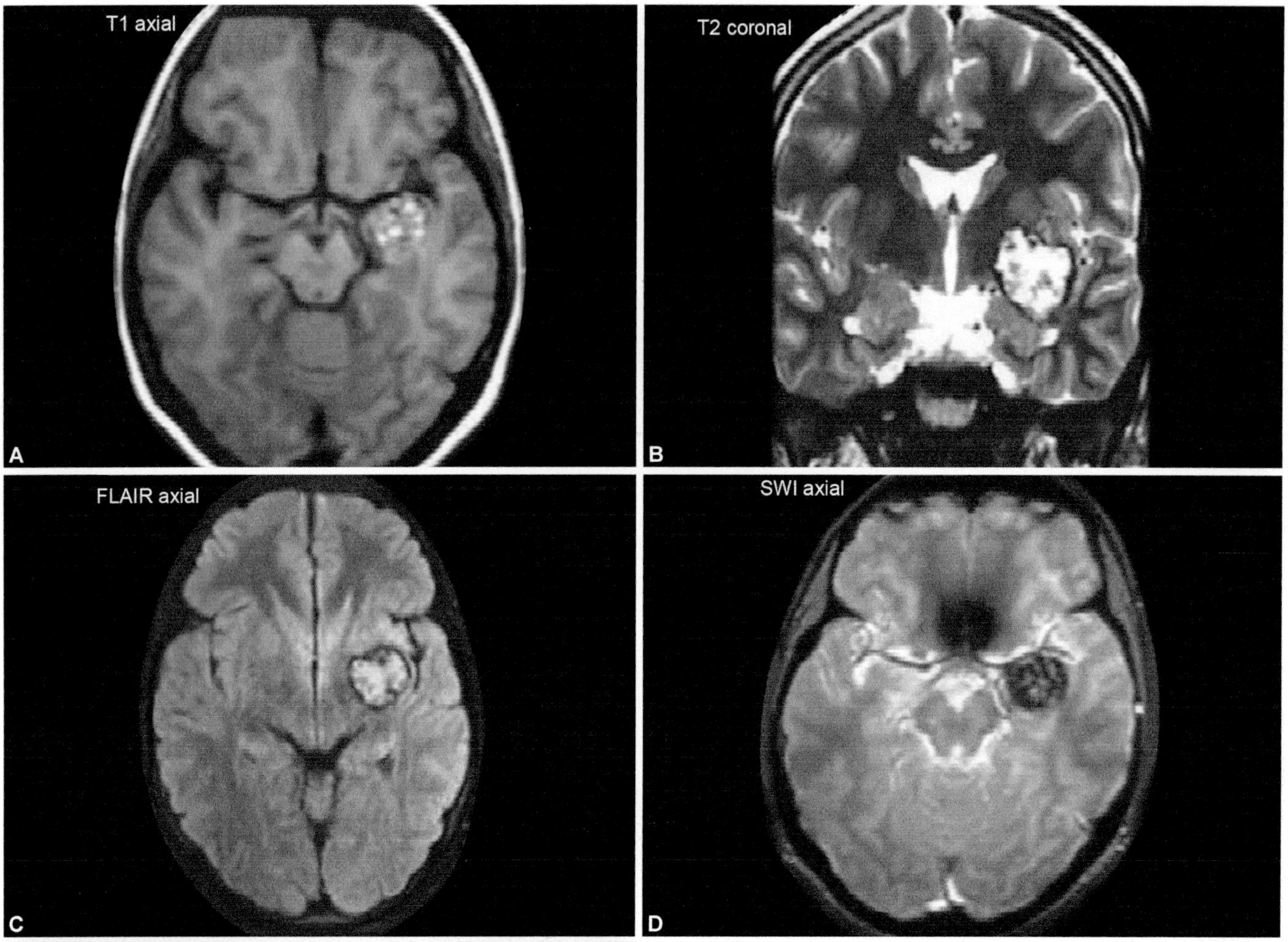

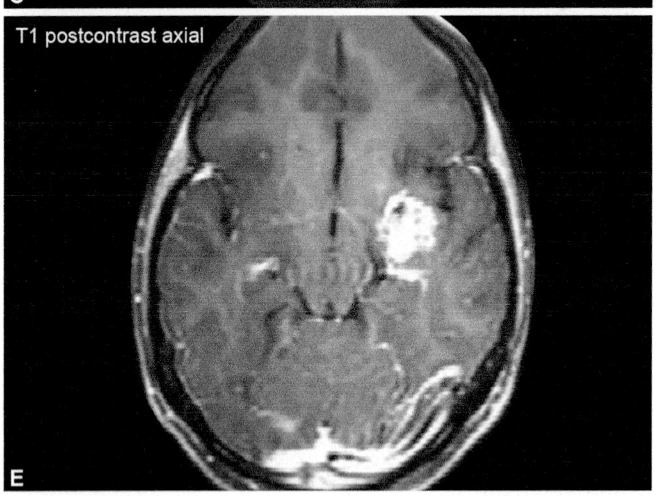

FIGS. 12A TO E: Cavernoma—presented with seizures. MRI showed T1-hyperintense dots (A), T2-mixed density hyper- and hypointense regions (B), FLAIR showing popcorn calcification (C). SWI showing blooming (D) and diffuse enhancement of postcontrast (E).

(FLAIR: fluid-attenuated inversion recovery; SWI: susceptibility-weighted imaging)

Spinal Cord Disorders

Spinal MRA along with MRI helps in localizing the vascular pathology. It may give valuable information before performing digital subtraction angiography.[25] **(Fig. 14)**. TOF pulse sequence MRA is better in visualizing abnormally enlarged and tortuous veins draining DAVFs and intramedullary AVMs.

Vessel Wall Imaging

Newer pulse sequences and specifically black blood sequence MRI of intracranial vessels are very important in understanding the pathophysiology of many vasculopathy and differentiate intracranial atherosclerosis **(Figs. 15A and B)**, aneurysms, vasculitis [reversible cerebral vasoconstriction syndrome (RCVS)] and vasculopathy,

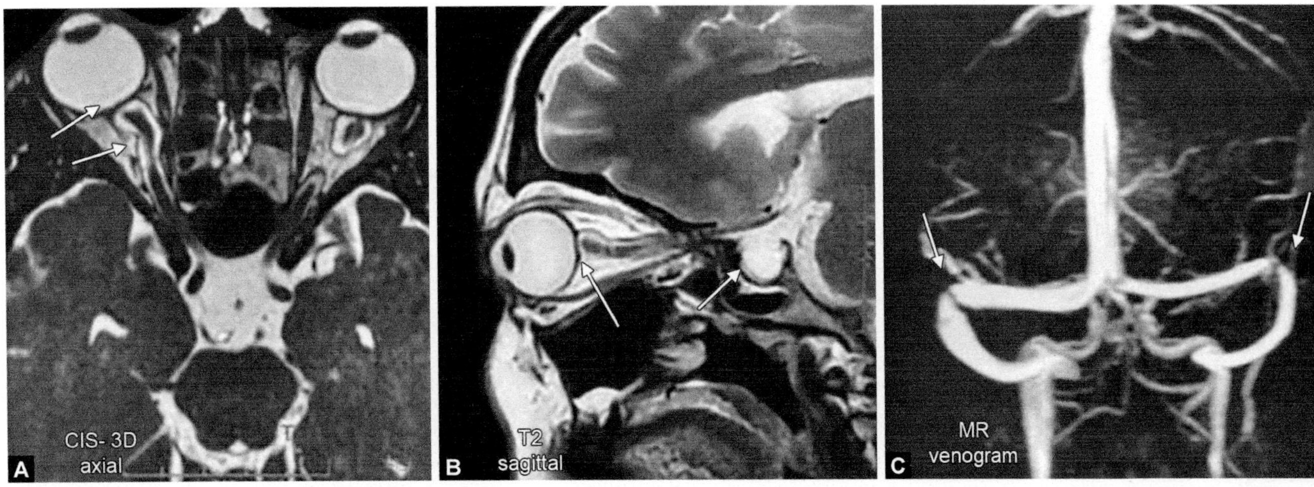

FIGS. 13A TO C: MRI in IIH: Signs of raised ICP like flattening of optic disk, prominent optic nerve sheath, kinking of optic nerve (A) white arrow (B), and empty sella on T2 orbital cuts (C) white arrow, and MR venogram showed absent flow in bilateral transverse sigmoid junction white arrows.

(ICP: intracranial pressure; IIH: idiopathic intracranial hypertension)

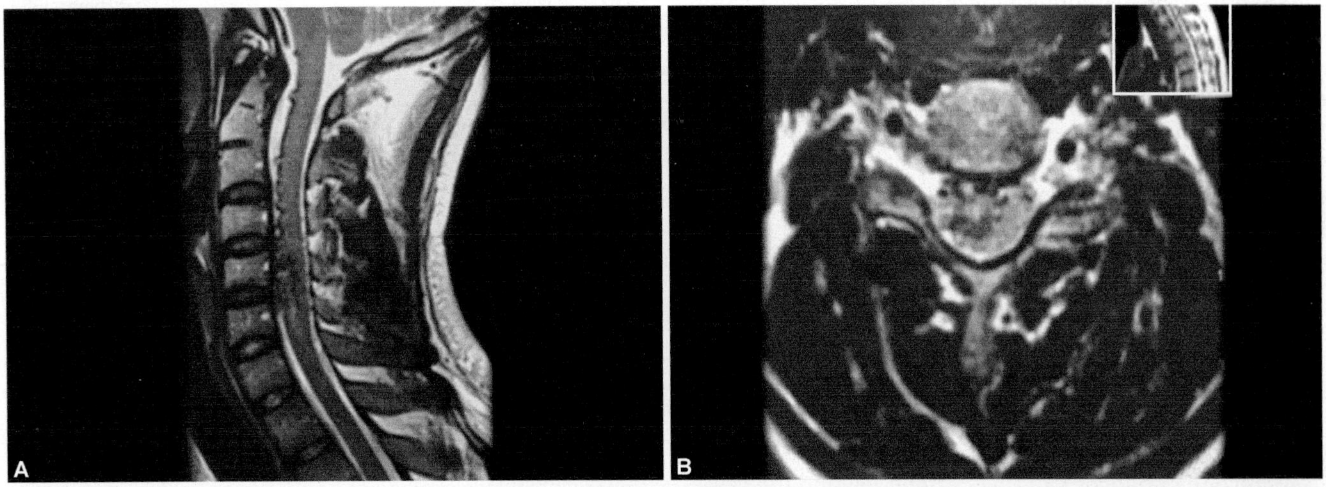

FIGS. 14A AND B: MRI T2 cervical spine sagittal and axial sections showing flow voids on anterior aspect extending from C1 to C4 region with glomus like vascular network suggestive of AVM.

(AVM: arteriovenous malformation)

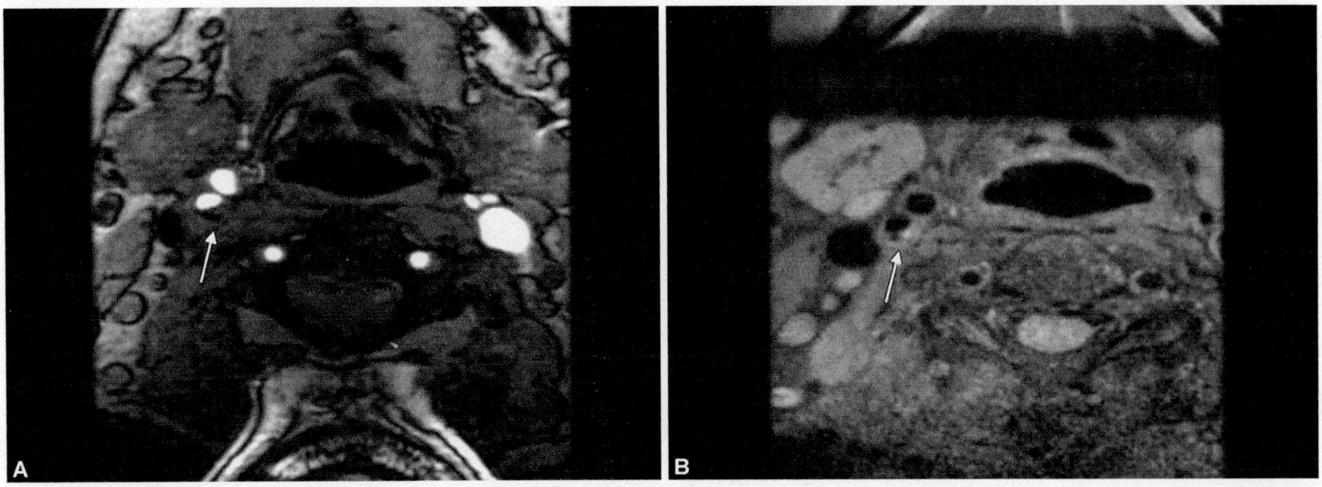

FIGS. 15A AND B: Vessel wall imaging showing right-sided ICA atherosclerotic plaque with intraplaque hemorrhage (shown by right arrow).

(ICA: internal carotid artery)

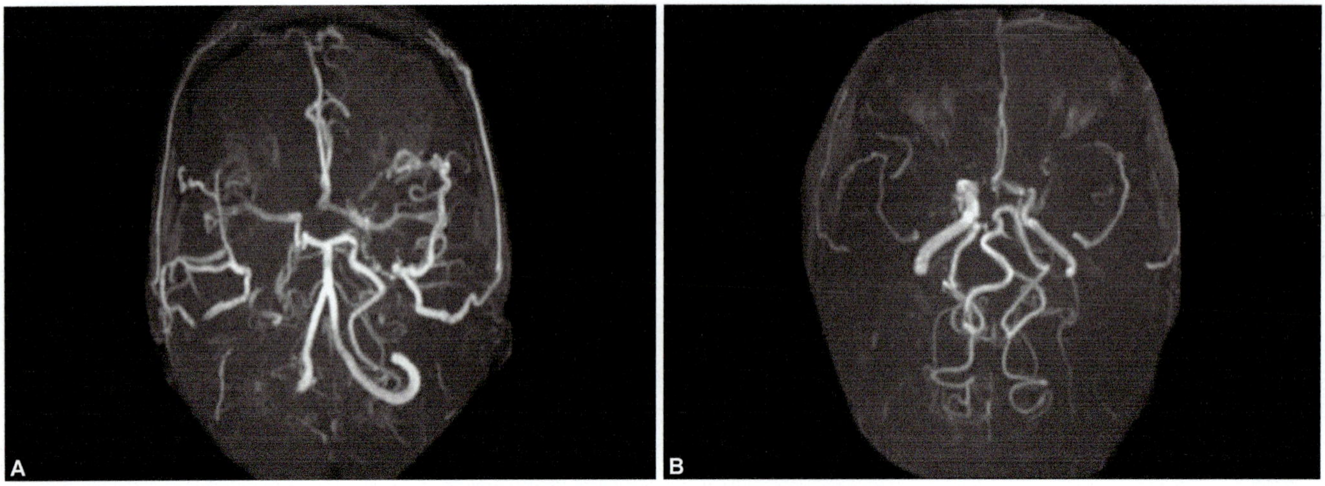

FIGS. 16A AND B: MRA of moyamoya showing supraclinoid ICA stenosis with collaterals from ECA and PCA (via PCOM) supplying the MCA. (ECA: external carotid artery; MCA: middle cerebral artery; ICA: internal carotid artery; PCA: posterior cerebral artery; PCOM: posterior communicating artery)

radiation-induced vasculitis, moyamoya disease, dissection, vertebrobasilar hypoplasia.[26] Various research articles are available to show the role of vessel imaging in evaluation of intracranial aneurysms and its various components, such as the vasa vasorum, the aneurysm wall, and mural hematoma which identify an aneurysm led to SAH among patients with multiple aneurysms. **Figure 16** is showing the moyamoya pattern.

- *Moyamoya disease*: Vascular enhancement can be seen in secondary causes of Moyà Moyà syndrome
- *RCVS*: No vessel wall enhancement, multifocal concentric/circumferential wall thickening
- *Dissection*: Eccentric wall thickening with enhancement and presence of a false lumen
- *Vasculitis*: Smooth, concentric/circumferential thickening and enhancement (may extend beyond the vessel wall into the surrounding perivascular soft tissue)
- *Aneurysm wall*—predictors for rupture, growth, etc. role of steroids for treatment in case of vessel wall inflammation (case reports). Aneurysm-aneurysm wall inflammation, aneurysm growth and rupture.

Plaque Imaging

High resolution images can be obtained and postprocessing software allows for semi and fully automated quantitative analysis. By using dedicated hardware high-resolution MRI, high-resolution images can be obtained and postprocessing software allows for semi- and fully-automated quantitative analysis.[27]

Combining pre- and postcontrast T1, T2, proton-density, and magnetization-prepared rapid acquisition GE-weighted fat-saturation imaging, atherosclerotic plaque components and total plaque burden within the carotid arteries can be delineated **(Table 2).**[28,29]

"Vulnerable plaque" is an unstable plaque which is more prone to rupture and distal embolization. Vulnerable plaques parameters include the presence of a thin fibrous cap (FC) with a large lipid core, intraplaque hemorrhage (IPH), and the presence of intraplaque active inflammation.[30] Unstable plaques (due to hemodynamic changes and shear stress) morphology shows an eccentric distribution, superficial ulcerations with intimal exposure, or an irregular surface without erosion of the intimal layer. Unstable plaques can show either positive or negative remodeling. Positive remodeling is a dilation of the vessel wall in response to an increase in the plaque/wall volume in order to maintain sufficient lumen diameter whereas negative remodeling is characterized by luminal stenosis.[31]

TABLE 2: MRI plaque imaging component.

	T1 pre	T1 post	T2	PD	TOF
Fibrous cap	Iso	Iso	Mixed	Mixed	Low
Fibrous tissue	Iso/high	Very high	Iso/high	Iso/high	Low
Hemorrhage	Very high		Variable	Variable	Variable
Calcification	Low	Low	Low	Low	Low
Lipid core	Iso/high	Low		Low	Low

(MRI: magnetic resonance imaging; Iso: isointense to skeletal muscle; PD: proton density; TOF: time-of-flight)

Atherosclerotic plaque [intracranial atherosclerotic disease (ICAD)]: Eccentric wall thickening/enhancement. T2-bright FC (mostly enhanced) and dark lipid core (between the vessel wall and FC). It may be heterogenous in presence of plaque hemorrhage.

Limitations

Metallic materials (clips, stents, coils, and FDs) remain a common concern in patients undergoing vascular imaging as a source of an artifact. Artifact sizes may increase at 3T compared with 1.5T, depending on various implant characters.[32] An uncommon and serious complication associated with gadodiamide (Omniscan) contrast dye is nephrogenic systemic fibrosis (NSF). Specific consideration should be done to patients with low GFR and CKD.[33]

ULTRASOUND

Ultrasound (US) is based on Doppler shift principle, which calculates transmitted and reflected wave frequencies difference. US transducer with the frequency of 2–10 Hz is being used for vascular imaging. US should be performed in gray scale US, color Doppler, power Doppler, and spectral Doppler. Brightness—B-mode (gray scale) imaging is a 2D structural and anatomical pattern based on acoustic properties.[34] Duplex imaging is a combination of B-mode and power Doppler, which shows anatomic and hemodynamic correlations. Color Doppler is a technique in which arteries are visualized depending upon flow direction and speed (Doppler flow velocity with gray scale mode). Power Doppler imaging is a type of color Doppler imaging to demonstrate amount of blood flow at each point by integrating amplitude or intensity in color Doppler.

Contrast-enhanced ultrasound (CEUS) is a noninvasive method for the evaluation of vascularity of plaque by vasa vasorum detection. Various US contrast agents are there with different compositions (protein, lipid, phospholipid, or sulfur hexafluoride microbubbles). By showing arterial lumen enhancement, it can measure stenosis, vessel irregularities, ulcers, or dissections.

Techniques

Carotid Ultrasound

Carotid duplex examination of the carotid arteries includes evaluation of the proximal, mid, and distal CCAs, proximal and distal ICAs, and the external carotid arteries (ECAs) bilaterally and proximal great vessels if visible **(Figs. 17A to C)**. The patient should be examined preferably in the supine position with the neck extended and slightly turned to the contralateral side with either a posterior or an anterior

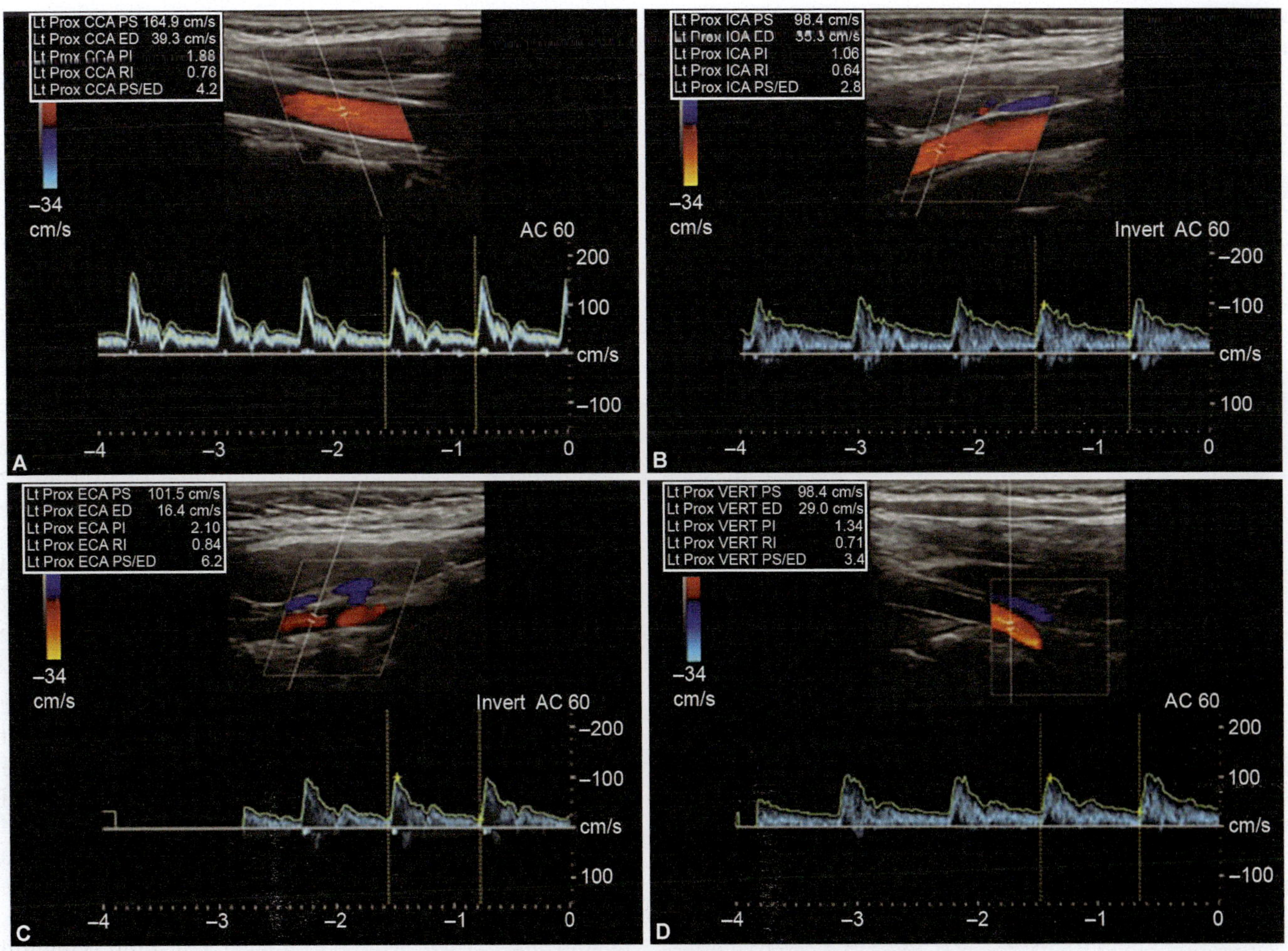

FIGS. 17A TO D: Carotid Doppler images showing normal CCA (A), ICA (B), ECA (C), and VA (D) flow.
(CCA: common carotid artery; ECA: external carotid artery; ICA: internal carotid artery; VA: vertebral artery)

TABLE 3: Differentiation between ECA and ICA.

	ICA	ECA
Size	Usually larger	Usually smaller
Branches	Rare	Present
Orientation	Posterior	Anterior
Pulse Doppler	Low resistance	High resistance
Temporal tap	Negative	Positive

(ECA: external carotid artery; ICA: internal carotid artery)

approach and angle of insonation is 45-60°. Transducer frequency ranges from 4 to 7.5 Hz (7 Hz for high resolution to look for plaque morphology). **Table 3** gives the identification of ECA and ICA by different US parameters. US evaluation of the carotid arteries needs evaluation of plaque, estimation of ICA stenosis by velocity criteria, and waveform analysis.

Vertebral Ultrasound

The vertebral artery is seen as low-resistance artery at pre- and intertransverse segment at C5-6 level. Doppler spectral pattern similar to that is seen with the ICA **(Fig. 17D)**. There are no widely accepted criteria for vertebral artery stenosis. Because of low sensitivity (40.7%), it is a poor tool for screening vertebral artery diseases.

TRANSCRANIAL DOPPLER

Transcranial Doppler ultrasonography (US) is a bedside technique that is noninvasive, inexpensive, real-time, easy to availability, and no exposure to contrast or ionizing radiation can be used in critical patients.[35,36]

Techniques

Nonduplex (nonimaging) and duplex (imaging) devices are available for TCD. In nonduplex imaging, the identification of arteries is done on spectral display and audible shift. Emitted US beam from the TCD probe crosses the skull and is reflected from the erythrocytes at the target location of vessels and signals are recorded. In B-mode transcranial color-coded duplex (TCCD) imaging, there is combination of pulsed wave Doppler US, which helps in identification of the arteries in relation to various anatomic locations.

Transcranial Doppler is usually performed using the 2 MHz frequency probe for better penetration through skull bones. TCCD is performed with a 2.25-MHz phased array and 2.5-MHz 90° sector transducers which provide color-coded imaging of intracranial arterial blood flow. There are blue and red colors indicating toward and away from the probe.

Cerebral blood flow velocity (CBFV) in a cerebral artery is inversely proportional to the diameter of that artery, which is the basic principle of TCD. TCD helps in the measurement of peak systolic velocity (PSV), end-diastolic velocity (EDV),

TABLE 4: Spectral Doppler parameters.

Artery	Window	Flow direction	Depth (mm)	Mean velocity (cm/s)
MCA	Transtemporal	Toward	30–60	55 ± 12
ACA	Transtemporal	Away	60–80	50 ± 11
ICA	Transtemporal/ transorbital	Toward/ bidirectional	55–60	39 ± 9
PCA	Transtemporal	Away—P2	60–70	39 ± 10
		Toward—P1		
OA	Transorbital	Toward	40–60	21 ± 5
VA	Transforaminal	Away	60–90	38 ± 10
BA	Transforaminal	Away	80–120	41 ± 10

(ACA: anterior cerebral artery; BA: basilar artery; ICA: internal carotid artery; MCA: middle cerebral artery; OA: ophthalmic artery; PCA: posterior cerebral artery; VA: vertebral artery)

pulsatility index (PI), and resistance index (RI). The PI is an indicator of the amount of vascular resistance in distal intracranial pressure (ICP) and it is used as an indirect evaluation of ICP.

The commonly used four windows are—trans-transtemporal, transorbital, submandibular, and suboccipital/transforaminal. Vessel identification is done by various criteria such as cranial window used, depth, angle of insonation, the direction of flow (as shown in **Table 4**), and relationship to other vessels, and maneuvers like CCA compression.

Clinical Applications

Subarachnoid Hemorrhage and Cerebral Vasospasm

Angiographic cerebral vasospasm occurs in two-thirds of patients with aneurysmal SAH with half becoming symptomatic (delayed cerebral infarction or mortality). Vasospasm develops after 3 or 4 days of the hemorrhage and usually resolves after day 12. Delayed cerebral ischemia can be prevented by early detection of vasospasm and appropriate treatment. In general, according to Spencer and Reid's curve, there is high-flow velocity when the vessel diameter is narrow and severe vasospasm.[37] TCD helps in monitoring of the early diagnosis of vasospasm, which helps in timely early treatment and prevention of complications. TCD monitoring should start as soon as aneurysmal SAH is diagnosed. Serial monitoring rather than random measurement helps in the detection of vasospasm as baseline values are available. Interpretation of the velocities should be done cautiously as affected by the changes with ICP, age, hematocrit, mean arterial pressure, technical expertise, arterial CO_2 level, collateral flow, and other interventions and has great intraobserver variability. TCD is more sensitive for detecting proximal than distal vasospasm. Proximal vasospasm in any intracranial artery

TABLE 5: Vasospasm criteria.

MCA vasospasm		
MFV (cm/s)	**Lindegaard ratio (MCA/ICA MFV ratio)**	**Severity**
<120	3	Mild
121–150	3–5.99	Moderate
151–200	>6	Severe
>200	>6	Critical
BA vasospasm		
	Modified Lindegaard ratio (BA/EVA MFV ratio)	
70–85	2–2.49	Mild
>85	2.5–2.99	Moderate
>85	>3	Severe

(BA: basilar artery; EVA: extracranial vertebral artery; ICA: internal carotid artery; MCA: middle cerebral artery; MFV: mean flow velocity)

results in a segmental or diffuse increase in the mean flow velocities (MFVs) without a parallel flow velocity increase in the neck vessel such as ICA and VA.

The Lindegaard ratio (LR) is the ratio between the MFV of the MCA and ICA.[38] The modified LR is the ratio between the MFV of posterior cerebral artery (PCA) and extracranial vertebral artery. These ratios help to differentiate between hyperemia from vasospasm as given in **Table 5**.

The sensitivity and specificity of the detection of vasospasm in the MCA are 66.7% and 89.5%, respectively.[39] Basilar artery vasospasm detection has a sensitivity of 75% and specificity of 80%.[40] However, the sensitivity of TCD is very inferior for vasospasm of the anterior cerebral artery (ACA) and PCA.[41]

Flow velocities usually decrease after medications and endovascular management. Persistent high flow velocities may indicate hyperaemia of treated vessel or vasospasm spreading into new segments. This dilemma can be resolved by cerebral angiography.

Acute Ischemic Stroke

Transcranial Doppler may diagnose acute MCA occlusions with high sensitivity (>90%), specificity, and positive and negative predictive values.[42,43] TCD can also detect occlusion in the ICA siphon, VA, and BA with reasonable (70–90%) sensitivity and positive predictive value and excellent specificity and negative predictive value (>90%).[44] TCD is useful in monitoring the effectiveness of thrombolysis. Few recent studies showed that the US has an additional effect on thrombolysis via significantly increased tissue plasminogen activator-induced arterial recanalization in the CLOTBUST trial. TCD is helpful in prognostication in patients presenting with AIS by using contrast-enhanced color-coded duplex sonography.

Transcranial power motion-mode Doppler (PMD-TCD) is a technique that provides additional displays of real-time flow signal intensity and direction over 6 cm of intracranial space along with spectral information.[45] PMD-TCD demonstrated higher sensitivity and specificity compared to posterior circulation.

Intracranial Stenosis

Transcranial Doppler helps in identifying stenosis and occlusion of the carotid siphon, proximal MCA, ACA, PCA, BA, and intracranial VA. The sensitivity, specificity, positive predictive value, and negative predictive value of TCD are generally higher in the anterior circulation compared to PC, as it has greater tortuosity and anatomic variability.

Diagnosis of stenosis (>50%) by TCD is based on the following criteria:[46]

1. Increase in flow velocity through the stenotic segment
2. Poststenotic dilatation
3. Side-to-side differences in MFVs
4. Flow disturbances (i.e., turbulence and murmurs)

Cerebrovascular reactivity identifies patients at an increased risk of recurrent stroke. Both IV acetazolamide administration and carbon dioxide inhalation are used to assess cerebrovascular reactivity by evaluating the presence of abnormal cerebral hemodynamic changes. In individuals with exhausted cerebrovascular reactivity reserves, MFV fails to adequately increase after the IV administration of acetazolamide or has a decreased response to hypercapnia and hypocapnia. There is impaired TCD cerebrovascular reactivity in patients with severe ICA stenosis or occlusion which is independently associated with ipsilateral stroke. Further investigation is mandatory for confirmation and may benefit from a revascularization procedure. **Figures 18 and 19** are showing normal and abnormal findings in MCA.

Extracranial Lesions and Plaque Imaging

Ultrasound is a noninvasive method for monitoring symptomatic or asymptomatic patients with carotid or vertebral artery disorders.[47] Early identification of atherosclerotic changes will allow interventions to prevent stroke/transient ischemic attack (TIA). Periodic evaluation according to severity and type of lesion may help in assessing the progression or regression of existing plaques or the development of new lesions. US is helpful in asymptomatic patients who are at high risk of stroke by demonstrating absence of vasomotor reactivity and presence of micro-emboli signals. Few studies have documented the association between risk factors and carotid intima-media thickening on B-mode imaging. With the development of new symptoms, there is a need to do an urgent re-evaluation. Carotid artery stenosis can be calculated by different parameters using Society of Radiologists in Ultrasound Consensus Conference criteria and has sensitivity of 95.5% and specificity of 94.3% as compared to CTA.[48] After carotid intervention (CEA), a repeat of the US is usually done at approximately 1 month after surgery and then yearly to identify restenosis. Duplex US is really helpful

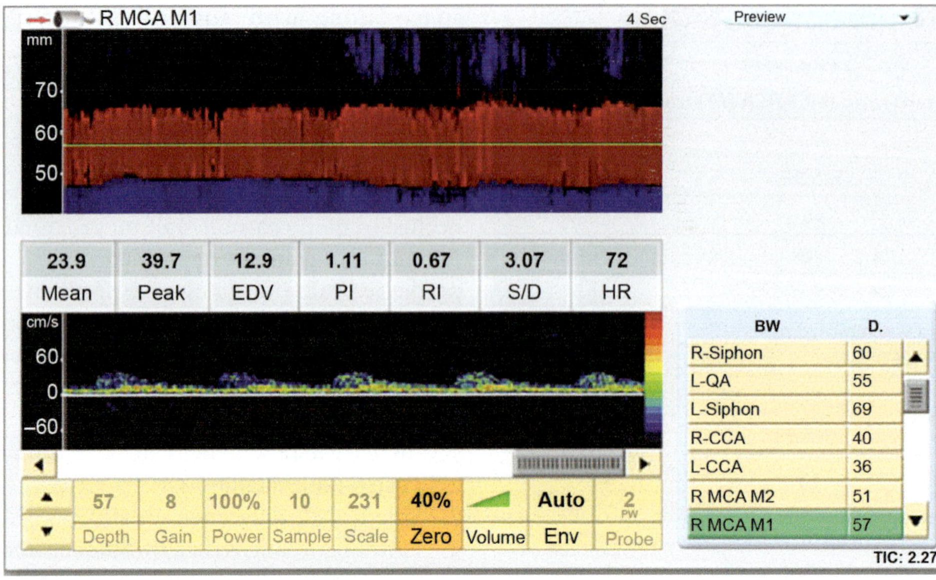

FIG. 18: TCD showing normal MCA flow.
(MCA: middle cerebral artery; TCD: transcranial Doppler)

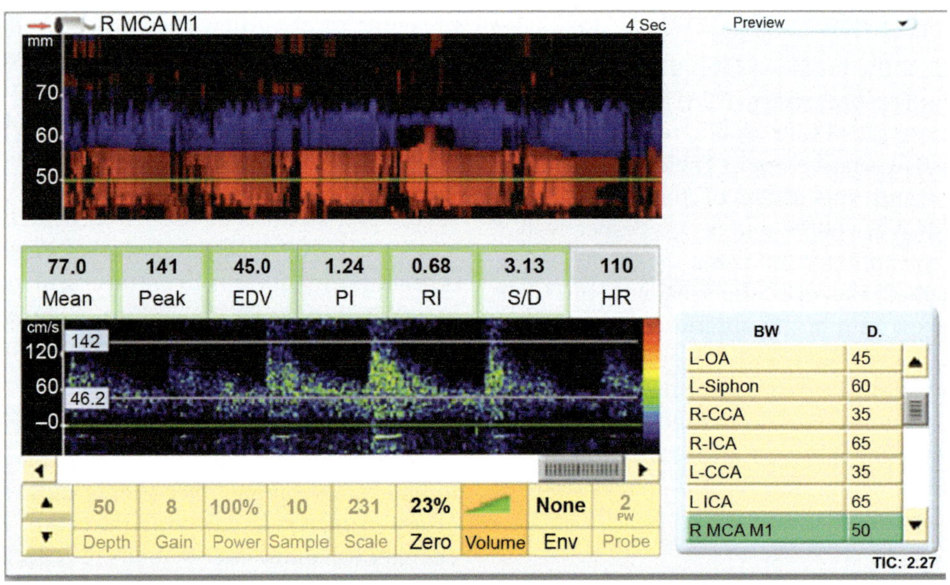

FIG. 19: TCD in patient with mild MCA stenosis.
(MCA: middle cerebral artery; TCD: transcranial Doppler)

in identification of in-stent restenosis or thrombosis. **Figures 20 and 21** are showing atherosclerotic plaque and **Figure 22** is showing poststenting follow-up.

Stable plaques are homogeneous or echogenic and less likely to embolize. Anechoic or hypoechoic focus in the plaque may suggest intra-plaque haemorrhage, deposits of lipid or cholesterol. Strong echolucent component of the plaque (heterogeneous plaque) and ulcerated plaque (focal depression or break) is unstable and more likely to embolize. Calcification is seen as both homogeneous and heterogeneous plaques.[49] CEUS may be helpful in showing neovascularization (adventitial vasa vasorum and intraplaque angiogenesis) seen in vulnerable plaques.

Microemboli Detection and Patent Foramen Ovale

Transcranial Doppler is a real-time technique that detects circulating cerebral microemboli, both solid and gaseous. Backscattering of the US waves from the emboli resulting in high-intensity transient signals (HITS) depends on the components of emboli.[50] Embolic signals using TCD US have been present in patients with atrial fibrillation, carotid stenosis, myocardial infarction, and mechanical cardiac valves. The microemboli detection by TCD may be useful in identifying the patients with asymptomatic carotid stenosis who are at high risk of stroke and TIA.

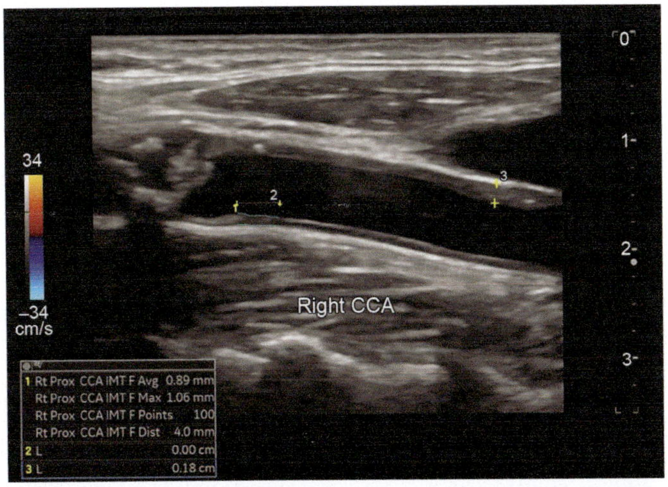

FIG. 20: Carotid Doppler image showing carotid intima media thickness (CIMT) of right CCA.
(CCA: common carotid artery)

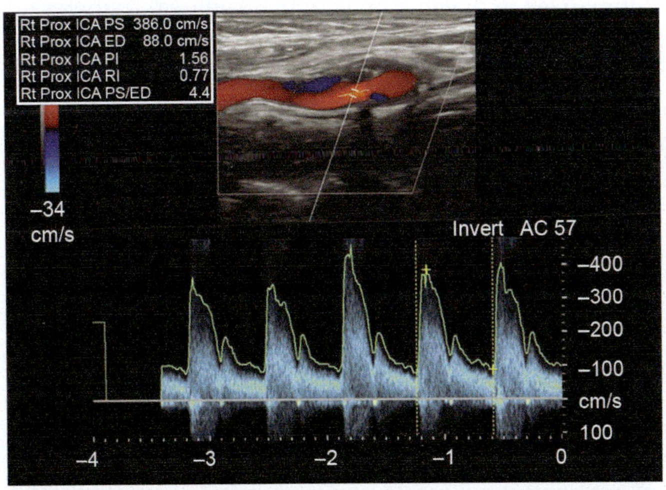

FIG. 21: Carotid image showing right ICA atherosclerotic plaque with increase in velocities.
(ICA: internal carotid artery)

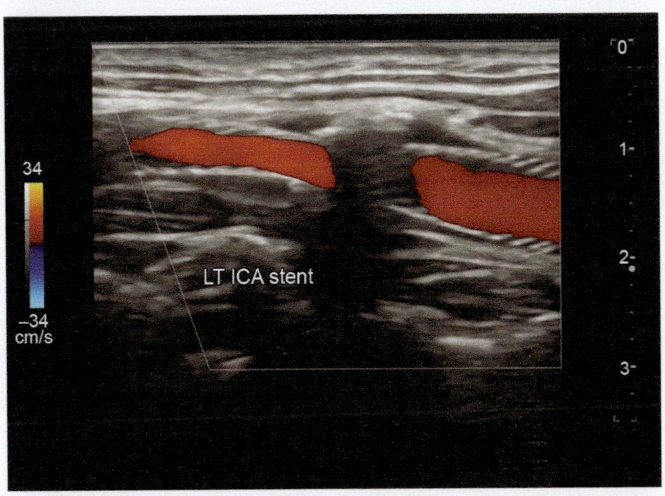

FIG. 22: Carotid Doppler image showing carotid stent in situ with normal color flow with signal drop in mid segment due to calcified plaque.

In suspected patients of patent foramen ovale (PFO), TCD with bubble study is very useful. Microembolic signal (MES) detection is done using microparticle contrast agents or simple agitated saline with microbubbles injected with continuous TCD monitoring of the MCA. The Valsalva maneuver after a few seconds of contrast helps in the arrival of microbubbles into the right atrium and the left atrium if a shunt is existent. It is comparable with transesophageal echocardiograms with little lower sensitivity and specificity.[51]

Sickle Cell Disease

Transcranial Doppler is an important tool in determining the need for prophylactic blood transfusion to prevent stroke in children with sickle cell disease (SCD). In patients with SCD, there is the development of occlusive vasculopathy characterized by fibrous proliferation of the intima, which often involves the basal cerebral arteries that often lead to cerebral infarction and has a frequency of approximately 5–15%. Children with SCD have chronic hemolysis resulting in chronic anemia and hypoxia-triggering angiogenesis, endothelial inflammation (via interaction of sickled red blood cells with endothelium), intracranial stenosis, and neovascularization. This altered hemodynamics leads to ischemic and hemorrhagic stroke. An MFV of ≥200 cm/s in the distal ICA and proximal MCA identifies neurologically asymptomatic children at an increased risk of ischemic stroke.[52]

In the Stroke Prevention Trial in Sickle Cell Disease (STOP), children between 2 and 16 years old without a history of stroke and an MCA velocity threshold of 200 cm/s were randomized for standard care or to periodic blood transfusion therapy to decrease the hemoglobin S concentration to <30% of total hemoglobin.[53] Blood transfusion based on MFV resulted in 92% stroke risk reduction. The STOP II trial assessed the safety of stopping long-term blood transfusion in children who had normal MFV and who had received blood transfusions for 30 months or more.[54]

Early TCD screening with prophylactic transfusion reduces overt stroke in children with SCD, TCD assessment should be a routine assessment of preventive care. The effect of blood transfusion and TCD in relation to stroke is not available in adults. It is better to avoid TCD. The impact of transfusion and subsequent stroke risk study is not available for adults.

India has the second highest number of SCD patients and mostly in communities living in a horizontal belt from Gujarat to Odisha state. Recently, one observational study was published on SCD patient's cerebral hemodynamics via TCD.[55]

Others

Transcranial Doppler remains a novelty in the field of periprocedural monitoring and provides valuable information on cerebrovascular complications. TCD monitoring detects microembolism and is very important because the majority of perioperative infarcts are thought to be secondary to cerebral embolism.

Transcranial Doppler remains useful as an ancillary test for brain death confirmation as it is noninvasive, portable, and relatively safe.[56] The pattern of TCD changes is not specific to a braindead and may occur in a variety of conditions related to raised ICP.

Limitations

Transcranial Doppler is very useful in intensive care, however, its limitations are operator-dependent, poor for distal vessels (apart from MCA and ICA), cataract with repeated use,[57] difficulty in differentiating vasospasm from edema, difficulty to get a view (thick skull or absent window), and confounders such as BP, hematocrit, fever, and hypo-/hypercapnia.[4,58]

DIGITAL SUBTRACTION ANGIOGRAPHY

Digital subtraction angiography is the gold standard for visualization of cerebral and spinal vasculature. Antonio de Egas Moniz was a Portuguese neurologist who first introduced cerebral angiography in 1920s.

Digital subtraction angiography is an invasive technique. It involves getting an arterial access and injecting intra-arterial contrast to visualize vessels. It needs proper training of performing interventionists to minimize complications. Diagnostic angiography may sometime be required for planning endovascular procedures.

Digital subtraction angiography has an overall complication rate of 2% with 1% chance of permanent neurological deficit. Non-neurological complications have been reported around 0.2–0.5% including puncture site, contrast-related complications, and thromboembolic phenomena at non-neurological sites.

Digital subtraction angiography resolves discrepancies between inconclusive findings of the other noninvasive methods in many conditions and serves as an integral part of endovascular interventional procedures.

In the last few decades, the spatial resolution of DSA imaging has improved and better images are available. Newer advances in DSA include rotational angiography, flat-panel detectors, and 3D and 4D angiography. A biplane angiography unit allows simultaneous acquisition of two projections [such as anteroposterior (AP) and lateral or two oblique views] during a single injection limiting the quantity of contrast medium injections and procedural time. Biplane imaging is preferred over monoplane imaging. Flat detector-equipped angiography helps in obtaining high-quality 3D rotational angiography and CT-like images (FD-CT) of brain parenchyma. The use of cone-beam CT technology is useful for the detection of intraparenchymal and SAHs in perioperative planning of endovascular treatment of complex aneurysms or AVMs. This ability to obtain CT images reduces the need to transfer patients from the catheterization laboratory to a separate CT facility.

Technique

Most often, diagnostic angiography is done under local anesthesia or mild sedation. Preprocedure patient should be kept fasting for 3 hours for diagnostic angiography and at least 6 hours before general anesthesia. Radiation safety measures including wearing lead aprons, thyroid collar, goggles, cap, etc. should be stringently followed. Minimizing personals in catheterization laboratory is also important. Use of transfemoral, transradial, or transbrachial routes for arterial access may sometimes be operator dependent or guided by anatomy of vessels to be studied. Seldinger technique is used for puncturing the artery. A trocar (hollow needle) is used to puncture the artery, followed by guidewire, and finally guide catheter is introduced, exchanging the trocar in the artery. The technique can be summarized as "needle in, wire in, needle off, catheter on wire, catheter in, catheter advance, and wire off." Doppler or USG may help in cases where it is difficult to find access to a vessel and prevent complication rates. Allen's test, previously used for assessing completeness of palmar arch before radial access, is hardly in use now. Different diagnostic catheters and guidewires are used depending on the individual expertise and vascular anatomy. Intraprocedure heparin is used to prevent clot formation and embolization in intracranial vessels. It is administered at the beginning of procedure at 40–50 U/kg. For an extended procedure, anticoagulant effect can be monitored by checking the activated coagulation time (ACT), with a target of ACT level of 1.5–2.5 times the baseline value. Advantage of the use of heparin is that its effect can be reversed immediately by protamine sulfate (1 mg protamine neutralizes 100 units of heparin). **Figures 23 to 26** are showing normal angioarchitecture of vessels.

Conventionally, in four-vessel DSA, both common carotids and both vertebral arteries/subclavian arteries are studied during diagnostic angiography. The study can be tailored depending on the diagnosis, curtailing to minimum number of vessels studied. Extensive study, involving selective catheterization of both external carotid arteries, internal carotid arteries, and both vertebral arteries, may be required in case of dural arteriovenous fistula. Contrast medium can be injected manually (handheld injections) or by pump injector. Injector offers a benefit of preventing air embolism. There are prespecified norms available for volume of contrast and flow rate to be injected for each vessel for angiography. Acquisition of images can be done with different views, e.g., Towne, AP, oblique, and caudal, for different vessels and site of pathology. Relation to the bony structures can be noted with different viewing angles. Postprocedure, puncture site should be carefully observed for local complications and sheath/catheter removal should be planned accordingly. Manual compression or

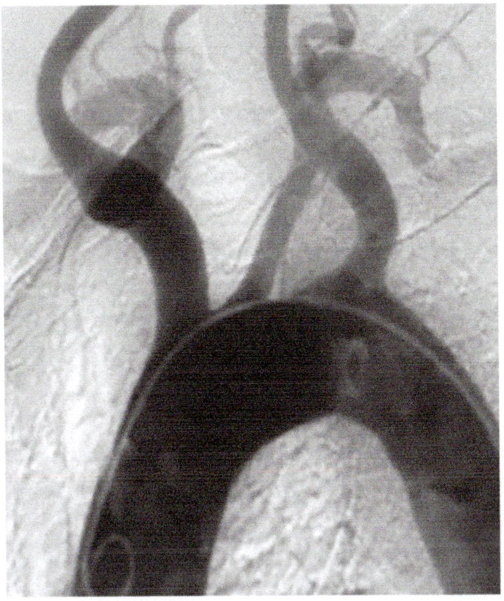

FIG. 23: Aortic arch angiogram showing right innominate, left CCA, and left subclavian artery origin from right to left.

(CCA: common carotid artery)

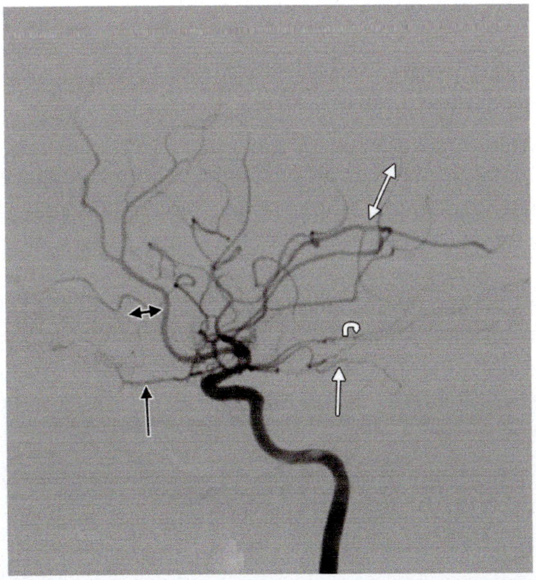

FIG. 24: Lateral view of CCA injection showing ACA (double black arrow), MCA (white double arrow), PCOM (white arrow), anterior choroidal (white arrow with turn), and ophthalmic artery (black arrow).

(ACA: anterior cerebral artery; CCA: common carotid artery; MCA: middle cerebral artery; PCOM: posterior communicating artery)

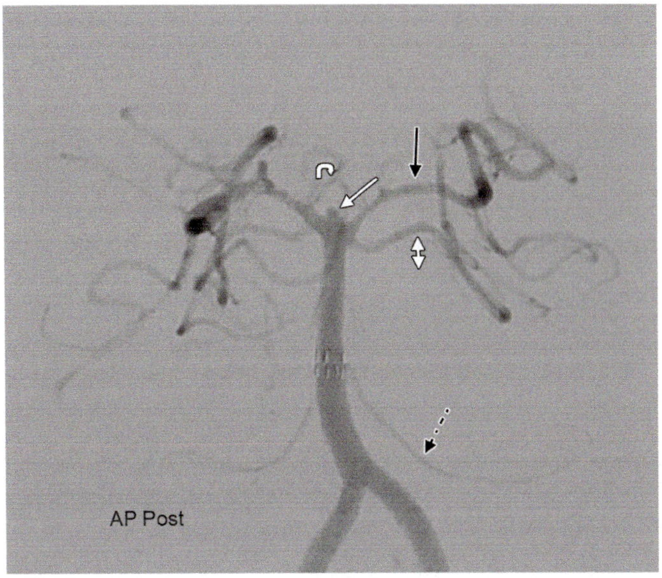

FIG. 25: Anteroposterior view of VA showing SCA (white double arrow), PCA (black arrow), AICA (arrow in dash), thalamic perforators (white arrow with turn), and top of basilar aneurysm (white arrow).

(AICA: anterior inferior cerebellar artery; PCA: posterior cerebral artery; SCA: superior cerebellar artery; VA: vertebral artery)

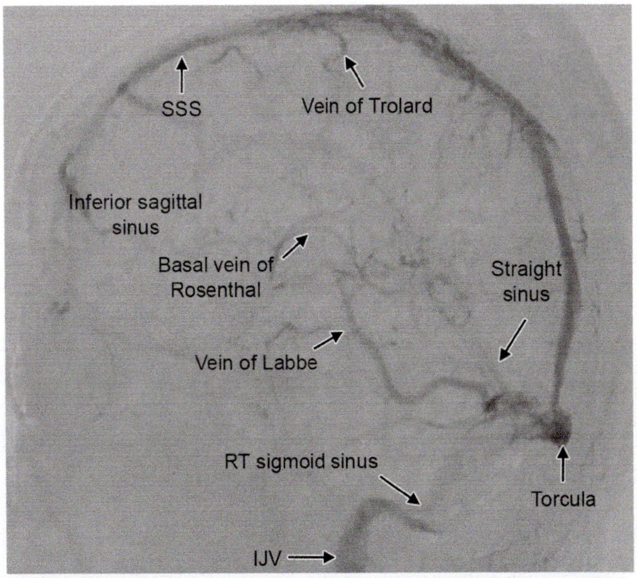

FIG. 26: Normal venous anatomy of the brain showing both deep and superficial venous system.

(IJV: internal jugular vein; RT: right; SSS: superior sagittal sinus)

closure devices, which occlude the puncture site, are used after removing catheter. Careful monitoring of patients for 12–24 hours should be done for local and/or neurological complications.

Special Considerations

- *Spinal angiography*: It is required for diagnosis of various spinal cord vascular malformations such as dural AV fistula or AVM. Detailed spinal cord vascular anatomy and diseases are described in chapter "Vascular Diseases of Spinal Cord". Preprocedure bowel preparation with laxatives or carminatives and antispasmodic medications is used for better visualization. Diagnostic angiography is done under local anesthesia. Vertebral bodies are marked on skin with radiopaque markers for counting levels during procedure. Special diagnostic catheters are used for spine angiography. They differ in shape and length compared to cerebral DSA. Thorough evaluation of all segmental arteries on both sides, both subclavian, vertebral, internal, and external iliac arteries may be necessary for dural AV fistula to demarcate the site of fistula.

- *Pediatric patients*: Small caliber arteries, superficial location, and higher chances of vasospasm are important considerations for arterial access. Developmental anomalies, narrow aortic arch with sharp bends may complicate the procedure. Small/narrow caliber femoral sheaths, short catheters (length ≤60 cm), and lower dose of heparin (30 U/kg) are used for pediatric DSA. Diagnostic angiography may be done under general anesthesia as pediatric patients may not co-operate during the procedure.
- *Diabetic patients*: Diagnosing and managing hypoglycemia are important for patients who are kept fasting for the procedure. Metformin is avoided to prevent risk of lactic acidosis.[59] In patients who are receiving neutral protamine Hagedorn (NPH) insulin, protamine sulfate should be avoided.[60]
- *Patients who are taking anticoagulants*: It is necessary to stop heparin 6 hours before the procedure to avoid hematoma at puncture site. Patients who are taking oral anticoagulants can be shifted to heparin or low molecular weight heparin perioperatively.
- *Thrombocytopenia*: Avoid angiography if platelet count is <75,000/µL.
- *Pregnant patients*:[61] Current recommendations for radiation exposure to the fetus include a maximum dose of 0.5 rem. Risk-benefit of diagnostic angiography should be weighed accordingly. In pregnant patients, angiography may be considered for planning procedure deemed necessary during pregnancy. Ruptured aneurysm/AVM/AV fistula and AIS are common indications. Radiation safety measures including protective shields, lead aprons, minimizing procedure time, collimation, and reducing frame rate reduce the radiation exposure to the fetus. Adequate hydration is important to reduce contrast-related complications.

Complications

Common complications of diagnostic angiography are as follows:[62]

- *Puncture site*: Local sites—groin or retroperitoneal hematoma, pseudoaneurysm, infection, avulsion of vessel, vasospasm, occlusion of the distal vessel are rare complications. Prompt diagnosis with use of USG or Doppler may prevent catastrophic outcomes.
- *Contrast-induced nephropathy*:[63] It may present usually within 3–4 days of procedure. It is defined by increase in serum creatinine by 25–50% over baseline, or absolute increase by 0.5–1 mg/dL. Pre-existing renal failure, diabetes, dehydration, use of diuretics, cardiovascular diseases, paraproteinemia, hyperuricemia, and age >60 years are important risk factors. Special measures such as using Iodixanol (Visipaque™) with osmolality 270 mL I/mL instead of Omnipaque™, oral hydration (water, 500 mL before the procedure and 2,000 mL after the procedure), intravenous hydration with 0.9% sodium chloride and sodium bicarbonate, and antioxidant acetylcysteine 600 mg (3 mL) PO BID on the day before and the day of the procedure in high-risk patients may be helpful in preventing nephropathy.
- *Anaphylactic reaction*: The patient can have various degrees of manifestations ranging from mild urticaria to respiratory distress. History of prior reaction, allergy, or asthma should be enquired. Oxygen, alpha- and beta-agonists, steroids, and H1 blockers may be required in a severe reaction.
- *Neurological complications*: Most of the neurological complications are related to thromboembolism, air embolism, vessel dissection, or perforation. Some of neurological deficits are transient, while 1% patients may have residual deficit. Adequate training of the interventionist and reasonable precautions are important for prevention.

Clinical Applications

Acute Ischemic Stroke and Intra- and Extracranial Circulation

Digital subtraction angiography is very helpful in localizing exact site of occlusion, collaterals, clot morphology, presence of plaques, and stenotic site calcifications. Newer approaches including direct to angio suite are being implemented to reduce door to puncture time in cases where LVO is contemplated. Treatment of underlying intra- or extracranial steno-occlusive disease can be planned accordingly. **Figures 27 and 28** show angiography in acute stroke and **Figures 29 and 30** show intra- and extracranial stenosis.

Subarachnoid Hemorrhage and Cerebral Vasospasm

Diagnostic cerebral angiography is helpful in localizing site, size, and morphology of aneurysm. It offers advantage over CTA for demonstrating precise vessel anatomy in planning endovascular treatment with FD, stent-assisted coiling, or flow disrupters like Web or Contour devices. Demonstration of vasospasm in patients with SAH and injection of intra-arterial vasodilators such as nimodipine, nitroglycerine, and milrinone can be done **(Figs. 31 to 33)**. It can be used as intraoperative assistance with aneurysm surgery. In smaller aneurysms, particularly <3 mm, DSA can better demarcate aneurysm anatomy compared to CTA and MRA. 3D DSA is very important in better visualization of morphological parameters of aneurysm and details of parent artery. DSA is also important in follow-up imaging after treatment (e.g., after aneurysm coiling or clipping).

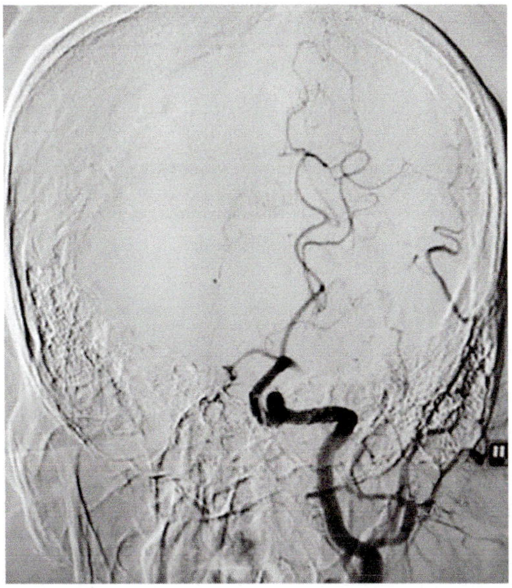

FIG. 27: DSA showing left MCA (M1) occlusion in patients with AIS.
(AIS: acute ischemic stroke; DSA: digital subtraction angiography; MCA: middle cerebral artery)

Vascular Malformations

In young or nonhypertensive ICH patients, DSA is mandatory to rule out AVM. For the diagnosis of vascular malformations (AVM and AVF; **Figs. 34 to 37**), DSA is the gold standard as it can show feeding artery, nidus or fistula and draining veins and collaterals. Follow-up imaging by DSA post-treatment is better as there are no artifacts compared to CTA or MRA.

Venous Disorders

Digital subtraction angiography is useful in venous disorders such as cerebral venous sinus thrombosis (CVST) **(Figs. 38A to D)**, vein of Galen malformation (VOGM) **(Fig. 39)**, and IIH as diagnostic (thrombus or stenosis) and for planning treatment such as thrombolysis, thrombectomy, or stenting.

Spinal Vascular Malformations

Spinal DSA is very useful in the evaluation of suspected vascular malformations and vascular neoplasms, blood supply, and embolization of vessels in highly vascular tumor

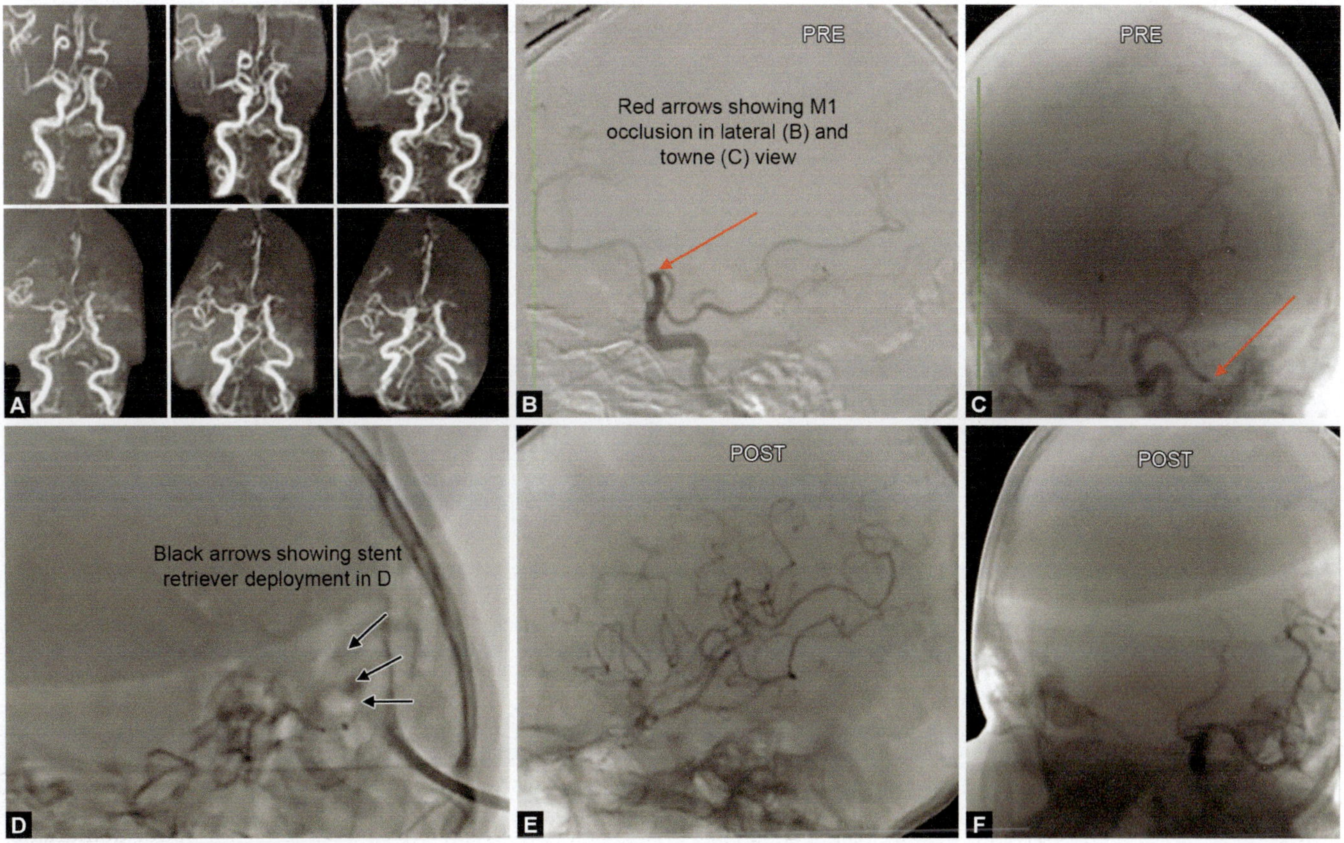

FIGS. 28A TO F: MRA and DSA (pre- and postprocedure) in patients with MCA occlusion.
(DSA: digital subtraction angiography; MCA: middle cerebral artery; MRA: magnetic resonance angiography)

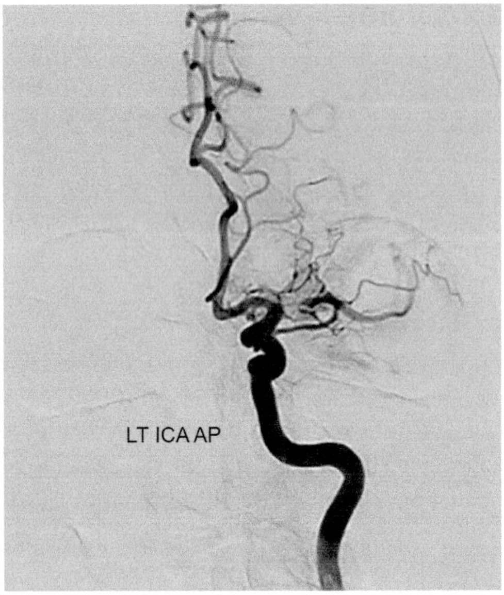

FIG. 29: DSA showing severe intracranial MCA narrowing.
(DSA: digital subtraction angiography; ICA: internal carotid artery; MCA: middle cerebral artery)

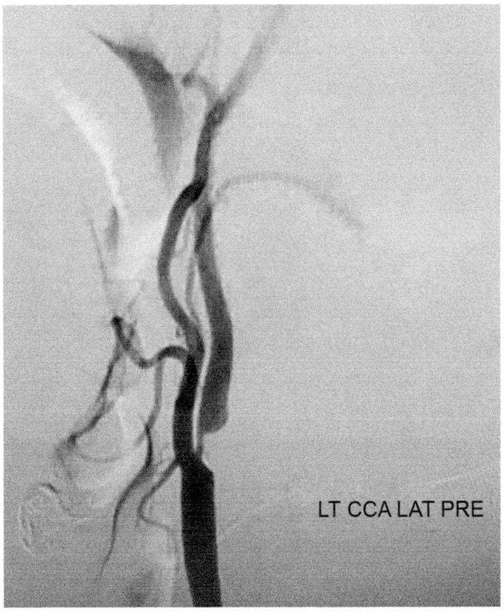

FIG. 30: DSA showing severe extracranial ICA and intracranial MCA narrowing.
(CCA: common carotid artery; DSA: digital subtraction angiography; ICA: internal carotid artery; MCA: middle cerebral artery)

(Figs. 40A and B). The goal of spinal DSA (in AVM or AVF) is to demonstrate the angio-architecture of the pathology and also the normal neural structure blood supply above and below the lesion including demonstration of the anterior and posterior spinal arteries.

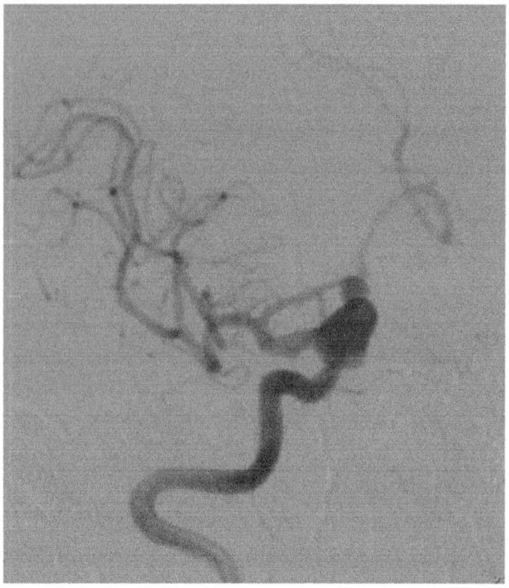

FIG. 31: Right ICA run showing right supraclinoid ICA aneurysm.
(ICA: internal carotid artery)

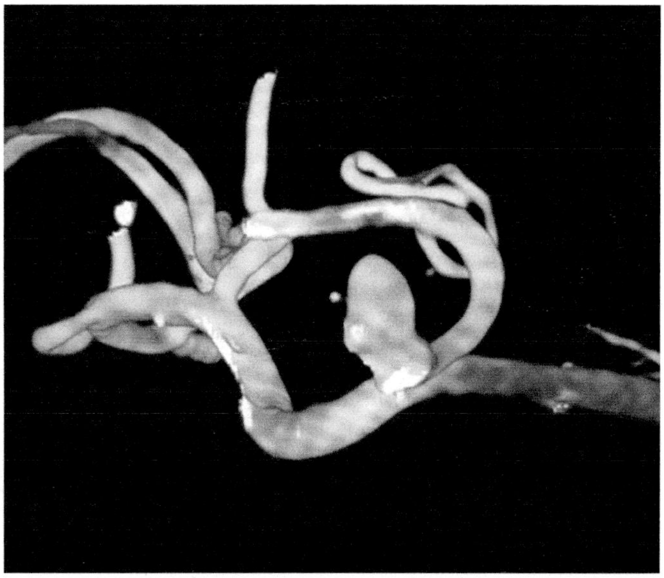

FIG. 32: 3D DSA showing right MCA bifurcation aneurysm.
(DSA: digital subtraction angiography; MCA: middle cerebral artery)

Others

Digital subtraction angiography is sometimes performed in meningioma, glomus tumor **(Fig. 41)**, or any vascular tumor to assess vascularity and may be combined with preoperative embolization to reduce subsequent intra-operative blood loss. DSA is also very important in diagnosis and follow-up of vasculopathies **(Figs. 42 and 43)**.

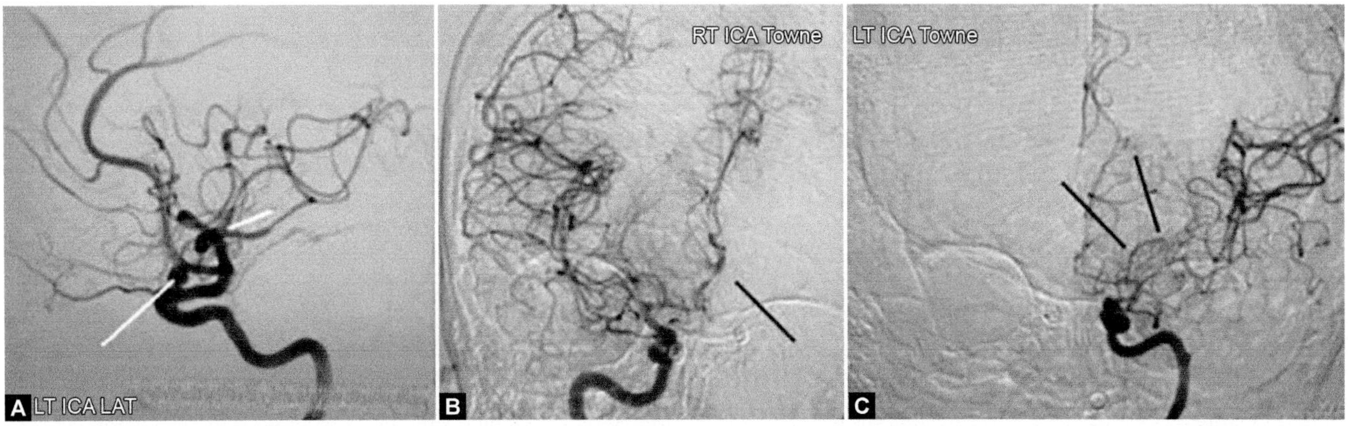

FIGS. 33A TO C: Bilateral mirror aneurysm in a patient with ruptured left para-ophthalmic aneurysm (A). There is secondary vasospasm to SAH with beading in the ACA and severe vasospasm in MCA territory respectively (B and C).

(ACA: anterior cerebral artery; ICA: internal carotid artery; MCA: middle cerebral artery; SAH: subarachnoid hemorrhage)

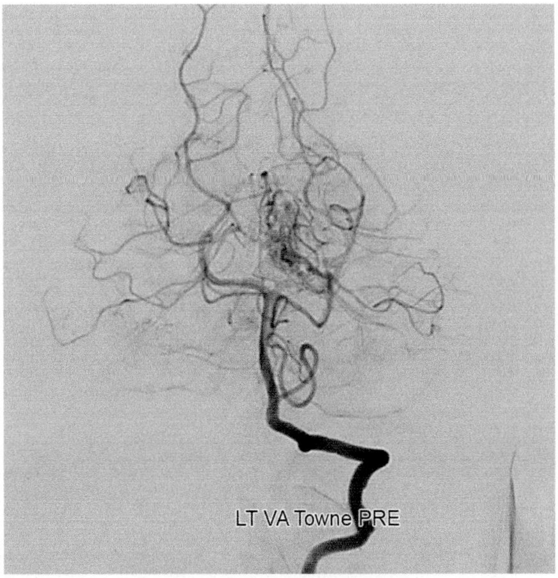

FIG. 34: Left VA Towne run showing AVM.

(AVM: arteriovenous malformation; VA: vertebral artery)

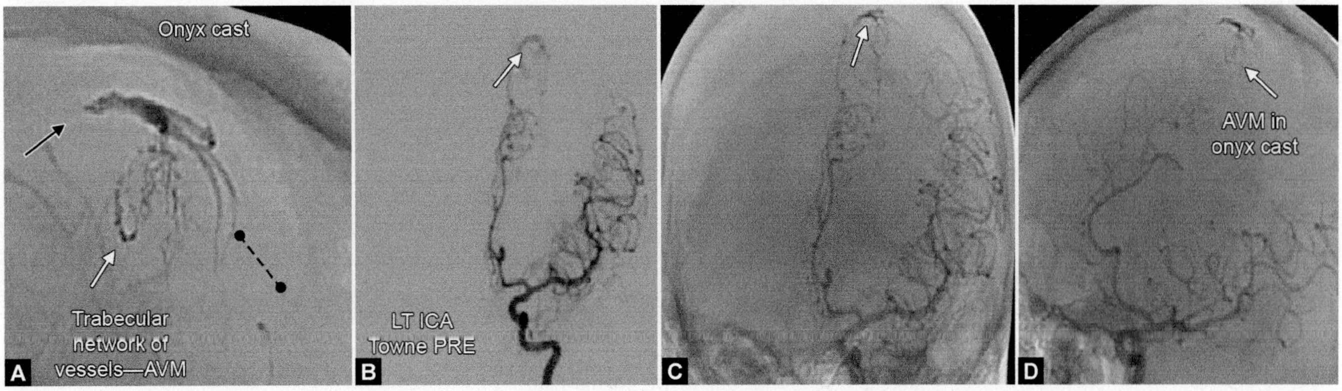

FIGS. 35A TO D: Eloquent cortex AVM presenting as right complete hemiplegia and left frontal bleed. Initial DSA on day 3 has not revealed AVM. Interval DSA after 6 weeks showed small cortical AVM with arterial supply from 2 branches of callosomarginal arteries (black dotted line). Trabecular network of AVM with early draining vein (black arrow) is seen in onyx cast zoomed (A). Early/prominent draining vein (white arrow) helped in identification of AVM (B). Unsubtracted images showing complete AVM with arterial supply and draining vein in Towne and lateral view (C and D).

(AVM: arteriovenous malformation; DSA: digital subtraction angiography)

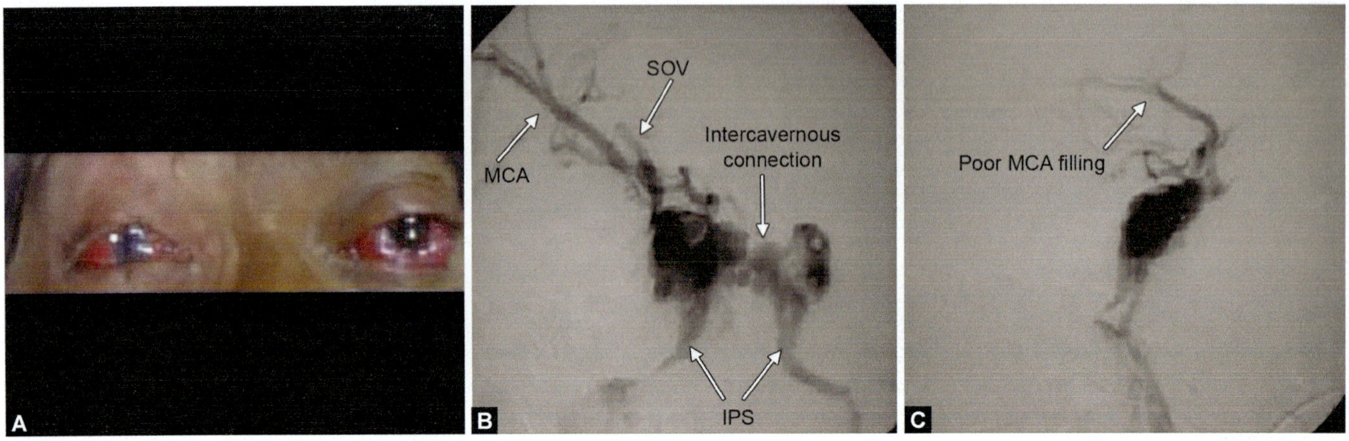

FIGS. 36A TO C: DSA image showing CCF in patients with bilateral redness and proptosis of eyes.
(CCF: carotid cavernous fistula; DSA: digital subtraction angiography; IPS: inferior petrosal sinus; MCA: middle cerebral artery; SOV: superior ophthalmic vein)

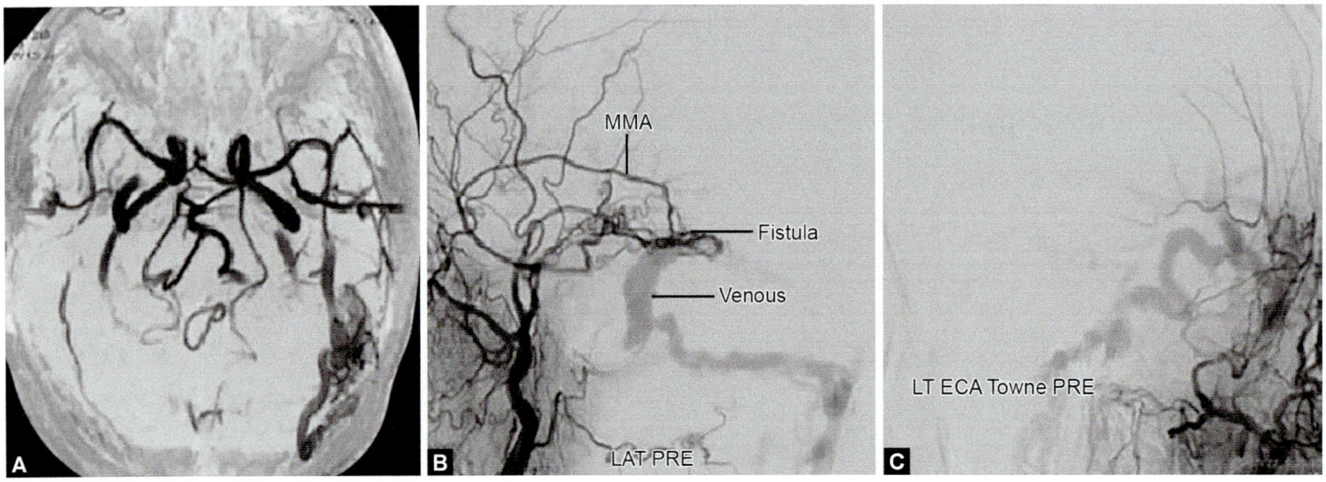

FIGS. 37A TO C: DSA image showing DAVF with feeding artery, fistulous connection, and draining vein.
(DAVF: dural arteriovenous fistula; DSA: digital subtraction angiography; MMA: middle meningeal artery)

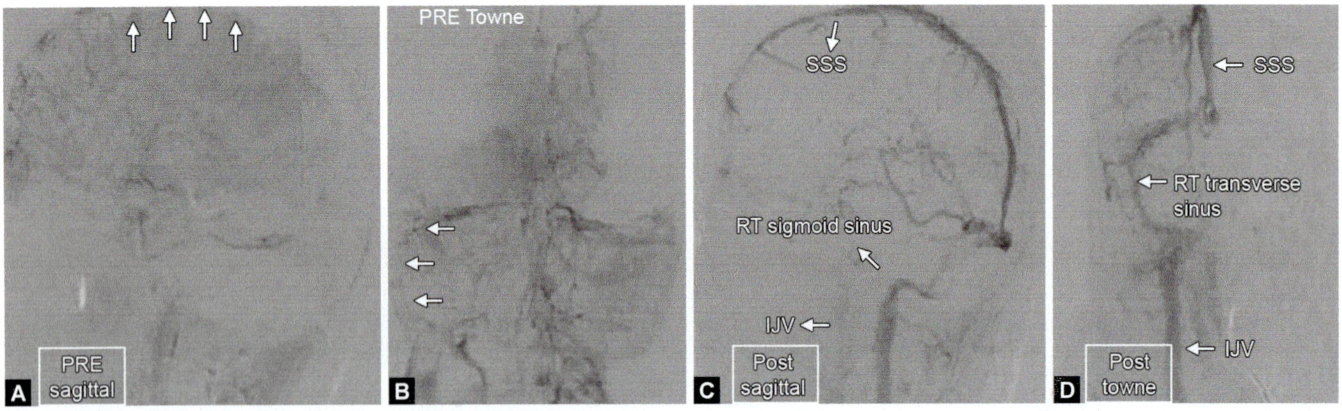

FIGS. 38A TO D: DSA showing pre (A and B) and post (C and D) in patient with CVST who received intrasinus thrombolysis.
(CVST: cerebral venous sinus thrombosis; DSA: digital subtraction angiography; IJV: internal jugular vein; RT: right; SSS: superior sagittal sinus)

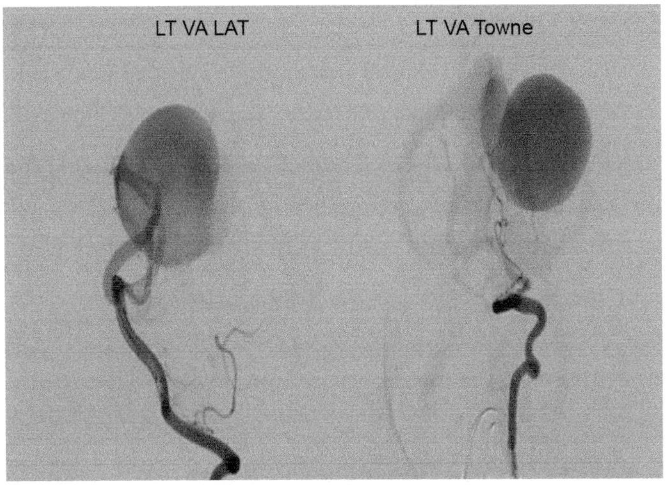

FIG. 39: Left VA run showing VOG malformation.
(VA: vertebral artery; VOG: vein of Galen)

MISCELLANEOUS

Positron emission tomography (PET), single-photon emission computed tomography (SPECT), and photoacoustic vascular imaging may be helpful in better visualization and understanding of angioarchitecture and pathophysiology.

ARTIFICIAL INTELLIGENCE

The artificial intelligence has potential in clinical decision making by identification of disease, image interpretation, and assessment of treatment which reduces interobserver variability.[64]

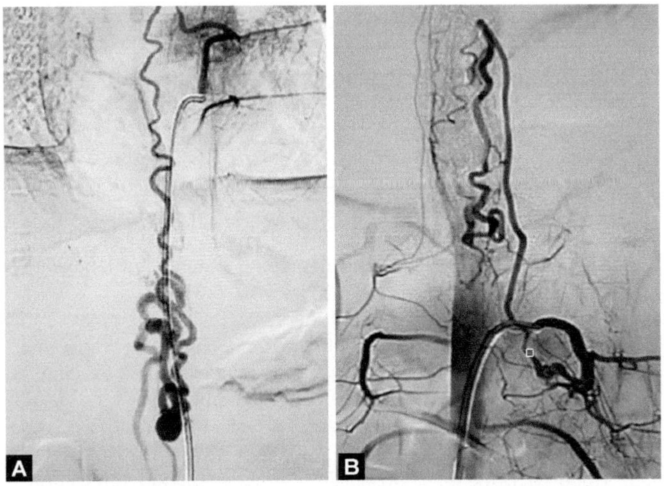

FIGS. 40A AND B: DSA spinal angiography showing pial AVF pre- (A) and postprocedure (B).
(AVF: arteriovenous fistula; DSA: digital subtraction angiography)

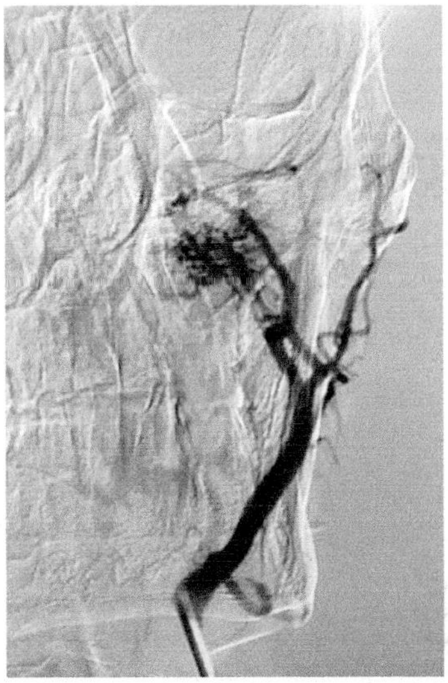

FIG. 41: DSA suggestive of glomus tumor with vascular blush.
(DSA: digital subtraction angiography)

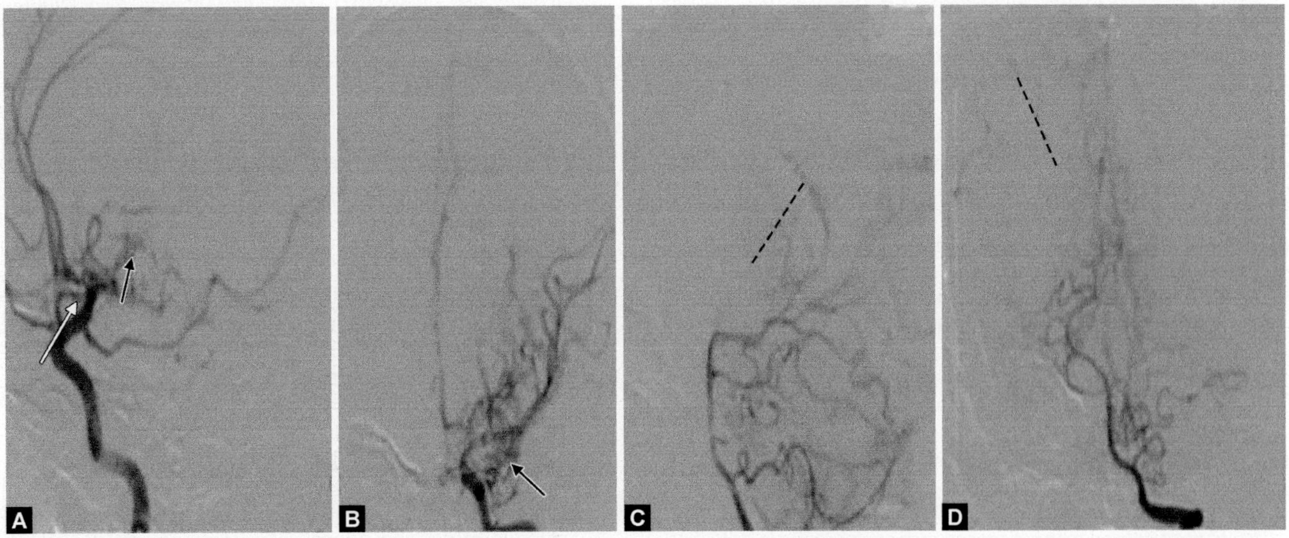

FIGS. 42A TO D: Moyamoya disease: DSA of ICA lateral view showing supraclinoid ICA stenosis (white bar) with "corkscrew" moyamoya vessels (black arrow) (A and B). Collaterals at splenium of the corpus callosum between posterior and anterior choroidal branches (C), black dots. Pial collaterals supplying the MCA territory from PCA (D), black dots.
(DSA: digital subtraction angiography; ICA: internal carotid artery; MCA: middle cerebral artery; PCA: posterior cerebral artery)

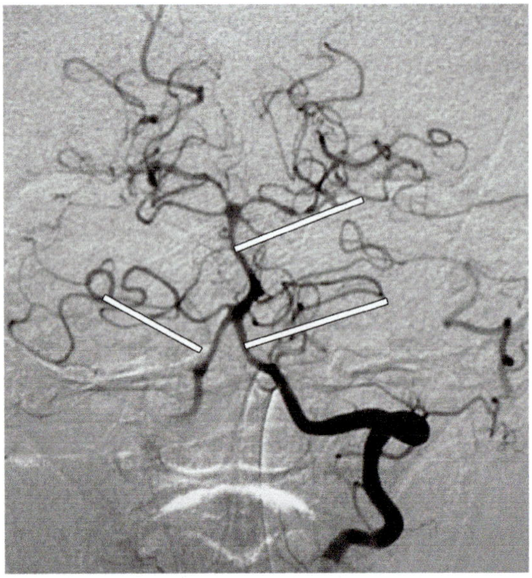

FIG. 43: Vasospasm of V4 segment of vertebral artery and mid-basilar giving beaded appearance in a patient of RCVS (white lines). (RCVS: reversible cerebral vasoconstriction syndrome)

CONCLUSION

- The CTA or MRA may be the modality in patients with AIS depending upon patient's status and availability of modality.
- The CTA and Doppler are better in showing stent thrombosis compared to MRA.
- Flow proximal and distal to vessel in poststenting can be seen better with MRA.
- Aneurysm features are best seen with DSA.
- Vascular malformation needs detailed evaluation with DSA.
- Venous hypoplasia versus thrombosis needs MR venography with contrast or DSA.
- Artificial intelligence will be very helpful in vascular imaging and specifically in stroke management in near future.

ACKNOWLEDGMENTS

Dr Anil Karapurkar, Dr Pawan Oza, Dr Neha Shah, Dr Lulla, and Dr Jagdish Annapureddy.

REFERENCES

1. Tan IY, Demchuk AM, Hopyan J, Zhang L, Gladstone D, Wong K, et al. CT angiography clot burden score and collateral score: correlation with clinical and radiologic outcomes in acute middle cerebral artery infarct. Am J Neuroradiol. 2009;30(3):525-31.
2. Kawiorski MM, Martínez-Sánchez P, García-Pastor A, Calleja P, Fuentes B, Sanz-Cuesta BE, et al. Alberta Stroke Program Early CT Score applied to CT angiography source images is a strong predictor of futile recanalization in acute ischemic stroke. Neuroradiology. 2016;58(5):487-93.
3. Menon BK, O'brien B, Bivard A, Spratt NJ, Demchuk AM, Miteff F, et al. Assessment of leptomeningeal collaterals using dynamic CT angiography in patients with acute ischemic stroke. J Cereb Blood Flow Metab. 2013;33(3):365-71.
4. Sloan MA, Alexandrov AV, Tegeler CH, Spencer MP, Caplan LR, Feldmann E, et al. Assessment: Transcranial Doppler ultrasonography: Report of the therapeutics and technology assessment subcommittee of the American Academy of Neurology. Neurology. 2004;62(9):1468-81.
5. Wang H, Li W, He H, Luo L, Chen C, Guo Y. 320-detector row CT angiography for detection and evaluation of intracranial aneurysms: comparison with conventional digital subtraction angiography. Clin Radiol. 2012;68:15-20.
6. Latchaw RE, Alberts MJ, Lev MH, Connors JJ, Harbaugh RE, Higashida RT, et al. Recommendations for imaging of acute ischemic stroke: a scientific statement from the American Heart Association. Stroke. 2009;40(11):3646-78.
7. Blacquiere D, Demchuk AM, Al-Hazzaa M, Deshpande A, Petrcich W, Aviv RI, et al. Intracerebral hematoma morphologic appearance on noncontrast computed tomography predicts significant hematoma expansion. Stroke. 2015;46(11):3111-6.
8. Linn J, Brückmann H. Cerebral venous and dural sinus thrombosis. Clin Neuroradiol. 2010;20(1):25-37.
9. Gross BA, Frerichs KU, Du R. Sensitivity of CT angiography, T2-weighted MRI, and magnetic resonance angiography in detecting cerebral arteriovenous malformations and associated aneurysms. J. Clin. Neurosci. 2012;19:1093-5.
10. Spetzler R, Martin N. A proposed grading system for arteriovenous malformations. J Neurosurg. 1986;65(4):476-83.
11. Cronin RE. Contrast-induced nephropathy: pathogenesis and prevention. Pediatr Nephrol. 2010;25(2):191-204.
12. Nael K, Michaely HJ, Villablanca P, Salamon N, Laub G, Finn JP. Time-resolved contrast-enhanced magnetic resonance angiography of the head and neck at 3.0 Tesla: initial results. Investig Radiol. 2006;41:116-24.
13. Hope TA, Hope MD, Purcell DD, von Morze C, Vigneron DB, Alley MT, et al. Evaluation of intracranial stenoses and aneurysms with accelerated 4D flow. Magn Reson Imaging. 2010;28:41-6.
14. Marks MP, Olivot JM, Kemp S, Lansberg MG, Bammer R, Wechsler LR, et al. Patients with acute stroke treated with intravenous tPA 3-6 hours after stroke onset: correlations between MR angiography findings and perfusion- and diffusion-weighted imaging in the DEFUSE study. Radiology. 2008;249:614-23.
15. Bash S, Villablanca JP, Jahan R, Duckwiler G, Tillis M, Kidwell C, et al. Intracranial vascular stenosis and occlusive disease: evaluation with CT angiography, MR angiography, and digital subtraction angiography. Am J Neuroradiol. 2005;26:1012-21.
16. Nael K, Meshksar A, Ellingson B, Pirastehfar M, Salamon N, Finn P, et al. Combined low-dose contrast-enhanced MR angiography and perfusion for acute ischemic stroke at 3T: a more efficient stroke protocol. Am J Neuroradiol. 2014;35:1078-108.
17. Kollias SS, Binkert CA, Ruesch S, Valavanis A. Contrast-enhanced MR angiography of the supra-aortic vessels in 24 seconds: a feasibility study. Neuroradiology. 1999;41:391-400.
18. Willoteaux S, Faivre-Pierret M, Moranne O, Lions C, Bruzzi J, Finot M, et al. Fibromuscular dysplasia of the main renal arteries: comparison of contrast-enhanced MR angiography with digital subtraction angiography. Radiology. 2006;241:922-9.
19. Cho YD, Lee JY, Kwon BJ, Kang HS, Han MH. False-positive diagnosis of cerebral aneurysms using MR angiography: location, anatomic cause, and added value of source image data. Clin Radiol. 2011;66:726-31.

20. Cirillo M, Scomazzoni F, Cirillo L, Cadioli M, Simionato F, Iadanza A, et al. Comparison of 3D TOF-MRA and 3D CE-MRA at 3T for imaging of intracranial aneurysms. Eur J Radiol. 2013;82:853-9.
21. Schaafsma JD, Velthuis BK, Vincken KL, de Kort GA, Rinkel GJ, Bartels LW. Artifacts induced by coiled intracranial aneurysms on 3.0-Tesla versus 1.5- Tesla MR angiography—an in vivo and in vitro study. Eur J Radiol. 2014;83:811-6.
22. Machet A, Portefaix C, Kadziolka K, Robin G, Lanoix O, Pierot L. Brain arteriovenous malformation diagnosis: value of time-resolved contrast-enhanced MR angiography at 3.0T compared to DSA. Neuroradiology. 2012;54:1099-108.
23. Farb RI, Agid R, Willinsky RA, Johnstone DM, Terbrugge KG. Cranial dural arteriovenous fistula: diagnosis and classification with time-resolved MR angiography at 3T. Am J Neuroradiol. 2009;30:1546-51.
24. Ayanzen RH, Bird CR, Keller PJ, McCully FJ, Theobald MR, Heiserman JE. Cerebral MR venography: normal anatomy and potential diagnostic pitfalls. Am J Neuroradiol. 2000;21:74-8.
25. Saraf-Lavi E, Bowen BC, Quencer RM, Sklar EM, Holz A, Falcone S, et al. Detection of spinal dural arteriovenous fistula with MR imaging and angiography: sensitivity, specificity, and prediction of vertebral level. Am. J. Neuroradiol. 2002;23:858-67.
26. Chaganti J, Woodford H, Tomlinson S, Dunkerton S, Brew B. Black blood imaging of intracranial vessel walls. Pract Neurol. 2021;21:101-7.
27. Singh N, Moody AR, Roifman I, Bluemke DA, Zavodni AE. Advanced MRI for carotid plaque imaging. Int J Cardiovasc Imag. 2016;32(1), 83-9.
28. Watanabe Y, Nagayama M. MR plaque imaging of the carotid artery. Neuroradiology. 2010;52(4):253-74.
29. Bitar R, Moody AR, Symons S, Leung G, Crisp S, Kiss A, et al. Carotid atherosclerotic calcification does not result in high signal intensity in MR imaging of intraplaque hemorrhage. AJNR Am J Neuroradiol. 2010;31(8):1403-7.
30. Naghavi M, Libby P, Falk E, Casscells SW, Litovsky S, Rumberger J, et al. From vulnerable plaque to vulnerable patient: a call for new definitions and risk assessment strategies: Part I. Circulation. 2003;108(14):1664-72.
31. Virmani R, Burke AP, Kolodgie FD, Farb A. Pathology of the thin-cap fibroatheroma: A type of vulnerable plaque. J Interv Cardiol. 2003;16(3):267-72.
32. Olsrud J, Latt J, Brockstedt S, Romner B, Björkman-Burtscher IM. Magnetic resonance imaging artifacts caused by aneurysm clips and shunt valves: dependence on field strength (1.5 and 3 T) and imaging parameters. J Magn Reson Imaging. 2005;22:433-7.
33. Kuo PH, Kanal E, Abu-Alfa AK, Cowper SE. Gadolinium-based MR contrast agents and nephrogenic systemic fibrosis. Radiology. 2007;242:647-9.
34. Tegeler CH, Ratanakorn D, Kim J. Advances in carotid ultrasound. Semin Cerebrovasc Dis Stroke. 2005;5:74-82.
35. Lupetin AR, Davis DA, Beckman I, Dash N. Transcranial Doppler sonography. Part 1. Principles, technique, and normal appearances. Radiographics. 1995;15(1):179-91.
36. Aaslid R, Markwalder TM, Nornes H. Noninvasive transcranial Doppler ultrasound recording of flow velocity in basal cerebral arteries. J Neurosurg. 1982;57(6):769-74.
37. Spencer MP, Reid JM. Quantitation of carotid stenosis with continuous-wave (C-W) Doppler ultrasound. Stroke. 1979;10(3): 326-33.
38. Lindegaard KF, Nornes H, Bakke SJ, Sorteberg W, Nakstad P. Cerebral vasospasm diagnosis by means of angiography and blood velocity measurements. Acta Neurochir (Wien). 1989;100(1-2): 12-24.
39. Yoo SJ, Sohn YH, Choi SE, Oh HB. Meta-analysis for the pooled sensitivity and specificity of anti-human immunodeficiency virus Ab rapid tests. Korean J Lab Med. 2009;29(4):345-52.
40. Soustiel JF, Shik V, Shreiber R, Tavor Y, Goldsher D. Basilar vasospasm diagnosis: investigation of a modified "Lindegaard Index" based on imaging studies and blood velocity measurements of the basilar artery. Stroke. 2002;33(1):72-7.
41. Wozniak MA, Sloan MA, Rothman MI, Burch CM, Rigamonti D, Permutt T, et al. Detection of vasospasm by transcranial Doppler sonography. The challenges of the anterior and posterior cerebral arteries. J Neuroimaging. 1996;6(2):87-93.
42. Camerlingo M, Casto L, Censori B, Ferraro B, Gazzaniga GC, Mamoli A. Transcranial Doppler in acute ischemic stroke of the middle cerebral artery territories. Acta Neurol Scand. 1993;88(2):108-11.
43. Baumgartner RW, Mattle HP, Schroth G. Assessment of >/= 50% and < 50% intracranial stenoses by transcranial color-coded duplex sonography. Stroke. 1999;30(1):87-92.
44. Demchuk AM, Christou I, Wein TH, Felberg RA, Malkoff M, Grotta JC, et al. Accuracy and criteria for localizing arterial occlusion with transcranial Doppler. J Neuroimaging. 2000;10(1):1-12.
45. Brunser AM, Lavados PM, Hoppe A, Lopez J, Valenzuela M, Rivas R. Accuracy of transcranial Doppler compared with CT angiography in diagnosing arterial obstructions in acute ischemic strokes. Stroke. 2009;40:2037-20.
46. Rasulo FA, De Peri E, Lavinio A. Transcranial Doppler ultrasonography in intensive care. Eur J Anaesthesiol Suppl. 2008;42(42): 167-73.
47. Qureshi AI, Alexandrov AV, Tegeler CH, Hobson RW 2nd, Dennis Baker J, Hopkins LN, et al. Guidelines for screening of extracranial carotid artery disease: a statement for healthcare professionals from the Multidisciplinary Practice Guidelines Committee of the American Society of Neuroimaging. J Neuroimaging. 2007;17: 19-47.
48. Grant EG, Benson CB, Moneta GL, Alexandrov AV, Baker JD, Bluth EI, et al. Carotid artery stenosis: grayscale and Doppler ultrasound diagnosis—Society of Radiologists in Ultrasound consensus conference. Radiology. 2003;19(4):190-8.
49. Shah F, Balan P, Weinberg M, Reddy V, Neems R, Feinstein M, et al. Contrast-enhanced ultrasound imaging of atherosclerotic carotid plaque neovascularization: a new surrogate marker of atherosclerosis? Vasc Med. 2007;12(4):291-7.
50. Markus H, Pereira A, Cloud G. Stroke Medicine. 1. New York: Oxford University Press; 2010.
51. Kobayashi K, Iguchi Y, Kimura K, Okada Y, Terasawa Y, Matsumoto N, et al. Contrast transcranial Doppler can diagnose large patent foramen ovale. Cerebrovasc Dis. 2009;27(3):230-4.
52. Adams RJ, McKie VC, Hsu L, Files B, Vichinsky E, Pegelow C, et al. Prevention of first stroke by transfusions in children with sickle cell anemia and abnormal results on transcranial Doppler ultrasonography. N Engl J Med. 1998;339:5-11.
53. Lee MT, Piomelli S, Granger S, Miller ST, Harkness S, Brambilla DJ, et al. Stroke Prevention Trial in Sickle Cell Anemia (STOP): extended follow-up and final results. Blood. 2006;108(3):847-52.
54. Optimizing Primary Stroke Prevention in Sickle Cell Anemia (STOP 2) Trial Investigators. Discontinuing prophylactic transfusions used to prevent stroke in sickle cell disease. N Engl J Med. 2005:353;2769-78.
55. Gajjar B, Sharma S, Khan E, Sharma P, Jain P, Goel V, et al. Cerebral hemodynamics in children with sickle cell disease in India: An observational cohort study. Medicine. 2022;101(27):e29882.
56. Sharma D, Souter MJ, Moore AE, Lam AM. Clinical experience with transcranial doppler ultrasonography as a confirmatory test for brain death: a retrospective analysis. Neurocrit Care. 2010;14: 370-6.
57. Do Y, Kim YJ, Lee JH. Transcranial Doppler: examination techniques and interpretation. Ann Clin Neurophysiol. 2019;21(2):71-8.
58. Sloan MA, Alexandrov AV, Tegeler CH, Spencer MP, Caplan LR, Feldmann E, et al. Therapeutics and Technology Assessment Subcommittee of the American Academy of Neurology.

Assessment: transcranial Doppler ultrasonography: report of the Therapeutics and Technology Assessment Subcommittee of the American Academy of Neurology. Neurology. 2004 May 11;62(9):1468-81.
59. Lalau JD, Race JM. Lactic acidosis in metformin therapy: searching for a link with metformin in reports of 'metformin-associated lactic acidosis'. Diabetes Obes Metab. 2001;3:195-201.
60. Stewart WJ, McSweeney SM, Kellett MA, Faxon DP, Ryan TJ. Increased risk of severe protamine reactions in NPH insulin-dependent diabetics undergoing cardiac catheterization. Circulation. 1984;70:788-92.
61. Piper J. Fetal toxicity of common neurosurgical drugs. In: Loftus C (Ed). Neurosurgical Aspects of Pregnancy. Park Ridge, IL: American Association of Neurological Surgeons; 1996. pp. 1-20.
62. Citron SJ, Wallace RC, Lewis CA, Dawson RC, Dion JE, Fox AJ, et al. Quality improvement guidelines for adult diagnostic neuroangiography: cooperative study between ASITN, ASNR, and SIR. J Vasc Interv Radiol. 2003;14:S257-62.
63. Morcos SK. Contrast media-induced nephrotoxicity—questions and answers. Br J Radiol. 1998;71:357-65.
64. Bivard A, Churilov L, Parsons M. Artificial intelligence for decision support in acute stroke - current roles and potential. Nature reviews. Neurology. 2020;16(10):575-85.

117

CHAPTER

Neuroimmunological Tests

R Sureshkumar, Minu George, Annamma Mathai, Sudheeran Kannoth

INTRODUCTION

Autoimmune neurology is an upcoming developing area in the field of neurosciences which involves immune-inflammatory diseases of the central nervous system (CNS). This subspecialty of neurology has developed more recently with discoveries of multiple autoantibodies that target proteins in the CNS. These discoveries helped to increase recognition of autoimmunity as the cause of neurological conditions misdiagnosed as primarily psychiatric disorders, degenerative diseases such as dementia or infections.

It can encompass a wide array of diseases like autoimmune encephalitis, paraneoplastic syndromes, neuromyelitis optica spectrum disorder (NMOSD) and myelin oligodendrocyte glycoprotein (MOG) other than multiple sclerosis (MS), movement disorders like stiff person syndrome or cerebellar ataxias, and newer disease like IgLON 5, etc.

Mostly the clinical symptoms may be nonspecific and transgress the boundaries of psychiatry, oncology, gastroenterology, rheumatology, etc.

It may become extremely challenging to diagnose these diseases unless we sent the appropriate panel of antibodies. The varied clinical presentations, unique pathophysiology, and the complexity of available treatments bring the need of a dedicated multidisciplinary team to diagnose and manage patients.

One of the earliest autoimmune tests we all came across was the acetylcholine receptor (AChR) antibody and cerebrospinal fluid (CSF) oligoclonal bands (OCBs). Since then neuroimmunology testing has developed in leaps and bounds.

Subsequently with the discovery of newer antibody testing, the field of neuroimmunology has progressed at an astonishingly fast pace. Many of these test improved technically, thereby helping clinicians to make the diagnosis with more confidence.

Many of these tests are commercially available now. However their interpretation may need to be monitored carefully.

In this chapter, we attempt to give the readers a brief overview of the neuroimmunological test commonly used in clinical practice.

NEUROIMMUNOLOGICAL TESTS IN CLINICAL PRACTICE AND THEIR UTILITY

Autoimmune disorders may be classified into peripheral and central. Central autoimmune disorders include autoimmune encephalitis, paraneoplastic syndromes, MS, and other autoimmune demyelinating disorders which include NMOSD and MOG antibody-related diseases.

There is a wide array of autoimmune encephalitis caused by humoral or cellular responses against specific neuronal antigens. Neuronal surface receptors and synaptic proteins have been identified as autoantigens of some of these disorders. They can be paraneoplastic or nonparaneoplastic based on the type of autoantibody involved.[1,2] Paraneoplastic syndromes can also be central or peripheral. They can be associated with cancer, but are not caused by the direct tumor invasion, metastasis, or consequences of treatment.[3]

Multiple sclerosis is a chronic inflammatory and demyelinating neurodegenerative disease of CNS. Differentiating MS from other relapsing inflammatory conditions such as NMOSD is important because treatment for both diseases differs and determines the clinical outcome.[4] In clinical practice, AQP4-ab-negative NMOSD patients are a diagnostic challenge.

Peripheral autoimmune disorders discussed in this chapter include Guillain-Barré syndrome (GBS), myasthenia gravis (MG)-related syndromes and antibodies related to various myositis.

Antiganglioside antibodies (AGAs) have been reported in the patients with GBS, particularly in acute motor axonal neuropathy (AMAN), acute motor sensory axonal neuropathy (AMSAN), and Miller Fisher syndrome (MFS). Distinct subtypes of MG are classified according to the clinical phenotypes, as it dictates the clinical approach.[5] Anti-acetylcholine receptor (Anti-AchR) antibodies are seen in 85% of patients with early and late onset MG.[6] In 15% of patients with MG, anti-AchR antibodies are not detected. Of these 15%, almost half are seronegative, but other half are positive for anti-muscle-specific kinase (anti-MuSK) antibodies. Muscle-specific kinase (MuSK) is a transmembrane polypeptide that is expressed at neuromuscular junction and has a fundamental role in AChR clustering.[7] Antibodies against lipoprotein receptor-related protein 4 (LRP4) are detected in patients with anti-AChR MG and anti-MuSK MG, but in 1–2% of all patients with MG, anti-LRP4 antibodies are the only detectable antibodies. Patients with these antibodies have mild symptoms, lack of a unique phenotype, and respond well to anticholinesterase or low-dose corticosteroids.[8]

Autoantibodies specific for idiopathic inflammatory myopathy, i.e., myositis-specific autoantibodies (MSAs) are clinically useful biomarkers to help the diagnosis of polymyositis/dermatomyositis (PM/DM). Many of these are also associated with a unique clinical subset of PM/DM, making them useful in predicting and monitoring certain clinical manifestations.

Autoimmune diseases based on their neuroimmunological testing can be divided to four broad subdivisions.

Autoimmune Encephalitis

Clinical Case

A 14-year-old female was referred from psychiatry department with acute onset psychosis characterized by paranoid delusions, thought disorder and auditory hallucinations. She had few facial automatisms. On examination, her symptoms were characterized by thought disorder and hypomania. There was no history of seizures. Hematological, biochemical, and septic screening were performed and yielded unremarkable results. Electroencephalogram (EEG) showed delta slowing with delta brushes. MRI brain was normal. CSF study done turned positive for anti-N-methyl-d-aspartate receptor (anti-NMDAR) antibodies. Her paraneoplastic workup for underlying malignancy was normal. She was given intravenous immunoglobulin (IVIG) with steroids followed by which there was mild improvement. Later she received rituximab with significant improvement.

Autoimmune encephalitis consists of a group of disorders in which the host immune system targets the self-antigens expressed in the CNS.[9] People with autoimmune encephalitis may have various neurologic and psychiatric symptoms **(Table 1)**.

TABLE 1: Autoimmune encephalitis—clinical features.

Neuronal antibody	Median age	Clinical symptomatology—when to suspect
NMDAR[14-16]	21 (2 months to 85 years)	Encephalitis with prominent neuropsychiatric presentation, polymorphic movement disorder, language disorder, autonomic dysfunction, coma, and central apnea. MRI normal in 70–80%. CSF shows lymphocytic pleocytosis in 80%. EEG shows slowing in 90% of patients. Evaluate for ovarian teratoma in female patients. Post-HSV, NMDAR encephalitis can develop, especially in children
LG1[17-19]	64 years	Limbic encephalitis with frequent focal seizures, including characteristic faciobrachial dystonic seizures. Forty percent show increased signal and swelling in medial temporal lobe. CSF pleocytosis in 25%. EEG abnormal in 50%. Hyponatremia in 70% of patients
CASPR2[20,21]	66 years	Peripheral nerve hyperexcitability, limbic encephalitis and Morvan's syndrome. Thirty percentage show increased signal in medial temporal lobe. CSF pleocytosis in 30% and EEG abnormality in the form of epileptiform abnormality in 40%. Electromyography can demonstrate hyperexcitability (fasciculations, myokymia)
GABA A receptor[22,23]	40 years	Encephalitis with frequent status epilepticus. Eighty percentage of patients show cortical and subcortical FLAIR signal abnormalities. Lymphocytic pleocytosis in 50%. EEG shows epileptiform abnormalities in 80%. Thymoma detected in 30%
GABA B receptor[24]	61 years	Limbic encephalitis with prominent seizures. Forty five percentage of patients show abnormal signal in medial temporal lobe. CSF show lymphocytic pleocytosis in 80% and EEG shows epileptiform abnormalities in 75 %. Tumors in 50% (mostly SCLC)
AMPAR[25]	53 years	Limbic encephalitis with prominent confusion, amnesia, seizures, and psychiatric/behavioral symptoms. MRI abnormal in 85% and CSF in 70% with lymphocytic pleocytosis. EEG abnormal in 45% of patients. Tumors identified in ~70% (thymus, SCLC, breast, ovary)

Continued

Continued

Neuronal antibody	Median age	Clinical symptomatology—when to suspect
DPPX[26]	53 years	Multifocal encephalitis with myoclonus, tremors, and hyperekplexia, prominent diarrhea/weight loss. MRI will be mostly normal. CSF shows pleocytosis in 30% and EEG abnormalities in 70%. Ten percentage of patients present with B-cell neoplasm (gastrointestinal follicular lymphoma, leukemia)
GlyR[27]	50 years	Three main syndromes: (1) Stiff-person spectrum disorder, (2) PERM (progressive encephalopathy with rigidity and myoclonus), and (3) limbic encephalitis. MRI shows nonspecific brain lesions in 30% and spinal lesions in 20% of patients. CSF pleocytosis in 40% and EEG abnormalities in 70% of patients. EMG is abnormal in 60% (continuous motor unit activity, spontaneous or stimulus-induced activity, neuromyotonia). Thymoma in 15%
IgLON5[28,29]	64 years	Four main syndromes: (1) Sleep disorder (REM and NREM parasomnias, sleep apnea), (2) Bulbar syndrome, (3) Progressive supranuclear palsy-like syndrome, and (4) Cognitive syndrome±chorea. Eighty percent show normal MRI. Thirty percent show lymphocytic pleocytosis. Fifty percent show elevated protein. EEG abnormalities not seen
Neurexin-3α[30]	44 years	Encephalitis. MRI shows abnormal mesial temporal T2/FLAIR hyperintensities in 20%. CSF shows pleocytosis in 100% of cases
GFAP-α1 antibody[31]	44–50 years	Encephalitis, meningoencephalitis or meningoencephalomyelitis

(AMPA1R: α-amino-3-hydroxy-5-methyl-4-isoxazolepropionic acid receptor; AMPA2R: α-amino-3-hydroxy-5-methyl-4-isoxazolepropionic acid receptor; CASPR2: contactin-associated protein-2; CSF: cerebrospinal fluid; DPPX: dipeptidyl-peptidase-like protein-6; EEG: electroencephalogram; FLAIR: fluid-attenuated inversion recovery; GABABR: gamma aminobutyric acid type B receptor; GFAP-α1: glial fibrillary acidic protein alpha-1; HSV: herpes simplex virus; IgLON5: immunoglobulin-like cell adhesion molecule 5; LGI1: leucine-rich, glioma inactivated 1; NMDAR: N-methyl-D-aspartate receptor; SCLC: small-cell lung cancer; VGKC: voltage-gated potassium channel)

Autoimmune encephalitis is a condition that is relatively difficult to diagnose. It has clinical, imaging, and laboratory similarities to many other autoimmune and infectious conditions of the brain. Some of them present early to psychiatrists with neuropsychiatric manifestations. The initial symptoms may be very nonspecific pertaining to the CNS.

Some of the best-characterized diseases are associated with autoantibodies that target neuroglial antigens. These autoantibodies are considered pathogenic because they are directed against the extracellular—and hence in vivo exposed—domains of their target antigens.[10-12] While the clinical features of these disorders span the spectrum of neurological symptomatology, for patients with autoantibodies against any individual target there is often a characteristic set of core phenotypic manifestations, which may relate to the regional expression, function and relative susceptibility of the target protein. In leucine-rich glioma-inactivated 1 (LGI1)-antibody encephalitis, the amnesia characteristically affects both anterograde memories and loss of autobiographical retrograde epochs.[13] Test for autoimmune encephalitis panel are elaborated in **Table 2**.

The antibodies may be divided into four groups. The first group includes the classic paraneoplastic disorders associated with antibodies to intracellular antigens, such as anti-Hu. These disorders are strongly cancer associated and involve T-cell responses targeting neurons. The prognosis tends to be poor due to irreversible neuronal killing by these mechanisms, the severity of associated cancers, and difficulty in controlling these types of immune responses. The second group involves autoantibodies to extracellular epitopes of ion channels, receptors and other associated proteins, such as the N-methyl-D-aspartate (NMDA) receptor. The cancer associations are variable, and the prognosis tends to be much better. The third group is the diseases with autoantibodies to intracellular synaptic proteins such as GAD65. A final group includes other forms of autoimmune encephalitis in which precise antigens are less clearly established, such as lupus cerebritis or acute disseminated encephalomyelitis (ADEM). Some diseases in this group have systemic manifestations outside the nervous system.

The diagnosis is mostly based on exclusion and also confirmation by the presence of specific antibodies in serum or CSF.

Treatment for suspected autoimmune encephalitis is often given empirically prior to specific antibody test results. This may include steroids and/or IVIG. If a cell-surface/synaptic antibody disorder is diagnosed, initial treatments may include IVIG, plasmapheresis, and/or steroids. Steroids may be beneficial in a range of autoimmune disorders but could potentially create problems with the diagnosis of certain disorders such as CNS lymphoma. IVIG and plasmapheresis are other modalities of treatment that offers an important advantage.

Pitfalls

N-methyl-D-aspartate receptor-antibodies are also detected in clinical syndrome of neuropsychiatric systemic lupus erythematosus. However, by contrast to antibodies which target native neuronal surface epitopes, those from patients with neuropsychiatric systemic lupus erythematosus have been found to show intrinsic "stickiness", which is not NMDAR-specific, and hence have limited diagnostic value.[32]

TABLE 2: Test in autoimmune encephalitis panel and methodology.

Tests in autoimmune encephalitis antibody panel	Sampling material	Methodology
NMDA receptor antibody—subunit-NR1	CSF/serum	CBA, IFA
LGI1 protein antibody	CSF/serum	CBA, IFA
CASPR2 protein antibody	CSF/serum	CBA, IFA
AMPA1 receptor antibody	CSF/serum	CBA, IFA
AMPA2 receptor antibody	CSF/serum	CBA, IFA
GABAB receptor antibody	CSF/serum	CBA, IFA
DPPX receptor antibody	CSF/serum	TBA - IFA and confirmation by CBA-IFA
IgLON5 antibody	CSF	CBA- IIF microscopy on fixed cell
IgLON5 antibody	Serum	TBA by IIF and positivity confirmed by CBA by IFA
GFAP-α1 antibodies	CSF	TBA by IIF
GFAP-α1 antibodies	Serum	TBA by IIF

(AMPA1: α-amino-3-hydroxy-5-methyl-4-isoxazolepropionic acid; AMPA2: α-amino-3-hydroxy-5-methyl-4-isoxazolepropionic acid; CASPR2: contactin-associated protein-2; CBA: cell-based assay; CSF: cerebrospinal fluid; DPPX: dipeptidyl-peptidase-like protein-6; GABAB: gamma aminobutyric acid type B; GFAP-α1: glial fibrillary acidic protein alpha-1; IFA: immunofluorescence assay; IgLON5: immunoglobulin-like cell adhesion molecule 5; IIF: indirect immuno-fluorescence; LGI1: leucine-rich, glioma inactivated 1; NMDA: N-methyl-D-aspartate; TBA: tissue-based assay)

Instructions (CSF)

- Preferred volume: 0.5 mL in sterile leak proof, polypropylene/plastic tube
- Pediatric preferred volume: 0.1 mL in sterile leak proof, polypropylene/plastic tube

Collection Instructions: Serum

- Collect 5 mL blood in golden top or red top Vacutainer
- Centrifuge and aliquot serum in polypropylene/plastic leak proof tubes within 2 hours of collection
- *Preferred volume*: 1 mL in leak proof, polypropylene/plastic tube
- *Pediatric preferred volume*: 0.5 mL in leak proof polypropylene/plastic tube

DPPX Antibody/IgLON 5 Antibody/GFAP-α1 Antibodies

Collection instructions: CSF

- *Preferred volume (CSF)*: 1 mL in sterile leak proof, polypropylene/plastic tube
- *Pediatric preferred volume*: 1 mL in sterile leak proof, polypropylene/plastic tube

Collection instructions: Serum

- Collect 4 mL blood in golden top or red top Vacutainer
- Centrifuge and aliquot serum in polypropylene/plastic leak proof tubes within 2 hours of collection
- *Preferred volume*: 1 mL in leak proof, polypropylene/plastic tube
- *Pediatric preferred volume*: 0.5 mL in leak proof, polypropylene/plastic tube

Specimen Stability during Transport

- *Room temperature*: 72 hours
- *Refrigerated*: 14 days
- *Frozen*: 28 days
- *Frozen at 70°C*: 1 year

Oncological Association of Paraneoplastic Syndromes[33,34]

Clinical Case

A 68-year-old chronic heavy smoker presented with recent onset memory impairment, personality changes, and behavior problems of 1 month duration. He reported recent weight loss also. Examination revealed a mini-mental state examination (MMSE) 20, and there was spasticity in lower limbs with extensor plantar. While undergoing evaluation in hospital, he developed seizures and altered sensorium. His MRI brain revealed bilateral mesial temporal lobe swelling with T2 hyperintense signal changes. CSF study revealed pleocytosis 25 cell/mm^3 with 100% lymphocytosis. Serum paraneoplastic antibody testing revealed antineuronal nuclear antibody 1 (ANNA-1) antibody positive. Considering the diagnosis of paraneoplastic encephalomyelitis, a whole body positron emission tomography-computed tomography (PET-CT) was done which showed a metabolically active lung mass. Fine needle aspiration cytology (FNAC) of the lesion revealed small cell carcinoma.

Paraneoplastic neurological syndromes (PNS) are rare, but are potentially treatable **(Table 3)**. These disorders are associated with cancer, but are not caused by the direct tumor invasion, metastasis or consequences of treatment. They can affect any area of the nervous system, including the central, peripheral and autonomic nervous system. Mainly, the PNS precede or follow the cancer diagnosis, although, in some cases, the primary cancer is not found even at autopsy.[33] The most commonly associated malignancies include small cell lung cancer, breast cancer, gynecologic tumors, and hematologic malignancies. Although the system involvement is often multifocal, like encephalomyelitis, it can involve a single system, e.g., cerebellar degeneration. The clinical symptoms may present even years before the primary malignancy manifests. Hence, a high index of suspicion is needed by the clinician to send these antibodies. Many a times there are no other specific investigations which make the diagnosis difficult. Sometimes a PET scan may reveal the malignancy. Early diagnosis can help in early treatment either by removal of primary tumor, immune-mediated therapies or chemotherapy. Early detection also improves the morbidity and mortality. The tests performed in this group of diseases are summarized in **Table 4**.

When the body tries to eliminate tumor cells, it launches an immune response, and this response can target normal neural tissues.[56] This could be mediated by antibodies or by T-cells. Thus, most of the PNS reflect a nervous system-specific autoimmune attack initiated by onconeural antigens released to the peripheral lymphoid tissue from an unsuspected primary or recurrent neoplasm.[33] Frequently, a CSF study in these patients reveals lymphocytic pleocytosis, elevated protein, increased immunoglobulin G (IgG) synthesis, and OCBs, supporting the immunological pathology.

TABLE 3: Paraneoplastic syndromes—clinical features.

Antibody	Neoplasm predicted by autoantibody	Clinical features
Neuronal antibodies		
Antineuronal nuclear antibody 1 (ANNA-1) (anti-Hu)[35]	Small cell lung cancer (SCLC), neuroblastoma, thymoma	PEM-limbic, cortical, brainstem encephalitis, PCD, myelitis, PSN, autonomic dysfunction
ANNA-2 (Ri)[36]	Lung carcinoma, breast carcinoma	Brainstem encephalitis, opsoclonus myoclonus, PCD
ANNA-3[37]	Lung carcinoma, upper airway carcinoma	Sensory/sensorimotor neuropathy, cerebellar ataxia, myelopathy, brainstem and limbic encephalopathy
Antiglial nuclear antibody (AGNA-1)[38]	SCLC	LEMS, PCD, sensory neuronopathy, limbic encephalitis, sensory motor neuropathy
Anti-Ma[39]	Germ cell tumor of testis, lung, GIT, breast, NHL	Cerebellar/brainstem syndrome limbic encephalitis. Narcolepsy like cataplexy, hypnagogic hallucination
Zic[40]	SCLC	Limbic encephalitis > cerebellar/ brainstem syndrome
Cytoplasmic antibodies		
Purkinje cell cytoplasmic antibody PCA-1[41]	Ovarian, Fallopian, endometrial and breast carcinoma	PCD
PCA-2[42]	SCLC	Brainstem/limbic encephalitis, PCD, LEMS, motor neuronopathy
PCA-Tr[43]	Hodgkin's lymphoma	PCD, limbic encephalopathy
Amphiphysin[44]	Breast carcinoma lung carcinoma	Stiff-man syndrome, PEM
CRMP-5 (collapsin response mediator protein-5)[45]	SCLC, thymoma, thyroid, renal carcinoma	PEM, PCD, chorea, optic neuropathy, myelopathy, and peripheral neuropathy
Striational (sarcomeric proteins)	SCLC, thymoma, breast carcinoma	Myasthenia gravis
Cell membrane antibodies		
Voltage-gated calcium channel (VGCC) N27	Lung, breast, ovarian carcinoma	LEMS, cerebellar degeneration
VGCC P/Q[46]	SCLC	LEMS, cerebellar degeneration
AChR, muscle[47]	Thymoma, SCLC	Myasthenia gravis
AChR, ganglionic[48]	Thymoma, SCLC	Autonomic neuropathy
Voltage-gated potassium channel (VGKC) related protein[49,50]	Thymoma, SCLC	Limbic encephalitis, Morvan's syndrome, PCD, GI dysmotility, parkinsonism, tremor, chorea, sensory motor neuropathy, hyponatremia, dyssomnia, and hyperphagia
NMDA receptor[51,52]	Thymoma, SCLC	Psychiatric features and memory loss, orofacial dyskinesia, choreoathetoid movements, abnormal posturing or increased tone, catatonic state, and central hypoventilation
AMPA receptor[53]	SCLC, thymoma, breast	Limbic encephalitis, atypical psychosis
GABAB receptor[24]	SCLC	Limbic encephalitis
Glycine receptor[54]	Lung cancer	Progressive encephalomyelitis with rigidity and myoclonus (PERM)
mGluR1[55]	Hodgkin's lymphoma	PCD

(AChR: acetylcholine receptor; AMPA: α-amino-3-hydroxy-5-methylisoxazole-4-propionic acid; GABAB: gamma-aminobutyric acid type B; GI: gastrointestinal; GIT: gastrointestinal tract; GluR1: metabotropic glutamate receptor 1; LEMS: Lambert–Eaton myasthenic syndrome; NHL: non-Hodgkin's lymphoma; NMDA: N-methyl-D-aspartate; PCD: paraneoplastic cerebellar degeneration; PEM: paraneoplastic encephalomyelitis; PSN: parasympathetic nerve)

TABLE 4: Tests in paraneoplastic neuronal autoantibody evaluation panel.

Tests in paraneoplastic neuronal autoantibody evaluation panel	Sampling material	Methodology
ANNA-1 (anti-Hu)—antineuronal nuclear antibody-1	CSF/serum	IIFA and confirm with dot-blot
ANNA-2 (anti-Ri)—antineuronal nuclear antibody-2	CSF/serum	IIFA and confirm with dot-blot
ANNA-3—antineuronal nuclear antibody-3	CSF/serum	IIFA
PCA-1-(anti-Yo)—anti-Purkinje cell cytoplasmic antibody-1	CSF/serum	IIFA and confirm with dot-blot
PCA-2—anti-Purkinje cell cytoplasmic antibody-2	CSF/serum	IIFA
PCA-Tr—anti-Purkinje cell cytoplasmic antibody-Tr	CSF/serum	IIFA
AGNA-1—anti-glial nuclear antibody-1	CSF/serum	IIFA
CRMP-5 (collapsin response mediator protein-5) (anti-CV-2) antibody	CSF/serum	IIFA and confirm with dot-blot
Anti-amphiphysin antibody	CSF/serum	IIFA and confirm with dot-blot
Anti-Ma/Ta antibody	CSF/serum	IIFA and confirm with dot-blot

(IIFA: indirect immunofluorescence assay)

Collection Instructions: CSF

- *Preferred volume*: 0.5 mL in sterile leak proof, polypropylene/plastic tube
- *Pediatric preferred volume*: 0.1 mL in sterile leak proof, polypropylene/plastic tube

Collection Instructions: Serum

- Collect 5 mL blood in golden top or red top Vacutainer
- Centrifuge and aliquot serum in polypropylene/plastic leak proof tubes within 2 hours of collection
- *Preferred volume*: 1 mL in leak proof, polypropylene/plastic tube
- *Pediatric preferred volume*: 0.5 mL in leak proof, polypropylene/plastic tube

Specimen Stability during Transport

- *Room temperature*: 72 hours
- *Refrigerated*: 14 days
- *Frozen*: 28 days
- *Frozen at 70°C*: 1 year

Multiple Sclerosis and Disorders

Clinical Case

A 14-year-old female presented in the year 2010 with instability of gait and visual loss in left eye of 2 weeks duration. She had history of hiccups with vomiting 12 days ago. On examination, the visual acuity in left eye was 2/60 with a hyperemic disk and left pupil mid dilated with RAPD, she also had a defective tandem walking. MRI *brain* with *contrast* showed hyperintensity of left optic nerve with contrast enhancement and multiple diffuse white matter lesions in brainstem. She was treated with steroids and had a partial improvement in left eye vision.

Four years later she again presented with visual loss in right eye. This time her right eye vision was 1/60 and left eye 6/60. Left eye fundus showed optic nerve atrophy. This time serum neuromyelitis optica (NMO) was sent and was positive. She was again treated with steroid and then put on azathioprine. She had no further attacks for next 8 years and is clinically stable and she also delivered a baby girl.

The clinical features of MS and related disorders are summarized in **Table 5**. Multiple sclerosis is a chronic inflammatory and demyelinating neurodegenerative disease of CNS. Both experimental and clinical evidence suggest that MS is an autoimmune disease driven by dysregulation of the adaptive immune response. The plaques that are present in the CNS of patients with MS contain inflammatory infiltrates composed mainly of lymphocytes and myeloid cells,[57] and a substantial fraction of T and B cells isolated from CNS lesions and the CSF of these patients are derived from clonal expansion.[58] Intrathecally produced oligoclonal antibodies are present in the CSF of patients with MS and these antibodies show evidence of antigen-dependent affinity maturation.[59] Oligoclonal bands of the CSF have been important in the diagnosis of MS for many years. Oligoclonal bands are nothing but immunoglobulins which are abnormally synthesised in CSF. The McDonald's diagnostic criteria for MS has been evolving since 2001. Initially, CSF OCB was an integral part of diagnosis of MS. However, in McDonald's revised criteria of 2010 CSF OCB was left out only to be included back in 2017 criteria where it was taken as a marker to prove dissemination in time.

The recent classification of NMOSD are divided based on aquaporin antibody positivity into NMO positive and NMO negative spectrum. Those with NMOSD antibody positive have therapeutic implication too. These patients are usually given long-term immune suppression to prevent relapses.

TABLE 5: Multiple sclerosis and related syndromes.

OCB	Multiple sclerosis	Sudden visual loss, motor weakness, sensory symptoms, bladder involvement, diplopia, trigeminal pain
NMO	NMOSD	Bilateral visual loss, paraplegia due to spinal cord involvement, Urinary symptoms
MOG	MOGAD	• Optic neuritis, transverse myelitis, brainstem encephalitis, encephalitis. Brain: ~75% abnormal (bilateral poorly demarcated subcortical lesions), ~30% brainstem involvement. Cord: ~50% abnormal, mixed STM/LTM with frequent conus medullaris involvement. Orbit: extensive, often bilateral, optic nerve lesions with frequent chiasmal involvement. 60% lymphocytic pleocytosis. OCB uncommon • Visual evoked potentials may show evidence of previous optic neuritis

(MOG: myelin oligodendrocyte glycoprotein; MOGAD: myelin oligodendrocyte glycoprotein-associated disease; NMO: neuromyelitis optica; NMOSD: neuromyelitis optica spectrum disorder; OCB: oligoclonal band)

Neuromyelitis optica spectrum disorder is a rare autoimmune disease mediated by recurrent inflammatory attack against the aquaporin-4 (AQP4) water channel on astrocytes primarily in the optic nerves and spinal cord, often leading to blindness and paralysis.[60] NMOSD is less prevalent than MS, and is distinguished by a highly specific serological marker, AQP4 immunoglobin G (IgG), in 70–80% of patients.[61] Since the discovery of a specific serum marker for NMO in 2004, and its subsequent identification as an antibody to AQP4, various methods have been developed to test for the antibodies in patient's sera. Antibodies against the astrocyte water channel protein, AQP4, were first described in 2004 in patients with the rare inflammatory demyelinating disease, NMO (Lennon et al., 2004).

Patients who test positive for antimyelin oligodendrocyte glycoprotein antibody (anti-MOG-Ab) present with a diversity of clinical and radiologic features, including manifestations suggestive of NMO spectrum disorder, as well as variability regarding disease course and response to disease modifying therapy. As well as in disease course and management as well. The investigative features of these diseases are summarized in **Tables 6 to 9**.

TABLE 6: Tests in multiple sclerosis evaluation panel.

Tests in multiple sclerosis evaluation panel	Sampling material	Methodology
Serum albumin quantitation	Serum	Colorimetric, BCG
Serum IgG quantitation	Serum	Colorimetric, BCG
CSF albumin quantitation	CSF	Turbidimetry
CSF IgG quantitation	CSF	Turbidimetry
CSF IgG index	NA	Calculation using the formula
CSF IgG synthesis rate	NA	Calculation using the formula
Albumin index	NA	Calculation using the formula
Intrathecal IgG synthesis rate	NA	Calculation using the formula
Serum oligoclonal bands	Serum	Isoelectric focusing and immunofixation
CSF oligoclonal bands	CSF	Isoelectric focusing and immunofixation

(BCG: bromocresol green; CSF: cerebrospinal fluid; IgG: immunoglobulin G)

Specimen Required

- Paired serum and CSF has to be collected at same time and labeled properly.
- *CSF volume*: 1 mL in sterile leak proof, polypropylene/plastic tube
- *Serum volume*: 2 mL in leak proof, polypropylene/plastic tube

Collection Instructions

- 4 mL of blood to be collected in golden top or red top Vacutainer
- Centrifuge and aliquot serum in polypropylene/plastic leak proof tubes within 2 hours of collection

Method of Sample Transportation

Use small leak proof, polypropylene/plastic tube. Sample is stable at ambient temperature for 72 hours. Samples refrigerated at 4°C are stable up to 14 days. It should reach the laboratory within 72 hours.

TABLE 7: CNS inflammatory panel evaluation.

CNS inflammatory evaluation panel includes	Preferred specimen	Methodology
Serum albumin quantitation	Serum	Colorimetric, BCG
Serum IgG quantitation	Serum	Colorimetric, BCG
CSF albumin quantitation	CSF	Turbidimetry
CSF IgG quantitation	CSF	Turbidimetry
CSF IgG index	NA	Calculation using the formula
CSF IgG synthesis rate	NA	Calculation using the formula
Albumin index	NA	Calculation using the formula
Intrathecal IgG synthesis rate	NA	Calculation using the formula
Serum oligoclonal bands	Serum	IEF and IF
CSF oligoclonal bands	CSF	IEF and IF

(BCG: bromocresol green; CNS: central nervous system; CSF: cerebrospinal fluid; IEF: isoelectric focusing; IF: immunofixation; IgG: immunoglobulin G)

Collection Instructions: Serum

- Collect 4 mL blood in golden top or red top Vacutainer
- Centrifuge and aliquot serum in polypropylene/plastic leak proof tubes within 2 hours of collection
- *Preferred volume*:
  - *Serum*: 2 mL in leak proof, polypropylene/plastic tube
  - *CSF*: 1 mL in sterile leak proof, polypropylene/plastic tube
- *Pediatric preferred volume*:
  - *Serum*: 1 mL in leak proof, polypropylene/plastic tube
  - *CSF*: 1 mL in sterile leak proof, polypropylene/plastic tube

Specimen Stability during Transport

- *Room temperature*: 72 hours
- *Refrigerated*: 14 days
- *Frozen*: 28 days
- *Frozen at 70°C*: 1 year

TABLE 8: NMO-IgG (AQP4) antibody in CSF/serum.

Test name: NMO- IgG (AQP4) antibody	Sampling material	Methodology
NMO-IgG	CSF/serum	CBA-IIF microscopy on fixed cell

(CBA-IIF: cell-based assay-indirect immunofluorescence; NMO-IgG: neuromyelitis optica-immunoglobulin G)

Collection Instruction: CSF

- *Preferred volume*: 1 mL in sterile leak proof, polypropylene/plastic tube
- *Pediatric preferred volume*: 0.5 mL in sterile leak proof, polypropylene/plastic tube

Collection Instructions: Serum

- Collect 5 mL blood in golden top or red top Vacutainer
- Centrifuge and aliquot serum in polypropylene/plastic leak proof tubes within 2 hours of collection
- *Preferred volume*: 1 mL in leak proof, polypropylene/plastic tube
- *Pediatric preferred volume*: 0.5 mL in leak proof, polypropylene/plastic tube

Specimen Stability during Transport

- *Room temperature*: 72 hours
- *Refrigerated*: 14 days
- *Frozen*: 28 days
- *Frozen at 70°C*: 1 year

TABLE 9: Neuromyelitis optica spectrum disorders (CSF/serum).

Neuromyelitis optica spectrum disorders antibody screen panel	Sampling material	Methodology
Neuromyelitis optica	CSF/serum	CBA, IFA
Myelin oligodendrocyte glycoprotein (MOG)	CSF/serum	CBA, IFA

(CBA, IFA: cell-based assay on transfected cell and detection by indirect immunofluorescence method; CSF: cerebrospinal fluid)

Collection Instruction: CSF

- *Preferred volume*: 1 mL in sterile leak proof, polypropylene/plastic tube
- *Pediatric preferred volume*: 0.5 mL in sterile leak proof, polypropylene/plastic tube

Collection Instructions: Serum

- Collect 4 mL blood in golden top or red top Vacutainer
- Centrifuge and aliquot serum in polypropylene/plastic leak proof tubes within 2 hours of collection
- *Preferred volume*: 1 mL in leak proof, polypropylene/plastic tube
- *Pediatric preferred volume*: 0.5 mL in leak proof, polypropylene/plastic tube

Specimen Stability during Transport

- *Room temperature*: 72 hours
- *Refrigerated*: 14 days
- *Frozen*: 28 days
- *Frozen at 70°C*: 1 year

Interpretation

The negative predictive value of OCB in neurological patients in CSF was 90%,[62] and even in patients with clinically isolated syndromes (CIS) negative predictive value of OCB was 88%.[63] So whenever we suspect MS and CSF shows OCB negative then one must workup for other differential diagnosis. Several authors found OCB in CSF highly sensitive and specific for MS.[64] Apart from a diagnostic role OCB are of prognostic value in CIS patients with a hazard ratio of 2.18 (95% confidence interval 1.71–2.77) for the prediction to convert to clinically definite MS.[65]

Antibodies to aquaporin-4 (called NMO-IgG or AQP4-Ab) constitute a sensitive and highly specific serum marker of NMO that can facilitate the differential diagnosis of NMO and classic MS. Anti-AQP4 antibody titers declined following treatment with high-dose methylprednisolone and remained low during periods of remission induced by immune suppression. These observations provide supportive evidence that the anti-AQP4 antibody is also a biomarker for disease activity in NMO.

Pitfalls

Apart from MS, there is a long list of diagnoses with CSF OCBs reported: systemic lupus erythematosus, neurosyphilis, neurological paraneoplastic disorders, Behçet's disease neuroborreliosis, aseptic meningitis, neurosarcoidosis, human immunodeficiency virus (HIV) infection, cerebral tumors including lymphomas, Sjögren's syndrome, herpes encephalitis, Morvan syndrome, anti-NMDA and other autoimmune encephalitis, neurotuberculosis, anticardiolipin syndrome, human T-lymphotropic virus (HTLV) myelopathy, prion disease, schistosomiasis, stiff-person syndrome, cerebral cysticercosis, GBS, and CNS vasculitis.[66]

However, AQP4-antibody positivity differs widely between studies (33–90%), suggesting either poor sensitivities of some tests or false positives in patients with clinically definite NMO.[17,18,67,68] False positives, which could lead to a diagnosis of NMO in patients with less requirement for aggressive/maintenance immunotherapies, have potential management implications.

Myelin oligodendrocyte glycoprotein IgG antibody titers may assist in monitoring disease course and prognosis, but their role is imperfect. Antibody titers may increase but may not be predictive of relapses or attacks. MOG IgG antibodies may become undetectable with immunosuppression, but this does not necessarily indicate clinical response. Results should not be used as a diagnostic procedure without confirmation of the diagnosis by another medically established diagnostic product or procedure. Children can be found to have the MOG antibody in the setting of ADEM; however, a positive MOG antibody test in the setting of ADEM does not necessarily imply a course of MOGAD. In many children, the MOG antibody disappears within 1 year, and relapses do not occur. In some cases, the MOG antibody persists, and relapses may occur. When a relapse occurs, the diagnosis of MOGAD is confirmed.

Muscle, Nerve, and Neuromuscular Diseases

Clinical Case

A 30-year-old female, postdelivery 1 week, history of coronavirus disease (COVID) vaccination taken 3 weeks back, presented with history of difficulty in walking associated with weakness of upper limbs, proximal > distal. She had history of headache and vomiting associated with neck muscle weakness and pharyngeal weakness in the form of difficulty in swallowing. On examination, she was conscious and oriented. She had neck muscle weakness with single breath count (SBC) of 25. Her gag was preserved. Fundus examination showed features of papilledema in both eyes. She had flaccid quadriparesis with flexor plantar response and spared sensory. Her nerve conduction study (NCS) was initially normal. MRI brain was unremarkable. CSF study showed CSF pressure of 32 cm of water with features of albuminocytological dissociation. Her NCS repeated after 3 days showed mild prolongation of F latency. In view of dilemma in diagnosis, serum ganglioside antibody panel was send which showed IgG-GQ1b antibody positivity which suggests possibility of variant of acute inflammatory demyelinating polyradiculoneuropathy (AIDP). She was started on plasmapheresis followed by which there was improvement of symptoms. Five cycles of PLEX was given. In this case, though the clinical scenario resulted in dilemma in diagnosis, the antibody positivity confirmed the diagnosis.

Guillain–Barré syndrome is an acute immune-mediated inflammatory polyneuropathy. Currently, two methodological approaches are available for AGAs detection; enzyme-linked immunosorbent assay (ELISA) (either in-house or commercial) and line-/dot-blot (commercial).[69]

The most common subtypes of the GBS include AIDP, AMAN, and AMSAN.[70-73] Other rare variants have also been described such as acute pandysautonomia, paraparetic variant, ptosis without ophthalmoplegia, acute ophthalmoparesis, and facial diplegia or sixth nerve palsy with paresthesias.[10-13] These subtypes are associated with distinct antiganglioside antibodies **(Tables 10 and 11)**.[10-13,74,75]

TABLE 10: Association of IgG antiganglioside antibodies with Guillain–Barré syndrome subtypes.

Subtypes/variants	IgG antibodies against	When to suspect
Acute inflammatory demyelinating polyradiculoneuropathy (AIDP)	None	Proximal > distal, ascending type of weakness
Acute motor axonal neuropathy (AMAN)	GM1 and GD1a	Pure motor variant, poor recovery
Acute motor sensory axonal neuropathy (AMSAN)	GM1 and GD1a	Motor and sensory axonal type of neuropathy, poor recovery
Acute motor conduction block neuropathy	GM1 and GD1a	Motor neuropathy with conduction block
Pharyngeal cervical brachial variant	GT1a (less frequently with GQ1b and GD1a)	Proximal muscle involvement, pharyngo-cervico-brachial weakness
Miller Fisher syndrome	GQ1b and GT1a	Ophthalmoplegia, areflexia, ataxia
Acute ataxic neuropathy	GQ1b and GT1a	Acute onset monophasic sensory neuropathy with diminished tendon reflexes, loss of proprioception, positive Romberg sign and nerve conduction features of demyelination
Pure sensory ataxic variant	GD1b (less frequently with GQ1b and GT1a)	Monophasic illness with exclusive sensory symptoms and signs, with evidence of widespread sensory neuropathy, in absence of systemic disorders that may cause acute sensory peripheral neuropathy
Bickerstaff brainstem encephalitis	GQ1b and GT1a	Ataxia, ophthalmoplegia, alteration in level of consciousness, hyperreflexia

(IgG: immunoglobulin G)

TABLE 11: Tests in ganglioside antibody evaluation panel.

Tests in ganglioside antibody evaluation panel	Sampling material	Methodology
GM1-IgG	Serum	ELISA
GD1b-IgG	Serum	ELISA
GQ1b-IgG	Serum	ELISA
GM1-IgM	Serum	ELISA
GD1b-IgM	Serum	ELISA
GQ1b-IgM	Serum	ELISA

(ELISA: enzyme-linked immunosorbent assay; GD1b: ganglioside-di-sialic acid; GM1: ganglioside-monosialic acid; GQ1b: ganglioside-tetra-sialic acid; IgG: immunoglobulin G; IgM: immunoglobulin M)

Preferred Specimen: Serum

Collection instructions

- Collect 5 mL blood in golden top or red top Vacutainer
- Centrifuge and aliquot serum in polypropylene/plastic leak proof tubes within 2 hours of collection
- *Preferred volume*: 1 mL in leak proof, polypropylene/plastic tube
- *Pediatric preferred volume*: 0.5 mL in leak proof, polypropylene/plastic tube

Specimen Stability during Transport

- *Room temperature*: 72 hours
- *Refrigerated*: 14 days
- *Frozen*: 28 days
- *Frozen at 70°C*: 1 year

Antiganglioside antibodies play an important role in the immunopathogenesis of GBS.[13] The most common antibodies that are identified are against GM1, GD1a, GD1b, GT1a, and GQ1b gangliosides. One of the proposed mechanisms is molecular mimicry in which antecedent infection produces specific antibodies, which in turn cross-reacts with peripheral nerve components because of the sharing of cross-reactive epitopes.[10] These antibodies can be directed against myelin or the axon. Antecedent infection with *Campylobacter jejuni* produces high titers of antibodies to GM1, GD1a, GalNAc-GD1a, and GD1b, which are strongly associated with the AMAN variant.[14] Similar association with *C. jejuni* infection and antibodies to GQ1b ganglioside has been reported in MFS.[15] Antibodies are more associated with the AMAN variant of GBS than with acute inflammatory demyelinating polyneuropathy.[76] Antiganglioside antibodies bind to the nodal axolemma or the paranodal myelin, thus leading to axonal degeneration or demyelination. Research has shown that the clinical features of GBS and its subtypes are closely associated with some specific antiganglioside antibodies.[10,77,78] Four gangliosides—(1) GM1, (2) GD1a, (3) GT1a, and (4) GQ1b—described in GBS differ with regard to the number and position of their sialic acids, in which M, D, T, and Q represent mono, di, tri, and quadri—sialosyl groups, respectively. IgG antiganglioside antibodies to GM1 and GD1a are more commonly associated with AMAN, AMSAN, and acute motor conduction block neuropathy, but not with AIDP.[76,79] Motor and sensory nerves express similar quantities of GM1 and GD1a; however, their expression within various tissues may differ.[80] It has been suggested that IgG anti-GD1a antibodies bind to the motor nerve terminals where the blood nerve barrier is deficient and cause pure motor neuropathy.[81] This could explain the preferential motor axon injury seen in AMAN. Testing AGAs panels by immunoblotting is simpler and more cost-effective than ELISA. The most common IgG antiganglioside antibodies observed in the acute demyelinating variant were anti-GT1b, followed by anti-GM2, anti-GD1a, anti-GD1b, anti-GQ1b, anti-GM1, and anti-GM3 antibodies and in the acute axonal variant were anti-GM1, anti-GM2, anti-GD1b, and anti-GT1b antibodies, followed by anti-GQ1b, anti-GM3, and anti-GD1a antibodies. The presence of antiganglioside antibodies in AIDP is not common. However, one study showed that, in AIDP, antiganglioside antibodies against GM3, GD3, and GT3 can be seen, which may produce an inhibitory effect on the spontaneous muscle action potential at the neuromuscular junctions.[82]

Disorders Involving Neuromuscular Junction

Clinical Case

A 52-year-old female, case of post-polio residual paralysis presented with generalized weakness and difficulty in walking which aggravated since 3–4 months. No history of diplopia/drooping of eyelids. History suggestive of symptoms getting exacerbated toward evening. On examination she has weakness of all four limbs with fatigability. NCS with repetitive nerve stimulation (RNS) done which showed evidence of decremental response. Acetylcholine receptor antibody level was done which was positive. She was started on pyridostigmine with steroids followed by which there was improvement of symptoms.

The clinical features of this group of disorders are summarized in **Table 12**. Majority of patients with neuromuscular junction (NMJ) dysfunction have either MG or Lambert-Eaton myasthenic syndrome (LEMS).[83,84] Both diseases are autoimmune in nature and each results from a T cell-directed antibody (Ab)-mediated attack on ion channels that are crucial for neuromuscular transmission via the NMJ. For MG, the target of the autoantibody attack is the nicotinic AChR in the postsynaptic membrane, whereas for LEMS the target is the P/Q-type voltage-gated calcium channel (VGCC) located in the presynaptic motor nerve terminal membrane. Currently, two well-characterized autoantibodies are known to be specific for, and to play a causative role in MG; namely, the anti-AChR and the anti-MuSK autoantibodies. Muscle-specific tyrosine kinase (MuSK) is a surface membrane enzyme that is essential in aggregating AChR during the development of the neuromuscular junction **(Table 13)**. The frequency of anti-MuSK antibodies in generalized but seronegative MG has been reported as between 40 and 70% in Caucasian populations.[85,86] The frequency of these antibodies in purely ocular MG is likely to be much lower.

In a third disorder, autoimmune neuromyotonia, antibody-mediated attack on the nerve terminal (rectifying) voltage-gated potassium channel results in spontaneous firing of the synapse.[87]

TABLE 12: Disorders involving neuromuscular junction (NMJ)—clinical features.

NMJ disorder	Autoantibody involved	When to suspect
Autoimmune MG AChR MG	Postsynaptic nicotinic AchR	• Ocular myasthenia, early and late onset MG—85% of patients are positive for anti-AChR antibodies). Major symptoms include fatigability, ptosis, diplopia, muscle weakness, dysarthria, dysphagia, and dyspnea
MuSK-MG	Postsynaptic MuSK	• In fifteen percentage of patients with MG, anti-AchR antibodies are not detected. 50% of these will be positive for anti-MuSK antibodies. These patients can have same presentation as anti-AchR MG, but with selective weakness and atrophy of neck, tongue, shoulder, and bulbar muscles[86]
Lrp4-MG	Postsynaptic LRP4	• Have mild symptoms, lack unique phenotype and respond well to anticholinesterases. Anti-LRP4 antibody positive patients comprise 6–8% of all patients with MG
LEMS	Presynaptic P/Q and N type VGCC	Present with proximal muscle weakness, absent DTR, oculobulbar weakness, and autonomic dysfunction. Postactivation facilitation of DTR is a characteristic feature[88]
Acquired peripheral nerve hyperexcitability syndrome	Presynaptic VGKC	The acquired peripheral nerve hyperexcitability syndromes include autoimmune neuromyotonia and cramp-fasciculation syndrome characterized by muscle cramps, weakness, fasciculations, and increased sweating. 20% of cases have been associated with thymoma[87]

(AChR: acetylcholine receptor; DTR: deep tendon reflex; LEMS: Lambert–Eaton myasthenic syndrome; LPR4: lipoprotein receptor-related protein-4; MuSK-MG: muscle-specific kinase myasthenia gravis; NMJ: neuromuscular junction; VGCC: voltage-gated calcium channel; VGKC: voltage-gated potassium channel)

TABLE 13: Muscle-specific kinase antibody.

Test name: Muscle-specific kinase antibody	Sampling material	Methodology
Muscle-specific kinase antibody	Serum	Quantitative sandwich ELISA

(ELISA: enzyme-linked immunosorbent assay)

Collection Instructions
- Collect 5 mL blood in golden top or red top Vacutainer
- Centrifuge and aliquot serum in polypropylene/plastic leak proof tubes within 2 hours of collection
- *Preferred specimen*: Serum
- *Preferred volume*: Serum 1 mL in leak proof, polypropylene/plastic tube
- *Pediatric preferred volume*: 0.5 mL in leak proof, polypropylene/plastic tube

Specimen Stability during Transport
- *Room temperature*: 72 hours
- *Refrigerated*: 14 days
- *Frozen*: 28 days
- *Frozen at 70°C*: 1 year

Utility

While very useful for diagnostic purposes, these autoantibodies have questionable utility for disease monitoring, with the possible exception of anti-MuSK antibodies.[89,90] AchR binding and blocking antibodies have high sensitivity and specificity. They are less sensitive in ocular myasthenia (~50%) compared with generalized MG (85–90%).[91,92] False positive test are seen infrequently in nonmyasthenic patients like those with amyotrophic lateral sclerosis (ALS).[93] Thymoma without MG, neonates to AchR antibodies positive mothers with myasthenia.[33] Acetylcholine receptor antibodies hence have diagnostic value and sometimes may also indicate the severity of the disease,[94] The identification of anti-MuSK antibodies effectively confirms the diagnosis of MuSK MG, as false positive results have not been reported and anti-MuSK antibodies are very seldom found in patients with anti-AChR antibodies.[95] Anti-MuSK and anti-striational antibodies (titin and ryanodine receptor) are correlated with disease severity and may predict treatment response but have not been studied in large enough patient numbers to recommend their use as disease biomarkers.

Myositis and Muscle-specific Antibodies

Autoantibodies specific for idiopathic inflammatory myopathy [myositis-specific autoantibodies (MSAs)] are clinically useful biomarkers which help in the diagnosis of PM/DM. Many of these are also associated with a unique clinical subset of PM/DM, making them useful in predicting and monitoring certain clinical manifestations. Classic MSAs known for over 30 years include antibodies to Jo-1 [histidyl transfer RNA (tRNA) synthetase] and other aminoacyl-tRNA synthetases (ARSs), anti-Mi-2, and anti-signal recognition particle (SRP). Anti-Jo-1 is the first autoantibodies to ARS detected in 15–25% of patients (**Tables 14 and 15**).

TABLE 14: Myositis antibodies and associations.

Autoantibodies	Disease association	Clinical association
Aminoacyl-tRNA synthetases Jo-1 antibody	PM, DM	Antisynthetase syndrome (myositis, ILD, polyarthritis, Raynaud's phenomenon, mechanic's hands)
PL-7 antibody	PM, DM	
PL-12 antibody	PM, DM	
EJ antibody	PM, DM	
OJ antibody	PM, DM	
KS	PM, DM	ILD
ZO		Myositis
YRS		Myositis
SRP antibody	PM	Myositis (necrotizing)
Mi2β antibody	DM	DM with typical skin lesions and mild myositis
MDA5/CADM-140	CADM/ADM	CADM, rapidly progressive ILD, severe skin manifestations
TIFIγ/α	DM	Malignancy-associated DM
MJ/NXP-2	DM	Adult and juvenile DM with severe skin disease
SAE	DM	DM

(ADM: amyopathic dermatomyositis; CADM: clinically amyopathic dermatomyositis; DM: dermatomyositis; ILD: interstitial lung disease; PM: polymyositis; SAE: small ubiquitin-like modifier activating enzyme)

TABLE 15: Tests in myositis antibody panel.

Tests in myositis antibody panel	Sampling material	Methodology
Mi-2β antibody	Serum	Qualitative line blot
Ku antibody	Serum	Qualitative line blot
PM-Scl100 antibody	Serum	Qualitative line blot
PM-Scl75 antibody	Serum	Qualitative line blot
Jo-1 antibody	Serum	Qualitative line blot
SRP antibody	Serum	Qualitative line blot
PL-7 antibody	Serum	Qualitative line blot
PL-12 antibody	Serum	Qualitative line blot
EJ antibody	Serum	Qualitative line blot
OJ antibody	Serum	Qualitative line blot
Ro-52 antibody	Serum	Qualitative line blot

Notes:
- Mi-2β: Recombinant Mi-2β protein. The corresponding human cDNA has been expressed with the baculovirus system in insect cells.
- Ku: Recombinant Ku protein. The corresponding human cDNA has been expressed with the baculovirus system in insect cells.
- PM-Scl100: Recombinant PM-Scl protein (100 kDa). The corresponding human cDNA has been expressed with the baculovirus system in insect cells.
- PM-Scl75: Recombinant PM-Scl protein (75 kDa). The corresponding human cDNA has been expressed with the baculovirus system in insect cells.
- Jo-1: Native Jo-1 protein (histidyl-tRNA synthetase), purified by affinity chromatography from calf and rabbit thymus.
- SRP: Recombinant SRP protein (54 kDa, signal recognition particle). The corresponding human cDNA has been expressed with the baculovirus system in insect cells.
- PL-7: Recombinant PL-7 protein (threonyl-tRNA synthetase). The corresponding human cDNA has been expressed with the baculovirus system in insect cells.
- PL-12: Recombinant PL-12 protein (alanyl-tRNA synthetase). The corresponding human cDNA has been expressed with the baculovirus system in insect cells.
- EJ: Recombinant EJ protein (glycyl-tRNA synthetase). The corresponding human cDNA has been expressed in *Escherichia coli*.
- OJ: Recombinant OJ protein (isoleucyl-tRNA synthetase). The corresponding human cDNA has been expressed in *E. coli*.
- Ro-52: Recombinant Ro-52 (52 kDa). The corresponding human cDNA has been expressed with the baculovirus system in insect cells.

Collection Instructions: Serum
- Collect 5 mL blood in golden top or red top Vacutainer
- Centrifuge and aliquot serum in polypropylene/plastic leak proof tubes within 2 hours of collection
- Preferred volume: 2 mL in leak proof, polypropylene/plastic tube
- Ped*iatric preferred volume*: 1 mL in leak proof, polypropylene/plastic tube

Specimen Stability during Transport
- Room temperature: 72 hours
- Refrigerated: 14 days
- Frozen: 28 days
- *Frozen at 70°C*: 1 year

CONCLUSION

Autoimmune neurology is a rapidly developing subspecialty in the field of neurology. Familiarity and awareness of different antibody-associated phenotypes can help to ensure prompt diagnosis and treatment. Clinical monitoring and treatment must expand beyond the acute care setting. A growing body of literature illustrates prolonged periods of recovery complicated by behavioral dysfunction and neuropsychiatric symptoms that can happen months to years after the diagnosis. The ultimate aim should be to provide optimal, long-term outpatient care in the field of autoimmune neurology.

REFERENCES

1. Graus F, Dalmau J. Paraneoplastic neurological syndromes. Curr Opin Neurol. 2012;25:795-801.
2. Lancaster E, Dalmau J. Neuronal autoantigens: pathogenesis, associated disorders and antibody testing. Nat Rev Neurol. 2012;8:380-90.
3. Dalmau J, Rosenfeld MR. Paraneoplastic neurologic syndromes. In: Fauci A, Braunwald E, Kasper D, Hauser S, Longo D, Jameson JL (Eds). Harrison's Principles of Internal Medicine, 17th edition. New York: McGraw Hill Medical; 2008. p. 623.
4. Palace J, Leite MI, Nairne A, Vincent A. Interferon beta treatment on neuromyelitis optica: increase in relapses and aquaporin 4 antibody titers. Arch Neurol. 2010;67:1016-7.
5. Gilhus NE. Myasthenic Gravis. N Engl J Med. 2016;375:2570-81.
6. Gilhus NE, Verschuuren JJ. Myasthenia gravis: subgroup classification and therapeutic strategies. Lancet Neurol. 2015;14:1023-36.
7. Guptil JT, Soni M, Meriggioli MN. Current treatment, emerging translational therapies, and new therapeutic targets for autoimmune myasthenia gravis. Neurotherapeutics. 2016;13:118-31.

8. Benatar M, Mcdermott MP, Sanders DB, Wolfe GI, Barohn RJ, Nowak RJ, et al. Efficacy of prednisone for the treatment of ocular myasthenia (EPITOME): A randomized, controlled trial. Muscle Nerve. 2016;53:363-9.
9. Dalmau J, Graus F. Antibody-Mediated encephalitis. N Engl J Med. 2018;378:840-51.
10. Sun B, Ramberger M, O'Connor KC, Bashford-Rogers RJM, Irani SR. The B cell immunobiology that underlies CNS autoantibody-mediated diseases. Nat Rev Neurol. 2020;16:481-92.
11. Ramanathan S, Al-Diwani A, Waters P, Irani SR. The autoantibody-mediated encephalitides: from clinical observations to molecular pathogenesis. J Neurol. 2021;268:1689-707.
12. Varley J, Taylor J, Irani SR. Autoantibody-mediated diseases of the CNS: structure, dysfunction and therapy. Neuropharmacology. 2018;132:71-82.
13. Miller TD, Chong TT, Aimola Davies AM, Ng TWC, Johnson MR, Irani SR, et al. Focal CA3 hippocampal subfield atrophy following LGI1 VGKC-complex antibody limbic encephalitis. Brain. 2017;140: 1212-9.
14. Al-Diwani A, Handel A, Townsend L, Pollak T, Leite MI, Harrison PJ, et al. The psychopathology of NMDAR-antibody encephalitis in adults: a systematic review and phenotypic analysis of individual patient data. Lancet Psychiatry. 2019;6:235-46.
15. Varley JA, Webb AJS, Balint B, Fung VSC, Sethi KD, Tijssen MAJ, et al. The Movement disorder associated with NMDAR antibody-encephalitis is complex and characteristic: an expert video-rating study. J Neurol Neurosurg Psychiatry. 2019;90:724-6.
16. Titulaer MJ, McCracken L, Gabilondo I, Armangué T, Glaser C, Iizuka T, et al. Treatment and prognostic factors for long-term outcome in patients with antiNMDA receptor encephalitis: an observational cohort study. Lancet Neurol. 2013;12:157-65.
17. Van SA, Thijs RD, Coenders EC. Anti-Lgi1 encephalitis: clinical syndrome and long-term follow-up. Neurology. 2016;87:1149-56.
18. Binks S, Varley J, Lee W, Makuch M, Elliott K, Gelfand JM, et al. Distinct HLA associations of LGI1 and CASPR2-antibody diseases. Brain. 2018;141:2263-71.
19. Ariño H, Armangué T, Petit-Pedrol M, Sabater L, Martinez-Hernandez E, Hara M, et al. Anti-LGI1-associated cognitive impairment: presentation and long-term outcome. Neurology. 2016;87:759-65.
20. van Sonderen A, Ariño H, Petit-Pedrol M, Leypoldt F, Körtvélyessy P, Wandinger KP, et al. The clinical spectrum of Caspr2 antibody-associated disease. Neurology. 2016;87:521-8.
21. Irani SR, Pettingill P, Kleopa KA, Schiza N, Waters P, Mazia C, et al. Morvan syndrome: clinical and serological observations in 29 cases. Ann Neurol. 2012;72:241-55.
22. Petit-Pedrol M, Armangue T, Peng X, Bataller L, Cellucci T, Davis R, et al. Encephalitis with refractory seizures, status epilepticus, and antibodies to the GABAA receptor: a case series, characterization of the antigen, and analysis of the effects of antibodies. Lancet Neurol. 2014;13:276-86.
23. Spatola M, Petit-Pedrol M, Simabukuro MM, Armangue T, Castro FJ, Barcelo Artigues MI, et al. Investigations in GABAA receptor antibody-associated encephalitis. Neurology. 2017;88:1012-20.
24. Lancaster E, Lai M, Peng X, Hughes E, Constantinescu R, Raizer J, et al. Antibodies to the GABA(B) receptor in limbic encephalitis with seizures: case series and characterisation of the antigen. Lancet Neurol. 2010;9:67-76.
25. Laurido-Soto O, Brier MR, Simon LE, McCullough A, Bucelli RC, Day GS. Patient characteristics and outcome associations in AMPA receptor encephalitis. J Neurol. 2019;266:450-60.
26. Tobin WO, Lennon VA, Komorowski L, Probst C, Clardy SL, Aksamit AJ, et al. DPPX potassium channel antibody: frequency, clinical accompaniments, and outcomes in 20 patients. Neurology. 2014;83:1797-803.
27. Carvajal-González A, Leite MI, Waters P, Woodhall M, Coutinho E, Balint B, et al. Glycine receptor antibodies in PERM and related syndromes: characteristics, clinical features and outcomes. Brain. 2014;137:2178-92.
28. Cabezudo-García P, Mena-Vázquez N, Estivill Torrús G, Serrano-Castro P. Response to immunotherapy in anti-IgLON5 disease: a systematic review. Acta Neurol Scand. 2020;141:263-70.
29. Gaig C, Compta Y. Neurological profiles beyond the sleep disorder in patients with anti-IgLON5 disease. Curr Opin Neurol. 2019;32:493-9.
30. Gresa-Arribas N, Planagumà J, Petit-Pedrol M, Kawachi I, Katada S, Glaser CA, et al. Human neurexin-3α antibodies associate with encephalitis and alter synapse development. Neurology. 2016;86:2235-42.
31. Kunchok A, Zekeridou A, McKeon A. Autoimmune glial fibrillary acidic protein astrocytopathy. Curr Opin Neurol. 2019;32(3):452-8.
32. Varley JA, Andersson M, Grant E, Berretta A, Zandi MS, Bondet V, et al. Absence of neuronal autoantibodies in neuropsychiatric systemic lupus erythematosus. Ann Neurol. 2020;88:1244-50.
33. Lachance DH, Lennon VA. Paraneoplastic neurological autoimmunity. In: Kalman B, Brannagan TH 3rd (Eds). Neuroimmunology in Clinical Practice. Oxford: Blackwell Publishing; 2008. pp. 210-7.
34. Rosenfeld MR, Dalmau J. Update on paraneoplastic and autoimmune disorders of the central nervous system. Semin Neurol. 2010;33:320-31.
35. Lucchinetti CF, Kimmel DW, Lennon VA. Paraneoplastic and oncological profiles of patients seropositive for type 1 anti-neuronal nuclear autoantibodies. Neurology. 1998;50:652-7.
36. Pittock SJ, Lucchinetti CF, Lennon VA. Anti-neuronal nuclear autoantibody type 2: Paraneoplastic accompaniments. Ann Neurol. 2003;53:580-97.
37. Chan KH, Vernino S, Lennon VA. ANNA-3 anti-neuronal nuclear antibody: Marker of lung cancer-related autoimmunity. Ann Neurol. 2001;50:301-11.
38. Graus F, Vincent A, Pozo-Rosich P, Sabater L, Saiz A, Lang B, et al. Anti-glial nuclear antibody: Marker of lung cancer-related paraneoplastic neurological syndromes. J Neuroimm. 2005;165:166-71.
39. Dalmau J, Graus F, Villarejo A, Posner JB, Blumenthal D, Thiessen B, et al. Clinical analysis of anti-Ma-2 associated encephalitis. Brain. 2004;127:1831-44.
40. Bataller L, Wade DF, Graus F, Stacy HD, Rosenfeld MR, Dalmau J. Antibodies to Zic4 in paraneoplastic neurological disorders and small-cell lung cancer. Neurology. 2004;62:778-82.
41. Peterson K, Rosenblum MK, Kotanides H, Posner JB. Paraneoplastic cerebellar degeneration. I. A clinical analysis of 55 anti-Yo antibody-positive patients. Neurology. 1992;42:1931-7.
42. Vernino S, Lennon VA. New Purkinje cell antibody (PCA-2): Marker of lung cancer-related neurological autoimmunity. Ann Neurol. 2000;47:297-305.
43. Bernal F, Shams'ili S, Rojas I, Sanchez-Valle R, Saiz A, Dalmau J, et al. Anti-Tr antibodies as markers of paraneoplastic cerebellar degeneration and Hodgkin's disease. Neurology. 2003;60:230-4.
44. Pittock SJ, Lucchinetti CF, Parisi JE, Benarroch EE, Mokri B, Stephan CL, et al. Amphiphysin autoimmunity: Paraneoplastic accompaniments. Ann Neurol. 2005;58:96-107.
45. Yu Z, Kryzer TJ, Griesmann GE, Kim K, Benarroch EE, Lennon VA. CRMP-5 neuronal autoantibody: Marker of lung cancer and thymoma-related autoimmunity. Ann Neurol. 2001;49:146-54.
46. Lennon VA, Kryzer TJ, Griesmann GE, O'Suilleabhain PE, Windebank AJ, Woppmann A, et al. Calcium-channel antibodies in the Lambert-Eaton syndrome and other paraneoplastic syndromes. N Engl J Med. 1995;332:1467-74.

47. Vernino S, Lennon VA. Autoantibody profiles and neurological correlations of thymoma. Clin Can Res. 2004;10:7270-5.
48. Vernino S, Adamski J, Kryzer TJ, Fealey RD, Lennon VA. Neuronal nicotinic ACh receptor antibody in subacute autonomic neuropathy and cancer-related syndromes. Neurology. 1998;50:1806-13.
49. Thieben MJ, Lennon VA, Boeve BF, Aksamit AJ, Keegan M, Vernino S. Potentially reversible autoimmune limbic encephalitis with neuronal potassium channel antibody. Neurology. 2004;62: 1177-82.
50. Vincent A, Buckley C, Schott JM, Baker I, Dewar BK, Detert N, et al. Potassium channel antibody-associated encephalopathy: A potentially immunotherapy-responsive form of limbic encephalitis. Brain. 2004;127:701-12.
51. Vitiliani R, Mason W, Ances B, Zwerdling T, Jiang Z, Dalmau J. Paraneoplastic encephalitis, psychiatric symptoms, and hypoventilation in ovarian teratoma. Ann Neurol. 2005;58:594-604.
52. Irani SR, Bera K, Waters P, Zuliani L, Maxwell S, Zandi MS, et al. N-methyl-D-aspartate antibody encephalitis: Temporal progression of clinical and paraclinical observations in a predominantly nonparaneoplastic disorder of both sexes. Brain. 2010;133:1655-7.
53. Lai M, Hughes EG, Peng X, Zhou L, Gleichman AJ, Shu H, et al. AMPA receptor antibodies in limbic encephalitis alter synaptic receptor location. Ann Neurol. 2009;65:424-34.
54. Hutchinson M, Waters P, McHugh J, Gorman G, O'Riordan S, Connolly S, et al. Progressive encephalomyelitis, rigidity, and myoclonus: A novel glycine receptor antibody. Neurology. 2008;71:1291-2.
55. Sillevis Smitt P, Kinoshita A, De Leeuw B, Moll W, Coesmans M, Jaarsma D, et al. Paraneoplastic cerebellar ataxia due to autoantibodies against a glutamate receptor. N Engl J Med. 2000;342:21-7.
56. Pittock SJ, Kryzer TJ, Lennon VA. Paraneoplastic antibodies coexist and predict cancer, not neurological syndrome. Ann Neurol. 2004;56:715-9.
57. Lucchinetti C, Brück W, Parisi J, Scheithauer B, Rodriguez M, Lassmann H. Heterogenicity of multiple sclerosis lesions: implications for the pathogenesis of demyelination. Ann Neurol. 2000;47:707-17.
58. Babbe H, Roers A, Waisman A, Lassmann H, Goebels N, Hohlfeld R, et al. Clonal expansions of CD8(+) T cells dominate the T cell infiltrate in active multiple sclerosis lesions as shown by micromanipulation and single cell polymerase chain reaction. J Exp Med. 2000;192;393-404.
59. Obermeier B, Mentele R, Malotka J, Kellermann J, Kümpfel T, Wekerle H, et al. Matching of oligoclonal immunoglobulin transcriptomes and prteomes of cerebrospinal fluid in multiple sclerosis. Nat Med. 2008;14:688-93.
60. Oh J, Levy M. Neuromyelitis optica: n antibody mediated disorder of central nervous system. Neurol Res Int. 2012;2012:460825.
61. Lennon VA, Wingerchuk DM, Kryzer TJ, Pittock SJ, Lucchinetti CF, Fujihara K, et al. A serum autoantibody marker of neuromyelitis optica: distinction from multiple sclerosis. Lancet. 2004;364: 2106-12.
62. Bourahoui A, de Seze J, Guttierez R, Onraed B, Hennache B, Ferriby D, et al. CSF isoelectrofocusing in a large cohort of MS and other neurological diseases. Eur J Neurol. 2004;11:525-9.
63. Tintore M, Rovira A, Brieva L, Grive E, Jardi R, Borras C, et al. Isolated demyelinating syndromes: comparison of CSF oligoclonal bands and different MR imaging criteria to predict conversion to CDMS. Mult Scler. 2001;7:359-63.
64. Freedman MS, Thompson EJ, Deisenhammer F, Giovannoni G, Grimsley G, Keir G, et al. Recommended standard of cerebrospinal fluid analysis in the diagnosis of multiple sclerosis: a consensus statement. Arch Neurol. 2005;62:865-70.
65. Kuhle J, Disanto G, Dobson R, Adiutori R, Bianchi L, Topping J, et al. Conversion from clinically isolated syndrome to multiple sclerosis: a large multicentre study. Mult Scler. 2015;2015;21:1013-24.
66. Petzold A. Intrathecal oligoclonal IgG synthesis in multiple sclerosis. J Neuroimmunol. 2013;262:1-10.
67. Waters PJ, Pittock SJ, Bennett JL, Jarius S, Weinshenker BG, Wingerchuk DM. Evaluation of aquaporin-4 antibody assays. Clin Exp Neuroimunol. 2014;5:290-303.
68. Jarius S, Wildemann B. Aquaporin-4 antibodies (NMO-IgG) as a serological marker of neuromyelitis optica: a critical review of the literature. Brain Pathol. 2013;23:661-83.
69. Franciotta D, Gastaldi M, Biagioli T, Benedetti L, Giannotta C, Bedin R, et al. Anti-ganglioside antibodies: experience from the Italian Association of Neuroimmunology External Quality Assessment Scheme. Clin Chem Lab Med. 2018;56:1921-5.
70. Yuki N, Hartung HP. Guillain–Barré syndrome. N Engl J Med. 2012;366:2294-304.
71. Hughes RA, Cornblath DR. Guillain–Barré syndrome. Lancet. 2005;366:1653-66.
72. Dimachkie MM, Barohn RJ. Guillain–Barré syndrome and variants. Neurol Clin. 2013;31:491-510.
73. Hartung HP, Pollard JD, Harvey GK, Toyka KV. Immunopathogenesis and treatment of the Guillain–Barré syndrome—Part I. Muscle Nerve. 1995;18:137-53.
74. Ogawara K, Kuwabara S, Mori M, Hattori T, Koga M, Yuki N. Axonal Guillain–Barré syndrome: Relation to anti-ganglioside antibodies and *Campylobacter jejuni* infection in Japan. Ann Neurol. 2000;48:624-31.
75. Jacobs BC, Hazenberg MP, van Doorn PA, Endtz HP, van der Meché FG. Cross-reactive antibodies against gangliosides and Campylobacter jejuni lipopolysaccharides in patients with Guillain–Barré or Miller Fisher syndrome. J Infect Dis. 1997;175: 729-33.
76. Sekiguchi Y, Uncini A, Yuki N, Misawa S, Notturno F, Nasu S, et al. Antiganglioside antibodies are associated with axonal Guillain–Barré syndrome: A Japanese–Italian collaborative study. J Neurol Neurosurg Psychiatry. 2012;83:23-8.
77. Yuki N. Guillain–Barré syndrome and anti-ganglioside antibodies: A clinician-scientist's journey. Proc Jpn Acad Ser B Phys Biol Sci. 2012;88:299-326.
78. Kaida K, Ariga T, Yu RK. Antiganglioside antibodies and their pathophysiological effects on Guillain–Barré syndrome and related disorders—a review. Glycobiology. 2009;19:676-92.
79. Capasso M, Caporale CM, Pomilio F, Gandolfi P, Lugaresi A, Uncini A. Acute motor conduction block neuropathy, another Guillain–Barré syndrome variant. Neurology. 2003;61:617-22.
80. Lopez PH, Zhang G, Zhang J, Lehmann HC, Griffin JW, Schnaar RL, et al. Passive transfer of IgG anti-GM1 antibodies impairs peripheral nerve repair. J Neurosci. 2010;30:9533-41.
81. Yuki N, Yoshino H, Sato S, Shinozawa K, Miyatake T. Severe acute axonal form of Guillain–Barré syndrome associated with IgG anti-GD1a antibodies. Muscle Nerve. 1992;15:899-903.
82. Usuki S, Sanchez J, Ariga T, Utsunomiya I, Taguchi K, Rivner MH, et al. AIDP and CIDP having specific antibodies to the carbohydrate epitope (-NeuAcalpha2-8NeuAcalpha2-3Galbeta1-4Glc-) of gangliosides. J Neurol Sci. 2005;232:37-44.
83. Mareska M, Gutmann L. Lambert–Eaton myasthenic syndrome. Semin Neurol. 2004;24:149-53.
84. Newsom-Davis J. Lambert–Eaton myasthenic syndrome. Rev Neurol. 2004;160:177-80.
85. Hoch W, McConville J, Helms S, Newsom-Davis J, Melms A, Vincent A. Auto-antibodies to the receptor tyrosine kinase MuSK in patients with myasthenia gravis without acetylcholine receptor antibodies. Nat Med. 2001;7:365-8.

86. Sanders DB, El-Salem K, Massey JM, McConville J, Vincent A. Clinical aspects of MuSK antibody positive seronegative MG. Neurology. 2003;60:1978-80.
87. Newsom-Davis J. Neuromyotonia. Rev Neurol. 2004;160:S85-9.
88. Jayarangaiah A, Theetha Kariyanna P. Lambert Eaton Myasthenic syndrome. In: StatPearls. [online]. Treasure Island (FL): StatPearls Publishing; 2022.
89. Lindstrom JM, Seybold ME, Lennon VA, Whittingham S, Duane DD. Antibody to acetylcholine receptor in myasthenia gravis. Prevalence, clinical correlates, and diagnostic value. Neurology. 1976;26(11):1054-9.
90. Vincent A, Newsom-Davis J. Acetylcholine receptor antibody as a diagnostic test for myasthenia gravis: results in 153 validated cases and 2967 diagnostic assays. J Neurol Neurosurg Psychiatry. 1985;48(12):1246-52.
91. Vincent A, Newsom-Davis J. Acetylcholine receptor antibody characteristics in myasthenia gravis, I: patients with generalized myasthenia or disease restricted to ocular muscles. Clin Exp Immunol. 1982;49(2):257-65.
92. Grob D, Brunner N, Namba T, Pagala M. Lifetime course of mysasthenia gravis. Muscle Nerve. 2008;37(2):141-9.
93. Mittag TW, Caroscio J. False-positive immunoassay for acetylcholine-receptor antibody in amyotrophic lateral sclerosis. New Engl J Med. 1980;302:868.
94. Tindall RS. Humoral immunity in myasthenia gravis: clinical correlations of anti-receptor antibody avidity and titer. Ann N Y Acad Sci. 1981;377:316-31.
95. Ohta K, Shigemoto K, Kubo S, Maruyama N, Abe Y, Ueda N, et al. MuSK antibodies in AChR Ab-seropositive MG vs AChR Ab-seronegative MG. Neurology. 2004;62(11):2132-3.

118

CHAPTER

Muscle and Nerve Biopsies

Megha S Uppin, Kiran Preet Malhotra, Afshan Jabeen

INTRODUCTION

The diagnostic platforms available for the evaluation of neuromuscular disorders (NMDs) include laboratory testing, electrophysiology, and histopathologic analysis in the form of invasive muscle and nerve biopsies. The diagnostic algorithms are revised with advances in non-invasive means such as genetics in hereditary NMDs as well as myositis antibodies in acquired inflammatory myopathies (IM). Nevertheless, muscle and nerve biopsies offer substantial diagnostic clues when the genetic testing does not yield a positive result or shows a "variant of unknown significance".[1,2] Similarly, many cases of IM can be seronegative requiring the help of a biopsy. This chapter emphasizes the utility of biopsies in the diagnosis of NMDs. Since the processing and interpretations are different, the chapter will be divided into two separate sections dealing with muscle and nerve biopsies, respectively. The biopsy-based diagnosis requires planning and a team-based approach involving a clinician, surgeon, and pathologist for optimal utility.

MUSCLE BIOPSY BASICS FOR CLINICIANS

Technique

The most appropriate site of the biopsy depends on the extent and distribution of the muscle weakness. CT and MRI may aid in selecting the muscle to be biopsied.[3-5] Generally, a moderately affected muscle is selected to be biopsied. The biopsy site should be superficial and easily accessible. Vastus lateralis and biceps brachialis are the most commonly biopsied muscles. However, according to the selectivity of the involvement, other sites including deltoid, triceps, brachialis, rectus femoris, soleus, tibialis anterior, and gastrocnemius are also chosen for biopsy. Tibialis anterior and gastrocnemius are biopsied in patients with predominant distal myopathy.[6,7]

The biopsy should be performed from the belly of the muscle since a biopsy close to the tendinous insertional zone may harbor changes such as endomysial fibrosis and fiber splitting which may result in a false diagnosis of muscular dystrophy.

There are two methods of performing muscle biopsy—needle biopsy and open biopsy. An open biopsy requires a larger incision, but a larger sample can be obtained. Needle biopsy is less invasive, and results in a smaller scar, but the sample size is smaller when compared to open biopsy. Needle biopsy is particularly useful in infants and children.[8,9]

Handling of Muscle Biopsy

The biopsied fresh muscle is wrapped in gauze moistened with a few drops of normal saline to prevent drying and immediately despatched to the laboratory. Care should be taken to ensure too much saline is not used to prevent saline artifacts. Upon receiving the muscle biopsy, the initial step is to prioritize the distribution of the sample. The frozen section is the most important aspect since frozen muscle is used for enzyme histochemistry, immunohistochemistry (IHC), western blot, and molecular studies. After assigning the portion for the frozen section, the rest of the muscle can be divided for glutaraldehyde fixation for electron microscopy and formalin fixation.

For the frozen section, the muscle biopsy is snap-frozen in isopentane cooled to −160°C in liquid nitrogen. Cryosections are used for both enzyme histochemistry (8–10 μm) and IHC (7–8 μm). After the sections are cut, the rest of the muscle can be stored at −80°C for further studies.

Stains

The muscle biopsy cryosections are processed for routine histochemistry, enzyme histochemistry, and special stains. Routinely, hematoxylin and eosin (H&E), modified

Gomori trichrome (MGT), reduced nicotinamide adenine dinucleotide tetrazolium reductase (NADH-TR), succinate dehydrogenase (SDH), combined cyclooxygenase and succinate dehydrogenase (COX-SDH), and adenosine triphosphatase (ATPase) at pH 9.4 and 4.6 are performed. In addition, for fiber typing fast and slow myosin, IHC is used. Additional stains such as periodic acid–Schiff (PAS), oil red O, and Congo red can be performed as required after assessing the biopsy with the routine stains.

The detailed protocols for enzyme histochemistry and IHC are described by Dubowitz V.[10]

Histochemistry

Hematoxylin and eosin: This stain gives the most important preliminary assessment of the architecture of the muscle. The muscle fibers are polygonal with subsarcolemmal nuclei and are arranged in fascicles which form the endomysium. The peripheral layer of connective tissue around each fascicle is perimysium whereas the outermost covering of connective tissue and vessels forms the epimysium.

The H&E stain helps in understanding:
- The general fascicular arrangement of the muscle
- Infiltration by adipose tissue and fibrosis
- Fiber size and shape variation with structural changes like vacuoles and whorling
- Presence of inflammation
- Changes in nuclear position
- Interstitial changes

The fascicular arrangement is lost in chronic long-standing myopathies of any cause and can lead to adipose tissue infiltration as well as fibrosis. Diffuse involvement is usually a feature of muscular dystrophy whereas focal involvement can be seen in neurogenic diseases or IM.

Fiber size: Its variation including hypertrophy and atrophy is a feature of many common myopathies; predominantly dystrophy; however, can be seen in long-standing neurogenic diseases. Hypertrophy can lead to fiber splitting. Fiber atrophy is a common feature of congenital myopathies and myotonic dystrophy. Perifascicular atrophy is an unequivocal feature of dermatomyositis (DM).

Fiber shape: The variations in fiber shape include rounded fibers in dystrophies and angulated atrophic fibers in denervation.

Nuclear changes: The nuclei of the skeletal muscle fiber are subsarcolemmal. Around 3% fibers showing the internalization of nuclei is considered nonpathogenic. However, internalization can be seen in chronic myopathies, particularly dystrophies. Centronuclear myopathies show >30% fibers with central nuclei. Fibers near the tendinous junctions show more internal nuclei. Regenerating fibers show bluish cytoplasm with plump vesicular nuclei unlike the slender ones in mature fibers.

Necrotic and degenerating fibers: These fibers show pale cytoplasm sometimes infiltrated by lymphocytes which is called myophagocytosis. These can be seen in dystrophies, IM, rhabdomyolysis, etc. The presence of significant fiber necrosis and regeneration in absence of inflammation is a characteristic of necrotizing myopathies. Perifascicular necrosis is one of the features of antisynthetase syndrome. A group of necrotic fibers within a fascicle forming a microinfarct is reported in DM associated with NXP2 antibodies.

Vacuoles: Rimmed and nonrimmed vacuoles can be seen in fibers. The rimmed vacuoles usually show granular eosinophilic rimming. These are usually seen in inclusion body myositis, GNE myopathies, and oculopharyngeal muscular dystrophy. However, the occasional rimmed vacuole is not specific and can be seen in any chronic myopathy with muscle degeneration. Nonrimmed vacuoles are seen in metabolic myopathies such as lipid and glycogen storage. The vacuoles of lipid myopathies are smaller and finer than those of glycogen storage which are bigger and coarser. Special stains with oil red O and PAS with diastase treatment (PAS-D) are used for staining lipid and glycogen, respectively.

Inflammation: This is mainly seen in all types of IM and some types of muscular dystrophies such as dysferlinopathies, calpainopathies, and facioscapulohumeral muscular dystrophies (FSHD). Perivascular inflammation is a characteristic feature of DM whereas endomysial inflammation around nonnecrotic fibers is seen in polymyositis and inclusion body myositis.

Modified Gomori's Trichrome: This is a special stain used for the demonstration of nemaline rods, red ragged fibers in mitochondrial myopathies and tubular aggregates. All these structures appear in red on MGT. MGT stains the nucleus of the fiber and the myelin of the interstitial nerve fibers; pink in color.

Masson trichrome: This is used as a connective tissue stain for highlighting the collagen. Fibrosis and collagen deposition in chronic myopathies stains blue/green on Masson trichrome.

Enzyme Histochemistry

Various enzyme histochemical stains aid in identification of fiber types as well as many structural abnormalities. Enzyme histochemical analysis can only be performed in fresh frozen muscle biopsies which emphasize the need for meticulous preservation of the biopsy in cold chain and immediate processing. It is recommended to have a muscle lab close to the procedure room to avoid artifacts caused due to delay.

Adenosine triphosphatase: At ATPase of pH 9.4, the type 1 fibers are pale and type 2 fibers are dark. This reaction is reversed at ATPase 4.6 and 4.3. This staining helps in characterizing specific fiber type changes.

Fiber type predominance: The presence of >55% of the type 1 fibers and 85% of the type 2 fibers is called type 1 and 2 fiber type predominance, respectively. Type 1 fiber predominance is a feature of myopathy whereas type 2 fiber predominance is seen in motor neuron disease. These percentages apply to vastus lateralis and biceps. In the gastrocnemius and deltoid, it cannot be used since there is usually more type 1 fibers in these muscles.

Fiber type atrophy: Type 1 fiber atrophy is a common feature for all congenital myopathies and myotonic dystrophy. Type 2 fiber atrophy is a nonspecific feature seen in disuse atrophy and following long-term steroid use, collagen vascular diseases, and myasthenia gravis.

Specific fiber type hypertrophy is not known.

Fiber type grouping: The type 1 and 2 fibers are arranged in a checkerboard pattern in a normal muscle. Loss of this pattern causing grouping of both types of fibers is a specific feature of neurogenic atrophy/spinal muscular atrophy.

Succinate dehydrogenase and NADH: These are oxidative enzymes that bring about mitochondrial and structural abnormalities in muscle fibers. The abnormal mitochondrial fibers show a classic blue ragged appearance. Other abnormalities such as central cores (central area of absence of oxidative enzyme activity), minicores, whorled fibers, and lobulated fibers are highlighted on these stains. The necrotic fibers have a peculiar moth-eaten appearance on NADH. This results due to the disruption of the myofibrillar network. These can be seen in any myopathic conditions with necrotic fibers such as dystrophy, IM, necrotizing myopathy.

Target fibers are characterized by three distinct zones. The central zone is devoid of oxidative enzyme activity, the middle zone of intense activity, and the outer zone of intermediate activity. They are usually seen in type 1 fibers. Target fibers are a feature of chronic neuropathies. Ring fibers with loss of oxidative enzyme activity in the center appear like a ring is seen in myotonic dystrophies.

Cyclooxygenase (COX): This is an important enzyme in mitochondrial respiratory chain and COX negative fibers are a hallmark of mitochondrial myopathies. A combined COX-SDH stain helps in picking up the negative fibers on COX. The percentage of COX negative fibers should be 1–2% in <30 years, >2% between 30 and 50 years and >5% in patients beyond 50 years. This is necessary for the correct diagnosis of mitochondrial diseases.

All these changes described so far are the foundation of the interpretation of muscle biopsy for beginners. These changes in various combinations are used for the diagnosis of specific entities which have been highlighted through some case-based examples.

Cai et al. have reported a pattern-based approach to the diagnosis of muscle diseases wherein they describe six different patterns[11]—(1) active myopathic damage and inflammation which is typical for IM; (2) active myopathic damage without associated inflammation as seen in necrotizing autoimmune myopathies, toxic, and metabolic myopathies; (3) chronic myopathic changes particularly seen in dystrophies, congenital and few metabolic myopathies; (4) myopathies with distinctive inclusions or vacuoles as seen in mitochondrial myopathies and storage diseases; (5) biopsies mainly showing atrophic changes; and (6) biopsies that appear normal.

It is important to note that finding a normal biopsy is not an insignificant finding. This helps the clinician to shift the focus away from a myopathic condition. The involvement of muscle in IM can be focal yielding a negative biopsy. Image guidance can help in such situations. Many metabolic myopathies can show normal biopsy.

Immunohistochemistry

Immunohistochemistry or immunofluorescence in frozen sections is the antibody-based techniques used to demonstrate the presence or absence of a particular protein. IHC can be used in diagnosis of muscular dystrophies and IM and myofibrillar myopathies.[10,12,13] The list of all the immunohistochemical markers and their applications is enlisted in **Table 1**. It is important to run controls alongside the test for comparison of the intensity of staining which can assess the presence, absence, or reduction of protein. The positive reaction on IHC depends on the location of the protein. Accordingly, it can stain positive on the sarcoplasmic membrane, blood vessels, nuclear membranes, or contractile proteins of the sarcoplasm. It is important to note that the IHC can show the absence of protein expression in primary as well as secondary deficiencies. The loss of expression in secondary deficiencies particularly in the case of dysferlin protein can result in a discrepant diagnosis of limb-girdle muscular dystrophy type 2B (LGMD2B). This is an important reason that the biopsy and IHC should always be interpreted in the light of complete clinical details.

Electron Microscopy

Ultrastructural study of cellular components including sarcolemma, sarcomere, nucleus, mitochondria, and blood vessels is necessary when routine enzyme histochemistry and histochemistry do not reveal definite abnormalities. It is useful in the diagnosis of congenital and metabolic myopathies, particularly glycogen storage disorders and mitochondrial myopathies.[14,15]

OTHER TECHNIQUES

Muscle tissue can be submitted for analysis by other techniques such as western blot, mitochondrial genome

TABLE 1: List of immunohistochemical stains and interpretation on muscle biopsy.

Antibody	Expression	Diagnosis
• Dystrophin rod domain (DYS1) • Dystrophin carboxy-terminal (DYS2) • Dystrophin amino-terminal (DYS3)	Complete absence along sarcolemmal membrane	Duchenne Muscular dystrophy
• Dystrophin rod domain (DYS1) • Dystrophin carboxy-terminal (DYS2) • Dystrophin amino-terminal (DYS3)	Variable expression along sarcolemmal membrane	Becker's muscular dystrophy
Alpha, beta, gamma, and delta sarcoglycans	Absent expression along sarcolemma	Sarcoglycanopathies 2C–2F
Dysferlin	Absent/reduced along sarcolemma	Dysferlinopathies/limb-girdle muscular dystrophy type 2B (LGMD2B)
Caveolin	Absent along sarcolemma	LGMD1C
Telethonin	Absent	LGMDR7
Emerin	Absent nuclear membrane	
Collagen VI	Absent/reduced along sarcolemma	Ullrich muscular dystrophy
Laminin-alpha 2 (merosin)	Absent/reduced along sarcolemma	Merosin deficient congenital muscular dystrophy
CD3, CD4, and CD8	Positive	T lymphocytes
CD20	Positive	B lymphocytes
CD68	Positive	Macrophages
MHC class 1	Positive along sarcolemma	Inflammatory myopathies
MHC class 2	Positive along sarcolemma	Antisynthetase syndrome
Myxovirus 1	Perifascicular, diffuse or focal along sarcolemma	Dermatomyositis
C5b-9	Positive capillary wall	Dermatomyositis
P62	Aggregates	Sporadic inclusion body myositis
Ubiquitin	Positive in sarcoplasm	Sporadic inclusion body myositis
Desmin	Positive in sarcoplasm	Desminopathy
Myotilin		Myotilinopathies

analysis, and mitochondrial respiratory chain enzymatic activity.[7,16]

Western blot is particularly useful in the diagnosis of muscular dystrophies such as calpainopathy, dysferlinopathy, and telethoninopathies.

ILLUSTRATIVE CASES

Case 1: Dermatomyositis

A 57-year-old woman presented for a neurologic consultation reporting 2–3 months of mild proximal muscle weakness of her legs and arms. Upon questioning, she reported myalgia, fatigue, and a 15-lb weight loss in the preceding few months but denied fevers, cough, or arthralgias. She also had recent mild erythema on her face that she attributed to sun exposure. On examination, she was found to have erythematous skin changes on her scalp, malar region of her face, eyelids, anterior neck (V sign), elbows, and metacarpophalangeal joints (Gottron's sign). On strength testing, she had weakness predominantly in the following areas: neck flexors 4+/5, shoulder abductors 4/5, elbow flexors and extensors 4/5, hip flexors 4/5, and knee extensors 4+/5. Creatine kinase level was mildly elevated at 389 U/L. Needle electromyography (EMG) showed fibrillation potentials with short-duration, low-amplitude motor unit potentials, and an early recruitment pattern in proximal muscles **(Figs. 1A to D)**.

Case 2: Sporadic Inclusion Body Myositis

A 68-year-old man was referred for weakness after a fall and poor response to physical therapy. The patient described difficulty getting up off the couch for the past 3 years and noted that he avoided sitting in some chairs at home. Over the past 6 months, he also noted that he could no longer loosen the lid of jars. Muscle strength testing showed—neck flexors 4+/5, bilateral deltoid 4/5, wrist extensor, and wrist flexor strength were both 5/5 but strength was 3/5 in bilateral finger flexors, and notably, he was unable to bury his fingernails when making a fist. In the lower extremities, there was asymmetric quadriceps weakness (4/5 on the right and 3/5 on the left) with obvious wasting of the medial and lateral aspects of his quadriceps bilaterally

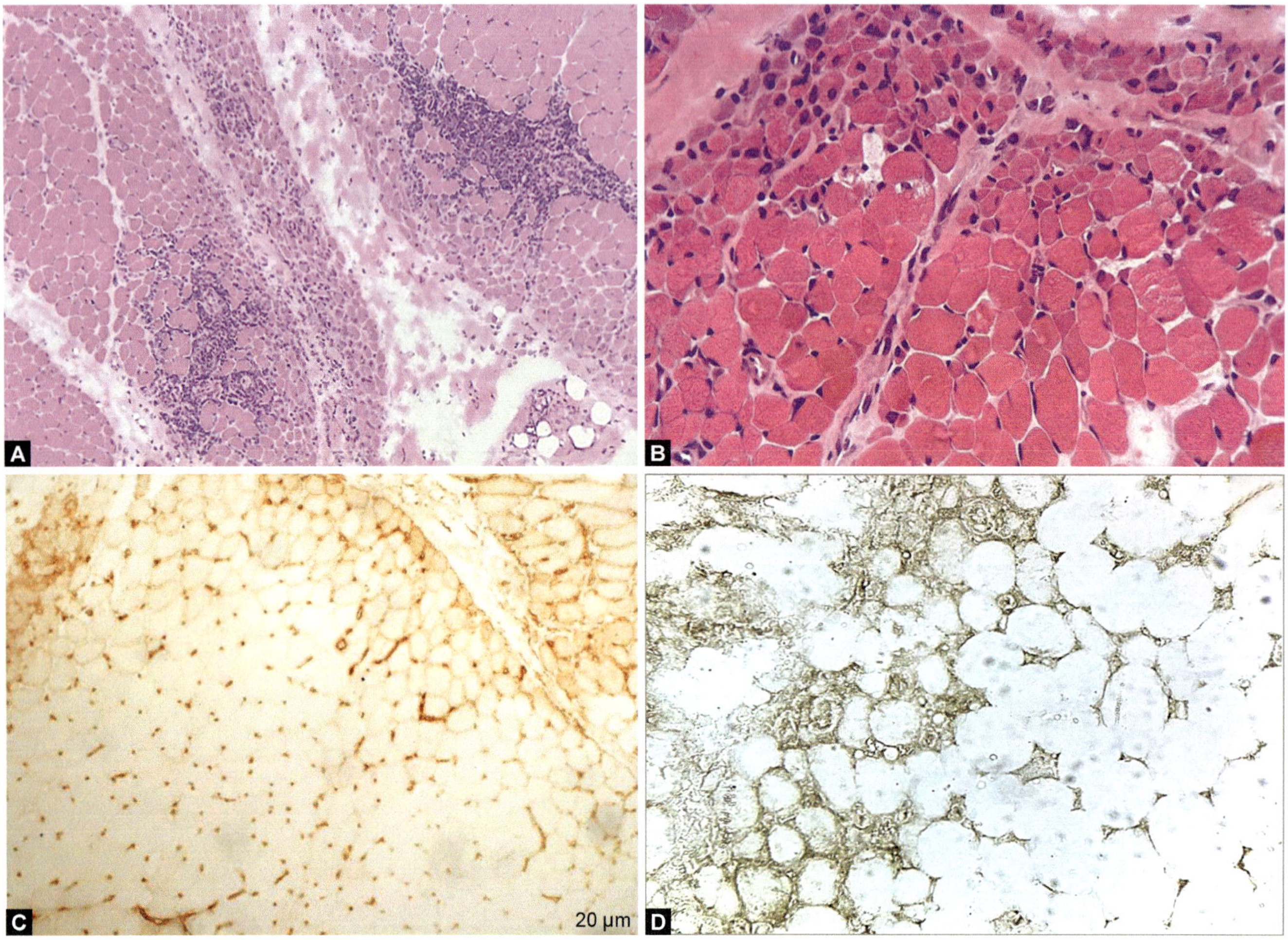

FIGS. 1A TO D: (A) Dense perivascular lymphocytic infiltrate with (B) prominent perifascicular atrophy; (C) The major histocompatibility complex (MHC) class 1 immunohistochemical expression along the sarcolemma in perifascicular fibers; (D) Immunoexpression of myxovirus antibody in perifascicular fibers.

with tibialis anterior muscle weakness of 4+/5. His reflexes were normal. Laboratory studies revealed a mildly elevated creatine kinase level of 479 U/L. EMG and electrodiagnostic studies were consistent with an irritable myopathy—abnormal spontaneous activity and myopathic motor unit potentials were observed in most tested muscles. An MRI of his lower extremities revealed prominent atrophy and T1 signal abnormalities in the vastus medialis and lateralis with sparing of the posterior compartment of the thigh **(Figs. 2A to F)**.

Case 3: Nemaline Myopathy

A 12-month-old boy was brought for evaluation of hypotonia and poor feeding, which he had experienced from birth. He had been born at 37 weeks of gestational age by induced vaginal delivery because of preeclampsia. He was in the neonatal intensive care unit for 2 weeks with stridor due to vocal cord paresis, feeding difficulties, micrognathia, and concern for aspiration. He had persistent failure to meet normal developmental milestones but had no regression. He was making age-appropriate progress in speech and language. He had made some gains in motor skills and was able to sit and roll front to back, but he could not pull himself up to stand or bear weight on his own. The general examination also at 12 months of age was significant for a high-arched palate, micrognathia, and pectus excavatum. Neurologic examination at this time was significant for low tone with decreased resistance to passive range of motion in all extremities and prominent head lag with facial weakness. His reflexes were normal. CPK was 530 U/L. Electromyoneurography (EMNG) showed myopathic potentials **(Figs. 3A to F)**.

Case 4: Mitochondrial Myopathy

A 15-year-old girl with normal cognitive function presented because of a 2-year history of slowly progressive ataxia and dysarthria. Her elder sister had early normal development but then developmental language declined. This sister died due to status epilepticus at age 3 years. Examination demonstrated mild ataxia involving the patient's limbs and trunk, absent muscle stretch reflexes, poor position sensation, poor vibratory sensation, and dysarthria. She

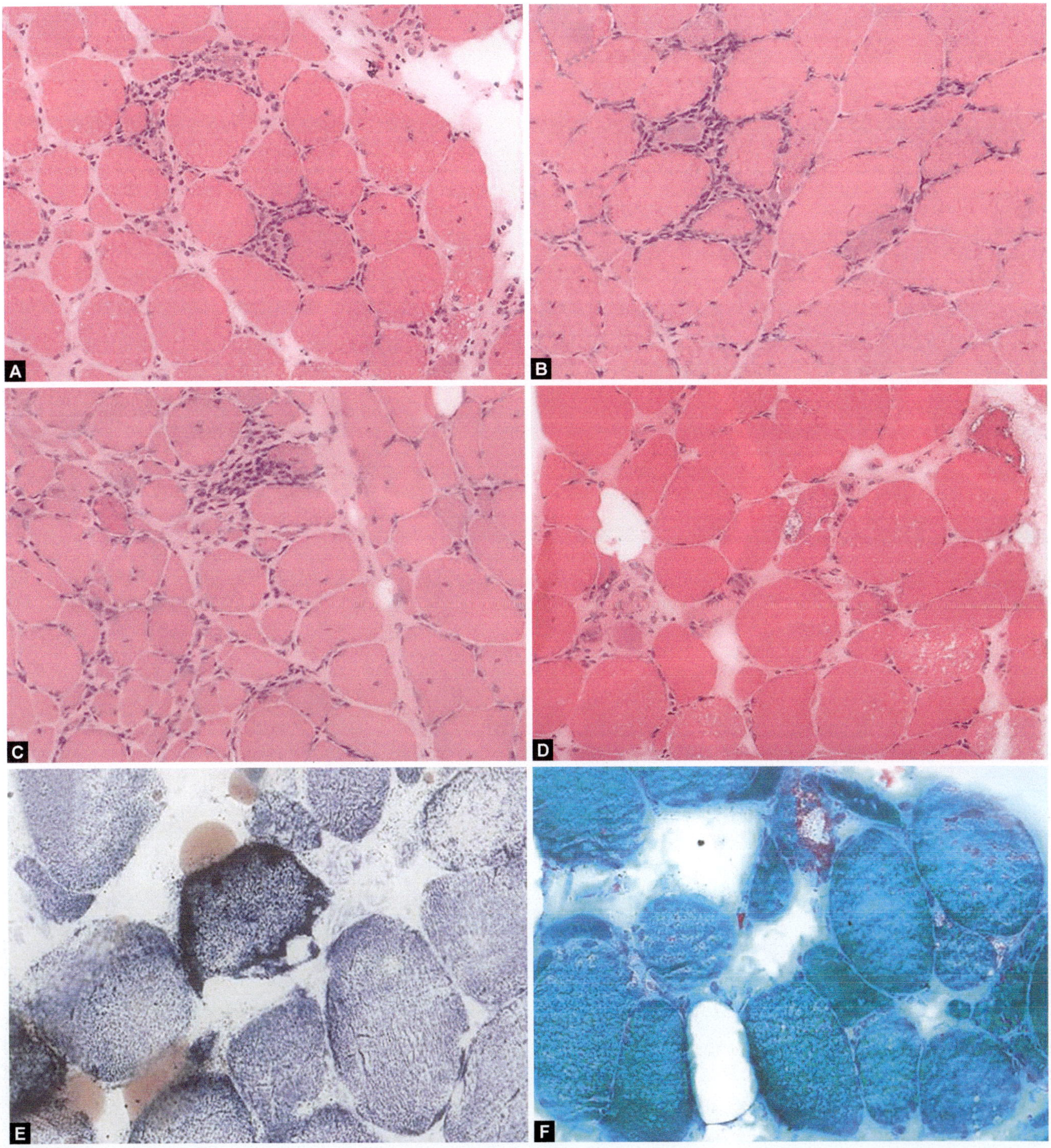

FIGS. 2A TO F: (A and B) Significant fiber size variation with atrophy, hypertrophy and internalization of nuclei. Endomysial lymphocytic inflammation around non-necrotic fibers. (C) The infiltrate is seen invading the muscle fibers; (D) Presence of rimmed vacuoles in the center as well as subsarcolemmal region; (E) The rimming of the vacuoles show red granular appearance on modified Gomori trichrome (MGT); (F) The biopsy also showed mitochondrial abnormalities in the form of blue ragged fibers highlighted on succinate dehydrogenase (SDH).

also had external ophthalmoplegia and mild proximal weakness in both lower limbs. Brain magnetic resonance imaging (MRI) and electroencephalogram (EEG) were normal. Her creatine phosphokinase (CPK) was 500 U/L. EMNG showed myopathic potentials. Nerve conduction study (NCS) showed sensory motor axonal neuropathy. Serum lactate to pyruvate ratio was elevated (25:1) **(Figs. 4A to F)**.

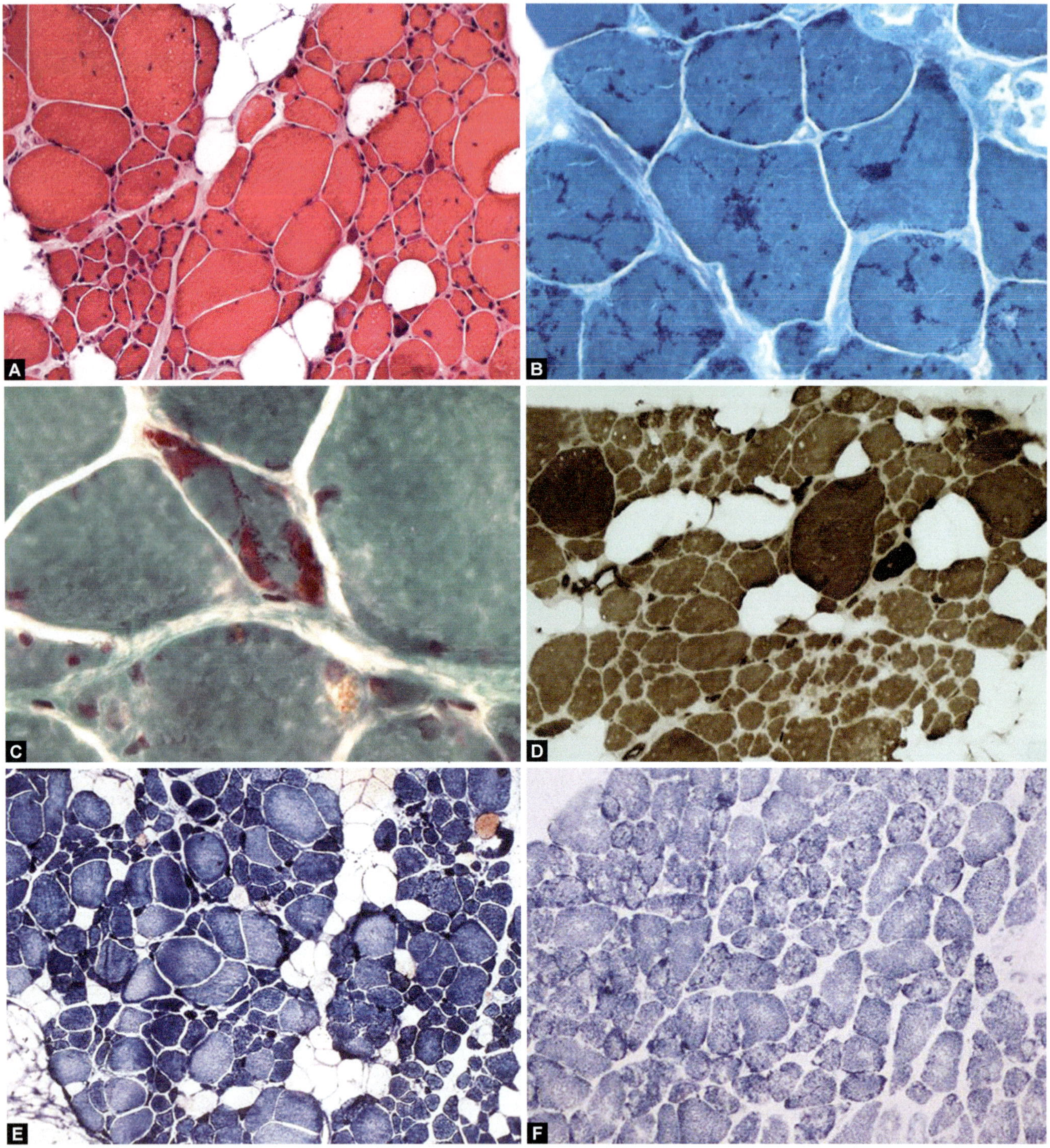

FIGS. 3A TO F: (A) Significant adipose tissue infiltration and fiber size variation; (B and C) The nemaline rods were seen in almost all the fibers and are highlighted as red-colored rods on MGT. (D) The ATPase at pH 9.4 showed type 1 fiber atrophy and predominance; (E and F) The SDH and NADH did not show any evidence of central cores or minicores.

(MGT: modified Gomori trichrome; NADH: nicotinamide adenine dinucleotide; SDH: succinate dehydrogenase)

Case 5: Glycogen Storage Disorder—Adult Onset Pompe Disease

A 32-year-old male was admitted to the intensive care unit with history of acute onset of breathlessness. He had developed easy fatigability and reduced exercise tolerance 1 year before the presentation. He has also noticed difficulty in getting up from a sitting position and performing overhead activities due to proximal muscle weakness for 1 year. The patient was born of a nonconsanguineous marriage, and there was no history of similar illness in the family. There was no history of fluctuations, fatigability,

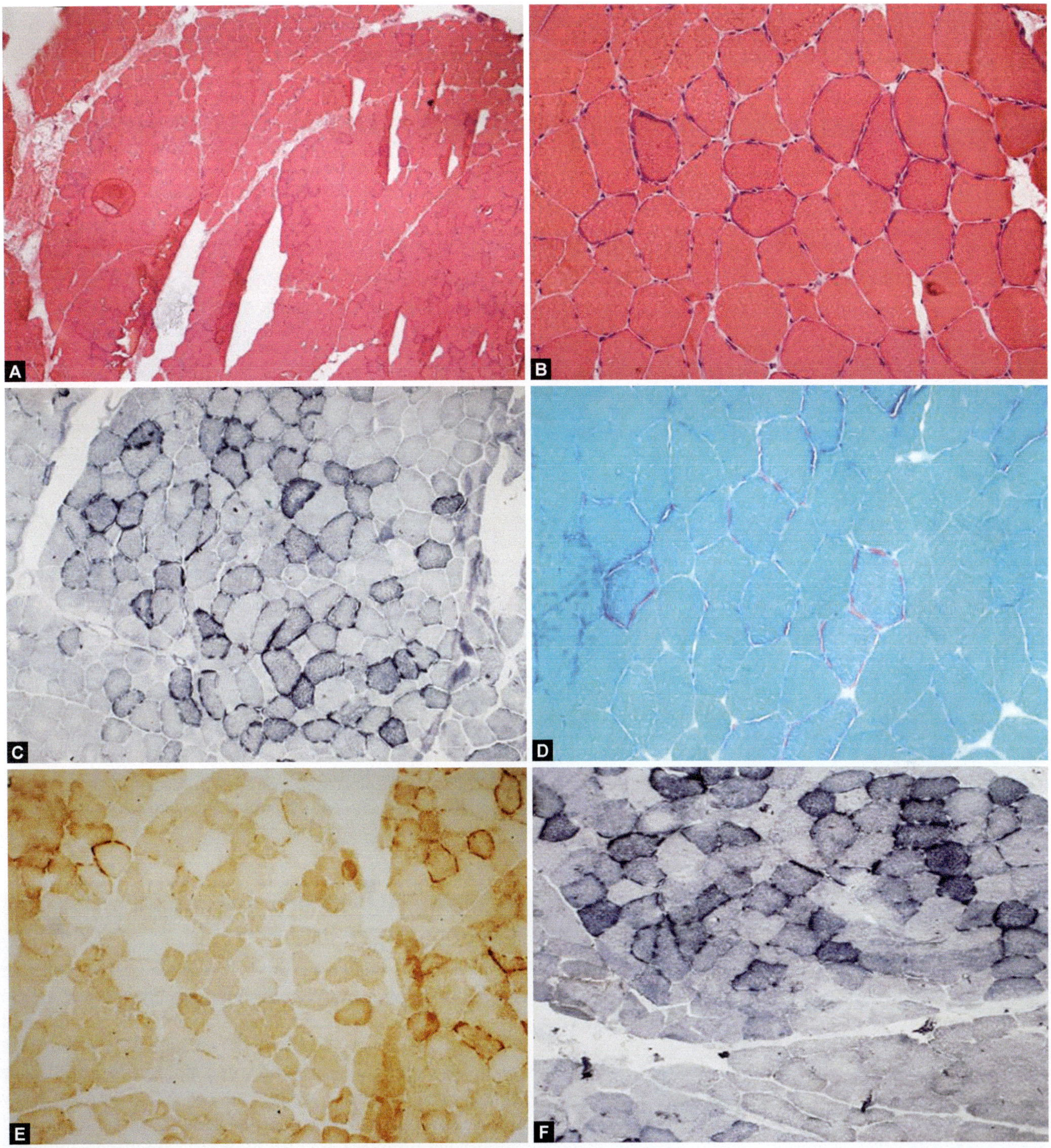

FIGS. 4A TO F: (A) Maintained fascicular architecture with many (B) red granular fibers; (C) The SDH showed many blue ragged fibers; (D) The MGT showed red ragged fibers; (E) Many fibers appear negative on COX and are highlighted on (F) COX-SDH stain.
(COX: cytochrome c oxidase; MGT: modified Gomori trichrome; SDH: succinate dehydrogenase)

diplopia, ptosis, bulbar weakness, or dark-colored urine. On examination, the patient was breathless and needed invasive ventilatory support due to poor respiratory efforts. There was symmetrical proximal (lower limbs 3/5; upper limbs 4/5) muscle weakness. Respiratory muscle weakness, out of proportion to limb weakness presents. CK levels were 1250 IU and ENMG confirmed myopathy. ECG and 2D ECHO were normal **(Figs. 5A to D)**.

Case 6: Becker's Muscular Dystrophy

A 14-year-old male presented with a history of proximal muscle weakness for 3 years. His parents informed that

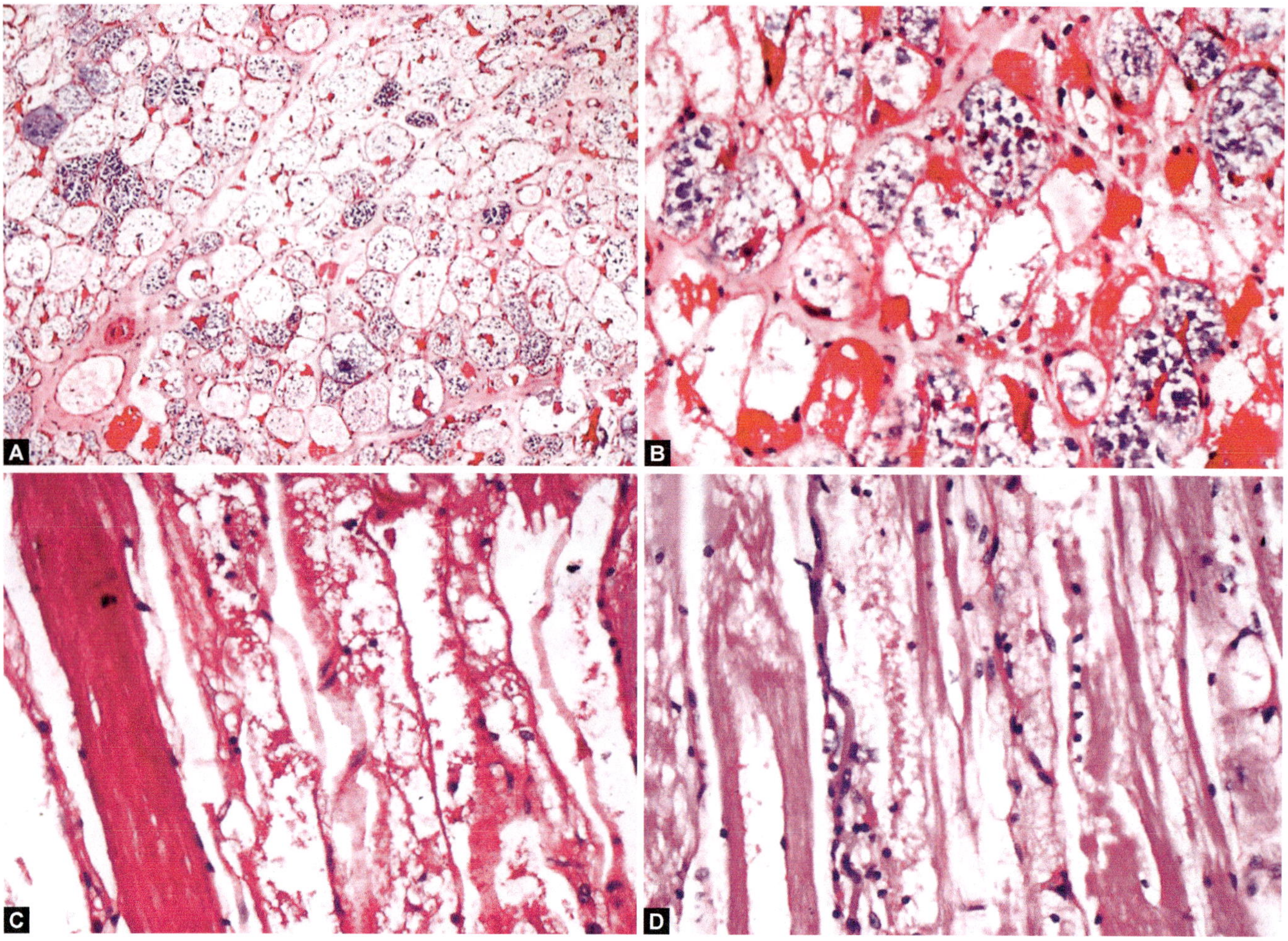

FIGS. 5A TO D: (A and B) Presence of large intrasarcoplasmic vacuoles with bluish granular material. (C) The periodic acid-Schiff stain shows positivity for this material. However, (D) The positive reaction fades away on diastase treatment confirming the content to be glycogen. The further genetic analysis confirmed glycogen storage disease type II.

he sustained a fall after playing resulting in a fracture of the femur about 3 years back. Now the weakness is worsening and he is not able to walk without support. Creatine kinase was 6,408 IU. The initial MLPA (multiplex ligation-dependent probe amplification) analysis for dystrophinopathy was negative and a muscle biopsy was done **(Figs. 6A to F)**.

NERVE BIOPSY BASICS FOR CLINICIANS

Introduction

Peripheral nerve biopsy remains an important investigation to aid any neurological workup. It requires specialized processing and expertise in interpretation. We review the status of nerve biopsies as an essential neurologic aid. Every clinician must understand the importance and drawbacks of performing a nerve biopsy and have valid expectations from the procedure. Important technical aspects of the nerve biopsy procedure, its processing, and its utility in facilitating a neurologic diagnosis and management are detailed.

Technical Aspects

Selection of Site

A moderately affected sensory nerve is the preferred choice for nerve biopsy. Severely affected or unaffected nerves add little to the diagnostic yield. Pure sensory nerves are preferred to avoid motor deficits. Distal nerves generally show more pathologic changes. Based on these factors, the sural nerve is the most commonly biopsied nerve.[17] It is also easily accessible. Other nerves such as the superficial radial and superficial peroneal are also biopsied sometimes, followed by other nerves in rarer instances. Neuroma formation and significant infections of the biopsy site are rare.[18] **Table 2** details the nerves biopsied and their advantages and disadvantages.

Fixation and Handling

The ideal length of sural nerve to be retrieved on biopsy is 4–5 cm. Minimal handling and compression of the tissue is of utmost importance. A 5 mm to 1 cm portion of the fresh unfixed tissue is cut off from one end for frozen sectioning,

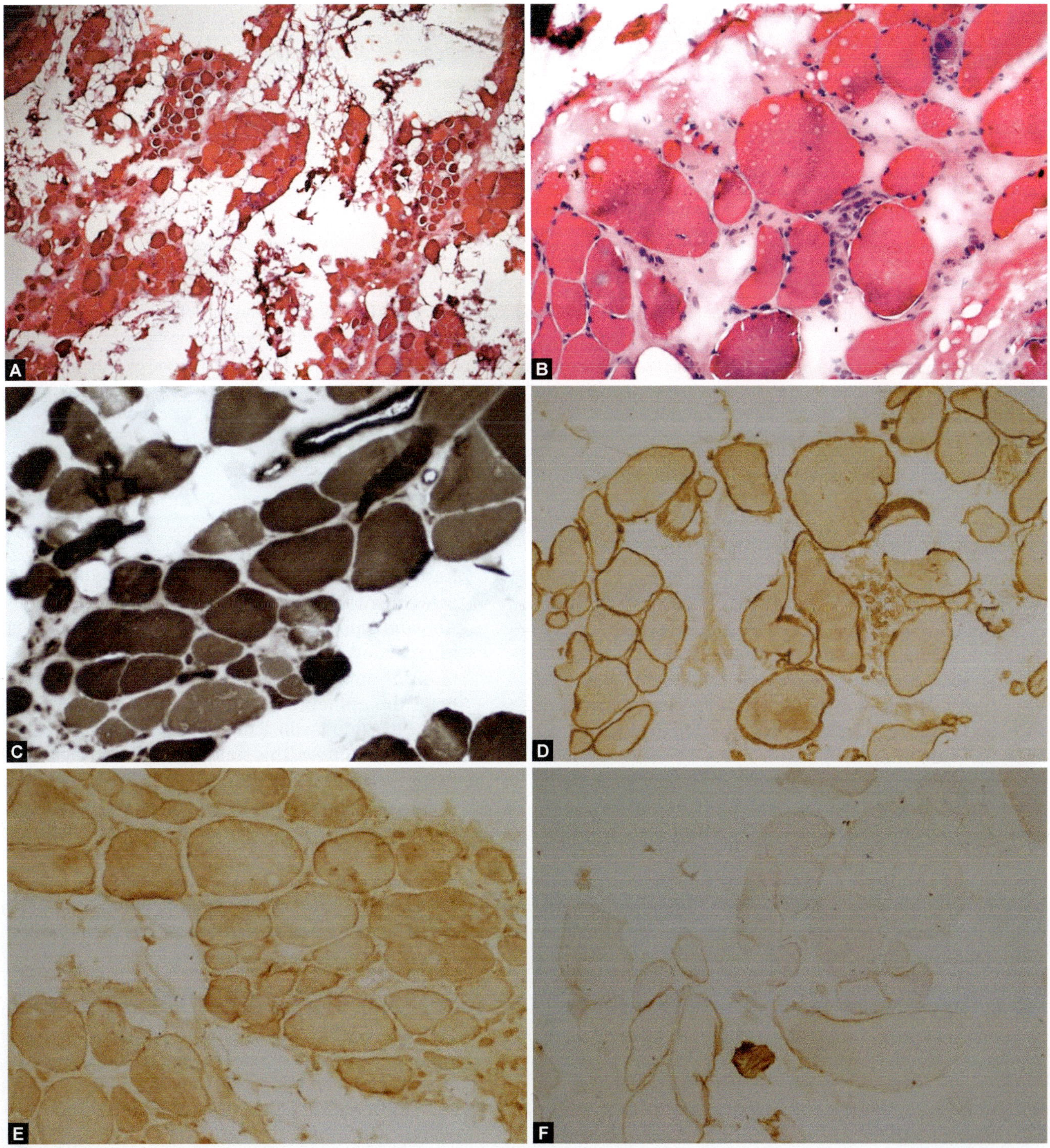

FIGS. 6A TO F: (A and B) Completely effaced architecture with adipose tissue infiltration. There is marked fiber size variation with atrophy, hypertrophy and hyalinized fibers. (C) The ATPase at pH 9.4 showed loss of checkerboard pattern. The Immunohistochemistry with dystrophin showed (D) intact expression of Dystrophin 1 along sarcolemma. (E) The dystrophin 2 showed weaker staining and (F) dystrophin 3 showed absent expression along sarcolemma.

wrapped in saline-moistened gauze and packed in an air-tight container. The rest of the nerve is immersed in a container with cool 2.5% glutaraldehyde.[18] Both containers are shipped without delay to the pathology laboratory.

- *Specimen processing*:
    - The *fresh unfixed tissue* is immediately frozen in isopentane cooled in liquid nitrogen. Cryostat sections of frozen tissue are cut. H&E staining can be performed within minutes for a quick diagnosis of vasculitis. Crystal violet staining of frozen tissue is helpful if metachromatic leukodystrophy is considered.[19] DNA can be extracted from this tissue for molecular studies and IHC or immunofluorescence studies performed.[20]

TABLE 2: Selection of site for peripheral nerve biopsy.

Nerve biopsied	Advantages	Disadvantages
Sural nerve	Purely sensory in 90% individuals; ease of access	Sensory loss. Post biopsy discomfort which generally improves with time.[18] May induce chronic pain
Superficial radial nerve	Preferred for upper limb involvement	Sensory loss in hand
Superficial peroneal nerve	Peroneus brevis muscle can be concomitantly biopsied. This may increase diagnostic yield specially in vasculitic neuropathy[44]	
Obturator nerve, motor branches of deep peroneal nerve	May help differentiate motor neuropathy from lower motor neuron disease	Weakness of muscle supplied by the nerve
Skin biopsy for intraepidermal nerve fiber analysis	Small fiber neuropathy diagnosis	Tissue processing and interpretation require expertise. Not widely available
Affected mixed motor and sensory nerves under MRI or USG guidance	Tumors like schwannomas, lymphomatous infiltrate or hypertrophic neuropathies[20]	Weakness of muscle supplied by the nerve
Affected sensory nerves: Superficial femoral, superficial radial, antebrachial cutaneous nerves, greater auricular nerve	Sensory nerves	

  - The *glutaraldehyde fixed tissue* is divided into two halves. One half is fixed in 10% buffered formaldehyde for H&E, amyloid, lepra staining, and other stains (*vide infra*). If electron microscopy facility is available, the glutaraldehyde fixed tissue can be plastic embedded for electron microscopic analysis. If not, the tissue is fixed in Flemming's solution overnight (and sections can be used for Kulchitsky Pal stain for myelin).
- *Routine stains*: Formaldehyde fixed tissue is processed routinely and transverse and longitudinal sections of paraffin-embedded tissue are cut. H&E staining is performed and is valuable in the assessment of adequacy, number of fascicles, epineurial and perineurial changes, vasculitis, endoneurial inflammation, and fibrosis. It is also essential to identify schwannomas or traumatic neuromas.[21]
- *Special stains*: Depending upon the preliminary findings in the H&E stained sections any or all of the following special stains may be of utility in the evaluation of nerve biopsies.
  - *Myelin stains*: The Kulchitsky Pal stain is of immense help in defining the myelinated fibers, their density and thickness. It cannot be performed on formaldehyde-fixed tissue and requires pretreatment of the tissue in Flemming's solution. Loyez and Luxol fast blue stains can be used if only formaldehyde fixed tissue is available.[20,22]
  - *Toluidine blue*: Toluidine blue staining on plastic-embedded semi-thin sections (cut at 1–2 μm thickness) is a valuable resource, but its availability is limited to high-end laboratories. It helps identify myelin changes, onion bulbs, and axonal degeneration with clarity.[20,22]
  - *Modified Gomori trichrome*: This is performed on fresh frozen tissue sections and can provide a quick assessment of myelinated fibers.[23]
  - *Amyloid stains*: Congo red staining with polarized microscopy can be used to identify apple green birefringent deposits of amyloid in the endoneurium or in the epineurial blood vessels. Other amyloid stains like thioflavine S may also be used.[24]
  - *Masson trichrome*: This stain highlights collagen and helps in identifying endoneurial fibrosis. Myelin is stained red and myelin ovoids can be identified.[23]
  - *Wade–Fite staining*: This is a modified acid-fast staining used for identifying lepra bacilli and helps in diagnosing multibacillary leprosy cases.
  - *Perl's stain*: This stain highlights hemosiderin deposits in the epineurial vessels and is helpful in identifying vasculitic neuropathy cases.[25]
- *Immunohistochemistry*: This is performed on formalin-fixed paraffin embedded nerve tissue and can help subtype the inflammatory infiltrate, e.g., leucocyte common antigen, CD3 (for T cells), CD20 (for B cells), and CD68 (for macrophages). Axons can be stained with PGP9.5 and neurofilament protein whereas myelin is stained by myelin basic protein and P0. IHC for axonal and myelin sheath markers is more distinctive than special stains.[20] S-100 for Schwann cells (to identify schwannomas) and epithelial membrane antigen (to highlight the perineurium or perineuriomas) are also useful markers.[20]
- *Electron microscopy*: Transmission electron microscopy is performed on glutaraldehyde fixed tissue, especially processed and embedded in resin. Ultrathin sections are stained with uranyl acetate and lead citrate. The peripheral nerve society guideline recommends

electron microscopy only in selective nerve biopsy cases where diagnosis is not established by routine testing. It is nevertheless a valuable investigation for visualizing unmyelinated fibers or those with focally folded myelin. Rare instances of subtle deposits of amyloid, mitochondrial neuropathy, and metachromatic leukodystrophy may be resolved by EM studies.[20,26]

- *Nerve fiber teasing*: This is a labor intensive procedure and is currently limited to research settings. Teased fiber analysis can demonstrate active degeneration and regeneration of axons and myelin abnormalities such as tomaculae, swellings, and demyelination.[26]
- *Polymerase chain reaction (PCR)*: This is a useful technique especially in suspected cases of pure neuritic leprosy, especially where nerve biopsy histopathology and lepra staining results are noncontributory.[27,28] PCR can be performed on tissue salvaged from paraffin blocks of nerve tissue and can help raise the sensitivity of biopsy diagnosis.[28] DNA amplification using PCR has similarly been used for identifying Lyme disease and human immunodeficiency virus (HIV).[29,30]

Interpretations

- *Inflammation*: Inflammatory infiltrates may be seen in any compartment of the peripheral nerve and may be lymphocytic, eosinophilic, granulomatous, etc. The type and distribution of the infiltrate along with concomitant axonal or myelination abnormalities help identify the underlying pathology. Epineurial and perineurial infiltrates are generally lymphocytic and may be associated with predominant endoneurial infiltrates as in leprosy, sarcoidosis, or chronic inflammatory demyelinating neuropathies (CIDP). Epineurial vessels may also be involved.
  - *Infectious causes:*
    - Leprosy is the leading cause of endoneurial inflammation and must be excluded before any other inflammatory disorder is diagnosed in the peripheral nerve. The inflammation centers on the endoneurium and may vary from pure epithelioid granulomas (with or without caseous necrosis) in tuberculoid leprosy, epithelioid cells with foamy histiocytes and lymphocytes in borderline leprosy to diffuse foam cell infiltrates in lepromatous leprosy **(Figs. 7A and B)**.[31] Stains for lepra bacilli if positive provide a definitive diagnosis; but up to half of the leprous neuritis cases may not show bacilli on staining. Substantial endoneurial inflammation, perineurial fibrosis, and loss of myelinated fibers are other supportive findings to suspect leprosy.[32]
    - HIV-associated neuropathy increases in incidence with the progression of HIV disease. In early stages, Guillain-Barré syndrome or CIDP like features are seen. In later stages, a distal symmetric polyneuropathy with sensory predominance occurs. In such cases, the nerve biopsy shows perivascular lymphocytic infiltration in the epineurial and endoneurial vessels along with axonal loss and macrophage infiltration.[18]
    - Rarer infectious causes of neuropathy include HTLV-1, Lyme disease, cytomegalovirus, herpes zoster, and syphilitic neuropathy.[18]
  - *Vasculitic neuropathy*: Vasculitic neuropathy can be primary or secondary to systemic vasculitis. The International Chapel Hill Consensus Conference classification (updated 2012) and Peripheral Nerve Society Task Force classification are useful schemes for classification. Epineurial arterioles can be affected by various idiopathic systemic vasculitides including those with predominantly small vessel involvement (microscopic polyangiitis, Churg-Strauss syndrome, Wegener's granulomatosis, essential mixed cryoglobulinemia, and Henoch-Schönlein purpura-IgA vasculitis); predominantly medium vessel vasculitis (polyarteritis nodosa) and predominantly large vessel vasculitis (Giant cell arteritis). Secondary systemic disorders affecting the epineurial arterioles include infections, malignancies, connective tissue diseases, and drugs. Involvement of endoneurial microvessels is seen in cases of nonsystemic vasculitic neuropathy (NSVN), diabetic neuropathy, cutaneous polyarteritis nodosa, viral infections, and Sjögren Syndrome. The diagnostic hallmark is the presence of transmural vessel wall inflammation along with karyorrhexis, usually seen in epineurial arterioles. Cases with perivascular cuffing with vessel wall thickening or sclerosis and lack of transmural inflammation are regarded as suspicious for vasculitis. Supportive features include the presence of active axonal degeneration and selective or central nerve fascicular degeneration. Electron microscopy may be of help in disclosing basal lamina disruption or necrosis of endothelium which are not evident by light microscopy alone.[33,34]
  - Idiopathic inflammations of the peripheral nerve: Involvement of the peripheral nerve by sarcoidosis shows presence of endoneurial epithelioid cell granulomas without lymphocytic collars or caseation necrosis. Axonal loss and regenerating clusters are often associated.[35]
- *Inflammatory demyelinating disorders*:
  - Guillain-Barré syndrome may manifest as acute inflammatory demyelinating polyneuropathy, or less commonly as acute axonal neuropathy. Though the clinical manifestations are suggestive of the diagnosis in most cases, rarely GBS can present as asymmetric or axonal pathology and require a nerve biopsy to exclude vasculitic neuropathy. The endoneurium

shows macrophage and less commonly lymphocyte infiltration along with cell debris and active demyelination.[18]

- Chronic inflammatory demyelinating pathology: The European Federation of Neurological Societies/Peripheral Nerve Society suggests electron microscopy and teased fiber studies to identify demyelination or remyelination as diagnostic features of CIDP. However, in resource-limited settings, the presence of onion bulbs, thinly myelinated fibers, endoneurial edema, and mild endoneurial lymphocytic infiltrate are supportive features on light microscopy **(Fig. 7C)**. These are, however, diagnostic only in the appropriate clinical context and their absence does not exclude a diagnosis of CIDP.[22,36]

- *Hereditary neuropathies*: Hereditary neuropathies may be isolated or a part of a syndrome with ataxia, spasticity, and other neurologic manifestations. The common subtypes include Charcot–Marie–Tooth disease (CMT) or hereditary motor and sensory neuropathy (HMSN); hereditary neuropathy with liability to pressure palsies (HNPP); hereditary sensory and autonomic neuropathy (HSAN); and distal hereditary motor neuropathy (dHMN). Genome sequencing and electrophysiology studies are less invasive and diagnostic methods of choice in hereditary neuropathies. However, nerve biopsy can aid in diagnosing sporadic cases or those with variants of unknown significance detected on sequencing analysis. Myelinated fibers generally show a diffuse loss. *PMP22* gene duplication causes the common form of demyelinating CMT (CMT1A) which is characterized by repeated demyelination and remyelination forming onion bulbs. Axonal variants of CMT show axon loss and regenerating clusters of three or more fibers. Tomaculae are sausage-shaped thickly myelinated fibers seen in HNPP. Gigaxonin gene mutations lead to large giant axons which can be highlighted by neurofilament staining **(Fig. 7D)**. Autosomal recessive metachromatic leukodystrophy is characterized by the deficiency of arylsulfatase A and deposition of metachromatic sphingolipids in frozen peripheral nerve biopsy sections which stain positive with Cresyl violet staining.[37,38]
- *Deposition disorders*:
  - *Amyloid neuropathy*: Deposition of amyloid in the peripheral nerve can be seen in about a quarter of cases with acquired primary amyloidosis, most cases of familial amyloidosis and rarely in secondary forms of amyloidosis. Amyloid deposits appear as weakly positive on PAS staining and give apple green birefringence on the polarization of Congo Red stained sections **(Figs. 7E and F)**. The deposits are usually seen in vessel walls, epineurium, or endoneurium. IHC can be used to characterize the type of amyloid deposits, AA (in secondary amyloid), Kappa or Lambda monotypic deposits (in primary amyloid) and transthyretin, etc. in specific familial forms. Electron microscopy is diagnostic and reveals typical beta pleated sheath configuration of amyloid fibrils.[18,34,37]
  - *Paraprotein deposits*: About half the cases with paraproteinemia show presence of a neuropathy. The type of paraprotein present determines the clinical manifestations. IgM monoclonal gammopathies associated with antimyelin-associated glycoprotein show the presence of abnormal myelin with splitting, the presence of folded myelin and tomaculae. All of these are best visualized using electron microscopy or teased fiber analysis.[38]
  - *Polyglucosan body disease*: Adult polyglucosan body disease can be diagnosed on axillary skin biopsies. Peripheral nerve biopsies show the presence of rounded PAS-positive inclusions within the axons.[39]
- *Endocrine related neuropathies*: At diagnosis, about 7.5% of diabetics show the presence of peripheral neuropathy, and the incidence increases with time. Distal symmetric sensorimotor neuropathy is commonly seen. Biopsy findings are not specific and include loss of myelinated axons and the presence of regenerating clusters. Vessels in the endoneurium may show hyaline deposition.[40]
- *Neoplasms*:
  - Lymphomas, leukemias, and multiple myeloma may infiltrate peripheral nerves. Nerve biopsy may help detect an undiagnosed lymphoma or its recurrence. Infiltration of epineurium, perineurium, and rarely endoneurium by typical malignant cells is seen, which can be typed using IHC.[41]
  - Schwannoma, traumatic neuroma, malignant peripheral nerve sheath tumors, and neurofibroma present as lesions arising from nerves with typical morphology.[42]

Diagnostic Utility of Nerve Biopsies

- Nerve biopsy is an invasive procedure that may cause sensory loss, pain, and paresthesia in the territory supplied by the biopsied nerve. Motor nerve biopsies are avoided. The performance of nerve biopsies should hence be justified and have clear diagnostic and therapeutic utility. Nerve biopsies have been reported to affect the management of neuropathy patients in about 60% of cases and change the clinical diagnosis in 14%. Performance of the nerve biopsy leads to biopsy site pain in 33% of cases.[43]
- In NSVN, Collins reported a diagnostic sensitivity of 58% for combined superficial peroneal nerve and peroneus brevis muscle biopsy while sensitivity was 47% for sural nerve biopsy alone.[44] In CIDP nerve biopsies are not indicated if the diagnosis can be made using serology and cerebrospinal fluid (CSF) examinations. The Peripheral Nerve Society recommends nerve biopsies in CIDP only when a patient is not responding to treatment or there is aggravation despite treatment.

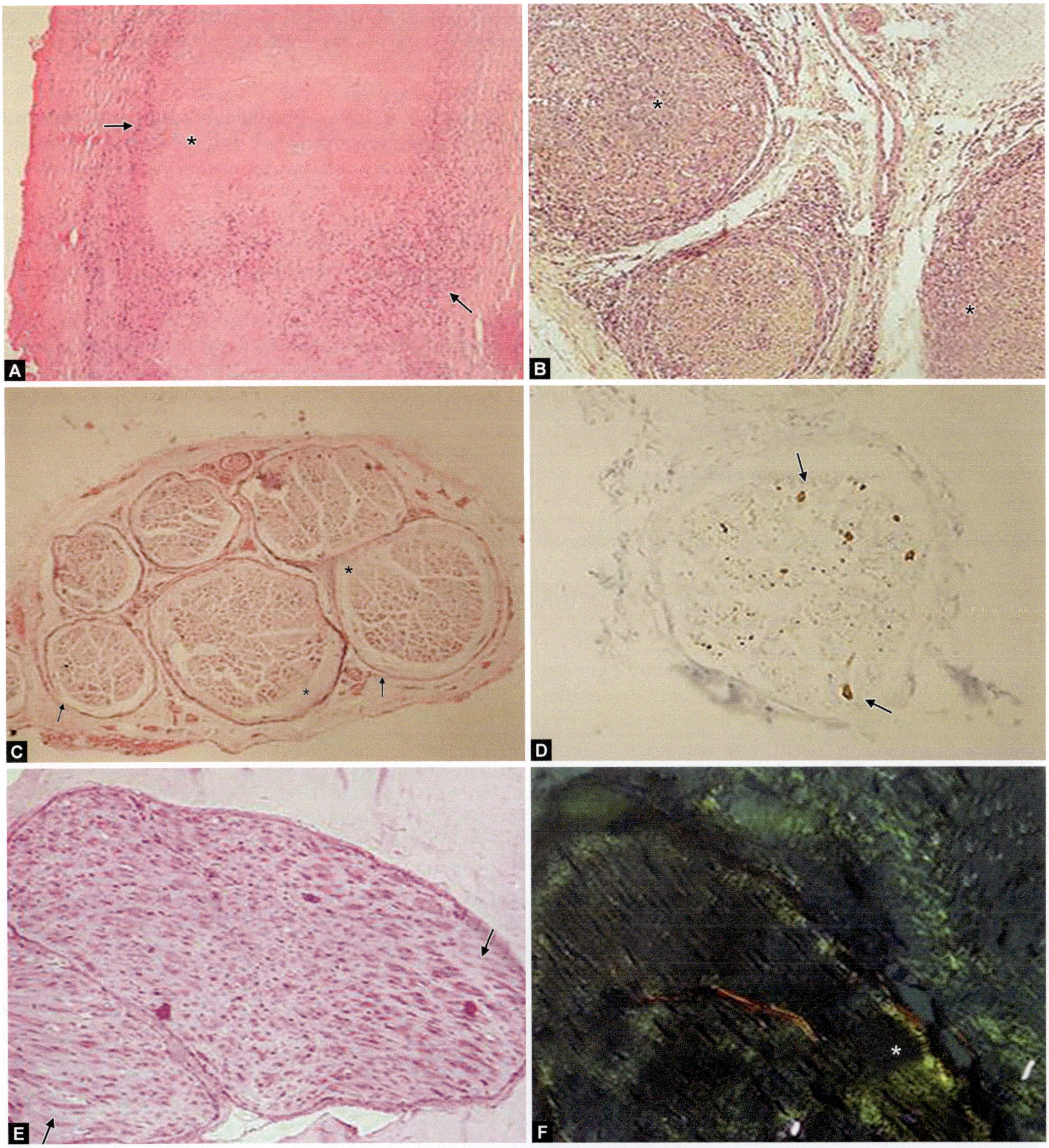

FIGS. 7A TO F: (A) Tuberculoid leprosy with central necrosis (asterisk) and peripheral epithelioid cell granuloma (arrows) in the endoneurium. (hematoxylin and eosin, × 200). (B) Enlarged nerve fascicles with epithelioid cells and foamy histiocytes (asterisk) in a case of borderline leprosy (hematoxylin and eosin, ×100). (C) Subperineurial edema (asterisk) and few lymphocytes (arrows) in a case of chronic inflammatory demyelinating neuropathy (CIDP) (hematoxylin and eosin, ×100). (D) Giant axons (arrows) highlighted by neurofilament immunohistochemistry in a case of giant axonal neuropathy (diaminobenzidine, ×200). (E) Endoneurial deposits of amyloid appearing as weakly eosinophilic substance (arrows) (hematoxylin and eosin, ×200). (F) Apple green birefringence (asterisk) in the endoneurium in a case of amyloid neuropathy (Congo red with polarization, ×200).

In a study on 84 neuropathy patients, nerve biopsy helped confirm a clinical suspicion in 51% of cases, including vasculitic neuropathy, CIDP, and leprosy. The clinical diagnosis was changed postnerve biopsy in 12% of cases, and in 19% cases, nerve biopsy was able to provide a diagnosis where no clear clinical diagnosis was possible.[45] In a study on childhood neuropathies from India, nerve biopsy proved most useful in inflammatory (vasculitis, leprosy) and demyelinating neuropathies. It helped identify unsuspected HNPP cases and those of metachromatic leukodystrophy where access to enzyme and genetic studies was not financially feasible. Biopsies in neuropathies with axonal degeneration did not offer many advantages and could be avoided.[46]

ILLUSTRATIVE CASES

Case 1: Hereditary demyelinating Neuropathy

A 16-years-old female presented with complaints of progressive weakness of all four limbs with sensory loss for 1 year. Weakness initially started in the right hand followed by the left hand, and bilateral legs. She also complained of diminished sensation. There was history of cataract surgery at 4 years of age. There was no history of bowel bladder involvement, fasciculations, or diurnal variation in symptoms, rash, or joint pains. There was no history suggestive of cranial nerve involvement, fever, trauma, or convulsions. No suggestive family history was present. On examination, there was weakness and atrophy of small muscles of her hands and feet, her deep tendon reflexes were absent. The sensory loss was present in glove and stocking pattern. Her plantar response was flexor. The rest of the CNS examination including higher mental functions, cranial nerves, cerebellar, and extra pyramidal system was normal. No signs of autonomic disturbances were present. Her NCS was suggestive of demyelinating sensory motor polyneuropathy. Her sural nerve biopsy **(Figs. 8A and B)** showed severe fiber loss, onion bulbs, and thinly myelinated fibers. No subperineurial edema or endoneurial inflammation was present. A diagnosis of demyelinating neuropathy with onion bulb formation, likely hereditary was made.

Chronic inflammatory demyelinating neuropathy can also present as slowly progressive neuropathy in childhood; however, diffuse rather than multifocal involvement and lack of endoneurial inflammation helped exclude it. Nerve biopsy helped confirm a clinical suspicion of hereditary neuropathy. The patient was referred for sequencing studies which showed duplication of *PMP22* gene confirming a diagnosis of CMT (CMT1A).

Case 2: Vasculitic Neuropathy

A 30-year-old female complained of tingling in right lower limb and right upper limb followed by weakness in both feet for ten days. On examination, ankle jerks were absent. No thickened nerves were seen. Erythrocyte sedimentation rate (ESR) was 109 mm and C-reactive protein (CRP) and rheumatoid factor analysis was positive. A diagnosis of acute neuropathy was entertained. Sural nerve biopsy **(Figs. 9A and B)** showed a perivascular infiltrate of lymphocytes around epineurial vessels. No transmural vessel wall infiltration was seen. Endoneurium showed patchy fiber loss and myelin ovoids. No endoneurial inflammation or regenerating clusters were seen. A diagnosis of probable acute vasculitic neuropathy was made on biopsy. A complete vasculitic profile was performed postbiopsy which revealed ANA and dsDNA positivity. The patient was treated with steroids in view of acute vasculitic neuropathy associated with lupus erythematosus to which she responded well. Nerve biopsy may not always detect

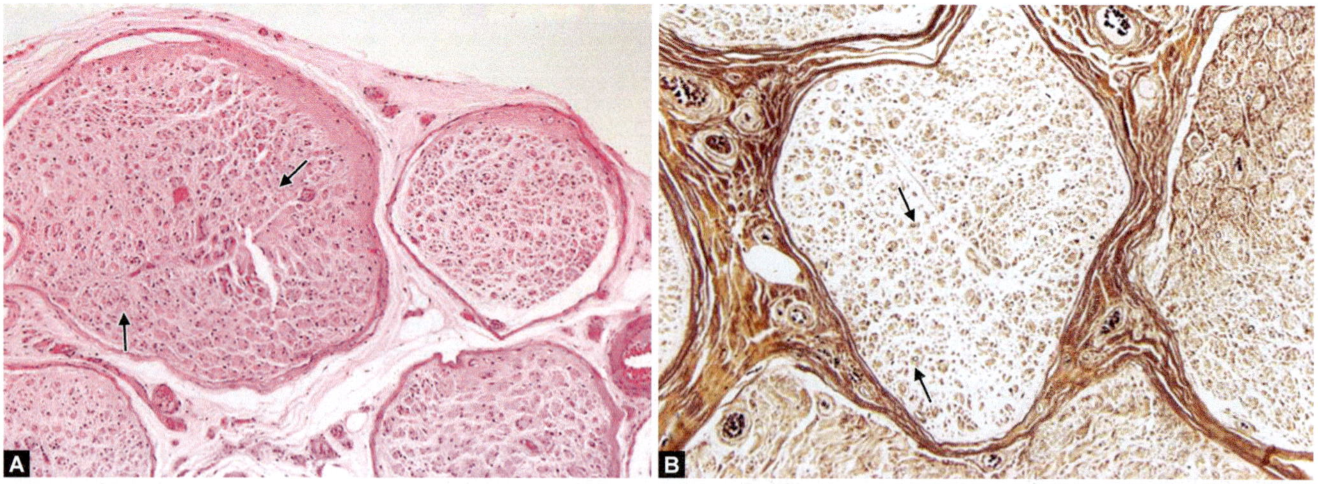

FIGS. 8A AND B: Case 1: (A) Peripheral nerve with numerous onion bulbs (arrows) (hematoxylin and eosin, ×200). (B) Severe diffuse fiber loss with few thinly myelinated fibers (arrows) (Kulchitsky Pal, ×200).

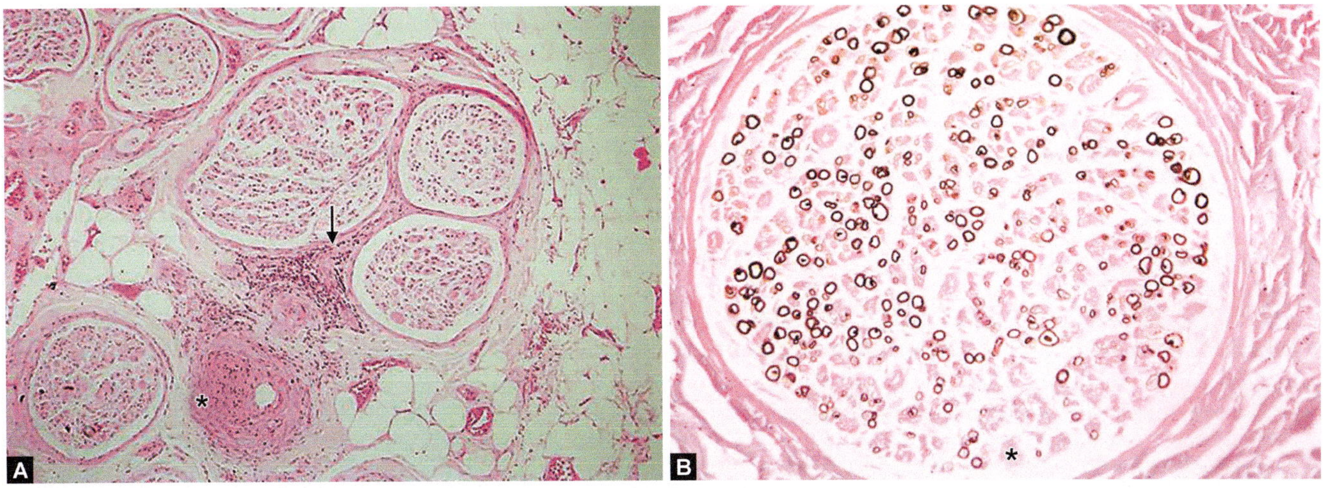

FIGS. 9A AND B: Case 2: (A) Epineurial vessel with perivascular lymphocytic infiltrate (arrow) and another vessel with concentric wall thickening (asterisk) (hematoxylin and eosin, ×100). (B) Patchy loss of myelinated fibers (asterisk) (Kulchitsky Pal, ×200).

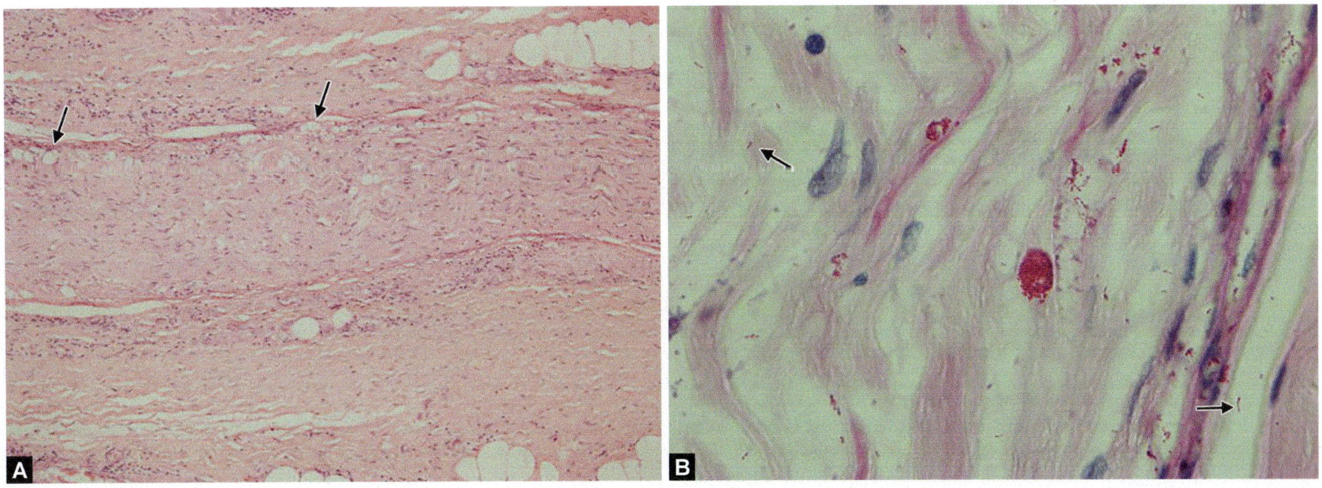

FIGS. 10A AND B: Case 3: (A) Numerous foamy histiocytes (arrows) and lymphocytes infiltrating the endoneurium (hematoxylin and eosin, ×100). (B) Numerous lepra bacilli lying singly (arrows) and in globi (Wade Fite, ×1,000).

active vasculitis. However, perivascular inflammation and patchy fiber loss should raise a suspicion of probable vasculitis and should direct a complete vasculitic profile workup.

Case 3: Pure Neuritic Leprosy

A 50-year-old male presented to the neurology OPD with history of decreased sensation in right followed by left lower limb since 1 year. He gave a history of slippage of slippers and tingling over medial aspect of left forearm. Symptoms were asymmetric in onset and progressing. On leading questions, he gave a history of occasional numbness in left inner forearm territory for 1 year. No joint pains or swelling, skin lesions, or rash was present. Motor nerve conduction velocities (NCVs) were normal. He showed a predominantly sensory axonopathy presenting as mononeuritis multiplex with clinical differentials of vasculitis and leprosy. Sural nerve biopsy **(Figs. 10A and B)** showed enlarged funicles with diffuse infiltration of admixed epithelioid and foamy histiocytes. Wade Fite stain revealed numerous lepra bacilli. He was diagnosed as a case of pure neuritic leprosy, borderline lepromatous type. The patient showed good response to multidrug therapy. Nerve biopsy proved diagnostic importantly in the absence of skin lesions of leprosy.

FUTURE TRENDS

Assessment of interepidermal and dermal nerve fiber twigs in skin biopsies is currently being researched as a means to study nonmyelinated and myelinated nerve fibers. IHC for axons using PGP9.5 and confocal microscopy are being utilized for the same.[47] Promising results are expected in small fiber sensory neuropathy as seen in Diabetes. IHC for myelin basic protein (highlights myelin sheaths) and neurofilament protein (highlights axons) is also becoming commonly used. They are expected to benefit laboratories where access to fiber teasing and electron microscopy is limited.

CONCLUSION

To conclude, muscle and nerve biopsies are essential investigations in the work of genetic and acquired neuromuscular disorders. These are minimally invasive and safe procedures which offer important diagnostic clues with the help of ancillary techniques. Despite advances in molecular testing, muscle and nerve biopsies remains the investigation of choice in cases with overlapping clinical phenotypes and cryptogenic neuropathies and in those which do not respond to treatment. Clinical, electrophysiology, and serology coordination is a prerequisite before proceeding to biopsy a peripheral nerve. Though nerve fiber teasing and electron microscopy are labor intensive investigations available sparingly, routine evaluation of nerve biopsies is of utmost utility in guiding further workup. It is desirable to have expertise for muscle and nerve biopsy processing and interpretation along with every clinical neurology set up.

REFERENCES

1. Yang K, Iannaccone S, Burkhalter LS, Reisch J, Cai C, Schindel D. Role of nerve and muscle biopsies in pediatric patients in the era of genetic testing. J Surg Res. 2019;243:27-32.
2. Nilipour Y. The art of muscle biopsy in the new genetic era: A narrative review. Iran J Child Neurol. 2019;13(4):7-17.
3. Caetano AP, Alves P. Advanced MRI patterns of muscle disease in inherited and acquired myopathies: What the radiologist should know. Semin Musculoskelet Radiol. 2019;23(3):e82-e106.
4. Ten Dam L, van der Kooi AJ, Verhamme C, Wattjes MP, de Visser M. Muscle imaging in inherited and acquired muscle diseases. Eur J Neurol. 2016;23(4):688-703.
5. Wattjes MP, Kley RA, Fischer D. Neuromuscular imaging in inherited muscle diseases. Eur Radiol. 2010;20(10):2447-60.
6. Joyce NC, Oskarsson B, Jin LW. Muscle biopsy evaluation in neuromuscular disorders. Phys Med Rehabil Clin N Am. 2012;23(3): 609-31.
7. Cotta A, Carvalho E, da-Cunha-Júnior AL, Valicek J, Navarro MM, Junior SB, et al. Muscle biopsy essential diagnostic advice for pathologists. Surg Exp Pathol. 2021;4:3.
8. Skram MK, Gulati S, Larsson E, Lindal S, Torp SH. Muscle biopsies in children--an evaluation of histopathology and clinical value during a 5-year period. Ups J Med Sci. 2009;114(1):41-5.
9. Barthelemy F, Woods JD, Nieves-Rodriguez S, Douine ED, Wang R, Wanagat J, et al. A well-tolerated core needle muscle biopsy process suitable for children and adults. Muscle Nerve. 2020;62(6):688-98.
10. Dubowitz V, Sewry CA, Oldfors A. Muscle Biopsy: A Practical Approach, 5th edition. China: Saunders Elsevier; 2020. pp. 1-600.
11. Cai C, Anthony DC, Pytel P. A pattern-based approach to the interpretation of skeletal muscle biopsies. Mod Pathol. 2019;32(4): 462-83.
12. Paciello O, Papparella S. Histochemical and immunohistological approach to comparative neuromuscular diseases. Folia Histochem Cytobiol. 2009;47(2):143-52.
13. Nix JS, Moore SA. What every neuropathologist needs to know: The muscle biopsy. J Neuropathol Exp Neurol. 2020;79:719.
14. Goebel HH, Stenzel W. Practical application of electron microscopy to neuromuscular diseases. Ultrastruct Pathol. 2013;37(1):15-8.
15. Santhoshkumar R, Narayanappa G. Electron microscopy in the diagnosis of skeletal muscle disorders: Its utility and limitations. Indian J Pathol Microbiol. 2022;65(Suppl S1):291-9.
16. Bernier FP, Boneh A, Dennett X, Chow CW, Cleary MA, Thorburn DR. Diagnostic criteria for respiratory chain disorders in adults and children. Neurology. 2002;59:1406.
17. Amoiridis G, Schöls L, Ameridis N, Przuntek H. Motor fibers in the sural nerve of humans. Neurology. 1997;49:1725-8.
18. Bilbao JM, Schmidt RE. Biopsy diagnosis of peripheral neuropathy. Switzerland: Springer; 2014.
19. Bindu PS, Mahadevan A, Taly AB, Christopher R, Gayathri N, Shankar SK. Peripheral neuropathy in metachromatic leucodystrophy. A study of 40 cases from south India. J Neurol Neurosurg Psychiatry. 2005;76(12):1698-701.
20. Weis J, Brandner S, Lammens M, Sommer C, Vallat JM. Processing of nerve biopsies: a practical guide for neuropathologists. Clin Neuropathol. 2012;31(1):7-23.
21. Mellgren SI, Lindal S. Nerve biopsy--some comments on procedures and indications. Acta Neurol Scand Suppl. 2011;(191):64-70.
22. Kulkarni GB, Mahadevan A, Taly AB, Nalini A, Shankar SK. Sural nerve biopsy in chronic inflammatory demyelinating polyneuropathy: are supportive pathologic criteria useful in diagnosis? Neurol India. 2010;58(4):542-8.
23. Oh SJ. Color Atlas of Nerve Biopsy Pathology, 1st edition. Delhi: CRC Press; 2001.
24. Vital C, Vital A, Bouillot-Eimer S, Brechenmacher C, Ferrer X, Lagueny A. Amyloid neuropathy: a retrospective study of 35 peripheral nerve biopsies. J Peripher Nerv Syst. 2004;9(4):232-41.
25. Dhinakaran S, Mahadevan A, Unchagi A, Kulkarni GB, Nagappa M, Chickabasaviah YT, et al. Is perls prussian blue stain for hemosiderin a useful adjunct in the diagnosis of vasculitic neuropathies? Neurol India. 2021;69(1):140-6.
26. Sommer CL, Brandner S, Dyck PJ, Harati Y, LaCroix C, Lammens M, et al; Peripheral Nerve Society. Peripheral Nerve Society Guideline on processing and evaluation of nerve biopsies. J Peripher Nerv Syst. 2010;15(3):164-75.
27. Malhotra KP, Husain N. Laboratory perspectives for Leprosy: Diagnostic, prognostic and predictive tools. Indian J Pathol Microbiol. 2022;65(Supplement):S300-9.
28. Tiwari V, Malhotra K, Khan K, Maurya PK, Singh AK, Thacker AK, et al. Evaluation of polymerase chain reaction in nerve biopsy specimens of patients with Hansen's disease. J Neurol Sci. 2017;380: 187-90.
29. Schwartz I, Wormser GP, Schwartz JJ, Cooper D, Weissensee P, Gazumyan A, et al. Diagnosis of early Lyme disease by polymerase chain reaction amplification and culture of skin biopsies from erythema migrans lesions. J Clin Microbiol. 1992;30(12):3082-8.
30. Winer JB, Bang B, Clarke JR, Knox K, Cook TJ, Gompels M, et al. A study of neuropathy in HIV infection. Q J Med. 1992;83(302): 473-88.
31. Kulshreshtha D, Malhotra KP, Malhotra HS, Thacker AK, Garg RK, Singh AK, et al. Mandating nerve biopsy: A step towards personalizing therapy in pure neuritic leprosy. J Peripher Nerv Syst. 2018;23(3):190-6.

32. Hui M, Uppin MS, Challa S, Meena AK, Kaul S. Pure neuritic leprosy: Resolving diagnostic issues in acid fast bacilli (AFB)-negative nerve biopsies: A single Centre experience from South India. Ann Indian Acad Neurol. 2015;18:292-7.
33. Gwathmey KG, Burns TM, Collins MP, Dyck PJ. Vasculitic neuropathies. Lancet Neurol. 2014;13(1):67-82.
34. Blaes F. Diagnosis and therapeutic options for peripheral vasculitic neuropathy. Ther Adv Musculoskelet Dis. 2015;7(2):45-55.
35. Said G. Sarcoidosis of the peripheral nervous system. Peripheral nerve disorders. In: Said G, Krarup C (editors). Handbook of clinical neurology, Volume 115 (3rd series). BV, Amsterdam: Elsevier; 2013. pp. 485-95.
36. Joint Task Force of the EFNS and the PNS. European Federation of Neurological Societies/Peripheral Nerve Society Guideline on management of chronic inflammatory demyelinating polyradiculoneuropathy: report of a joint task force of the European Federation of Neurological Societies and the Peripheral Nerve Society--First Revision. J Peripher Nerv Syst. 2010;15(1):1-9.
37. Lacomis D. Clinical utility of peripheral nerve biopsy. Curr Neurol Neurosci Rep. 2005;5(1):41-7.
38. Cai Z, Cash K, Swift J, Sutton-Smith P, Robinson M, Thompson PD, et al. Focal myelin swellings and tomacula in anti-MAG IgM paraproteinaemic neuropathy: Novel teased nerve fiber studies. J Periph Nerv Syst. 2001;6:95-101.
39. Milde P, Guccion JG, Kelly J, Locatelli E, Jones RV. Adult polyglucosan body disease – diagnosis by sural nerve and skin biopsy. Arch Pathol Lab Med. 2001;125:519-22.
40. Malik RA, Tesfaye S, Thompson SD, Veves A, Sharma AK, Boulton AJ, et al. Endoneurial localization of microvascular damage in human diabetic neuropathy. Diabetologia. 1993;36:454-9.
41. Krendel DA, Stahl RL, Chan WC. Lymphomatous polyneuropathy. Biopsy of clinically involved nerve and successful treatment. Arch Neurol. 1991;48:330-2.
42. Belakhoua SM, Rodriguez FJ. Diagnostic pathology of tumors of peripheral nerve. Neurosurgery. 2021;88(3):443-56.
43. Gabriel CM, Howard R, Kinsella N, Lucas S, McColl I, Saldanha G, et al. Prospective study of the usefulness of sural nerve biopsy. J Neurol Neurosurg Psychiatry. 2000;69:442-6.
44. Collins MP, Periquet MI, Mendell JR, Sahenk Z, Nagaraja HN, Kissel JT. Nonsystemic vasculitic neuropathy: Insights from a clinical cohort. Neurology. 2003;61(5):623-30.
45. Goel J, Anadure RK, Nair MD, Nair S, Yasha TC. A study correlating nerve biopsy with clinical diagnosis and its impact on improving management in peripheral neuropathies. Interdisciplinary Neurosurgery. 2021;25:101237.
46. Krishnan P, Mahadevan A, Bindu PS, Chickabasaviah YT, Taly AB. Etiologic spectrum of biopsy-proven peripheral neuropathies in childhood from a resource-poor setting. J Child Neurol. 2015;30(6): 707-15.
47. Narasimhaiah D, Mahadevan A. Role of skin punch biopsy in diagnosis of small fiber neuropathy-A review for the neuropathologist. Indian J PatholMicrobiol. 2022;65(Supplement):S329-36.

119 CHAPTER

Ultrasound of the Nervous System

Junling Dong, John C Klick, Vanessa Baute, Aarti Sarwal

INTRODUCTION

Echoencephalography to visualize signals from echoic parts of the brain was the original application of ultrasound and clinical medicine.[1] This single-dimension sonar-based technology then gave way to two-dimensional (2D) B-mode scanning. The addition of color Doppler and spectral Doppler further added the ability to insonate the cerebral vasculature. Many evolving clinical applications for ultrasound were described in neurology in the 1970s and 80s but the evolution of computed tomography (CT) and magnetic resonance imaging (MRI) revolutionized clinical applications of neuroimaging and allowed new therapeutic strategies. Despite the widespread availability of these diagnostics, ultrasound applications continue to be a major area of research. Ultrasound has several advantages for clinical applications in neurology. It is noninvasive, free of radiation and can be performed at the bedside. It also renders itself to serial imaging since multiple scans can be done to follow up patient's natural history of disease over time. In critical care and emergency settings, in particular, ultrasound has several benefits where it allows imaging where it might be unsafe to move patients for traditional neuroimaging modalities.[2] It can be an important supplement to the neurological examination in patients where lack of consciousness or delirium impairs the ability to perform a comprehensive clinical neurological evaluation. With improving technology, the availability of point-of-care and hand-held devices, the cost-effectiveness of ultrasound as a neuroimaging modality is also a significant consideration. In this chapter, we describe a few key clinical applications where ultrasound has clinical applications in the evaluation of patients with neurological disorders.

TRANSCRANIAL DOPPLER ULTRASOUND

Transcranial Doppler (TCD) is an ultrasound modality that uses spectral pulse Doppler waveforms to insonate the vessels in the circle of Willis to assess for blood flow velocities through different segments of the intracranial vasculature. Doppler effect has been used in vascular ultrasound to calculate the blood flow velocity by measuring the frequency shift of moving red blood cells through the vessel segment being insonated. The blood flow velocities are a surrogate for blood flow and can help detect the hemodynamic phenomena related to stenosis, spasm or hyperemic perfusion which define most vascular pathologies.

The clinical utility of TCD ultrasonography was first introduced by Aaslid et al. in 1982 to estimate cerebral perfusion pressure based on TCD flow velocity and arterial pressure.[3] Since then, utilization of TCD has expanded to include monitoring of vasospasm after subarachnoid hemorrhage (SAH), evaluation of cerebral circulatory arrest, noninvasive monitoring of intracranial pressure (ICP), and diagnosis of intracranial stenosis. TCD is a dynamic physiological modality where blood flow velocities can be affected in real-time by different factors such as blood pressure, carbon dioxide levels, anemia, and pre-existing cerebrovascular disease hence the contextual information of the clinical settings in which TCD is performed is extremely important.[4] Perfusion changes detected via TCD are typically very sensitive but may lack specificity to discern the differential diagnosis unless the clinical setting, results of previous vascular imaging, if available and the knowledge of the underlying natural history of the disease being investigated is considered. TCD has been extremely useful in the noninvasive evaluation of ischemic stroke for the diagnosis of large vessel occlusions where patients may not be able to receive CT contrasted scans, screening of vasospasm in aneurysmal SAH, noninvasive measurements of ICP in traumatic brain injury, and evaluation of cerebral circulatory arrest for patients who need ancillary testing for evaluation of death by neurological criteria. This section details the image acquisition techniques for TCD images, waveform interpretation, and key clinical applications in both outpatient and inpatient settings.[5]

Technical Aspects

The skull in general does not allow easy insonation of the intracranial structures but the temporal bone in a majority of patients is thin enough to allow transmission of sound.[4,6] The temporal window allows insonation of the anterior, middle, and posterior cerebral artery and approximately 85% of the patients **(Fig. 1A)**.[7] Some patients may have a unilateral window hence insulating both sides is key before ruling out presence of a dose. TCD typically utilizes a low-frequency 1-3 Hz phased array probe placed on the temple to insonate the brain through the temporal window. Nonimaging TCD probes use knowledge of vessel depth from the temporal bone and direction of flow to guide insonation. Imaging TCD uses B-mode color-coded duplex imaging to visualize the segments of circle of Willis which guides placement of sampling gate for pulse Doppler insonation **(Fig. 1A)**. The TCD probe is placed to insonate the brain to yield an axial section at the level of the basal cistern. On B-mode Doppler, this can be confirmed by visualizing the opposite skull and the midbrain **(Fig. 1A)**. On M-mode guided nonimaging Doppler, appearance of consistent signals toward the probe at the expected depth of the MCA help identify the vessel with further anterior and posterior adjustments of the probe direction to acquire anterior and posterior cerebral artery, respectively **(Figs. 1A and B)**.

Insonation through the foramen magnum using the suboccipital windows facilitates the insonation of vertebrobasilar circulation. In the suboccipital windows, the probe is placed few centimeters lateral to the midline pointed towards the forehead to align the line of insonation along the clivus.[4] Transorbital windows are used to assess ophthalmic artery which serves as a major channel of collateralization between the external and internal carotid artery (ICA). Orbital insonation requires the ultrasound to be reduced to 10% of the usual to prevent adverse effects to the eye. Most machines are specifically designed with an orbital preset which must be used for insonation across the eye. Submandibular windows, classically described with TCD use the TCD probe to insonate the extracranial ICA in the neck. This window is only used to get extracranial ICA to provide Lindegaard ratios described below.

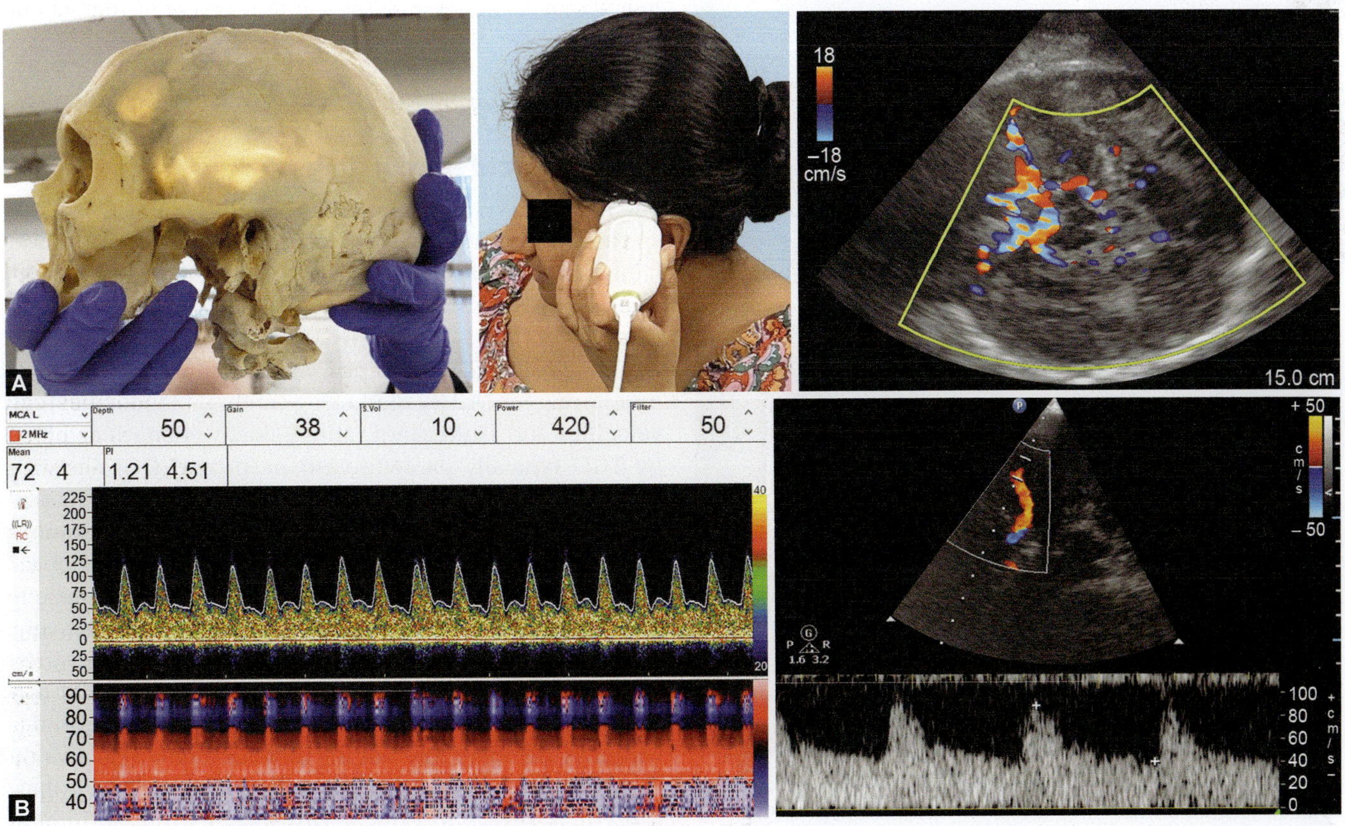

FIGS. 1A AND B: (A) Skull held against light to show presence of temporal windows that allow insonation of the brain through an intact cranium (left). Probe placement on the temporal bone with index marker pointed anteriorly and line of insonation aligned with basal cisterns (middle). B-mode transcranial ultrasound showing axial section at midbrain level with color Doppler highlighting the Circle of Willis (right); (B) Nonimaging Doppler guided by M-mode shows a band of signal coming toward the probe between the depth of 50 and 70 mm most consistent with the ipsilateral middle cerebral artery (left). The gate is placed at 50 mm depth (white line) to yield pulse Doppler waveforms in the upper panel. Imaging Doppler on the other hand uses B-mode guided color duplex (right) to identify the middle cerebral artery and then pulse Doppler sampling gait is placed at 3.2 cm depth to yield the waveforms.

Interpretations

Despite the difference in the way, signals are acquired on imaging and nonimaging TCD, the actual interpretation of the waveforms on pulse Doppler and clinical applications are the same. Detailed practice parameters for TCDs have been published by the American Society of Neuroimaging both details of insonation as well as waveform interpretation which can be great resource for readers interested in developing expertise on this topic.[4,8]

Intracranial circulation has classical low-resistance waveforms with each waveform representing a rapid systolic upstroke, stepwise the examination during systolic down stroke, and a robust diastolic flow where end-diastolic velocity typically a third or more of the peak systolic velocity **(Figs. 2A and 3)**.[4] This represents the need for brain tissue to receive consistent blood flow throughout systole and diastole. In contrast, peripheral vascular circulation including external carotid artery has high resistance patterns on vascular Doppler examination with each cardiac cycle who presents in rapid upstroke, a rapid systolic deceleration, and diastolic flow well below a fourth of the peak systolic flow **(Figs. 3A to E)**. Some vessels may show late systolic reversal. When intracranial resistance increases due to focal mural stenosis in the blood vessel or extramural compression from increased ICP waveforms in the intracranial circulation can change from low resistance **(Figs. 2 and 4C)** to high-resistance waveforms **(Figs. 3C and 4A)**. If this transition is caused by a focal stenosis, insonation of the vessel further downstream will show parvus at the tardus waveforms **(Figs. 3 and 4D)**. Increasing ICP may cause further increase in resistive patterns with oscillating flow with forward flow during systole and backward flow during diastole **(Figs. 3 and 4B)**. In contrast to increase in diastolic flow relative to the systolic flow may be a sign of low cerebrovascular resistance or hyperemia **(Figs. 2D and 4F)**. Recognition of such waveforms in the context of patient's presentation can help diagnose the underlying cerebrovascular hemodynamic state. The Spencer Reid curve is a robust hemodynamic model that explains the relationship between blood flow and velocity changes that occur in the cerebral circulation leading to evolution of such waveforms **(Figs. 3A to E)**.

Figures 4A to J represent various waveform morphologies that can help in assessment of cerebral hemodynamics in various clinical settings.[4]

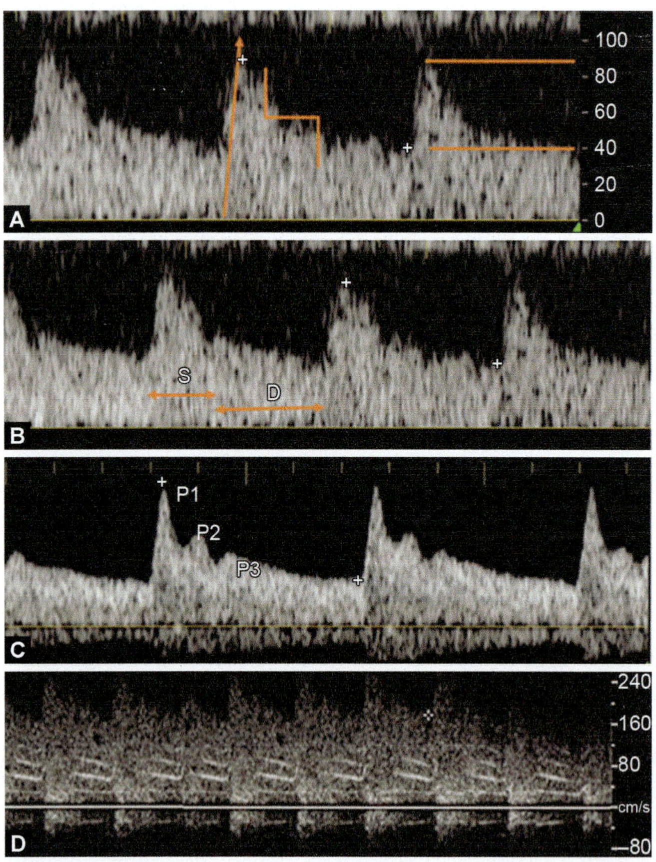

FIGS. 2A TO D: (A) A normal low resistance waveforms on cerebrovascular ultrasound has a rapid systolic upstroke, stepwise systolic deceleration with a robust diastolic flow that is more than a one-third of systolic flow. (B) For each cardiac cycle, systole represents the initial third of the waveform and diastole represents the latter two-thirds. (C) Three notches on the systolic deceleration represent the compliance of the brain similar to waveforms created by intracranial pressure tracing. (D) Hyperemic flow can be detected by relatively high diastolic flow.

Utility

Subarachnoid Hemorrhage

The most well-known and accepted utility of TCD is vasospasm monitoring in SAH.[9] In patients with an impaired clinical examination, there is significant need for cerebrovascular hemodynamic monitoring for prediction of delayed cerebral ischemia (DCI) before it manifests as focal neurological deficits. TCD provides a noninvasive means of monitoring for DCI by measuring cerebral blood mean flow velocities and Lindegaard ratio. Velocity changes detected by TCD typically precede vasospasm and DCI allowing the clinician to escalate frequent neuromonitoring and potentially treat the patient before clinical deterioration. Insonation of the middle cerebral artery has the best negative and positive predictive value to predict DCI especially if mean flow velocity <120 cm/s or >200 cm/s, respectively. The Lindegaard ratio, is the ratio of MCA velocity measured through temporal windows to ipsilateral extracranial ICA measured with the same probe using submandibular windows, can help rule out the increased flow velocity due to systemic hypertension or hyperemia. Ratio more than 6 predicts severe to critical vasospasm while additional <3 minutes signify increased MCA velocities related to systemic causes. The trend of velocities on serial daily testing is also a significant predictor for developing vasospasm and a velocity increase of >50 cm/s is significant. Serial monitoring of TCD velocity in high-grade subarachnoid patients can also risk stratify patients for intensive care monitoring facilitating triage of patients demonstrating normal velocities for lesser intensity in patient care.

Noninvasive Measure of Increased Intracranial Pressure

As ICP increases, flow in intracranial vessels changes. In the initial phase, the systolic velocity increases as the cerebral vessels are narrowed due to ICP signifying high resistance flow. With further increase, the ICP approaches diastolic pressure and obliterates the diastolic flow **(Figs. 3A to E)**.[2,6,10] Further increase in ICPs will cause diastolic flow reversal **(Figs. 3 and 4B)**. Raised ICP can be estimated by qualitative review of waveforms showing transition of normal cerebral low-resistance waveforms to high-resistance waveforms on serial testing. This can also be done quantitatively using the pulsatility index (PI), the difference between the peak systolic velocity and end-diastolic velocity divided by mean blood flow velocity.[10,11] Also call the Gosling index, this parameter represents a sensitive measure of distal cerebral vascular resistance and hold normal values between 0.6 and 1.2. Increased PI may be caused by distal atherosclerotic disease or increased ICP hence measurement of baseline values to facilitate further serial comparisons can be extremely helpful. A PI of >2.1 correlates with increased ICP >22.[12] Several attempts have been done to measure cerebral perfusion pressure quantitatively using TCD metrics with a recent trial IMPRESSIT-2 showing good predictive value of TCD in predicting increased ICPs.[13] TCD waveforms can also be a sensitive biomarker for ruling out perfusion limiting cerebral edema by demonstrating normal intracranial waveforms.[13] Presence of normal low-resistance waveforms can rule out presence of cerebral edema although hyperperfusion state causing increased ICPs should be considered in the differential diagnosis in these cases.

Cerebral Circulatory Arrest

Malignant cerebral edema is caused by a no-salvageable acute brain injury causing increased ICP eventually leading to cerebral circulatory arrest and brain death. Brain death is a clinical diagnosis marked by irreversible loss of brain and brainstem function confirmed with a physical examination and apnea test. In patients where such examination is confounded further ancillary testing may be needed to confirm cerebral circulatory arrest. When presence of temporal windows can be documented with prior TCD's, this test can provide a noninvasive means of confirming brain death.[14] Oscillating flow, small systolic spikes of

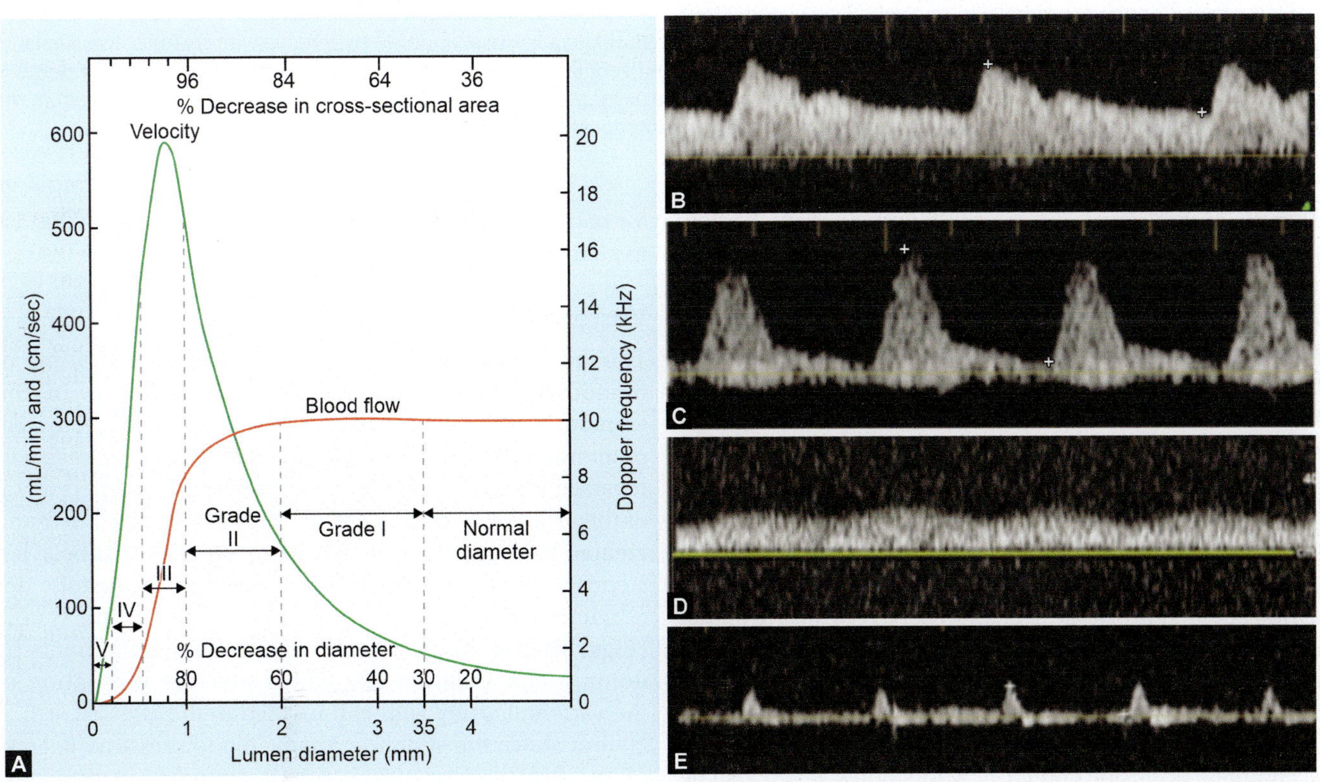

FIGS. 3A TO E: (A) Spencer Reid curve is the hemodynamic model that combined Hagen–Poiseuille law, continuity principle, and cerebrovascular resistance to show the relationship between the blood flow and velocity changes in cerebral circulation in response to changed in diameter of the vessel (left). (B) Doppler waveforms on cerebrovascular ultrasound show low resistance, good flow waveforms with normal diameter, (C) High resistance waveforms compromising blood flow with stenosis, (D) Poststenotic waveforms with reduced velocities and (E) Low flow low velocity waveforms seen in very high grade stenosis.

Source: Spencer MP, Reid JM. Quantitation of carotid stenosis with continuous wave Doppler ultrasound. Stroke. 1979;10:326-30.

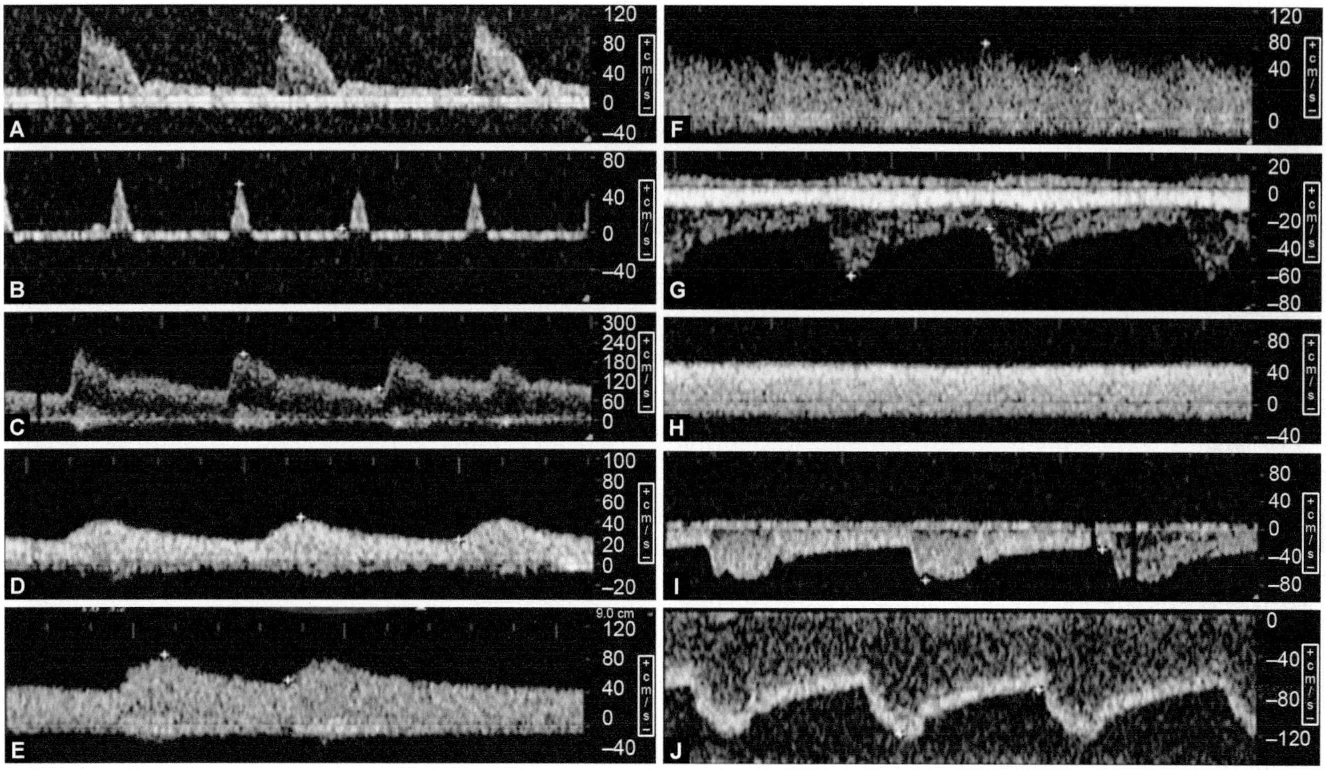

FIGS. 4A TO J: Waveform analysis can be useful in assessing cerebral hemodynamics. (A) High resistance waveforms seen in distal atherosclerotic disease or increased intracranial pressure. (B) To and fro waveforms with forward systolic flow and reversed diastolic flow that is sustained portends progression to cerebral circulatory arrest. (C) Normal low resistance cerebral artery waveforms. (D) Poststenotic waveforms also called parvus et tardus. (E) Irregular heart rate captured during cranial insonation. (F) Hyperemia with diastolic flow similar to systolic flow. (G) Posterior cerebral artery waveforms with superimposed venous waveforms from basilar vein of Rosenthal. (H) Nonpulsatile waveforms seen in a patient on venoarterial extracorporeal membrane oxygenation. (I) Vertebral artery waveforms with flow away from the probe on suboccipital views. (J) High velocity high flow waveform of anterior cerebral artery.

<200 ms duration and <50 cm/s PSV with no diastolic flow or disappearance of intracranial flow must be present on two examinations at least 30 minutes apart.[15,16] Physicians planning to incorporate TCD's as part of their ancillary testing and brain death evaluation and encouraged to follow a standardized imaging protocol based on institutional guidelines which can be informed by published national and international organizations.[17]

Acute Ischemic Stroke

Transcranial Doppler continues to have an important role in the evaluation of patient with acute ischemic stroke despite significant increase in the availability of CT, MRI, and digital subtraction angiography.[18,19] TCD is the only dynamic study that is able to elucidate collateral pathways and can demonstrate active microembolization.[20] It can also help to distinguish near occlusions that may be misdiagnosed as complete occlusions on CT or MRI studies. It can also be complementary to existing radiological studies by confirming hemodynamic significance of stenosis.[21] Physiological testing for vasomotor reactivity is also a distinct advantage for patients with intracranial stenosis or Moyamoya disease to guide further management strategies.[22]

Vertebral Steal

The dominant nature of TCD allows visualization of hemodynamic phenomena like reversed flow in the vertebral arteries that is a hallmark feature of subclavian steal phenomena.[23] While some patients may have a consistent reversed vertebral artery in other patients dynamic reversal of the artery may only occur in times of increased demand created by use of the ipsilateral arm affected by subclavian stenosis. Vertebral artery waveforms showing systolic deacceleration **(Fig. 5A)** or reversal of flow during systole **(Figs. 5B and C)** can also be elicited in such patients by doing a cuff inflation test which involves insonation of the vertebral artery with cuff inflated in the affected arm at 20 mm above the systolic systemic blood pressure. Release of the cuff creates postischemic reperfusion and may uncover a latent steal. Vertebral steal phenomenon is a surrogate marker for cerebrovascular disease and independently predicts morbidity and mortality.

CRANIAL B-MODE ULTRASOUND

B-mode ultrasound of the brain parenchyma using the temporal windows can be a surrogate for assessing midline shift, hemorrhage and ventricular measurements in patients that are unstable or unable to get traditional neuroimaging such as CT or MRI. While the diagnostic accuracy of cranial ultrasound in comparison to CT scan is not perfect when intracranial pathology is visible through temporal windows this can be important diagnostic modality to rule out major pathological status such as malignant cerebral edema causing midline shift or large-volume hemorrhage or expanding hydrocephalus.

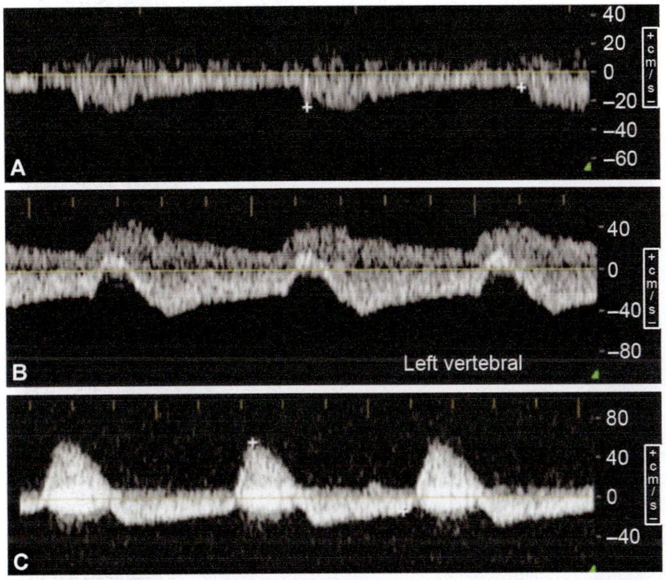

FIGS. 5A TO C: (A) Vertebral artery waveforms with flow away from the probe on suboccipital views. The systolic deceleration after initial systolic upstroke may be a sign of latent vertebral steal or subclavian stenosis. (B and C) Reversed flow in the vertebral artery during systole and forward flow during diastole consistent with overt steal phenomena. Flow toward the probe in suboccipital windows is shown above the baseline (positive Doppler effect) and represents flow from vertebral to the subclavian artery.

Technical Aspects

The low frequency 1–3 MHz echo probe can be placed on the temporal bone to visualize the axial section of the brain at the level of the basal cisterns.[24] The typical landmarks include the opposite skull visible at 12–15 cm depth, hypoechoic area representing the midbrain with 2 hyperechoic markings anterior to the midbrain representing the clinoid processes and the convex ridge created by the petrous part of the temporal bone and lesser wing of the sphenoid outlining the middle cranial fossa **(Figs. 6A to D)**. Midbrain often has a hyperechoic shadows around it created by the arachnoid and the trailing shadow caused by posterior through transmission normally seen in many patients. Falx cerebri and septum pellucidum can also be visualized to serve as midline structures for the calculation of midline shift **(Figs. 7A and B)**. Both the third and the fourth ventricle can be visualized in plane superior to the basal cistern and the size can be measured in the axial as well as coronal planes.

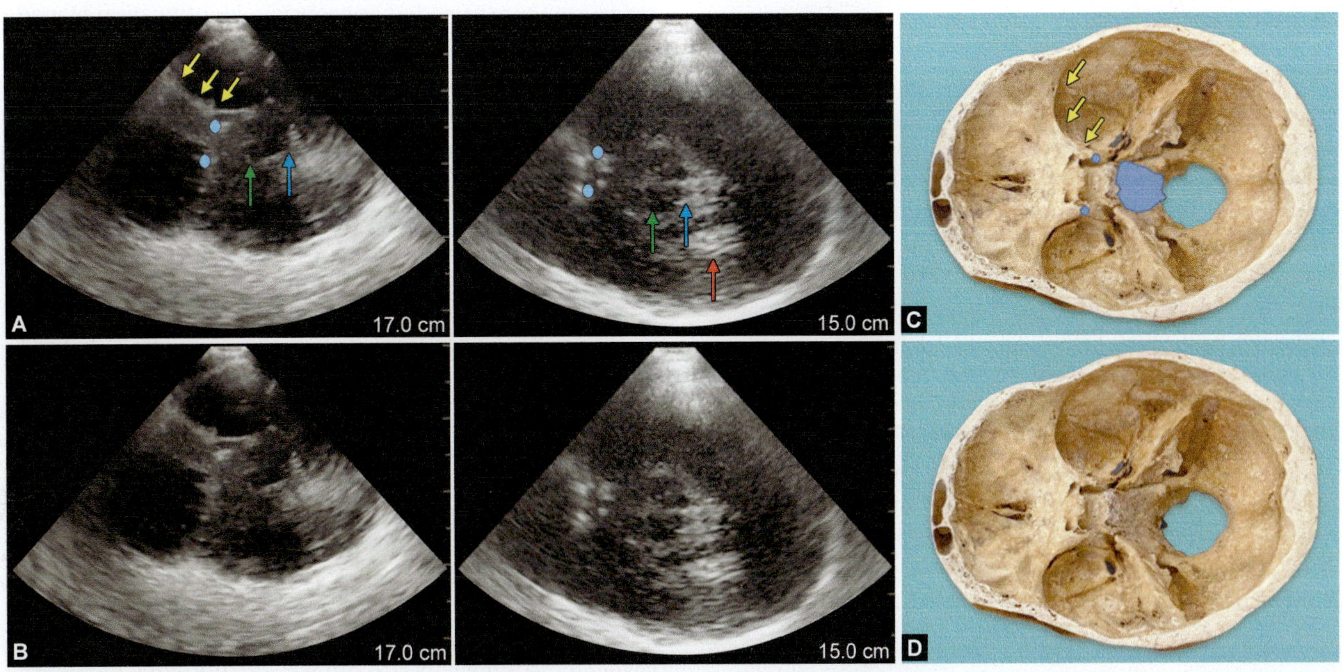

FIGS. 6A TO D: Transcranial B mode ultrasound showing the clinoid processes [blue dots, sphenoid wing (yellow arrows), midbrain green arrow and basal cisterns (blue arrow)]. Choroid plexus in the temporal horn is visible as hyperechoic signal (red arrow). Corresponding view of the base of the skull showing clinoid processes [blue dots, sphenoid wing (yellow arrows), midbrain (blue shape)].

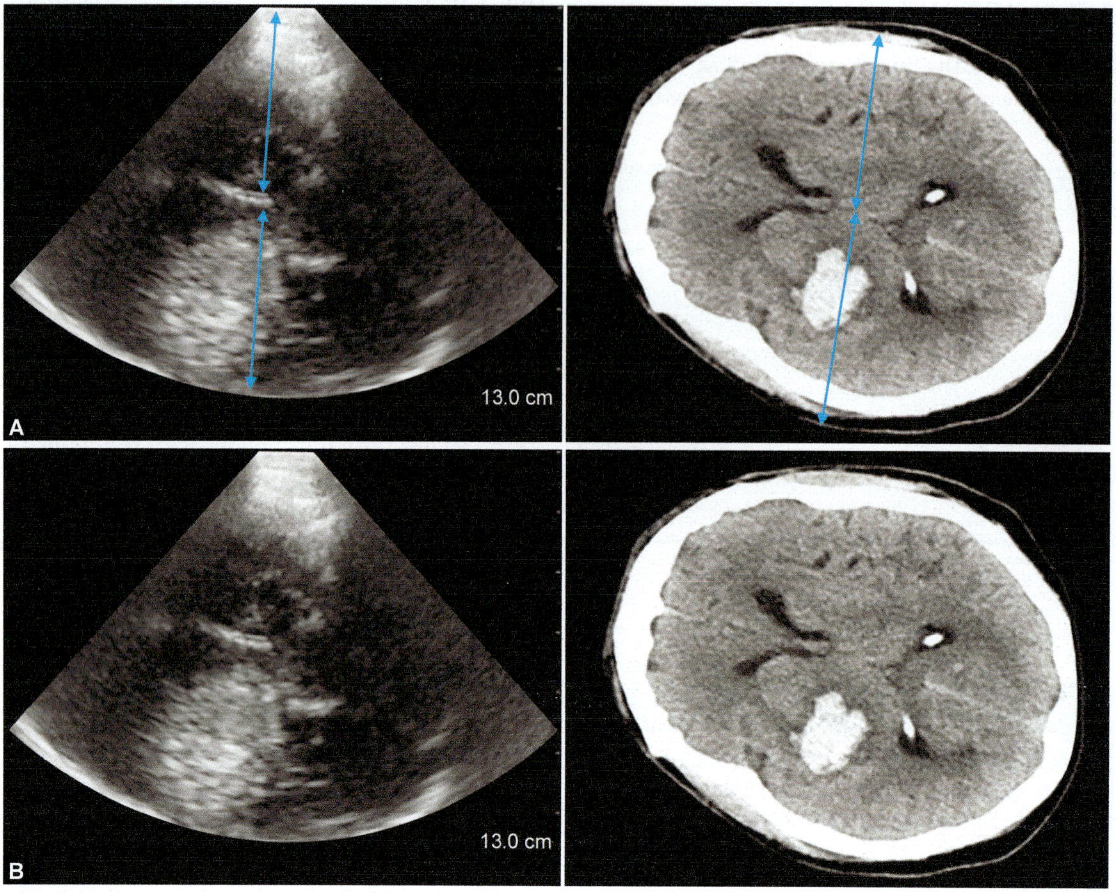

FIGS. 7A AND B: Measurement of the midline shift in the axial plane (left image) through the temporal windows on transcranial B mode ultrasound with ipsilateral and contralateral measurements in the same plane. Corresponding images of the computer tomography are shown in the right image.

Interpretation

Midline Shift Assessment

On cranial ultrasound, midline shift can be calculated by measuring the distance from the ipsilateral temporal bone as well as contralateral temporal bone to the third ventricle on the septum pellucidum as the midline structure.[25,26] The difference between the ipsilateral displacement and contralateral displacement is divided by 2 to calculate midline shift. Displacement of the third ventricle on ultrasound correlates well with CT findings and is an alternative method for patients not amenable to CT imaging.[27]

Intracranial Hemorrhage Measurements

In some patients, acute intracranial hemorrhage <5 days old can be visible as a hyperechoic shadow on the side opposite to the window being insonated. When hemorrhage is clearly visible, ultrasound can be used to measure the dimensions of the hemorrhage in axial and coronal planes and allow serial testing **(Figs. 8A and B)**.[28]

Hydrocephalus

Third ventricular measurements on ultrasound have been described to have good correlation to CT-based measurements provided appropriate identification is made **(Figs. 9A and B)**.[29,30] The accuracy of lateral ventricular measurements has not been investigated rigorously.

Hemicraniectomy

In patients after hemicraniectomy, cranial imaging is facilitated by lack of bone.[31] In this scenario, the abdominal preset can be used to distinguish parenchymal details and follow these serially in a critically ill patient. **Figures 10A and B** demonstrate the topography of brain ultrasound B-mode images in hemicraniectomy patient showing ipsilateral hemorrhagic conversion of an ischemic stroke that required decompressive hemicraniectomy.

Caution must be exercised in over interpreting hyperechoic shadows using TCD windows on cranial B-mode ultrasound imaging in patients with intact skulls. Several hyperechoic artifacts including posterior through transmission and ring artifacts are common on cranial B-mode imaging and require expertise to distinguish it from hemorrhage. In addition, extensive white matter disease and vasogenic edema can also appear hyperechoic. Familiarity with the expected topography of the brain on B-mode ultrasound is key to his clinical application in patients not able to undergo traditional neuroimaging.[24]

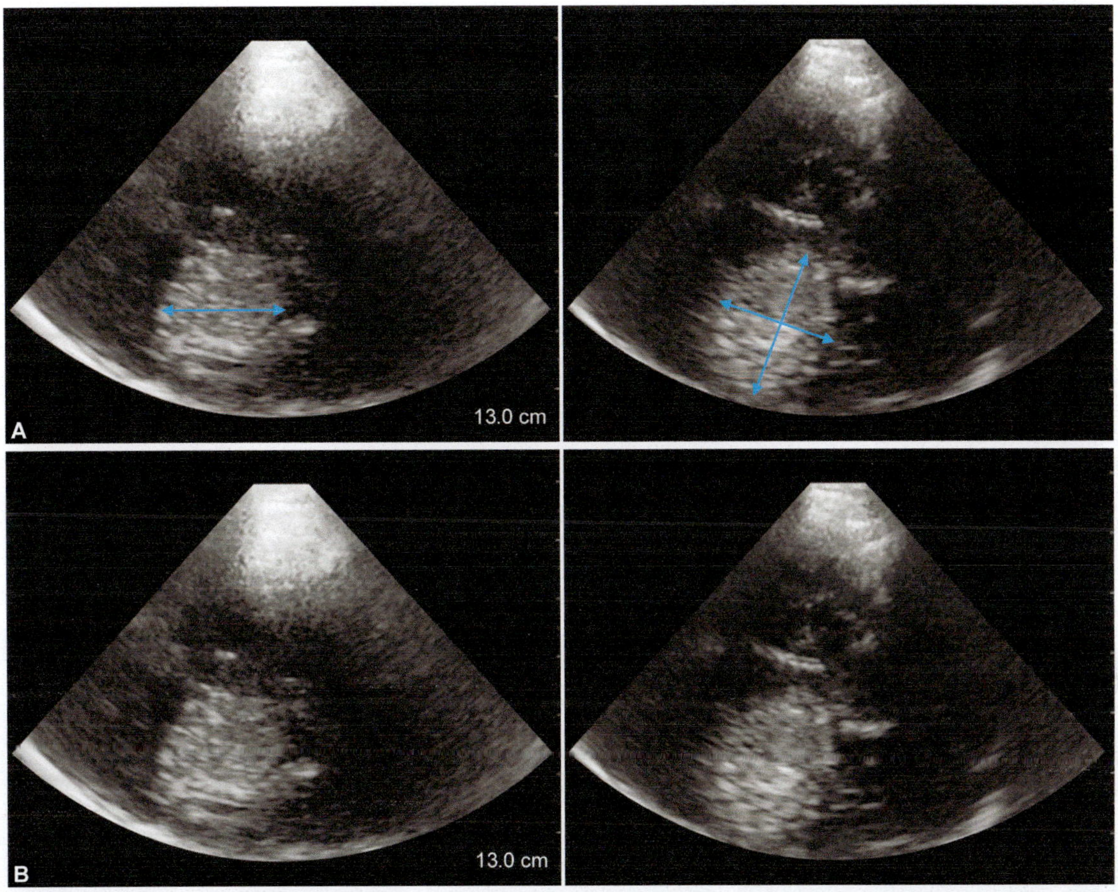

FIGS. 8A AND B: An acute intracranial hemorrhage when seen distinctly on transcranial B mode ultrasound can be measured in the coronal plane (left) and axial plane (right) through the temporal windows to render the volume of the hemorrhage similar to measurements performed on a computer tomography scan.

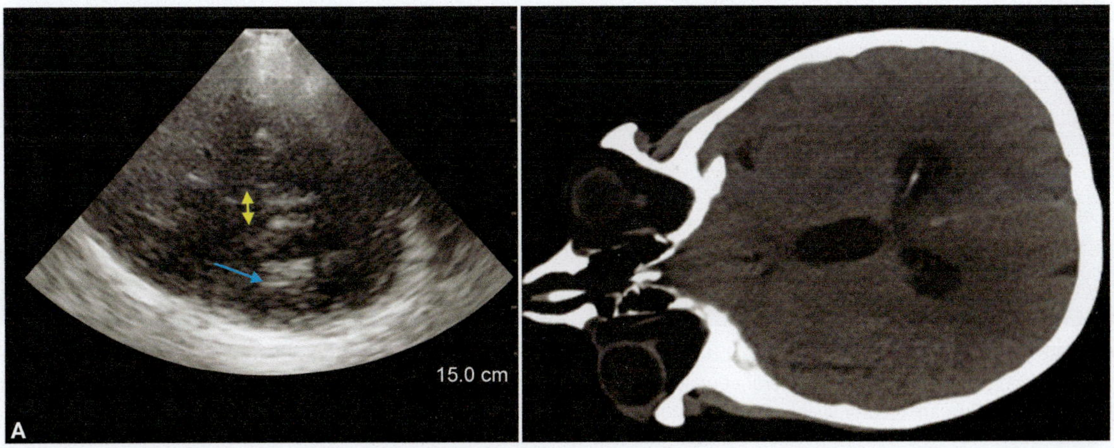

FIGS. 9A AND B: *Continued*

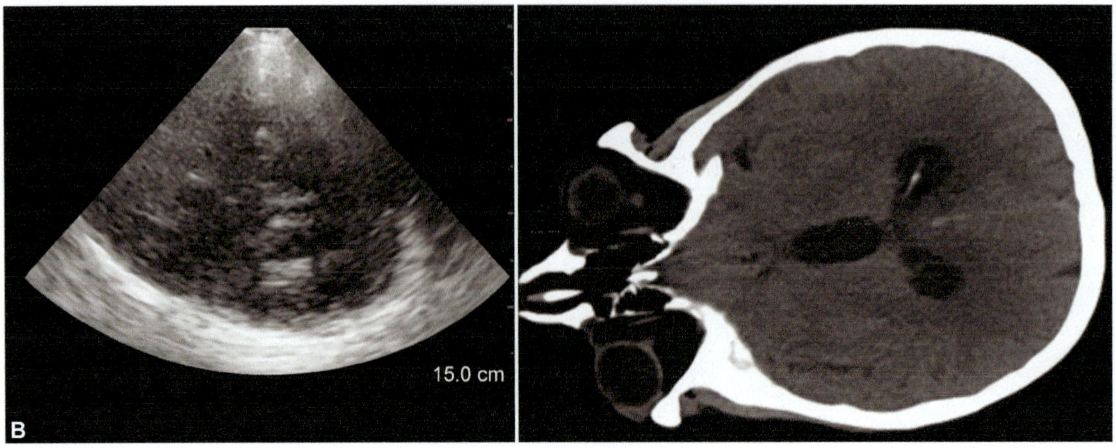

FIGS. 9A AND B: Left image shows enlargement of the third ventricle (double headed yellow arrow) seen on the axial section on cranial ultrasound. The choroid plexus in the temporal horn of lateral ventricle is also visible as a hyperechoic signal (blue arrow). Corresponding computed tomography images on the right side.

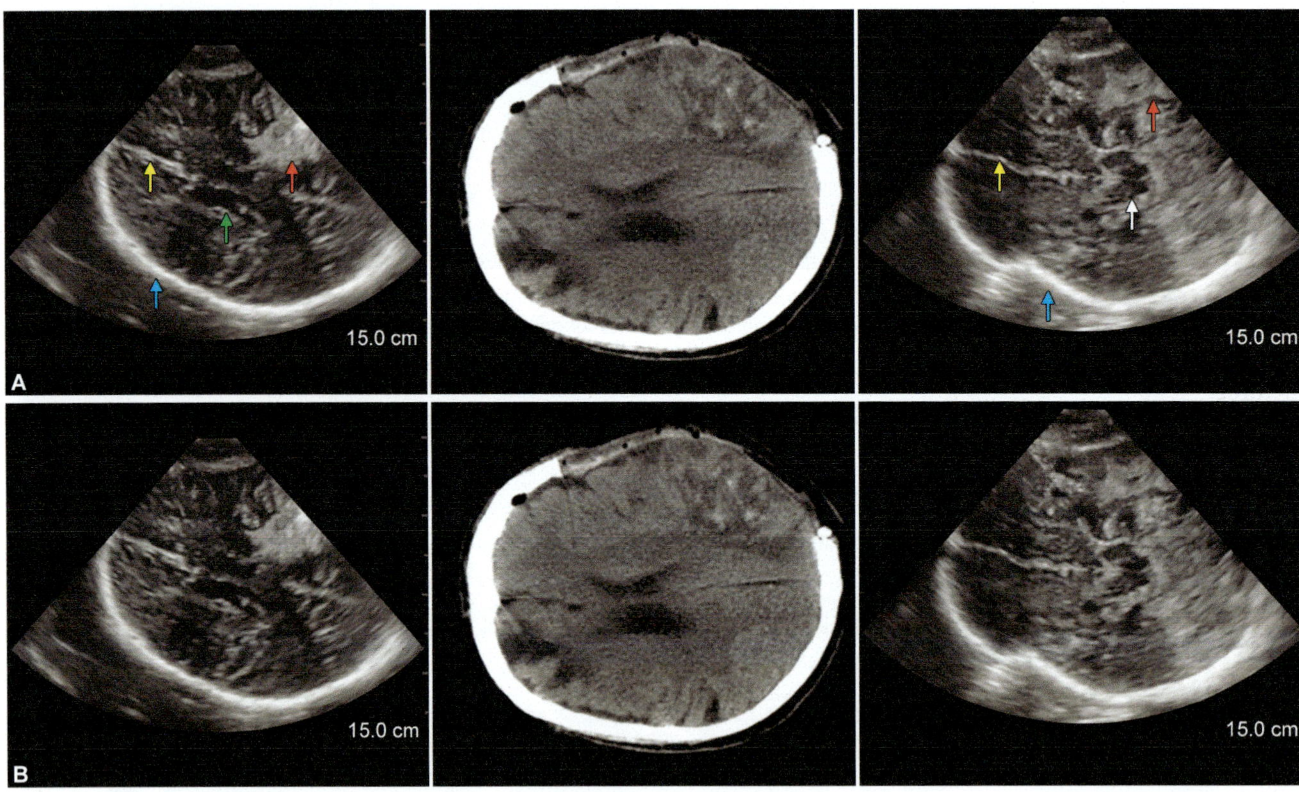

FIGS. 10A AND B: Cranial ultrasound B mode in abdominal present in a patient with hemicraniectomy. In addition to the opposite skull (blue arrow), the falx cerebri (yellow arrow), lateral ventricles (green arrow), midbrain (white arrow), vasogenic edema (red arrow) related to hemorrhage after evacuation are clearly visible. Middle image shows the computed tomography image.

Clinical Utility

Ultrasound can aid in diagnosis of massive hydrocephalus or measurements of intracranial hemorrhage when visualized. In addition serial measurements on ultrasound can help measure third ventricular enlargement and weaning of external ventricular drain (EVD). Kiphuth et al. demonstrated that an increase of 5.5 mm in ventricle width after clamping had a sensitivity, specificity positive predictive value, and negative predictive value of 100%, 83%, 81%, and 100%, respectively in needing a permanent shunt.[32] Serial imaging in hemicraniectomy patients can help diagnose an incidental subdural or epidural contralateral to the insonation. While the resolution of ultrasound does not allow it to be used in replacement of CT scans such

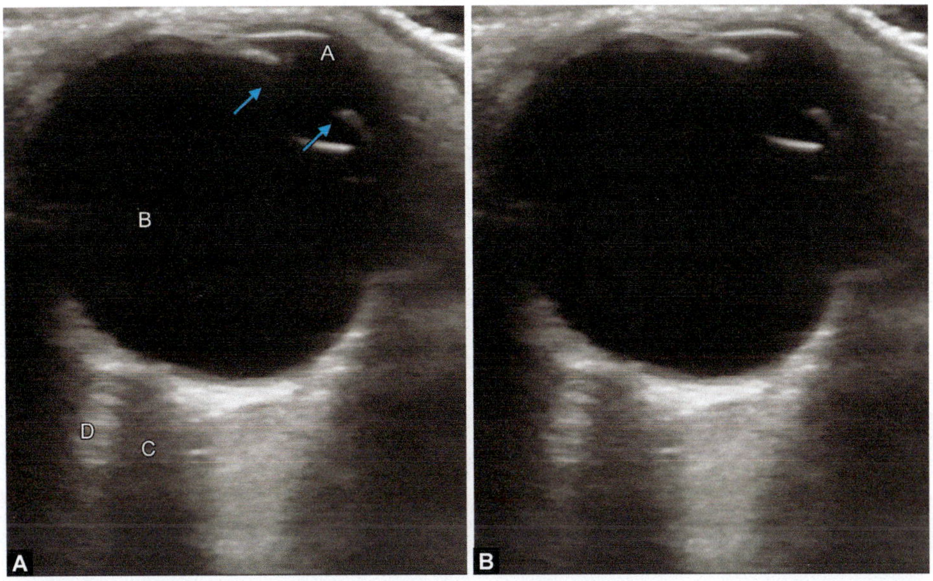

FIGS. 11A AND B: Axial section of the eyeball can be insonated using high frequency probe (5–15 MHz) using orbital preset (MI 0.2, TI 0) placed on a closed eye. A anterior chamber, B posterior chamber lined by the retina, C optic nerve and D represents the optic nerve sheath with cerebrospinal fluid surrounding the nerve.

clinical indications can help point-of-care assessment in clinical situations where CT is inaccessible.

OCULAR ULTRASOUND

B-mode ultrasound using high-frequency probe adjusted to orbital preset can be used to visualize the anterior and posterior chamber of the eye as well as retrobulbar structures including optic nerve sheath and central retinal artery **(Figs. 11A and B)**. Such clinical applications can help assess patients with acute brain injury as well as patients presenting with visual symptoms with unclear etiology.[33]

Technical Aspects

High-frequency linear probe is placed on the closed eyelid using gel to insonate the globe while preventing pressure on the eye. Care must be taken to prevent exposure of the eye to the gel which can be discomforting. Hypoallergenic gel is not available for pediatric population. Orbital preset on ultrasound that reduces the mechanical index and thermal index of insonation facilitates safe imaging of the eye which is more sensitive to the mechanical and thermal adverse effect of ultrasound.

Assessment of pupillary reaction can be a key surrogate for uncal herniation.[34] When access to the pupil is restricted by eyelid edema or injury, pupillary reflex can be tested by insonating the eye to assess for movements of the iris in response to consensual light reflex shown on the opposite eye **(Figs. 12A to D)**. Pupillary reflex can be tested both on transverse and coronal views. Qualitative assessment of the pupillary reactivity can be done on B-mode which also facilitates quantitative measurements.

Ultrasound can also be used to assess for presence of papilledema **(Figs. 13A to C)** which is visible as protrusion of the optic nerve into the posterior vitreous chamber also another "crescent "sign.[35]

Optic nerve sheath diameter (ONSD) can be visualized behind the retina when optic nerve can be visualized along the longitudinal axis.[36,37] The probe is pointed medially posteriorly to follow the direction of the optic nerve. Measurements are taken 3 mm behind the retina ensuring a long axis view of the optic nerve.[38] This facilitates a transverse diameter measurement of the optic nerve sheath. Such measurements can be inaccurate due to inherent variability in the optic nerve anatomy and may be difficult in patients with nystagmus, involuntary ocular movements or tonic gaze deviation.

Interpretations

Pupillary Reflex

Absence of pupillary reactivity can be a clinical sign of uncal herniation and serial ultrasound testing can be helpful in patients with routine pupillary testing when using penlight is not feasible. Quantitative pupillometry using M-mode has been described but needs widespread validation. Presence of the crescent sign can be a marker of papilledema in a patient with recent increased intracranial pressure.

Noninvasive Surrogate for Increased ICP

Optic nerve sheath diameter has shown strong correlation with elevated ICP. The optic nerve is surrounded by subarachnoid space and is distensible as ICP increases. Large ONSDs have been associated with increased ICP but wide

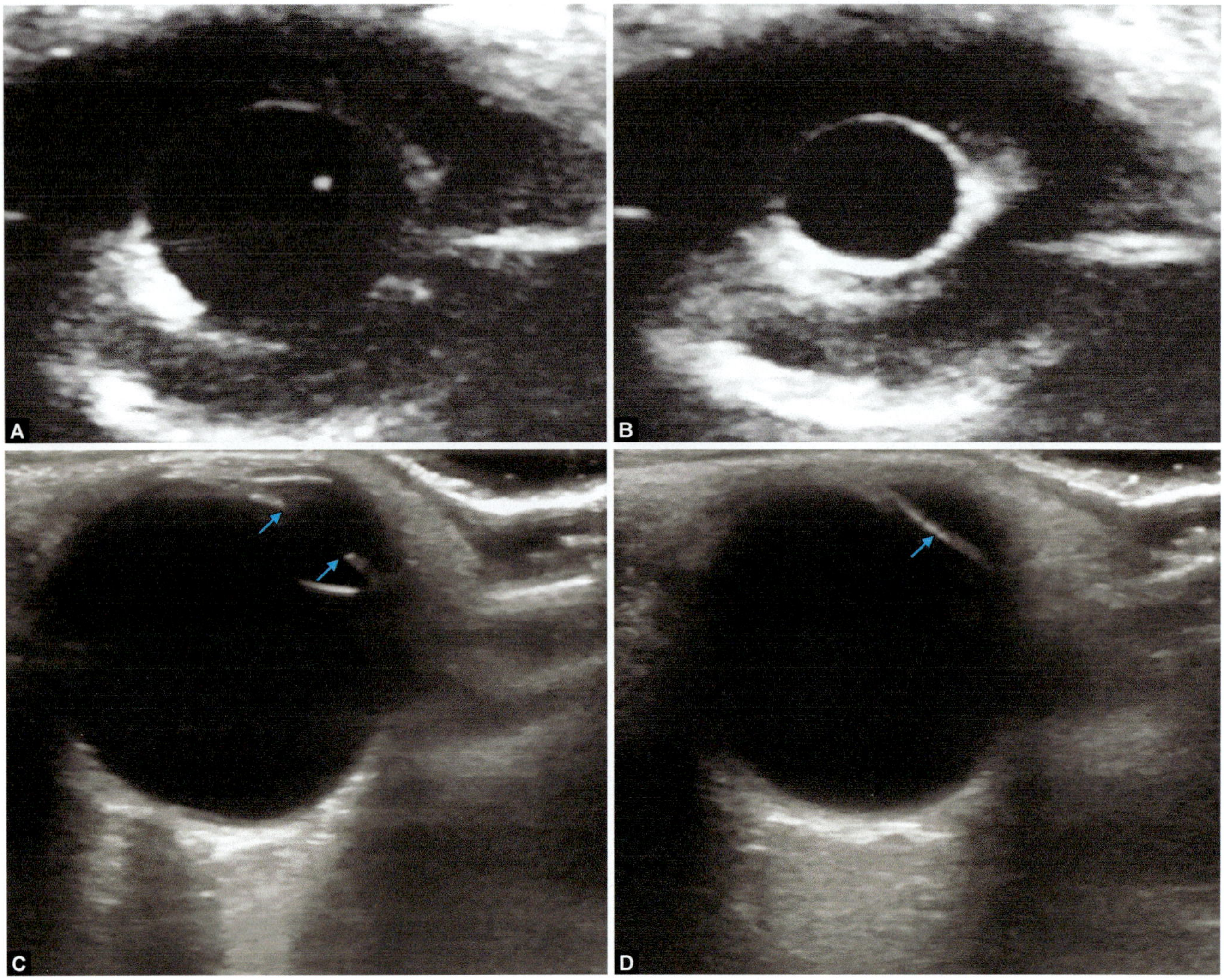

FIGS. 12A TO D: Demonstration of consensual light reflex when high frequency (5–15 MHz) probe using orbital preset (MI 0.2, TI 0) is placed on a closed eye and light is shown on opposite eye. (A and B) Coronal view of the eye at the level of the iris showing pupillary size changes. (C and D) Axial section views with similar dilation and constriction of the pupil.

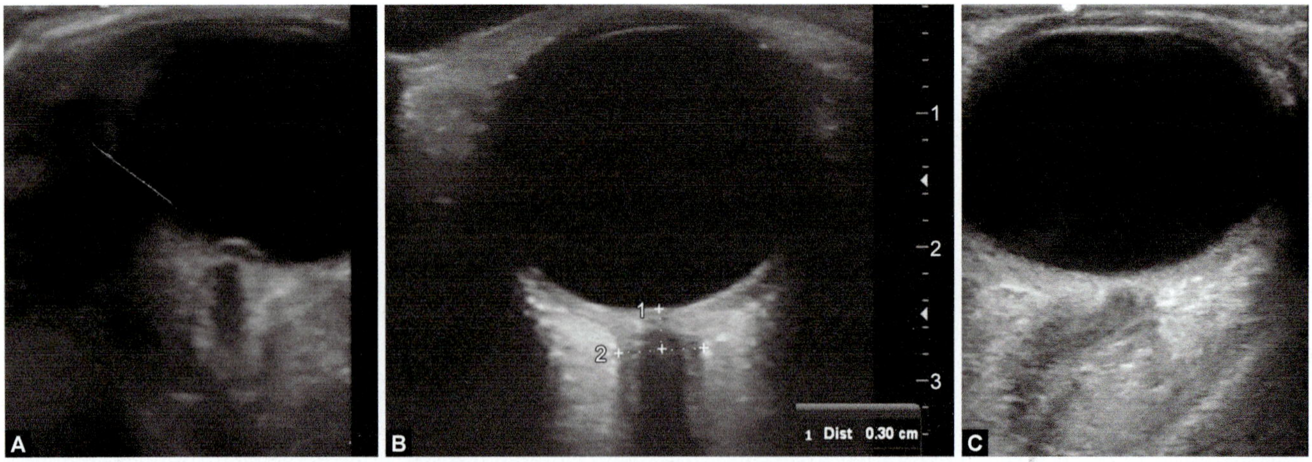

FIGS. 13A TO C: (A) Axial section on ocular ultrasound showing raised optic nerve protruding into the posterior chamber consistent with papilledema; (B) The measurement of optic nerve sheath diameter (ONSD) 3 mm behind the retina. Anatomical variations in course of optic nerve; (C) and inability to insonate a true long axis to yield transverse diameter limit widespread scalability of ONSD.

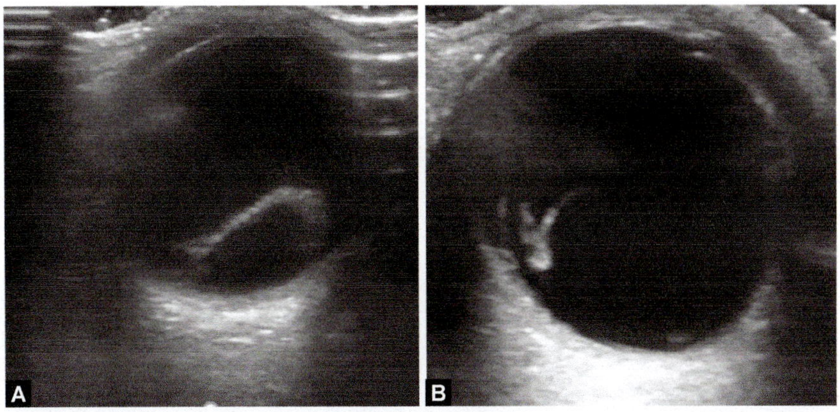

FIGS. 14A AND B: Ocular ultrasound may show retinal detachment as well as vitreous hemorrhage in the posterior chamber. Retinal detachment respects the optic nerve and flap can be seen attached to posterior wall at optic nerve while vitreous hemorrhage typically crosses the optic nerve.

optic nerves have been known to occur in normal healthy volunteers. Unilateral cerebral pathology also causes inconsistent increases in ONSD. While exact cutoff for using ONSD in predicting ICPs is fraught with several challenges, serial imaging using standardized image acquisition protocol can be extremely helpful to predict increased ICPs in a patient with widening optic nerve sheath. Sudden increase in ICP that obliterates the basal cisterns may also not manifest in wide optic nerve sheaths. ONSD reduction also lags in normalization after a bout of increased ICP crisis. Other limitations include anatomical variability contributing to inaccuracy.

Orbital Pathology

The posterior chamber can be further visualized and may show changes of retinal detachment which can be distinguished by vitreal hemorrhage in respecting the optic nerve boundaries **(Figs. 14A and B)**.[39]

Utility

Ocular ultrasound allows evaluation of the pupillary light reflex through the eyelids. In most patients, the pupillary size and reactivity can be assessed through bedside examination and newer tools such as pupillometry.[34] However, in a subset of patients, such as those with trauma or recent craniotomy when it is near impossible to visualize the pupil, ultrasound allows visualization of the pupil through the eyelids, and reactivity can be assessed via the consensual light reflex. Ultrasound markers of papilledema or wide ONSD can be important surrogates of increased ICP specially on serial testing in patients who otherwise cannot receive an invasive ICP monitor.[36] Patients with visual symptoms can be evaluated for posterior orbital pathology to diagnose retinal detachment or vitreous hemorrhage which can also be seen in patients with Terson syndrome.

CAROTID AND VERTEBRAL ARTERY ULTRASOUND

Ultrasound has significant utility in identifying the hemodynamic significance of carotid artery stenosis, a major cause of cerebrovascular disease. Published guidelines recommend a carotid ultrasound as the first-line imaging in screening for severe carotid stenosis in a patient suspected of cerebrovascular disease as well as asymptomatic carotid stenosis patients in high-risk groups. The hemodynamic significance of the luminal stenosis diagnosed on radiological imaging is a key parameter diagnosed only on ultrasound that has informed multiple clinical trials and management strategies for carotid artery stenosis.[40]

Technical Aspects

Carotid ultrasound is performed using a high-frequency linear probe to visualize the common carotid artery, ICA, and external carotid artery in both the short axis **(Figs. 15A to F)** and with the long axis **(Figs. 16A to F)**.[41] Color Doppler is used to identify any areas of major luminal stenosis **(Figs. 17A and B)**. Pulse Doppler measurements using the gate align with the vessel lumen is used to measure the peak and end-diastolic velocity standardized in the angle of insonation at 60° **(Figs. 18A to D)**.[42] The insonation is done to visualized three segments of the common carotid artery from its origin to the bifurcation, three segments of the ICA from the bifurcation to its disappearance under the mandible and at least one segment of the external carotid artery. At each designated segment of the vessel pulse Doppler waveforms are captured to measure the peak flow velocity and end-diastolic velocity in centimeters per second **(Figs. 19A and B)**. The highest velocity insonated in the ICA is compared to the distal CCA velocity to provide the carotid index or the ICA:CCA ratio.

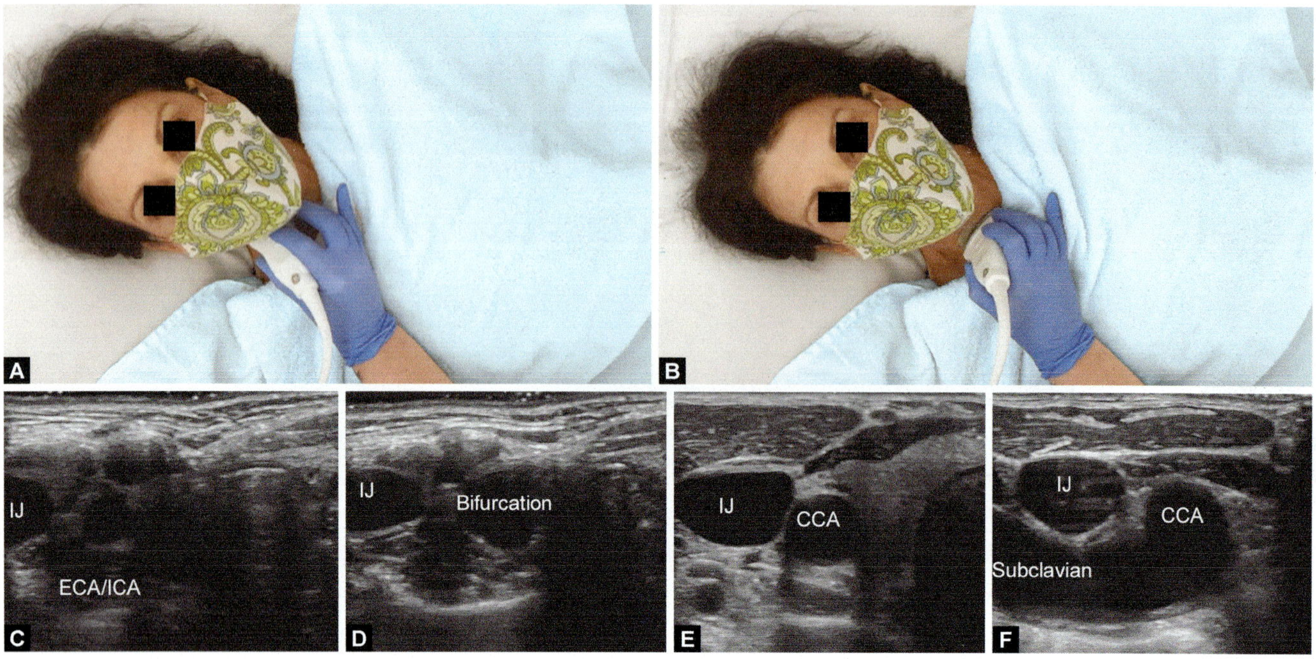

FIGS. 15A TO F: The short axis view of the carotid system (right to left) showing the origin of the common carotid artery (CCA) close to the subclavian artery and its course through the neck with bifurcation into the internal (ICA) and external carotid artery (ECA). The internal jugular can be appreciated as well as a collapsible vessel. The probe is held in short axis.

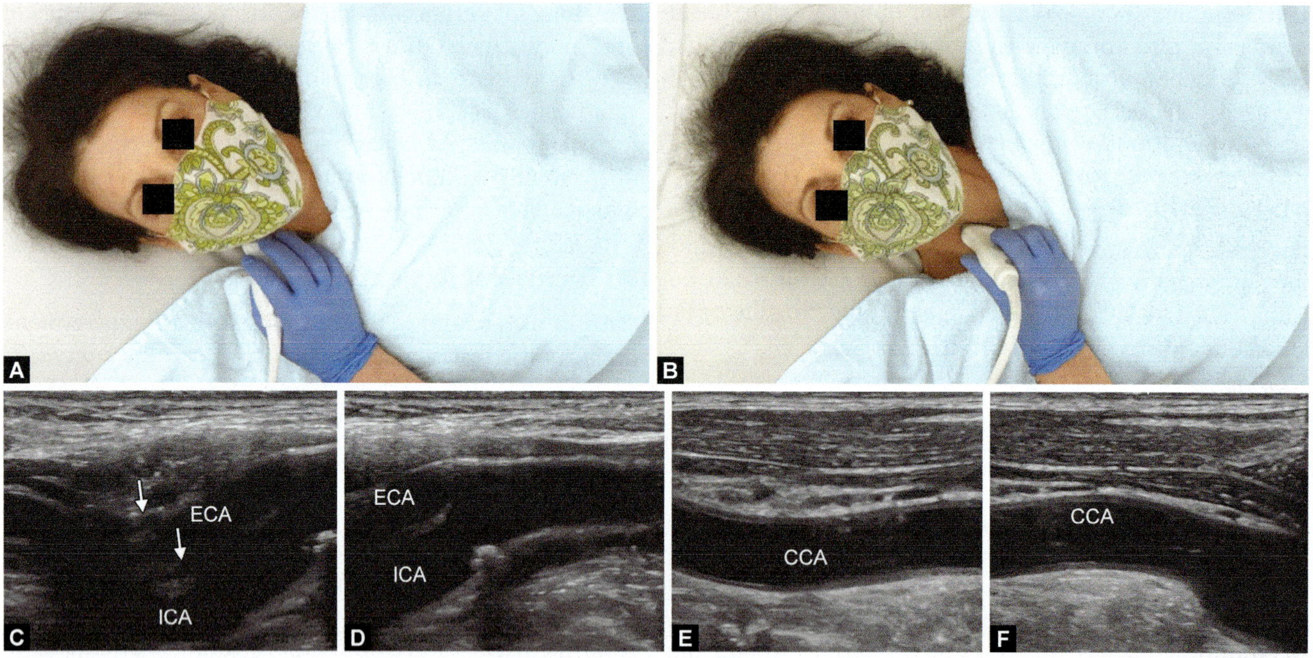

FIGS. 16A TO F: The long axis view of the carotid system (right to left) showing the origin of the common carotid artery (CCA) close to the subclavian artery and its course through the neck with bifurcation into the internal (ICA) and external carotid artery (ECA). The internal jugular can be appreciated as well as a collapsible vessel. ECA is remarkable for branches in the neck (white arrows). The probe is held in the long axis.

While in the long axis, the probe placed on the anterior neck can then be pointed a few centimeters lateral to the midline to visualize the V2 segment of the vertebral artery passing through the transverse foramina of the transverse processes of the cervical vertebra **(Figs. 20A to D)**.

Interpretations

The external carotid artery can be distinguished from the ICA by presence of branches in the neck, its anteromedial location, high-resistance waveforms with minimal diastolic flow as well as presence of temporal tap where periodically

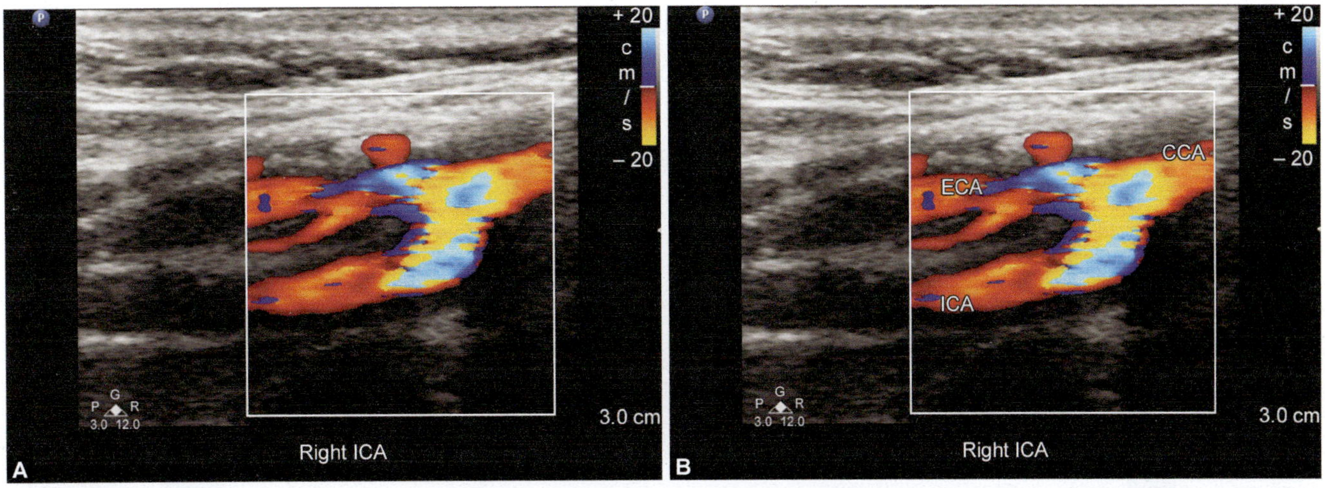

FIGS. 17A AND B: Long axis view of the carotid system showing the common carotid artery (CCA), external carotid artery (ECA) and its branches and internal carotid artery (ICA) in color Doppler mode. The color Doppler scale assigns color based on Doppler shift. Negative Doppler shift in this image is assigned red color and will denote all flow going away from the probe. The probe direction is pointing cranially towards left of the screen that by convention always represents the cranial side.

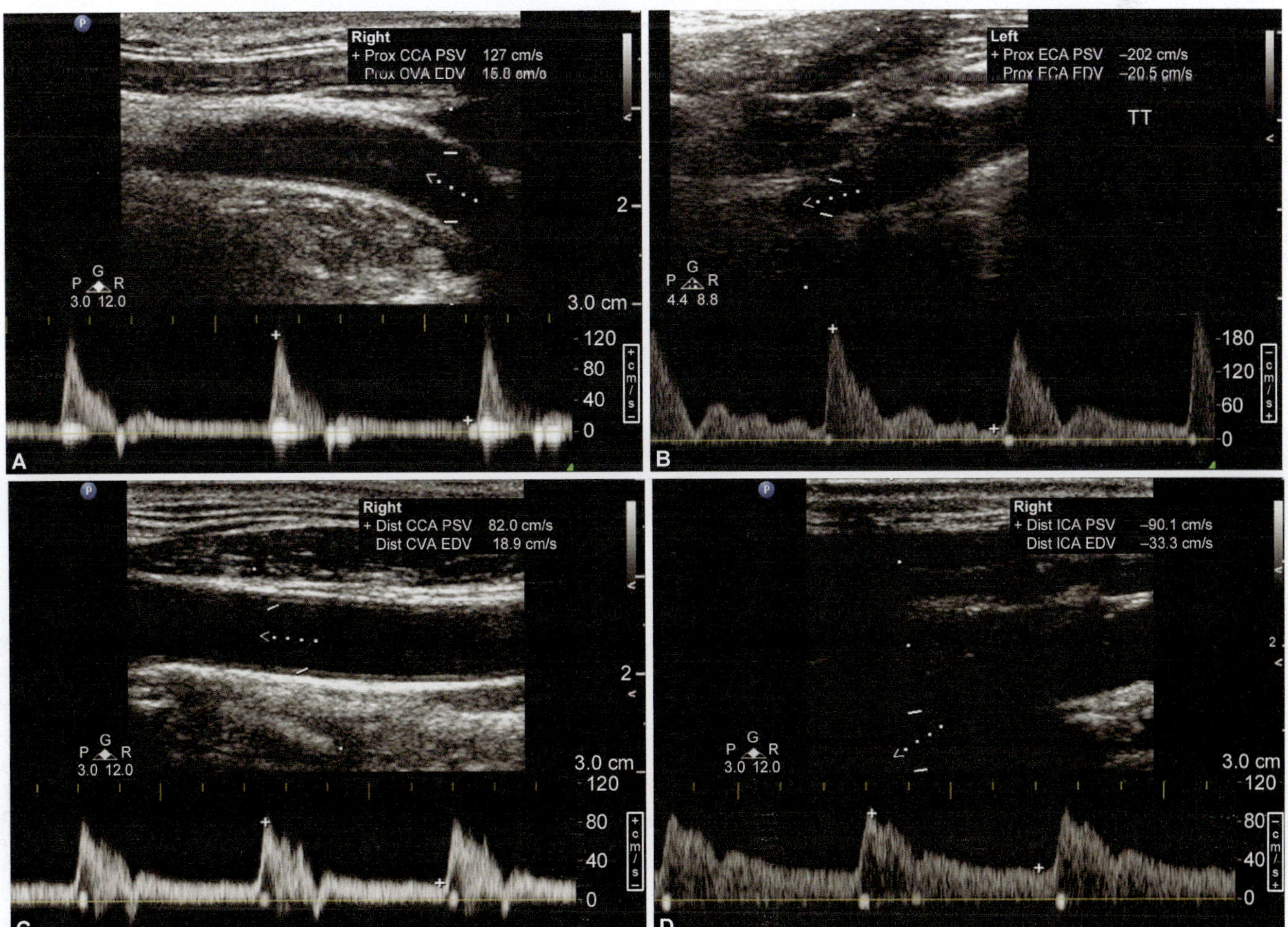

FIGS. 18A TO D: (A) Proximal common carotid artery waveforms and external carotid artery waveforms; (B) show high resistance. Distal CCA waveforms; (C) typically show variable resistive patterns suppling blood into the flow divider at bifurcation. Internal carotid artery waveforms; (D) are typically low resistance with robust diastolic flow.

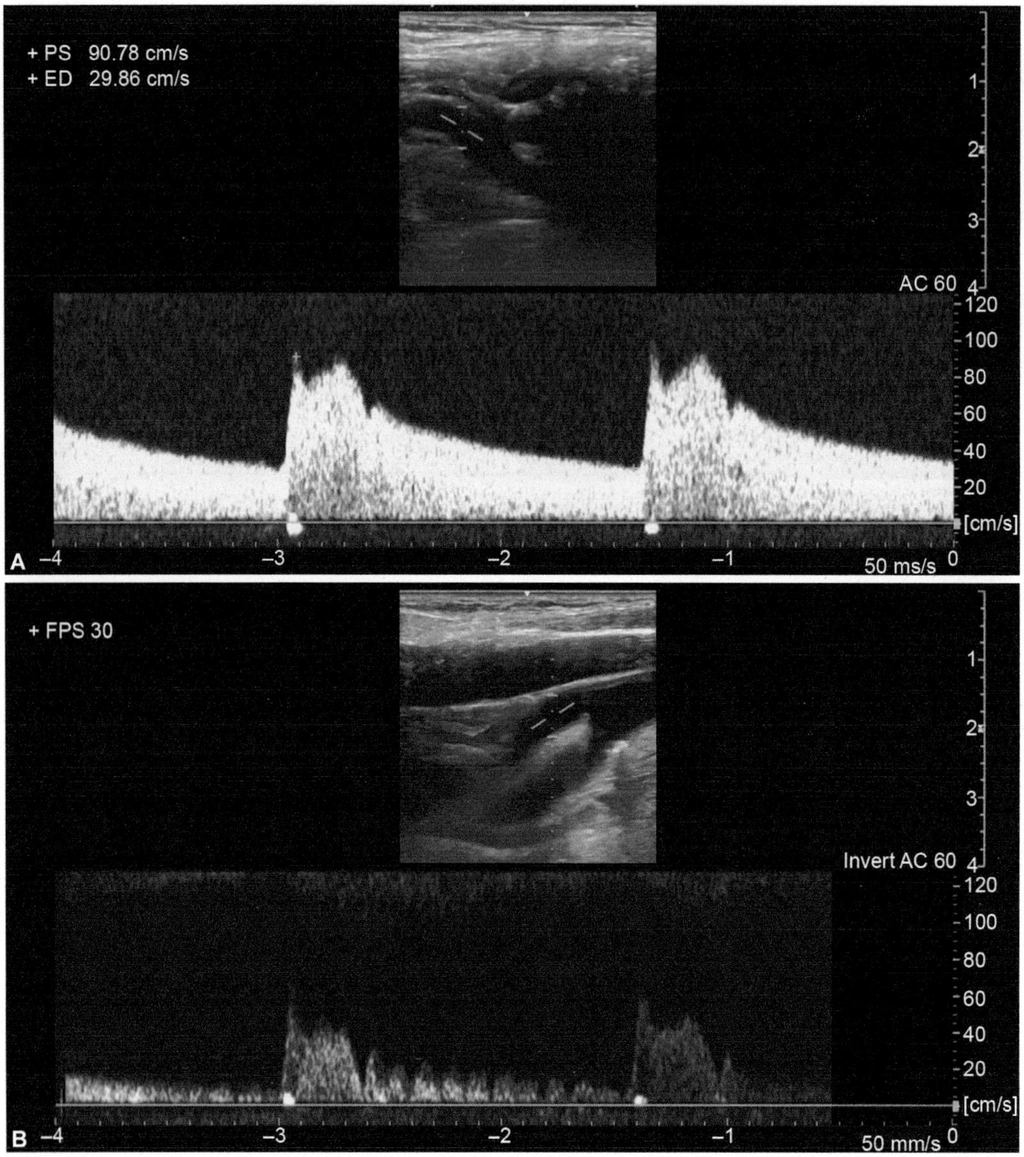

FIGS. 19A AND B: Insonation of the internal carotid artery shows low resistance waveforms with a peak flow velocity of 90.78 cm/s and end diastolic velocity of 29.86 cm/s (A). External carotid artery (ECA) confirmed by temporal tap in contrast has a high resistance waveform (B). Tapping the superficial temporal artery shows transmitted taps in the ECA waveforms.

pressing the superior temporal artery will transmit the pulsations to the external carotid artery **(Figs. 19A and B)**. ICA is posterolateral and has no resistance waveforms since it supplies the low resistance cerebrovascular bed intracranially **(Figs. 19A and B)**. Low-resistance waveforms of the ICA have a rapid upstroke, stepwise deceleration and robust diastole more than a third of the peak systolic flow.

The Society of Radiologists in Ultrasound Consensus Conference has published criteria for using ICA ultrasound measurements for the diagnosis of carotid stenosis.[42] High peak flow velocities >125 cm/s predict carotid stenosis >50%. An end-diastolic flow of 40–100 cm/s classifies the stenosis in the 50–69% range while end-diastolic flow of >100/s places the stenosis at a >70% range.[43] In cases where clear-cut distinction of degree of carotid stenosis not feasible using peak and end-diastolic criteria, the carotid index of 2–4 for 50–69% range and >4 to designate carotid stenosis >70% range is used. Such criteria are typically validated with a local CT angiograms and digital subtraction angiography. The degree of stenosis may be underestimated in the case of advanced age with severe arterial rigidity as well as tandem lesions. Carotid stenosis may be overestimated in younger patients and patients with hyperdynamic states such as anemia or arteriovenous malformations.

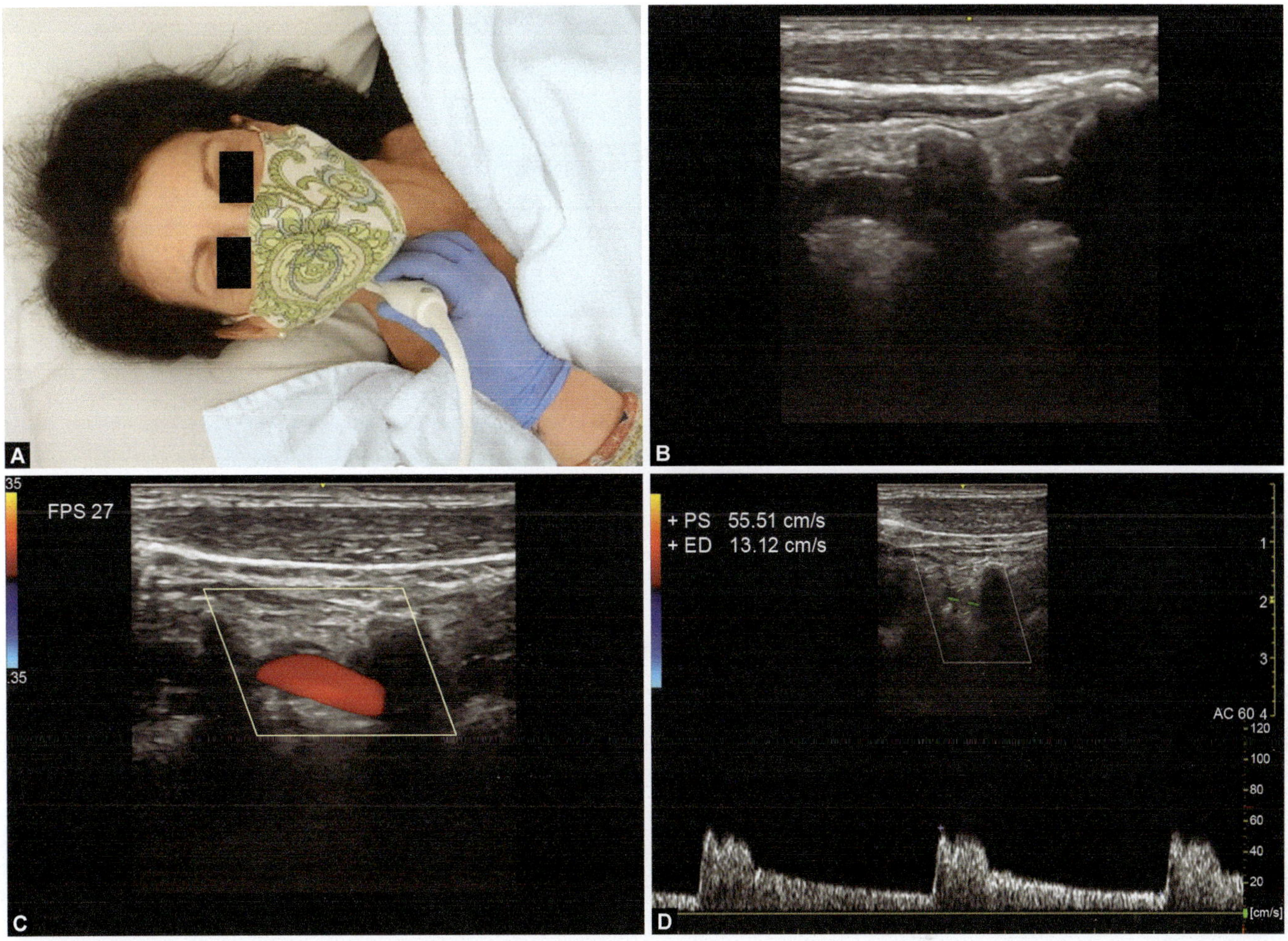

FIGS. 20A TO D: (A) Insonation of the neck in the sagittal plane; (B) to visualize the vertebral artery travelling in the transverse foramina; (C) on B mode and color Doppler; (D) pulse Doppler insonation @60° yields the peak and end diastolic velocity with caudal to cranial flow. The probe is held in the long axis similar to carotid scanning but depth is adjusted to scan the posterior part of the neck and line of insonation pointing lateral to the midline.

Carotid waveforms also show effects of intramural stenosis based on the Spencer Reid curve **(Fig. 3A)**. Hemodynamically significant stenosis can cause resistive waveforms with parvus et tardus waveforms insonated downstream to the area of highest stenosis **(Figs. 21A to C)**. Such waveform transitions may guide sonographer to perform a more thorough search for an area of high velocity and point to a stenosis segment where initial search may have missed high velocity area. In cases of severe stenosis affecting blood flow and drop in velocities (far left of the Spencer Reid curve, **Fig. 3A**), such waveforms can also provide indirect evidence of stenosis.

Utility

Carotid stenosis is a first-line imaging in the screening of patients with suspected carotid stenosis as cause of cerebrovascular disease. The degree of carotid stenosis > 70% informs indications for carotid endarterectomy (CEA) for long-term prevention of stroke and death. Diagnosis of carotid stenosis can also be extremely valuable in patients with transient ischemic attacks or amaurosis fugax which also may be amenable to CEA. Carotid ultrasound can be useful tool for screening high-risk patients undergoing coronary artery bypass grafting with concomitant CEA may be needed to reduce cerebrovascular risk related to the surgery. Other high-risk patients that may benefit from carotid screening for stenosis if otherwise an operative candidate include patients with lower extremity peripheral arterial disease and multiple cerebrovascular risk factors including older patients with smoking diabetes hypertension coronary artery disease. Carotid ultrasound also has value in elucidating the nature and size of plaques. When performed with a thorough standardized protocol in an accredited lab, high location of carotid bifurcation, presence of heavily calcified carotid lesions, and demonstration of complex bifurcation stenosis can guide choice of revascularization surgical technique between CEA, carotid stenting, and transcarotid artery revascularization.

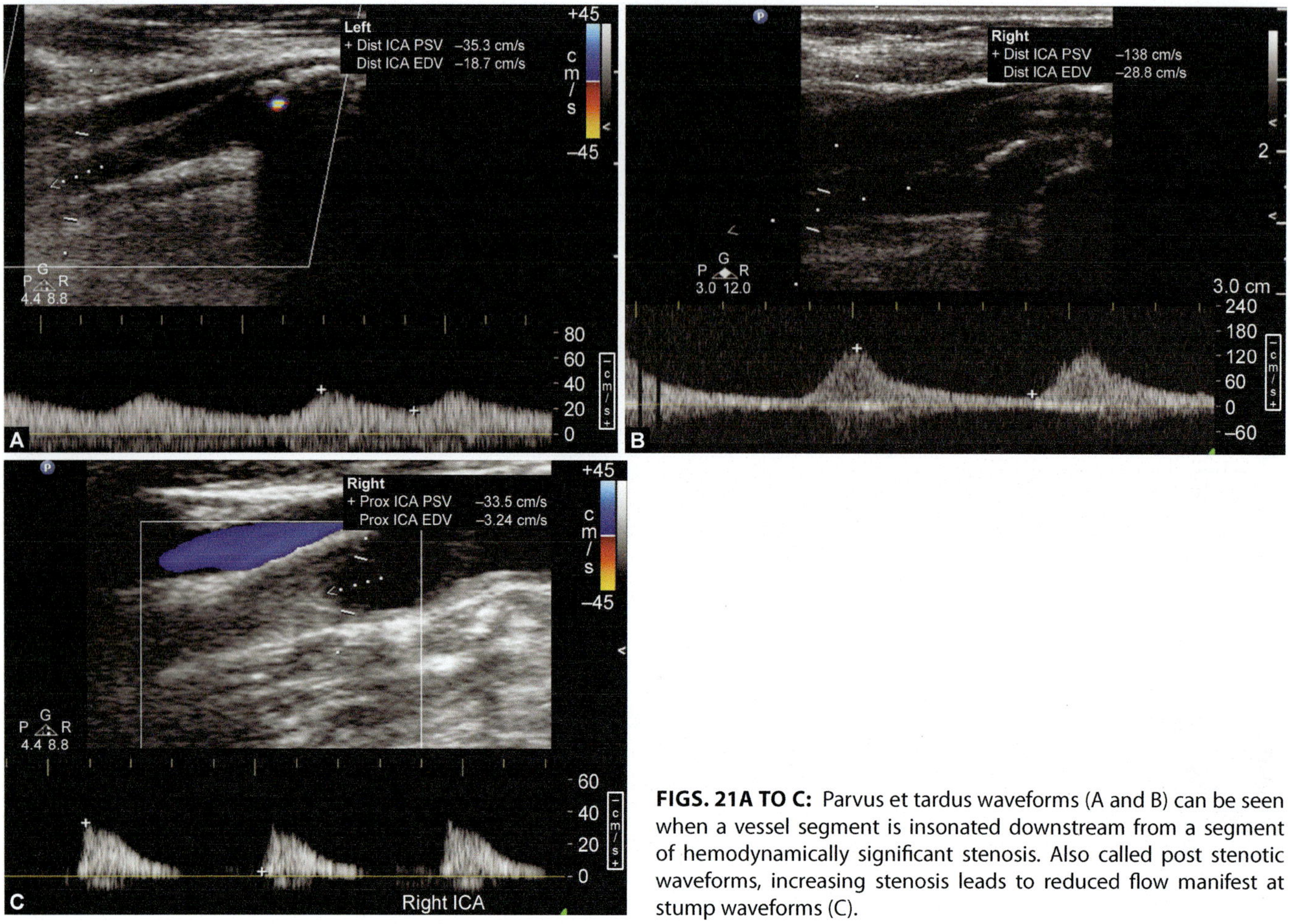

FIGS. 21A TO C: Parvus et tardus waveforms (A and B) can be seen when a vessel segment is insonated downstream from a segment of hemodynamically significant stenosis. Also called post stenotic waveforms, increasing stenosis leads to reduced flow manifest at stump waveforms (C).

DIAPHRAGM ULTRASOUND

Dysfunction of the diaphragm, the major muscle of inspiration, may lead to respiratory failure, prolonged mechanical ventilation, and potential failure to wean from mechanical ventilation. Multiple clinical conditions can affect diaphragm structure and function including major thoracoabdominal surgery, cervical spinal cord injury, critical illness polyneuropathy, direct phrenic nerve injury, polyradiculoneuritis as well as ventilator induced diaphragm dysfunction.[44] Paralysis of the diaphragm is often underdiagnosed due to its variable presentation. Clinical findings range from unexplained dyspnea, particularly when supine asymmetric breathing pattern, recurrent pneumonia, recurrent unilateral lung collapse to difficult ventilator weaning in patients intubated for unrelated causes.[45] Current mainstream evaluation of diaphragm muscle and movement is facilitated via chest X-rays, sniff test under fluoroscopy, spirometry, dynamic CT or MRIs or electromyography (EMG), and nerve conduction velocity.[46] The gold standard for the diagnosis of bilateral diaphragmatic paralysis remains measurement of transdiaphragmatic pressure (Pdi) using esophageal balloon catheters; this unfortunately has poor sensitivity, depends on patient cooperation, requires invasive catheters and remains ineffective for diagnosis of unilateral diaphragmatic paralysis. One functioning hemidiaphragm is generally sufficient to generate clinically adequate transdiaphragmatic pressure during quite breathing hence elevated hemidiaphragm on chest X-ray may or may not be accompanied with clinical symptoms. In fact, up to 6% of asymptomatic patients may have a dyskinetic diaphragm. Fluoroscopic examinations have a high false negative rate, while chest radiography has poor specificity for unilateral paralysis of the hemidiaphragm. Dynamic CT or MRI allows evaluation of the excursion, synchronicity, and velocity of diaphragmatic motion but is not easily applicable to the ICU patient who is intubated and mechanically ventilated.[44] Phrenic nerve conduction studies coupled with EMG can detect evidence of denervation and can be performed on full ventilator support, but it is uncomfortable for patients, technically challenging to perform and interpret, and does carry a risk of pneumothorax.[45] These diagnostic modalities are limited by the risks of ionizing radiation, transportation of critically ill patients to the radiology suite, or by the need for highly specialized equipment and training. Most of these modalities also focus only on the structure or function and fail to provide comprehensive evaluation of diaphragm muscle and tendon.

Technical Aspects

There are four anatomical components to the diaphragm—(1) the transverse septum, (2) pleuroperitoneal folds, (3) esophageal mesentery, and (4) the muscular body wall laterally. Evaluation of the diaphragm is performed from two locations.[47] The diaphragm tendon is evaluated in the mid-clavicular line below the right and left costal margins using the low-frequency probe. The right and left anterior axillary line to visualize the diaphragm muscle in the coronal plane **(Figs. 22 and 23)**.

Intercostal Approach

Using a high-frequency linear probe (>10 MHz), thickness of the diaphragm can be evaluated (Tdi, mm) in the zone of apposition of the diaphragm to the rib cage **(Figs. 22A to D)**. The zone of apposition is defined as the area of the chest wall where the abdominal contents reach the lower rib cage. Here the diaphragm is seen as a structure with three distinct layers—two echogenic layers of peritoneum and pleura sandwiching a more hypoechoic line of diaphragm muscle. The muscle is visualized in the coronal plane in the intercostal space usually along the mid axillary line **(Figs. 22A to D)**. The patient is scanned along the intercostal spaces in the long axis with probe pointed medially. The liver is used as an acoustic window to the right and the spleen provides an acoustic window on the left. Diaphragmatic thickness is measured during quiet spontaneous breathing and during maximal inspiratory and expiratory efforts. The sonographer must have complete visualization of both

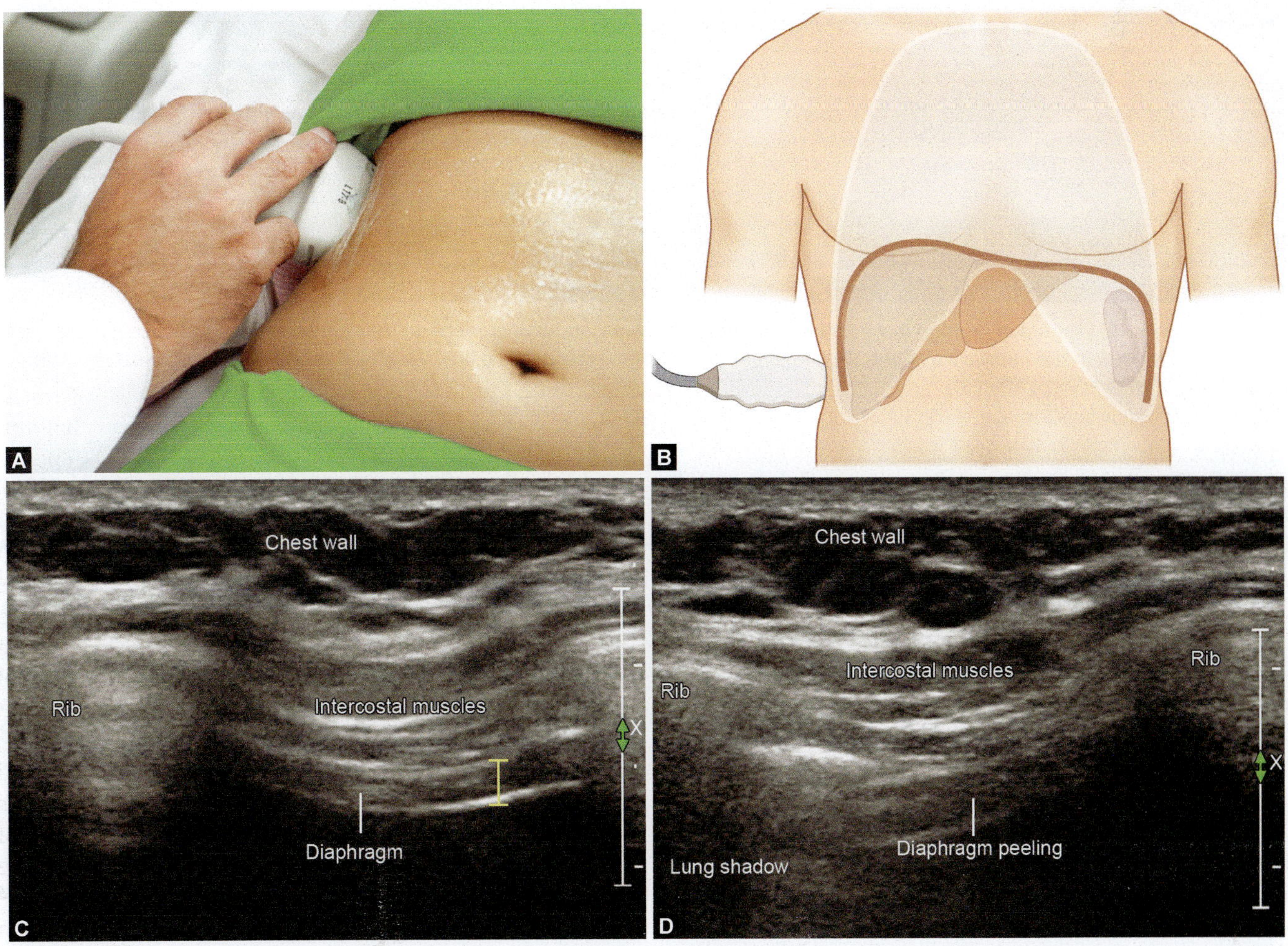

FIGS. 22A TO D: (A) Diaphragm muscle insonation using high frequency linear probe in the midaxillary line; (B) showing the diagram muscle in a coronal plane; (C) at the end of expiration; and (D) inspiration. Lung shadow in seen to cover the cranial portion as diaphragm thickens and moves caudally (right).

Source: With permission from Sarwal, et al (2013).[45]

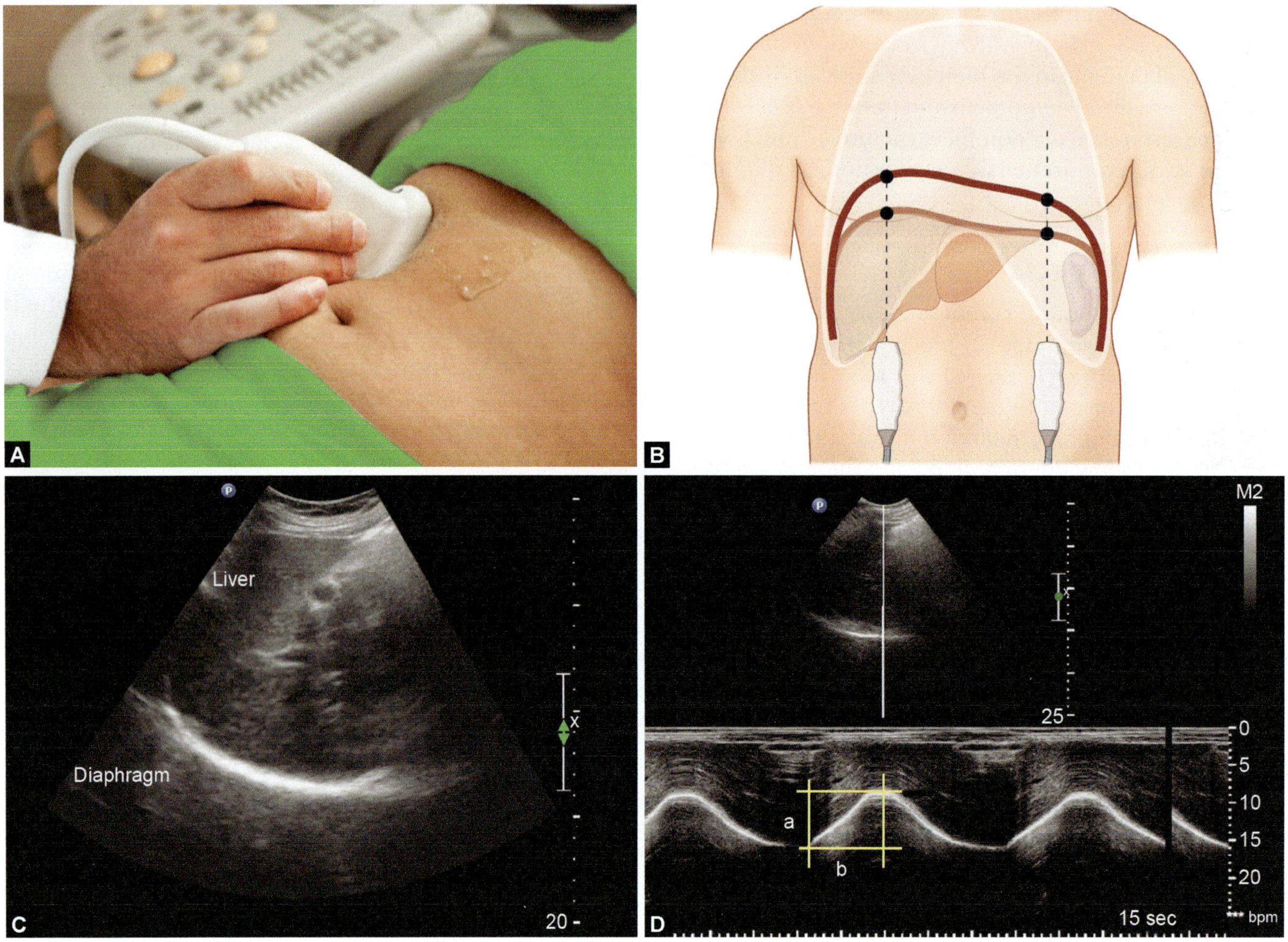

FIGS. 23A TO D: (A) Diaphragm tendon insonation using a low frequency abdominal probe to (B) insonate the cranial caudal movements of the central tendon in the midclavicular line. (C) The tendon is visualized through the liver (D) and M mode is used to assess excursion of the diaphragm (a) over inspiration (b).

Source: With permission from Sarwal, et al (2013).[45]

the pleural and peritoneal membranes at all times while imaging the diaphragm for thickness measurements. This allows reproducible images for quantitative analysis.[45] The thickening fraction (TF) can be calculated using M-mode (TF = thickness at end-inspiration thickness at end-expiration/thickness at end-expiration) **(Figs. 24A and B)**. The TF reflects the efficiency of the diaphragm as a pressure generator.[44] The presence of pleural effusions, atelectasis, or lung consolidation may enhance the ultrasound imaging of the diaphragm.

Subcostal Approach

The diaphragm tendon can be visualized using the low-frequency abdominal or echo probe placed in the subcostal space as a hyperechoic line distal to the spleen or liver moving cranial to caudal with respiration. The probe is directed medially, cephalad, and dorsally so the ultrasound beam perpendicularly intersects the posterior third of the corresponding hemidiaphragm.[44] 2D B-mode imaging is used initially to find the best imaging plane and M-mode is then used to show the motion of the diaphragm along the selected line. The M-mode cursor should always be as perpendicular as possible to the middle or posterior parts of the diaphragm.[44] M-mode ultrasound can display the peak convexity of the tendon dome on the Y-axis and tendon excursion can be seen as tendon moves with respiration. In a spontaneously breathing patient, normal inspiratory motion of the diaphragm is caudal as the diaphragm moves toward the probe while normal expiratory movement is cranial as the diaphragm moves away from the probe. Using M-mode, diaphragmatic excursion (displacement, cm), speed of diaphragmatic contraction (slope, cm/s), inspiratory time (Tinsp, s), and duration of the cycle (T tot, s) can be measured **(Figs. 24A and B)**. Evaluation of diaphragm tendon excursion can be paired with transmagnetic or needle phrenic nerve stimulation to assess response. Since ultrasound images the posterior and lateral parts of the diaphragm, the muscular crural components innervated by the phrenic

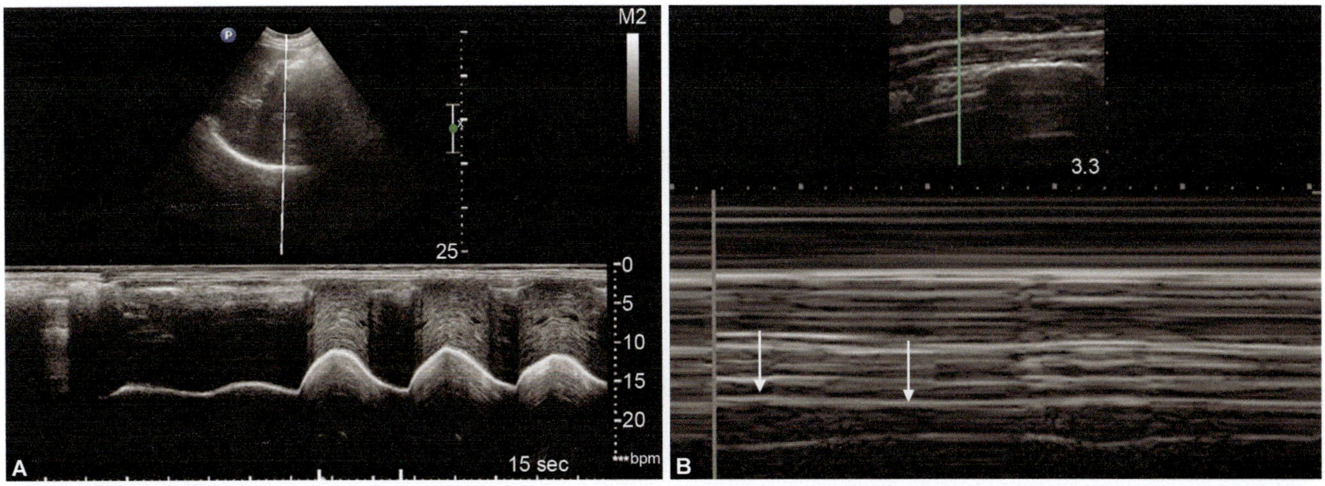

FIGS. 24A AND B: (A) M mode measurements of the diaphragm tendon excursion depend on the tidal volume with initial resting breaths followed by deep breaths. (B) Diaphragm muscle thickening can be demonstrated in M mode to yield thickening fraction with respiration.

nerve,[45] it shows higher correlation with diaphragm dysfunction than sniff test that assesses the anterior dome with less excursion.

Interpretations

Diaphragm Muscle Thickness

In normal individuals, there is a wide range of tdi at functional residual capacity (FRC) between 1.8 and 3 mm. As the lung expands from residual volume (RV) to total lung capacity (TLC) the tdi increases on average 54% (range 42–78%). The diaphragm also thickens during a maximal inspiratory pressure (Pi-max) maneuver at FRC. A normal thickening ratio is 2.6, measured by dividing the diaphragmatic thickness during Pi-max at FRC by the diaphragm thickness while relaxing at FRC. Studies have shown a high degree of intraobserver and interobserver reproducibility of these measurements.[44] Thickening of the diaphragm is only affected by active contraction, however, the thickness measurements during spontaneous ventilation may be influenced by lung volume. Above 50% of the vital capacity diaphragmatic thickening is more pronounced, and there is a large increase in thickness between relaxation and 10% of the inspiratory effort.[44] Extremely thin or atrophied diaphragm can be seen in denervated diaphragm as in phrenic nerve injury or amyotrophic lateral sclerosis **(Figs. 25A to C)**.

Diaphragm Tendon Excursion

Normal reference values for diaphragmatic excursion in healthy individuals are reported as 1.8 ± 0.3, 7.0 ± 0.6, and 2.9 ± 0.6 cm for males and 1.6 ± 0.3, 5.7 ± 1.0, and 2.6 ± 0.5 cm for females during quiet, deep breathing, and voluntary sniffing respectively. The slope or speed of diaphragmatic contraction during quite breathing has been measured at 1.3 ± 0.4 cm/s in healthy males and females.[44]

Evaluation of excursion should first be done qualitatively to assess, if the respective domes of the diaphragm are moving in the physiological direction with inspiration. Qualitative assessment and excursion measurements should be performed during spontaneous breaths. Any degree of assistance with positive pressure ventilation noninvasive or invasive can affect these assessments. For the diaphragmatic excursion measurement patients under assisted modes of ventilation, the clinician must keep in mind that the measured excursion will represent the sum of two forces working in the same direction. The force of the diaphragmatic contraction is one force, while the passive displacement of the diaphragm by the ventilator applied pressure represents the second force. There is no means to determine which part of the diaphragmatic displacement is passive versus active. Patients on mechanical ventilation can be assessed during their spontaneous breathing trial or changing to spontaneous modes to assess for excursion patterns and velocity. Placing the patient in the supine position or 30° head elevation is preferred due to less variability, and greater reproducibility of measurements. Diaphragm excursion is greater in the supine position for the same inspired tidal volume when compared to upright positioning, and the relationship between inspired volume and movement of the diaphragm has been demonstrated to correlate better in the supine position.[45]

Clinical translation of single cutoffs for quantitative diaphragm measurements is limited by significant variability in thickness of diaphragm muscle within the same intercostal space **(Figs. 26A and B)**, change in muscle thickness with generalized edema or anasarca, dependence of excursion amplitude on inspiratory volumes, and change in measures with body habitus. A standardized protocol highlighting image acquisition details with patients used as their own controls for serial measures can help obviate few of these limitations.

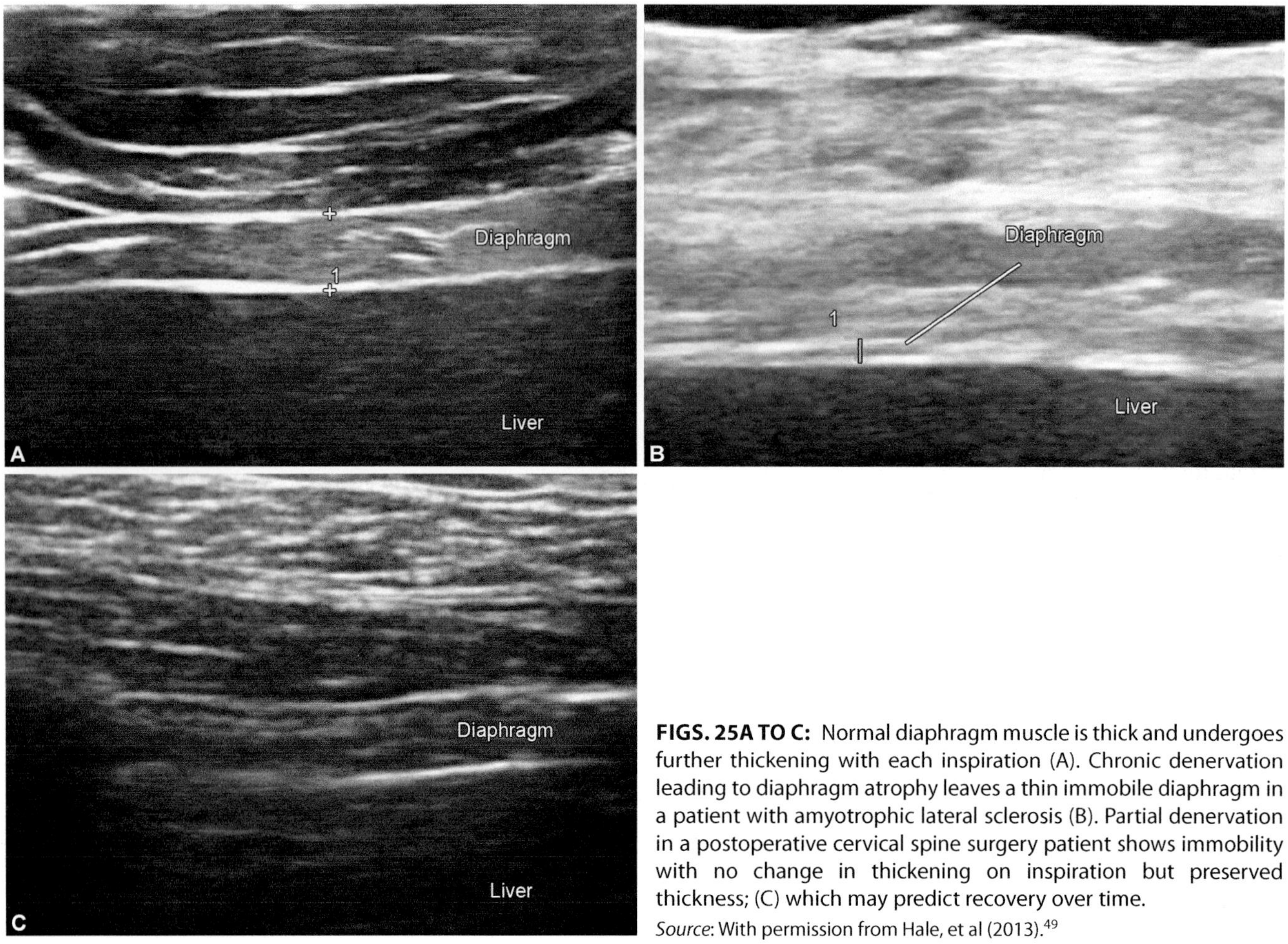

FIGS. 25A TO C: Normal diaphragm muscle is thick and undergoes further thickening with each inspiration (A). Chronic denervation leading to diaphragm atrophy leaves a thin immobile diaphragm in a patient with amyotrophic lateral sclerosis (B). Partial denervation in a postoperative cervical spine surgery patient shows immobility with no change in thickening on inspiration but preserved thickness; (C) which may predict recovery over time.

Source: With permission from Hale, et al (2013).[49]

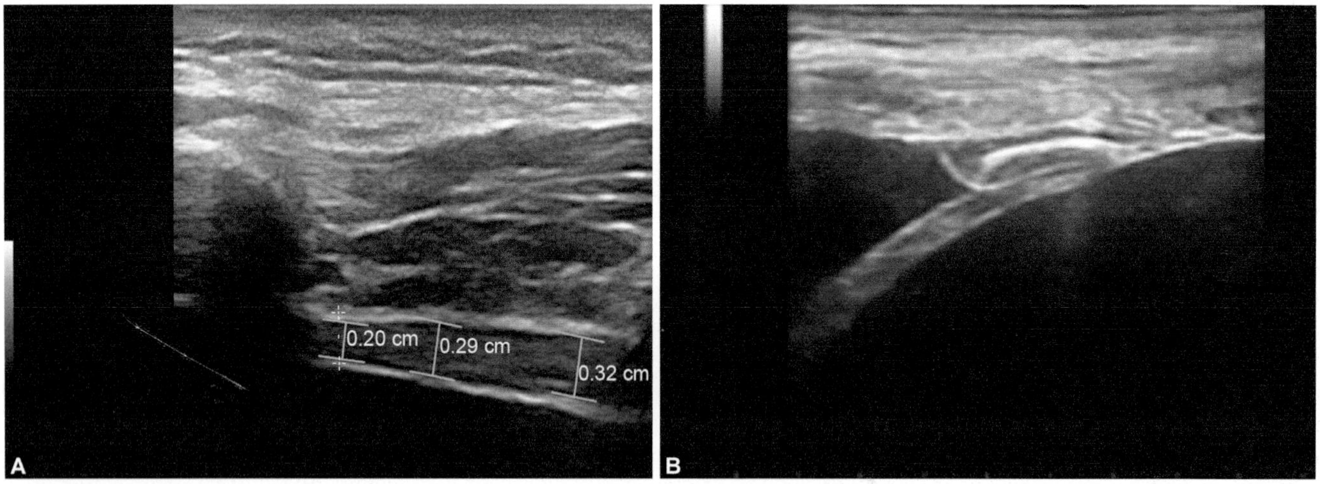

FIGS. 26A AND B: Diaphragm muscle has heterogeneous thickness (A) making single measures of thickness an imperfect measure. Hypertrophied diaphragm in a patient with emphysema may be in-effective in contributing to lung volumes with no lung excursions seen in costophrenic space (B).

Utility

Ultrasound can help in fast and accurate noninvasive bedside assessment of diaphragm movements to assess for paralysis and has the advantage that it does not depend on patient cooperation. Ultrasound-based diaphragm parameters can be measured with high reproducibility and reliability to follow serial examinations on patients with neuromuscular disease.[44,48] A combined approach to assess for diaphragm muscle thickness, changes in diaphragm thickness during inspiration, patterns of motion of central diaphragmatic tendon with respiration, and inspiratory amplitude of tendon excursion can allow rapid evaluation of patients suspected of diaphragmatic weakness and may provide insight into etiology of respiratory failure. Normal diaphragm muscle is thick and undergoes further thickening with each inspiration **(Figs. 24A and B)**. Chronic denervation leading to diaphragm atrophy leaves a thin immobile diaphragm in a patient with amyotrophic lateral sclerosis. Partial denervation, e.g., phrenic nerve injury in a postoperative cervical spine surgery patient may show immobility of the diaphragm with no change in thickening on inspiration but preserved thickness. Preservation of diaphragm thickness in an immobile diaphragm may mean early injury that has not manifest in atrophy yet or persistence preservation on serial testing may denote a partial injury with possibility of reinnervation that may predict recovery over time **(Figs. 25A to C)**.[49] Diaphragm ultrasound may also show structural abnormalities such as hypertrophied diaphragm in a patient with emphysema that may be in-effective in contributing to lung volumes with no lung excursions seen in costophrenic space **(Figs. 26A and B)**. Such visualization can help elucidate the natural history of respiratory failure in chronic obstructive pulmonary disease. Diaphragm muscle ultrasound visualization with B mode to guide needle placement can also facilitate safe needle EMG by preventing the complication of pneumothorax and lover hematoma.[50,51]

MEDIAN NERVE ULTRASOUND

Nerve and muscle pathologies can be easily identified with high-resolution ultrasound facilitating early diagnosis. Median nerve at the level of the carpal tunnel is the most common entrapment neuropathy that can be improved if a surgically amenable cause is found. Nerve ultrasound can be complementary test to electro diagnostic examinations in facilitating correct diagnosis or visualizing the cause of nerve entrapment. We describe the use of high-resolution ultrasound to visualize the median nerve in the carpal tunnel, to evaluate medial nerve entrapment neuropathy causing carpal tunnel syndrome (CTS).

Technical Aspects

A high-frequency (12–18 MHz) linear array transducer in musculoskeletal preset is used to evaluate the median nerve through its course in the forearm in two distinct planes, cross-sectional and sagittal. Knowledge of the relative anatomical positioning of the median nerve at different levels of the arm is key to the identification of the nerve. In addition, the surrounding anatomical structures to the median nerve should be assessed to determine if there are anatomical explanations for the entrapment such as cysts, tumors, or aberrant muscles.

To image the median nerve **(Figs. 27A to C)**, the patient can be either seated with palms upward and resting on a pillow or supine if they are unable to sit for several minutes. A cross-sectional view is obtained, with the transducer placed at the thenar crease of the wrist. Flexor retinaculum can be seen as a band-like structure across the wrist superficially and hyperechoic line of the lunate forms the most posterior boundary of the volar wrist. Nerve is visible as a honeycomb fascicular structure in the transverse axis medial to the flexor carpi radialis tendon that can be confirmed by asking patient to flex the wrist. The tendons of the wrist also appear as gray oval structures that show anisotropy, their appearance changes with direction of the probe. Nerve is distinguished from tendons since its appearance stays the same with changing direction of the probe relative to the skin and its constant position when finger or wrist movements occur. Once the nerve is visualized, the transducer is slowly moved proximally from the wrist to the mid-forearm keeping the median nerve within sight toward the middle of the ultrasound screen. At this proximal forearm location, the median nerve takes on a more triangular appearance and lies deep to the flexor digitorum superficialis muscles and superficial to the flexor digitorum profundus muscles. Next, the transducer is turned 90° and aligned with the third digit and the distal wrist crease to obtain a sagittal view. Median nerve here appears a straw-like fascicular structure lying on the top of the flexor tendons. Flexing the third and fourth finger can help differentiate between the moving tendon and the median nerve. Identification of the ulnar artery as hypoechoic pulsatile structures can be helpful in relative anatomy identification since median nerve runs along the medial aspect of this artery.

Interpretations

Median nerve compression at the wrist (CTS) typically causes nerve enlargement proximal to the carpal tunnel or flexor retinaculum. Measurements of the nerve cross-sectional area can be obtained by using the drawing tool to trace along the inner epineurial rim of the nerve **(Fig. 28)**. Angling the transducer so that it is perpendicular to the nerve will avoid overestimating the cross-sectional area. Maximum cross-sectional area with a cut-off of >12 mm^2 is sensitive for the diagnosis of CTS.[52] A wrist-to-forearm area ratio of cross-sectional area >1.4 is also sensitive and specific for the diagnosis of CTS.[53,54] The reference values used to define nerve cross-sectional area enlargement

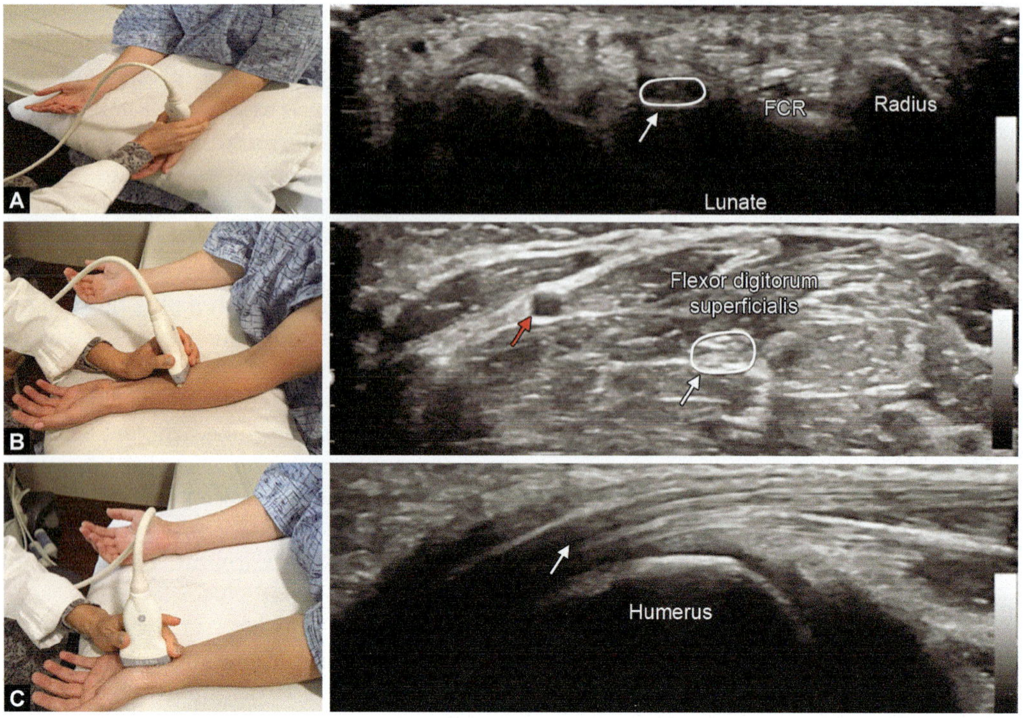

FIGS. 27A TO C: Insonation of the median nerve (white arrow) at the wrist (A) in the short axis using a high frequency linear probe. Median nerve is then traced proximally through the forearm (B) where it can be seen deep to the flexor digitorum superficialis. Sagittal view of the median nerve at the wrist (C) and medial to the ulnar artery (red arrow).

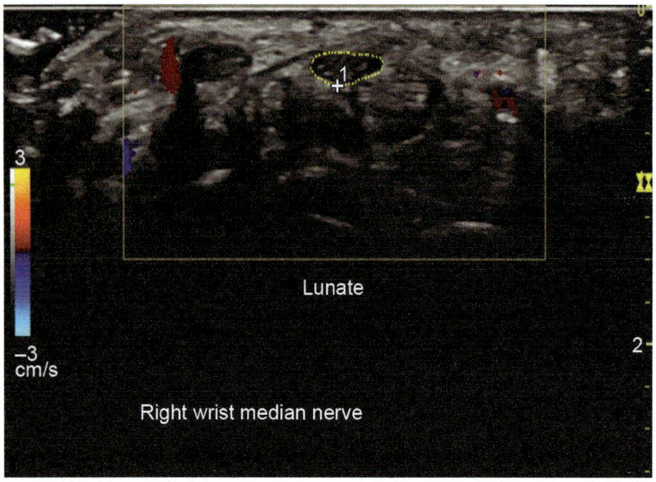

FIG. 28: Cross-section area of median nerve at the level of the wrist outlined to measure the surface area.

include—(1) an area >2 standard deviations above the mean reference value and (2) an area 1.5 times or greater than an unaffected portion of the same nerve.[1] In CTS, enlargement of the median nerve cross-sectional area at the distal wrist crease is an accurate parameter for diagnosis. The proposed mechanism for enlargement is an inflammatory and/or vascular process that contributes to nerve enlargement, as corticosteroids injected near an enlarged nerve can reverse some degree of enlargement within a week of injection.[55]

Other changes seen are in entrapment neuropathies include nerve echogenicity, nerve shape, fascicle size, and vascularity.[52] Hypoechogenicity of the median nerve is less well characterized although often seen in CTS. Dynamic testing to look for decreased nerve mobility in carpal tunnel is also emerging as a possible diagnostic modality in CTS with dynamic testing. There are also reports of increased nerve vascularity as detected with Doppler ultrasound in CTS.[56]

Utility

Neuromuscular ultrasound has revolutionized the evaluation of CTS.[57] Ultrasound can be helpful is visualizing some anomalies that may be associated with CTS. About 10–15% of all individuals assessed with neuromuscular ultrasound have bifid median nerves at the wrist, and 5–10% have persistent median arteries running through the carpal tunnel.[58] Bifid median nerves and persistent median arteries are not more common in CTS, but they are important to identify especially when considering a perineural injection. Anatomic abnormalities that may contribute to CTS include traumatic neuromas, schwannomas, lipofibromatous hamartomas, ganglion cysts, thrombosed persistent median arteries, abscesses, and compressive gouty tophus.[59,60] These structures can be visualized with neuromuscular ultrasound and change clinical management. Ultrasound is also very helpful in therapeutic management of CTS by providing visual guidance for steroids injections.

CONCLUSION

Ultrasound in neurology is a rapidly expanding field and with advancement of technology, it is bound to be an invaluable tool for any neurologist. This is especially true in low resource settings with limited access to advanced neuroimaging. The noninvasive, radiation free, bedside tool that can facilitate repeated examination can allow an ultrasound to be the neurologist's stethoscope.

REFERENCES

1. Brown RE. A standardized procedure for echoencephalography and for analyzing echoencephalograms. Can Med Assoc J. 1967; 96(20):1349-54.
2. Robba C, Goffi A, Geeraerts T, Cardim D, Via G, Czosnyka M, et al. Brain ultrasonography: methodology, basic and advanced principles and clinical applications. A narrative review. Intensive Care Med. 2019;45(7):913-27.
3. Aaslid RLT, Lindegarrd KF. Estimation of cerebral perfusion pressure from arterial blood pressure and transcranial Doppler recordings. Intracranial Pressure VI. 1986:226-9.
4. Alexandrov AV, Sloan MA, Wong LK, Douville C, Razumovsky AY, Koroshetz WJ, et al. Practice standards for transcranial Doppler ultrasound: part I–test performance. J Neuroimaging. 2007;17(1): 11-8.
5. Robba C, Citerio G. Echography and Doppler of the Brain. India: Springer; 2020.
6. Sarwal A. Neurocritical Care Ultrasound. Comprehensive Critical Care Ultrasound, 2nd edition. India: Society of Critical Care Medicine; 2020.
7. Marinoni M, Ginanneschi A, Forleo P, Amaducci L. Technical limits in transcranial Doppler recording: inadequate acoustic windows. Ultrasound Med Biol. 1997;23(8):1275-7.
8. Alexandrov AV, Sloan MA, Tegeler CH, Newell DN, Lumsden A, Garami Z, et al. Practice Standards for Transcranial Doppler (TCD) Ultrasound. Part II. Clinical Indications and Expected Outcomes. J Neuroimaging. 2012;22(3):215-24.
9. Gyanendra K, Reza Bavarsad S, Mark RH. Vasospasm on transcranial Doppler is predictive of delayed cerebral ischemia in aneurysmal subarachnoid hemorrhage: a systematic review and meta-analysis. J Neurosurg. 2016;124(5):1257-64.
10. Cardim D, Robba C, Bohdanowicz M, Donnelly J, Cabella B, Liu X, et al. Non-invasive Monitoring of Intracranial Pressure Using Transcranial Doppler Ultrasonography: Is It Possible? Neurocrit Care. 2016;25(3):473-91.
11. Bellner J RB, Reinstrup P, Kristiansson KA, Rydig E, Brandt L. Transcranial sonography pulsatility index (PI) reflects intracranial pressure (ICP). Surg Neurol. 2004;62(1):45-51.
12. de Riva N, Budohoski KP, Smielewski P, Kasprowicz M, Zweifel C, Steiner LA, et al. Transcranial Doppler Pulsatility Index: What it is and What it Isn't. Neurocrit Care. 2012;17(1):58-66.
13. Rasulo FA, Calza S, Robba C, Taccone FS, Biasucci DG, Badenes R, et al. Transcranial Doppler as a screening test to exclude intracranial hypertension in brain-injured patients: the IMPRESSIT-2 prospective multicenter international study. Crit Care (London, England). 2022;26(1):110.
14. Greer DM, Shemie SD, Lewis A, Torrance S, Varelas P, Goldenberg FD, et al. Determination of Brain Death/death by neurologic criteria: The World Brain Death Project. JAMA. 2020;324(11): 1078-97.
15. Ducrocq XBM, Debouverie M, Junges C, Hummer M, Vespignani H. Brain death and transcrannial Doppler: experience in 130 cases of brain dead patients. J Neurolog Sci. 1998;160(1):41-6.
16. Ducrocq X, Hassler W, Moritake K, Newell DW, von Reutern GM, Shiogai T, et al. Consensus opinion on diagnosis of cerebral circulatory arrest using Doppler-sonography: Task Force Group on cerebral death of the Neurosonology Research Group of the World Federation of Neurology. J Neurol Sci. 1998;159(2):145-50.
17. Chang JJ, Tsivgoulis G, Katsanos AH, Malkoff MD, Alexandrov AV. Diagnostic Accuracy of transcranial Doppler for brain death confirmation: Systematic review and meta-analysis. Am J Neuroradiol. 2016;37(3):408-14.
18. Brunser AM, Mansilla E, Hoppe A, Olavarría V, Sujima E, Lavados PM. The Role of TCD in the Evaluation of Acute Stroke. J Neuroimaging. 2016;26(4):420-5.
19. Gomez JR, Hobbs KS, Johnson LL, Vu QD, Bennett J, Tegeler C, et al. The clinical contribution of neurovascular ultrasonography in acute ischemic stroke. J Neuroimaging. 2020;30(6):867-74.
20. Huang G, Johnson LL, Peacock JE Jr, Tegeler C, Davis K, Sarwal A. Transcranial Doppler Emboli monitoring for infective endocarditis. J Neuroimaging. 2020;30(4):486-92.
21. Gomez J, Wolfe S, Sarwal A. Sonographic demonstration of a perfusion-dependent stroke with negative MRI and a flow-limiting stenosis. Neurocritical Care. 2020;32(3):883-8.
22. Ringelstein EB, Sievers C, Ecker S, Schneider PA, Otis SM. Noninvasive assessment of CO_2-induced cerebral vasomotor response in normal individuals and patients with internal carotid artery occlusions. Stroke. 1988;19(8):963-9.
23. Kliewer MA, Hertzberg BS, Kim DH, Bowie JD, Courneya DL, Carroll BA. Vertebral artery Doppler waveform changes indicating subclavian steal physiology. Am J Roentgenol. 2000;174(3):815-9.
24. Kapoor S, Offnick A, Allen B, Brown PA, Sachs JR, Gurcan MN, et al. Brain topography on adult ultrasound images: Techniques, interpretation, and image library. J Neuroimaging. 2022;32(6): 1013-26.
25. Robba C, Wong A, Poole D, Tayar AA, Arntfield RT, Chew MS, et al. Basic ultrasound head-to-toe skills for intensivists in the general and neuro intensive care unit population: Consensus and expert recommendations of the European Society of Intensive Care Medicine. Intensive Care Med. 2021;47(12):1347-67.
26. Tang SC, Huang SJ, Jeng JS, Yip PK. Third ventricle midline shift due to spontaneous supratentorial intracerebral hemorrhage evaluated by transcranial color-coded sonography. J Ultrasound Med. 2006;25(2):203-9.
27. Seidel GGT, Kaps M, Missler U. Dislocation of the third ventricle due to space-occupying stroke evaluated by transcranial duplex sonography. J Neuroimaging. 1996;6(4):227-30.
28. Ovesen C, Christensen AF, Krieger DW, Rosenbaum S, Havsteen I, Christensen H. Time course of early postadmission hematoma expansion in spontaneous intracerebral hemorrhage. Stroke. 2014;45(4):994-9.
29. Stolz E, Gerriets T, Fiss I, Babacan SS, Seidel G, Kaps M. Comparison of transcranial color-coded duplex sonography and cranial CT measurements for determining third ventricle midline shift in space-occupying stroke. Am J Neuroradiol. 1999;20(8):1567-71.
30. Caricato A, Ioannoni E, Gelormini C. Is It Really Third Ventricle? A Pitfall in the Diagnosis of Hydrocephalus by Brain Ultrasound. Neurocritical Care. 2020;33(3):844-6.
31. Sarwal A, Elder NM. Point-of-care Cranial Ultrasound in a Hemicraniectomy Patient. Clin Pract Cases Emerg Med. 2018;2(4): 375-7.

32. Kiphuth IC HH, Struffert T, Schwab S, Kohrmann M. Sonographic monitoring of ventricle enlargement in posthemorrhagic hydrocephalus. Neurology. 2011;76(10): 858-62.
33. Mohson KI, Auday N. Role of orbital ultrasound in the assessment of clinically detected papilledema. J Med Ultrasound. 2019;27(3): 135-40.
34. Farina F, Vosko MR, Baracchini C, Ermani M, Sommer P, Greisenegger S, et al. Ultrasound Examination of the Pupil: A New Tool for the Neuro-Ophthalmological Assessment. Ultraschall Med. 2021;42(1):84-91.
35. Bhosale A, Shah VM, Shah PK. Accuracy of crescent sign on ocular ultrasound in diagnosing papilledema. World J Methodol. 2017;7(3):108-11.
36. Koziarz A, Sne N, Kegel F, Nath S, Badhiwala JH, Nassiri F, et al. Bedside optic nerve ultrasonography for diagnosing increased intracranial pressure: A systematic review and meta-analysis. Ann Intern Med. 2019;171(12):896-905.
37. Wang J, Li K, Li H, Ji C, Wu Z, Chen H, et al. Ultrasonographic optic nerve sheath diameter correlation with ICP and accuracy as a tool for noninvasive surrogate ICP measurement in patients with decompressive craniotomy. J Neurosurg. 2020;133(2):514-20.
38. Helmke KH, Hansen HC. Fundamentals of transorbital sonographic evaluation of optic nerve sheath expansion under intracranial hypertension II. Pediatr Radiol. 1996;26(10):706-10.
39. Lahham S, Shniter I, Thompson M, Le D, Chadha T, Mailhot T, et al. Point-of-Care ultrasonography in the diagnosis of retinal detachment, vitreous hemorrhage, and vitreous detachment in the emergency department. JAMA Network Open. 2019;2(4): e192162.
40. AbuRahma AF, Avgerinos ED, Chang RW, Clement Darling 3rd R, Duncan AA, Forbes TL, et al. The Society for Vascular Surgery implementation document for management of extracranial cerebrovascular disease. J Vasc Surg. 2022;75(1s):26s-98s.
41. Beach KW, Bergelin RO, Leotta DF, Primozich JF, Sevareid PM, Stutzman ET, et al. Standardized ultrasound evaluation of carotid stenosis for clinical trials: University of Washington Ultrasound Reading Center. Cardiovasc Ultrasound. 2010;8:39.
42. Grant EG, Benson CB, Moneta GL, Alexandrov AV, Baker JD, Bluth EI, et al. Carotid artery stenosis: gray-scale and Doppler US diagnosis–Society of Radiologists in Ultrasound Consensus Conference. Radiology. 2003;229(2):340-6.
43. Reutern G-Mv, Goertler MW, Bornstein NM, Sette MD, Evans DH, Hetzel A, et al. Grading carotid stenosis using ultrasonic methods. Stroke. 2012;43(3):916-21.
44. Matamis D, Soilemezi E, Tsagourias M, Akoumianaki E, Dimassi S, Boroli F, et al. Sonographic evaluation of the diaphragm in critically ill patients. Technique and clinical applications. Intensive Care Med. 2013;39(5):801-10.
45. Sarwal A, Walker FO, Cartwright MS. Neuromuscular ultrasound for evaluation of the diaphragm. Muscle Nerve. 2013;47(3):319-29.
46. ATS/ERS Statement on respiratory muscle testing. Am J Respir Crit Care Med. 2002;166(4):518-624.
47. Sarwal A, Serfas JD, Mitchell E, Mitchell E, Buj-Bello A, Beggs AH, et al. Neuromuscular ultrasound for diaphragm assessment following gene replacement therapy in a canine model of X-Linked myotubular myopathy (XLMTM) (P05.083). Neurology. 2013;80:P05-083.
48. Parry S, Sarwal A, Cartwright M, Morris P, Denehy L. Reliability of quantitative muscle ultrasound analysis in the critically ill population. Critical Care Med. 2013;1:A108.
49. Hale J, Dowlen H, Cartwright M, Sarwal A. Neuromuscular Ultrasound for Evaluation of the Normal and Abnormal Diaphragm (P05.084). Neurology. 2013;80:P05-084.
50. Sarwal A, Serfas JD, Mitchell E, Cartwright M, Beggs A, Buj-Bello A, et al. A novel method for targeting intramuscular diaphragm injections using ultrasound and electromyography (P02.220). Neurology. 2013;80:P02-220.
51. Sarwal A, Cartwright MS, Mitchell E, Williams K, Walker FO, Childers MK. Guiding intramuscular diaphragm injections using real-time ultrasound and electromyography. Muscle Nerve. 2015;51(2): 287-9.
52. Nulle K, Jaudzema A. Ultrasonographic evaluation of the median nerve: normal and variant anatomy and appearance. J Ultrasound. 2021;21(87):e318-25.
53. Hobson-Webb LD, Massey JM, Juel VC, Sanders DB. The ultrasonographic wrist-to-forearm median nerve area ratio in carpal tunnel syndrome. Clin Neurophysiol. 2008;119(6):1353-7.
54. Wiesler ER, Chloros GD, Cartwright MS, Smith BP, Rushing J, Walker FO. The use of diagnostic ultrasound in carpal tunnel syndrome. J Hand Surg Am. 2006;31(5):726-32.
55. Cartwright MS, White DL, Demar S, Wiesler ER, Sarlikiotis T, Chloros GD, et al. Median nerve changes following steroid injection for carpal tunnel syndrome. Muscle Nerve. 2011;44(1):25-9.
56. Mallouhi A, Pülzl P, Trieb T, Piza H, Bodner G. Predictors of carpal tunnel syndrome: accuracy of gray-scale and color Doppler sonography. Am J Roentgenol. 2006;186(5):1240-5.
57. Cartwright MS, Hobson-Webb LD, Boon AJ, Alter KE, Hunt CH, Flores VH, et al. Evidence-based guideline: Neuromuscular ultrasound for the diagnosis of carpal tunnel syndrome. Muscle Nerve. 2012;46(2):287-93.
58. Padua L, Liotta G, Di Pasquale A, Granata G, Pazzaglia C, Caliandro P, et al. Contribution of ultrasound in the assessment of nerve diseases. Eur J Neurol. 2012;19(1):47-54.
59. Shekhani HN, Hanna T, Johnson JO. Lipofibromatous Hamartoma of the Median Nerve: A Case Report. J Radiol Case Rep. 2016; 10(11):1-7.
60. Therimadasamy A, Peng YP, Putti TC, Wilder-Smith EP. Carpal tunnel syndrome caused by gouty tophus of the flexor tendons of the fingers: sonographic features. J Clin Ultrasound. 2011;39(8): 463-5.

120

CHAPTER

Cerebrospinal Fluid

Heli Shah, Varsha A Patil

INTRODUCTION

Cerebrospinal fluid (CSF) examination has been an integral and important part of the evaluation of various neurological disorders. The earliest mention of CSF comes from the seventeenth century BC in the Edwin Smith Surgical Papyrus.[1] Centuries later, in 1825, Magendie described the "CSF" and its pathways comprising of the intercommunicating ventricles and the subarachnoid spaces around the brain and the spinal cord.[2] The popular concept of the "Monro-Kellie doctrine" that "the blood, brain, and CSF volumes can change reciprocally", was reported by Burton (1846), much later after Monro (1783) and Kellie (1824) had hypothesized that the contents of the cranium have a nearly fixed volume. Later, the CSF anatomic pathways were described in detail by Weed (1935).[2] The credit for a first successful lumbar puncture (LP) goes to Heinrich Quincke, who further described the technique using a percutaneous needle with a stylet, manometry, and the biochemical parameters of CSF evaluation.[3]

Traditionally, the most common indication for an LP is to evaluate a central nervous system (CNS) infection or to measure the CSF opening pressure. The utility of LP has further expanded to diagnosing subarachnoid hemorrhage (SAH), CNS inflammatory disorders, meningitis, neoplastic lesions, neurodegenerative disorders like dementia, and therapeutically for the administration of certain drugs (chemotherapeutics, antibiotics, analgesics, antisense oligonucleotides, and enzyme replacement therapies) intrathecally.

CEREBROSPINAL FLUID (COMPOSITION, PATHWAY OF CIRCULATION AND ABSORPTION)

Cerebrospinal fluid is a clear and colorless fluid, which is an ultrafiltrate of blood, secreted by the choroid plexus.[4] The choroid plexus consists of projections of vessels and pia mater that protrude into the ventricular cavities as villi containing capillaries in the loose connective stroma. A specialized layer of ependymal cells known as choroidal epithelium overlies these villi.[5] The major site of production of CSF is by the choroid plexus in the ventricles, the remainder is produced by the interstitium and the meninges. CSF formation is an active secretory process, as the blood passes through the large fenestrated capillaries of the choroid plexus.[4]

The CSF formation rate in healthy adults is around 0.3–0.4 mL/min (around 450–550 mL/day).[4] The rate of CSF formation in children is lower than in adults and depends on the height and weight of the child. The rate of CSF formation in newborns is further low, around 25 mL/day. The total CSF volume space in an adult is about 90–150 mL, the volume of spinal CSF space being 30 mL.[6,7] The CSF is actively reabsorbed so that the complete CSF volume gets replaced three to four times a day.[2]

The CSF is produced by the choroid plexi in the lateral ventricles, passes through the foramina of Monro into the third ventricle and then through the aqueduct of Sylvius into the fourth ventricle **(Fig. 1)**.[2,8] From the fourth ventricles, it further exits through the lateral foramina of Luschka to the prepontine cistern and cerebellopontine angles. The alternate route is via the foramen of Magendie centrally to the cisterna magna and flows upward over the cerebellar hemispheres or downward into the spinal subarachnoid spaces, brainstem, and then into the basal cisterns (including the interpeduncular cistern). Around the spinal cord, the flow is predominantly downward posteriorly and upward in the anterior compartment. Finally, the fluid reaches the basal cisterns and then flows upward over the brain convexity. The circulation of CSF is a complex process, contrary to the prior belief of bulk (unidirectional flow). There appears to be a combination of directed bulk flow, pulsatile to-and-fro movement, and continuous bi-directional fluid exchange at the blood-brain barrier

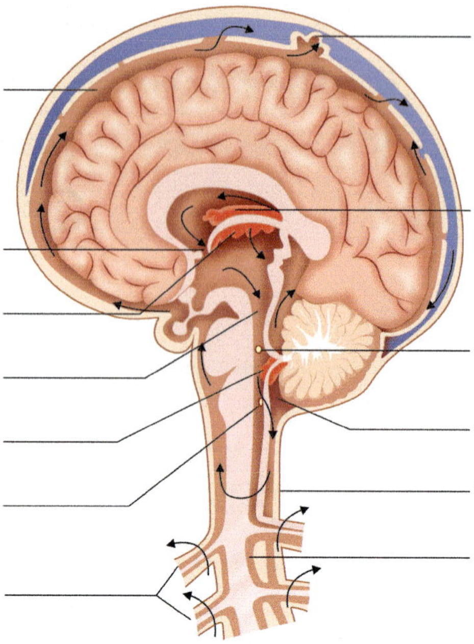

FIG. 1: Cerebrospinal fluid (CSF) pathway- production, circulation and absorption (Arrows indicate the direction of CSF circulation).
Source: Adapted from Tille PM. Bailey & Scott's Diagnostic Microbiology. St Louis: Elsevier; 2013.

(BBB) and the cell membranes at the borders between CSF and interstitial fluid (ISF).[4]

The CSF is absorbed across the arachnoid villi and granulations (arachnoid membrane invaginations through the dural lining of the sinuses that are concentrated near the sagittal sinus). Absorption across the arachnoid villi occurs by vesicular transport. The villi act as a one-way pressure valve that opens above a threshold pressure, usually 20–50 mm of water. The remainder of CSF gets reabsorbed via the peripheral lymphatic vessels (10–15%) of the nasal mucosa and neck along the perineural spaces surrounding cranial nerves.[9,10]

The extracellular space surrounding the brain is separated from the circulating blood by the BBB, which comprises the brain capillary endothelial cells, the basal lamina, pericytes, the perivascular layer of astrocytic end-feet, interacting microglial cells, and neurons. The BBB has a large surface area (12–18 m^2) in adults.[11] The exchange of ions across the barrier occurs through passive diffusion (small molecules and lipophilic substances) or facilitated transport (glucose and amino acids). Immune cells may invade the barrier at times.[4]

FUNCTIONS OF CEREBROSPINAL FLUID

Cerebrospinal fluid provides buoyancy to support the weight of the brain and acts as a protective layer to cushion it from injury. It serves regulatory functions like the distribution of neurotrophic factors and stabilization of brain pH and chemical gradients.[12] The direct transfer of brain metabolites into the CSF provides excretory function. An essential function of CSF is the provision and maintenance of an appropriate chemical environment for neural tissue.

Cerebrospinal fluid protects the brain from changes in arterial and central venous pressure associated with posture, respiration, and exertion.

Technical Aspects

The various indications and contraindications for LP are listed in **Boxes 1 and 2**.

Many institutes follow a protocol for withholding anticoagulants prior to LP [low-molecular-weight heparin (LMWH) for 24 hours and unfractionated heparin (UH) for 4 hours] and restarting several hours afterward (4–6 hours for UH and 6–9 hours for LMWH), with a low risk of complications reported.[13]

There is a considerable fear that LP in patients with a CSF obstruction can disturb the pressure across the area of obstruction and contribute to cerebral herniation or spinal cord compression **(Box 2)**.

Neuroimaging, usually with cranial computed tomography (CT) or magnetic resonance imaging (MRI), is often performed before LP, especially in patients with suspected meningitis. Patients are considered to be at an increased risk for cerebral herniation if neuroimaging reveals a focal mass lesion or signs of impending herniation, such as severe cerebral edema with obliteration of the fourth ventricle or basal cisterns. Clinical guidelines have recommended that children with suspected meningitis who have a history of immunodeficiency, CNS disease, or congenital heart disease, or who present with seizures, papilledema, abnormal level of consciousness, or a focal

BOX 1 Indications for lumbar puncture.

Diagnostic
- Suspected CNS infections
- Subarachnoid hemorrhage with negative CT scan
- Carcinomatous meningitis
- CNS vasculitis
- Primary CNS demyelinating disorders: MS, NMOSD, MOGAD, neurosarcoidosis
- Acute and chronic inflammatory demyelinating polyneuropathy
- Injection of contrast media for myelography or cisternography

Therapeutic:
- Idiopathic intracranial hypertension
- Cryptococcal meningitis in HIV infection
- Normal pressure hydrocephalus
- Spinal anesthesia
- Delivery of intrathecal drugs like chemotherapeutics, antibiotics, nusinersen (an antisense oligonucleotide in spinal muscular atrophy)

(CNS: central nervous system; CT: computed tomography; HIV: human immunodeficiency virus; MOGAD: myelin oligodendrocyte glycoprotein-associated disease; MS: multiple sclerosis; NMOSD: neuromyelitis optica spectrum disorder)

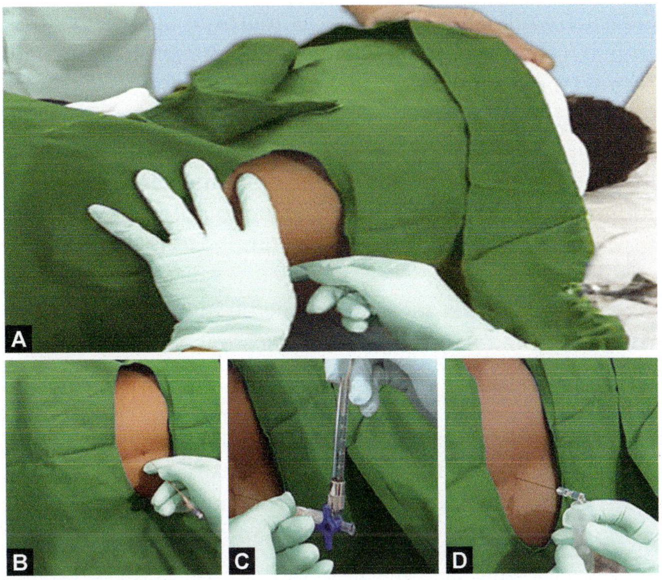

FIGS. 2A TO D: Clinical photograph depicting the technique of lumbar puncture. (A) Position for lumbar puncture. (B) Technique of inserting the needle (to be inserted in the L3–L4 intervertebral space). (C) CSF manometry. (D) Collection of CSF in a tube.

(CSF: cerebrospinal fluid)

BOX 2 Contraindications of lumbar puncture.

Relative contraindication:
- Platelet counts of 20,000–40,000/mm^3

Absolute contraindication:
- Uncorrected bleeding diathesis including platelet counts <20,000/mm^3
- Noncommunicating obstructive hydrocephalus
- Possible raised intracranial pressure with risk of cerebral herniation due to cerebral edema or space-occupying lesion
- Spinal epidural abscess
- Spinal cord compression above the level of puncture

neurologic abnormality, should undergo neuroimaging before LP.[14]

Technique

Lumbar puncture is a simple bedside procedure, which if performed correctly (in indicated patients), has minimal complications. A successful procedure depends on two factors—the positioning of the patient (which largely depends on the assistant who gives position to the patient, especially in young children) and the level of relaxation of the patient, rather than the expertise of the person performing the test.[2] Patients with spine deformity may require prior imaging of the spine additionally. Local analgesia, with or without anxiolytics may be necessary in older children and adults. Deep sedation may be needed in younger children.

The position for LP is usually lateral decubitus or sitting (the former being the preferred position for manometry) **(Fig. 2)**. The conus medullaris ends at L1-L2 interspace. Hence, in a patient with a normal spinal curvature, the interspace below L3 is considered safe for an LP.[15] The L3-L4 interspace can be found at the level of the superior iliac crests, in a patient lying in a lateral recumbent position **(Fig. 2B)**. If the patient is instructed to flex the neck and hips, this interspace becomes more prominent. After carefully palpating and locating the space, it can be marked prior to the preparation of the local area. The physician performing the test should be comfortable and the patient should be placed with their back near the edge and at a proper height above the ground **(Figs. 2A and B)**. Prior to the procedure, the patient's skin should be prepared using a microbiocidal agent (10% solution of povidone-iodine), allowed to dry then wiped clean with sterile towels. A local anesthetic (1% solution of lidocaine) may be injected or alternatively a topical analgesic cream (5% emulsion of lidocaine and prilocaine) may be applied 20–30 minutes prior to the procedure.[2,16]

The various types of spinal needles available are: Quincke (commonly used), Whitacre, and Sprotte needles **(Fig. 3)**. The most commonly used needles are 2.5 or 5 cm long, 20- or 22-gauge Quincke needles. These have a sharply beveled tip and a stylet **(Fig. 3)**. The beveled tip should be turned to face the patient so that the cutting-edge pushes in between and does not tear the dura. Whitacre and Sprotte needles are more flexible needles with dull tips and require an introducer. These needles have a lesser propensity to cause spinal dural tears.[17,18]

After local anesthesia is given, the spinal needle is gently and gradually advanced. As the ligamentum flava and dura are pierced, a popping sensation can be felt. Once inside the subarachnoid space, the stylet is removed and clear fluid drains in the needle. The needle position may be adjusted (rotated for a quarter) if no fluid is seen till the needle hub. Sometimes, if this maneuver does not yield fluid, the needle may not have reached the subarachnoid space. Hence, an attempt may be made to further advance the needle by a few millimeters. If both these maneuvers do not yield CSF, the needle may need to be withdrawn and a second puncture may be needed.

Once the CSF is seen in the needle hub, a manometer may be applied with an intervening stopcock **(Fig. 2C)**. It is essential that the patient is relaxed while the pressure is measured. The rise of CSF in the manometer is recorded. If the CSF flow is slow, slight pressure may be applied to the patient's abdomen. If there is truly a slow flow or obstruction, and the assembly is well placed, there should be rapid rise and fall correlating with application and release of abdominal pressure, respectively. The Queckenstedt test was earlier used for identifying CSF obstruction. It involved the application of pressure on the jugulars and is somewhat obsolete now.[19]

The normal opening pressure in adults and older children is between 120 and 200 mm H_2O. In an obese individual, a pressure as high as 250 mm H_2O may be considered normal.[2] Moderate to deep anesthesia may cause the pressure to be additionally higher by 35 mm H_2O.[2] After the opening pressure is recorded, CSF should be collected for analysis. At least 5 mL of CSF should be collected. The initial three tubes of 1–2 mL are sufficient for routine studies including microbiology (Gram-stain and bacterial culture) and biochemistry (cell count and differential, glucose, and protein concentrations). When the first tubes are grossly bloody or blood-stained, the fourth tube of at least 2 mL should be collected to aid in the differentiation of SAH from a traumatic tap. The fourth tube may be additionally used for further studies such as specialized microbiological tests [gene expert or tuberculosis (TB) mycobacteria growth indicator tube (MGIT), etc.], immunological, metabolic tests, or analysis for malignant cells. Transfer of the tubes of CSF to the laboratory should be expedited because sitting for 2 hours at room temperature can cause lysis of up to 40% of white blood cells (WBC). This is especially important when we test for malignant cells in the CSF.

If indicated therapeutically, some fluid (about 25 mL) may be drained especially when IIH is suspected or a strong suspicion for cryptococcal meningitis. After draining/collecting the necessary samples, the stylet should be replaced before withdrawing the needle. This prevents the risk of CSF leak or significant postprocedural headache. The entire procedure should be carefully documented in the medical records.

In young children or neonates with suspected ventriculitis, CSF can be obtained by a ventricular or cisternal puncture, which is ideally a surgical procedure.

Complications

Lumbar puncture, if performed after due screening for possible contraindications, is generally a safe procedure. However, some complications may occur **(Table 1)**.[17] Most of the complications of LP can be regarded as minor (like back pain or local nerve root irritation) or moderately severe (like postdural puncture headache). The potentially severe or life-threatening complications that can occur after an LP are spinal hematoma, bacterial meningitis, cerebral venous sinus thrombosis (CVST), or cerebral herniation **(Table 1)**.[17]

Postdural puncture headache is an orthostatic headache caused by CSF leakage that may occur within 72 hours after an LP.[2,20] It may be accompanied by nausea, neck stiffness, tinnitus, or photophobia. The potential patient-related factors for a postdural puncture headache are young age, female sex, low body-mass index, and medical

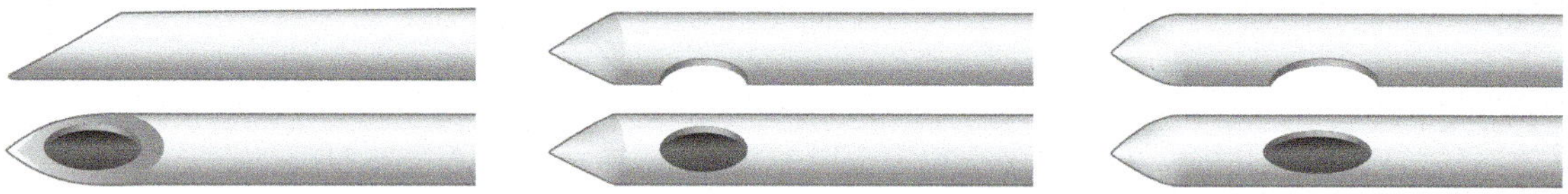

FIG. 3: Types of needles used for lumbar puncture.

TABLE 1: Complications of lumbar puncture.

Transient	Common	Serious
Pain and paresthesia in the distribution of a lumbar nerve root resulting from contact with the needle	Back pain (10%)	*Hematomas*: Subarachnoid, subdural, and epidural
	Postprocedural headache (1–50%)	*Infectious complications (if not performed in aseptic condition)*: Meningitis, epidural abscess, and osteomyelitis
		Spontaneous intracranial hypotension **(Fig. 4A)**
		Cerebral herniation (3–7%) (life-threatening) **(Fig. 4B)**
		Cerebral venous sinus thrombosis

history of headache, as well as technical factors such as needle tip design or performing the puncture in a sitting position.[21-25] It can be treated conservatively with analgesics combined with bed rest since pain is exacerbated by sitting and standing.[25] Although, the use of caffeine has shown some effectiveness, but the evidence is lacking.[25] The other drugs helpful are hydrocortisone, theophylline, and gabapentin, but the evidence for the same is not very robust.[26] A postprocedure fluid supplementation or bed rest does not prevent headaches but may be helpful if a headache has occurred due to multiple predisposing factors mentioned earlier.[27] After 5 days of conservative therapy, if no improvement is seen, a therapeutic blood patch may be done.[28,29] MRI study may reveal diffuse meningeal and dural venous sinus contrast enhancement which is known as spontaneous intracranial hypotension **(Fig. 4A)**, due to low CSF volume which induces a painful compensatory venous sinus engorgement.[30] An identical clinical and radiologic picture is occasionally seen in patients with a documented low CSF pressure (<60 mm H_2O) and no history of an LP or other known source of a dural tear, such as head trauma or surgery.[31]

Cerebral herniation following LP is a rare complication **(Fig. 4B)**, seen in patients with severe cerebral edema or brain abscess, or focal mass lesions prior to performing the LP.[17] The other rare complications of LP include bacterial meningitis, spinal hematoma, and CVST. Possible causes for post LP infection include contamination of the puncture site by skin bacteria or aerosolized mouth commensals from medical personnel, with the most commonly reported causative organisms being *Streptococcus salivarius* and viridans streptococci.[32] The risk of spinal hematoma is most likely to occur in patients taking anticoagulant therapy or in those with an uncorrected coagulopathy prior to LP. It may cause cauda equina compression with a poor outcome.[33] CVST is hypothesized to be a complication of intracranial hypotension following LP. The exact incidence of CVST is unknown, although certain case reports hypothesize risk factors like prothrombotic diseases, such as factor V Leiden mutation or protein C deficiency or pregnancy.[17,34]

CSF ANALYSIS AND INTERPRETATIONS

Appearance

Normal appearance of CSF is clear and colorless when held up to white light in identical tubes. Xanthochromia, a yellowish discoloration of the CSF, is seen with the presence of red blood cell (RBC) breakdown products such as oxyhemoglobin, bilirubin, and methemoglobin, each of which can be quantified by spectrophotometry.[2] With RBC counts between 500 and 6,000 cells/mm^3, color of CSF becomes pink or xanthochromic. Other causes of orange to brown discoloration of the CSF include hypercarotenemia, malignant meningeal melanomatosis, and drug treatment with rifampin.[2] Moreover, protein concentrations >150 mg/dL can also give CSF a mildly yellowish tint.

Opening Pressure

The normal opening pressure (upper limit of normal) with the patient in the lateral recumbent position is 110 mm H_2O in infants, 150 mm H_2O in children, 180 mm H_2O in adults, and 200–250 mm H_2O in obese adults **(Table 2)**.[35]

Cells

The normal CSF WBC count ranges from 0 to 5 mononuclear cells (lymphocytes and monocytes) per mm^3. There should

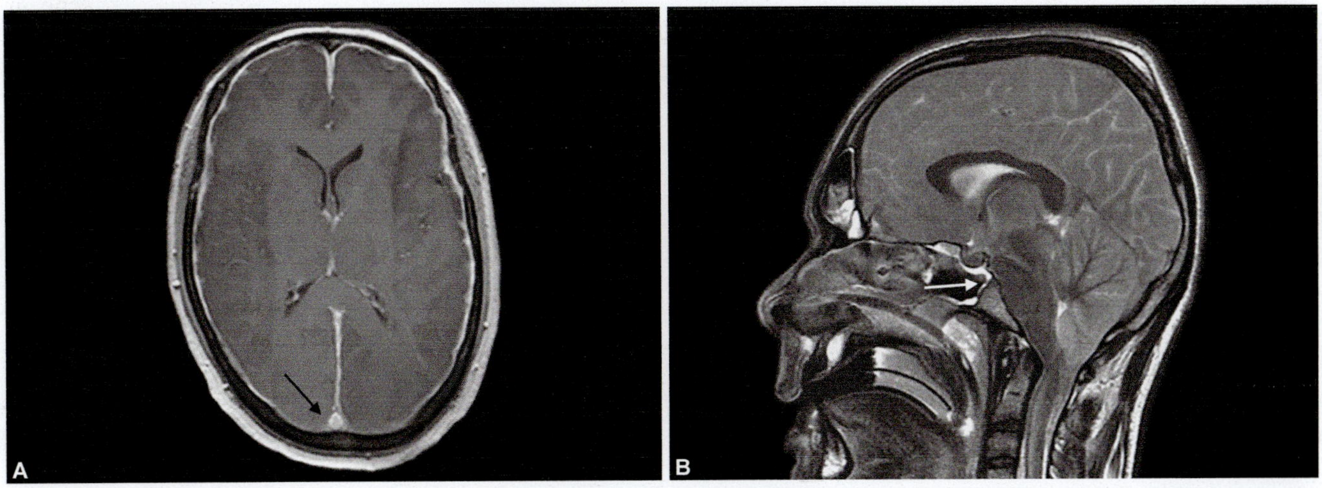

FIGS. 4A AND B: (A) Magnetic resonance imaging (MRI) brain images of spontaneous intracranial hypotension (SIH)—axial T1-weighted MRI of the brain after intravenous gadolinium contrast injection shows diffuse, abnormal pachymeningeal thickening along bilateral cerebral convexity and enlargement of the sagittal venous sinus (arrow). (B) MRI brain images of cerebral herniation—sagittal image reveals caudal herniation of cerebellar tonsils in upper cervical spinal canal with compression and distortion of brainstem (arrow) and effacement of cerebral sulci.

Image courtesy: Dr Ankur Shah, Consultant Radiologist, Gujarat Imaging Centre, Ahmedabad.

TABLE 2: Normal CSF composition in a healthy adult.

CSF composition	Normal range
Color	Clear
Opening pressure	50–200 mm H_2O
Specific gravity/pH	1.006–1.007/7.4
WBC count	0–5 (up to 30 in neonates)
RBC count	Nil
CSF proteins	15–40 mg/dL
CSF glucose	50–80 mg/dL (two-thirds of blood glucose)
CSF lactate	1–3 mmol/L
Microbial examination	No microorganism

(CSF: cerebrospinal fluid; RBC: red blood cell; WBC: white blood cell)

be no polymorphonuclear leukocytes in normal uninfected CSF. However, if the total WBC count is less than five, the presence of a single polymorphonuclear leukocyte may be considered normal.[36]

After a traumatic tap or if the CSF is contaminated with blood, the WBC count needs to be corrected by one WBC/mm^3 for every 700 red blood cells/mm^3.[2,36]

After 2 months of age, the normal range of CSF WBC count is 0–5/mm^3; in all ages, the CSF ANC should be <1/mm^3.[37] The CSF becomes grossly opalescent when there are 200–500 WBCs/mm^3 present.[37]

Glucose

The normal CSF glucose concentration is between 45 and 80 mg/dL when the serum glucose is 70–120 or approximately 65% (two-thirds) of the serum glucose. CSF glucose concentrations below 45 mg/dL are abnormal.[38]

A serum glucose concentration should always be obtained at the time of LP to determine the CSF: serum glucose ratio. The normal CSF: serum glucose ratio is 0.6. The CSF glucose concentration is low when the CSF: serum glucose ratio is <0.6 (CSF hypoglycorrhachia).[36,38]

Proteins

The upper range of normal for the lumbar CSF protein concentration is 50 mg/dL in the adult and 45 mg/dL in the child. The upper range of normal for the cisternal CSF protein concentration in children and adults is 30 mg/dL.[2,36]

Traumatic Lumbar Puncture

A traumatic tap occurs when the spinal needle penetrates a radicular artery or vein. In the collection tube, a clot or thread of blood appears in the CSF.[37] A sample of the bloody CSF should be centrifuged. In a traumatic tap, the supernatant is colorless, whereas in a SAH, the supernatant is yellow (xanthochromic).[2]

When CSF pleocytosis precedes traumatic LP, the CSF ratio of WBC:RBC should exceed that of peripheral blood. When CSF pleocytosis is associated with traumatic LP, it should be possible to use this relationship to distinguish the contribution of contaminating blood elements and to determine if the pretap CSF WBC was abnormally elevated.[37] The common formula for this relationship is:

$$\text{Predicted CSF WBC} = \text{CSF RBC} \times \frac{\text{CBC WBC}}{\text{CBC RBC}}$$

Cerebrospinal Fluid Lactate

In children with suspected inborn errors of metabolism, CSF lactate and/or glycine are calculated, although abnormal levels may not be specific for these conditions.[39,40] CSF lactate may also be used to investigate mitochondrial disorders.[41]

Microbiology and Immunological Testing

A normal CSF is generally sterile. CSF may be sent for additional microbiological testing and immunological testing, depending on the indication.

Utility

Cerebrospinal fluid analysis is vital for the diagnosis of various infectious, neuroinflammatory disorders, neurodegenerative conditions as well as for the prognosis of some of these conditions. The therapeutic role of CSF is also well known in certain disorders, e.g., IIH, cryptococcal meningitis, etc. CSF being much more accessible, less costly than imaging, and reflecting metabolic and pathological states of the CNS more directly than any other body fluids is an ideal source for biomarker discovery. CSF may be helpful in the diagnosis of following diseases:

- Subarachnoid hemorrhage (SAH)
- *Intracranial CNS infections*: Meningitis, encephalitis, and meningoencephalitis
- *Inflammatory and demyelinating central neurological disorders*: Multiple sclerosis (MS), neuromyelitis optica spectrum disorder (NMOSD), myelin oligodendrocyte glycoprotein-associated disorder (MOGAD), and acute disseminated encephalomyelitis (ADEM)
- *Inflammatory neuropathies*: Chronic relapsing inflammatory optic neuropathy (CRION), acute inflammatory demyelinating polyradiculoneuropathy (AIDP), and chronic acute inflammatory demyelinating polyradiculoneuropathy (CIDP)
- Autoimmune encephalitis
- CNS vasculitis
- *Neurodegenerative disorders*: Alzheimer's dementia (AD), Parkinson's disease (PD)
- Creutzfeldt-Jakob disease (CJD) and other prion disorders
- Normal pressure hydrocephalus (NPH)
- Idiopathic intracranial hypertension (IIH)
- Brain and spinal cord neoplasm

- Traumatic spinal cord injury
- Neurometabolic disorders in children

ROLE IN NEUROLOGICAL DISORDERS AND CLINICAL APPLICATION

Subarachnoid Hemorrhage

Subarachnoid hemorrhage is one of the acute neurological emergencies requiring intensive care. CSF analysis by LP is indicated if there is high clinical suspicion of SAH, but a negative CT finding. The presence of RBCs (more than 1,000 cells/mm^3) or xanthochromia confirms the diagnosis of SAH.[42,43] To distinguish a traumatic tap from SAH, CSF is collected in three test tubes and by counting the red cells in the consecutive tubes. A fourth tube may be collected, which persists to remain blood stained in SAH. A decrease in the red cells would usually indicate a traumatic tap. Another method is to centrifuge the CSF and look for xanthochromia of the supernatant fluid. Spectrophotometry is recommended for xanthochromia detection. Xanthochromia could be seen as early as 12 hours which is due to the lysis of RBCs in CSF and the release of pigments like oxyhemoglobin, methemoglobin, and bilirubin.[44] For the diagnosis of rebleeding of SAH, LP is not useful due to the presence of pigments till 3 weeks of first SAH.[45] Elevated CSF ferritin concentrations can be found in patients with SAH when examined at least 3 days after the ictus because it takes approximately 3 days for the CSF ferritin levels to increase, but spectrometric analysis of CSF hemoglobin and bilirubin concentrations is considered more accurate and can be assessed at least 12 hours after the ictus.[46]

Intracranial CNS Infections

Cerebrospinal fluid analysis is the gold standard for diagnosis of meningitis as well as to identify its etiology. CSF parameters in conjunction with the clinical presentation provide an initial impression of the possible microbiological diagnoses to guide empiric therapy. However, they cannot be relied on because they may change after the initiation of antimicrobial therapy and over the course of the illness.[47]

Gram staining of CSF **(Table 3)** remains a quick and easy way to guide antimicrobial therapy[48] whereas CSF culture is considered the gold standard for the diagnosis of bacterial meningitis. CSF samples are also used for gram stains, microbial culture, venereal disease research laboratory (VDRL), antibodies against antigens using polymerase chain reaction (PCR), and immunohistochemistry analysis. Multiplex PCR has emerged as the gold standard for the detection of viruses[49] and is also increasingly used for the detection of bacteria.

A neutrophilic predominance is generally seen in bacterial infections, whereas a lymphocytic predominance is seen in viral, fungal, and mycobacterial infections. However, a neutrophilic predominance may be seen early in the course of viral infections and throughout the course of West Nile virus encephalitis. CSF glucose

TABLE 3: CSF analysis in meningitis.

	Type of central nervous system infection				
CSF analysis	**Bacterial**	**Tuberculosis**	**Viral**	**Fungal**	**Aseptic**
Pressure	Increased	Increased	Normal to increased	Normal to mild increased	Increased
Color	Turbid	Turbid	Clear	Clear	Clear/Turbid
Proteins	↑↑	↑↑↑	Normal/↑	Normal/↑	↑
Glucose	<40 mg/dL	Low	Normal	Low to normal	Low
WBCs	10–2,000/mm^3	Elevated, <500	>100/mm^3	10–50/mm^3	Mildly elevated
RBCs	Elevated	Elevated	Normal	Normal	Elevated
Lactate	Elevated (>6 mmol/L)	Elevated	0–6 mmol/L	Normal	Normal
WBC types	Neutrophils	Lymphocytes	Lymphocytes	Lymphocytes	Neutrophils
Gram-stain	Positive	Acid fast bacilli	Negative	India ink for spores/fungi	Negative
Microbial culture	Positive	Positive (high yield in early stage)	Negative	Positive	Negative
PCR test	—	Identification of organisms even after antibiotics started	Helps in identification of organisms	—	—
BioFire	Positive	—	Positive	—	—
Biomarkers	↑CRP	↑ CSF procalcitonin, ADA	↓CRP and ADA		Seen following neurosurgery or antibiotic use

(↑: mildly elevated; ↑↑: elevated; ↑↑↑: highly elevated; ADA: adenosine deaminase; CRP: C reactive protein; CSF: cerebrospinal fluid; PCR: polymerase chain reaction; RBC: red blood cell; WBC: white blood cell)

is decreased in bacterial (including mycobacterial) and fungal infections and generally normal in viral infections, but it may be decreased in mumps, herpes simplex virus 2, cytomegalovirus, and Eastern equine encephalitis-infection, as well as in meningitis associated with leptomeningeal metastases and sarcoidosis.[47]

Cerebrospinal fluid serology is considered a more sensitive test than PCR for certain viruses [arbovirus immunoglobulin M (IgM); varicella-zoster virus IgG in myelitis and vasculitis], and serology is also the test of choice for Lyme disease (IgG) and neurosyphilis. Lumbar puncture can itself be used therapeutically in patients with cryptococcal meningitis by relieving headaches as a result of lowering of CSF pressure.[50] In an observational cohort study, including 248 patients with HIV-associated cryptococcal meningitis, therapeutic LPs were associated with a 69% relative improvement in survival.[51]

Metagenomic next-generation sequencing of CSF is an emerging new technique that evaluates all genetic material in a sample to detect any nonhost sequences and identify them through computational algorithms using bioinformatic libraries.[52] This technique has identified novel or unexpected pathogens in patients with neurologic infections that were unable to be diagnosed with conventional microbiological testing.[53]

Central Nervous System Demyelinating Disorders

The basic parameters of CSF [WBC and RBC counts, protein, glucose, and oligoclonal bands (OCBs)/IgG index] are helpful to show evidence of inflammation. Most of these conditions are responsive to therapy and hence early diagnosis and treatment lead to better outcomes for the patient. CSF analysis gives valuable information regarding the diagnosis, progression, or relapse of the disease as well as the effect of treatment. CSF findings used in the routine diagnosis of MS serve two aims—(1) to confirm a diagnosis of MS early in the disease course; and (2) to rule out differential diagnoses. Typical CSF findings in MS include a slightly elevated leukocyte count (5–50 cells/μL, compared with a normal range of <5 cells/μL), the presence of activated B cells or plasma cells on routine cytological analysis, elevated IgG synthesis, OCBs, and increased synthesis of intrathecally produced immunoglobulins against measles, rubella, and varicella zoster (MRZ) viruses.[54] However, up to 10% of patients with MS can present with normal CSF findings.

Cerebrospinal fluid findings are of value in the differentiation between patients with MS and those with anti-aquaporin-4-negative neuromyelitis optica. The leukocyte count in CSF is usually higher in patients with neuromyelitis optica than in those with MS, and shows a high frequency of neutrophils and eosinophils. Furthermore, the CSF of patients with neuromyelitis optica usually tests negative for OCBs and the MRZ reaction (MRZR).[55] The majority of patients with ADEM also test negative for OCB.[56] In MOG-IgG antibody-associated syndromes the frequency of OCB of 13% is similarly low as in NMO spectrum disorders.[57] A positive MRZR is shown in about 70–90% of patients with clinically definite MS.[58] A positive MRZR in patients with optic neuritis or with clinically isolated syndrome (CIS)[59] predicts conversion to definite MS with a higher specificity than does the presence of OCBs and can be detected even in patients with early-stage MS who test negative for OCBs.[60] The presence or absence of OCBs and the MRZR in patients with CIS can, therefore, be used for counseling patients about the course of their disease, and may also support treatment decisions.

Detection of oligoclonal IgG bands and elevated CXCL13 levels in the CSF can be used to make a prognosis and predict subsequent relapse in patients with the CIS.[54] Of all CSF parameters, CXCL13 has the best positive predictive value for conversion of CIS to MS.[61]

Prognostic CSF markers may influence the choice of therapy for MS. For example when it is possible to distinguish between a very active disease course and a mild progression.[62] Protein chitinase 3-like1 (CHI3L1) and neurofilament light protein (NfL) are the most promising prognostic CSF markers to predict conversion of MS on the one hand and disability on the other.[63]

Immune-mediated Neuropathies

The classic immunologic alteration of CSF in AIDP is high CSF protein with normal cell count (albuminocytologic dissociation), although pleocytosis may rarely also occur. CSF sphingomyelin (SM) levels are higher in AIDP and CIDP, than in various non-inflammatory neurological disorders and axonal neuropathies including acute motor axonal neuropathy (AMAN).[64] CSF SM level is a diagnostic and staging wet biomarker for acquired demyelinating neuropathies and may effectively improve the management of patients affected by AIDP and CIDP.[64] While SM shows promise as a diagnostic and possibly prognostic biomarker, the results need to be replicated in other studies.[65]

Autoimmune Encephalitis

Cerebrospinal fluid analysis is the most important test for the diagnostic workup of AE which usually follows neuroimaging. Common CSF findings in AE include mild-to-moderate lymphocytic pleocytosis, hyperproteinorrachia, and elevated IgG index and/or IgG synthesis rate and positive intrathecal OCBs (unmatched in the serum) in some cases.[66] CSF detection is more sensitive for some antibodies (e.g., NMDAR and GFAP antibodies) while serum is more sensitive for other antibodies (e.g., onconeuronal, LGI1, and AQP4 antibodies).[67] It is important to note that if the clinical picture is highly suggestive of an antibody with a higher serum sensitivity [e.g., faciobrachial dystonic seizure (FBDS) suggestive of LGI1-antibody encephalitis], then it might be reasonable to avoid CSF testing in clinical situations where CSF sampling is challenging.[68] Inclusion of both CSF and serum is recommended for neuronal antibody testing in suspected anti-NMDAR encephalitis.[67]

Central Nervous System Vasculitis

Primary angiitis of the central nervous system (PACNS) is an inflammatory disease affecting the brain and spinal cord. Stroke, encephalopathy, headache, and seizures are major clinical manifestations.[69] The diagnosis of PACNS is based on the combination of clinical presentation, imaging findings (MRI and angiography), and laboratory, CSF, and brain biopsy. Typically, CSF examinations show inflammatory findings, mild lymphocytic pleocytosis combined with an elevated protein level. CSF examination is abnormal in 80–90% of patients.[70]

Alzheimer's Dementia

The best-established fluid biomarkers for AD are the core CSF Aβ1–42 that reflects Aβ plaque formation in the brain, CSF phospho-tau 181 (P-tau) that reflects neurofibrillary tangle pathology in AD, and CSF total-tau (T-tau) that is a marker of axonal degeneration **(Table 4)**. A large number of studies show that the typical Alzheimer's disease biomarker signature in CSF (elevated levels of T-tau and P-tau181 and reduced levels of $A\beta_{42}$) mirrors Alzheimer's disease neuropathology.[71] These biomarkers have been validated against pathology and are 85–95% sensitive and specific for AD in both dementia and prodromal mild cognitive impairment stages of the disease.[72] In research settings, CSF biomarkers have good diagnostic accuracy on a group level for Alzheimer's disease but are not yet recommended for routine diagnostic purposes at clinical level.[73]

TABLE 4: Cerebrospinal fluid (CSF) biomarkers in various neurological disorders.

Neurological disorder	CSF biomarker
Alzheimer's dementia	↑t-tau and ↑P tau181, ↓$A\beta_{42}$
Parkinsonian syndromes	α-synuclein, sAPP-α, and NfL
Multiple sclerosis	Oligoclonal bands, IgG index, MRZR, CXCL13, and CHI3L1
Neuromyelitis optica	AQP4-IgG
Acute and chronic inflammatory demyelinating polyneuropathies	Sphingomyelin
Motor neuron disease	NfL, pNfH
Huntington's disease	NfL
Narcolepsy	Hypocretin-1
Neurosarcoidosis	Soluble IL-2 receptor
Prion diseases	14-3-3
Cerebral folate deficiency	5-methyltetrahydrofolate

[AQP4-IgG: aquaporin-4 immunoglobulin G antibodies; $A\beta_{42}$: amyloid-β 1-42; CXCL: chemokine (C-X-C motif) ligand; NfL: neurofilament light protein; YKL-40: chitinase-3-like protein 1; t-tau: total tau; p-tau 181: phosphorylated tau181; pNfH: phosphorylated neurofilament heavy chain; MRZR: measles, rubella, and varicella zoster viruses' reaction]

Parkinson's Disease

Parkinson's disease is a common neurodegenerative disorder; however, well-established biochemical markers are yet to be identified.[74] Several studies have demonstrated that CSF α-synuclein decreased early in the disease, preceding motor PD.[75-78] Alpha synuclein in the CSF is a promising candidate as a biomarker for the diagnosis of PD as its concentrations may reflect the accumulation and aggregation of misfolded α-synuclein in Lewy bodies and Lewy neurites that neuropathologically characterize PD.[79] CSF α-synuclein levels do not correlate with measures of disease severity, including striatal dopaminergic deficit.[80] A prospective cohort study of 160 patients with parkinsonian syndromes and 30 healthy controls found a role for CSF NfL protein, soluble amyloid precursor protein α, and α-synuclein concentrations in predicting diagnosis of PD versus atypical parkinsonian syndromes.[81]

Motor Neuron Disease

Several CSF biomarker candidates (both diagnostic and prognostic) have been proposed for amyotrophic lateral sclerosis (ALS) and primary lateral sclerosis (PLS), the most promising candidate biomarkers are phosphorylated neurofilament heavy chain **(Table 4)** and NfL chain,[82,83] which have been found to be increased in patients with motor neuron diseases compared with healthy controls. However, further studies are required to provide evidence to support their use as a marker of disease progression. Furthermore, intrathecal delivery of a novel drug nusinersen, an antisense oligonucleotide by LP that increases the amount of functional survival motor neuron protein, which is deficient in patients with spinal muscle atrophy is fascinating. A phase 2 randomized controlled study in 20 patients aged 3–7 months showed acceptable safety of nusinersen in this previously untreatable disease and an encouraging clinical response.[84]

Normal Pressure Hydrocephalus

The classic presentation of NPH is that of an insidiously progressive gait syndrome, urinary urgency followed by incontinence, and cognitive impairment. This clinical triad is thought to occur because of impairment of periventricular frontal cortical–basal ganglia–thalamocortical circuitry in the setting of CSF hypervolemia.[85] Anecdotal case reports have recently demonstrated that patients with idiopathic NPH show hypometabolism in the caudate nucleus, and have shown functional recovery of the supplementary motor area after CSF drainage.[86,87] In hydrocephalus with normal CSF opening pressure, the CSF tap test can be done by removal of 30–50 mL CSF to predict efficacy of CSF catheter placement.[88] In a prospective case series including 115 patients with idiopathic NPH, the tap test had a positive predictive value of 88% and a negative predictive value of 18% for clinical improvement especially in gait after catheter placement.[89]

Idiopathic Intracranial Hypertension

In most patients, IIH manifests with severe headache, transient visual obscuration, pulsatile tinnitus, and bilateral papilledema. LP is essential in the diagnosis of IIH because the diagnostic criteria include a raised CSF opening pressure (>25 cmH_2O) and normal CSF composition.[90] Serial CSF drainage by LP can be useful as a temporizing measure to preclude surgery. However, it might not be useful for long-term management of IIH.

Creutzfeldt–Jakob Disease and Other Prion Disorders

Currently, the detection of increased 14-3-3 protein in CSF is used as a molecular diagnostic criterion for patients that are clinically compatible with sporadic CJD (sCJD). The gamma-isoform of the 14-3-3 protein (14-3-3 gamma) expressed in neurons could be a specific marker for neuronal damage and is useful for sCJD diagnosis.[91,92] It has high sensitivity (86–97%) for sCJD.[93] Its combination with t-tau and the ratio of t-tau/p-tau has very good sensitivity and specificity and is more accessible compared to other techniques, such as RT-QuIC.[94,95] Diagnostic performance improves for both genetic and sporadic CJD if above CSF biomarkers are used in combination.

Brain and Spinal Cord Neoplasm

Neoplasms of CNS in which CSF analysis are helpful is usually due to primary CNS lymphoma or secondary leptomeningeal deposits.[45] After initial neuroimaging tests, centrifuged CSF can be used for presence or absence of malignant cells. CSF cytology is used to detect malignant cells in suspected CNS lymphoma, leukemia, leptomeningeal dissemination of metastatic tumors, and spread of primary brain tumors.[96] Immunophenotyping by multiparameter flow cytometry of CSF cells can add to the diagnostic sensitivity in hematological malignancies[97] such as primary CNS lymphoma.

Spinal Cord Traumatic Injury

Analysis of various biomarkers in the CSF in patients who has sustained injury to spinal cord can help in assessing the severity of injury as well as in prognostication of patients.[98,99] Spinal cord injury can cause elevation of various biomarkers including microRNA (mRNA), neuron-specific enolase (NSE), glial fibrillary proteins, interleukin-6 (IL-6), and cleaved tau proteins. These represent different components of damage like neurons, axons, glial cells, and vascular injury.[45]

Cerebrospinal Fluid in Children with Neurometabolic Disorders

Pediatric neurotransmitter disorders should be suspected in patients with unexplained seizures, encephalopathy, dysautonomia, extrapyramidal symptoms, or intermittent ocular abnormalities, such as oculogyric crises or convergence spasms.[2] Cerebral folate deficiency (CFD) syndrome is a rare treatable neurometabolic disorder with low levels of the active form of folate in CSF.[100] It occurs due to different causes such as *FOLR1* gene mutations or autoantibodies against the folate receptor-alpha (FR) protein that can block folate transport across the choroid plexus. The level of CSF 5-MTHF is low, while the active form of folate concentration in plasma is normal. Another clue for the important treatable disorder is an isolated low CSF glucose in combination with a low to normal CSF lactate, which is the diagnostic marker for glucose transporter 1 deficiency syndrome and should not be missed.[38]

NOVEL CEREBROSPINAL FLUID BIOMARKERS

The study of molecular biomarkers in CSF constitutes an emerging field of neurological research, with many candidates being investigated **(Table 3)**. It can be used potentially to study fundamental biological processes, for early diagnosis, monitoring of therapy, and personalized medicine.[101] Commercial immunoassays on biomarkers of neurodegeneration have been developed and are being validated to standardize analytical methods and improve diagnostic accuracy.[102] Several such biomarkers have been under investigation including NSE, S-100 beta, tau protein, neurogranin, synaptosomal-associated protein 25 (SNAP-25), glial fibrillary acidic protein (GFAP), micro-RNA (miRNA), IL-6, and NfL chain.[103] Detailed CSF analysis of a variety of small molecules is advancing our understanding of the pathophysiology of CNS disorders and holds great potential for future clinical use in the diagnosis, future therapeutics, and prognosis. Once validated, CSF biomarkers could be used to subcategorize individuals on the spectrum of each neurological disease, into several biological endophenotypes necessitating targeted drug therapies.[104]

FUTURE APPLICATIONS

"Omics" technologies offer another potential tool to identify candidate CSF biomarkers for monitoring both disease progression and the response to therapy in patients with MS. Many of these markers, however, require validation in independent clinical studies before they can be implemented in routine clinical practice.[54] Potential biomarkers need to be rigorously validated in combination with clinical and MRI data, and preferably require the development of quantitative detection assays. Shotgun metagenomic sequencing of total DNA and RNA from host and pathogen is a newer technique that has successfully identified new and known viral pathogens in patients with encephalitis of unknown origin.[104] Another recently advanced technique is Matrix-assisted laser desorption or ionization time-of-flight mass spectrometry (MALDI-TOF MS) which can detect pathogens based on protein fragments released from the bacterial cell surface.[105] This novel technique requires only minutes to deliver a final result and its ability to identify microorganisms is not limited to prespecified targets. Intrathecal gene therapy has shown promising results in experimental models of malignant leptomeningeal neoplasia, ALS, and neurological manifestations of mucopolysaccharidoses suggesting a ray of new hope.[46]

CONCLUSION

Early detection will be crucial to prevent or intervene in the early phase of neurological disorders and CSF diagnostic biomarkers are expected to play a central role. The newer laboratory techniques have widened the horizons of indications for CSF examination in many neurological disorders, e.g., biomarkers of neurodegenerative diseases, neuronal autoantibodies in autoimmune encephalitis, and discovery of previously unidentified pathogens by sequencing. The assessment and evaluation of CSF have an irreplaceable and vital role in the diagnostics of both the central and peripheral nervous system disorders; from inflammatory processes, to infectious and autoimmune, to tumorous infiltrations of CSF and neurodegenerative diseases. CSF biomarkers would aid in understanding the pathophysiological mechanisms, improve diagnostic accuracy, and facilitate the future development of novel therapies, including disease-modifying drugs.[74]

REFERENCES

1. Sakula A. A hundred years of lumbar puncture: 1891–1991. J R Coll Physicians Lond. 1991;25:171-5.
2. Michelson DJ. Spinal fluid examination. In: Swaiman KF, Ashwal S, Ferriero DM, Schor NF, Finkel RS, Gropman AL, et al. Swaiman's Pediatric Neurology: Principles Practice, 6th edition. India: Elsevier; 2017. pp. 160.
3. Pearce JM. Walter Essex Wynter, Quincke, and lumbar puncture. J Neurol Neurosurg Psychiatry. 1994;57(2):179.
4. Tumani H, Huss A, Bachhuber F. The cerebrospinal fluid and barriers - anatomic and physiologic considerations. Handb Clin Neurol. 2017;146:21-32.
5. Brinker T, Stopa E, Morrison J, Klinge P. A new look at cerebrospinal fluid circulation. Fluids Barriers CNS. 2014;11:10.
6. Davson H, Hollingsworth G, Segal MB. The mechanism of drainage of the cerebrospinal fluid. Brain. 1970;93(4):665-78.
7. Nakada T. Virchow-Robin space and aquaporin-4: new insights on an old friend. Croat Med J. 2014;55(4):328-36.
8. Sakka L, Coll G, Chazal J. Anatomy and physiology of cerebrospinal fluid. Eur Ann Otorhinolaryngol Head Neck Dis. 2011;128(6): 309-16.
9. Aspelund A, Antila S, Proulx ST, Karlsen TV, Karaman S, Detmar M, et al. A dural lymphatic vascular system that drains brain interstitial fluid and macromolecules. J Exp Med. 2015;212(7):991-9.
10. Louveau A, Smirnov I, Keyes TJ, Eccles JD, Rouhani SJ, Peske JD, et al. Structural and functional features of central nervous system lymphatic vessels. Nature. 2015;523(7560):337-41.
11. Abbott NJ, Patabendige AA, Dolman DE, Yusof SR, Begley DJ. Structure and function of the blood-brain barrier. Neurobiol Dis. 2010;37(1):13-25.
12. Simon MJ, Iliff JJ. Regulation of cerebrospinal fluid (CSF) flow in neurodegenerative, neurovascular and neuroinflammatory disease. Biochim Biophys Acta. 2016;1862(3):442-51.
13. Avila ML, Macartney CA, Hitzler JK, Williams S, Kiss A, Brandão LR. Assessment of the outcomes associated with periprocedural anticoagulation management in children with acute lymphoblastic leukemia. J Pediatr. 2014;164(5):1201-7.
14. Le Saux N; Canadian Paediatric Society, Infectious Diseases and Immunization Committee. Guidelines for the management of suspected and confirmed bacterial meningitis in Canadian children older than one month of age. Paediatr Child Health. 2014;19(3):141-52.
15. Rahmani M, Vaziri Bozorg SM, Ghasemi Esfe AR, Morteza A, Khalilzadeh O, Pedarzadeh E, et al. Evaluating the reliability of anatomic landmarks in safe lumbar puncture using magnetic resonance imaging: does sex matter? Int J Biomed Imaging. 2011;868632:2011.
16. Weise KL, Nahata MC. EMLA for painful procedures in infants. J Pediatr Health Care. 2005;19(1):42-7.
17. Costerus JM, Brouwer MC, van de Beek D. Technological advances and changing indications for lumbar puncture in neurological disorders. Lancet Neurol. 2018;17(3):268-78.
18. Nigrovic LE, Kuppermann N, Neuman MI. Risk factors for traumatic or unsuccessful lumbar punctures in children. Ann Emerg Med. 2007;49:762.
19. Pearce JM. Queckenstedt's manoeuvre. J Neurol Neurosurg Psychiatry. 2006;77(6):728.
20. Leblanc A, Catrevaux O, Guillaumat C, Robin L, Foucaud P. Post lumbar puncture headache in general pediatrics: a prospective multicenter study. Arch Pediatr. 2005;12(8):1199-203.
21. Nath S, Koziarz A, Badhiwala JH, Alhazzani W, Jaeschke R, Sharma S, et al. Atraumatic versus conventional lumbar puncture needles: a systematic review and meta-analysis. Lancet. 2018;391(10126):1197-204.
22. van Oosterhout WP, van der Plas AA, van Zwet EW, Zielman R, Ferrari MD, Terwindt GM. Postdural puncture headache in migraineurs and non headache subjects: a prospective study. Neurology. 2013;80:941-8.
23. Crock C, Orsini F, Lee KJ, Phillips RJ. Headache after lumbar puncture: randomised crossover trial of 22-gauge versus 25-gauge needles. Arch Dis Child. 2014;99:203-7.
24. de Almeida SM, Shumaker SD, LeBlanc SK, Delaney P, Marquie-Beck J, Ueland S, et al. Incidence of post-dural puncture headache in research volunteers. Headache. 2011;51:1503-10.
25. Basurto Ona X, Osorio D, Bonfill Cosp X. Drug therapy for treatingpost-dural puncture headache. Cochrane Database Syst Rev. 2015;7:CD007887.
26. Amorim JA, Gomes de Barros MV, Valenca MM. Post-dural (post-lumbar) puncture headache: risk factors and clinical features. Cephalalgia. 2012;32:916-23.
27. Arevalo-Rodriguez I, Ciapponi A, Figuls MR, Munoz L, Bonfill Cosp X. Posture and fluids for preventing post-duralpuncture headache. Cochrane Database Syst Rev. 2016;3:CD009199.

28. van Kooten F, Oedit R, Bakker SL, Dippel DW. Epidural blood patch in post dural puncture headache: a randomised, observer-blind, controlled clinical trial. J Neurol Neurosurg Psychiatry. 2008;79:553-8.
29. Boonmak P, Boonmak S. Epidural blood patching for preventing and treating post-dural puncture headache. Cochrane Database Syst Rev. 2010;1:CD001791.
30. Urbach H. Intracranial hypotension: clinical presentation, imaging findings, and imaging-guided therapy. Curr Opin Neurol. 2014;27(4):414-24.
31. Gordon N. Spontaneous intracranial hypotension. Dev Med Child Neurol. 2009;51:932.
32. Baer ET. Post-dural puncture bacterial meningitis. Anesthesiology 2006;105:381-93.
33. van Veen JJ, Nokes TJ, Makris M. The risk of spinal haematoma following neuraxial anaesthesia or lumbar puncture in thrombocytopenic individuals. Br J Haematol. 2010;148:15-25.
34. Kate MP, Thomas B, Sylaja PN. Cerebral venous thrombosis in post-lumbar puncture intracranial hypotension: case report and review of literature. F1000Res. 2014;3:41.
35. Corbett JJ, Mehta MP. Cerebrospinal fluid pressure in normal obese subjects and patients with pseudotumor cerebri. Neurology. 1983;33:1386-8.
36. Roos KL. Lumbar puncture. Semin Neurol. 2003;23(1):105-14.
37. Bonadio W. Pediatric lumbar puncture and cerebrospinal fluid analysis. J Emerg Med. 2014;46(1):141-50.
38. Leen WG, de Wit CJ, Wevers RA, van Engelen BG, Kamsteeg EJ, Klepper J, et al. Child neurology: differential diagnosis of a low CSF glucose in children and young adults. Neurology. 2013;81(24): e178-81.
39. Chow SL, Rooney ZJ, Cleary MA, Clayton PT, Leonard JV. The significance of elevated CSF lactate. Arch Dis Child. 2005;90(11): 1188-9.
40. Aburahma S, Khassawneh M, Griebel M, Sharp G, Gibson J. Pitfalls in measuring cerebrospinal fluid glycine levels in infants with encephalopathy. J Child Neurol. 2011;26(6):703-6.
41. Schmiedel J, Jackson S, Schafer J, Reichmann H. Mitochondrial cytopathies. J Neurol. 2011;250(3):267-77.
42. Vivancos J, Gilo F, Frutos R, Maestre J, García-Pastor A, Quintana F, et al. Guía de actuación clínica en la hemorragia subaracnoidea. Sistemática diagnóstica y tratamiento. Neurología. 2014;29(6): 353-70.
43. Carpenter CR, Hussain AM, Ward MJ, Zipfel GJ, Fowler S, Pines JM, et al. Spontaneous subarachnoid hemorrhage: A systematic review and meta-analysis describing the diagnostic accuracy of history, physical examination, imaging, and lumbar puncture with an exploration of test thresholds. Acad Emerg Med. 2016;23(9): 963-1003.
44. Vermeulen M, van Gijn J. The diagnosis of subarachnoid haemorrhage. J Neurol Neurosurg Psychiatry. 1990;53(5):365-72.
45. Hrishi AP, Sethuraman M. Cerebrospinal fluid (CSF) analysis and interpretation in neurocritical care for acute neurological conditions. Indian J Crit Care Med. 2019;23(Suppl 2):S115-9.
46. Jm C, Mc B, van de DB. Technological advances and changing indications for lumbar puncture in neurological disorders. Lancet Neurol. 2018;17(3):267-78.
47. Berkowitz AL. Approach to neurologic infections. Continuum (Minneap Minn). 2021;27(4):818-35.
48. McGill F, Heyderman RS, Panagiotou S, Tunkel AR, Solomon T. Acute bacterial meningitis in adults. Lancet. 2016;388(10063): 3036-47.
49. Kleines M, Scheithauer S, Schiefer J, Häusler M. Clinical application of viral cerebrospinal fluid PCR testing for diagnosis of central nervous system disorders: a retrospective 11-year experience. Diagn Microbiol Infect Dis. 2014;80(3):207-15.
50. Chang CC, Perfect JR. Repeated therapeutic lumbar punctures in cryptococcal meningitis - necessity and/or opportunity? Curr Opin Infect Dis. 2016;29(6):539-45.
51. Rolfes MA, Hullsiek KH, Rhein J, Nabeta HW, Taseera K, Schutz C, et al. The effect of therapeutic lumbar punctures on acute mortality from cryptococcal meningitis. Clin Infect Dis. 2014;59(11): 1607-14.
52. Ramachandran PS, Wilson MR. Metagenomics for neurological infections—expanding our imagination. Nat Rev Neurol. 2020;16 (10):547-56.
53. Wilson MR, Sample HA, Zorn KC, Arevalo S, Yu G, Neuhaus J, et al. Clinical Metagenomic Sequencing for Diagnosis of Meningitis and Encephalitis. N Engl J Med. 2019;380(24):2327-40.
54. Stangel M, Fredrikson S, Meinl E, Petzold A, Stüve O, Tumani H. The utility of cerebrospinal fluid analysis in patients with multiple sclerosis. Nat Rev Neurol. 2013;9(5):267-76.
55. Jarius S, Franciotta D, Bergamaschi R, Rauer S, Wandinger KP, Petereit HF, et al. Polyspecific, antiviral immune response distinguishes multiple sclerosis and neuromyelitis optica. J Neurol Neurosurg Psychiatry. 2008;79(10):1134-6.
56. Dale RC, de Sousa C, Chong WK, Cox TC, Harding B, Neville BG. Acute disseminated encephalomyelitis, multiphasic disseminated encephalomyelitis and multiple sclerosis in children. Brain. 2000;123 Pt 12:2407-22.
57. Jarius S, Ruprecht K, Kleiter I, Borisow N, Asgari N, Pitarokoili K, et al. MOG-IgG in NMO and related disorders: a multicenter study of 50 patients. Part 2: Epidemiology, clinical presentation, radiological and laboratory features, treatment responses, and long-term outcome. J Neuroinflammation. 2016;13(1):280.
58. Reiber H, Ungefehr S, Jacobi C. The intrathecal, polyspecific and oligoclonal immune response in multiple sclerosis. Mult Scler. 1998;4(3):111-7.
59. Tumani H, Tourtellotte WW, Peter JB, Felgenhauer K. Acute optic neuritis: combined immunological markers and magnetic resonance imaging predict subsequent development of multiple sclerosis. The Optic Neuritis Study Group. J Neurol Sci. 1998;155(1):44-9.
60. Brecht I, Weissbrich B, Braun J, Toyka KV, Weishaupt A, Buttmann M. Intrathecal, polyspecific antiviral immune response in oligoclonal band negative multiple sclerosis. PLOS One. 2012;7(7):e40431.
61. Serafini B, Rosicarelli B, Magliozzi R, Stigliano E, Aloisi F. Detection of ectopic B-cell follicles with germinal centers in the meninges of patients with secondary progressive multiple sclerosis. Brain Pathol. 2004;14(2):164-74.
62. Deisenhammer F, Zetterberg H, Fitzner B, Zettl UK. The Cerebrospinal Fluid in Multiple Sclerosis. Frontiers in Immunology. 2019;10:726.
63. Comabella M, Sastre-Garriga J, Montalban X. Precision medicine in multiple sclerosis: biomarkers for diagnosis, prognosis, and treatment response. Curr Opin Neurol. 2016;29(3):254-62.
64. Capodivento G, De Michelis C, Carpo M, Fancellu R, Schirinzi E, Severi D, et al. CSF sphingomyelin: a new biomarker of demyelination in the diagnosis and management of CIDP and GBS. J Neurol Neurosurg Psychiatry. 2021;92(3):303-10.
65. Wieske L, Smyth D, Lunn MP, Eftimov F, Teunissen CE. Fluid biomarkers for monitoring structural changes in polyneuropathies: Their use in clinical practice and trials. Neurotherapeutics. 2021;18(4):2351-67.
66. Blinder T, Lewerenz J. Cerebrospinal fluid findings in patients with autoimmune encephalitis—A systematic analysis. Front Neurol. 2019;10:804.
67. Graus F, Titulaer MJ, Balu R, Benseler S, Bien CG, Cellucci T, et al. A clinical approach to diagnosis of autoimmune encephalitis. Lancet Neurol. 2016;15(4):391-404.
68. Abboud H, Probasco JC, Irani S, Ances B, Benavides DR, Bradshaw M, et al. Autoimmune encephalitis: proposed best practice recommendations for diagnosis and acute management. J Neurol Neurosurg Psychiatry. 2021;92(7):757-68.
69. Beuker C, Schmidt A, Strunk D, Sporns PB, Wiendl H, Meuth SG, et al. Primary angiitis of the central nervous system: diagnosis and treatment. Ther Adv Neurol Disord. 2018;11:1756286418785071.

70. Salvarani C, Brown RD, Calamia KT, Christianson TJH, Weigand SD, Miller DV, et al. Primary central nervous system vasculitis: analysis of 101 patients. Ann Neurol. 2007;62(5):442-51.
71. Zetterberg H. Cerebrospinal fluid biomarkers for Alzheimer's disease: Current limitations and recent developments. Curr Opin Psychiatry. 2015;28(5):402-9.
72. Blennow K, Dubois B, Fagan AM, Lewczuk P, Leon MJ, Hampel H. Clinical utility of cerebrospinal fluid biomarkers in the diagnosis of early Alzheimer's disease. Alzheimers Dementia. 2015;11(1): 58-69.
73. McKhann GM, Knopman DS, Chertkow H, Hyman BT, Jack CR, Kawas CH, et al. The diagnosis of dementia due to Alzheimer's disease: recommendations from the National Institute on Aging-Alzheimer's Association workgroups on diagnostic guidelines for Alzheimer's disease. Alzheimers Dement. 2011;7(3):263-9.
74. Katayama T, Sawada J, Takahashi K, Yahara O. Cerebrospinal fluid biomarkers in parkinson's disease: A critical overview of the literature and meta-analyses. Brain Sci. 2020;10(7):466.
75. Mollenhauer B, Locascio JJ, Schulz-Schaeffer W, Sixel-Döring F, Trenkwalder C, Schlossmacher MG. α-Synuclein and tau concentrations in cerebrospinal fluid of patients presenting with parkinsonism: A cohort study. Lancet Neurol. 2011;10(3):230-40.
76. Mollenhauer B, Trautmann E, Taylor P, Manninger P, Sixel-Döring F, Ebentheuer J, et al. Total CSF α-synuclein is lower in de novo Parkinson patients than in healthy subjects. Neurosci Lett. 2013;532:44-8.
77. Wennström M, Surova Y, Hall S, Nilsson C, Minthon L, Boström F, et al. Low CSF levels of both α-synuclein and the α-synuclein cleaving enzyme neurosin in patients with synucleinopathy. PLoS One. 2013;8(1):e53250.
78. Shi M, Bradner J, Hancock AM, Chung KA, Quinn JF, Peskind ER, et al. Cerebrospinal fluid biomarkers for parkinson disease diagnosis and progression. Ann Neurol. 2011;69(3):570-80.
79. Gao L, Tang H, Nie K, Wang L, Zhao J, Gan R, et al. Cerebrospinal fluid alpha-synuclein as a biomarker for Parkinson's disease diagnosis: a systematic review and meta-analysis. Int J Neurosci. 2015;125(9):645-54.
80. van Dijk KD, Bidinosti M, Weiss A, Raijmakers P, Berendse HW, van de Berg WDJ. Reduced α-synuclein levels in cerebrospinal fluid in Parkinson's disease are unrelated to clinical and imaging measures of disease severity. Eur J Neurol. 2014;21(3):388-94.
81. Magdalinou NK, Paterson RW, Schott JM, Fox NC, Mummery C, Blennow K, et al. A panel of nine cerebrospinal fluid biomarkers may identify patients with atypical parkinsonian syndromes. J Neurol Neurosurg Psychiatry. 2015;86(11):1240-7.
82. Lu CH, Macdonald-Wallis C, Gray E, Pearce N, Petzold A, Norgren N, et al. Neurofilament light chain: A prognostic biomarker in amyotrophic lateral sclerosis. Neurology. 2015;84(22):2247-57.
83. Steinacker P, Feneberg E, Weishaupt J, Brettschneider J, Tumani H, Andersen PM, et al. Neurofilaments in the diagnosis of motoneuron diseases: a prospective study on 455 patients. J Neurol Neurosurg Psychiatry. 2016;87(1):12-20.
84. Finkel RS, Chiriboga CA, Vajsar J, Day JW, Montes J, De Vivo DC, et al. Treatment of infantile-onset spinal muscular atrophy with nusinersen: a phase 2, open-label, dose-escalation study. Lancet. 2016;388(10063):3017-26.
85. Curran T, Lang AE. Parkinsonian syndromes associated with hydrocephalus: case reports, a review of the literature, and pathophysiological hypotheses. Mov Disord. 1994;9(5):508-20.
86. Townley RA, Botha H, Graff-Radford J, Boeve BF, Petersen RC, Senjem ML, et al. 18F-FDG PET-CT pattern in idiopathic normal pressure hydrocephalus. Neuroimage Clin. 2018;18:897-902.
87. Lenfeldt N, Larsson A, Nyberg L, Andersson M, Birgander R, Eklund A, et al. Idiopathic normal pressure hydrocephalus: increased supplementary motor activity accounts for improvement after CSF drainage. Brain. 2008;131(Pt 11):2904-12.
88. Williams MA, Malm J. Diagnosis and treatment of idiopathic normal pressure hydrocephalus. Continuum (Minneap Minn). 2016;22 (2 Dementia):579-99.
89. Wikkelsø C, Hellström P, Klinge PM, Tans JTJ, European iNPH Multicentre Study Group. The European iNPH Multicentre Study on the predictive values of resistance to CSF outflow and the CSF Tap Test in patients with idiopathic normal pressure hydrocephalus. J Neurol Neurosurg Psychiatry. 2013;84(5):562-8.
90. Markey KA, Mollan SP, Jensen RH, Sinclair AJ. Understanding idiopathic intracranial hypertension: mechanisms, management, and future directions. Lancet Neurol. 2016;15(1):78-91.
91. Matsui Y, Satoh K, Miyazaki T, Shirabe S, Atarashi R, Mutsukura K, et al. High sensitivity of an ELISA kit for detection of the gamma-isoform of 14-3-3 proteins: usefulness in laboratory diagnosis of human prion disease. BMC Neurology. 2011;11(1):120.
92. Castellani RJ, Colucci M, Xie Z, Zou W, Li C, Parchi P, et al. Sensitivity of 14-3-3 protein test varies in subtypes of sporadic Creutzfeldt-Jakob disease. Neurology. 2004;63(3):436-42.
93. Leitão MJ, Baldeiras I, Almeida MR, Ribeiro MH, Santos AC, Ribeiro M, et al. CSF Tau proteins reduce misdiagnosis of sporadic Creutzfeldt-Jakob disease suspected cases with inconclusive 14-3-3 result. J Neurol. 2016;263(9):1847-61.
94. Zanusso G, Fiorini M, Ferrari S, Gajofatto A, Cagnin A, Galassi A, et al. Cerebrospinal fluid markers in sporadic Creutzfeldt-Jakob disease. Int J Mol Sci. 2011;12(9):6281-92.
95. Lattanzio F, Abu-Rumeileh S, Franceschini A, Kai H, Amore G, Poggiolini I, et al. Prion-specific and surrogate CSF biomarkers in Creutzfeldt-Jakob disease: diagnostic accuracy in relation to molecular subtypes and analysis of neuropathological correlates of p-tau and Aβ42 levels. Acta Neuropathol. 2017;133(4):559-78.
96. Scott BJ, Douglas VC, Tihan T, Rubenstein JL, Josephson SA. A systematic approach to the diagnosis of suspected central nervous system lymphoma. JAMA Neurol. 2013;70(3):311-9.
97. Hoang-Xuan K, Bessell E, Bromberg J, Hottinger AF, Preusser M, Rudà R, et al. Diagnosis and treatment of primary CNS lymphoma in immunocompetent patients: guidelines from the European Association for Neuro-Oncology. Lancet Oncol. 2015;16(7): e322-32.
98. Tigchelaar S, Gupta R, Shannon CP, Streijger F, Sinha S, Flibotte S, et al. MicroRNA Biomarkers in Cerebrospinal Fluid and Serum Reflect Injury Severity in Human Acute Traumatic Spinal Cord Injury. J Neurotrauma. 2019;36(15):2358-71.
99. Yokobori S, Zhang Z, Moghieb A, Mondello S, Gajavelli S, Dietrich WD, et al. Acute diagnostic biomarkers for spinal cord injury: review of the literature and preliminary research report. World Neurosurg. 2015;83(5):867-78.
100. Kanmaz S, Simsek E, Yilmaz S, Durmaz A, Serin HM, Gokben S. Cerebral folate transporter deficiency: a potentially treatable neurometabolic disorder. Acta Neurol Belg. 2021;123(1):121-7.17.
101. Patti GJ, Yanes O, Siuzdak G. Innovation: Metabolomics: the apogee of the omics trilogy. Nat Rev Mol Cell Biol. 2012;13(4): 263-9.
102. van Waalwijk van Doorn LJC, Kulic L, Koel-Simmelink MJA, Kuiperij HB, Versleijen AAM, Struyfs H, et al. Multicenter Analytical Validation of Aβ40 Immunoassays. Front Neurol. 2017;6:179.
103. Gaetani L, Paolini Paoletti F, Bellomo G, Mancini A, Simoni S, Di Filippo M, et al. CSF and blood biomarkers in neuroinflammatory and neurodegenerative diseases: Implications for treatment. Trends Pharmacol Sci. 2020;41(12):1023-37.
104. Houldcroft CJ, Beale MA, Breuer J. Clinical and biological insights from viral genome sequencing. Nat Rev Microbiol. 2017;15(3): 183-92.
105. Angeletti S. Matrix assisted laser desorption time of flight mass spectrometry (MALDI-TOF MS) in clinical microbiology. J Microbiol Methods. 2017;138:20-9.

121
CHAPTER

Genetic Investigations

Avni Anand, Mohammed Faruq

INTRODUCTION

The discovery of nucleic acids by Miescher in conjunction with its discovery as the genetic material and the elucidation of key features by combined efforts of scientists like Watson, Crick,[1] Franklin, and Chargaff led to a long road of combinatorial research efforts across multiple interdisciplinary fields to gain a more fundamental understanding of the basis of life. With the recent advances in the field of genetics, the quest to satiate the desire to understand disease mechanisms and heritability has continued.[2,3]

In particular, the field of neurology has benefited from advances in fields of genetics along with neuroscience. In a clinical context, adjunct research in these fields aids in establishing causal relations between the molecular machinery as well as its dysfunctions. Before the use of recent genetic techniques to aid in clinical diagnosis, it was difficult to establish etiology for most disorders. A large degree of phenotypic heterogeneity is observed in neurological disorders and with no gold standard other than the clinicians' opinions, high rates of inaccuracy are usually observed. Consequently, vague descriptors have been used throughout history, and not much contribution to diagnostic, prognostic, and therapeutic information could be provided. However, more efficient techniques for genetic investigations have led to greater avenues for genetic testing and allow for genotype-phenotype correlation possibilities to help in evaluation and in the long run management of these clinical disorders to offer not only a better quality of life to patients, but also offer hope of disease modification. However, this is not without its own challenges. While some disorders are believed to arise due to mutations in particular genes (monogenic), most complex disorders such as Parkinson's disease (PD) and Alzheimer's disease (AD) have complex pathogenic mechanisms that result from an interplay between genetic and environmental factors. Even where monogenic forms of these disorders are concerned, a large range of variation is observed in terms of phenotype, age at onset, as well as severity.[4] Thus, the boundaries of sporadic or idiopathic and familial are constantly challenged. In view of the expanding horizons of genetic testing and its role in dissection of brain function and disease, it is imperative for neurologists to gain a deep understanding of human genetics to become equipped with a repertoire of tools to face clinical challenges. Here, we aim to prime the readers to certain essentials, including the wide-varying genetic mechanisms that are crucial to understand complex neurological problems, highlight some important technologies at our disposal to aid in diagnosis, and present a few examples of how these can be incorporated to achieve diagnostic accuracy. The chapter also aims to highlight certain challenges that arise in this crusade for establishing a diagnosis and how solving these would pave the way for genomic medicine.

HISTORY OF GENETIC INVESTIGATIONS IN NEUROLOGY

Historically, the interest in genetics around neuroscience began as early as in the 1970s and before that much of neuroscience pertains to neurophysiological research for synapse, neurotransmission-related studies, and neuropathology at large. The genetic research for gene mapping in neuromuscular disease, i.e., Duchenne muscular dystrophy (DMD) (mapped in 1979) and neurodegenerative disorder, i.e., Huntington's disease (HD) (mapped in 1983) opened up avenues for solving other related disorders and also paved the way for the Human Genome Sequencing Project. Like HD, the importance of tandem nucleotide repeats (TNRs) in causing neurodegenerative disorders and thus proteinopathies helped in the identification of spinocerebellar ataxias and spinobulbar muscular atrophy. Akin to the later identification of the causal defect in DMD, i.e., deletion, identification of PMP22 deletion with Charcot Marie tooth Disease took place in 1994. The two decades following the HGP have witnessed rapid expansion in the interest to solve a variety of neurogenetic disorders and it

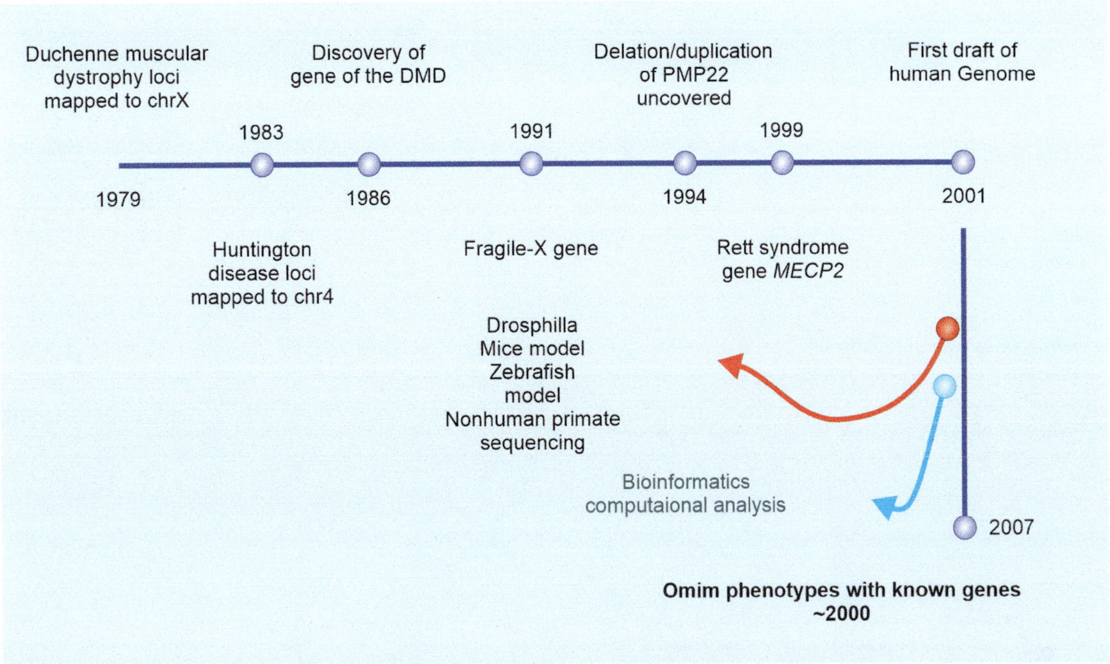

FIG. 1: Timeline detailing history of genetic investigation in neurology starting with mapping of DMD to chromosome X. The years after the HGP have witnessed vast improvements in the field of neurogenetics. As advancement in fields of experimental and computational neuroscience ushers in an era of rapid gene and phenotype discovery, it is imperative to incorporate genetic investigations into clinical neurology.

(DMD: Duchenne muscular dystrophy; HGP: Human Genome Project)

continues with more advancement in the field. The period after drafting of human genome sequencing has seen newfound interest in the development of the animal models of respective genetic disorders for better insights into the mechanism of the disease to understand the large spectrum of sporadic cases of each neurodegenerative disorder (AD, PD, motor neuron disease, and cerebellar ataxias). Time since 2007, the evolution of DNA sequencing methodologies to the next-generation sequencing (NGS) platforms allowed rapid growth in the discovery of novel genes and neurogenetic disorders. This eventually has brought the scope for computational research (Bioinformatics) in genetics for the extensive analysis of big data. The NGS methodologies allow parallel sequencing of hundreds of human genomes and thousands of coding regions of the genomes on a single run and with a rapid turnaround time. The expansion in the nucleotide data generation brings several challenges, not only the interpretations but also the annotations. The science of DNA variation and its correct interpretation needs a next-phase revolution for understanding the new scope of therapeutic developments and disease modification **(Fig. 1)**.

VARIATIONS IN THE HUMAN GENOME

Following the discernment of DNA structure and replication by DNA polymerase enzyme, it was noted that although DNA replication machinery is quite precise and efficient and there are numerous surveillance mechanisms involving cellular preventive proofreading and repair, the process of replication allows for DNA damage to be incorporated with an error rate of approximately $1–1.8 \times 10^{-8}$ per nucleotide, resulting in about 50 de novo point mutations and a smaller number of larger mutations with each genome replication. As these mutations are not uniformly distributed in the genome, subject to sequence complexity with some areas having a greater propensity for mutation, and do not contribute to disease risk in a uniform way, a deeper, more fundamental understanding of these mutations underpins the clinical evaluation and in the long run management of neurological disorders.[5]

TYPES OF DNA SEQUENCE VARIATIONS

Typically, a human genome exhibits 4–5 million variations of which 99.9% are single nucleotide change or small insertion or deletions. The remaining DNA changes are contributed by structural variations, i.e., large deletion, duplication, rearrangements, and repetitive regions nucleotide sequence alterations.

Single-nucleotide variations (SNVs) occur due to transition (T>C/A>G) or transversion (purines > pyrimidines) changes at the nucleotide level giving rise to alternative alleles. They are exceedingly common and occur with a frequency of 1 every 300–1000[6] base pairs in the human genome with a cumulative count of 4–5 million/genomes

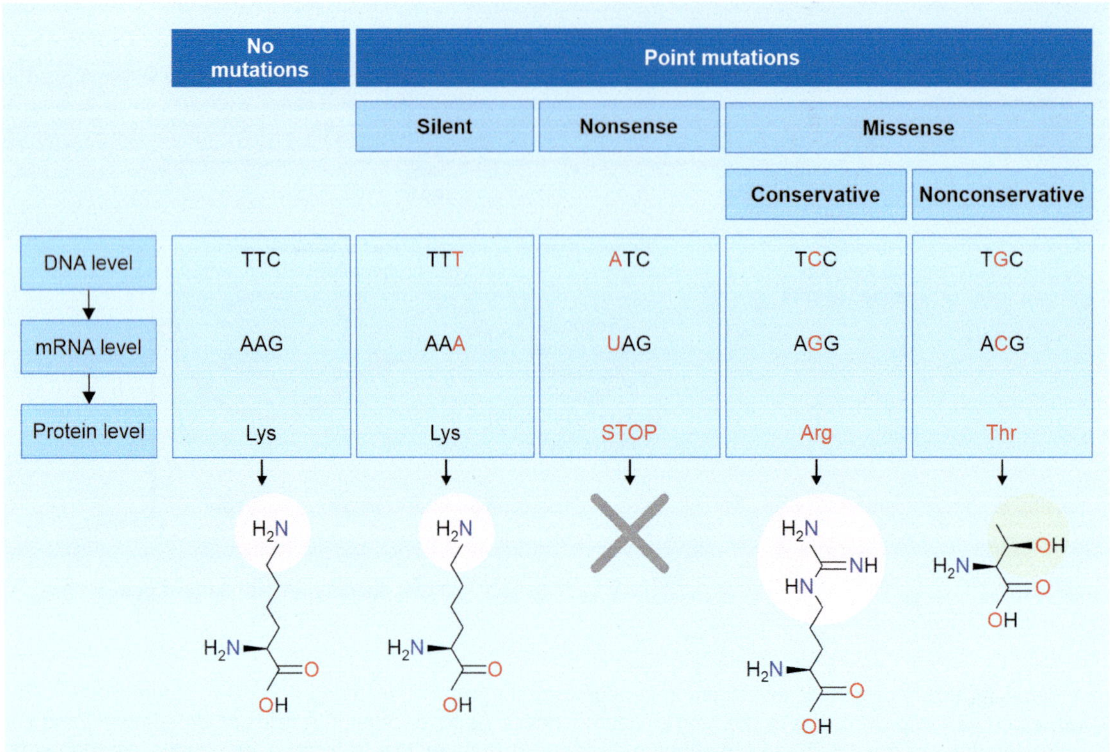

FIG. 2: Types of point mutations: Note that conservative mutations refer to the replacement of an amino acid with similar properties while nonconservative mutations result in a completely different type of amino acid being added and thus may produce more severe changes.

and the majority of them reside in noncoding region of the DNA (junk DNA) as SNVs in expressed content of genome (2% gene coding regions).

Variations in the genic regions are broadly categorized as exonic, intronic, and promoter region variations. SNVs particularly in coding regions are associated with the majority of the Mendelian (monogenic) disorders observed in numbers 12,000/genome, meaning not all SNVs in coding regions are pathogenic and those with pathogenicity are termed commonly as mutations **(Fig. 2)**.

Exonic Region Variations

- Missense (nonsynonymous) variations—leading to a change in the amino acid sequence. [HGVS nomenclature: These are represented in the diagnostic setting at DNA level with reference to coding reference sequence denoted by the prefix "c", followed by the start codon (ATG). The first base is numbered 1 and CDS that ends at the last position of the stop codon. A reference sequence ID of gene transcript has to be provided that starts with NM_001875, for example, ARSA (NM_001085425.3): c.1296G>T (p.Asp432Tyr). If c. nucleotide position (if it is the last base of a codon) is divided by 3, then we can get the reference amino acid position p.432 in this case.] *Source*: *https://varnomen.hgvs.org*
- Nonsense variations leading to a premature stop codon and thus a truncated protein (PTC) [HGVS nomenclature: denoted by *, e.g., c.4375C>T and p.Gln1459*]
- Silent variations (synonymous) are coding region variations that do not alter the amino acid sequence and thus the resulting protein but in some instances may influence transcript level expression or RNA splicing. [HGVS: denoted by the same scheme as for missense but without amino acid change, NM_001005484:exon1:c.G462C:p.Ala154Ala
- Untranslated region (UTR) variations are those variations that are found in the untranslated sequence of mRNA that flanks the coding sequence, i.e., 5′ upstream region and 3′upstream region, respectively. The UTR region variations can affect mRNA stability, mRNA expression regulation, as well as binding of regulatory proteins and miRNAs. In a genome, nearly 37,000 UTR site variations are observed. [HGVS nomenclature: UTR region comes after CDS hence denoted by * after c. position, i.e., c.*49C>G]

Intronic Regions Variations

Introns are larger than exonic regions and harbor a great number of variations, i.e., 2.6 million/genome. SNVs at canonical splice sites (GT-AG) on exon-intron boundaries affect splicing of the exons (skipping of the exon) and thus would result in a change in the length of protein sequence (truncated or elongated).

Other intronic variations may be associated with the disease if they affect gene expression through mechanisms such as alternative splicing. Splicing defects are exceedingly common in neurodegenerative disorders. One such example is that of amyotrophic lateral sclerosis (ALS) wherein aberrant splicing in EAAT2 (excitatory amino acid transporter 2) leads to a decrease in the amount of functional protein and thus the disease phenotype.[7] [HGVS nomenclature: denoted by "-" sign or plus sign depending upon the proximity to the nearest c. position. If proximal to upstream exon then the distance from the last base of exon, e.g., c.342 base is added with "+" sign, i.e., c.342+30 C>A or if the intronic variation is proximal to downstream exon then the distance from the first base of that exon c.343 is placid with "-" sign, i.e., c.343-5 G>A. Splice site variations are located ±2 position, e.g., ;NM_199349:exon9:c.749-1G>A.].

Single-nucleotide variations in promoter regions of the genes have regulatory consequences and alter the level of gene expressions. [HGVS nomenclature: located upstream of the first base of coding sequence (c.), hence gets a minus sign, e.g., c.–35 C>A].

Small Insertion and Deletion Variations

Deletion or insertion involving few base pairs (1–10 kb) coding regions may lead to frame shift variations (non-multiples of 3) and may result in either premature truncating mutations or extension of the protein sequence. These frameshift variations are most regarded as disease-causing as they often lead to absent or nonfunctional truncated proteins, premature stop codons lead to nonsense-mediated mRNA decay, and dominant negative effect. However, in a human genome, 100–200 occurrences are observed and not all have functional consequences, implying alternative mechanisms at the transcript level (alternate splice isoforms), stop codon read-through, or limited functional loss. However, often the functional implications of these variants are difficult to establish without experimental validation or strong statistical evidence as even the complete knockout of one allele by a premature stop codon, which is known as haploinsufficiency, may not lead to disease[8] [HGVS nomenclature: refer https://varnomen.hgvs.org].

Chromosomal Abnormalities and Errors of Copy Number Variations (Structural Variations)

The newfound knowledge obtained from sequencing of the human genome formed the basis for the discovery of copy number variations (CNVs) and their ubiquitous nature. Since then, improvements in technology such as the incorporation of microarray in the genomic investigation have indicated that CNVs are more common than previously believed and may comprise as much as 12–18% of the human genome with 3–7 rare variations being present in an average genome.[9]

Despite the relatively benign nature of the majority of CNVs, numerous of these variations have been linked to a wide variety of disorders including intellectual disability, congenital anomalies, and neurodegenerative as well as neuropsychiatric problems.[10,11]

Errors of chromosomal replication and recombination can result in large duplications, deletions, inversions, translocations, or insertions via mechanisms such as nonallelic homologous recombination, nonhomologous end joining and replication error mechanisms including fork stalling, and template switching. These structural variations that can range from kilobases to megabases and are hard to detect via chromosomal banding are termed CNVs.[10]

Copy number variations affect disease states through a variety of mechanisms that vary depending on their size, genomic location, as well as gene content. Most often, the alteration of dosage-sensitive genes affects disease phenotype, as seen in Charcot–Marie–Tooth disease type 1A/hereditary neuropathy with pressure palsies (CMT1A/HNPP) as well as DMD and spinal muscular atrophy (SMA). Other mechanisms include disruption of gene expression through disruption of regulatory elements as well as haploinsufficiency **(Fig. 3)**.[12-17]

Tandem Nucleotide Repeats

With more than a million annotated tandem repeats present, TNRs constitute a large portion of the human genome. These repeats have a mutational rate and are usually used as markers (microsatellite or minisatellite) in genetic linkage analyses. In healthy subjects, most of these TNRs exhibit a length polymorphism and have a range (locus specific), and once cross a threshold that is also locus specific, these result in pathologies, e.g., Huntington disease, spinocerebellar ataxias, spinobulbar muscular dystrophies, etc. **(Table 1)**. Owing to the dynamic nature of TNRs, dominant repeat expansion disorders show expansion across generations known as anticipation, which results in clinical manifestation at earlier ages.[18] These repeat expansions can occur in coding as well as noncoding regions, and when present in coding regions, these lead to the production of long tracts of polyglutamine (CAG) or may be translated into alternative reading frames to give other peptide species (polyserine, polyalanine, or dipeptide repeats) which ultimately lead to protein oligomerization and formation of protein aggregates (toxic gain-of-function).[19]

Noncoding repeat expansions exhibit a wider range and variability in terms of location, length, and type of repeat motif, with more GC-rich repeat motifs present in regulatory regions which are often linked to hypermethylation and gene silencing.[20] There are several other mechanisms by which these repeats can cause disease **(Fig. 4)**.

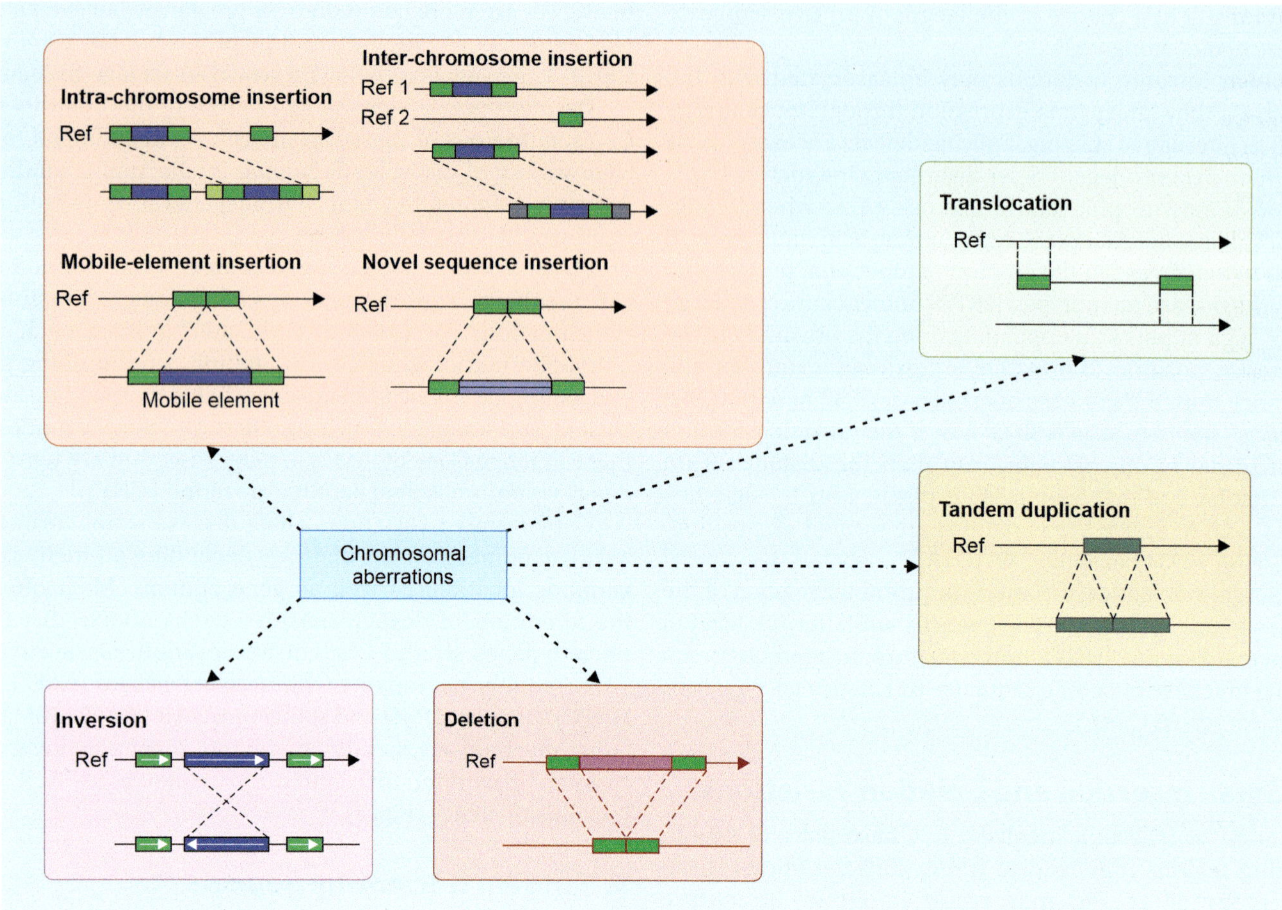

FIG. 3: Types of chromosomal aberrations include insertions, translocations, duplications, deletions, and inversions.

TABLE 1: List of some recently identified repeat expansion disorders.

Disorder	Type of inheritance	Gene	Location	Repeat motif
Fragile X syndrome (FXS)	XLD	*FMR1*	5'UTR	CGG (>200)
Myotonic dystrophy type 1 (DM1)	AD	*DMPK*	3'UTR	CTG
Fragile XE syndrome (FRAXE)	XLR	*AFF2*	5'UTR	CCG
Friedreich ataxia (FRDA)	AR	*FXN*	Intron	GAA
Spinocerebellar ataxia 8 (SCA8)	AD	*ATXN8*	3'UTR	CTG/CAG
Spinocerebellar ataxia 12 (SCA12)	AD	*PPP2R2B*	5'UTR	CAG
Spinocerebellar ataxia 10 (SCA10)	AD	*ATXN10*	Intron	ATTCT
Fragile X-associated tremor ataxia syndrome (FXTAS)	XLR	*FMR1*	5'UTR	CGG (>50–200)
Frontotemporal dementia/amyotrophic lateral sclerosis (FTD/ALS)	AD	*C9ORF72*	5'UTR/intron	GGGGCC
Cerebellar ataxia, neuropathy and vestibular areflexia syndrome (CANVAS)	AR	*RFC1*	Intron	AAGGG
Neuronal intranuclear inclusion disease (NIID)	AD	*NOTCH2NLC*	5'UTR	CGG
Huntington disease (HD)	AD	*HTT*	Exon	CAG
Spinocerebellar ataxia 1 (SCA1)	AD	*ATXN1*	Exon	CAG
Spinocerebellar ataxia 2 (SCA2)	AD	*ATXN2*	Exon	CAG
Spinocerebellar ataxia 3 (SCA3)	AD	*ATXN3*	Exon	CAG
Spinocerebellar ataxia 6 (SCA6)	AD	*CACNA1A*	Exon	CAG

Continued

Continued

Disorder	Type of inheritance	Gene	Location	Repeat motif
Spinocerebellar ataxia 7 (SCA7)	AD	*ATXN7*	Exon	CAG
Spinocerebellar ataxia 17 (SCA17)	AD	*TBP*	Exon	CAG
Spinal and bulbar muscular atrophy (SBMA)	XLR	*AR*	Exon	CAG
Dentatorubral–pallidoluysian atrophy (DRPLA)	AD	*ATN1*	Exon	CAG
Synpolydactyly type 1 (SPD1)	AD	*HOXD13*	Exon	GCG
Oculopharyngeal muscular dystrophy (OPMD)	AD	*PABPN1*	Exon	GCG

[AD: autosomal dominant; AR: autosomal recessive; UTR: untranslated region; CAG: polyQ (polyglutamine); GCG: polyA (polyalanine); XLD: X-linked dominant; XLR: X-linked recessive]

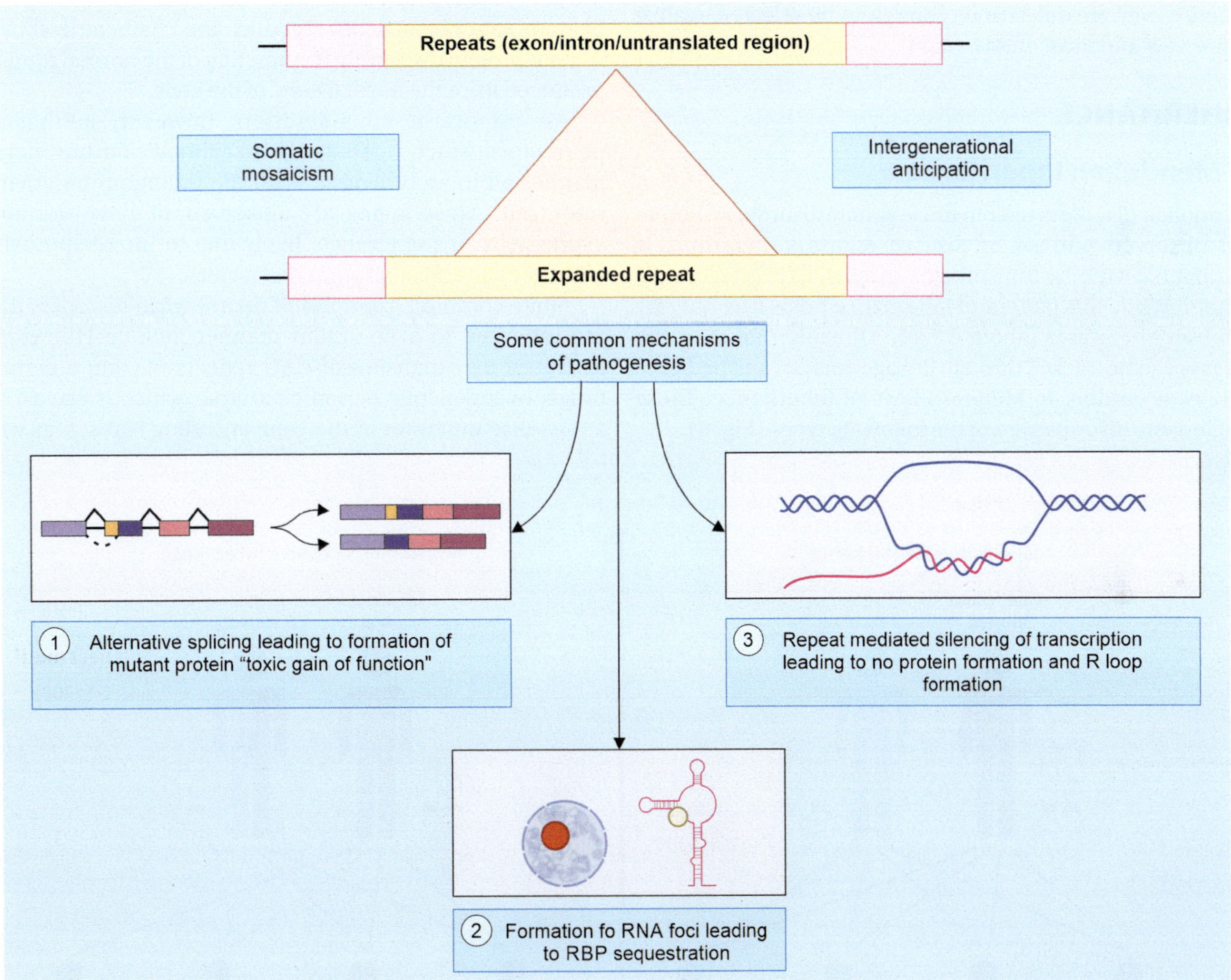

FIG. 4: Repeat expansion disorders: Varied disease mechanisms include repeat-mediated toxicity and protein-mediated toxicity.

Rare and Common Variations

The genetic basis of disorders including neurological diseases has been the topic of much debate in the past decades. Recent advances in molecular biology techniques and the advent of NGS have been instrumental in discerning the genetic architecture of complex disorders. The most common mutations in the human genomes are point mutations or SNVs, with an estimated of about 3.5 million SNVs reported in the human genome and around 30,000–40,000 SNVs in the coding region (2% region that codes for genes/proteins) of the genome.[21] While other mutations such as TNR length polymorphisms expansions and structural variants (deletions, duplications, and inversions) are relatively rarer. In accordance with the principles of natural selection, most genetic mutations are not deleterious, and the resulting phenotype often acts as a source of evolution. For clinical application, it is often helpful to classify variants as rare and common by setting an arbitrary cut off (often 1% of the population frequency) while still appreciating that genetic variation is a continuum and any clean-cut categorical classification is not fruitful to the overall dissection of disease understanding. Common variants, often termed polymorphisms, occur with a frequency of >1% in the population and are not deleterious enough to cause disease. These are, therefore, adaptive and not subjected to very strong negative selection pressure. Contrary to these, rare variants are less prevalent in the population either because they are deleterious enough to be selected against or are new and most often benign.

INHERITANCE

Mendelian Inheritance

Mendelian disorders refer to those simple disorders wherein the observed pattern of disease across generations is compatible with the transmission through alleles at a single locus.[22] While this pattern of inheritance holds true only for a subset of diseases (about 6,000),[23] the inheritance of the disease can be tracked through linkage analysis and pedigree studies according to Mendel's laws of inheritance. These single-gene disorders are of the following types **(Fig. 5)**.

Autosomal Dominant

Autosomal dominant inheritance refers to the pattern of transmission of disease which requires only one of the alleles of the gene to be mutated or dysfunctional for the individual (heterozygous) to show the phenotype. These pathogenic mutations are often associated with a toxic gain of function which imparts a new functionality. The risk of transmission in autosomal dominantly inherited disorders is 50% as only one deleterious copy of the gene is required to produce the disease phenotype in the offspring, with males and females being at equal risk. The disease may also occur through haploinsufficiency wherein inactivation of one allele of the gene is sufficient to produce the disease phenotype or by dominant negative effects which are characterized by a mutant protein disrupting the function of the normal protein produced from the normal copy of the gene.

An important consideration, however, is that of penetrance which refers to the likelihood of a trait being manifested in an individual with the mutation underlying said trait. Most genes are observed to have variable expressivity or penetrance, likely due to interaction with other genetic and environmental factors.

Some common examples of neurological disorders that are inherited in a dominant manner include HD which is caused by expansion of CAG repeats beyond a certain range, hyperkalemic periodic paralysis which is caused by a missense mutation in the gene encoding NaV1.4, as well

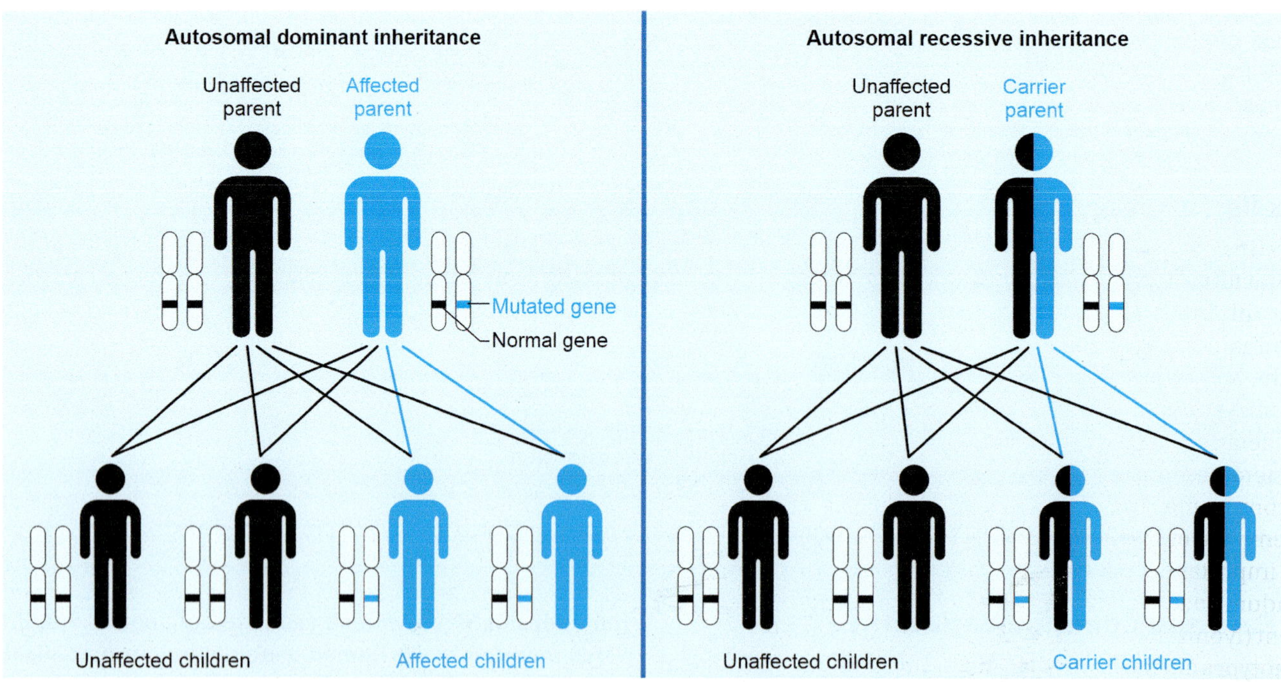

FIG. 5: Modes of inheritance in mendelian disorders—autosomal dominant and autosomal recessive.

as Charcot–Marie–Tooth type 1B caused by mutations in the *MPZ* gene.

Autosomal Recessive

Autosomal recessive inheritance refers to diseases that require two copies of the mutated allele to be present for the person to show the disease phenotype. An unaffected individual with just one copy of the mutated allele is called a carrier. To manifest the disease phenotype, an individual has to be either homozygous, i.e., two identical alleles, or compound heterozygous, i.e., two different pathogenic alleles. Autosomal recessive disorders usually manifest as a loss of function due to the loss of both copies of functional alleles and subsequently functional proteins.

Males and females tend to be equally affected and a loss of intergenerational transmission is observed. For an individual to be affected, both parents must at least possess one copy of the mutant allele, i.e., be carriers or be afflicted with the disease themselves. In rare cases, it is possible to observe cases of pseudodominance wherein a carrier parent has children with an afflicted parent resulting in a greater possibility of disease phenotype in children (0.5 compared to 0.25) resulting in horizontal transmission which can be differentiated from vertical transmission observed in autosomal dominant cases with the help of a pedigree.

Autosomal recessive cerebellar ataxias are examples of disorders exhibiting autosomal recessive inheritance involving both the central and peripheral nervous systems in most cases characterized by an early onset of phenotype. Other examples of such disorders include Friedreich ataxia caused by a GAA repeat expansion in *FXN* gene, SMA-1 caused by deletion of exon 7 in SMN1, and Wilson Disease caused by a mutation in ATP7B which leads to copper overload in affected individuals.

Sex-linked Disorders

Sex-linked disorders refer primarily to disorders characterized by a gene on the X chromosome in humans. The inheritance can either be sex chromosome linked dominant or recessive. Since males possess only one copy of the X chromosome and thus genes on this chromosome (hemizygous), any mutation on these genes is expressed by default in males leading to the disease phenotype. As females possess two copies of all genes on the X chromosome, they are usually carriers and express the phenotype only when both copies of the allele are mutated. An important consideration in females is the occurrence of random inactivation of X chromosomes during development (lyonization). Thus, females possess cells with different genotypes and are mosaics for these disorders.

X-linked recessive single-gene disorders are more frequently observed in men than women due to the presence of only one gene. For females to display the disease phenotype, both the inherited alleles need to carry the mutation which is rare and thus women are more likely to be carriers for the trait. Examples of XLR disorders include DMD which is caused by mutations in the dystrophin gene DMD as well hemophilia A which is caused by a mutation in the factor VIII gene.

In contrast, X-linked dominant disorders are equally likely in both males and females as only one mutated copy can affect the disease phenotype. Rett syndrome is a common example of XLD. It is a neurodevelopmental disease linked to dominant mutations in the *MECP2* gene (methyl-CpG-binding protein 2 gene). It is almost exclusively observed in females because male embryos with a dominant mutation in the gene do not survive.

Y-linked disorders are even more rarely observed than X-linked disorders and due to the characteristic presence of Y chromosomes, these are only observed in males and inherited from fathers. Unlike X-linked disorders, these mutations whether dominant or recessive are always linked to the disease phenotype as only one copy of the gene is present.

Linkage Analysis

As disorders are identified in individuals and added to rapidly expanding knowledge, the need to identify causal genes is impressed upon the scientific community. In cases of disorders that are inherited in accordance with Mendelian principles, linkage analysis is the main tool to help narrow down the possibilities and arrive at the insult-causing gene. Linkage analysis has been used for many years to examine the segregation of traits. This method relies on sufficient data being available from the family (minimum of 10 informative meiosis) to be able to trace the inheritance of the trait of interest across generations and is used to identify the area of chromosome likely to contain the gene responsible for a trait. It involves the identification of a region of DNA termed a marker (polymorphic) that segregates with the trait being studied. In principle, two loci on a chromosome segregate independently of one another. However, as recombination is less likely to occur between two points that are closer compared to those that are farther away, segments of DNA in close proximity with each other are said to be linked and thus segregate together. Disequilibrium refers to an increased degree of linkage observed than would be expected by chance. Subsequently, through this study, the disease can be narrowed down to a region of the chromosome (likely to contain more than one gene). Important to note is the fact that if the more informative meiosis is included (i.e., meiosis that occurs when a parent is heterozygous for the polymorphic marker as well as the disease allele so the inheritance of different alleles can be tracked in the offspring), the shared peak region can be narrowed down.[24] Subsequently, a more robust investigation employing DNA-sequencing techniques can help to identify the causal gene. Several disorders have been investigated this way including DMD, Wilson disease, Von Hippel–Lindau syndrome, as well as Friedreich ataxia. However, it is of limited utility in cases of complex traits or when insufficient family data is present.

Non-Mendelian Forms of Inheritance

In clinical genetic settings, it is common to come across cases that show a clear genetic component with familial inheritance and recurrence across generations, but the inheritance pattern cannot be clearly ascribed to Mendelian patterns of inheritance. These cases house an added degree of complexity in counseling and treatment. A few key mechanisms of non-Mendelian inheritance are highlighted here.

Mitochondrial Disorders

Mitochondria are double membrane-bound organelles primarily responsible for cellular energy production via the process of oxidative phosphorylation. Incorporated into eukaryotes because of an endosymbiotic event, mitochondria have their own genomes. These 37 genes encode proteins required for the normal functioning of the cell. These organelles are present in the cytoplasm and are inherited from the maternal line as most of the cytoplasm in the zygote is derived from the egg with sperm mitochondria being eliminated. Replicative segregation refers to the random distribution of these mitochondria during cell division and in presence of a mutation in some mitochondria can result in a state of homoplasmy, i.e., daughter cell receiving all wildtype or all mutant mitochondria or more commonly heteroplasmy, i.e., a mix of wildtype and mutant mitochondria. As a cell contains multiple mitochondria which divide independently of the nucleus, as cells continue to divide, this state of heteroplasmy is subject to change. Also, only 13 of the ~1,500 proteins required for mitochondrial function are encoded by mtDNA with nDNA coding for the rest. As a result, these disorders show Mendelian patterns of inheritance and can involve defects in mtDNA maintenance, translation, or mitochondrial homeostasis **(Fig. 6)**.[25]

As mitochondria are responsible for energy production to meet the cellular metabolic needs through the shuttling of electrons between several complexes, dysfunction in mitochondrial bioenergetics can lead to several disorders, including neurological problems. These diseases typically manifest as dysfunctional dynamics of high-energy consuming organs including the brain, heart, and kidneys. Poor growth in tandem with muscular atrophy or weakness and movement problems are warning signs. Some mitochondrial disorders are MELAS (mitochondrial encephalomyopathy, lactic acidosis, and stroke-like episodes) which is caused by mutations within the gene coding for mitochondrial tRNA, MERRF (myoclonic epilepsy with ragged-red fibers) which is characterized by clumps of diseased mitochondria accumulating in the subsarcolemmal region of the muscle fiber and visualized when the muscle is stained with modified Gömöri trichrome stain, and NARP (neuropathy, ataxia, retinitis pigmentosa, and ptosis).[26,27]

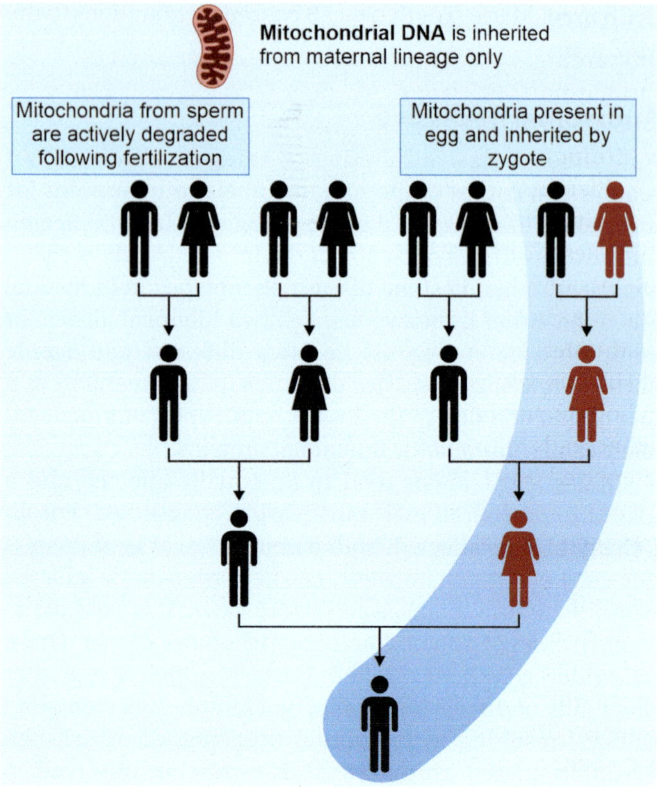

FIG. 6: Mitochondrial inheritance is maternal.

Epigenetics and Imprinting Disorders

Epigenetics refers to differences in gene expression caused by modifications other than sequence variations and refers to modifications of genes that determine whether the genes are expressed. The two most common types of epigenetic changes are methylation and acetylation. While the latter is invariably linked to expression upregulation, methylation can lead to both upregulation and downregulation.

Imprinting refers to the variation in expression of genes depending on whether it was inherited from the mother or the father and arises from epigenetic modifications which are parent specific. For example, some genes are silenced by DNA methylation during the formation of gametes in a sex-specific manner which allows the gene expression to be driven by the allele derived from the other parent. Two classic examples of disorders related to imprinting are Prader-Willi and Angelman syndromes which are characterized by loss of paternal and maternal patterning of the genes on chromosome 15q. Prader-Willi syndrome is characterized by hypotonia, low birth weight and later obesity as well as mental retardation and hypogonadism.[28] On the other hand, Angelman syndrome is characterized by mental retardation along with abnormal facies and seizures. A significant portion of both these disorders are due to uniparental disomy (UPD).[29]

Uniparental Disomy and Imprinting Disorders

Uniparental disomy refers to the occurrence of both chromosomes in a pair from one parent. It is of two types:

1. *Uniparental isodisomy*: Both chromosomes are identical.
2. *Uniparental heterodisomy*: Two chromosomes are different.

Uniparental disomy usually occurs due to resolved trisomies wherein the zygote is usually initially trisomic but the loss of extra chromosome results in two chromosomes from the same parent. Apart from Angelman and Prader-Willi syndromes, Beckwith-Wiedemann syndrome is an example of UPD, in which loss of maternal imprinting pattern due to both copies of chromosome 11 being received from the father leads to problems including neonatal hypoglycemia, lateralized overgrowth, and defects in the abdominal wall.[30]

COMPLEX DISEASE GENETICS

Unlike the previously discussed simple Mendelian disorders, most disorders that neurologists encounter in a clinical setting are unlikely to be explained by mutations in one gene. While most neurological disorders have a significant genetic contribution **(Table 2)**, it is difficult to establish a clear genetic cause in the majority of cases.

A more likely explanation is that most diseases have a genetic and an environmental component. While the relative degree of these might differ with different disorders, in the real world, interaction between genetic and environmental components drives pathogenesis.

While monogenic forms of disorders are characterized by mutations in a single causal gene, polygenic inheritance recognizes that the heritability (genetic influence) of a gene cannot be explained by a single gene, and it is likely several genes with variable effect size (risk alleles) that together contribute to the pathogenesis. This interplay between genetic and environmental factors, none of which can sufficiently affect the process of disease development to cause the phenotype but each of which confers a small risk and thus increases susceptibility, forms the basis of the common disease-common variant (CDCV) hypothesis **(Fig. 7)**.

Genome-wide association studies (GWAS), based on the CDCV hypothesis, are employed in identifying genetic risk factors and candidate genes over linkage analysis. The approach is based on the hypothesis that the major contributors to genetic susceptibility to disease are many common low-risk alleles or genetic variations with appreciable frequency and low penetrance.

These studies focus on genetic variation across the human genome to pinpoint genetic associations with the presence or absence of observable diseases or traits.[40]

The single nucleotide polymorphisms (SNPs) are thought of as markers for a particular genomic location or gene that influences the disease.

Genome-wide association studies present a useful tool in delineating causality to genes in neurological problems and have been utilized in ALS, multiple sclerosis (MS), PD, strokes, as well as AD. For example, some alleles of *IL2RA* and *IL7RA* genes have been strongly linked to MS with an odds ratio range of 1.11–1.36 and 1.11–1.26, respectively[41] **(Fig. 8)**.

It is important to note however that GWAS results only indicate genes that may be linked to disease and are not the equivalent of disease genes. GWAS helps to identify common variants with a reduced penetrance because if these variants had a big effect size, they would have been selected against by natural selection and the inheritance would follow Mendelian patterns. It is possible that these genes are associated with disease modifiers and instead of directly causing pathogenesis, their interaction with other genes

TABLE 2: Some complex neurological problems and their heritability: Despite the vast advancements, there are still significant gaps in our knowledge of these disorders and what exactly triggers them.

Disease	Heritability	Reference
Alzheimer disease	58%	31
Amyotrophic lateral sclerosis	21%	32
Attention-deficit hyperactivity disorder	68%	33
Autism spectrum disorder	53%	34
Epilepsy	26%	35
Multiple sclerosis	64%	36
Multiple system atrophy	2.09–6.65%	37
Obsessive compulsive disorder	56%	33
Parkinson disease	34%	38
Schizophrenia	41–87%	39

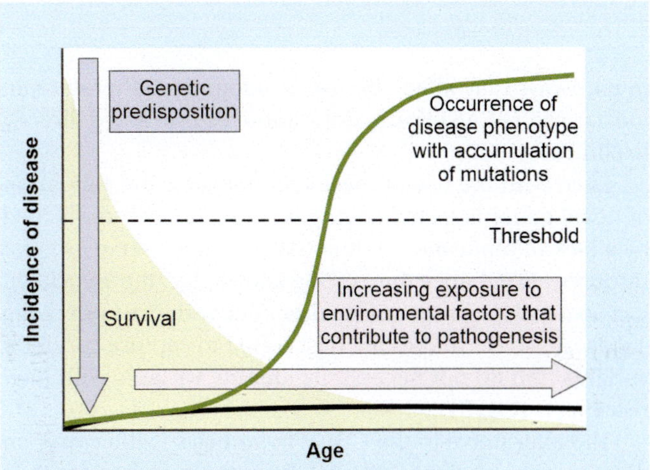

FIG. 7: Incidence of a disease increases exponentially as mutations (due to genetic and environmental factors) accumulate with age (quantitative model).

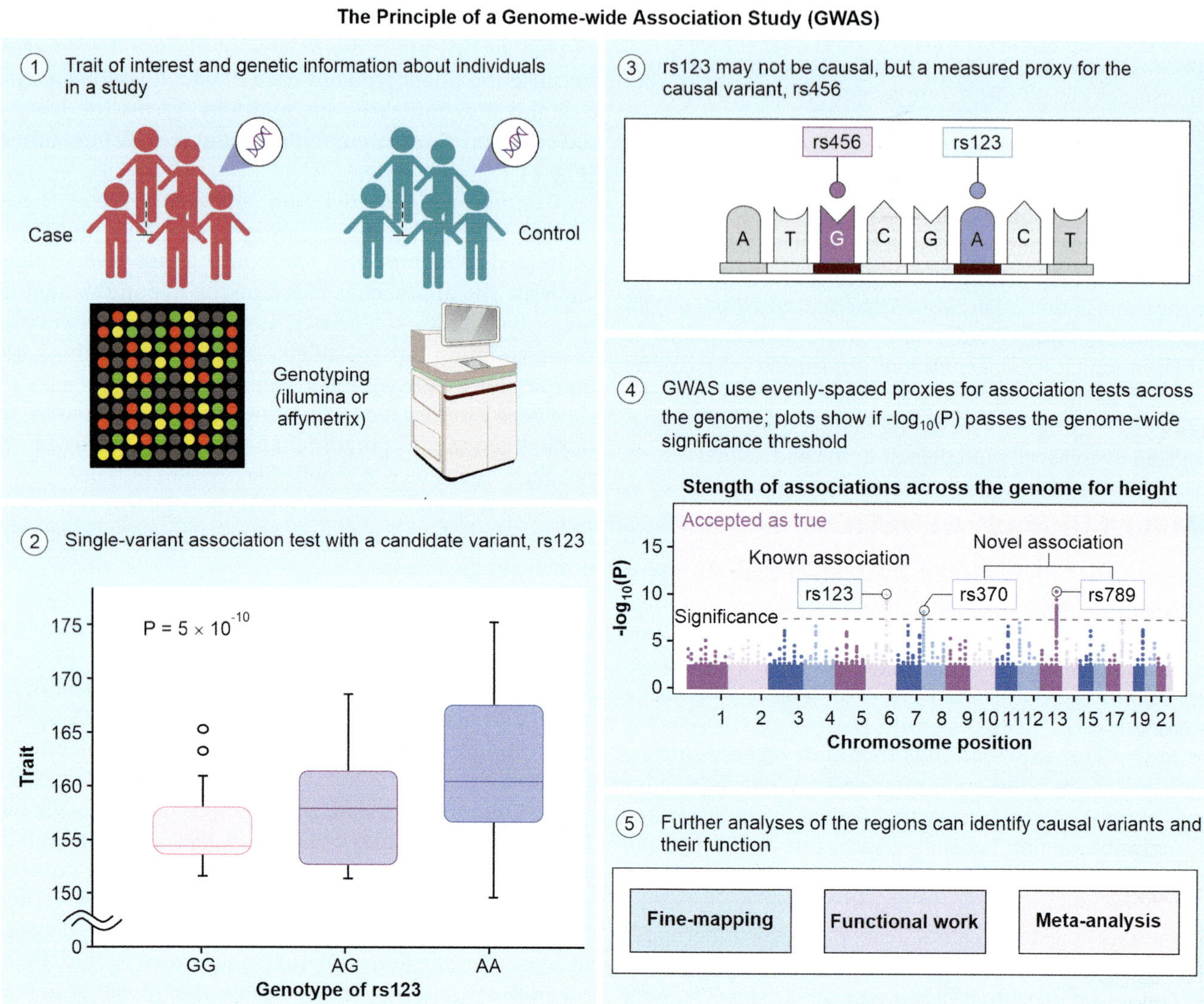

FIG. 8: GWAS helps to identify common variants that may be contributing to the disease through genotyping of diseases individuals and healthy controls by microarray or other technologies to aid in the detection of SNPs across the genome. This helps in identifying if any SNP could be associated with the disease (odds ratio >1).

(GWAS: genome-wide association study; SNP: single nucleotide polymorphism)

in pathways may affect disease development. Therefore, in most cases, GWAS information cannot be translated directly to clinical settings.

Even with the use of these technologies, the validation of novel genes is a challenging process, often complicated by a lack of replication. While GWAS studies serve as great resources to enhance the existing knowledge, the associated loci do not always account for all genetic variance underlying a disease. These studies are best suited to capture common variants and do not necessarily identify variants with low-risk effects **(Fig. 9)**.

The alternative to the CDCV hypothesis is the common disease–rare variant (CDRV) hypothesis wherein it is believed that instead of common SNPs with small effect size, it is the rare variant with intermediate to large effect size (or de novo mutations) that constitutes the genetic make-up of complex disorders. Common variants have only been able to explain a fraction of the genetic constituents and lead to the problem of missing heritability. In the CDRV model, it is the rare variant that occurs with a frequency of <1% that alone or in conjunction with other common variants causes the disease.[42] Identification of these variants depends on the resequencing of a number of candidate genes.

Next-generation sequencing (see Technical Aspects) technology facilitates gene identification through sequencing of the entire genome or exome and has been instrumental in identifying rare variants with a strong risk effect. This helps to provide genetic information which can be used to make a timely diagnosis and develop appropriate therapies, a process often complicated due to the genetically heterogeneous composition of most neurological disorders. However, considering the fact that compared

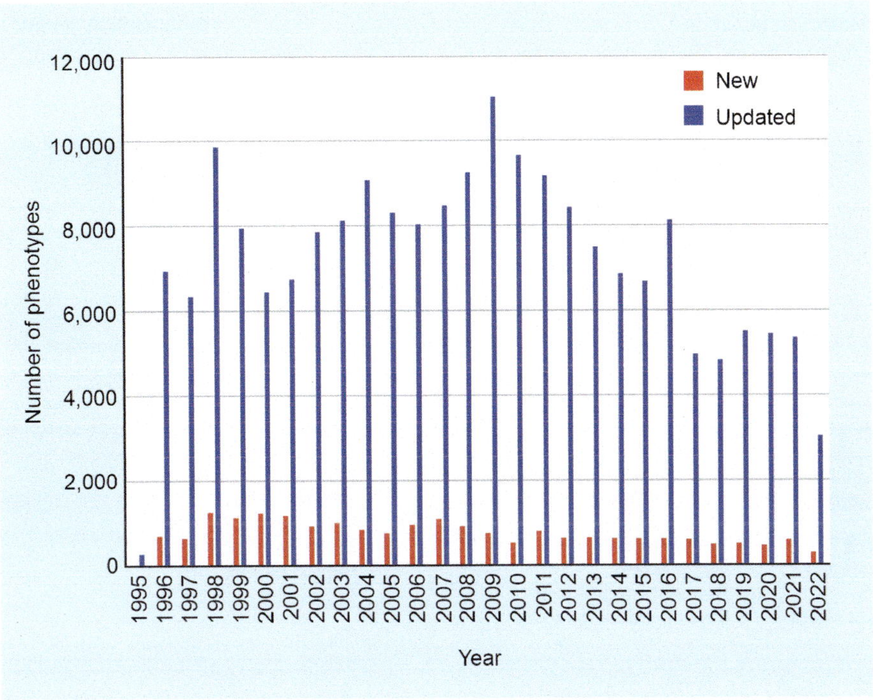

FIG. 9: Journey of gene discovery: As more phenotypes are identified and added to public databases (data from OMIM), the hunt for gene discovery continues, which necessitates the need for technological advancement to test different hypotheses.

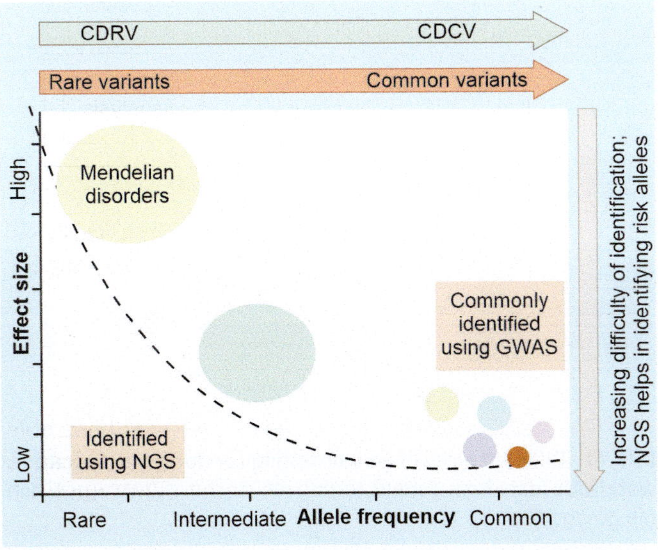

FIG. 10: Models for gene discovery: As CDCV and CDRV hypotheses outline different genes as being causal for disorders, methods for gene discovery also vary.

(CDCV: common disease–common variant; CDRV: common disease–rare variant; GWAS: genome-wide association study; NGS: next-generation sequencing)

to the reference genome, several differences exist in each individual out of which around 50–100 are considered putative, the process of establishing pathogenicity is complicated **(Figs. 10 and 11)**.

TECHNICAL ASPECTS

Following the identification of genes underpinning disorders, it is imperative for diagnostic screening techniques which can detect genetic abnormalities to maintain the pace for competent management as well as the development of treatments and interventions to limit disease severity or even prevent diseases. The genetic diagnosis workup in most laboratories across the world consists of techniques that fall into three main types:

1. *Molecular genetic testing*: It refers to the direct analysis of DNA for the presence of mutations. Several techniques employed are discussed below in greater length.
2. *Biochemical genetic testing*: It involves the wide range of biochemical reactions that occur in cells to maintain the living state. Proteins involved in these biochemical pathways are of innumerable types including enzymes, transporters, and structural as well as regulatory proteins, and a mutation in any of these increases the disposition to disease development. Thus, clinical testing under this category involves a detailed examination of the proteins to measure their activity, level or size, and quantity. It involves a tissue sample like blood, urine, cerebrospinal fluid (CSF), or amniotic fluid which must be stored properly and tested as soon as possible owing to the more dynamic and thus less stable nature of proteins.
3. *Cytogenetic testing*: It involves the examination of the entire chromosome to check for abnormalities.

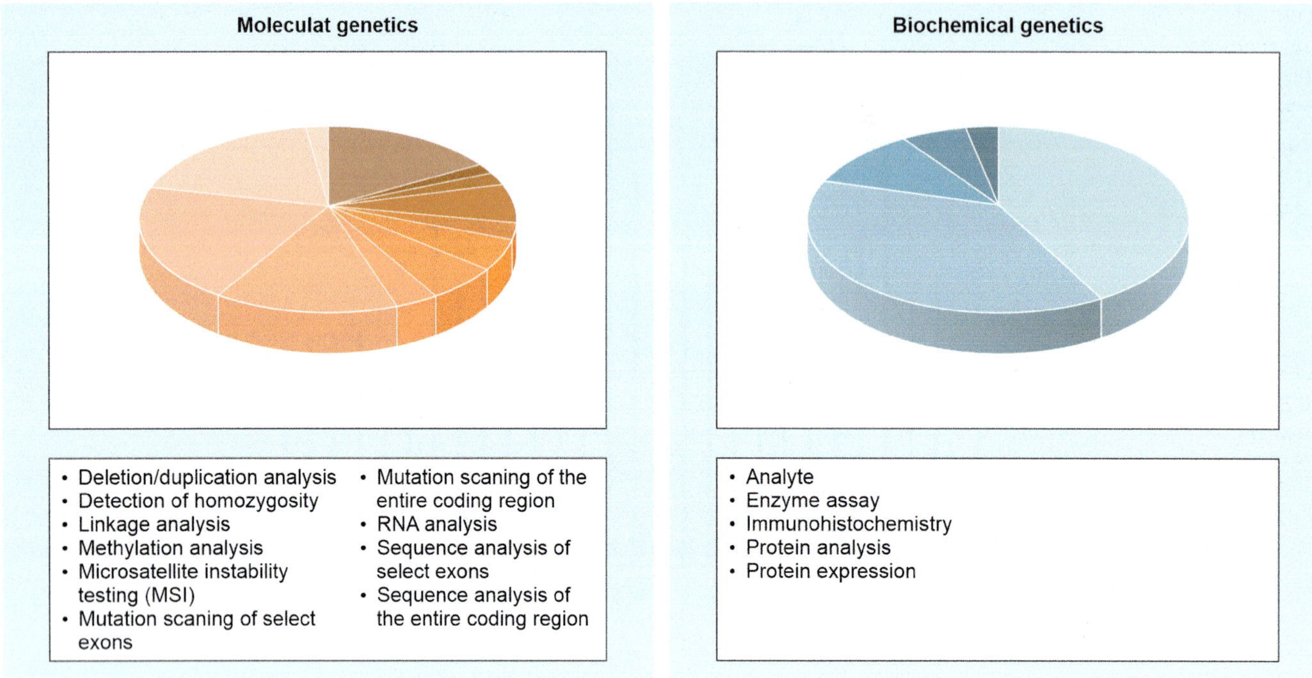

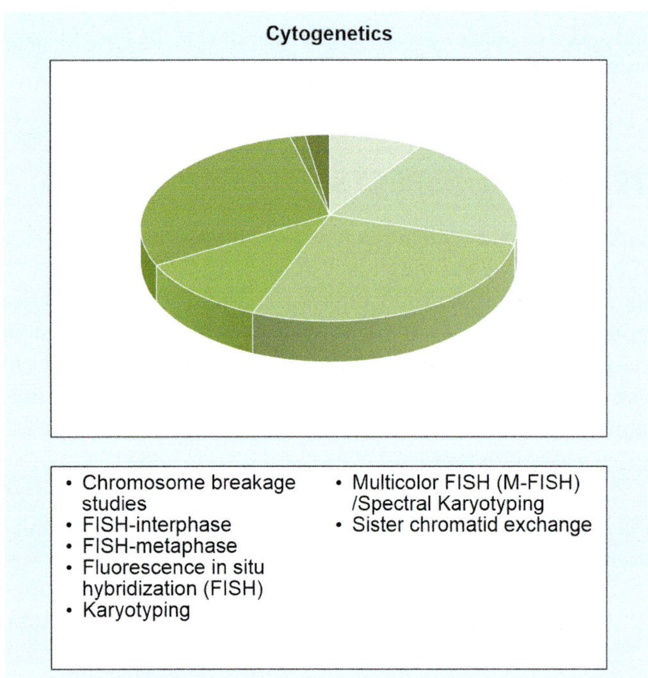

FIG. 11: Different types of genetic testing conducted in laboratories worldwide (data from genetic testing registry https://www.ncbi.nlm.nih.gov/gtr/).

It usually makes use of white blood cells due to the ease of collection and rapid dividing nature in cell culture but other tissue samples from biopsies can also be used. It involves culturing of the sample, chemical fixation, and then visualization using microscopes. Certain techniques used are discussed below in more detail.

As the technology available to aid diagnosis increases rapidly, it is important to keep in mind the advantages of each to be able to make decisions that would help the patient.

Sanger Sequencing

The standard method of DNA sequencing technology most familiar to physicians is Sanger sequencing that effectively and accurately determines the genetic sequence of small areas of the genome (<1 kb),[43] usually a gene or select regions of a gene. Principle of Sanger sequencing is based on di-deoxy chain termination chemistry with fluorescently labeled A, T, G, and C nucleotides. The first step for Sanger is the clonal amplification of regions of interest by polymerase chain reaction (PCR) and in the second step after purification of PCR product, the amplified fragments are subjected for the sequencing reaction (deploying fragment synthesis using fluorescent-labeled dideoxynucleotides) using one primer annealing on the region of interest **(Fig. 12A)**.

Sanger sequencing can help to identify most of the known variations in a gene including point mutations, small insertion-deletion mutations (INDELs), as well as mutations at splice site junctions **(Fig. 12B)**. Due to the limitation of size, this method is usually employed to check for a particular known mutation in a region or unknown mutations in a gene previously implicated in a disorder and is not of utility in the discovery of novel mutations.

While the method has been reliably used since its advent by Fred Sanger in the 1970s.[44]

Limitations

It is not useful or can prove to be too laborious or cost-ineffective when sequencing a large gene, or when searching for previously unknown mutations in which case NGS is employed. It cannot detect large deletions, copy number changes, and repetitive DNA regions.

PCR Fragment Size Analysis

Polymerase chain reaction enables the amplification of genomic regions of interest to aid in detection of

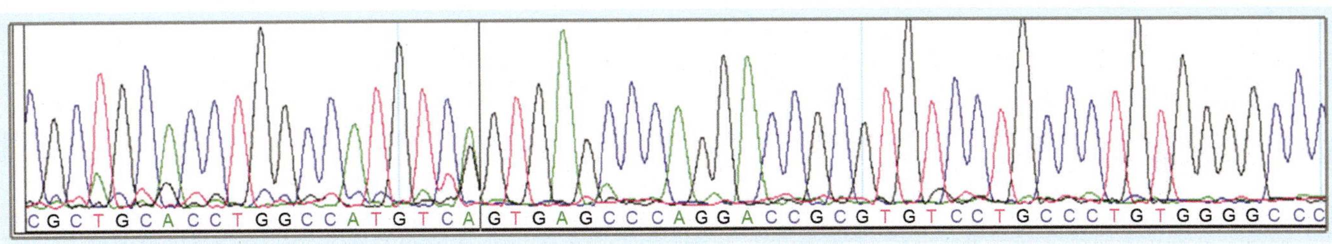

FIG. 12A: Depicting a typical electropherogram showing fluorescent signals representing nucleotide strings in a gene.

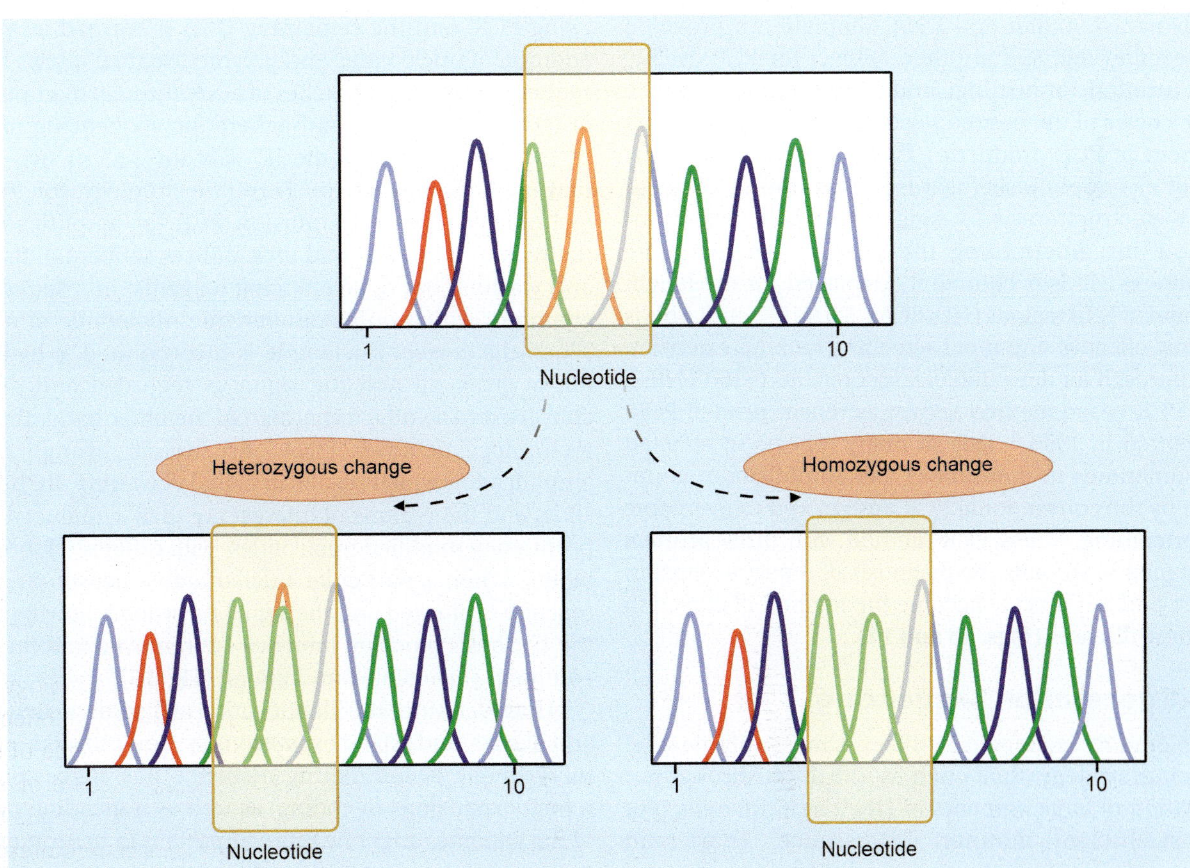

FIG. 12B: Detection of homozygous and heterozygous changes by Sanger sequencing.

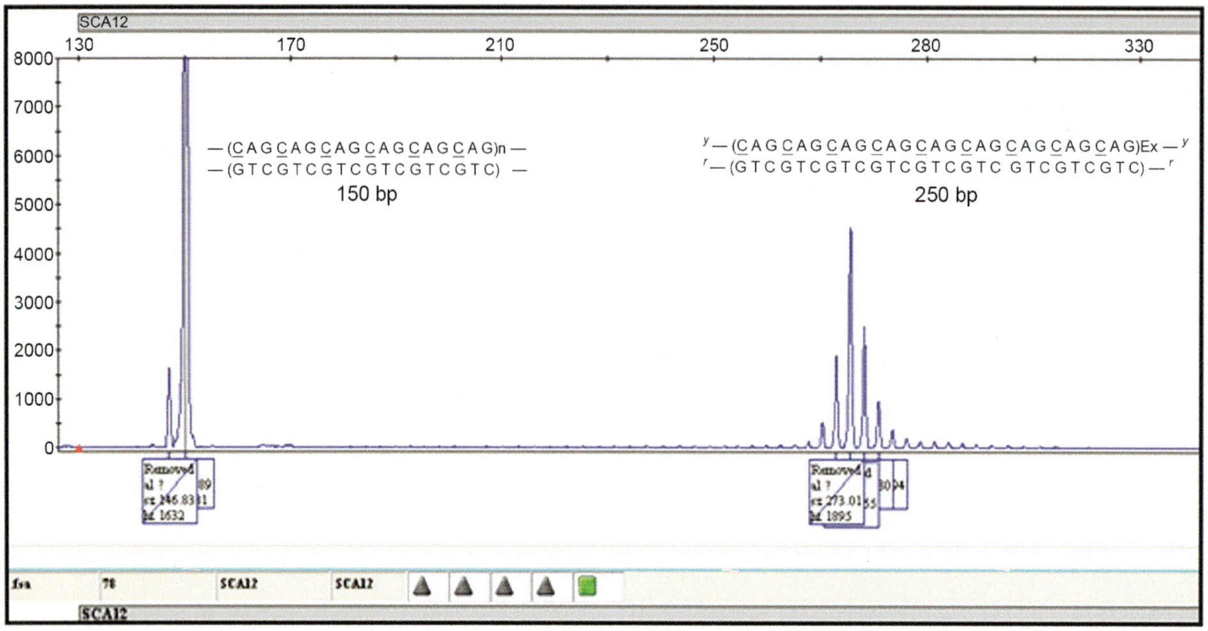

FIG. 13: Fragment analysis showing biallelic amplification of trinucleotide repeat regions depicting differences of 100 base pairs with alle size difference of 33 repeats and marks expansion.

genetic abnormalities. This method relies on synthetic oligonucleotide (primers) designed flanking the region of interest, deoxynucleoside triphosphates (dNTPs), and Taq polymerase, buffer and DNA template are provided in the reaction mix and are then subject for PCR cycling of denaturation, annealing, and extension to produce multiple copies of the desired region. Afterward, the length assessment of PCR product or fragment size analysis by means of electrophoresis (agarose resolution of 20 bp or capillary electrophoresis for single base pair resolution) can allow for determining the length change in the region interest. This is commonly deployed for the length assessment of TNR regions (HD, SCA1-3, DMPK, etc.). This is a very cost-effective and rapid screening tool. An extension of this approach for detection of larger repeats (>100 TNRs), a novel PCR-based method known as repeat-primed PCR, was invented in 1996.[45] Due to many repeats in affected areas (sometimes in thousands), the amplification is not possible by the conventional PCR design, and to overcome this shortcoming, a new PCR method with three primers was designed to simplify the diagnosis of repeat expansion disorders and has quickly become the method of choice to detect these diseases **(Figs. 13 and 14)**.

Next-generation Sequencing

Next-generation sequencing utilizes a massively parallel sequencing strategy that enables the high-throughput investigation of large amounts of DNA, in a time-efficient and cost-efficient manner. In essence, short-read sequencing (150–500 bp) relies on the fragmentation of genomic DNA into multiple segments known as a shotgun library, following which adaptors are ligated to the end which enable amplification of the region of interest as well as interaction with the solid substrate. Following this, the shotgun library is then enriched for the sequences of interest using PCR, and the remaining DNA is washed away. The addition of nucleotides and polymerase then allows for the sequencing of short stretches of DNA, through manipulation of chemistry. This second-generation sequencing method of "sequencing by synthesis" saw the rise of two major players: Illumina and Ion Torrent technology. Ion Torrent technology relies on emulsion PCR for amplification of the region of interest and then utilizes sequential flooding and washing out of sequencing reagents, in a sequencing chamber, which only contains one nucleotide at a time. When the correct nucleotide is incorporated, a hydrogen ion is given off and the signal is recorded and directly converted to a voltage change. On the other hand, Illumina technology achieves DNA enrichment through bridge amplification which results in clonal clustering on the glass slide, and the regions of interest are then sequenced using proprietary modified nucleotides, with different fluorescent labels. When a particular nucleotide is incorporated, the reaction is blocked and the signal recorded following which the synthesis blocking moieties are removed and the cycle continues (reversible terminators) **(Fig. 15)**.

However, since the identification of disorders such as HD and ataxias, and repeat expansions as their causative agents, increasingly accumulating evidence has suggested that repeat expansions in coding, as well as noncoding regions of the genome, might be more important in neuromuscular and neurodegenerative disorders than previously thought. Short-read sequencing is, however, of limited utility in the detection of these neurological problems owing to the

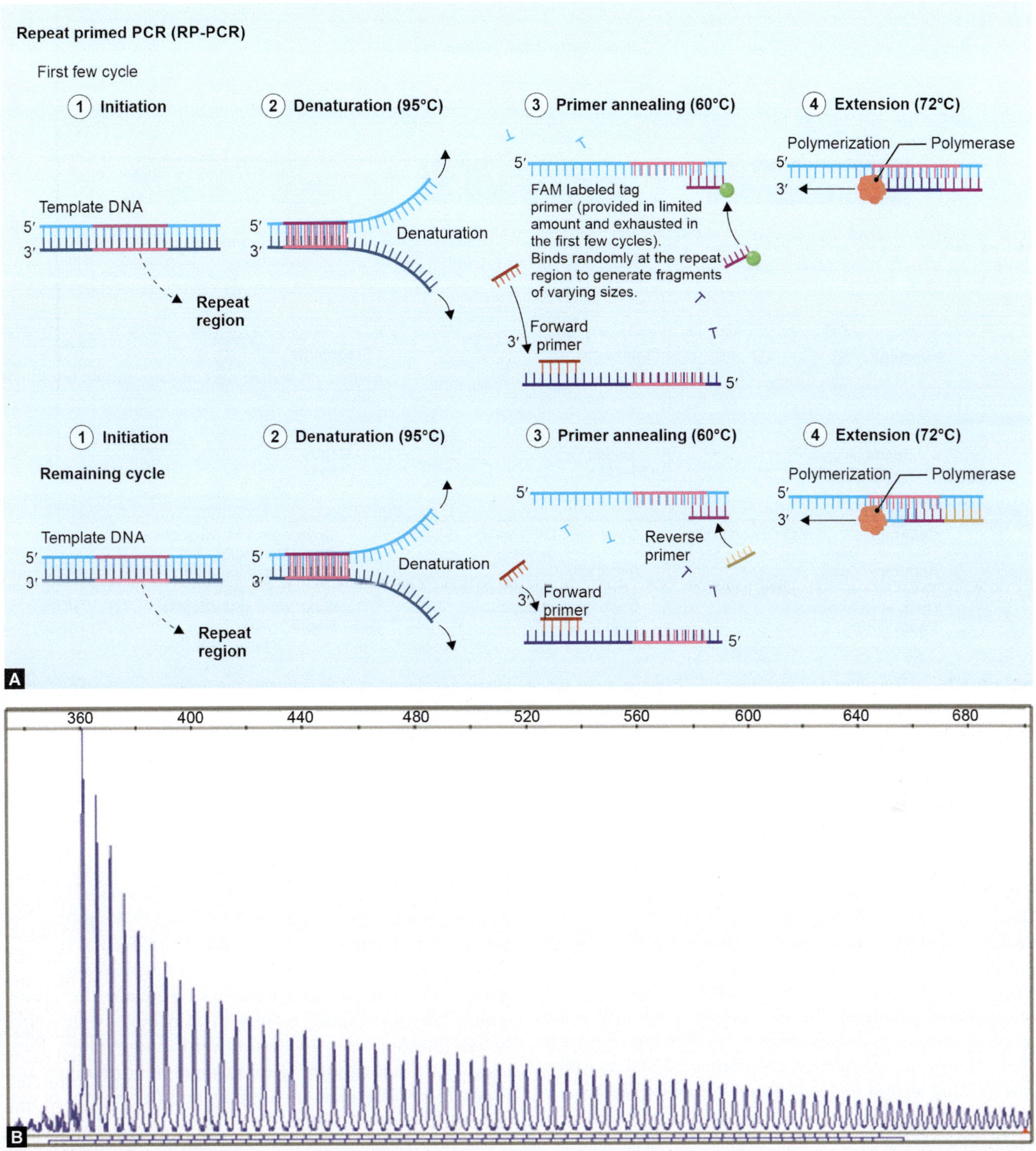

FIGS. 14A AND B: (A) Principle of tandem repeat-primed PCR; (B) Fragment analysis of the amplified product of tandem repeat-primed PCR by capillary electrophoresis.
(PCR: polymerase chain reaction)

limitation of short-read lengths and difficulty in sequencing GC-rich and repetitive regions in the genome. To this end, the discovery and incorporation of long-read sequencing or third-generation sequencing technologies in genetic testing have largely enabled the identification of novel repeats in previously unexplored regions of the genome, leading the way into third-generation sequencing. Of note, there are two technologies—single-molecule real-time (SMRT) sequencing developed by PacBio and Oxford Nanopore Technologies.

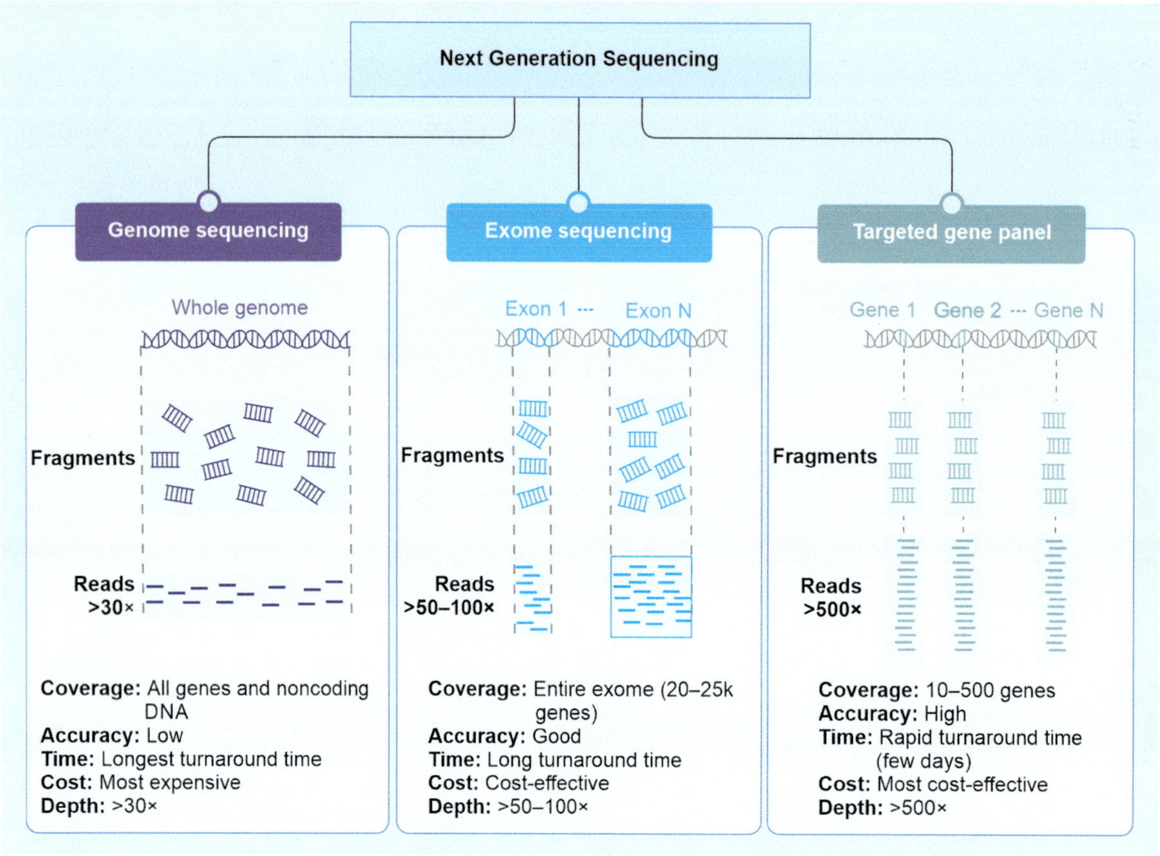

FIG. 15: NGS can be utilized to sequence the entire genome (whole-genome sequencing), the entire exome (whole-exome sequencing), as well as certain genes (targeted gene panel) depending upon the disorders and resource availability.
(NGS: next-generation sequencing)

Single-molecule real-time sequencing allows discernment of very long fragments in the range of 30-50 kb or even longer by reading in real time the signals emitted by nucleotides as they are being incorporated in a single circular DNA molecule via circular consensus sequencing. This is achieved by ligating circular adaptors to the end of a fragment of DNA to form what is known as a SMRT cell. The sample is then loaded onto an SMRT cell and diffuses into a zero-mode waveguide where DNA polymerase allows the incorporation of nucleotides and completes multiple passes of the molecules in a single read to achieve high coverage. This enables the methodical elucidation of STR as well as surrounding regions to detect genetic variants **(Fig. 16)**.

Microarray

Microarray was first introduced commercially in 1996 and is now widely used in genetic testing across the globe. It is utilized in genotyping in array comparative genomic hybridization or CGH to detect chromosomal abnormalities and structural variants and in SNP panels to detect genome-wide or phenotype-specific SNPs panels. Additionally, it is a useful tool to study expression, by quantifying RNA at the transcriptional level. Knowledge gained about differential expressed genes in this manner can provide clues about the diseased state.

For microarray, DNA or RNA from individuals is fluorescently labeled and allowed to hybridize to a slide that contains probes. As the sequences complementary to the probes bind and are imaged through laser-induced dye excitation, a map of the SNPs detected is prepared for each sample. For the detection of CNVs using CGH, probes are designed corresponding to specific chromosomal regions. Differences in fluorescence intensity are exploited to detect abnormalities. If both samples hybridize equally, the genetic content being evaluated is equal in both, but any difference in hybridization intensity hints toward abnormalities. Thus, array CGH can capture chromosomal abnormalities at a much finer scale than karyotyping and fluorescent in situ hybridization (FISH) **(Fig. 17)**.

Fluorescent In Situ Hybridization

Fluorescent in situ hybridization is a reliable method to detect a region of interest in the genome using a complementary probe that is fluorescently labeled. For hybridization to occur, the DNA of interest is first denatured and then mixed with the fluorescently labeled probe. It can help to detect deletions, duplications, translocations, as well as other chromosomal aberrations by helping to visualize interphase chromosomes.

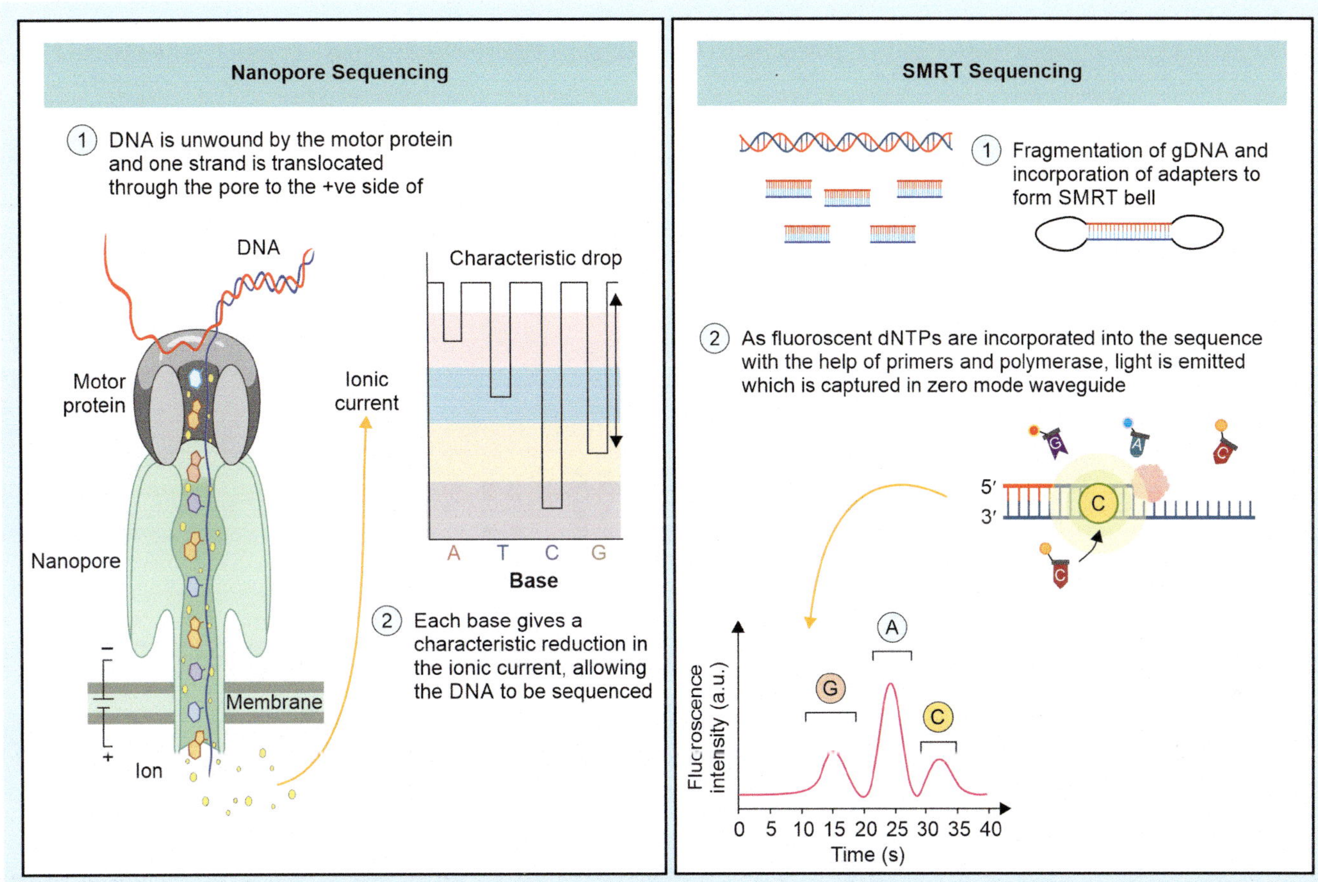

FIG. 16: Sequencing by nanopore and SMRT differs in the chemistry applied but is able to generate long reads ranging from a few thousand base pairs to mega base pairs.
(SMRT: single-molecule real-time)

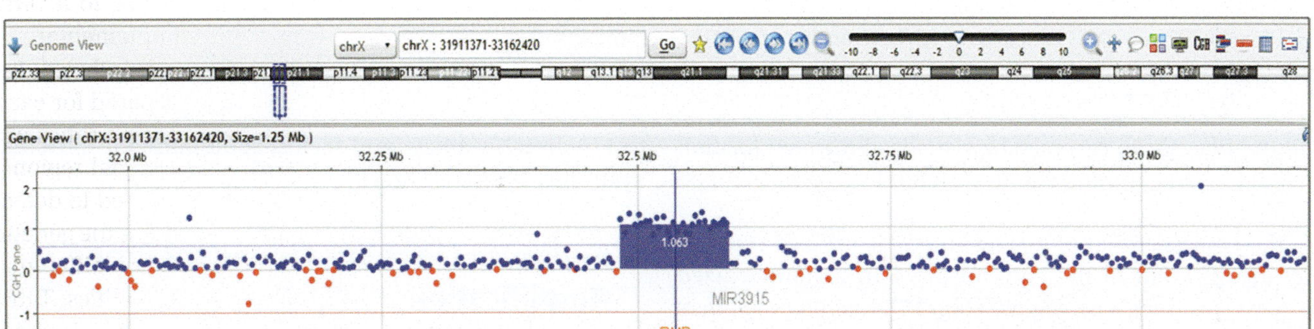

FIG. 17: Depicting differential probe ratio in a patient's microarray profile around *DMD* gene showing duplication.

Karyotyping

Karyotyping as a diagnostic method has been used for over 50 years to detect gross copy number variants. It has been utilized in genetic testing to reveal changes in chromosome numbers associated with aneuploidy (a condition in which an abnormal number of chromosomes is present).[46]

More meticulous analysis can also lead to the detection of structural changes including chromosomal deletions duplications, translocations, and inversions.[47] Karyotyping makes use of metaphase chromosomes because at this stage of cell division, chromosomes are at their most condensed state and can be visualized with ease. The procedure involves the short-term culture of cells following which they are suspended in metaphase with the help of colchicine poison which acts on the mitotic spindle. Next, the cells are suspended in a hypotonic solution which results in cell lysis

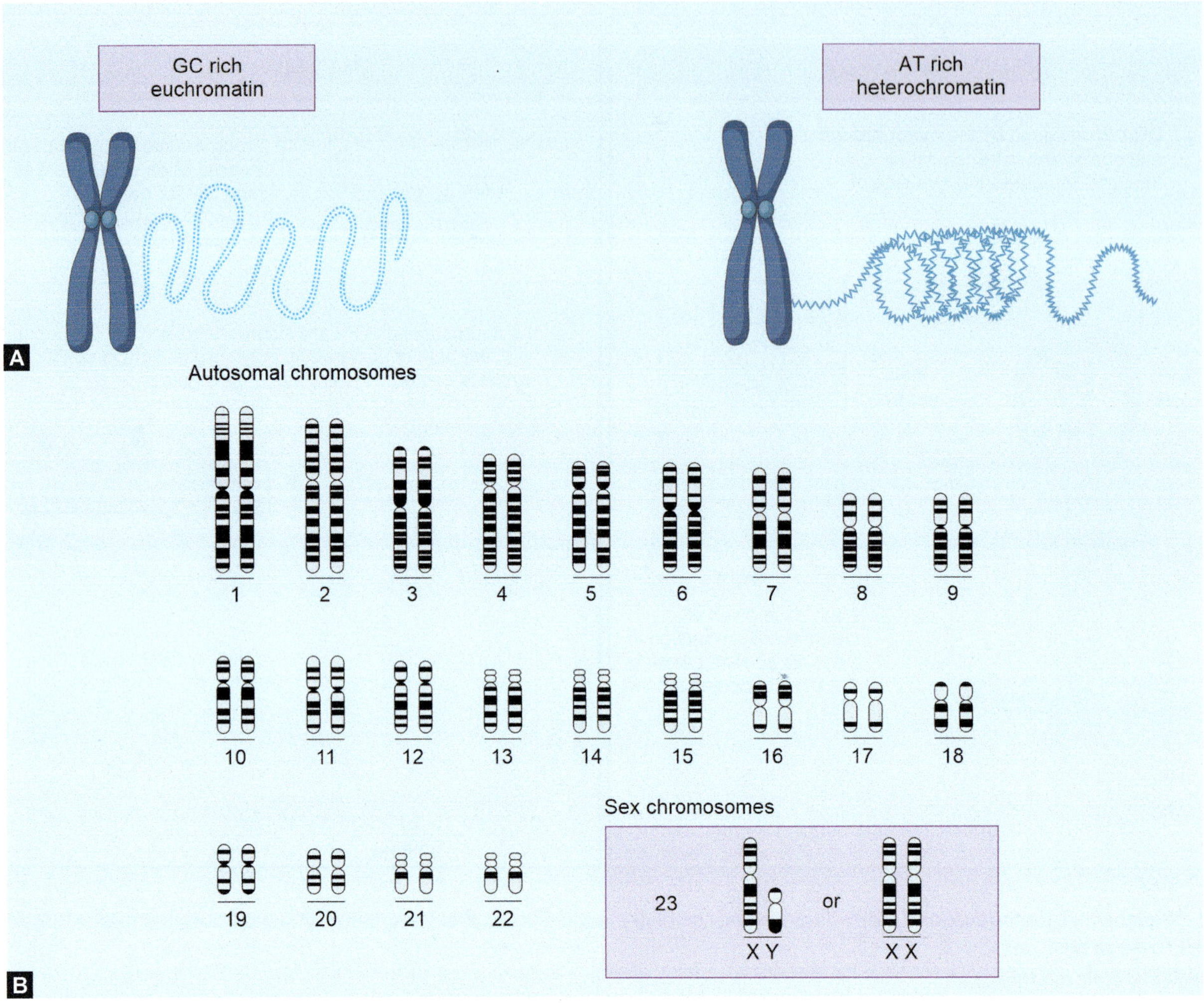

FIGS. 18A AND B: A typical karyogram showing all the chromosomes in the human genome which helps aid detection of chromosomal abnormalities. The most used method for karyotyping involves G banding wherein Giemsa dye is added to metaphase chromosomes after digestion with trypsin. In G banding, AT-rich heterochromatin DNA stains more darkly.

and the free nuclei can then be visualized through fixation on a glass slide and the subtle structural variations can be detected.

The true potential of this technique is utilized through the arrangement of the chromosomes in a standardized format to produce a karyogram **(Fig. 18)**. Karyotyping offers a diagnostic resolution of about 3 Mb.

Southern Blot

Southern blot is routinely incorporated into genetic testing for disorders, especially neuromuscular disorders. It involves the strategic digestion of genomic DNA by restriction enzymes and size-fractionation on an agarose gel. DNA is then denatured by treatment with an alkylating agent and transferred to a nylon membrane on which specific DNA sequences can be detected through hybridization with labeled probes and subsequent visualization. It has been the method of choice to detect disorders involving repeat number variation for several years, including but not limited to Friedreich's ataxia and facioscapulohumeral muscular dystrophy (FSHD) **(Fig. 19)**.

Multiplex Ligation-dependent Probe Amplification

It is a multiplex PCR assay that makes use of multiple probes (~40) which correspond to different DNA sequences or areas of interest to detect the relative copy number of each of these sequences. Each probe contains two half probes that correspond to a target-specific sequence and a universal primer sequence so that simultaneous PCR amplification of all probes can be achieved. First, the DNA is denatured which is followed by a period of incubation with the multiplex ligation-dependent probe amplification (MLPA) probes. The probes hybridize to target-specific sequences and get amplified. For PCR amplification, only one primer pair is used and one of them is fluorescently labeled. The PCR products are fractionated using capillary electrophoresis

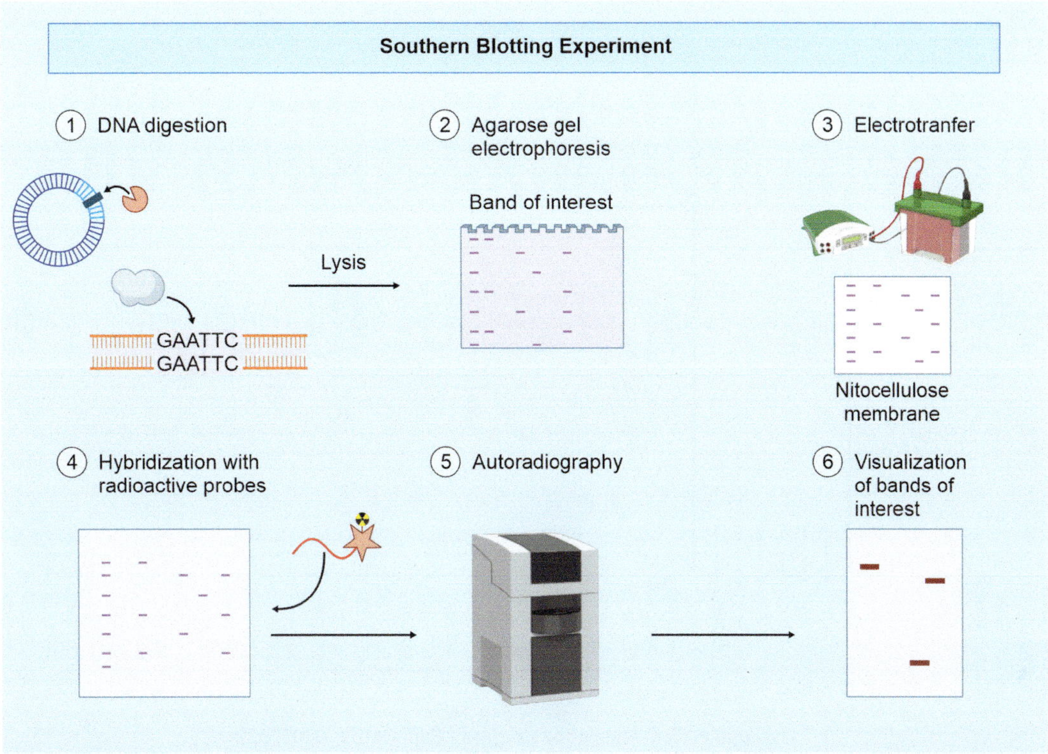

Note: Very large fragments cannot be sufficiently resolved by normal agarose gel electrophoresis and require pulsed field gel electrophoresis.

FIG. 19: Detailed account of genetic investigation using southern blot.

and the subsequent analysis of peaks helps in quantifying the amount of PCR product and thus the relative amount of target DNA through comparison with control DNA samples inferred as dosage quotient (DQ). CNVs considered normal copy if DQ is 0.8<DQ<1.20; homozygous deletion if DQ=0; heterozygous deletion if DQ is 0.4<DQ<.65; heterozygous duplication if DQ is 1.3<DQ<1.65, and homozygous duplication if 1.75<DQ<2.15.

Multiplex ligation-dependent probe amplification is a very reliable and commonly deployed test that can be utilized to detect gene level duplications or deletions, especially in neuromuscular disorders such as Duchenne muscular dystrophy, SMA, and Charcot-Marie-Tooth disease.[48] There are MLPA assays which cover multiple genes (e.g., CMT-PMP22, GJB1, and MPZ) **(Figs. 20A and B; Table 3)**.

INTERPRETATIONS

With the advent of NGS, the repertoire of tools at the clinician's disposal to be able to efficiently evaluate and diagnose individuals has dramatically improved. However, the technology presently is riddled with problems relating to data interpretation and analysis.[58] Depending upon the type of platform and sequencing done, i.e., targeted gene panel, exome sequencing, or genome sequencing, the number of identified variants can range from a few to tens of thousands or even millions. This necessitates the use of stepwise filtering in order to rule out possibilities. While the filtering algorithm may vary in an individual laboratory setting and depending upon case requirements, a strong hold over both clinical and genetic diagnosis is imperative.[59] Typically, in a single whole-exome sequencing (WES), 40–50 thousand variations are obtained in coding regions; of this, ~20% variations will affect protein sequence or length alterations (insertion/deletions). Of this filtered content typically ~10% variations will be very rare or novel comprising ~10% homozygous and the remaining heterozygous variations. The successful application of further filtration strategy, i.e., dominant or recessive inheritance model combined with in silico approach, helps deduce the likely causal variation in the case. Sometimes a supervised approach with variation search restricted to the candidate gene panel ascertains the genetic family. For the identification of compound heterozygous variations, a quick strategy can be to sequence parental samples. For the identification of de-novo variations, trio design is adopted (proband and both parents). Given all the scenarios described above, the diagnostic yield can be achieved in ~20–30% cases. Most often, the investigator may see a number of variations of uncertain significance (VUS). The filtered final variations will require both technical and computational validations. For technical validation, Sanger sequencing is the standard method. For analytical validation, a rigorous genotype–phenotype correlation and family-based segregation analysis and/or observation of similar variations in other patients with identical phenotypes add to the significance toward its causality. A typical monogenic variation of a Mendelian disease should have a high penetrance

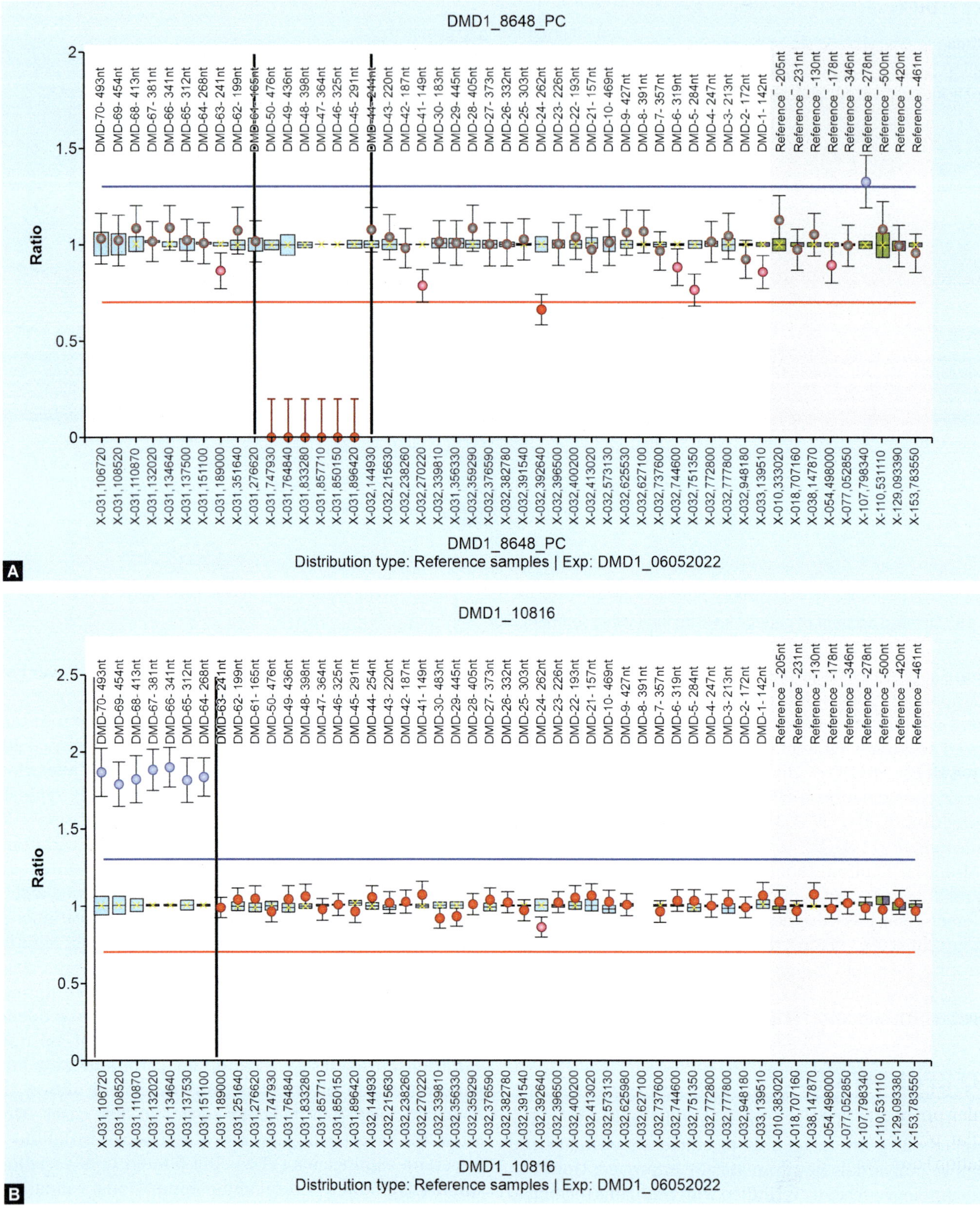

FIGS. 20A AND B: (A) Duchenne muscular dystrophy (DMD) hemizygous deletion; (B) DMD heterozygous deletion.

TABLE 3: Utility of different technologies.

Method	Advantages	Size resolution	Disadvantages	Examples
Whole-exome sequencing	Identification of rare variants with string risk effect in the coding region of the genome	Few base pairs	Short-read sequences fail to capture CNVs or repetitive elements with efficiency	Advantageous for coverage of all the expressed content of the genome. Cover all of the Mendelian repertoire of genes
Whole-genome sequencing	Captures the entire genome	Few base pairs	Short-read sequences fail to capture CNVs or repetitive elements with efficiency	Helps to detect mutations in noncoding regions of the genome including regulatory regions like enhancers and promoters[49]
Long-read sequencing	Captures structural variants and repetitive elements	Thousands of base pairs (single read length up to ~6 Mb)	Slower, lower accuracy compared to short-read sequencing reported	• Newer tandem nucleotide regions have been identified. NOTCH2NLC • Minisatellite repeats of ABCA7 can be sequenced.[50,51]
SNP array	Able to detect copy neutral loss of heterozygosity	Few base pairs	Unable to detect small rearrangements and is low throughput	Detection of a homozygous deletion c.483delG in CAPN3 as causal mutation for limb girdle muscular dystrophy[52]
Southern blot	Able to detect small rearrangements, deletions or expansions as well as mosaicism	Size limitation a few thousand bp	Laborious, time consuming, unable to detect copy neutral loss of heterozygosity and is not quantitative	Detection of repeat expansion disorders (REDs) like Friedreich's ataxia[53]
MLPA	• Able to detect small rearrangements and several targets (up to 40) • High throughput and cost-effective	Utilized to detect CNVs ~100 bp	• Unable to detect copy neutral loss of heterozygosity • Problems faced with mosaicism	Detection of DMD[54]
CGH array	Able to detect very small rearrangements and can investigate the entire genome, low cost	~40 kb	Unable to detect copy neutral loss of heterozygosity and is low throughput	Detection of disorders caused by genomic imbalances[55]
Karyotyping	First-line investigation for aneuploidies, large chromosomal abnormalities as it allows genome-wide detection of submicroscopic imbalances	Size limitation of ~5 Mb	Limited in its ability to detect cryptic aberrations, marker chromosomes and INDELs or small rearrangements	Detection of aneuploidies like Down's syndrome
FISH	Able to detect rearrangements, mosaicism, and tumor heterogeneity. Can help quantify multiple copies	Size limitation ~5–10 Mb (metaphase FISH)	Unable to detect copy neutral loss of heterozygosity, small rearrangements, or several targets at once	Helps detect chromosomal abnormalities like Philadelphia chromosome[56,57]

(CNV: copy number variation; DMD: Duchenne muscular dystrophy; FISH: fluorescent in situ hybridization; INDELs: insertion-deletion mutations; MLPA: multiplex ligation-dependent probe amplification)

(all subjects harboring the variation should exhibit the similar phenotype) and high detectance (all subjects with similar phenotypes in the family should carry the same variation) quotient **(Fig. 21 and Table 4)**.

Variants of Unknown Significance

A common problem faced in genetic testing is the discovery of novel mutations of unknown and uncertain significance. While in the case of known variations, it is easy to delineate pathogenicity, the same is not possible for VUS due to incomplete knowledge. This requires additional investigation into the variation to understand if it might be causative of the disease phenotype. This calls for the investigation of familial segregation along with computational modeling and experimental validation to establish pathogenicity. It is important to note that bioinformatic prediction is still mostly riddled with uncertainty due to existing gaps in our knowledge about how variants may cause disease and experimental validation is required. With advances in modeling software and prediction tools at our disposal along with an enhanced understanding of disease development, it will become easier to distinguish pathogenic variants from nondeleterious ones. Several tools exist presently that aid in the evaluation of such variants and in the future as new

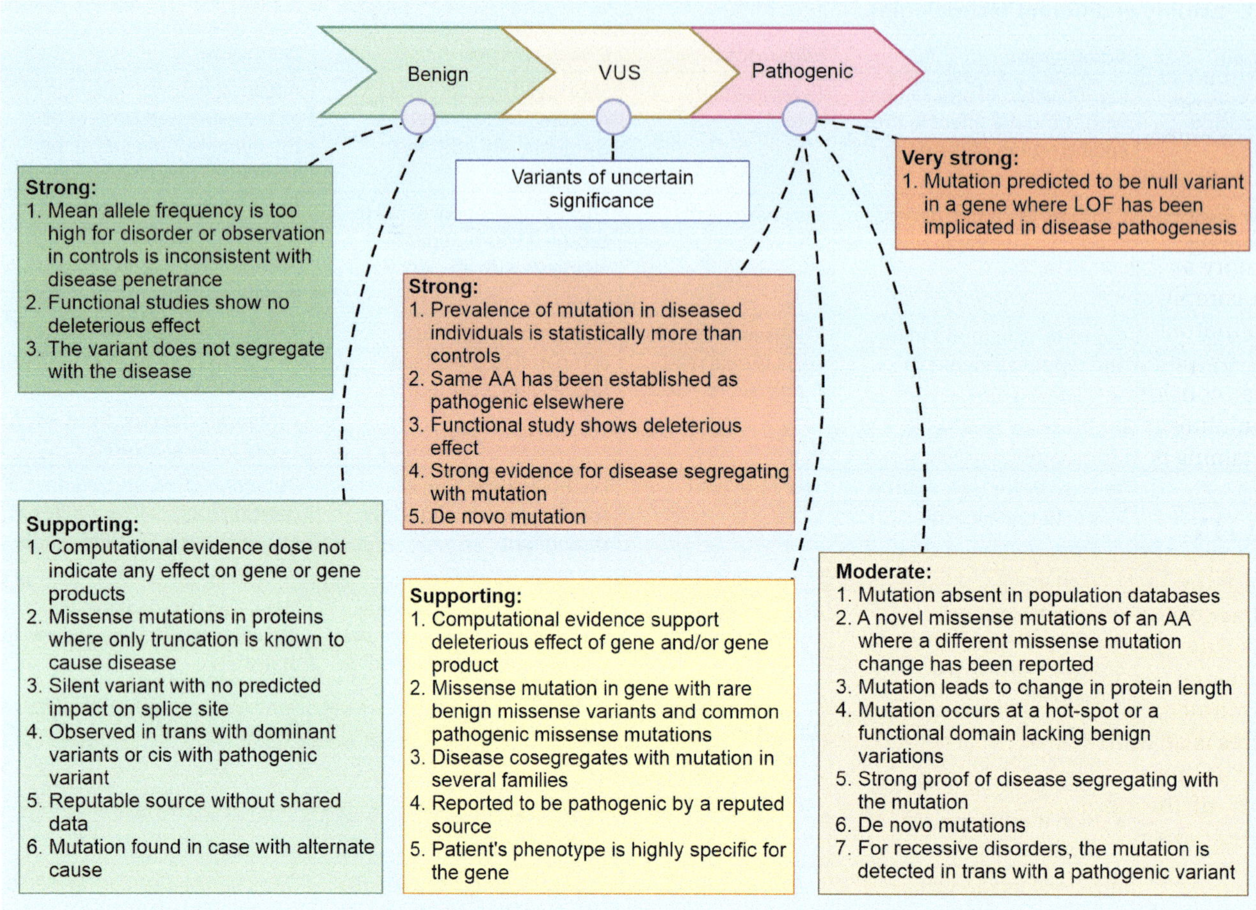

FIG. 21: ACMG criteria-guided variant classification: ACMG[60] highlights different criteria for delineating benign or pathogenic status. As highlighted above, evidence can be classified in various categories which can then pave the way for establishing pathogenicity.
(ACMG: American College of Medical Genetics and Genomics)

TABLE 4: List of resources for genetic investigation.

Population database	
Exome aggregation consortium	https://gnomad.broadinstitute.org/
Exome variant server	http://evs.gs.washington.edu/EVS
1000 Genomes	https://www.internationalgenome.org/
dbSNP	http://www.ncbi.nlm.nih.gov/snp
dbVar	http://www.ncbi.nlm.nih.gov/dbvar
Disease databases	
ClinVar	http://www.ncbi.nlm.nih.gov/clinvar
OMIM	http://www.omim.org
Human gene mutation database	http://www.hgmd.org
Locus/disease/ethnic/other-specific databases	https://www.hgvs.org/ http://www.lovd.nl
DECIPHER	http://decipher.sanger.ac.uk
National Heart, Lung, and Blood Institute (NHLBI)	https://www.nhlbi.nih.gov/
Genome sequence and variant classification databases	
GWAS studies catalog	https://www.ebi.ac.uk/gwas/
Database of genomic variants	http://dgv.tcag.ca/dgv/app/home
Ensembl database	https://asia.ensembl.org/index.html
UCSC genome browser	https://genome.ucsc.edu/
NCBI	https://www.ncbi.nlm.nih.gov/
RefSeq Gene	https://www.ncbi.nlm.nih.gov/refseq/rsg/
MitoMap	https://www.mitomap.org/MITOMAP

Continued

(GWAS: genome-wide association study; OMIM: Online Mendelian Inheritance in Man; UCSC: University of California Santa Cruz)

knowledge is deposited in repositories, it would be helpful to re-evaluate these variants to enhance the chances of potential diagnosis for patients. While American College of Medical Genetics and Genomics (ACMG) guidelines dictate that a VUS should not dictate clinical decision-making, it is somewhat used as a case of unconfirmed pathogenicity. VUS presents a dilemma for clinicians and often blurs the lines between research and diagnosis. Where clinicians are concerned, significant debate exists around best practices regarding disclosing the VUS. It is generally considered best practice to follow up closely with the patient and family members to try to establish any links to the disease phenotype by seeing if the variant is shared by any affected family member. They also present significant problems for the patients who are viewed as being placed in genetic purgatory as these variants can be hard to understand and often complicate decision-making for patients. Therefore, it is important for clinicians to keep in mind the problems faced by patients and family members and with these ethical considerations in mind, choose the way forward that minimizes the emotional burden on the patients while maintaining best management practices.

UTILITY

Despite the importance of genetic testing in establishing the diagnosis and subsequent management and treatment of disorders, it is important to not underestimate the importance of clinical evaluation of patients. Establishing an accurate phenotype based on an assessment of clinical features is an important cornerstone of diagnosis. Another important part of clinical evaluation is taking a thorough history of the patient and family. Prior to considering a genetic diagnosis, other nongenetic causes including environmental exposure should be able to start a treatment regime in a timely manner. If genetic testing is ordered to confirm a suspicion or in cases where physical examination is unable to lead to a conclusive diagnosis, genetic counseling should be provided to the patient and the family to ensure a proper understanding of the procedure and the possible results. In diseases with a classic presentation, with reduced expressivity like HD, it is easy to pinpoint the cause and thus reduce the time of diagnosis. However, in disorders such as spinocerebellar ataxias or PD wherein phenotype varies substantially, diagnosis is almost impossible to establish in absence of genetic testing. It is also important to note that neurological disorders, especially movement disorders, exhibit a marked similarity between phenotypes, and thus over-reliance on clinical features often leads to misdiagnosis.

With the introduction of NGS, it is increasingly becoming routine practice to order whole-exome or whole-genome test panels to identify the causative mutation in most cases, even when this practice may not be justified. No matter the disorder, the goal remains to establish a diagnosis in a time and cost-efficient manner which would require the establishment of a robust diagnostic decision-making tree. A better approach to achieve this goal would be to consider single gene testing wherever indicated through robust clinical evaluation to establish a genotype–phenotype correlation **(Fig. 22; Table 5)**.

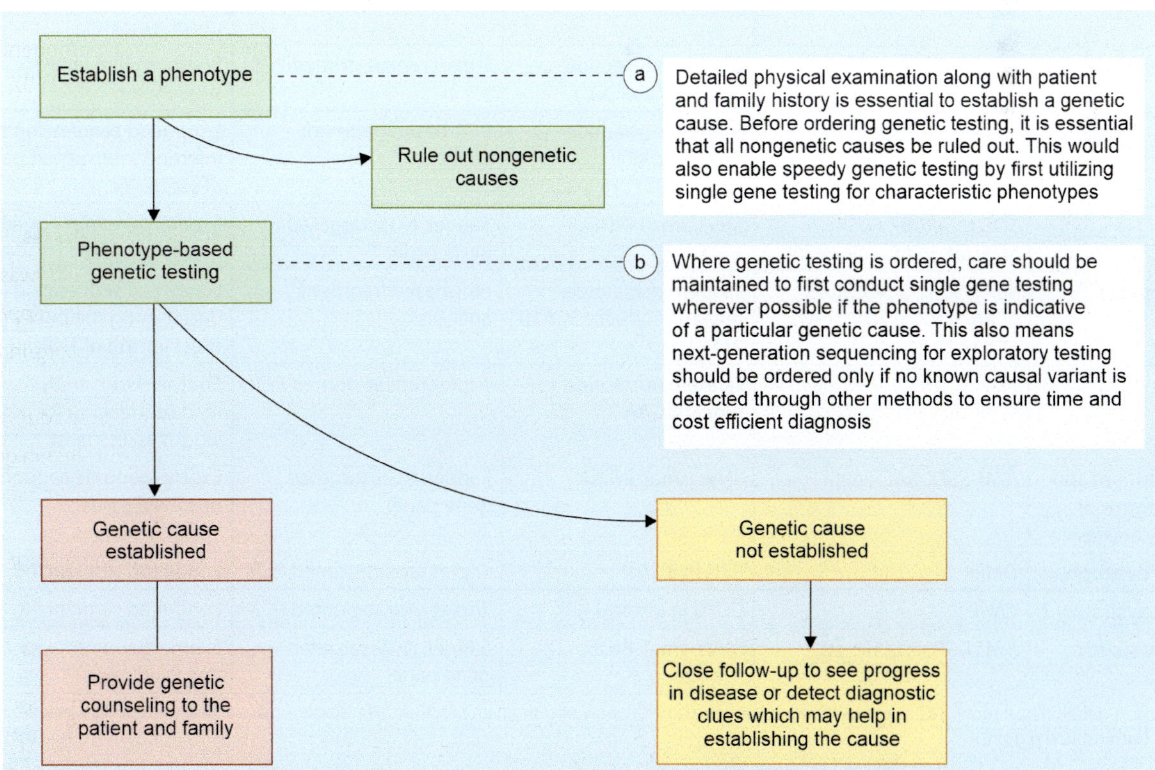

Note: Very large fragments cannot be sufficiently resolved by normal agarose gel electrophoresis and require pulsed field gel electrophoresis.

FIG. 22: Diagnostic Decision Making Tree: Diagnostic decision making in the clinic generally follows this workflow while deciding which patients to refer to genetic testing. This helps to ensure that the patient and family is not subjected to unnecessary inconvenience while still being able to establish a genetic basis for the disease, wherever possible.

TABLE 5: Some common neurological problems with their respective causes and technologies that are utilized in their detection.

Disorders	Gene/core genes	Common defects	Common and cost-effective detection tools for screening	Advance techniques
Duchenne muscular dystrophy	Dystrophin	Deletion/duplication (some exons are hot spot for deletions, i.e., 44–52 region)	Multiplex ligation probe assay (MLPA) or Multiplex PCR-based assays	Long-read genome sequencing or microarray for exact breakpoint detection
		SNVs, small INDEL	Sanger, NGS	NGS
Spinal muscular atrophy (SMA)	*SMN1*	Complete deletion of SMN1 and SMN2 duplication has modifier effects	MLPA, PCR-based gene copy number assessment	Long-read genome sequencing
Spinal muscular atrophy plus syndromes	Multiple genes	SNVs, small INDEL	Sanger, NGS	NGS
Charcot–Marie–Tooth disease	*PMP22*	Deletions are associated with Charcot–Marie–Tooth neuropathy, type 1A and duplications are associated pressure nerve palsy	MLPA, microarray	Genome sequencing for exact breakpoint determination
Charcot–Marie–Tooth disease	*GJB2/MPZ*	Deletion	MLPA, microarray	Genome sequencing for exact breakpoint determination
	GDAP1, GJB1, HINT1, MFN2, MPZ, PMP22, SH3CT2, and *SORD*	SNVs, small INDEL	Sanger, NGS	Genome sequencing for unsolved cases
Parkinson's disease	*LRRK2, PINK1, SNCA*	SNVs, small INDEL	Sanger, NGS	Exome/genome sequencing for unsolved cases
Motor neuron disease	c9ORF72	Tandem nucleotide repeats (GGGGCC)	Triplet repeat-primed PCR	Southern blot analysis, genome sequencing
	ATXN2	Tandem nucleotide repeats (CAG)	PCR-based fragment analysis	Long-read sequencing for inferring interrupted patterns of sequence
	SOD1, TARDBP, FUS, SQSTM1, VAPB, VCP, OPTN	SNVs, small INDEL	Sanger, NGS, targeted gene panel	Exome/genome sequencing for unsolved cases
Spinocerebellar ataxias	*SCA1, SCA2, SCA3, SCA6, SCA6, SCA7, SCA10, SCA12, SCA17*	Tandem nucleotide repeats (CNG) for SCA10 ATTCT	PCR-based fragment analysis	Long-read sequencing for deciphering the purity and exact length of TNRs
FRDA	*FXN*	Tandem nucleotide repeats, GAA	Triplet repeat-primed PCR	Southern blot analysis, long-read sequencing for accurate length assessment
Other dominant and recessive forms of hereditary ataxias	*ATM, SETX, SACS*, etc.	SNVs, small INDEL	Sanger, NGS, targeted gene panel	Exome/genome sequencing for unsolved cases
Myotonic dystrophy 1	*DMPK*	CTG in 3′ *UTR*	Triplet repeat-primed PCR	Long-read sequencing
Myotonic dystrophy 2	*CNBP*	CCTG in intron 1	Triplet repeat-primed PCR	Long-read sequencing
Hereditary spastic paraplegia	*SPAST, SPG7, SPG4*, etc.	SNVs, small INDEL	Sanger, NGS, targeted gene panel	Exome/genome sequencing for unsolved cases

(INDEL: insertion-deletion mutations; NGS: next-generation sequencing; PCR: polymerase chain reaction; SNV: single-nucleotide variation; TNR: tandem nucleotide repeat; UTR: untranslated region)

CONCLUSION

Genetic testing has become a routine part of neurological diagnostic workup with most neurologists availing resources like NGS to help identify causal variants. As such, there is still a lack of appreciation for and incorporation of the vast tools available at our disposal and over-reliance on WES and whole-genome sequencing (WGS). These tests should not be utilized when all existing resources have been exhausted and not as primary screening methods. Care should be taken to recognize the emotional and financial burden on the patient and family members.

Despite the significant advancement in the field of neurogenetics in India, progress has not kept up pace with other healthcare leaders in the world. One reason for this is that genetic testing is offered ordered very late in the diagnostic workup. Moreover, much of the big data generation of human genomes has happened in the western world and resulted in genetic mapping of several hundred new disorders; however, inequitable access to genome sequencing in low-resource countries faces a prolonged diagnostic odyssey and a slow rate of discoveries of new genetic defects.

In this situation, it is even more important for different stakeholders in the fields of neurology, neuroscience, genetics and genomics, medical practice, and public health to come together and foster an environment of knowledge sharing by creating publicly available knowledge repositories. Population-specific data would help to accelerate the process of gene discovery as well as progress in the field of disease management and treatment.

REFERENCES

1. Watson JD, Crick FHC. Molecular Structure of Nucleic Acids: A Structure for Deoxyribose Nucleic Acid. Nature. 1953;171(4356): 737-8.
2. Alberts B, Johnson A, Lewis J, Raff M, Roberts K, Walter P. Molecular biology of the cell, 5th edition. Biochem Mol Biol Edu. 2008;36(4):317-8. [online] Available from https://onlinelibrary.wiley.com/doi/full/10.1002/bmb.20192. [Last accessed March, 2023].
3. Griffiths AJF. Modern genetic analysis: integrating genes and genomes, 2nd edition. New York, NY: W.H. Freeman and Co; 2002. p. 736.
4. Fogel B. (2013). Clinical Neurogenetics: An Issue of Neurologic Clinics. [online] Available from https://books.google.com/books?hl=en&lr=&id=resBAgAAQBAJ&oi=fnd&pg=PP1&ots=vixBaClrcC&sig=aiPOd4oY6CemkwiZjYUQawFEcY4. [Last accessed March, 2023].
5. Acuna-Hidalgo R, Veltman JA, Hoischen A. New insights into the generation and role of de novo mutations in health and disease. Genome Biol. 2016;17(1):1-19.
6. Kruglyak L, Nickerson DA. Variation is the spice of life. Nat Genet. 2001;27(3):234-6.
7. Lin CLG, Bristol LA, Jin L, Dykes-Hoberg M, Crawford T, Clawson L, et al. Aberrant RNA processing in a neurodegenerative disease: the cause for absent EAAT2, a glutamate transporter, in amyotrophic lateral sclerosis. Neuron. 1998;20(3):589-602.
8. Lupski JR. Genomic rearrangements and sporadic disease. Nat Genet. 2007;39(7 Suppl):S43-6.
9. Harel T, Lupski JR. Genomic disorders 20 years on-mechanisms for clinical manifestations. Clin Genet. 2018;93(3):439-49.
10. Stankiewicz P, Lupski JR. Structural variation in the human genome and its role in disease. Annu Rev Med. 2010;61:437-55.
11. Girirajan S, Campbell CD, Eichler EE. Human copy number variation and complex genetic disease. Annu Rev Genet. 2011;45:203-26.
12. Chiang C, Scott AJ, Davis JR, Tsang EK, Li X, Kim Y, et al. The impact of structural variation on human gene expression. Nat Genet. 2017;49(5):692.
13. Zhang F, Lupski JR. Non-coding genetic variants in human disease. Hum Mol Genet. 2015;24(R1):R102.
14. Wiszniewska J, Bi W, Shaw C, Stankiewicz P, Kang SHL, Pursley AN, et al. Combined array CGH plus SNP genome analyses in a single assay for optimized clinical testing. Eur J Hum Genet. 2014;22(1):79.
15. Boone PM, Bacino CA, Shaw CA, Eng PA, Hixson PM, Pursley AN, et al. Detection of Clinically Relevant Exonic Copy-Number Changes by Array CGH. Hum Mutat. 2010;31(12):1326.
16. Carvalho CMB, Lupski JR. Mechanisms underlying structural variant formation in genomic disorders. Nat Rev Genet. 2016;17(4):224-38.
17. Shaikh TH. Copy number variation disorders. Curr Genet Med Rep. 2017;5(4):183.
18. Depienne C, Mandel JL. 30 years of repeat expansion disorders: What have we learned and what are the remaining challenges? Am J Hum Genet. 2021;108(5):764.
19. Stoyas CA, la Spada AR. The CAG-polyglutamine repeat diseases: a clinical, molecular, genetic, and pathophysiologic nosology. Handb Clin Neurol. 2018;147:143-70.
20. Colak D, Zaninovic N, Cohen MS, Rosenwaks Z, Yang WY, Gerhardt J, et al. Promoter-bound trinucleotide repeat mRNA drives epigenetic silencing in fragile X syndrome. Science. 2014;343(6174):1002-5.
21. Marian AJ. Clinical interpretation and management of genetic variants. Basic Transl Sci. 2020;5(10):1029-42.
22. Genetic Alliance; District of Columbia Department of Health. (2010). Understanding Genetics: A District of Columbia Guide for Patients and Health Professionals. [online] Available from https://www.ncbi.nlm.nih.gov/books/NBK132145/. [Last accessed March, 2023].
23. Online Mendelian Inheritance in Man (OMIM). (2022). OMIM Entry Statistics. [online] Available from https://www.omim.org/statistics/entry. [Last accessed March, 2023].
24. Teare MD, Koref MFS. Linkage analysis and the study of Mendelian disease in the era of whole exome and genome sequencing. Brief Funct Genomics. 2014;13(5):378-83.
25. Gorman GS, Chinnery PF, DiMauro S, Hirano M, Koga Y, McFarland R, et al. Mitochondrial diseases. Nat Rev Dis Primers. 2016;2(1): 1-22.
26. Massimo Zeviani, Stefano Di Donato, Mitochondrial disorders, Brain. 2004;127(Pt 10):2153-72. [online] Available from https://doi.org/10.1093/brain/awh259.
27. DiMauro S, Hirano M. Pathogenesis and treatment of mitochondrial disorders. Adv Exp Med Biol. 2009;652:139-70.
28. Cassidy SB, Schwartz S, Miller JL, Driscoll DJ. Prader-Willi syndrome. Genetics in Medicine. 2011;14(1):10-26.
29. Buiting K, Williams C, Horsthemke B. Angelman syndrome—insights into a rare neurogenetic disorder. Nat Rev Neurol. 2016;12(10):584-93.

30. Wang KH, Kupa J, Duffy KA, Kalish JM. Diagnosis and Management of Beckwith-Wiedemann Syndrome. Front Pediatr. 2019;7:562.
31. Gatz M, Reynolds CA, Fratiglioni L, Johansson B, Mortimer JA, Berg S, et al. Role of Genes and Environments for Explaining Alzheimer Disease. Arch Gen Psychiatry. 2006;63(2):168-74.
32. Keller MF, Ferrucci L, Singleton AB, Tienari PJ, Laaksovirta H, Restagno G, et al. Genome-wide analysis of the heritability of amyotrophic lateral sclerosis. JAMA Neurol. 2014;71(9):1123-34.
33. Mathews CA, Grados MA. Familiality of Tourette syndrome, obsessive-compulsive disorder, and attention-deficit/hyperactivity disorder: Heritability analysis in a large sib-pair sample. J Am Acad Child Adolesc Psychiatry. 2011;50(1):46-54.
34. Gaugler T, Klei L, Sanders SJ, Bodea CA, Goldberg AP, Lee AB, et al. Most genetic risk for autism resides with common variation. Nat Genet. 2014;46(8):881-5.
35. Speed D, O'Brien TJ, Palotie A, Shkura K, Marson AG, Balding DJ, et al. Describing the genetic architecture of epilepsy through heritability analysis. Brain. 2014;137(10):2680-9.
36. Westerlind H, Ramanujam R, Uvehag D, Kuja-Halkola R, Boman M, Bottai M, et al. Modest familial risks for multiple sclerosis: a registry-based study of the population of Sweden. Brain. 2014;137(3):770-8.
37. Federoff M, Price TR, Sailer A, Scholz S, Hernandez D, Nicolas A, et al. Genome-wide estimate of the heritability of multiple system atrophy. Parkinsonism Relat Disord. 2016;22:35-41.
38. Wirdefeldt K, Gatz M, Reynolds CA, Prescott CA, Pedersen NL. Heritability of Parkinson disease in Swedish twins: a longitudinal study. Neurobiol Aging. 2011;32(10):1923.e1-e8.
39. Cardno AG, Marshall EJ, Coid B, Macdonald AM, Ribchester TR, Davies NJ, et al. Heritability estimates for psychotic disorders: The Maudsley Twin Psychosis Series. Arch Gen Psychiatry. 1999;56(2):162-8.
40. Need AC, Goldstein DB. Whole genome association studies in complex diseases: where do we stand? Dialogues Clin Neurosci. 2010;12(1):37.
41. Hafler DA, Compston A, Sawcer S, Lander ES, Daly MJ, De Jager PL, et al. Risk alleles for multiple sclerosis identified by a genomewide study. N Engl J Med. 2007;357(9):851-62.
42. Schork NJ, Murray SS, Frazer KA, Topol EJ. Common vs. Rare Allele Hypotheses for Complex Diseases. Curr Opin Genet Dev. 2009;19(3):212.
43. Fogel BL, Geschwind DH. Clinical Neurogenetics. In: Daroff R, Fenichel G, Jankovic J, Mazziotta J (Eds). Neurology in Clinical Practice. Philadelphia, PA: Elsevier; 2012. pp. 704-34.
44. Sanger F, Nicklen S, Coulson AR. DNA sequencing with chain-terminating inhibitors. Proc Natl Acad Sci U S A. 1977;74(12):5463.
45. Warner JP, Barron LH, Goudie D, Kelly K, Dow D, Fitzpatrick DR, et al. A general method for the detection of large CAG repeat expansions by fluorescent PCR. J Med Genet. 1996;33(12):1022.
46. Santaguida S, Amon A. Short- and long-term effects of chromosome mis-segregation and aneuploidy. Nat Rev Mol Cell Biol. 2015;16(8):473-85.
47. Ozkan E, Lacerda MP. (2022). Genetics, Cytogenetic Testing and Conventional Karyotype. [online] Available from https://www.ncbi.nlm.nih.gov/books/NBK563293/. [Last accessed March, 2023].
48. Stuppia L, Antonucci I, Palka G, Gatta V. Use of the MLPA assay in the molecular diagnosis of gene copy number alterations in human genetic diseases. Int J Mol Sci. 2012;13(3):3245.
49. Alfares A, Aloraini T, Subaie LA, Alissa A, Qudsi AA, Alahmad A, et al. Whole-genome sequencing offers additional but limited clinical utility compared with reanalysis of whole-exome sequencing. Genet Med. 2018;20(11):1328-33.
50. Duchateau L, Küçükali F, Dongen J van, Bossaerts L, Hens E, Roeck A de, et al. Transcript analysis using long-read sequencing reveals the complex splicing profile of AD-associated gene ABCA7. Alzheimers Dement. 2020;16(S3):e042815.
51. Deng J, Gu M, Miao Y, Yao S, Zhu M, Fang P, et al. Long-read sequencing identified repeat expansions in the 5'UTR of the NOTCH2NLC gene from Chinese patients with neuronal intranuclear inclusion disease. J Med Genet. 2019;56(11):758-64.
52. Papić L, Fischer D, Trajanoski S, Höftberger R, Fischer C, Ströbel T, et al. SNP-array based whole genome homozygosity mapping: A quick and powerful tool to achieve an accurate diagnosis in LGMD2 patients. Eur J Med Genet. 2011;54(3):214.
53. Bidichandani SI, Purandare SM, Taylor EE, Gumin G, Machkhas H, Harati Y, et al. Somatic Sequence Variation at the Friedreich Ataxia Locus Includes Complete Contraction of the Expanded GAA Triplet Repeat, Significant Length Variation in Serially Passaged Lymphoblasts and Enhanced Mutagenesis in the Flanking Sequence. Hum Mol Genet. 1999;8(13):2425-36.
54. Verma PK, Dalal A, Mittal B, Phadke SR. Utility of MLPA in mutation analysis and carrier detection for Duchenne muscular dystrophy. Indian J Hum Genet. 2012;18(1):91.
55. Vissers LELM, Veltman JA, van Kessel AG, Brunner HG. Identification of disease genes by whole genome CGH arrays. Hum Mol Genet. 2005;14(suppl_2):R215-23.
56. Chrzanowska NM, Kowalewski J, Lewandowska MA. Use of Fluorescence In Situ Hybridization (FISH) in Diagnosis and Tailored Therapies in Solid Tumors. Molecules. 2020;25(8):1864.
57. Cui C, Shu W, Li P. Fluorescence in situ hybridization: Cell-based genetic diagnostic and research applications. Front Cell Dev Biol. 2016;4:89.
58. Ezewudo M, Zwic ME. Evaluating rare variants in complex disorders using next-generation sequencing. Curr Psychiatry Rep. 2013;15(4):349.
59. Koboldt DC. Best practices for variant calling in clinical sequencing. Genome Med. 2020;12(1):1-13.
60. Richards S, Aziz N, Bale S, Bick D, Das S, Gastier-Foster J, et al. Standards and guidelines for the interpretation of sequence variants: A Joint Consensus Recommendation of the American College of Medical Genetics and Genomics and the Association for Molecular Pathology. Genet Med. 2015;17(5):405.

122

CHAPTER

Neuropsychological Evaluations

Porrselvi AP, Elizabeth W Choi

INTRODUCTION

"Imaging is not enough."

—Mortimer Mishkin, 1988[1]

Neuropsychology is a specialized field of psychology that is concerned with the behavioral and cognitive expression of brain dysfunction.[1] Neuropsychological assessment is a means of measuring, in a quantitative, standardized fashion, the most complex aspects of human behavior—attention, perception, memory, speech and language, building and drawing, reasoning, problem-solving, judgment, planning, and emotional processing.[1]

Beginning in the 19th century, controlled observations about brain-behavior relationships became accepted, paving the way for psychometric assessment. In the early 20th century, studying war-damaged brains gave much impetus to the role of neuropsychometry. This gradually led to sophisticated examination and treatment techniques.[1]

Neuropsychology today is the product of a combined evolution of clinical neurosciences and psychology. Our knowledge comes from cognitive functions in both humans and other animals. The modern dynamic and functional neuroimaging techniques have given the neuropsychological constructs the neurological bases and support for the comprehension of the brain.

In neuropsychological assessment, answers and explanations to both neurological and psychological questions are sought. Findings from the neuropsychological assessment are interpreted by neuropsychologists within the clinical context of the patient's presentation, history, psychosocial circumstances, as well as other diagnostic information.[1]

There is an ever-growing sensitivity among neurologists, neurosurgeons, psychiatrists, psychologists, and counselors to ask for neuropsychology assistance in identifying candidates, who may have underlying neuropathology, for their services. Due to the advances in diagnostic technology, except in cases of early or mild or questionable cognitive impairments, neuropsychologists are no longer asked if there is a brain disorder but are asked to comment on the cognitive strengths and weaknesses of an individual, estimate their premorbid levels of functioning, their emotional functioning, contributions of different variables to the individual's cognitive concerns, and predict their capacity to function in their everyday world.

Often, neurologists and neurosurgeons request neuropsychometry to aid in the diagnosis and to document the course of brain disorders or the effects of treatment while rehabilitation specialists use neuropsychometry to assist in the planning and management of neurological conditions.[1] Recently, much work is being done in the field of positive neuropsychology to understand the clinical applications of our knowledge about aging. Child neuropsychology has also developed rapidly to understand neurodevelopmental conditions and children's behavior problems.

The use of technology in neuropsychological assessments is the future direction we are headed toward as it continues to proliferate due to the advantages it offers like the ease of standardized administration and scoring, the ability to record previously impossible data like accurate response latencies and error tracking algorithms, remote evaluation, etc. It can also help to address some of the limitations of neuropsychology like catering to patient capacities—ceiling and floor effects, problems with diversity, etc. However, in a humanistic field that requires the interpretation of trained professionals, neuropsychological assessment can only be computer-assisted and not computerized.[2] The use of virtual reality assessment programs, which simulate real-world conditions, could potentially increase the ecological validity of neuropsychological assessment and rehabilitation programs.

To sum up, the distinct purposes that prompt a neuropsychological examination are:

- Diagnosis
- Patient care—identifying treatment needs and planning individualized treatment programs and rehabilitation recommendations

- Evaluating treatment efficacy
- Predicting outcomes and everyday behavior
- Research
- Forensic assessments

UTILITY

There are many reasons for referral to neuropsychological evaluations. According to a research done in the United States, the most common reasons for referrals by medical providers include "establishing and confirming diagnosis" (64.5%), "establishing baseline cognitive functioning" (60.2%), "receiving treatment recommendations" (36.4%), "competency or legal issues" (29.8%), and "for a second opinion" (21.4%).[3] The utility of neuropsychological assessments referrals is outlined as follows with examples:

- *Differential diagnosis*: Assessment can reveal cognitive patterns, or lateralization of cognitive functions, which are consistent with certain etiologies or pathologies. For example, a recognition and rapid forgetting pattern reflected from a verbal learning and memory test is more likely to be associated with Alzheimer's disease pathology, whereas a retrieval deficit profile may be more likely associated with frontal-subcortical deficits commonly found in Huntington's disease, dementia with Lewy bodies, or other vascular etiologies.[4]
- *Establishing cognitive status*: Neuropsychologists help to illustrate a baseline of the patient's cognitive and emotional profiles. For instance, a patient with newly diagnosed relapsing-remitting multiple sclerosis (RRMS) may benefit from having a baseline evaluation as later changes are anticipated with future relapses and MS flare-ups.
- *Monitoring clinically significant changes in cognitive abilities over time*: The psychometrics of certain neuropsychological tests allow for repeated testing, as the test batteries may come in different forms (Form A *vs*. Form B; Standard Form *vs*. Alternate Form). Neuropsychologists also utilize the statistics of the reliable change index (RCI) made available from the normative data of the tests to discern clinically and statistically significant change.[5] This is particularly useful for tracking cognitive symptoms progression in dementia, and any pre- and post-changes of neurosurgical and cognitive interventions.
- *Presurgical evaluation*: Neuropsychological assessments are particularly crucial in many pre-neurosurgical procedures. For instance, a neuropsychological evaluation is helpful in detecting adverse cognitive and behavioral impairment after epilepsy surgery.[6] Neuropsychologists also play an intraoperative role in brain mapping procedures (e.g., Wada) to locate cognitive functions such as language, executive functions, and visuospatial awareness, with the goal to minimize patients' diminishing postoperative quality of life.[7] Neuropsychological evaluation also helps to facilitate the neurosurgical team's determination of patients' candidacy for deep brain stimulation (DBS). The patient's baseline cognitive and mood functionings were assessed to rule out the presence of dementia and depression, as cognitive and mood symptoms could likely exacerbate right after DBS placement surgery.[8,9]
- *Capacity evaluation*: Enquiry of decision-making capacity in patients is often a common reason for referrals, especially in the in-patient medical setting. Neuropsychologists use clinical interviews [at times semi-structure capacity interviews, e.g., MacArthur Competence Assessment Tool for Treatment (MacCAT-T)][10] and cognitive tests to describe patient's level of understanding of the situation, appreciation of the consequences and benefits, and ability to reason the choices and express their rationale and wishes.[11]
- *Inform rehabilitation and treatment directions*: Neuropsychological evaluations can identify cognitive strengths and weaknesses to help the medical team to perform determination of patient's disability, estimate the ability to return to work/school, and driving ability. Neuropsychological evaluations may also serve forensic (legal) purposes.[12]

TECHNICAL ASPECTS

Upon referral, neuropsychologists perform a comprehensive chart review that notes the patient's medical and psychiatric history, laboratory and neuroimaging results, and medications. When the patient comes in for an evaluation, the neuropsychologist performs a detailed clinical interview (usually an hour) and behavioral observations pertaining to the cognitive complaints and the referring provider's questions. Collateral information from education, employment records, and family/caregivers' reports will be collected. Next, the neurocognitive testing takes 2–5 hours of direct contact depending on the patient's physical and cognitive stamina. Typical outpatient evaluations tend to be longer and more comprehensive than inpatient evaluations. Test batteries can be "fixed" or "flexible" with the latter being more common as the neuropsychologists adopt the hypothesis testing approach to adjust and add necessary tests to elucidate certain cognitive domain performance in the process. Tests are always administered in a standardized manner (instructions are given according to the publishers' manual). Cognitive tests and behavioral and psychological measures are typically done in a paper-and-pencil manner, with the more recent incorporation of computerized and telehealth platforms. Basic and instrumental adaptive functionings are also assessed to understand the impact of cognitive factors on self-care abilities.

It should be noted that as many tests were first found in Western countries and later adopted in Asian countries, neuropsychologists pay attention to understand the patient's cultural and ethnic background, as well as their language proficiency, education, vocational attainment, and acculturation levels. The neuropsychologist also Reference the latest research data derived from cross-cultural studies and select the most appropriate normative information and test adaptation to suit the patient's cultural background for testing and later scoring and interpretation.

Scoring of the test is performed by comparing the patient's scores to the appropriate population-derived norms. Comparative scoring is in reference to the patient's demographic background—age, gender, education level, and ethnicity. In some occasions, subregions of the patient's home origin (e.g., rural *vs.* urban regions) are considered.

After completion of test administration and scoring, the neuropsychologist incorporates all of the above-mentioned components to write an integrated report. In some rehabilitation settings, the neuropsychologist provides feedback to the patient to highlight their strengths and limitations, with the goal to bridge them for further rehabilitation work.

INTERPRETATIONS

Neuropsychology reports vary with the neuropsychologists' reporting style, but they commonly covers these broad areas. **Table 1** outlines the subsections that typically appear on a report's interpretation portion, alongside a description of what data neurologists may find useful in their reading/interpretation of the report.

CASE EXAMPLES

Case 1

The first example illustrates an example of how neuropsychology can help in the differential diagnoses of mild cognitive impairment (MCI) versus mood-related cognitive deficiencies.

Mr R, a 69-year-old man, was referred to neuropsychological assessment to answer the referral question of whether the cognitive concerns he had expressed to the neurologist, especially with recent and autobiographical memory as well as some word finding difficulties, were due to MCI or dementia pathology. His presentation is a subjective opinion that his memory has gotten worse over the past 4 years, and he forgets about things like recent trips and has some word-finding difficulties. He was worried he might make mistakes while doing his finances and checks them repeatedly, though he has not made errors so far. His recent magnetic resonance imaging (MRI) of the brain was normal with age-related changes.

Mr R is a retired software engineer who used to be very proficient in business and software coding. He lives with his wife, and he is currently supporting her after her recent diagnosis of cancer. He takes care of his dog, does his finances, and manages his properties. He has been ambidextrous since childhood. He says he continues to think of software codes, likes to find information on the

TABLE 1: Outline of the subsections in a neuropsychology report and their descriptions.

Subsections of interpretation summary	Description
Estimated premorbid intellectual functioning	This data is helpful in putting the test scores into context. For example, an average range of test scores in an average premorbid functioning individual may mean relatively preserved cognitive levels. An average range of test scores in a superior premorbid functioning individual may suggest a possible cognitive decline from baseline
Test of effort	This data identifies any factors that may confound test performance, and hence the validity of the report. These can include a patient's level of fatigue, motivation, test-taking approach, and cooperation
Abilities within expectations	This data refers to the cognitive functions that remain unchanged, or less impacted by the existing known medical condition
Cognitive deficits	This data refers to any test scores that fell below expected of the patient's demographic background. Deficits are typically identified through test scores falling in the "borderline impaired", "mildly impaired", "moderately impaired", or "severely impaired" range
Inconsistent/equivocal findings	Inconsistency can be found in "intra-evaluation" (e.g., variable scores within the same domain) or in the form of test scores not consistent with the patient's or neurologist's observations (e.g., high average verbal memory test scores vs. patient's subjective memory decline). Findings can also be equivocal when neuropsychological data substantiates existing medical information. Neuropsychologists put forth their hypotheses on how inconsistency/equivocal findings occur
Lateralization/localization of impairments	Based on the deficits pattern, neuropsychologists conceptualize test findings in relation to neuroanatomy, or certain neuroanatomical structures. For example, identification of difficulties in set-shifting, impulsivity, and preservative behaviors during hours-long testing may point to possible frontal lobe dysfunctions
Emotional functioning/ personality traits	This data is helpful in understanding the patient's status of psychological disturbances, and any personality traits, which may serve as confounding variables in the test data. Having this data also allows the neuropsychologist to make recommendations for care management, e.g., referral for psychotropic medications, or psychotherapy, or other treatment considerations
Comorbid conditions that may affect cognition	Neuropsychologists comment on how existing comorbid medical conditions may contribute to cognitive functioning. For example, cerebrovascular events history, prediabetes, low vitamin B12/vitamin D, and white matter hyperintensities identified on neuroimaging

Continued

Continued

Subsections of interpretation summary	Description
Diagnostic possibilities/ rule-outs	This data explains what are the primary driving forces of cognitive deficits on a differential diagnosis framework. In some instances, neuropsychological data may shed light on possible pathologies and etiologies of diseases. Neuropsychologists determine if the patient meets the diagnostic criteria of a "neurocognitive disorder" based on the DSM-5 and ICD-10
Recommendations	Common recommendations on management may include, but are not limited to: • Medical referrals (laboratories, neuroimaging, and sleep study) • Educational (extended time, IEP/504, therapy, and summer school) • Driving safety evaluation • Sleep hygiene • Community support (social work referrals, caregiver's association, and services to promote safety and independence) • Mood management (psychiatry follow-up, psychotherapy, and support group) • Legal (advanced directives; discussion on attorney of power) • Referrals to other therapies (occupational, physical, speech, and vocational therapy) • Need for neuropsychological re-evaluation • Cognitive remediation (psychoeducation, cognitive rehabilitation, assess for return to work/school)[13-17]

(DSM-5: Diagnostic and Statistical Manual of Mental Disorders, Fifth Edition; ICD-10: International Statistical Classification of Diseases and Related Health Problems)

web, follows the news, and does DIY projects for home improvement.

When he was a teenager, he received some therapy for psychogenic tachycardia. His mother had memory concerns as she aged, though she did not have any formal diagnosis.

During the assessment, his mood was found to be low, and he was anxious. Though he is hopeful that she will recover, his wife's diagnosis has been making him worried.

He has a delayed onset of sleep and sleeps only about 2 hours in the night on some days which results in him feeling tired in the afternoons. He takes a nap at about 4–5 PM in the evening. His appetite is normal.

Neuropsychological Assessment

He was well-groomed, mild-mannered, and cooperative. During the testing, his behavior was noticed to be anxious, especially with regard to his performance. There was a consistent expression of frustration that he should be performing better, and frequent encouragement and urging were necessary to ensure he was putting in optimal levels of effort.

Insight

His insight is good.

Orientation

He was oriented to the date, time, place, and person. He could name the prime minister and discuss recent politics.

Mood

- *PHQ 9-17*: Moderately severe depressive features
- *GAD 7-19*: Severe anxiety features

Effort

The test performance is valid, and he put in optimal effort for completing the tests.

Estimated Premorbid Cognition and Current Intellectual Functioning

Using the estimate of his premorbid cognitive function (predicted estimate FSIQ-117.3), it was noticed that there is a decline in his cognitive functioning [prorated FSIQ-100 (-17.3); proration because all tests on the Wechsler Adult Intelligence Scale 4th Edition (WAIS-IV)[18] could not be administered in addition to the other tests required to get a complete current cognitive profile]. His score on the vocabulary subtest of the WAIS-IV was in the superior range.

Memory

His verbal memory was in the average and high average range with short delay recall being in the superior range. On the nonverbal memory test, his performance was on average for the short delay and low average for the long delay. This shows that currently, his verbal memory is better than his nonverbal memory. His recognition on the nonverbal memory test was in the average range indicating that his recognition was better than recall on nonverbal memory.

Language

Mild word-finding difficulties were observed in his conversations, but no paraphasia was noted. On the picture naming test from Brain Injury Rehabilitation Trust Memory and Information Processing Battery II (BMIPB-II), he performed in the average range.

Visuospatial Skills

His clock drawing was accurate. His scores were in the low average range on the matrix reasoning and symbol search subtests of the WAIS-IV. On block design and coding subtests, his performance was in the average range. It has to be noted that on the block design subtest, he was doing well until he was given 9 blocks to construct, and he was frustrated and did not want to attempt further.

Executive Function

His scores on all tests of executive function, information processing, and working memory are in the average or high average range except for the category switching task of the Delis–Kaplan Executive Function System (D-KEFS)[19] Verbal Fluency Test in which his performance was low average. It must be noted that during this subtest, he was observed to be frustrated. His speed of processing was found to be in the average range.

Summary and Recommendations from the Neuropsychologist

The neuropsychological assessment of Mr R shows a decline from his estimated premorbid levels of functioning. This decline in cognitive functioning, which he is also subjectively concerned about, could be exacerbated by his current mood, chronic pain, frustration to perform better, and the decrease in the amount of restful sleep he is getting every day.

It is recommended that Mr R:

- Receives support for better sleep management
- Receives support for mood management (talk therapy and counseling)
- Maintains a planner/journal for keeping track of his engagements and activities currently, in the future, and in the recent past
- *Emotional regulation*: Is mindful of the expectations he places on himself in consideration for the current life situations which seem to be adding to his feelings of frustration and anxiety.
- Is referred for follow-up neuropsychological assessment if his cognitive problems persist/decline if required.

Action Taken by the Neurologist

The neurologist made the informed decision to educate Mr R that given his family history and subjective concerns, it was considered if there was any underlying neuropathology but in the event of a normal neuroimaging and the above neuropsychological findings, it is more important to address his sleep and mood concerns currently.

Case 2

The second example illustrates the use of neuropsychological assessment in which the neurologist requested it to support his evidence in the case of a forensic evaluation in response to a legal suit filed by the individual against a heating solutions company demanding compensation.

Mrs B is a 57-year-old right-handed woman with a history of carbon monoxide exposure 2 years ago due to a boiler malfunction following which she developed tinnitus, loss of smell, vertigo, and balance issues. She suffers from frequent headaches that affect her functioning and she feels fatigued all the time. Her MRI brain is reported normal. She reports a previous back injury from a fall and hypothyroidism for which she is under medical management.

Subjectively, she reported that since the next day of the incident, she has been feeling like she is "constantly drunk" as she is not able to register anything, is not able to pay attention, forgets her words, loses her train of thought, cannot follow conversations, or remember them, even if she tries to write down information, she forgets them. She feels overwhelmed with everything and prefers to just be by herself without doing anything.

She used to work as a school services coordinator. She quit her job after the boiler malfunction incident as she could not perform on the job. She currently lives with her daughter who does all the domestic and financial activities for her. She does not have any routine, or hobbies, and does not like to socially interact or travel because of her current condition. She reports until the incident, she was active and very independent.

Her mother and grandfather were diagnosed with Alzheimer's disease and her father died after a diagnosis of motor neurone disease (MND). Considering her family history, she says since her young adulthood days, she has been proactive about reducing her risk factors.

Current Mood

She reports she does not feel anything and is emotionally numb since the episode and does not take pleasure in any activities nor does she feel low or angry about anything.

Sleep and Appetite

She reports poor quality of sleep with many nights spent with no sleep. Her appetite is poor, and she only eats rarely in small quantities.

Neuropsychological Assessment

She was well-groomed and mild-mannered. She did not want to do the assessments as she felt that she cannot register anything and switched off. She needed multiple reassurances and constant encouragement to get her to complete some of the tests that were planned to be administered. She refused to do some of the tests saying they were making her feel giddy and nauseous.

During the testing, it was noted that she was very sensitive to small sounds and changes in her environment. Her attention was hard to sustain and test instructions had to be repeated or shortened for her to follow them.

Insight

Her insight was partial but during the feedback, after the assessment, she seemed more willing to accept her concerns and what they may be caused by.

Orientation

She was not oriented to the date and day but was oriented to the time, place, and person.

Mood

- *PHQ9-21*: Severe depressive features
- *GAD7-15*: Severe anxiety features

Effort

Fluctuations in test performance is noted and hence discrepancy in outcome of the testing and her actual cognitive ability is expected.

Estimated Premorbid Cognition and Current Intellectual Functioning

Using the estimate of her premorbid cognitive function (predicted estimate FSIQ-109), it can be noticed that there is a significant decline in her cognitive functioning; however, it must be noted that her effort in test performance is questionable.

Memory

Her verbal memory was impaired in the logical memory subtest of the Wechsler Memory Scale® Fourth Edition (WMS-IV)[20] and in the California Verbal Learning Test, Third Edition (CVLT-3)[21] brief. She was not willing to do the nonverbal memory tests. Her recognition on all the verbal memory tests was better than recall but still in the impaired range indicating that there are impairments in both encoding and learning.

Language

Word-finding difficulties were observed in her conversations and during the testing with her performance on the picture naming test of the BMIPB-II being in the impaired range.

Visuospatial Skills

Her scores were in the average range on the block design subtest of the WAIS-IV. She refused to attempt a few other tests and said they made her dizzy.

Executive Function

Her scores on the verbal fluency subtest of the D-KEFS were impaired. She refused to attempt the other tests of executive function. It was noted that in the fluency tasks, digit span subtests that her self-inhibition and switching were error free.

Summary and Recommendations

The neuropsychological assessment of Mrs B shows a significant decline from her estimated premorbid levels of functioning but her effort in test performance is questionable. This decline in cognitive functioning which she is also subjectively concerned about and is reflecting in her real-world functioning could be exacerbated by her current mood, fatigue, and poor quality of sleep. Impairments in her vestibular function and headaches combined with depression and anxiety are contributing to her current cognitive concerns. Nevertheless, it is noted that since the boiler malfunction incident, Mrs B has been experiencing significant impairments to her everyday functioning and has had to leave active employment because of her inability to perform at her job.

It is recommended that Mrs B:

- Is referred to specialized acceptance and commitment therapy (ACT) for her mood.
- Receives support for better sleep management.
- Is referred to specialized cognitive rehabilitation.
- Adopts good sleep hygiene practices.
- Uses to do lists/calendar reminders/taking notes and other technological support to plan her day and activities.
- Uses visual cues and images to help her remember better.
- Completes most demanding tasks when she is at her best (e.g., morning).
- Allows extra time to complete cognitively demanding tasks.
- Breaks down tasks into smaller steps where needed.
- Paces her tasks so that she does not become overtired by taking sufficient breaks instead of forcing herself to continue when she is zoning out or tired.
- Engages in new hobbies, art, reading comics, and other cognitive stimulating leisure activities with some time spent outside her room and outdoors every day (e.g., short walks, short drives to the grocery, etc.), if possible.
- Uses ear defenders to help her with her sensitivity to sounds.

Action Taken by the Neurologist

The neurologist made the informed decision to inform the concerned authorities that it is reasonable that Mrs B received disability support and recommended that she be compensated for the life-changing circumstances caused by the boiler malfunction and carbon monoxide poisoning that followed.

Case 3

The third example illustrates the use of neuropsychological assessment for the purpose of gathering evidence during differential diagnosis in cases of atypical Parkinson's. The neurologist referred Mr F to psychometry to understand and gather evidence to diagnose him with multiple system atrophy (MSA) or progressive supranuclear palsy (PSP) in the circumstance of atypical clinical presentation.

Mr F, a 70-year-old man, reported that his memory is generally good, but he has difficulty remembering people's names, but this has always been the case. He does not remember birthdays and again he has never been good at this. He was a former bus driver. He can retain the main news items. He can follow the plot of TV programs. He rarely reads. He manages the household finances without difficulty. He has a good memory for events that happened in the past including his primary and secondary school. He reported that his main difficulties are to do with his physical ability which impacts his ability to do things.

He currently lives with his wife.

Mood

Mr F scored on the severe range on the PHQ-9.

Neuropsychological Assessment

On tests of general intellectual functioning, Mr F obtained scores in the low average range on verbal tests. On one visual test, his performance was in the borderline range. On the other (Matrix reasoning) test, he was unable to pass the example questions. He appeared to answer very quickly without fully considering all options.

On tests of verbal memory, his performance was variable. His story recall was in the average range. His list learning recall was impaired. His learning curve was in the average range as was his list recognition. This would indicate some variability in the retrieval of information which is seen in subcortical dementias. His performance on visual memory recognition was in the borderline range. His performance on a picture-naming test was below expectations. It was observed that he was showing high impulsivity and blurting out responses or choosing responses even before he had processed the test stimuli.

On tests of executive functioning, his performance was variable. Letter fluency was in the borderline range, category fluency was in the average range, and category switching in the low average range. On a test of inhibition, his performance was in the borderline range. When cognitive demand increased, his performance improved to the average range (color word interference test; D-KEFS). This is hypothesized to be because when tasks were more difficult, he could inhibit himself and concentrate on the task better. He made a high rate of errors on both conditions of the color word interference test, indicating some difficulties in monitoring his performance. On the Hayling sentence completion task, his performance on the inhibition condition was in the average range.

Summary and Recommendations

Overall, his performance on the tests indicates impulsivity, retrieval deficits in memory, and executive function difficulties along with depression. Performance on the remaining tests is broadly within expectations. Considering the current scientific literature,[8,9] absence of apathy and his engagement levels contraindicate PSP. The current neuropsychological findings support a diagnosis of MSA with predominant parkinsonism (MSA-P) subtype.

It is recommended that Mr F:

- Is referred to local psychology services for support with his mood difficulties.

Action Taken by the Neurologist

The neurologist made the informed decision for subsequent patient care including treatment planning.

CONCLUSION

"If a man has lost a leg or an eye, he knows he has lost a leg or an eye; but if he has lost a self—himself—he cannot know it, because he is no longer there to know it."

—Oliver Sacks

Neuropsychological evaluations attempt to uncover this. Neuropsychology is a distinct field within science, which has evolved out of the necessity to study brain function and how it relates to human behavior and thinking based on the scientific principles borrowed from clinical neurosciences and psychology.[22] "The competent practice of the field requires an in-depth understanding of psychometric techniques, principles of deficit measurement, theories of brain-behavior relationship, and effects of various brain diseases/injuries on cognitive and behavioral functioning."[23] As the field continues to grow, an accurate and timely referral of all patients who may benefit from neuropsychological evaluation and rehabilitation, and the application of the findings in clinical decision-making will result in better patient outcomes and their improved quality of life.

REFERENCES

1. Lezak MD, Howieson DB, Bigler ED, Tranel D. Neuropsychological Assessment, 5th edition. New York: Oxford University Press; 2012.
2. Porrselvi AP. TAM battery: Development and pilot testing of a Tamil computer-assisted cognitive test battery for older adults. Clin Neuropsychol. 2022;1-20: Online ahead of print.
3. Temple RO, Carvalho J, Tremont G. A national survey of physicians' use of and satisfaction with neuropsychological services. Arch Clin Neuropsychol. 2006;21(5):371-82.
4. Salmon DP, Bondi MW. Neuropsychological assessment of dementia. Annu Rev Psychol. 2009;60:257-82.

5. Duff K. Evidence-based indicators of neuropsychological change in the individual patient: relevant concepts and methods. Arch Clin Neuropsychol. 2012;27(3):248-61.
6. Wilson SJ, Baxendale S, Barr W, Hamed S, Langfitt J, Samson S, et al. Indications and expectations for neuropsychological assessment in routine epilepsy care: Report of the ILAE Neuropsychology Task Force, Diagnostic Methods Commission, 2013-2017. Epilepsia. 2015;56(5):674-81.
7. Landers MJF, Sitskoorn MM, Rutten GJM, Mandonnet E, de Baene W. A systematic review of the use of subcortical intraoperative electrical stimulation mapping for monitoring of executive deficits and neglect: what is the evidence so far? Acta Neurochir (Wien). 2022;164(1):177-91.
8. Santangelo G, Cuoco S, Pellecchia MT, Erro R, Barone P, Picillo M. Comparative cognitive and neuropsychiatric profiles between Parkinson's disease, multiple system atrophy and progressive supranuclear palsy. J Neurol. 2018;265(11):2602-13.
9. Nasri A, Gharbi A, Sghaier I, Mrabet S, Souissi A, Gargouri A, et al. Determinants of cognitive impairment in multiple system atrophy: Clinical and genetic study. PLoS One. 2022;17(12):e0277798.
10. Grisso T, Appelbaum PS, and Hill-Fotouhi C. The MacCAT-T: a clinical tool to assess patients' capacities to make treatment decisions. Psychiatr Serv. 1997;48(11):1415-9.
11. Appelbaum PS, Grisso T. Assessing patients' capacities to consent to treatment. N Engl J Med. 1988;319(25):1635-8.
12. Eliassen IV, Fladby T, Kirsebom BE, Waterloo K, Eckerström M, Wallin A, et al. Predictive and diagnostic utility of brief neuropsychological assessment in detecting Alzheimer's pathology and progression to dementia. Neuropsychology. 2020;34(8):851-61.
13. Chew KA, Chong EJY, Chen CLH, Xu X. Psychometric Properties of the National Institute of Neurological Disorders and Stroke and Canadian Stroke Network Neuropsychological Battery in an Asian Older Adult Sample. J Am Med Dir Assoc. 2020;21(6): 879-83.e1.
14. Donders J. The incremental value of neuropsychological assessment: A critical review. Clin Neuropsychol. 2020;34(1):56-87.
15. Heilbronner RL. American Academy of Clinical Neuropsychology (AACN) practice guidelines for neuropsychological assessment and consultation. Clin Neuropsychol. 2007;21(2):209-31.
16. Heilbronner RL. A status report on the practice of forensic neuropsychology. Clin Neuropsychol. 2004;18(2):312-26.
17. Kolitz BP, Kolitz Russell S. The usefulness of a validated neuropsychological test battery in scientifically supporting and communicating forensic evaluation results. The Scientific Foundation of Neuropsychological Assessment. Amsterdam: Elsevier; 2012. pp. 341-57.
18. Wechsler, D. (2008). Wechsler Adult Intelligence Scale (4th edition). San Antonio, TX: Pearson Assessment.
19. Delis DC, Kaplan E, and Kramer JH. (2001). Delis-Kaplan Executive Function System (D-KEFS). San Antonio, TX: The Psychological Corporation.
20. Wechsler, D. (2009). Wechsler Memory Scale (4th edition). San Antonio, TX: Pearson.
21. Delis DC, Kramer JH, Kaplan E, and Ober BA. (2017). California Verbal Learning Test-3 (3rd edition). San Antonio, TX: The Psychological Corporation.
22. Delis DC. Neuropsychological Testing. Encyclopedia of Neuroscience. Amsterdam: Elsevier; 2009. pp. 983-91.
23. Lucas JA, Mahone EM, Westerveld M, Bieliauskas L, Baron IS. The American Board of Clinical Neuropsychology and American Academy of Clinical Neuropsychology: updated milestones 2005-2014. Clin Neuropsychol. 2014;28(6):889-906.

6

SECTION

Principles of Management

123
CHAPTER

Principles of Drug Therapy

Sandeep Kaushal, Shalini Arora

INTRODUCTION

The central nervous system (CNS) is functionally more complex and least understood among all the organ systems of the human body. The number of neurological disorders is large, and so is the number of drugs used for these disorders. Pharmacological intervention plays a major key role in treating these disorders. Also, several other psychological conditions and symptomatic treatment of pain and pyrexia involve the use of pharmacotherapy. On top of that, a number of other nonmedicinal substances are used, as well as abused for their effects on CNS. These include tea, coffee, alcohol, cannabis, nicotine, and so on.

The complexity of the CNS and the effects of drugs at the biochemical and molecular levels make it furthermore difficult to understand the processes and circuitry in the brain. It becomes particularly challenging to understand the drug effects on CNS.

The primary goal of knowing the principles of drug therapy is to apply the information about the drugs and their mechanisms to develop safe and effective treatments, both preventive and curative, for the vast array of neurological problems. In this chapter, the general principles, which govern the action of drugs, will be discussed including the important aspects of pharmacokinetics and pharmacodynamics of the drugs acting on the CNS. The pharmacokinetic properties of a drug determine the concentration of the drug at the site of action which in turn determines the intensity of response to a drug. Pharmacokinetic considerations also determine the dose, duration of action, frequency, and route of administration of the given drug. Pharmacodynamics is the study of the effects of drugs on the human body and also how these effects are produced. It also includes the interaction of drugs, food, and other substances.

BLOOD–BRAIN BARRIER

The functional separation of the extracellular fluid of the brain from the blood in circulation is responsible for checking the penetration of drugs and other substances into the CNS. The endothelial cells of the capillaries have tight junctions with a covering of neural tissue **(Fig. 1)**. Only those drugs can enter the CNS, which either are lipid soluble or have a specific transport mechanism. For example, levodopa, a precursor of dopamine, is used in Parkinsonism, as dopamine cannot cross the blood–brain barrier (BBB). Levodopa enters the brain via an amino acid transporter. Gabapentin, a water-soluble drug, crosses BBB through a large neutral amino acid transporter (LAT1) as gabapentin has structure that mimics the endogenous substrate, neutral amino acids.[1] Drowsiness with older-generation antihistamines has led to the development of

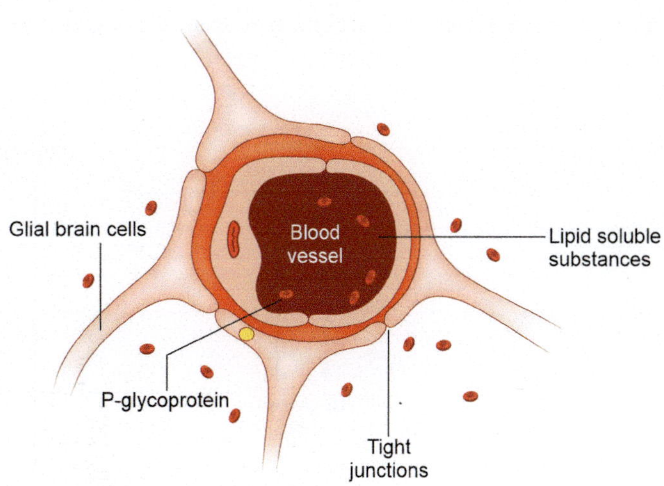

FIG. 1: Blood–brain barrier.

newer drugs that are less sedative, the change includes making them more polar and hence, they cannot cross the BBB freely.[2] Apart from lipid solubility, a number of other factors determine the rate of drug transport through the BBB. These include its protein binding, ionization, availability of transport carriers, and concentration in the blood. A number of nutrients such as glucose and essential amino acids have specific transporters to let these substances cross the CNS. Blood-brain barrier can be disrupted by infection, inflammation, and certain tumors, allowing easy permeability to many substances.[3] Therefore, penicillin, a large molecule, is able to achieve high concentration in cerebrospinal fluid (CSF) in a patient suffering from meningitis but not in case of any other systemic infection.

The normal BBB is deficient in the circumventricular organs, including area postrema, chemoreceptor trigger zone (CTZ), and anterior hypothalamus, and hence some drugs which are not lipid soluble can still act on CNS through these sites. Apomorphine though not lipid soluble can cause nausea because of CTZ stimulation, as CTZ lies outside the BBB.[4] Peptides such as desmopressin can be administered intranasally in patients with diabetes insipidus for direct delivery into CSF. In addition, there may be specific efflux transporters [e.g., P-glycoproteins(P-gp)] present which extrude the drugs entering the brain. Efflux transporter may be responsible for the reduced effectiveness of certain antiepileptic drugs such as phenytoin.

PHARMACOKINETICS

Pharmacokinetics is the quantitative description of what happens to a drug when it enters the body, including drug absorption, distribution, metabolism, and elimination or excretion. Absorption, to a great extent, is determined by the route of administration. A large number of drugs acting on the CNS are available for oral administration, although some have formulations that are also available for intravenous, intramuscular, intranasal, buccal, intrathecal, transdermal, or rectal administration.

Absorption

Absorption means the movement of the drug from its site of administration into circulation. The fraction of the drug reaching the circulation further determines the amount which reaches the site of action, i.e., the CNS. The measure of the fraction of administered dose of a drug that reaches the site of action in unchanged form is termed bioavailability. Bioavailability of drugs administered intravenously is usually 100%. But, as most of the drugs are administered orally, several factors determine the bioavailability of the drugs including its molecular size, solubility, ionization, plasma protein binding, and its ability to penetrate the BBB. Most antiepileptic drugs undergo complete or nearly complete absorption when given orally.[4]

Ionization changes lipid solubility; hence, drugs in unionized state are lipid soluble but become nonlipid soluble after ionization and, hence, are able to cross the membrane **(Fig. 2)**. For example, aspirin gets trapped in gastrointestinal mucosa as it is unionized in the acidic pH of the stomach and reaches gastric mucosa but the pH inside these cells is neutral and hence it ionizes and gets trapped and becomes lipid insoluble.

Most often, administration of these drugs with food slows absorption and can help to avert peak dose-related side effects. Moreover, food delays gastric emptying. Calcium-containing antacids may interfere with phenytoin absorption. Tricyclic antidepressants can also decrease gut motility and thus decrease the absorption of some drugs. Gabapentin is absorbed by a saturable amino acid transport system and does not get absorbed after a certain dose. Oral absorption of certain drugs can also be hindered by efflux transporters, such as P-gp, located in the gut epithelium which extrudes the absorbed drug back into the

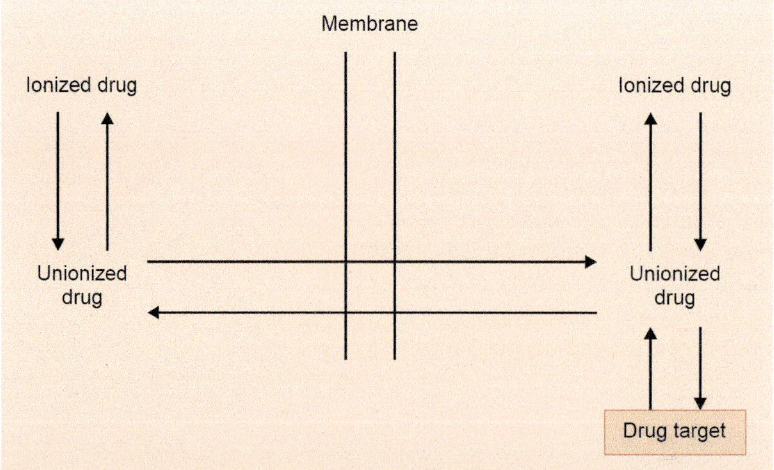

FIG. 2: Drug disposition across the biological membrane.

intestinal lumen.[5] Phenobarbitone is an inducer of P-gp and can reduce the oral bioavailability of certain drugs such as cyclosporine. Apart from incomplete absorption, the absorbed drug may also undergo the first-pass metabolism in the intestinal mucosa or liver or may be excreted in the bile. Rectal administration of diazepam (available as a rectal gel) has been shown to terminate repetitive seizures and can be administered by family members at home. The buccal route is used for the termination of febrile seizures (midazolam) to avoid rectal administration which is difficult and uncomfortable for patients to administer. This route is easier to follow, and the drug can be easily placed in the buccal cavity for better and safe administration.

The intramuscular route allows better bioavailability of drugs and more predictable and consistent plasma concentrations as compared to the oral route. Fosphenytoin may be administered intramuscularly if intravenous access cannot be established in cases of status epilepticus. The intravenous route is used for emergencies. Programmed intravenous pumps are used to deliver small fixed doses of opioid analgesics, such as fentanyl, for patient-controlled analgesia. The intravenous route is also used for fosphenytoin which is a prodrug and has been developed to overcome the difficulties in the intravenous administration of phenytoin.

Intrathecal baclofen is used for patients with severe spasticity and dystonia. Transdermal delivery also provides consistency in plasma concentration and is used for various drugs including clonidine, fentanyl, and rivastigmine. Because of its convenience, compliance is better and bioavailability is also improved as compared to oral route. Nasal spray for drugs such as butorphanol provides longer lasting effects.

Distribution

After reaching the systemic circulation, the drug gets distributed to the body tissues. A number of factors determine the extent and pattern of tissue distribution of a drug. These factors include the lipid solubility of the drug, its ionization at physiological pH, binding to plasma proteins and tissue proteins, the presence of membrane transporters in a tissue, and regional blood flow.[6]

Drug distributes in the body as the free drug and bound fractions. Drug movement occurs until an equilibrium is achieved between the free drug in the plasma and in the tissue fluids **(Fig. 3)**. Free drug is responsible for drug action. The molecular size of drug increases once it binds with plasma proteins and, hence, the transport across membrane is not possible. But, the drug in free form is able to move across the membrane and undergo changes, e.g., free phenytoin gets metabolized in the liver but bound form is not metabolized, though there is an equilibrium between bound form and free form. As the free form gets metabolized, the equilibrium shifts to unbind the drug bound with plasma proteins and overall metabolism/excretion takes place over time. This can result in high free drug concentration in malnourished patients/patients with hypoproteinemia.

Also, concurrent administration of two highly protein-bound drugs, e.g., phenytoin and valproic acid, can compete with each other and cause displacement, resulting in high free drug concentration and hence toxicity. Volume of distribution (Vd) is a parameter to determine the extent of drug distribution. It is defined as the amount of drug in the body in relation to the plasma concentration (Cp) of the drug.

$$Vd = Dose\ or\ amount\ of\ drug\ in\ body/Cp$$

Plasma protein binding and lipid solubility are the two major factors and determinants for the Vd of a drug.

The Vd can, sometimes, exceed the physical volume in the body. This occurs for drugs with high concentrations in extravascular tissue (drug sequestered in tissues due to high affinity) **(Fig. 4)**. Whereas, drugs that remain restricted to the vascular compartment have low values of "Vd". So, it is more appropriately termed as apparent volume of distribution (aVd) if the body is presumed to be a single homogenous compartment in which the drug gets

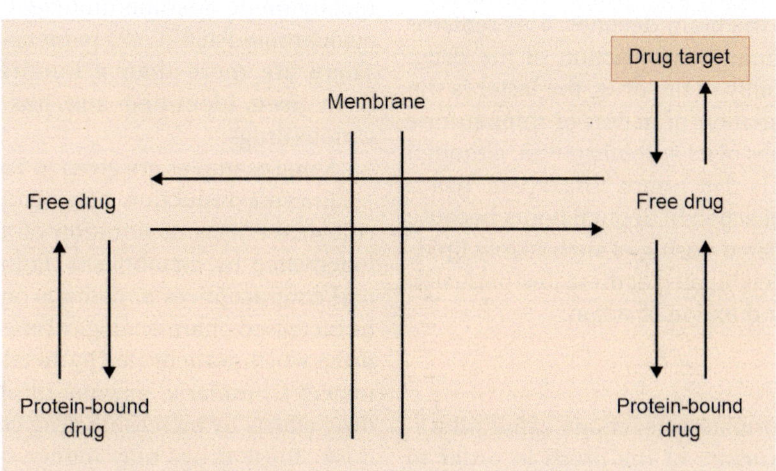

FIG. 3: Drug disposition of protein-bound drugs.

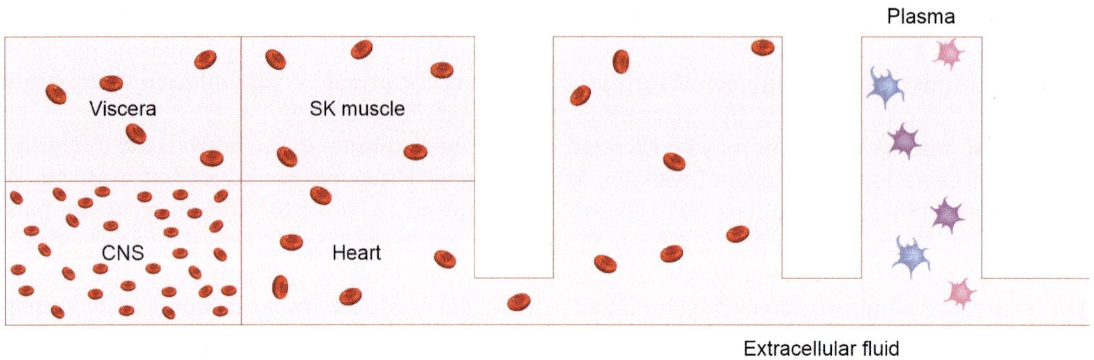

FIG. 4: Drug sequestration in body compartments.
(CNS: central nervous system; SK: skeletal)

uniformly distributed. aVd is an index of the distribution of a drug in the body by comparing the Vd of the drug to the physiological volumes of various water compartments of the body. High aVd also implies that this drug, in case of overdose and toxicity, cannot be easily removed by hemodialysis.[4]

The Vd also helps in calculating the loading dose needed to attain the required therapeutic plasma concentrations, especially in emergency situations like status epilepticus, to minimize the lag period for onset of drug action.

The Vd may change for the same person during physiological changes (e.g., it increases in pregnancy) and pathological states (e.g., Vd increases in patients with symptomatic congestive heart failure as compared to treated heart failure).

Redistribution

Highly lipid-soluble drugs get distributed initially to organs with high-blood flow including the brain and heart. The general anesthetic, thiopentone sodium, is highly lipid soluble. It rapidly reaches the brain which is the site of action of thiopentone. Later, the less vascular tissues, such as muscle and fat, take up the drug to maintain equilibrium and the concentration in the brain declines. This redistribution results in the termination of action of the drug. The higher the lipid solubility of the drug, the faster is the redistribution, e.g., termination of action of thiopentone occurs within a few minutes of its administration, although its elimination half-life is 3–8 hours. Diazepam has a relatively short duration of action of about 6 hours because of redistribution. On repeated dosing of such highly lipid-soluble drugs, these get accumulated at these low-perfusion sites, thus prolonging their duration of action.

Metabolism

Metabolism or biotransformation reactions cause alterations in the chemical structure of the drugs in order to convert the lipid-soluble compounds to polar compounds so that these can be excreted by the renal tubules. Hydrophilic drugs, such as pancuronium, do not require much biotransformation and are excreted as such. Most of the drugs used for neurological disorders are lipid soluble and require a metabolic transformation in the body. The primary site for drug metabolism is the liver, others include kidney, lungs, intestine, skin, brain, and plasma. Biotransformation results in either inactivation of the drugs, e.g., paracetamol, conversion of the drug into active metabolite, e.g., morphine to morphine-6-glucuronide, diazepam to oxazepam, imipramine to desipramine, amitriptyline to nortriptyline, or activation of the inactive drug, e.g., levodopa to dopamine, alpha methyldopa to alpha methylnorepinephrine. Biotransformation reactions can be Phase I (nonsynthetic) reactions in which a functional group (–OH, $–NH_2$, and –SH) is introduced or unmasked resulting in the formation of an active or inactive metabolite and the Phase II (synthetic/conjugation) reactions resulting in the formation of highly polar conjugates.[4]

Among the Phase I nonsynthetic reactions, oxidations are the major drug-metabolizing reactions that are carried out by monooxygenases or mixed function oxidases. These reactions involve a cytochrome P450 hemoprotein, nicotinamide adenine dinucleotide phosphate (NADPH), cytochrome P450 (CYP) reductase, and molecular oxygen. There are more than a hundred CYP isozymes which have been identified and have differing affinities for various drugs.

Some examples are given in **Table 1**.

Enzyme induction can result in decreased pharmacological effects or duration of action of drugs which get inactivated by metabolism (failure of contraception with oral contraceptives in patients on phenytoin) or there may be increased pharmacological effects or duration of action of drugs which get activated by metabolism (acute paracetamol toxicity). Similarly, enzyme inhibition causes increase in drug effects by increasing drug concentration for the same dose. These drugs may induce or inhibit the enzymes of their own metabolism and/or other CYP enzymes leading

TABLE 1: CYP isoenzyme, its substrates, inducers, and inhibitors.

CYP isozyme	Substrates	Inducers	Inhibitors
CYP3A4 and CYP3A5	Paracetamol, diazepam, carbamazepine, and buspirone	Phenytoin, carbamazepine, and barbiturates	Fluoxetine, erythromycin, and ketoconazole
CYP2D6	Fluoxetine, paroxetine, venlafaxine, clozapine, risperidone, clomipramine, amitriptyline, and haloperidol	Phenobarbitone and rifampicin	Fluoxetine and paroxetine
CYP2C8 and CYP2C9	Phenytoin, carbamazepine, and diclofenac	Phenytoin, carbamazepine, and rifampicin	Fluvoxamine and fluconazole
CYP2C19	Phenytoin, diazepam, amitriptyline, and citalopram	Carbamazepine and rifampicin	Fluconazole and omeprazole
CYP1A1 and CYP1A2	Carbamazepine, paracetamol, and theophylline	Carbamazepine, rifampicin, and smoking	Fluoxetine and fluvoxamine
CYP2E1	Paracetamol, halothane, and alcohol	Alcoholism and isoniazid	Disulfiram and fomepizole
CYP2B6	Sertraline and methadone	Phenobarbitone	Paroxetine and sertraline

(CYP: cytochrome P450)

to important considerations for their use in therapeutics. Hence, based on microsomal enzyme induction or inhibition, the doses of concomitant drugs need modification.[6]

This enzyme modulation is useful in patients with idiopathic generalized epilepsy when we combine valproate with lamotrigine, in case seizures are not controlled with valproate alone. As lamotrigine clearance is reduced by valproate due to decreased metabolism, it results in higher lamotrigine drug concentration and proportionally increasing therapeutic effect. But at the same time, the risk of skin rash, even leading to Stevens–Johnson syndrome, increases. Hence, to optimally use this synergistic relationship, lamotrigine should be started at half the dose and the subsequent dose escalation should be slow, caution the patient for rash and if any rash appears, advise him to stop lamotrigine at the earliest and add on another antiepileptic drug to maintain seizure control.[7]

The effect of microsomal enzyme induction or inhibition on various types of drugs is as given in **Table 2**.

First-pass Metabolism

On oral administration, the drugs are absorbed from the small intestine and transported to the liver via portal circulation. These drugs are exposed to the drug-metabolizing enzymes in the intestinal wall and the liver and can undergo extensive metabolism. This is called as first-pass or presystemic metabolism. Drugs such as clonazepam and chlorpromazine are extensively metabolized in the gut wall itself. Drugs such as morphine and pethidine must be given in high oral doses because of their extensive hepatic metabolism. This first-pass effect limits the oral bioavailability of drugs, requiring either a higher oral dose (morphine, pethidine, and propranolol) or using an alternative route of administration (lidocaine).

TABLE 2: Effect of microsomal enzyme induction and inhibition.

Drug	Microsomal enzyme induction	Microsomal enzyme inhibition
Prodrug	Increase effect	Decrease effect
Drug with inactive metabolite	Decrease effect	Increase effect
Drug with active metabolite	Increase effect	Decrease effect
Drug with toxic metabolite	Increase toxicity	Decrease toxicity

Excretion

Renal excretion is the primary route for majority of drugs, in addition to feces, saliva, sweat, exhaled air, and milk as other minor routes. The unchanged polar drugs and the lipophilic drugs, which have been biotransformed to their hydrophilic metabolites, get excreted in the urine. Renal excretion involves three distinct processes—(1) glomerular filtration, (2) active tubular secretion, and (3) passive tubular reabsorption. Glomerular filtration of a drug depends on the renal blood flow and plasma protein binding of the drug. Tubular reabsorption occurs by passive diffusion. It depends upon two factors—lipid solubility of the drug and ionization of the drug at the existing urinary pH. Most of the lipid-soluble drugs get reabsorbed whereas the nonlipid soluble and highly ionized drugs, e.g., aminoglycosides do not get reabsorbed, and their rate of excretion mainly depends on the glomerular filtration rate.[4]

The acidic drugs get ionized in alkaline urine and their reabsorption is less, while the weak bases get ionized in acidic urine, thus reducing the reabsorption. This forms the basis of enhancing the elimination of drugs in case of toxicity, i.e., urine is alkalinized in barbiturate and salicylate poisoning and can be acidified in case of overdose with morphine and amphetamine (acidification is not practiced clinically).

Tubular secretion involves the active transport of organic acids and bases in the proximal tubules. It also promotes the excretion of protein-bound drugs. Drugs eliminated by tubular secretion compete among themselves, hence can be used to increase the duration of action, e.g., probenecid and amoxicillin fixed dose combination reduces the frequency of administration from three times a day to two times a day.

Fecal excretion occurs for the unabsorbed fraction of drugs and for the actively secreted drugs and metabolites into the bile, e.g., benzodiazepines and cannabinoids. The free drug in the gut and the drug which is released by deconjugation of glucuronides by the enteric flora gets reabsorbed and is excreted in the urine. The remaining drug is excreted in feces. This enterohepatic cycling may prolong the presence of the drug and its effects in the body, e.g., erythromycin, ampicillin, and vecuronium.

Lungs are responsible for the elimination of volatile liquids such as general anesthetics and alcohol in the exhaled air. Saliva and sweat are minor routes for drugs such as lithium. Milk excretion is important because it exposes the infant to the drugs, as majority of the drugs can be present in milk. The risk of drugs crossing milk barrier exists when a breastfeeding mother is prescribed such drugs.

"Clearance" is a measure of the body's efficiency in eliminating the drug from the systemic circulation. It is defined as the volume of plasma from which the drug is completely removed per unit time. Clearance is important to be considered when we must devise a regimen for long-term use of a drug. The aim is to maintain the plasma concentration of the drug at a steady state which is within the therapeutic range of the drug, i.e., rate of elimination ~ rate of drug administration.[6]

Majority of the drugs follow first-order kinetics where the rate of elimination is directly proportional to the drug concentration, as the processes involved in elimination are not saturated. The clearances for such drugs remain constant or a constant fraction of the drug present in the body is eliminated per unit of time. Some drugs saturate the elimination processes of the body and follow zero-order kinetics where the rate of elimination remains constant irrespective of the drug concentration in the body. Clearance decreases with an increase in concentration or a constant amount of drug present in the body is eliminated per unit of time, e.g., ethyl alcohol. Drugs such as phenytoin and theophylline change their order from first order to zero order if dose escalation is done for therapeutic effect. Hence, caution is needed when we escalate the dose and a patient with no toxicity manifestation at a lower dose may suddenly develop toxicity manifestation with just a slight increase in dose,[8] e.g., no toxicity at 300 mg/day of phenytoin but toxicity manifestations are observed when the dose is increased to 350 mg/day.

"Half-life" is the time a drug takes for its plasma concentration to be reduced to half. Nearly 4–5 half-lives are required for the complete elimination of a drug from the body. Half-life, as clearance, remains constant for drugs following first-order kinetics. For those with zero-order kinetics, half-life gets prolonged with dose as the clearance also decreases.

Repeated drug administration at short intervals causes the accumulation of drug in the body till the time elimination balances the drug intake. This is the time when steady-state concentration is achieved **(Fig. 5)**.[6] If the target therapeutic drug concentration and clearance are known, the dose rate can be calculated as a product of the target steady-state concentration and clearance. For orally administered drugs, this value needs to be divided by the fraction of the drug reaching the site of action, i.e., bioavailability.

For drugs with longer half-lives, if a quick response is required, a higher dose may be given to attain the target concentration with a single dose. This is termed as loading dose (calculated as target plasma concentration × aVd/bioavailability). This can be followed by maintenance dose which can then be repeated at regular intervals to attain the steady-state concentration (calculated as target steady-state concentration × clearance/bioavailability). For this reason, oral loading with phenytoin is done by starting with 300 mg phenytoin in patients suspected to have cluster seizures.[9] For example, in patients with neurocysticercosis, the loading dose is given to achieve the target concentration at the earliest rather than waiting to achieve a steady state. Attainment of this target level can be assisted by therapeutic drug monitoring (TDM) which is particularly useful for drugs with low safety margins (e.g., anticonvulsants, tricyclic antidepressants, and lithium), for drugs with individual variations (e.g., lithium), to check compliance (psychoactive drugs), potentially toxic drugs, or in case of failure of response to a drug.[10] There is a risk

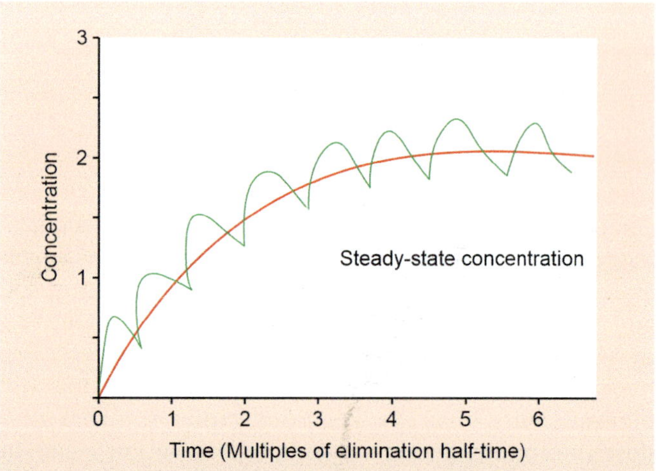

FIG. 5: Steady-state concentration after repeated doses.

of dose-dependent adverse effects when a loading dose is used, e.g., while using loading dose of phenytoin, the rate of administration should not exceed 25 mg/min and it should be administered under electrocardiographic (ECG) monitoring to prevent cardiac arrhythmias, if any.

DRUG TARGETS/PHARMACODYNAMICS

Drugs useful in neurological disorders act by enhancing or blunting the neurotransmission in CNS.

Neurotransmitters are the endogenous chemicals in the brain responsible for chemical signaling across a synapse. The nerve terminals contain multiple transmitter substances that are released with an action potential and act jointly on the postsynaptic membrane and on the presynaptic membrane to affect the release of the transmitter. The nerve conduction gets modulated by inputs from excitatory and inhibitory interneurons to get nerve response **(Fig. 6)**.

The drugs acting on CNS produce their effects mediated either through ion channels or receptors.[2]

Neuronal membranes have two types of ion channels—voltage-gated and ligand-gated. Sodium channels are an example of voltage-gated channels responsible for fast action potentials along the nerve axon. The calcium and potassium channels are responsible for much slower responses. Ligand-gated channels, also called as ionotropic receptors, involve the binding of neurotransmitter to the receptor to operate the channel, e.g., γ-aminobutyric acid type A ($GABA_A$) receptor chloride ion channel; receptors for the amino acids glycine, glutamate, and aspartate; the nicotinic acetylcholine (ACh) receptor; and the serotonin 5-HT_3 receptor. Benzodiazepines, for example, act through the $GABA_A$ receptor chloride ion channels **(Fig. 7A)**. Other classes of neurotransmitter receptors are the G-protein-coupled receptors or metabotropic receptors which act via second messengers to initiate a signaling cascade **(Fig. 7B)**.

Modifying the chemical synaptic transmission in one of the several ways is the major target of action of most of the drugs acting on CNS. These actions can be at the presynaptic or synaptic level. Presynaptic actions include those on synthesis, storage, metabolism, and release of the neurotransmitter while at the synapse, drugs can act by their agonistic or antagonistic actions on the receptors.

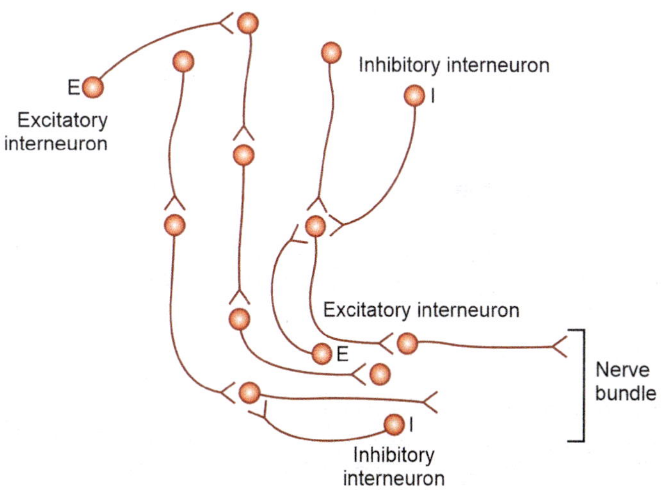

FIG. 6: Neuromodulation in nerve bundle.

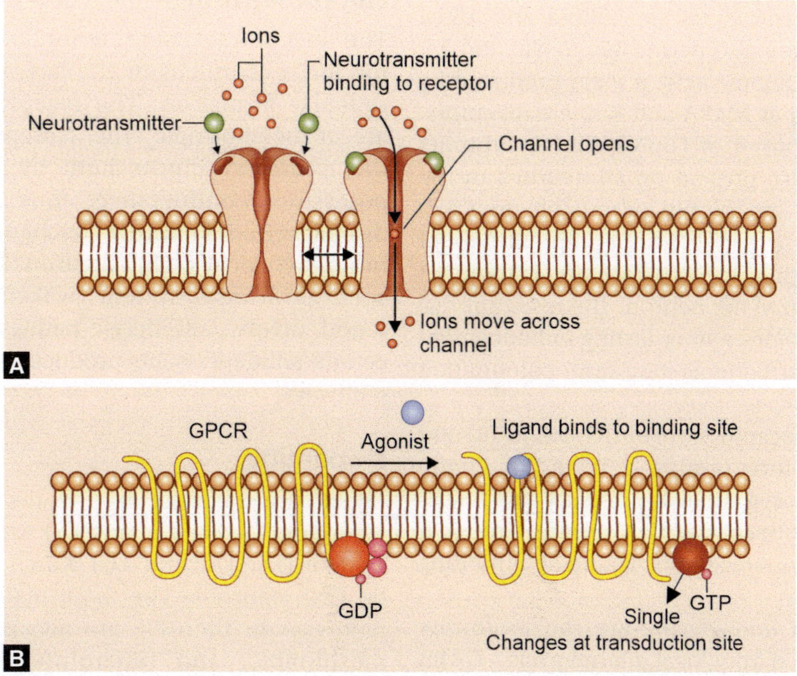

FIGS. 7A AND B: (A) Ion channel-coupled receptor. (B) Metabotropic receptors.
(GDP: guanosine diphosphate; GPCR: G-protein-coupled receptor; GTP: guanosine triphosphate)

- *At the presynaptic level*: Tetanus toxin can block the release of neurotransmitters while capsaicin enhances the release of substance P. Botulinum toxin prevents the release of ACh from axon ending at the neuromuscular junction, thus causing flaccid paralysis. The uptake of the neurotransmitter catecholamines, which is one of the mechanisms for the termination of their action, can be blocked by cocaine. Anticholinesterases inhibit the hydrolysis of ACh by acetylcholinesterase, thus prolonging its action.
- *At the receptor level*: Opioids act as agonists to mimic the actions of enkephalin, while they block certain receptors to act as analgesics.

NEUROTRANSMITTERS IN THE CNS

Several chemicals act as neurotransmitters in the brain. These include amino acids, monoamines, ACh, purines, neuropeptides, lipids, and gases.[11]

Amino Acid Neurotransmitters

Glutamate is responsible for mediating excitatory synaptic transmission. Released from the presynaptic terminal by calcium-dependent exocytosis, glutamate causes the excitation of both ionotropic and metabotropic receptors. The ionotropic receptors are of further three types—AMPA (α-amino-3-hydroxy-5-methylisoxazole-4-propionic acid), KA (kainic acid), and NMDA (N-methyl-D-aspartate). All these receptors are composed of four subunits. AMPA receptors (composed of GluA1–GluA4) are present on all neurons and are permeable to Na^+ and K^+, and not to Ca^{2+}. Kainate receptors (composed of GluK1–GluK5) are present mainly in the hippocampus, cerebellum, and spinal cord. Kainate receptors are also permeable to Na^+ and K^+, and some also to Ca^{2+}. Domoic acid, a toxin produced by algae, is a potent agonist at AMPA and Kainate receptors. NMDA receptors (composed of GluN1–GluN2 subunits GluN2A–GluN2D) are also present on all neurons in the CNS. NMDA receptors are highly permeable to Ca^{2+}, Na^+, and K^+. For NMDA channels to open up, binding of glutamate as well as glycine, at a separate site, is required along with depolarization of the neuron. The resultant rise in intracellular Ca^{2+} provides a long-lasting enhancement in synaptic strength, referred to as long-term potentiation (LTP).[12]

The metabotropic receptors (mGluR1–mGluR8) are also further divided into three groups—I, II, and III. Group I receptors are located postsynaptically and act via inositol triphosphate-mediated intracellular Ca^{2+} release. Groups II and III are presynaptic autoreceptors, acting by inhibiting neurotransmitter release.

γ-aminobutyric acid and glycine are the inhibitory neurotransmitters released from local interneurons—GABA throughout the CNS and glycine in the brainstem and spinal cord. Glycine receptors have a pentameric structure, selectively permeable to Cl^-. Strychnine, a convulsant, selectively blocks the glycine receptors. GABA receptors are of $GABA_A$ and $GABA_B$ types. $GABA_A$ are ion channel-coupled (ionotropic) receptors and mediate the fast responses. These are pentameric structures selectively permeable to Cl^-. Convulsants, such as bicuculline and picrotoxin, selectively inhibit $GABA_A$ receptors. $GABA_B$ receptors are metabotropic or the G-protein-coupled receptors and are responsible for mediating the slow responses. Baclofen, an antispastic drug, selectively activates $GABA_B$ receptors.

Acetylcholine

It is synthesized by choline acetyltransferase in the presynaptic nerve terminal and stored there in the vesicles. Following its release in the synapse, it produces its postsynaptic effects and is then degraded by acetylcholinesterase enzyme. Cholinergic receptors in the CNS mainly belong to the muscarinic type, which are the G-protein-coupled receptors. ACh is primarily found in the interneurons. The degeneration of certain cholinergic pathways is characteristic of Alzheimer's disease. Nicotinic receptors are ion channel-coupled receptors. These also have a therapeutic role in a number of neurological disorders and importantly, in smoking cessation.[12]

Monoamine Neurotransmitters

Monoamines include norepinephrine, dopamine, and 5-hydroxytryptamine (5-HT). These compounds are present in very small amounts in CNS.

Norepinephrine

The location of noradrenergic neurons is mainly in the locus coeruleus or the lateral tegmental area of the reticular formation. The receptors for norepinephrine are of metabotropic type. Norepinephrine can enhance the excitatory inputs both by direct (decreasing the potassium conductance, thus slowing the neuronal discharge) and indirect mechanisms (inhibition of the inhibitory local circuit neurons). Behavioral processes, such as arousal system (wakefulness) and control of mood, involve adrenergic pathways. Amphetamines and certain antidepressants produce their effects through these pathways.

Dopamine

Effects are mediated by five distinct G-protein-coupled receptors, D_1-like (D_1 and D_5) which are stimulatory and D_2-like (D_2, D_3, and D_4) which have inhibitory action on CNS neurons. The three main dopamine-containing pathways in the CNS are nigrostriatal, mesocortical or mesolimbic, and tuberoinfundibular. Dopaminergic pathways have a role in motivation and reward (for drugs of abuse), motor control, and for the release of various hormones. Parkinsonism is associated with a deficiency of dopamine in the nigrostriatal pathway. Schizophrenia may be associated with dopaminergic hyperactivity. Amphetamine and cocaine activate the mesocortical pathway. D_2 receptor blockers increase prolactin release via the tuberohypophyseal pathway. Dopamine agonist such as bromocriptine is used to suppress prolactin secretion. Phenothiazines have antiemetic activity by acting on dopamine receptors in the CTZ.[11]

5-hydroxytryptamine

5-hydroxytryptamine is contained in unmyelinated fibers innervating most of the regions of CNS. 5-HT neurons are concentrated in the midline raphe nuclei in the pons and medulla, projecting diffusely to the cortex limbic system, hypothalamus, and spinal cord. All 5-HT receptors are expressed in the CNS and influence several functions, including sleep, aggression, sensory perception, motor activity, cognition, mood, appetite, nociception, temperature regulation, and neuroendocrine control. Some of the major receptors and their function are shown in **Table 3**.

Neuropeptides

A large number of neuropeptides have been identified in the CNS. These include hypothalamic hormones (vasopressin and oxytocin), hypothalamic releasing and inhibitory hormones (e.g., somatostatin, corticotropin-releasing factor, growth hormone-releasing hormone), calcitonin, calcitonin gene-related peptide, neuropeptide Y, opioid peptides (e.g., β-endorphin), pituitary hormone [e.g., growth hormone, adrenocorticotropic hormone (ACTH)], glucagon-like peptide, vasoactive intestinal peptide, etc.[11] These peptides behave as neuromodulators in the CNS rather than true neurotransmitters.

Most neuropeptide receptors are G-protein-coupled receptors. They usually coexist with a conventional neurotransmitter and on release, they may act either locally or diffuse to a different site. These are involved in a number of modulatory functions in the CNS including appetite, social behavior, arousal, reproduction, learning, memory, and pain. Peptides, themselves, are inefficient as drugs because of the issues in permeability through the blood-barrier. Drugs acting as agonists or antagonists at peptide receptors have been under development, e.g., fentanyl has an agonistic effect on opioid receptors, naloxone is an antagonist on these receptors, and aprepitant antagonizes NK_1 receptors of tachykinin family.

Apart from these chemical mediators, some other signaling substances have also been identified in the CNS. Endogenous brain lipids, such as anandamide, activate cannabinoid CB_1. Cannabinoids influence memory, cognition, and pain perception. Nitric oxide has been implicated in long-term depression of synaptic transmission in the cerebellum. CNS also has receptors for various purines, including adenosine, adenosine triphosphate (ATP), and uridine triphosphate (UTP). ATP has been shown to have a role in several neuropsychiatric disorders, wakefulness, appetite, and memory.

DRUG BINDING AND DRUG RECEPTOR INTERACTION

The binding of drug to its neurotransmitter receptor initiates a signaling cascade which ultimately results in a change in the behavior of cells and the complex circuits in the CNS. In other words, binding of a drug to its target results in a biological effect. This delineates the two important aspects of drug action, i.e., *potency or affinity* and *efficacy or intrinsic activity*. The tendency of

TABLE 3: 5-HT receptor distribution with its ligands and role.

	5-HT_{1A}	5-HT_{1D}	5-HT_{2A}	5-HT_{2c}	5-HT_3
Location	• Limbic system • Hypothalamus • Cortex • Dorsal horn	• Cortex • Striatum • Dorsal horn	• Neocortex • Limbic system	• Choroid plexus • Substantia nigra • Basal ganglia	• Area postrema • Limbic system • Nucleus tractus solitarius
Function	• Mood/emotion • Temperature regulation • Nociception	Motor function	• Stereotype behavior • Mood/emotions • Hallucinations	CSF production	• Anxiety • Emesis • Nociception
Agonists	Buspirone	Sumatriptan		Lorcaserin	Quipazine
Antagonists			• Clozapine • Ketanserin • Risperidone • Methysergide	Mesulergine	Ondansetron

(5-HT: 5-hydroxytryptamine; CSF: cerebrospinal fluid)

a drug to bind to the receptor is governed by its affinity. It also denotes the strength with which the drug binds to its target. The affinity of a drug for a receptor determines the concentration of the drug required to form the drug receptor complex. The higher the affinity, the lower is the concentration of the drug required. Once bound to the target, the ability of this drug-receptor complex to evoke a biological response is termed as efficacy.[5]

When a drug is administered systemically, in most instances, the response produced is directly proportional to the plasma concentration of the drug which in turn depends on the drug dosage. This relationship is pronounced by the log dose-response curve, as shown in **Figure 8**.

The position of the curve on the dose axis is an index of potency, i.e., the amount of drug needed to produce a certain response. The upper limit of the curve is an index of drug efficacy or the maximal response which can be elicited by a drug. Efficacy is a deciding factor for the choice of a drug, e.g., morphine is more efficacious than aspirin. *Agonists* have both affinity and maximal intrinsic activity. Agonists can be in the form of drugs or endogenous regulatory molecules.

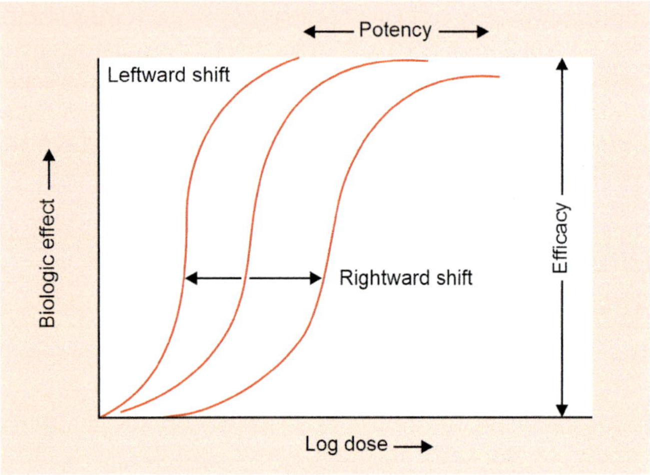

FIG. 8: Log dose-response curve modulation by change in dose.

The primary action of antagonists is to decrease the effects of agonists that, otherwise, activate the receptors. Receptor antagonists are further of two types: (1) competitive and (2) noncompetitive. A *competitive antagonist* competes with the agonist for occupying the receptor. If the agonist concentration is limited, increasing concentrations of competitive antagonists can progressively inhibit the response of agonist **(Fig. 9)**. However, increasing the concentration of the agonist can restore the response to an agonist. Therefore, this type of antagonism is also said to be reversible. In such a case, the log dose-response curve shifts to right without any change in the slope or the maximal effect. Naloxone is a competitive antagonist at all opioid receptors. The actions of *noncompetitive antagonists* are not reversible, irrespective of the concentration. Also, the binding of these antagonists to the receptor may be irreversible. In such a case, the duration of action is independent of its rate of elimination and may depend on the rate of turnover of receptor molecules. Problems may arise in case of an overdose of such drugs. Ketamine is a noncompetitive antagonist at the NMDA-glutamate receptor.

Chemically related agonist drugs acting on the same receptor may have varying maximal responses. The drug, which produces the largest response that the tissue is capable of, is called a *full agonist,* whereas a *partial agonist* produces a submaximal response at full receptor occupancy. The reason for this less than maximal response is that a partial agonist competitively inhibits the

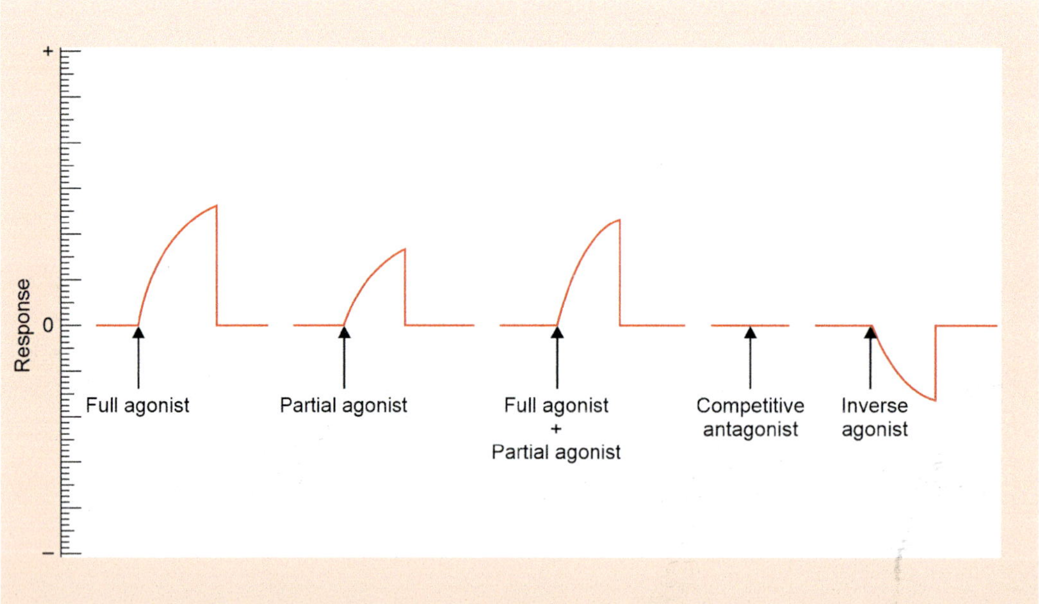

FIG. 9: Response of various types of ligands on receptor.

response of a full agonist, i.e., these have mixed agonistic-antagonistic activity **(Fig. 9)**. Buprenorphine is a partial agonist at μ-opioid receptors. It is safer than morphine as it produces less respiratory depression. However, when given in combination with an efficacious opioid, it will act as an antagonist resulting in antianalgesic effect.

Majority of the receptors are active only when an agonist molecule binds to them. But, there are receptors which have constitutive activation even in absence of a ligand, e.g., receptors for benzodiazepines, cannabinoids, and serotonin. Some ligands, called as *inverse agonists*, may reduce the level of constitutive activation of these receptors **(Fig. 9)**. The 6,7-dimethoxy-ethyl-carbomethoxy-β-carboline (DMCM) is an inverse agonist at benzodiazepine receptors and can cause convulsions.

THERAPEUTIC DRUG MONITORING

At present, it is not recommended to chase the plasma concentration for antiepileptic drugs so that if the patient is seizure free and tolerating the prescribed dose despite being lower than or higher than recommended plasma concentration, no dose alteration is recommended. However, in case there is a breakthrough seizure or toxicity manifestations, TDM is recommended to validate subtherapeutic plasma concentrations or high-plasma concentrations, respectively. This requires intervention in terms of increasing the dose of the antiepileptic or addition of another antiepileptic drug to control seizures in the first scenario and similarly reducing the dose in case of toxicity manifestation and try to cover the risk of breakthrough seizure by adding an additional antiepileptic drug on case-to-case basis. However, the variability could be due to age, gender, physiological conditions (pregnancy, lactation, and menstruation), pathological changes (hepatic or renal dysfunction), concomitant diseases, and even coadministration of drugs (drug–drug interactions with microsomal enzyme inducers and inhibitors).[10]

The children have high clearance and hence resultant half-life reduces. Also, the Vd changes. Hence, younger children often need higher doses as compared to older children and adults. In the elderly population, all the pharmacokinetics processes undergo a change, the absorption rate reduces, changes in drug distribution, reduced serum proteins, reduced metabolism, and elimination (reduced hepatic and renal clearance). Additionally, elderly patients have a number of comorbidities and concomitant administration of drugs which can affect the drug concentration.

In female patients, on administering microsomal enzyme-inducing drugs (antiepileptics), there could be a failure of contraception if she is using oral contraceptives. Similarly, the transplacental transfer of antiepileptics carries a risk of fetal anomalies (neural tube defects with valproate, fetal phenytoin syndrome with phenytoin, and risk of teratogenesis with other drugs) in newborn and sedative effects in children who are being breastfed due to drugs crossing milk barrier. One needs to infer the plasma concentration carefully especially in women if sampling is done during menstruation as they may be at risk of catamenial epilepsy during the menstrual cycle despite having plasma concentration in recommended range. Also, as the Vd changes during pregnancy, one needs to modify the dose accordingly.

Sampling time is very important for drawing the sample. If suspecting toxic manifestations, order mid dose level (peak level); if doing TDM for efficacy, get sample just before next dose (trough level); and if wish to check compliance, random sample is needed (detectable drug concentration would indicate that the patient is taking medicines).

The therapeutic effects are contributed by drug as well as its active metabolites, e.g., in case of carbamazepine, 10–11 epoxide, metabolite contributes to antiepileptic effects so the drug level of carbamazepine alone may not be responsible for the control of seizures. Pharmacogenomics can also affect drug levels as genetic polymorphism in microsomal enzymes can cause variability, especially for phenytoin and lamotrigine. But as the tests for genetic testing are not easily available, one must suspect genetic polymorphism as a contributing factor in case of an unexpected relationship between dosage used and drug levels.

In order to evaluate the drug concentration, it is very important to note the time of last dose of administration, time of blood sampling, serum proteins and hepatic and renal function along with the exact dosage being used, and body weight of the patient.

CONCLUSION

Thus, drug therapeutics are dependent on how the body treats the drug and also the effect of drug in terms of the response of the body. These effects get modulated by changes in kinetics based on age, gender, and genetics. Similarly, changes in drug target may also produce different effects with the same drug at various time points in the same patient based on the presence/absence of comorbidities and other changes. Understanding these principles, based on the need for a shorter lag period, a loading dose strategy can be used. In case the risk of dose related toxicity is not acceptable, the LD can be fractioned to split single high peak into multiple smaller peaks. Understanding previous use of similarly acting drugs can reduce response. Drug interaction due to concomitant drug use can increase/decrease drug effects. One needs to tailor therapies based on patient presentation and other drug factors.

REFERENCES

1. Pardridge WM. Drug transport across the blood-brain barrier. J Cereb Blood Flow Metab. 2012;32:1959-72.
2. Zastrow M. Drug receptors and pharmacodynamics. In: Katzung BG (Ed). Basic and Clinical Pharmacology, 14th edition. Chennai: McGraw Hill Education (India); 2018. pp. 20-40.
3. Johnston MV, Gross RA. Principles of drug therapy in neurology, 2nd edition. Oxford: Oxford University Press; 2008. pp. 3-32.
4. Buxton ILD. Pharmacokinetics: The dynamics of drug absorption, distribution, metabolism and elimination. In: Brunton L, Hilal-Dandan R, Knollmann B (Eds). Goodman & Gilman's The Pharmacological Basis of Therapeutics, 13th edition. New York: McGraw Hill; 2018. pp. 13-30.
5. Blumenthal DK. Pharmacodynamics: molecular mechanisms of drug action. In: Brunton L, Hilal-Dandan R, Knollmann B (Eds). Goodman & Gilman's The Pharmacological Basis of Therapeutics, 13th edition. New York: MacGraw Hill; 2018. pp. 31-54.
6. Holford NHG. Pharmacokinetics and Pharmacodynamics: Rational dosing & the time course of drug action. In: Katzung BG (Ed). Basic and Clinical Pharmacology, 14th edition. Chennai: McGraw Hill Education (India); 2018. pp. 41-55.
7. Baxter K. Stockley's Drug Interactions, 9th edition. London: Pharmaceutical Press. 2010.
8. Richens A, Dunlop A. Serum phenytoin levels in management of epilepsy. The Lancet. 1975;2(7928):247-8.
9. Van Der Velde EA, Driessen O. Prediction of phenytoin dosage in relation to the variability of phenytoin plasma concentration. Br J Clin Pharmac. 1981;91:41-52.
10. Landmark CJ, Johannessen SI, Patsalos PN. Therapeutic drug monitoring of antiepileptic drugs: current status and future prospects. Expert Opin Drug Metab Toxicol. 2020;16(3):227-38.
11. Rang HP, Ritter JM, Flower RJ, Henderson G. Chapter 37: Chemical transmission and drug action in the central nervous system. Rang & Dales Pharmacology, 8th edition. China: Elsevier Churchil Livingstone; 2016. pp. 449-53.
12. Gray JA. Introduction to the Pharmacology of CNS drugs. In: Katzung BG (Ed). Basic and Clinical Pharmacology, 14th edition. Chennai: McGraw Hill Education (India); 2018. pp. 41-55.

124
CHAPTER

Pain Management

Nagalaxmi Patnala

"Pain is a more terrible lord of mankind than death itself."

—Albert Schweitzer, Nobel Laurette

INTRODUCTION

The International Association for the Study of Pain defines pain as "an unpleasant sensory and emotional experience associated with actual or potential tissue damage or described in terms of such damage." Pain is a complex experience involving physical, emotional, and cognitive components. It is highly subjective.

Pain can be nociceptive, neuropathic, or mixed. Neuropathic pain is initiated or caused by a primary lesion or dysfunction in the nervous system. The pain can arise at any level—the peripheral nerves, spinal cord, and brain.

Neuropathic pain often feels like a shooting, stabbing, or burning sensation. People with neuropathic pain are often sensitive to touch or cold and can experience pain as a result of stimuli that would not normally be painful.

The adverse effects of unrelieved pain can be physiological, emotional, spiritual, economic, and sociocultural, affecting every part of a patient's well-being. Effective pain management helps in decreasing pain, improving functional status, increasing the ability to perform activities of daily living, and returning to employment.[1] In this chapter, we would be dealing with the treatment options for neuropathic pain.

ETIOLOGIES OF NEUROPATHIC PAIN

The most common cause of neuropathic pain is diabetes mellitus **(Fig. 1)**.

Other causes are as follows:
- Alcoholism
- Complex regional pain syndrome (CRPS)
- Postherpetic neuralgia (PHN)

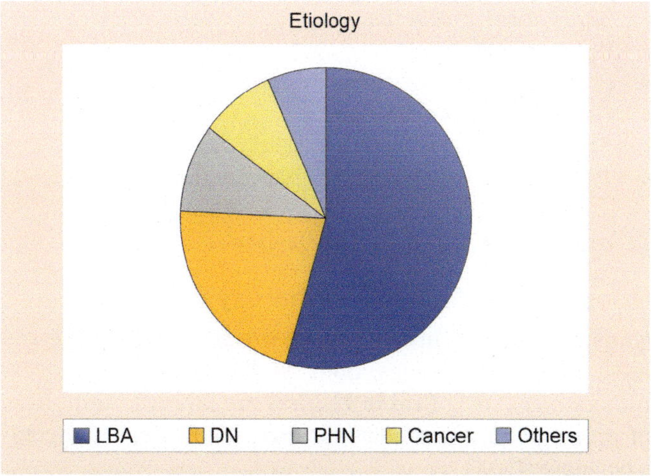

FIG. 1: Etiologies of neuropathic pain.
(DN: diabetic neuropathy; LBA: low backache; PHN: postherpetic neuralgia)

- Spinal cord injury
- Post-stroke pain
- Spine pain and radiculopathy
- Peripheral neuralgias
- Cancer
- Multiple sclerosis

TOOLS FOR NEUROPATHIC PAIN

- Neuropathic pain questionnaire
- Leeds assessment of neuropathic signs and symptoms
- Neuropathic pain symptom inventory

This classifies neuropathic pain into definitive, possible, and unlikely neuropathic pain. Definitive neuropathic pain has greater pain intensity and greater opioid usage.

GOALS OF NEUROPATHIC PAIN MANAGEMENT

Treating pain requires a multimodal approach including the psychological, physical, and emotional well-being of the patient in addition to pharmacology, surgical, and percutaneous options **(Flowchart 1)**.

PAIN TREATMENT PROTOCOL

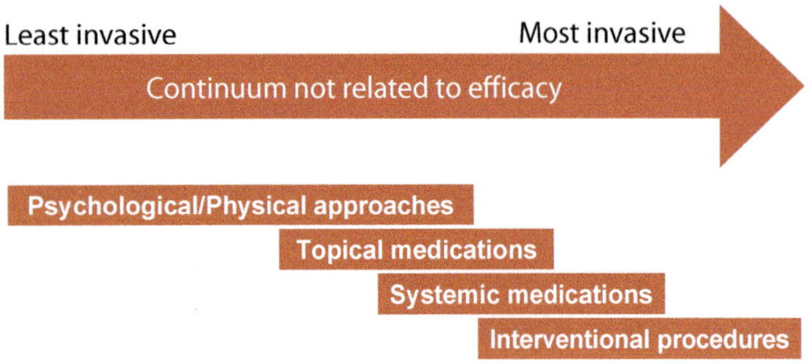

Nonpharmacological Methods

- Biofeedback mechanisms
- Relaxation therapy
- Physical and occupational therapies
- Cognitive behavioral therapy
- Acupuncture
- Transcutaneous electrical nerve stimulation (TENS)

Pharmacological Methods

Nonsteroidal Anti-inflammatory Drugs

Nonsteroidal anti-inflammatory drugs (NSAIDs) are the most widely used drugs, both on prescription and over-the-counter (OTC) **(Table 1)**. They are powerful inhibitors of prostaglandin synthesis through their effect on cyclo-oxygenase (COX).

They are used primarily to treat pain from inflammation and hyperalgesia. When used in conjunction with opioids, they decrease the dose of opioids and there by their side effects. Common side effects of NSAIDs include gastrointestinal (GI) toxicity, stomach ulcers, and gastric bleeding. Renal dysfunction can occur with prolonged and excessive use of NSAIDs. Particularly at risk are elderly patients with renal dysfunction, congestive heart failure, ascites, or hypovolemia.[2]

Antidepressants

Antidepressants include tricyclic antidepressants (TCAs), selective serotonin reuptake inhibitors (SSRIs), and serotonin and noradrenaline reuptake inhibitors (SNRIs).

Tricyclic antidepressants are the most commonly used medications in the treatment of chronic neuropathic pain **(Table 2)**. They alter the monoamine transmitter activity at the synapse by blocking the reuptake of serotonin and norepinephrine. Their sedating properties help people with insomnia. Anticholinergic properties of TCAs are tachycardia, dry mouth, sedation, urinary retention, and constipation. They should be avoided in patients with heart disease and closed-angle glaucoma.

Selective serotonin reuptake inhibitors selectively block the reuptake of serotonin by blocking the sodium/potassium adenosine triphosphate (ATP) pump, resulting in increased levels of serotonin at the synaptic cleft.

TABLE 1: Commonly used nonsteroidal anti-inflammatory drugs (NSAIDs).

Drug	Adult dosage
Acetaminophen	500–1,000 mg q4h
Acetylsalicylic acid	325–650 mg q4h
Celecoxib	200 mg q12h
Diclofenac sodium	25–75 mg q8–12h
Ibuprofen	400–800 mg q6–8h
Indomethacin	25–50 mg q8–12h
Ketoprofen	25–75 mg q6–8h
Ketorolac	10 mg q6–8h
Naproxen	275–500 mg q8–12h
Piroxicam	10–20 mg once daily

TABLE 2: Tricyclic antidepressants.

Drugs	Dosage (mg/day)
Amitriptyline	10–100
Clomipramine	25–200
Desipramine	10–200
Imipramine	10–200
Nortriptyline	10–150

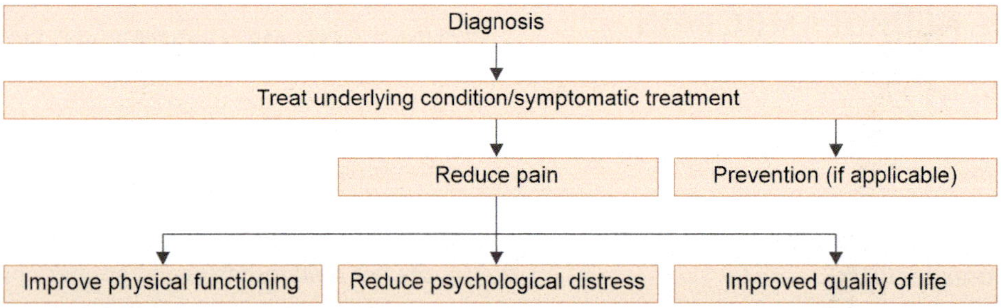

FLOWCHART 1: Treatment of pain.

Fluoxetine and paroxetine, once daily, have variable effects on neuropathic pain and are not commonly used.

Serotonin and noradrenaline reuptake inhibitors are effective in neuropathic pain and diabetic neuropathy. Duloxetine is started once daily with 20 mg and increased to 60 mg depending on the response.

Anticonvulsants

Anticonvulsants are believed to be particularly useful in treating lancinating, electrical, or tic-like neuropathic pain due to their membrane-stabilizing properties. They can be used in patients unresponsive to antidepressants.

Carbamazepine is the most commonly used drug for trigeminal neuralgia (TN). It is started at a dose of 100 mg at bedtime. Side effects include sedation, nausea, vomiting, bone marrow suppression, hyponatremia, and hepatic dysfunction. Rash, though rare, can be life-threatening causing Steven Johnson Syndrome in some patients.

Oxcarbazepine, a keto derivative of carbamazepine, has better tolerability and fewer side effects.

Valproic acid is effective in reducing the frequency of migraine attacks. It is also used in patients with PHN and diabetic neuropathy. Common side effects include tremors, ankle swelling, sedation, and GI discomfort. Weight gain and hair loss also occur.

Gabapentin modulates the function of voltage-dependent calcium channels in the dorsal horn of the spinal cord to decrease the release of excitatory neurotransmitters. It is the recommended first-line coanalgesic for treating nonmalignant neuropathic pain conditions. Side effects include drowsiness, dizziness, and unsteadiness. It is started at a dose of 100–300 mg at bedtime and increased to a maximum of 3,600 mg/day.

Pregabalin is a gamma-aminobutyric acid (GABA) analog similar to gabapentin. It has anxiolytic, analgesic, and antiepileptic effects. It seems to be more effective than other anticonvulsants in treating neuropathic pain. Common side effects include dizziness, sedation, dry mouth, and peripheral edema.

Lamotrigine stabilizes neural membranes by blocking the activation of voltage-sensitive sodium channels and inhibiting the presynaptic release of glutamate.

Topiramate is used in the prophylactic treatment in migraine. It is started as a dose of 25 mg twice a day and increased to 50–200 mg/day. Topiramate can induce memory loss, disorientation, and sedation.

Systemic Local Anesthetics

Intravenous (IV) lidocaine is used for the treatment of neuropathic pain as a second-line therapy in patients who failed to respond to anticonvulsants and antidepressants.

Topical Analgesics

A 5% lidocaine patch is used for the treatment of PHN and for those patients with trigger points in the myofascial pain syndrome. Minimal systemic absorption occurs. The patch is usually applied for 12 hours a day.

Capsaicin is the spicy ingredient in chili pepper. It can deplete substance P from the terminals of afferent C fibers, potentially leading to decreased pain perception. It is also effective in treating postsurgical pain in cancer patients.

N-methyl-D-aspartate Receptor Blockers

N-methyl-D-aspartate (NMDA) antagonists modulate central nervous system (CNS) function. Low-dose IV ketamine is used for pain relief in CRPS type I without significant psychomimetic side effects.

Opioids

Opioids are the major class of analgesics used to treat moderate-to-severe pain. They are used as adjuvants in the treatment of neuropathic pain. They produce analgesia by mimicking the action of endogenous opioids. Side effects include constipation, nausea and vomiting, respiratory depression, muscular rigidity, convulsions, and urinary retention.

The most commonly used oral opioid is tramadol. It has fewer side effects. The dose is 50–100 mg qid. Tapentadol is a nonracemic mixture of tramadol, having less nausea. The dose is 50–75 mg every 4–6 hours, to a maximum of up to 600 mg **(Table 3)**.

Pharmacoresistance: A neuropathic pain condition in which there is resistant to pharmacotherapy when mono or a rational combination treatment using drugs proved efficacious in randomized controlled trials (RCTs) fails in inducing useful pain relief from the patients'/physician's point of view after an appropriate duration of treatment with adequate dosage or if intolerable side effects occur. In cases of pharmacoresistance, interventional procedures play a major role.

Interventional Pain Management

Interventions for neuropathic pain are recommended for patients who have refractory pain despite maximum medical management **(Table 4)**. They are disease-specific, minimally invasive procedures including percutaneous precision needle placement, with the placement of drugs in targeted areas or ablation of targeted nerves.

TABLE 3: Equivalent doses of opioids.

	Oral	Parenteral
Codeine	30–60 mg qid	
Tramadol	1–2 mg/kg tds	1–2 mg/kg tds
Morphine	10–60 mg qid	0.1–0.15 mg/kg 6 hourly
Pethidine	25–300 mg qid	• 1–2 mg/kg 6 hourly • Infusion 0.1–0.5 μg/kg/h
Buprenorphine	0.3–0.6 mg tds	5–8 mg/kg tds

TABLE 4: Commonly used interventions indications and techniques for neuropathic pain.

Procedure	Indication
Discography	Diagnosis of anatomical localization of discogenic pain
Epidural corticosteroid injection	Lumbar or cervical radiculopathy, vertebral fractures
Facet joint block	Lumbar or cervical facet joint syndrome
Facet joint rhizotomy	Lumbar or cervical facet joint syndrome
Gasserian ganglion block	Trigeminal neuralgia
Greater occipital nerve block	Greater occipital neuralgia, headache
Intravenous regional block	Complex regional pain syndromes
Lumbar sympathetic block	CRPS of legs, Ischemic pain
Percutaneous disc decompression	Lumbar or cervical disc herniation
Sacroiliac joint injection	Sacroiliac joint pain
Sphenopalatine ganglion block	Headache and facial pain
• Spinal cord stimulator • Peripheral nerve blocks • Musculoskeletal interventions	• CRPS, PVD, low backache, angina • Meralgia paresthetica, supraorbital neuralgia knee and shoulder interventions carpal tunnel, tarsal tunnel syndrome, epicondylitis, plantar fasciitis
Stellate ganglion block	CRPS of arm, neck, and head, headache, poststroke pain
Suprascapular nerve block	Shoulder pain
Vertebroplasty	Vertebral fracture
Motor cortex stimulation	Neuropathic pain
• Deep brain stimulation • Regenerative therapy • Botulinum toxin injection	• Neuropathic pain • Musculoskeletal interventions • Spasticity, headache, neuropathic pain

(CRPS: complex regional pain syndrome; PVD: peripheral vascular disease)

HEADACHE

Headache is one of the most common complaints for which a patient seeks attention. Although it is benign at most of the times it can herald an ominous disorder. The "red flags" such as the worst possible headache, change in headache character, headache in elderly or immunocompromised patients, or headache with the presence of systemic features/neurological deficits triggered by cough or Valsalva definitely merit thorough evaluation.

A proper history, examination, and evaluation help in the diagnosis of secondary headache disorders. Among the primary headaches, though tension-type headache is the most common, patients seek attention for migraine as it causes significant disability. Among the trigeminal autonomic neuralgias cluster headache may present as a medical emergency that necessitates urgent abortive treatment.

The goals of acute treatment for migraine include fast and consistent relief with minimal adverse effects. With the availability of migraine-specific therapy, treatment of acute migraine including drugs and devices may undergo a sea change in the future.

The drugs used in the acute treatment are given in **Table 5**.

Clinical features such as speed of onset, the presence of visual aura, and vomiting may influence the choice of initial headache medication. Opioids should be discouraged as there is a chance of abuse and the problem of rebound headaches. Preventive medications are advised if the patient is disabled by headaches for ≥4 days a month.

Preventive medication should be initiated at a low dose and slowly uptitrated to avoid side effects and should be continued for an adequate time, possibly 3 months, so that the possible benefits of the medication are not missed **(Table 6)**.

Chronic migraine defined as a headache lasting more than 15 days of a month for more than 3 months is the most common headache seen in a tertiary headache center. There are a few treatment options including topiramate and nortriptyline. Onabotulinum toxin A is efficacious in decreasing the number of headaches per month.

Among the trigeminal autonomic cephalgia, cluster headache merits special attention because of its severe pain; in fact it is called a suicidal headache. Early recognition of the pattern and advising high-flow oxygen with a nonbreathing mask can go a long way in the management of repeated episodes. In refractory cluster headaches, sphenopalatine blockade should be tried. Paroxysmal hemicrania continua

TABLE 5: Drugs used in acute treatment.

Established efficacy	Probably effective
Migraine specific	
Triptans	Ergotamine
Ergotamine derivatives	Other forms of ergotamine
Lasmiditan	
Gepants	
Nonspecific	
NSAIDs: Aspirin, naproxen, diclofenac, ibuprofen, celecoxib oral solution	*NSAIDs*: Flurbiprofen, ketoprofen, IV and IM ketorolac
Combination analgesic	IV magnesium
	Isometheptene-containing compounds
	Antiemetics: Chlorpromazine, metoclopramide, promethazine

(IM: intramuscular; IV: intravenous; NSAIDs: nonsteroidal anti-inflammatory drugs)

TABLE 6: Drugs given for headaches.

Drug	Dosage (mg)	Remarks
Flunarizine	5–10	Weight gain, and parkinsonism may be precipitated
Propranolol	20–80	Avoid in migraine with aura, asthmatics
Metoprolol	25–100	Good choice in HTN, CAD patients
Atenolol	25–100	
Divalproex sodium	250–1,000	Choice in patients with depression
Topiramate	25–100	Good in overweight patients
Venlafaxine	37.5	Well tolerated
Gabapentin	300–100	Good SE profile
Verapamil	80–340	Vestibular migraine

(CAD: coronary artery disease; HTN: hypertension; SE: side effects)

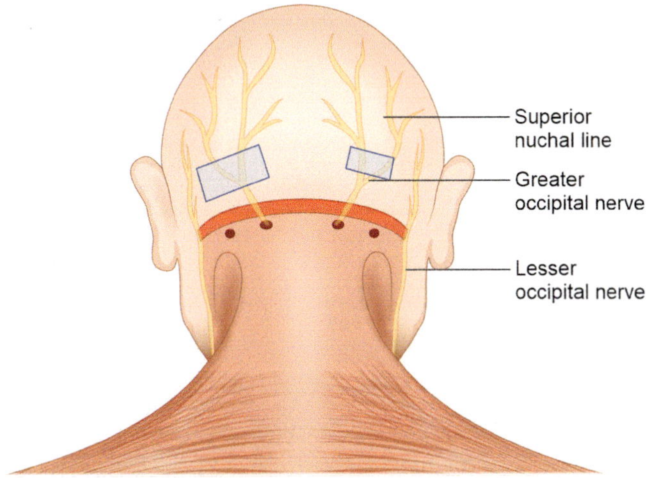

FIG. 2: Occipital nerve block.

respond to indomethacin magically, and an adequate dose should be tried before stopping its use.

Calcitonin Gene-related Peptide Antagonists

Calcitonin gene related peptide (CGRP) is considered to have a prominent role in pathogenesis of migraine and medications to antagonize CGRP are genuine migraine preventive medications.

Two classes of drugs-gepants which are small molecules which inhibit CGRP receptor and anti-CARP monoclonal antibodies(mAB). Among the mAB, ERENUMAB targets the CARP receptor, whereas galcanezumab, fremanezumab and eptinezumab target the CGRP Ligand.

The mABs have been successful in decreasing mean monthly migraine days over a 12 weeks study period also in real life situations.

The drugs are relatively safe but their long-term efficacy, wearing off effect needs to be assessed.

Medication Overuse Headache

Medication overuse headache should always be considered when a refractory headache patient is being treated. A careful history of usage of OTC drugs, pain balms, and aromatic oils should always be investigated as the patients may not consider it worthwhile mentioning about them. They may need hospitalization followed by weaning the offending drug and starting other abortive medications followed by preventive medications and lifestyle changes.

Peripheral Nerve Blocks in Headaches

Peripheral nerve blockade has a role in the management of acute and chronic migraines, trigeminal autonomic cephalgias, and other painful cranial neuralgias. The commonly used nerve blocks are greater and lesser occipital nerve blocks **(Fig. 2)**; supraorbital, supratrochlear **(Fig. 3)**, and auriculotemporal nerve blocks are used for specific indications. Usually, a combination of lidocaine and bupivacaine is used for nerve blocks, and corticosteroids are added for greater occipital nerve blocks. The nerve blocks are generally well tolerated, and the side effects, if present, such as giddiness or exacerbation of headache are usually transient in nature. Diagnostic blocks are followed by radiofrequency ablation for long-term effect.

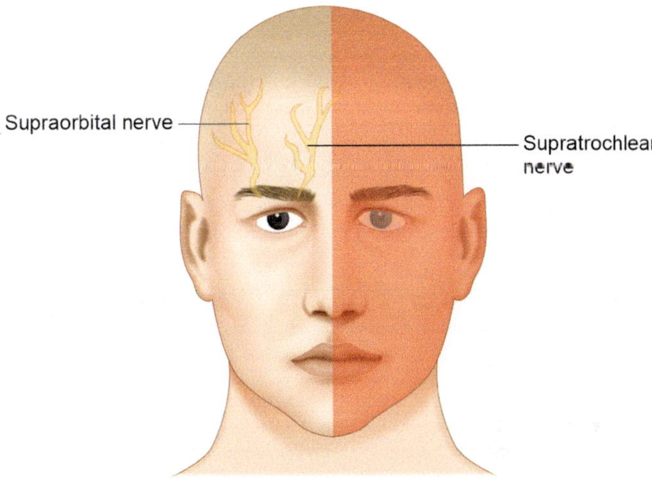

FIG. 3: Supraorbital nerve block.

TRIGEMINAL NEURALGIA

Trigeminal neuralgia is sudden, usually unilateral, severe electric shock-like, brief stabbing recurrent pain in the distribution of one or more branches of the V cranial nerve **(Fig. 4)**.

In approximately 90% of cases a vessel, usually an artery, is found in contact with the trigeminal nerve at the root entry zone as it exits the pons **(Fig. 5)**.

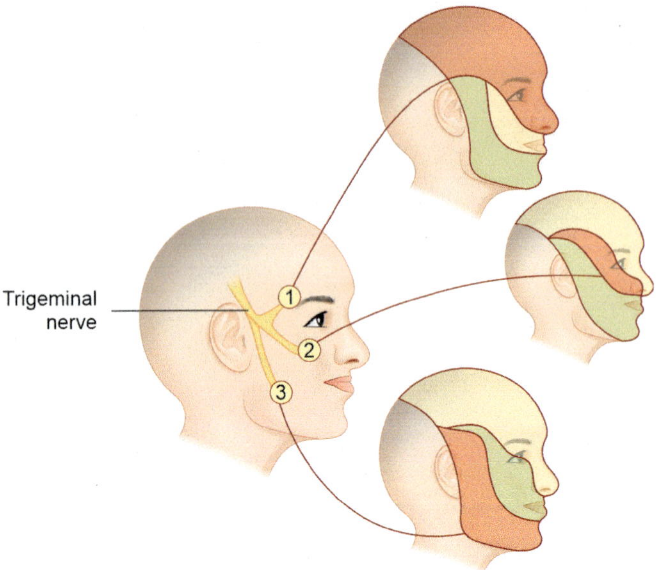

FIG. 4: Trigeminal nerve distribution.

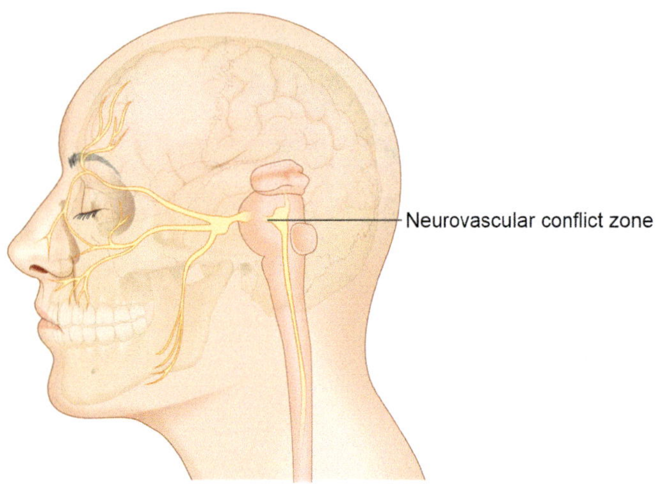

FIG. 5: Neurovascular conflict zone.

International Classification of Headache Disorders-3 Beta Diagnostic Criteria for Classical Trigeminal Neuralgia

Trigeminal neuralgia developing without apparent cause other than neurovascular compression:

A. At least three attacks of unilateral facial pain fulfilling criteria B and C
B. Occurring in one or more divisions of the trigeminal nerve, with no radiation beyond the trigeminal distribution
C. *Pain has at least three of the following characteristics*:
   - Recurring in paroxysmal attacks lasting from a fraction of a second to 2 minutes
   - Severe intensity
   - Electric shock-like, shooting, stabbing, or sharp in quality
   - Precipitated by innocuous stimuli to the affected side of the face
D. No clinically evident neurological deficit
E. Not better accounted for by another International Classification of Headache Disorders-3 (ICHD-3) diagnosis

Treatment

Medical Management

Carbamazepine is considered the drug of choice according to the European Federation of Neurological Society and the American Academy of Neurology. Oxcarbazepine can be considered the first-line agent in patients having intolerable side effects with carbamazepine.

The recommended starting dose is 100–200 mg twice daily with a gradual increase to 200 mg until pain relief or rashes appear. The typical maintenance dose is 600–1,200 mg/day in divided doses.

Lamotrigine also decreases the repetitive firing of sodium channels. It is used in a dose of 400 mg and has proved its efficacy when used versus placebo.

Phenytoin, one of the oldest anticonvulsants, has been used in refractory cases. It is given 3–5 mg/kg intravenously in acute therapy.

Baclofen can be used either as monotherapy or as an add-on to carbamazepine in patients with TN. The starting dose is 5–10 mg three times a day, with gradual titration to a maintenance dose of 50–60 mg/day.

Intranasal 8% lignocaine spray is sometimes effective in patients with V2 division TN. Relief lasted from 0.5 to 24 hours.

Gabapentin and phenytoin have been used as additive therapies to carbamazepine.

Treatment: Nerve and Neurolytic Blockade

Peripheral nerve blocks with local anesthetic and steroid, like mandibular or infraorbital nerve help relieve pain. 10% phenol or glycerol block helps relieve pain for a median time period of 9 months in most of the patients.

Microvascular Decompression

Microvascular decompression (MVD) is performed under general anesthesia using a microscope to visualize the trigeminal nerve as it leaves the pons via a suboccipital craniectomy. Compression of the nerve by an artery or vein is relieved by repositioning the artery or coagulating the vein. Although invasive, the recurrence rate and complications are low with MVD.

Gangliolysis

- *Percutaneous radiofrequency (RF) ablation/thermocoagulation* **(Figs. 6A and B)**: It involves the use of RF to create anatomically distinct lesions in cycles of 45–90 seconds at temperatures of 60–90°. It is performed under

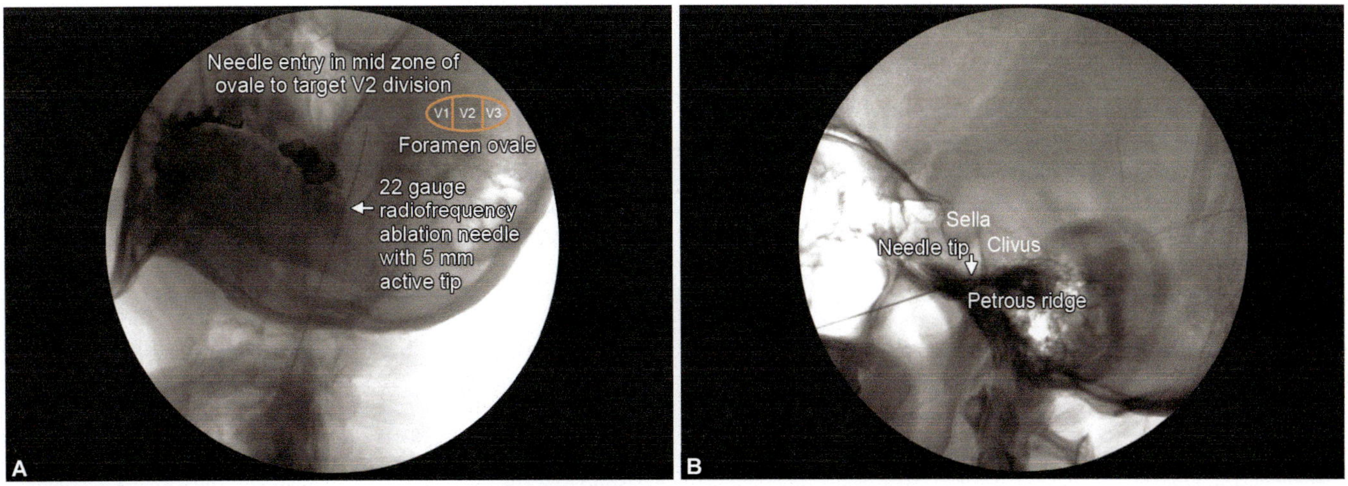

FIGS. 6A AND B: Fluoroscopy-guided needle placement in foramen ovale.

local anesthesia or mild sedation, thereby negating the risk of general anesthesia. It is particularly useful in patients where there is no neurovascular conflict and in cases of recurrence post-MVD. There is no surgical and anesthetic risk in the procedure, thereby very useful to high risk patients as first choice as well.

- Percutaneous trigeminal ganglion compression is performed under general anesthesia using Fogarty catheter that is inserted via a 14G catheter into the trigeminal cistern and inflated with radiocontrast to compress the gasserian ganglion. Hemodynamic alterations such as severe bradycardia and hypotension requiring atropine and vasopressors can occur.
- *Percutaneous glycerol rhizolysis*: With the patient in a sitting position, after confirmation of the position of the needle with radiocontrast, 01–0.4 mL of anhydrous glycerol is injected into the Meckel's cave.

The complications with gangliolysis are less. The initial response rate is very high with a recurrence rate of around 50% after 3–4 years.

Stereotactic Radiosurgery

Gamma knife stereotactic radiosurgery is another modality of treatment where pain relief occurs after a lag period of 1 month after the procedure. Up to 75% of patients receive complete pain relief within 3 months. Sensory disturbances are common.

CyberKnife radiosurgery is a more recently developed system to incorporate the time for a miniature linear accelerator mounted on a flexible, robotic arm. This system offers to target accuracy without the need for an invasive head frame. The median latency period to pain relief is 7 days. The time for the reoccurrence of pain is widely varied.

Peripheral Neurectomy

Surgical or cryoablation of the peripheral branches of the trigeminal nerve is indicated for patients who have failed medical therapy, gangliolysis, or who have a severe cardiopulmonary disease and are unable to undergo MVD **(Flowchart 2)**.

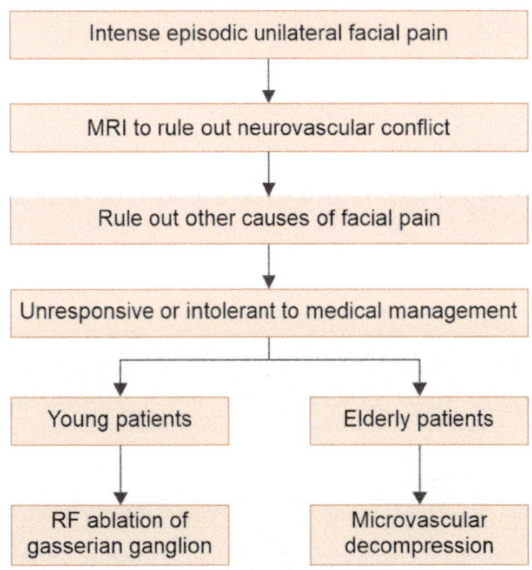

FLOWCHART 2: Peripheral neurectomy.
(MRI: magnetic resonance imaging; RF: radiofrequency)

GLOSSOPHARYNGEAL NEURALGIA

Glossopharyngeal neuralgia is defined as paroxysmal pain in the areas supplied by cranial nerves IX and X. The glossopharyngeal nerve supplies the posterior one-third of the tongue, the tonsils, pharynx, the middle ear, and the carotid body **(Fig. 7)**. The unbearable, electric lancinating pain is located unilaterally in the ear, larynx, tonsillar fossa, or the base of the tongue.

It may radiate toward the ear, the angle of the jaw, or the upper and lateral aspects of the neck. Paroxysms of pain are often triggered by swallowing, yawning, coughing, or talking.

Magnetic resonance imaging (MRI)/magnetic resonance angiography (MRA) is done to rule out a mass lesion.

Treatment

Treatment of glossopharyngeal neuralgia is similar to TN. When conservative therapy fails, surgical exploration and vascular decompression are shown to be effective. Percutaneous real-time image-guided pulsed RF ablation **(Figs. 8A and B)** is also highly effective with fewer side effects and less complications.

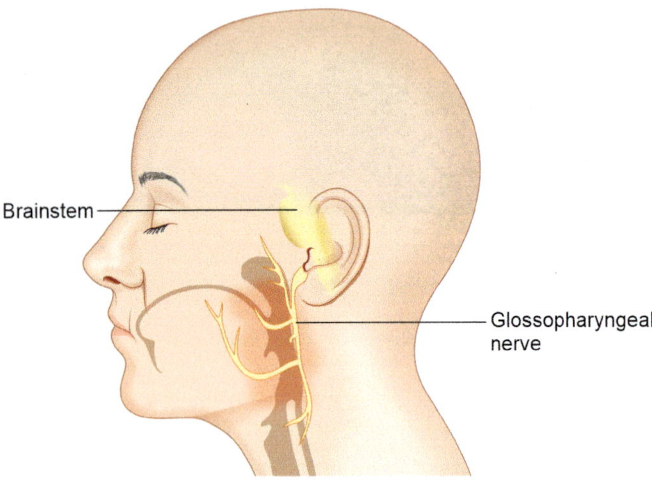

FIG. 7: Glossopharyngeal nerve.

NECK PAIN

Neck pain is a common complaint seen in most of the outpatient departments (OPDs). Around 25–76% of adult population experience neck pain or stiffness in their lifetime.

Causes:
- Cervical radiculopathy and spondylosis
- Polyneuropathy
- PHN and CRPS
- Vertebral fractures
- Cervical rib
- Myofascial pain syndrome
- Traction injuries to brachial plexus
- Malignancies

Cervical Radiculopathy

The symptoms depend on the level of the disc pathology. The patient complains of neck pain with tingling and numbness in the hands **(Table 7)**.

Magnetic resonance imaging helps in the diagnosis.

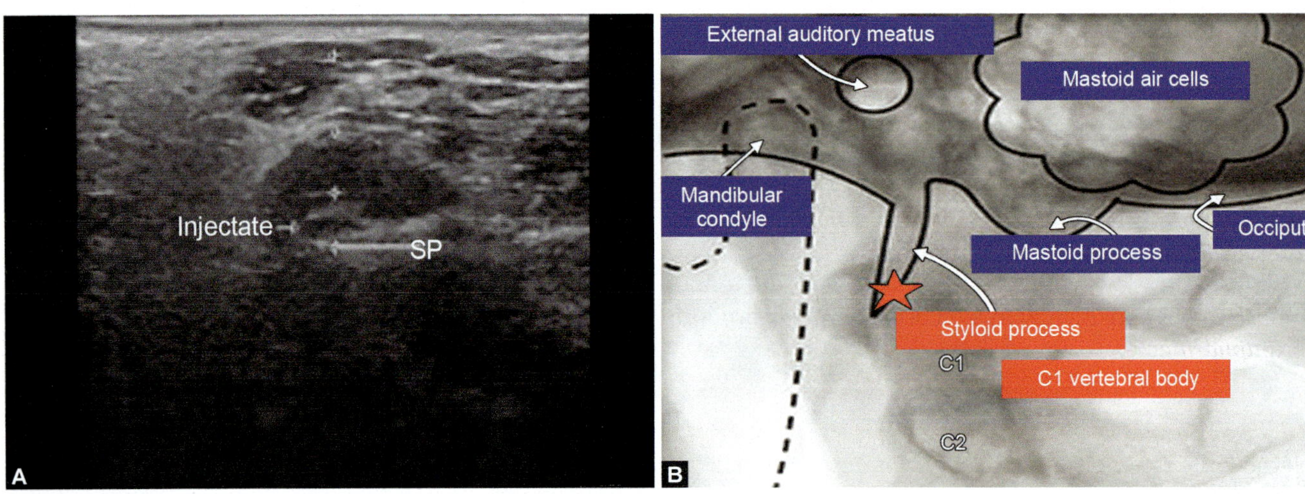

FIGS. 8A AND B: Glossopharyngeal nerve block ultrasound and fluoroscopy guided.
(SP: styloid process)

TABLE 7: Clinical findings.

Disc level	Root	Pain distribution	Weakness	Sensory root	Reflex loss
C4–C5	C5	Medial scapular border, lateral upper arm to the elbow	Deltoid, supraspinatus, infraspinatus	Lateral upper arm	Supinator
C5–C6	C6	Lateral forearm, thumb, and index finger	Biceps, wrist extensors, brachioradialis	Thumb and index finger	Biceps
C6–C7	C7	Medial scapula, posterior arm, dorsum forearm, third finger	Triceps, wrist flexors, finger extensors	Posterior forearm, third finger	Triceps
C7–T1	C8	Shoulder, medial side of forearm, fifth finger	Thumb flexors, abductors, intrinsic muscles of hand	Fifth finger	

Treatment

- *Preventive measures*: Proper posturing, exercises
- *Nonpharmacological*: Proper posturing, traction, physiotherapy
- *Pharmacological*: NSAIDs, anticonvulsants
- *Interventions*:
    - *Cervical epidural steroid injections (ESIs)* **(Figs. 9A and B)**: If the pain and neurological symptoms do not reduce on prolonged medical management or if the patient suffers from recurrent breakthrough pain, cervical epidural steroid injection should be considered.
    - *RF lesioning of dorsal root ganglion (DRG)*: Reserved for cases with upper extremity segmental pain secondary to radiculitis, mononeuropathies, postlaminectomy syndromes, etc. A selective nerve root block is performed with local anesthetic at the desired level; if the patient has pain relief, RF lesioning of DRG at that level is performed.
    - Botulinum toxin for subacute and chronic pain if there is spasm of the neck muscles unresponsive to medications and physiotherapy
    - *Surgery*:
        - Cervical disc replacement
        - Fusion techniques for degenerative disc disease

Facet Joint Pathology

Facet joints are meant to restrain excessive mobility and distribute axial loading over a broad area. Facetal arthropathy is most seen in degenerative diseases and motor vehicle trauma. Facet joint pathology presents with deep and aching pain over the corresponding nerve distribution area **(Fig. 10)**. Pressing firmly on the facet joint and rotating the cervical spine elicits pain.

Treatment

- *Nonpharmacological methods*: Rest, physiotherapy
- *Pharmacological*: NSAIDs, muscle relaxants
- *Interventional*: Facet joint injections, facet medial branch RF ablation

POSTHERPETIC NEURALGIA

Postherpetic neuralgia is the most common complication of shingles. The condition affects nerve fibers and skin, causing burning pain that lasts long after the rash and blisters of shingles disappear **(Fig. 11)**. Pain that lasts 3 months or more after the shingles rash has disappeared, associated with itching and numbness, and sensitivity to touch constitutes PHN.

Factors predisposing herpes zoster patients for PHN are elderly age patients, severe rash, severe acute pain, and the presence of a prodrome.

Prevention includes prompt treatment with antiviral medications and control of pain during the acute episode with TCAs and anticonvulsants.

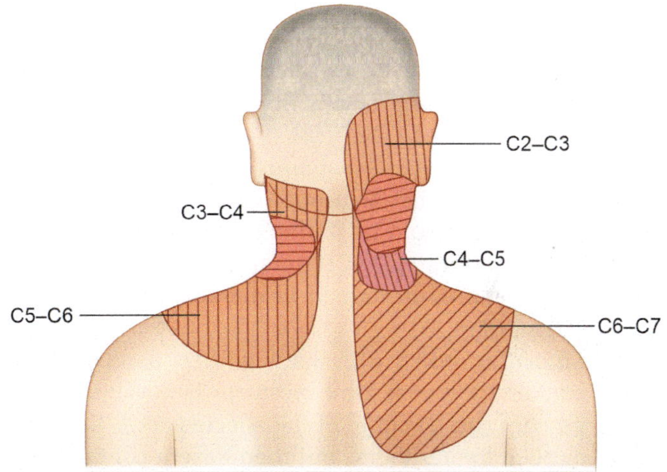

FIG. 10: Cervical facet dermatomal distribution.

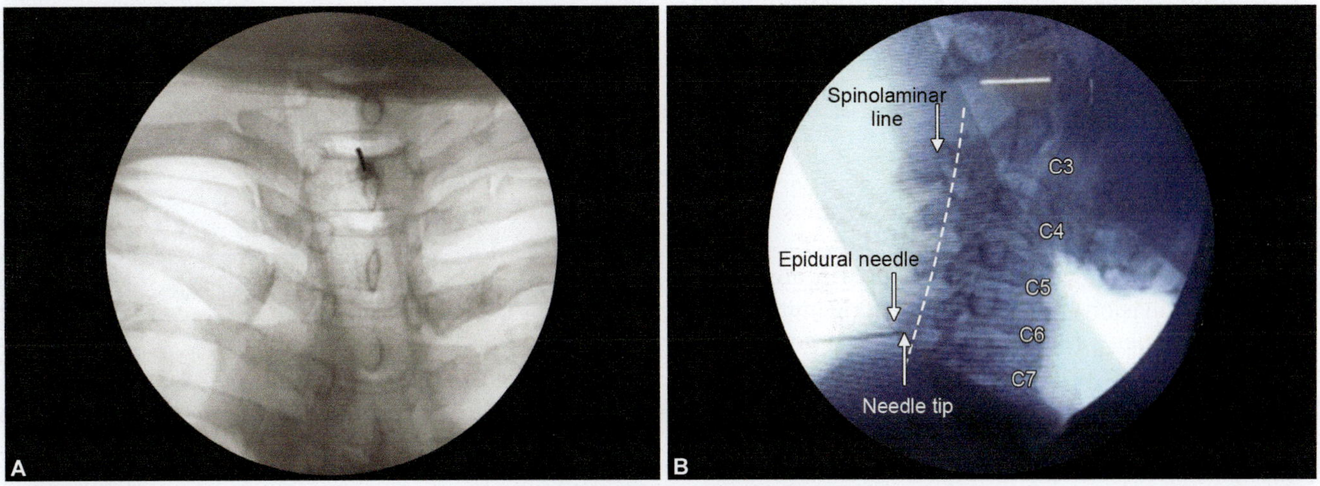

FIGS. 9A AND B: Fluoroscopy-guided cervical epidural injection anteroposterior (AP) view and oblique view.

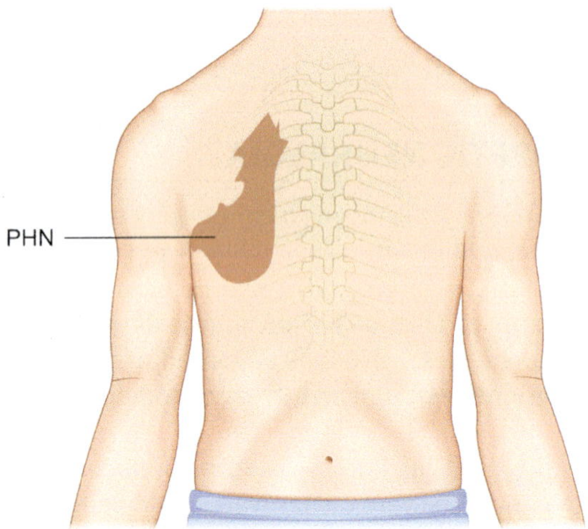

FIG. 11: Postherpetic neuralgia (PHN) in thoracic dermatomes.

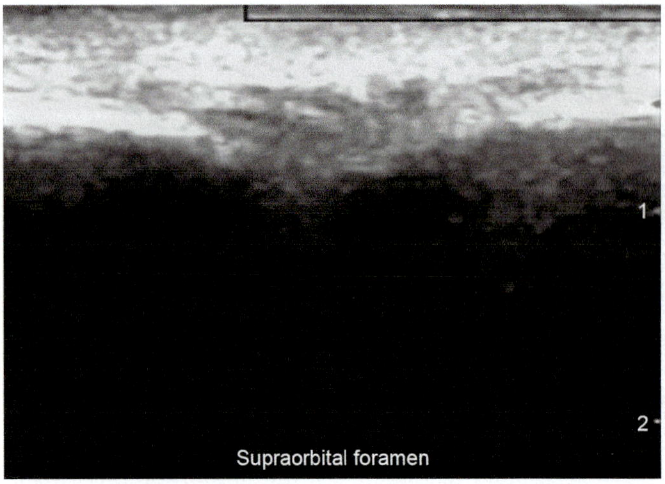

FIG. 12: Supraorbital block.

Treatment

- *Nonpharmacological*: TENS has been of some use in the long run but depends on there being sufficient innervation from normally conducting fast fibers.
- *Pharmacological*:
    - *TCAs*: They have been shown to provide moderate to excellent pain relief. Amitriptyline is the most commonly used TCA.
    - *Anticonvulsants*: Gabapentin and pregabalin are effective against neuropathic pain. Gabapentin treatment should be initiated at 900 mg/day, and additional titration to 1,800 mg/day is often necessary. Pregabalin is prescribed in divided doses of 150–600 mg/day.
    - *Lidocaine patch 5%*: Bandage-like patches that contain the topical local anesthetic lignocaine. These patches can be cut to fit the affected area. They are applied for 12 hours, and then have a contact-free period of 12 hours before the second application. They are Food and Drug Administration (FDA)-approved first-line agents along with gabapentin.
    - *Capsaicin patch*: A high concentration of an extract of chili peppers is available as a skin patch to relieve pain. Applied for over 2 hours by trained personnel, a single application can decrease pain for 3 months.

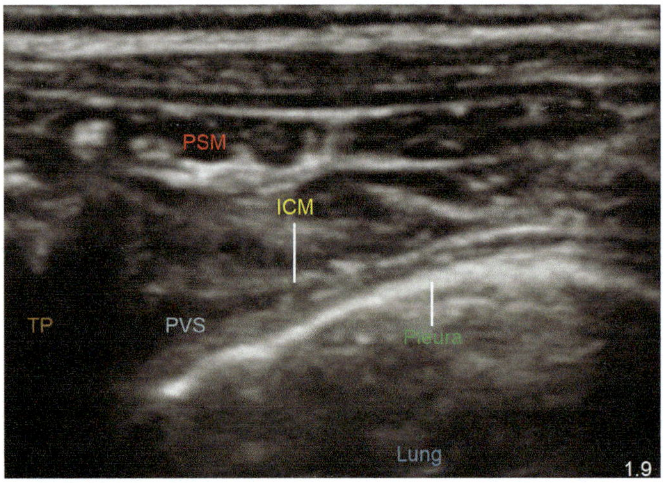

FIG. 13: Paravertebral block.
(ICM: internal intercostal membrane; PSM: paraspinal muscles; PVS: paravertebral space; TP: transverse process)

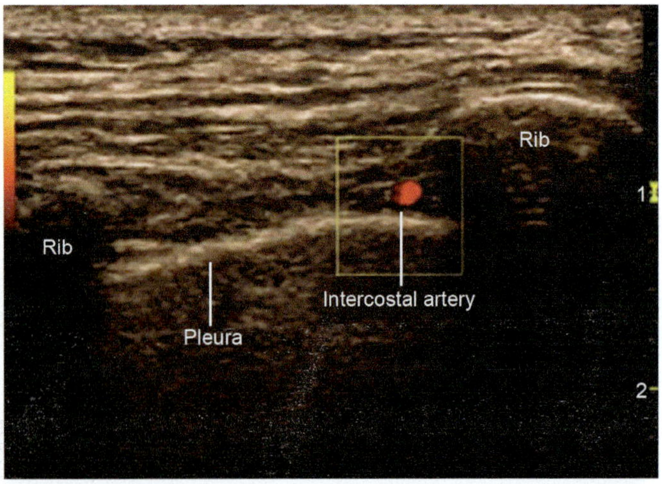

FIG. 14: Intercostal block.

Interventional Approach

The type of intervention is determined by the site of the lesion.

The most commonly occurring sites of PHN are the face (ophthalmic division) and chest wall. Trigeminal nerve or supraorbital nerve **(Fig. 12)** RF ablation is preferred for the PHN of the face. PHN of chest wall can be treated with paravertebral block **(Fig. 13)** and intercostal block **(Fig. 14)**.

In resistant cases, DRG pulsed radiofrequency (PRF) ablation can be done **(Fig. 15)**.

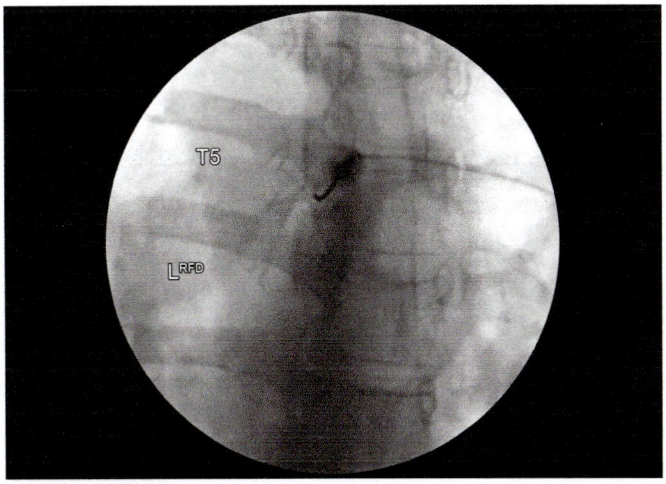

FIG. 15: Dorsal root ganglion (DRG) block.

7 days' conservative treatment of acute herpes
↓
Recurrence or inadequate relief
↓
Epidural or paravertebral steroid block
↓
Repeat the block or SCS

FLOWCHART 3: Treatment algorithm for PHN.
(PHN: postherpetic neuralgia; SCS: spinal cord stimulation)

Patients unresponsive to all the above treatments will need spinal cord stimulation (SCS) **(Flowchart 3)**.

COMPLEX REGIONAL PAIN SYNDROME

Complex regional pain syndrome is a distinct chronic pain syndrome previously known as causalgia, reflex sympathetic dystrophy, causalgia, Sudeck's dystrophy, shoulder-hand syndrome, neuroalgodystrophy, and reflex neurovascular dystrophy, commonly seen in females and upper extremities.

It is a form of chronic pain that usually affects an arm or leg. CRPS typically develops after an injury, a stroke, surgery, or a heart attack. The pain is out of proportion to the severity of the initial injury.

Signs and symptoms include:
- Continuous burning or throbbing pain usually in the arm, leg, hand, or foot
- Sensitivity to touch or cold
- Swelling of the painful area
- Changes in skin temperature, alternating between sweaty and cold
- Changes in skin color, ranging from white and blotchy to red or blue
- Changes in skin texture, which may become tender, thin, or shiny in the affected area

- Reactivation
- Desensitization
- Exposure therapy

↓

- Diagnosis and treatment of myofascial pain
- Edema control
- Isometric strengthening
- Correction of posture

↓ ← In unresponsive cases consider escalation of medications and increased psychological support

- Isotonic strengthening
- General aerobic conditioning
- Postural normalization and balanced use

↓

- Ergonomics
- Movement therapies
- Functional rehabilitation

FLOWCHART 4: Functional restoration algorithm.[3]

- Changes in hair and nail growth
- Joint stiffness, swelling, and damage
- Muscle spasms, tremors, weakness, and loss (atrophy)
- Decreased ability to move the affected body part

Symptoms may change over time and vary from person to person. Treatment would be effective when started early **(Flowchart 4)**.

Treatment Protocol

In treating CRPS, a drug regimen that draws two basic classes of medications needs to be given: prophylactic drugs (for maintenance, drugs used on a scheduled basis) to obtain baseline analgesia and abortive drugs (rescue agents, "as needed") for breakthrough pain or symptom flares.

Psychological Interventions

- Cognitive behavioral therapy principles
- Training in relaxation techniques

Interventional Therapies

- Sympathetic nerve blocks and surgical sympathectomies give significant relief of pain for patients with a subset of sympathetic-mediated pain.
- Axillary brachial plexus block with catheter technique is used for patients with upper extremity CRPS with intractable pain, which helps to break the pain cycle.
- Epidural steroids can be used empirically.
- IV regional anesthesia (IVRA) with lignocaine has been shown beneficial in some cases.
- Spinal cord stimulation for refractory cases
- DRG stimulation has variable results, tried in patients resistant to medical management and sympathectomy.
- Hyperbaric oxygen therapy

LOW BACK PAIN

Lumbar spinal pain is pain perceived anywhere in the region bounded by the lateral margins of the erector spinae muscles, an imaginary transverse line through the tip of the last thoracic spinous process, and an imaginary transverse line through the tip of the first sacral spinous process **(Fig. 16)**.

Chronic back pain is defined, by convention, as back pain that has persisted for longer than 3 months.

Somatic referred pain must be differentiated from radicular pain.

Causes: There are many pain-sensitive structures in the spine other than the annulus fibrosis of the intervertebral disc such as the vertebral body periosteum, dura, facet joints, epidural veins, and ligaments. **Flowchart 5** shows the management of lower backache.

ASSESSMENT

- The practitioner should not miss any serious causes of pain.
- Information should be gathered to formulate the type of diagnosis to form the base of treatment.
- Evaluate the physical and emotional state of the patients along with their social circumstances to formulate a management plan.
- History taking, clinical examination, identification of red flag signs, and investigations help in the diagnosis.
- Discography, selective nerve root sleeve blocks, lumbar medial branch blocks, sacroiliac joint injection, and lateral sacral nerve root blocks help in the diagnosis when cannot be established with history and investigations.

TREATMENT

Pharmacological:
- Paracetamol
- NSAIDs
- Muscle relaxants
- Pregabalin, gabapentin
- Opioids

Physical modalities: Physiotherapy, massage, traction, manual therapy, lumbar supports, exercise therapy

Simple Needle Therapies

- *Acupuncture*: It provides transient relief, and provides no better effect for improved function and long-lasting effect.
- *Trigger point injection*: Injecting local anesthetic with a small dose of steroid helps in transient pain relief.
- *Prolotherapy*: It involves the injection of sclerosing agents such as hypertonic dextrose or phenol into tender areas of the back muscles, possibly at the muscle attachment sites.
- 20% of patients have prolonged relief at 12 month intervals.

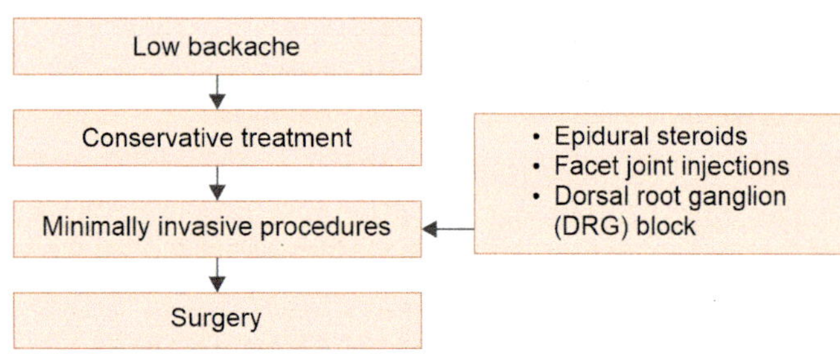

FLOWCHART 5: Management of lower backache.

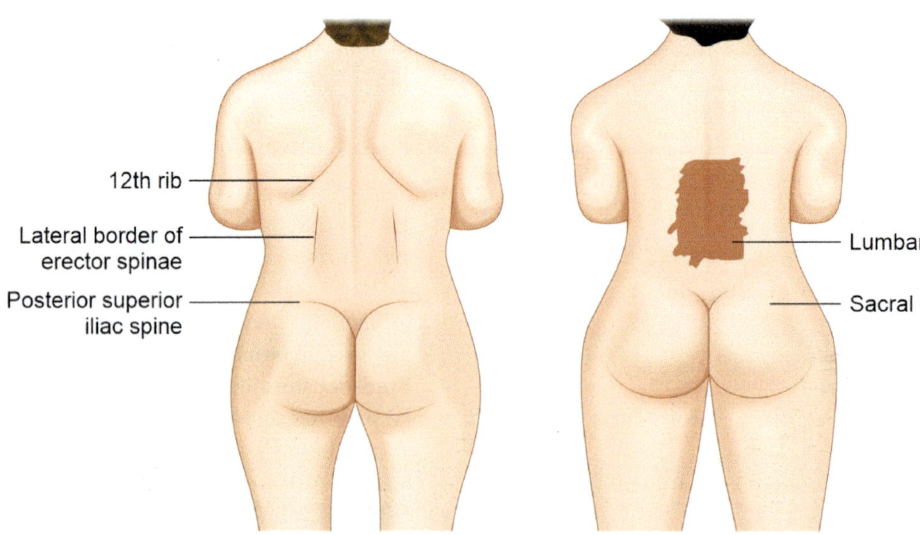

FIG. 16: Lower back anatomical distribution.

- *Psychological interventions*: Progressive relaxation, operant therapy, cognitive behavioral therapy.

Specific Targeted Therapies

Discogenic Pain

Discogenic low back pain is pain arising from an intervertebral disc. Intradiscal biacuplasty has been shown to provide some marginal benefit.

Epidural Steroid Injections

Epidural steroid injections **(Fig. 17)** are minimally invasive procedures designed to treat radicular pain. They involve inserting a needle into a location from which medication can be delivered onto the affected spinal nerve, the DRG, or its roots. The most commonly used drugs are corticosteroids as it is believed that radicular pain is caused not only by compression but also by inflammation of the target nerve.

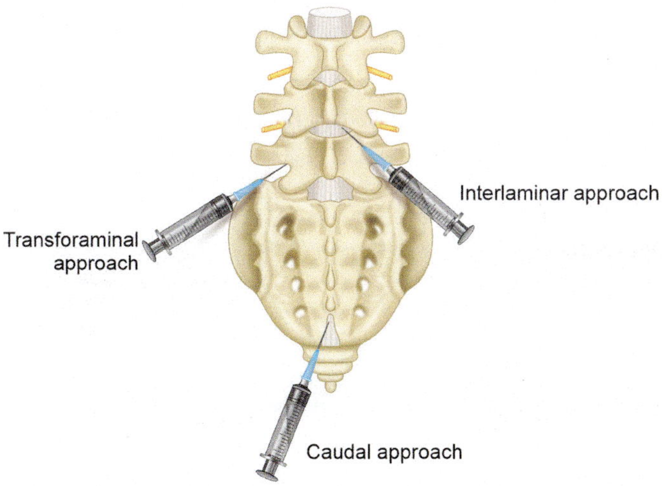

FIG. 17: Various approaches of epidural injections.

Technique

In the caudal route **(Figs. 18A to C)**, the needle is inserted through the sacral hiatus and the target is the epidural space. Multiple nerves can be targeted with a single injection. Adverse effects are uncommon but can occur, the most common being soreness at the injection site.

In the interlaminar route **(Figs. 19A and B)**, the needle is inserted between consecutive laminae that are closest to the target nerve, and the target is the dorsal epidural space. Minor complications such as dural puncture and vasovagal syncope can occur while major complications such as neurological injury and abscess are extremely rare in expert hands.

In the transforaminal route **(Figs. 20A to C)**, the needle is placed just inside the intervertebral foramen and the targets are the spinal nerve, the DRG, and its roots, which traverse the foramen. It is site- and side-specific, delivering the drug to the target nerve. It can combat the inflammatory effects of exudates from the disc into the retrodiscal, and epidural space, and epidural space and if they diffuse into the disc they could exert the same effects within the disc. It also blocks the sinuvertebral nerves that innervate the posterior disc.

Spinal Cord Stimulation

Spinal cord stimulation is a minimally invasive, reversible therapy implemented with sophisticated techniques and implanted equipment, including a variety of electrodes and multiple output pulse generators **(Fig. 21)**. It does not ablate the pain pathways or result in anatomic change. SCS also offers a screening trial with a temporary SCS system before proceeding to implantation. It can reduce, not eliminate, pain, particularly neuropathic pain. It is not expected to relieve nociceptive pain.

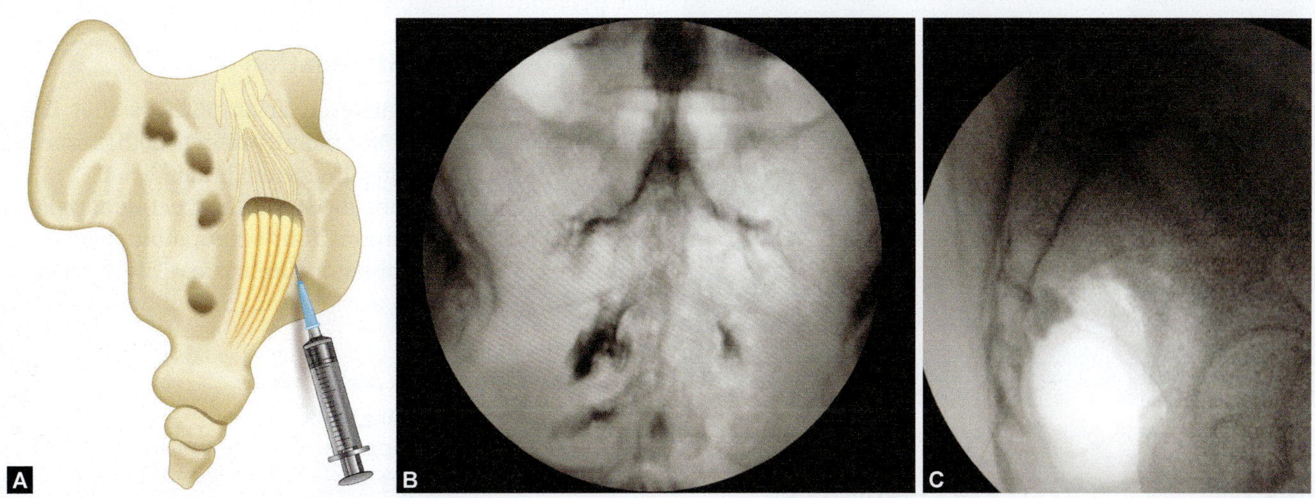

FIGS. 18A TO C: Caudal epidural injection.

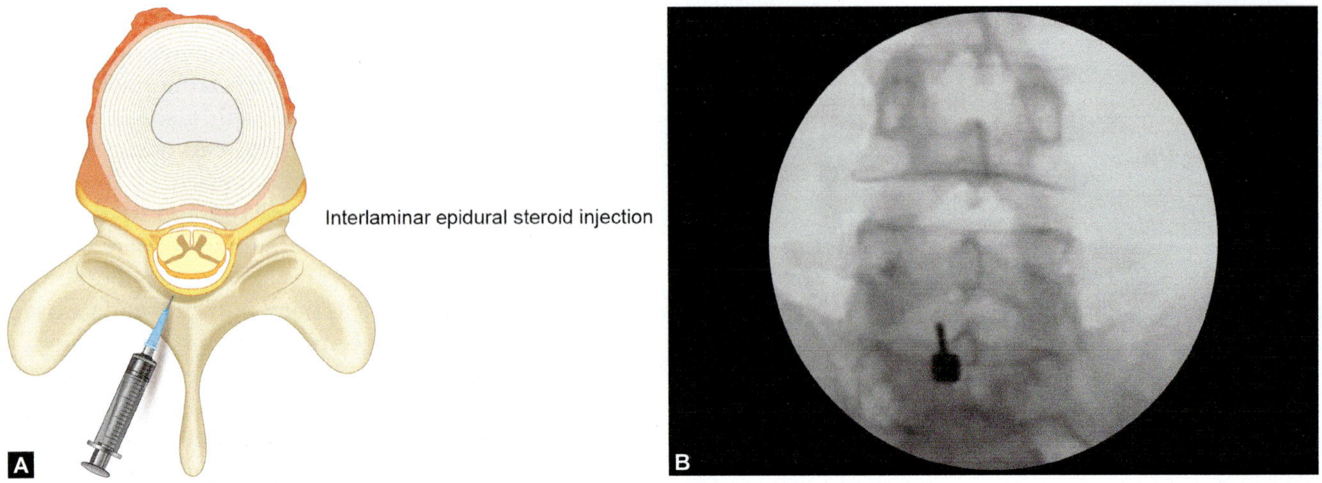

FIGS. 19A AND B: Interlaminar epidural injection.

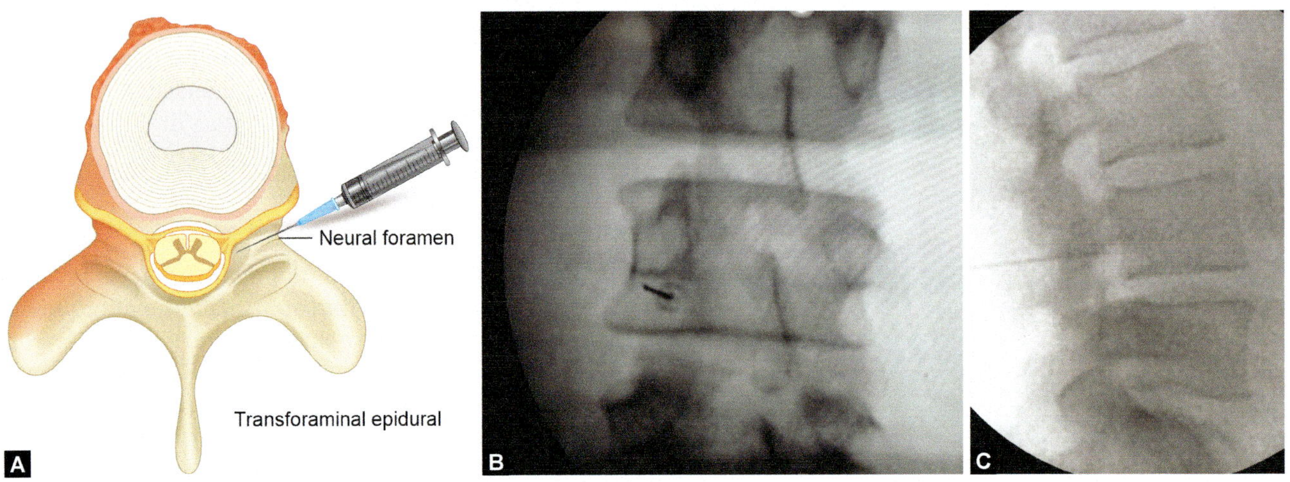

FIGS. 20A TO C: Transforaminal epidural injection.

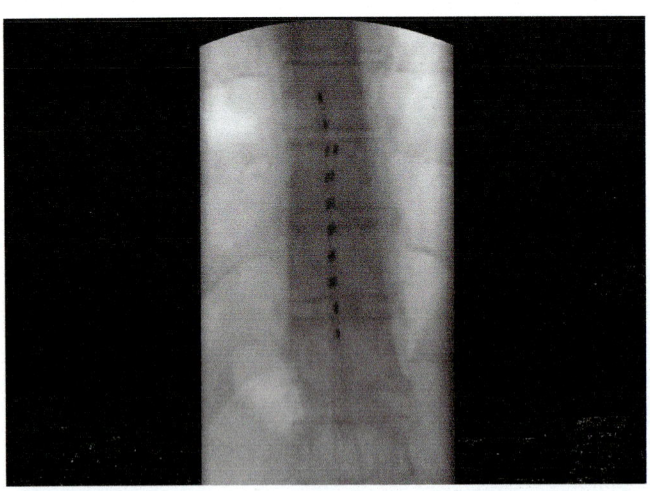

FIG. 21: Electrodes in spinal cord stimulation.

High-frequency Spinal Cord Stimulation

Clinical high-frequency (HF) SCS is applied via bipolar stimulation at a pulse repetition rate of 10 kHz and a short PW of about 30 microseconds at an amplitude that is below the perceptual threshold.

Burst Spinal Cord Stimulation

It is commonly administered at amplitudes that donot produce paraesthesias. Normally 5 pulses at 500Hz repeated with 40Hz rate at subparesthetic amplitude is used.

The major indications for SCS is the treatment of FBSS, particularly with a component of neuropathic pain. It can also be used for CRPS, phantom limb pain, PHN, Root injury pain, and pain/spasm arising from Spinal cord injury or lesion.

Goals: *The clinical goals are as follows—*
- Minimum of 50% pain relief
- Reduced consumption of medication and other healthcare resources
- Improved ability to engage in daily activities
- Return to work when uncontrolled pain was the only impediment

Screening Trial

A typical screening trial with a temporary percutaneous electrode lasts for a week and could be longer or shorter. A successful trial is defined by at least 50% patient-reported pain relief despite the appropriate (provocative) physical activity and stable or reduced analgesic consumption with patient satisfaction.

FACET JOINT PAIN

Facet joint arthropathy occurs as a result of degeneration of the joints that hold vertebrae together or the wear and tear of cartilages present between the joints. Patients often experience lower back pain **(Fig. 22)** that worsens with twisting, standing, or bending backward.

Treatment

Intra-articular Steroids

Intra-articular joint injection of steroids is sometimes used to treat pain arising from facet joints.

Lumbar Medial Branch Radiofrequency Neurotomy

For patients with facet joint pain, a diagnostic block of the medial branch of the dorsal spinal nerve is given. For patients having >50% pain relief thermal RF ablation is done, which involves coagulating the nerves that innervate the painful joint, using electrodes that generate a heat lesion around their tip **(Figs. 23A and B)**.

Flowchart 6 gives the algorithm for facetal arthropathy treatment.

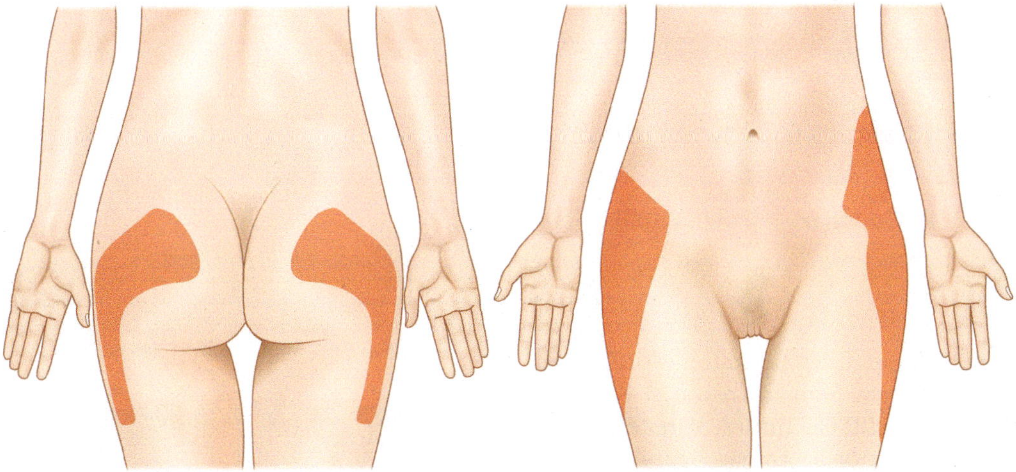

FIG. 22: Facet distribution of pain.

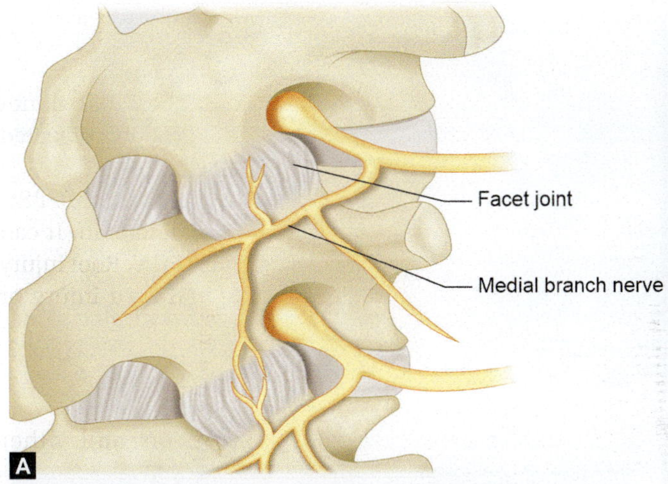

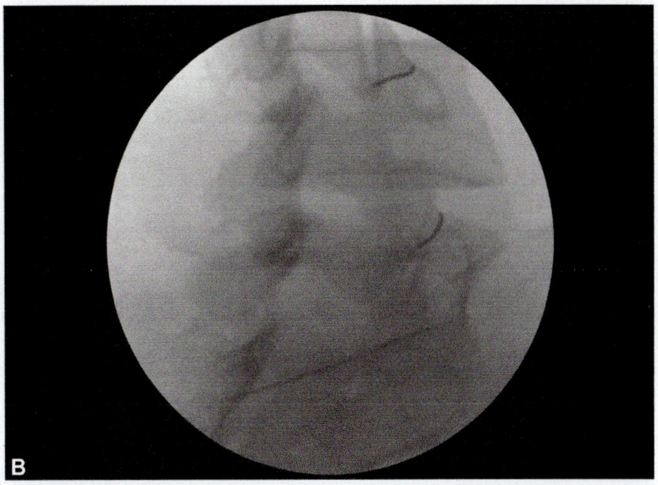

FIGS. 23A AND B: Facet medial branch rhizotomy.

Chronic low backache (LBA)

↓ ← Red flags ruled out

Signs and symptoms suggestive of facetal arthropathy

↓

Diagnostic facet joint block

↓ ← >50% pain relief

Radiofrequency ablation of medial branch

FLOWCHART 6: Algorithm for facetal arthropathy treatment.

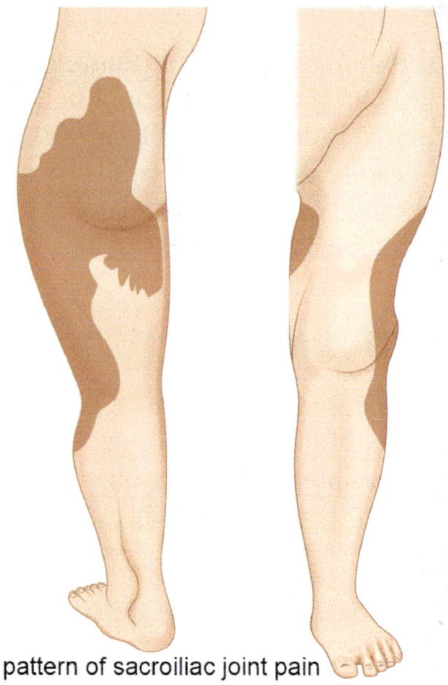

FIG. 24: Sacroiliac joint pain.

SACROILIAC PAIN

Sacroiliitis is an inflammation of one or both sacroiliac joints. Patients experience pain that is sharp, stabbing that radiates from the hips and pelvis up to the lower back and down to the thighs **(Fig. 24)**. Pain is worse on standing or walking. MRI is the diagnostic modality for the diagnosis.

Sacroiliac Joint Steroid Injections: Both Diagnostic and Therapeutic

Figures 25A and B and **Flowchart 7** show sacroiliac joint steroid injections.

Sacral Lateral Branch Neurotomy

Sacral lateral branch thermal RF neurotomy (RFN) is a procedure in which the lateral branches of the S1–S3 dorsal rami are coagulated with RF electrodes. It relieves pain stemming from the posterior sacroiliac ligaments, and the indication is complete pain relief following controlled diagnostic blocks of the target nerves **(Figs. 26A to C)**.

SI joint pain

↓ ← Red flags ruled out

Diagnostic SI joint injection

Positive	Negative
↓	↓
Cooled/PRF L5–S3 dorsal rami	Reconsider diagnosis

FLOWCHART 7: SI joint injection.
(PRF: pulsed radiofrequency; SI: sacroiliac)

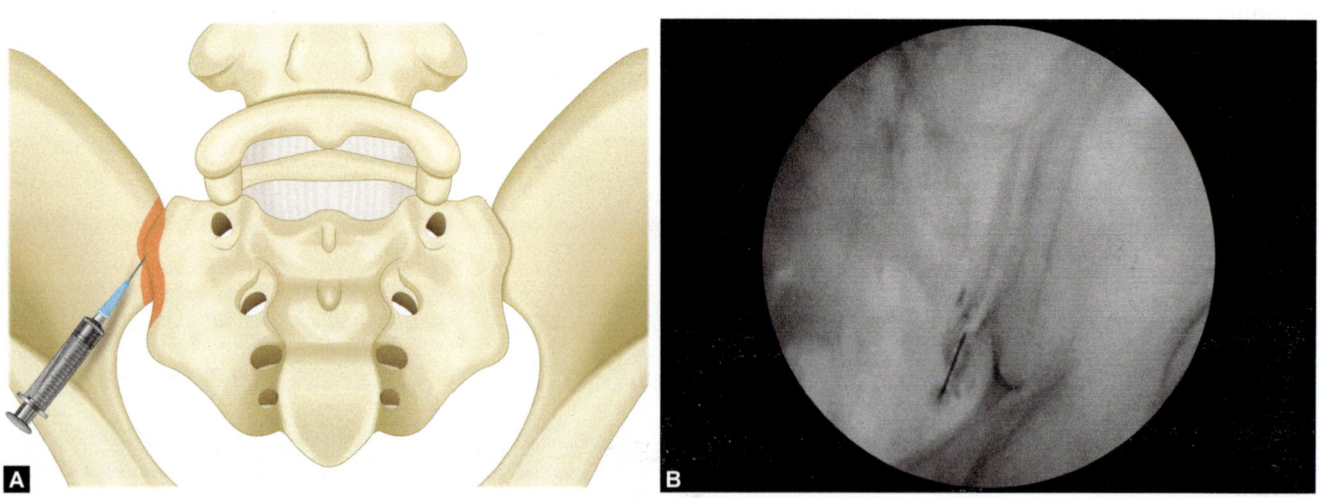

FIGS. 25A AND B: Sacroiliac joint injection.

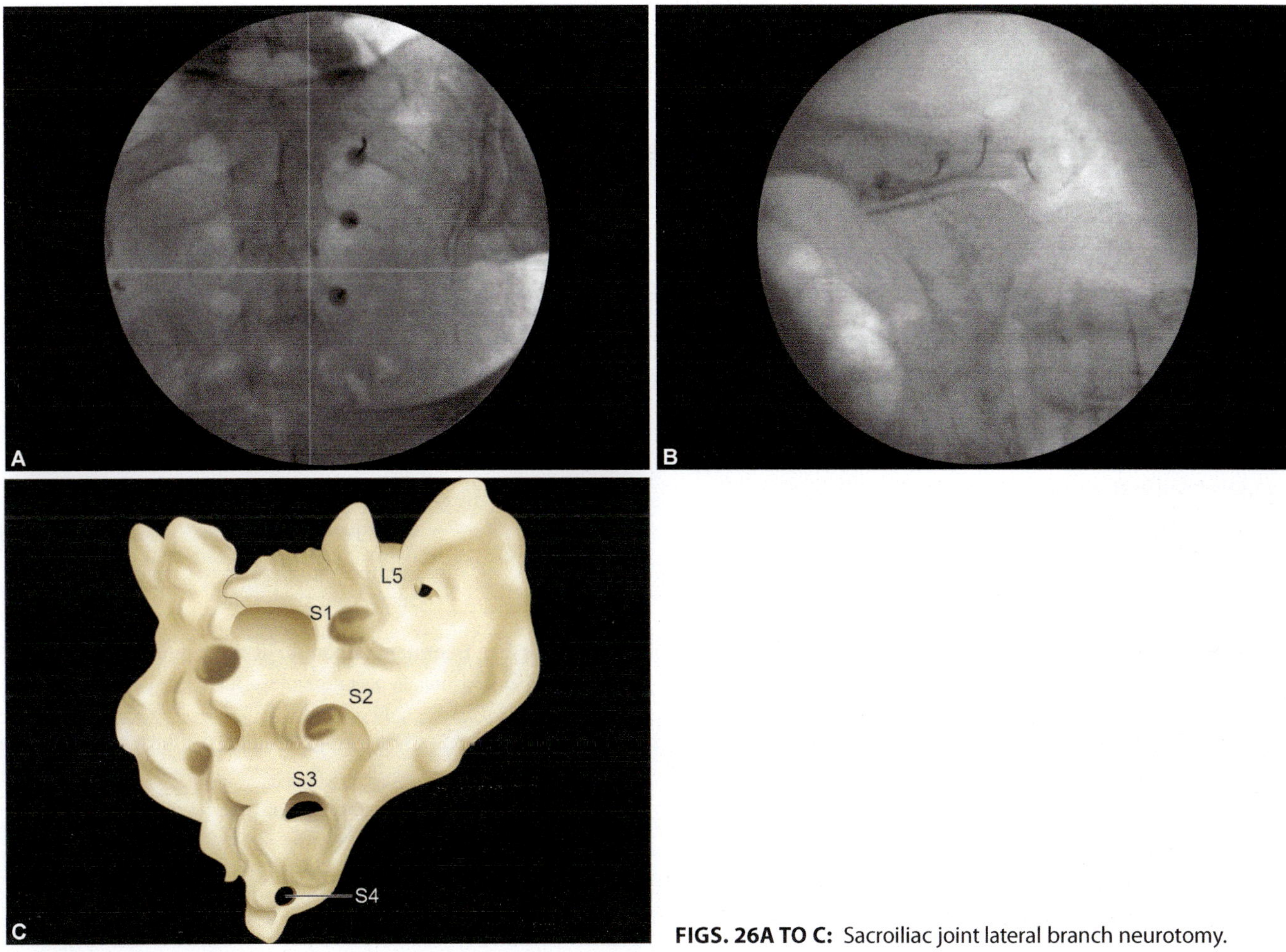

FIGS. 26A TO C: Sacroiliac joint lateral branch neurotomy.

INVASIVE TREATMENTS

Implanted Devices

Implanted devices are used for the control of severe, chronic low back pain unresponsive to any other treatment. Devices are implanted to deliver drugs intrathecally or to provide SCS. They are typically reserved for the treatment of patients with FBSS.

Spinal Surgery

Indications

- Neurological symptoms involving bowel and bladder sphincters
- Neurological symptoms such as numbness or weakness in lower limbs
- Conservative methods fail to relieve pain.
- Chronic disc prolapse characterized by nagging pain

The most common surgeries performed are discectomy and laminectomy. Discectomy involves removing the prolapsed disc, releasing the compressed roots, and restoring the mobility of the spine as early as possible. Laminectomy involves removing bony material, ligament, and cartilage pressing the nerves **(Flowchart 8)**.

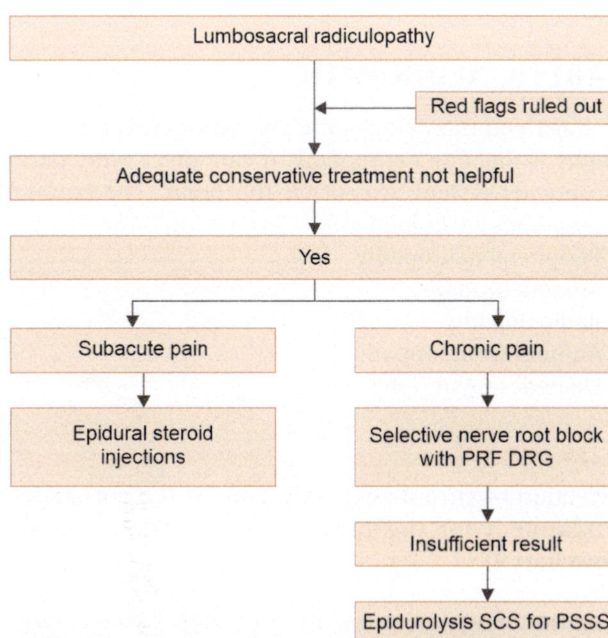

FLOWCHART 8: Lumbosacral radiculopathy.

(DRG: dorsal root ganglion; PRF: pulsed radiofrequency; PSSS: post-spine surgery syndrome; SCS: spinal cord stimulation)

POSTSPINE SURGERY SYNDROME

Postspine surgery syndrome (PSSS) is a nonspecific term that implies the outcome of spine surgery did not meet the expectations established before surgery of the patient and the surgeon.

Acute: Immediate postoperative period to 6 weeks postoperative.

Chronic: More than 6 weeks postoperatively.

It clinically determines any structural cause of pain and if it is a residual, recurrent or new problem.

Causes

- Lateral canal stenosis
- Painful disc
- Neuropathic pain
- Facet syndrome
- Recurrent herniated disc
- Sacroiliac joint pain

Failed Back Surgery Syndrome Stepladder Treatment Approach

Conservative: Rest, medicines, physiotherapy, and meditation.

Interventional: Facet joint block, epidural steroid injection, trigger point injection.

Surgery: Simple or instrumentation.

Advanced interventional: RF ablation, epidural adhesiolysis, intradiscal procedure, SCS, intrathecal pump.

DIABETIC NEUROPATHY

The most common cause of distal symmetrical polyneuropathy is diabetic neuropathy. It can affect every part of the nervous system, except for the brain. The common presentations are as follows:

- Peripheral neuropathy
- Mononeuropathy
- Radiculopathy
- Autonomic neuropathy
- Diabetic amyotrophy

Treatment

Correction of chronic hyperglycemia is the cornerstone of treatment for the preservation of nerve function **(Flowchart 9)**.

Pharmacology

- *Tricyclic agents*: Initiated at a dose of 10 or 25 mg bedtime
- *Alpha 2 ligands*: Pregabalin and gabapentin
- SSRIs and SNRI: Duloxetine and venlafaxine

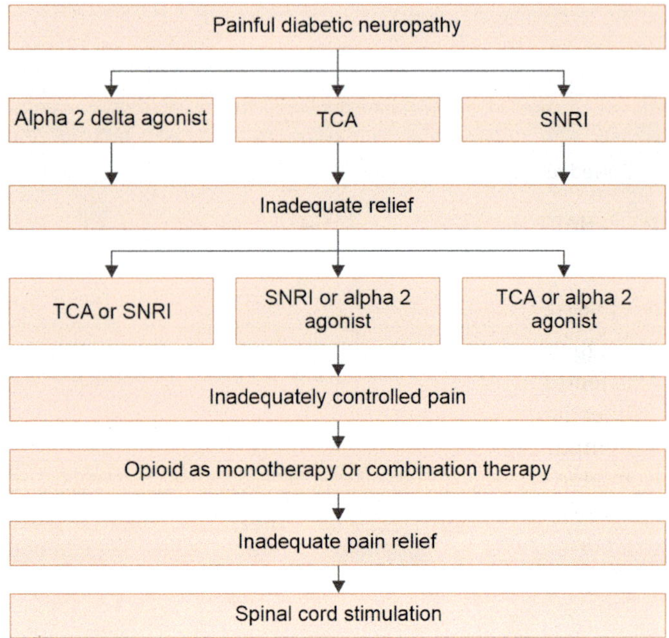

FLOWCHART 9: Treatment of painful diabetic neuropathy.
(SNRI: serotonin and noradrenaline reuptake inhibitor; TCA: tricyclic antidepressant)

- Opioids
- *Topical agents*: Capsaicin, lidocaine

PHANTOM LIMB PAIN

Phantom pain refers to pain perceived in a missing body part and may occur in 50–80% of all amputees. Pain may be related to certain positions or movements of the phantom and elicited or exacerbated by a range of physical and psychological factors. It seems to be more severe in distal portions of the phantom and can have several different characters.

Treatment

Treatment of phantom limb pain requires a multimodal approach including behavioral techniques **(Flowchart 10)**.

Pharmacology

- Antidepressants
- Antiepileptics
- NMDA receptor antagonists
- Opioids
- Calcitonin
- Modulators

Behavioral Therapies

Behavioral therapies include mirror therapy, biofeedback mechanisms, relaxation techniques, graded motor imagery, and eye movement desensitization and reprocessing (EMDR).

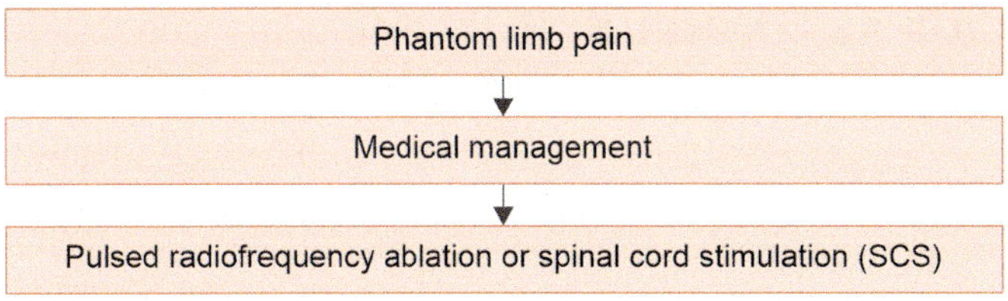

FLOWCHART 10: Management of phantom limb pain.

Interventional Therapy

- Trigger point injections, sympathetic blocks, stump injections, peripheral nerve blocks, and epidural injections all have been tried with variable results.
- Sympathetic blocks are successful if amputees are treated soon after the onset of phantom limb pain.
- Botulinum injection
- *Neuromodulation*: TENS
- SCS
- DRG stimulation

CENTRAL NEUROPATHIC PAIN

Central neuropathic pain is the pain caused by a lesion or disease of the central somatosensory system. It is mostly seen in stroke, multiple sclerosis, and spinal cord injury.

Central pain is characterized by spontaneous and/or evoked pain in an area with partial or complete sensory loss to one or more modalities. Decreased sensation to thermal or painful stimuli is more common. The location of pain and sensory abnormalities is compatible within the area of the CNS lesion **(Flowchart 11)**.

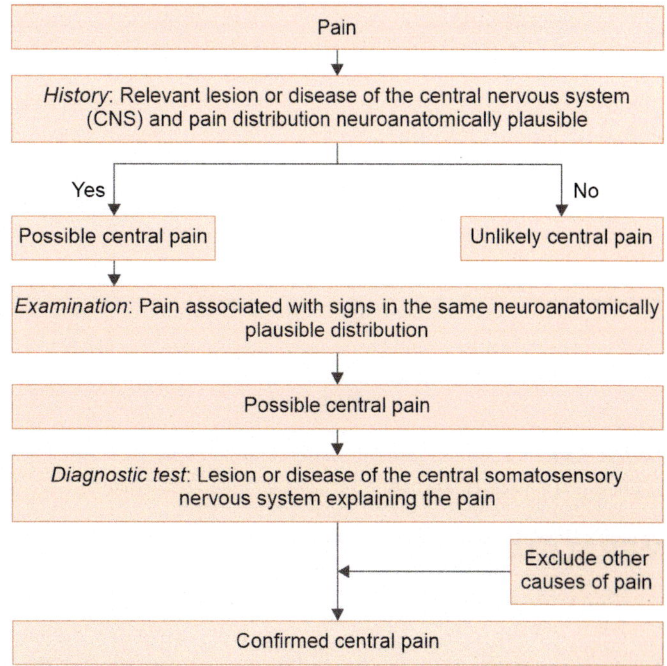

FLOWCHART 11: Central neuropathic pain.

CENTRAL POSTSTROKE PAIN

Central poststroke pain (CPSP) is pain arising after a cerebrovascular lesion including ischemic or hemorrhagic lesions of the thalamus, brainstem, and cerebral cortex. Central pain occurs in 3–8% of stroke patients. CPSP occurs on the contralateral side of the stroke.[4]

The diagnosis of central pain and the presumptive underlying mechanisms are the first important steps and require a thorough assessment.

The treatment of central pain is often symptomatic, but in some cases, the underlying cause of neuropathic pain can be treated, e.g., with the use of corticosteroids for the treatment of spinal cord compression. Consider the exacerbating factors.

Treatment

Psychological and Physiotherapy Treatment

These therapies help in early rehabilitation.

Pharmacology

- *First-line agents*: TCA/alpha 2 agonists/SNRI
- *Second-line agents*: Tramadol
- *Third-line agents*: Opioids

When treatment with a single drug is only partly effective, a combination with another drug of a complementary mechanism of action is included. Side effects should be carefully monitored, and sequential add-on therapy is recommended.

In refractory cases, intrathecal drug delivery systems are considered.

Neurosurgical Interventions

Targeted drug delivery into the subarachnoid space for the treatment of refractory central pain includes delivery most commonly via a catheter inserted into the intrathecal space in the spinal canal or less commonly directly into the brain via an intraventricular catheter. The catheters are connected to a subcutaneously implanted drug reservoir allowing the controlled infusion of various medications.

Neuroablation

It refers to the ablation of the thalamus in patients undergoing stereotactic or radiosurgical thalamotomy, and the spinothalamic and quintothalamic pathways in stereotactic mesencephalotomy are commonly used.

Neuromodulation

It includes motor cortex stimulation, deep brain stimulation (DBS), and SCS.

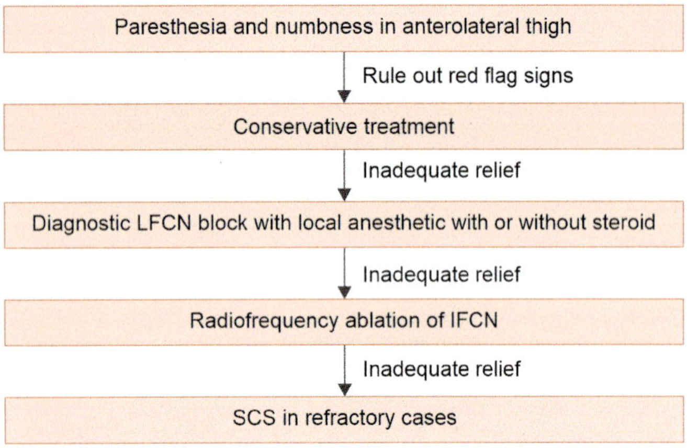

FLOWCHART 12: Management of meralgia paresthetica.
(LFCN: lateral femoral cutaneous nerve; SCS: spinal cord stimulation)

MERALGIA PARESTHETICA

Meralgia paresthetica is lateral femoral cutaneous nerve (LFCN) entrapment. LFCN is a purely sensory nerve originating from the lumbar plexus and supplying the anterolateral surface of the thigh. LFCN entrapment, therefore, causes unilateral sensory loss, paresthesias, or dysesthesias in the territory supplied by the nerve.

Treatment

Initial recommendations include advising the patients to avoid wearing tight-fitting garments or belts, advising obese patients to lose weight, and correcting limb length discrepancies, if any.

In cases where symptoms persist, ice, TENS, and analgesic medications can be tried.

In refractory cases, LFCN block is given under the guidance of ultrasound, which is followed by RF ablation or chemical neurolysis for prolonged results **(Flowchart 12)**.

CARPAL TUNNEL SYNDROME

Carpal tunnel syndrome (CTS) is an entrapment median neuropathy, causing paresthesia, pain, numbness, and other symptoms in the distribution of the median nerve due to its compression at the wrist in the carpal tunnel.

Numbness in the distribution of the median nerve, nocturnal symptoms, thenar muscle weakness/atrophy, positive Tinel's sign at the carpal tunnel, and abnormal sensory testing are considered for diagnosis.

Treatment

- *Supportive care*: Immobilizing braces, activity modification, physiotherapy, local massage therapy.
- *Pharmacological treatment*: Neuropathic drugs
- Localized corticosteroid injections
- Pulsed RF ablation
- Carpal tunnel release surgery

CONCLUSION

Neuropathic pain has clinical presentation and result of simple physical, neurological evaluation at the bedside compounded by few investigations for diagnosis. Despite newer drugs and the rationale of combination therapy, the response to treatment is mostly modest. Interventional pain procedures bridge the gap between medical therapy and surgery and are a boon in conditions where surgery is not advisable. They are minimally invasive procedures including percutaneous precision needle placement, with the placement of drugs in targeted areas or ablation of targeted nerves. Fluoroscopy or ultrasound-guided real-time imaging procedures have increased the accuracy of the procedures, thereby increasing the success rate and decreasing the complications. The management of neuropathic pain should include patient-centric care.

REFERENCES

1. Ballantyne JC, Fishman SM, Rathmell JP (Eds). Bonica's Management of Pain, 5th edition. Philadelphia: Wolters Kluwer; 2018.
2. Joshi M. Textbook of Pain Management, 3rd edition. New Delhi: Paras Publishers; 2014.
3. Van Zundert J, Hartrick C, Patijn J, Huygen F, Mekhail N, van Kleef M. Evidence-based interventional pain medicine according to clinical diagnoses. Pain Pract. 2011;11(5):423-9.
4. Jankovic J, Mazziotta JC, Pomeroy SL, Newman NJ. Bradley and Darroff's Neurology in Clinical Practice, 8th edition. Amsterdam: Elsevier Health; 2021.

125

CHAPTER

Neurorehabilitation

Nirmal Surya, Abhishek Srivastava, Guhan Ramamurthy

INTRODUCTION

Neurological diseases are common and often have a vital impact on the survivors and on society. They typically show up as a disabling illness, involving several aspects of the patient's life, especially, on the power to perform activities of daily living (ADLs) and walking. The aims of neurorehabilitation are to minimize the impact of the incapacity ensuing from medical illness and to optimize the standard of life for each patient and caregiver. Formal neurorehabilitation is economical and price effective and is best provided by well-organized multidisciplinary team in a patient friendly setting followed by regular follow-up and time of care.

NEED FOR NEUROREHABILITATION

With 90 million deaths and 16.5% of world deaths, disorders of the nervous system are the second leading reason for death behind cardiac causes, and with 276 million disability-adjusted life years (DALYs) and 11.6% of world DALYs, it is the leading reason behind incapacity. This prominence within the world burden of disease is because of increasing numbers of individuals tormented by disorders of the nervous system and also the longevity of affected people living with incapacity, therefore, inflicting an enormous monetary burden in the long run.[1]

The contribution of noncommunicable disorders of the nervous system to total DALYs in the Republic of India doubled from 4.0% in 1990 to 8.2% in 2019, and also the contribution of injury-related disorders of the nervous system tripled from 0.2 to 0.6%. In 2019, the most important contributors to the DALYs in the Republic of India were stroke (37.9%), headache disorders (17.5%), epilepsy (11.3%), cerebral palsy (5.7%), and encephalitis (5.3%).[2]

The burden of noncommunicable disorders is reaching a considerable proportion of the DALYs in the Republic of India, with a growing share of the aging population. The impact on human wellness and the economic burden of noncommunicable disorders of the nervous system in Republic of India is increasing significantly. The scientific and clinical care prices can shortly become unmanageable for all tiers of Indian society. This needs an appropriate pragmatic approach, with the institution of newer, realistic, and possible interventions for providing low-price but price-effective neurorehabilitation care.[3]

Neurological disease will have an effect on completely different components of the brain inflicting multiple deficits together with, cognitive, behavioral, visual, speech, language, swallowing, sensation, movement, tone and sphincter, and sexual functions.

There are two completely different approaches of neurorehabilitation: First is the compensatory approach, as an example, if somebody does not have movements in the leg, inflicting issues in walking, we gave him an aid to walk. Second is the remediation approach, within which we tend to attempt to minimize the impairment or improve power within the leg muscles thus an individual will walk and cut down the possibilities of employing aid to walk. This ability of the brain to revive the functions is by minimizing the impairment and depends upon the formation of other circuits within the brain. This inherent however not wide proverbial ability of the brain to adapt in response to stimulus information is named as neuroplasticity.

INTERNATIONAL CLASSIFICATION OF FUNCTIONING MODEL

These are key ideas that forge the essential principles of neurorehabilitation. The ideas were developed by the World Health Organization in 1980. Though the terms have recently been modernized, the three original terms—impairment, disability, and handicap—are thus standard and still utilized in the philosophy of neurorehabilitation.[4]

Impairment is simply a descriptive term. It implies nothing concerning consequence. Examples are right hemiparesis, left-sided sensory loss, or homonymous visual defect. However, a right hemiparesis may be comparatively minimal and cause nearly no significant consequence or will be severe and cause an entire inability to steer. The consequence of impairment is a disability. However, neuro-rehabilitation goes on the far beyond the impairment and appears to minimize the impact of the incapacity on the individual. Handicap is the description of the social context of incapacity. An individual with right hemiparesis, as an example, might have a comparatively minimal weakness, however, even a minimal weakness might have profound social consequences for a few individuals. Neuro-rehabilitation clearly must take into consideration not solely the disability but conjointly the actual handicap for the individual, whereas bearing in mind that several social and physical barriers rely upon social attitudes and also the physical surroundings and will be outside the management of the rehabilitation team **(Table 1)**.

The WHO has made a new classification that has fewer negative connotations. Disability is currently termed activity and handicap is currently termed participation. The principles are identical; however, the classification currently places additional stress on the individual's skills instead of disabilities and additional stress is given to social context **(Flowchart 1)**.

NEURAL PLASTICITY

There are two different but related ways that patients improve after stroke.[5] The first type of recovery, a reduction in the extent of neurological impairment, can result from natural spontaneous recovery, which usually accounts for early spontaneous improvement after stroke within the first 3–6 months. This form of recovery manifests as improvement in motor control, language ability, or other primary neurological functions.[6] The underlying mechanisms include the resolution of local edema, resorption of local toxins, restoration of circulation in the ischemic penumbra, and recovery of partial damaged ischemic neurons.[7] This sequence of recovery, however, can stop at any stage.

The second type of recovery demonstrated in stroke patients is the improved ability to perform daily functions in their environment, within the limitation of their physical impairment. The underlying mechanism to explain the second type of recovery is neuroplasticity. Brain plasticity is the ability of the nervous system to modify its structure and functional organization. The two most plausible forms of plasticity are the collateral sprouting of new synaptic connections and the unmasking of previous latent pathways. Other mechanisms of plasticity include the assumption of function by undamaged pathways, reversibility from diaschisis, denervation supersensitivity, remyelination, and regenerative proximal sprouting of transacted neuronal

TABLE 1: New classifications of the International Classification of Functioning and Disability: ICIDH II (WHO, 1998).

Classification	Definition
Impairment	The loss or abnormality of a body structure or of a physiological or psychological function
Activity	The nature and extent of functioning at the level of the person. Activities may be limited in nature, duration, and quality
Contextual factors (participation)	Include the features, aspects and attributes of objects, structures, human made organizations, service provision, and agencies in the physical, social, and attitudinal environment in which people live and conduct their lives. Contextual factors include both environmental factors and personal factors

(ICIDH: International Classification of Impairments, Disability, and Handicaps)

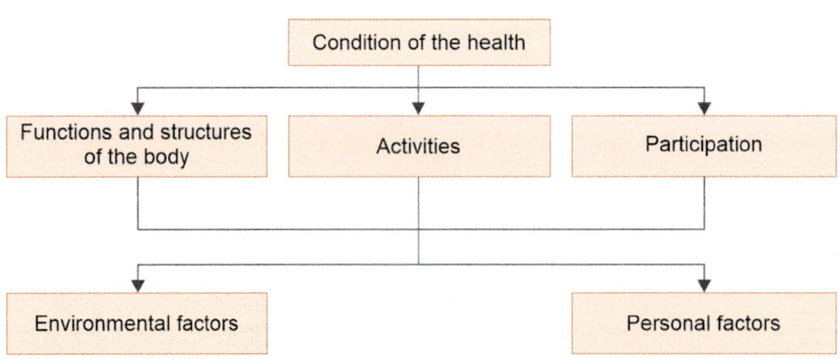

FLOWCHART 1: International classification of function, disability, and health proposed by World Health Organization.

axons.[8,9] Experimental evidence suggests that this plasticity can be altered by several external conditions, including pharmacological agents, electrical stimulation, intensive training, and environmental manipulation.[10] The ability to perform the task can improve through adaptation and training, despite the presence or absence of natural neurological recovery. It is the element of recovery on which rehabilitation is believed to exert the greatest effect. The degree of recovery in independent functioning that occurs during rehabilitation is often greater than expected by the reduction in neural impairments alone, which suggests that timely rehabilitation intervention probably plays important role in recovery.[11]

GOALS OF NEUROREHABILITATION

Neurological rehabilitation is as much a philosophy as it is a set of tasks to carry out. Roth enumerated five major goals of neurorehabilitation program which are enumerated in **Box 1**.[12]

Brandstater and Basmajian (1987) laid down the guidelines for neurorehabilitation of stroke patients **(Box 2)**.[13]

BOX 1 Goals of neurorehabilitation program.

Goals:
1. Prevention, recognition, and management of comorbid illness and intercurrent medical complications
2. Training for maximal functional independence in all respective domains or impairments
3. Facilitating psychosocial copping and adaptation by patient and the family
4. Promoting community reintegration, including resumptions of home, family, recreational, and vocational activities
5. Enhancing quality of life

BOX 2 Guidelines for neurorehabilitation of stroke patients.

Guidelines:
- Committed medical direction to provide continuity of care from acute phase to rehabilitation and long-term follow-up
- Use of a team approach with staff that is knowledgeable of, experienced in, and dedicated to patient care
- Goal-directed treatment
- Early initiation of treatment
- Emphasis on patient education
- Intensive focus on training of skills
- Focus on facilitating adaptation
- Early discharge planning
- Involvement of family members in the management program
- Attention to psychosocial issues
- Introduction of the patient to community resources
- Preparing the patient to resume optimal life roles at home, in the family, and in the community

INDICATIONS FOR NEUROREHABILITATION AND SELECTION OF PATIENTS

There are essentially five categories of people with disabilities summarized in **Box 3**.[4]

There is enough evidence to show that persons with neurologic diseases in all these five categories benefit from neurorehabilitation interventions.

Prognostication regarding the outcome for a patient is often expressed in the simple question: "Is this patient a good candidate for rehabilitation?" Patients and family members need to know the prospects for survival, the degree of recovery that may be expected, and the extent of possible residual disability following rehabilitation.

It is important to distinguish between prognostic and outcome variables. Prognostic variables influence the survival, recovery, and ultimate outcome of an individual **Box 4**.[14]

Outcome variables on the other hand describe different aspects of the status of the patient at a particular endpoint. Typical outcome variables are survival, impairment—neurologic deficit in the form of degree of paralysis, speech or visual field defect, disability—in ADLs and ambulation, and social variables—discharge destination, living arrangements, and social integration.

TEAM MODELS IN NEUROREHABILITATION

Neurorehabilitation is done with the patient, rather than to the patient. This requires a dedicated, comprehensive, and multidisciplinary rehabilitation team **(Fig. 1)**. The

BOX 3 Categories of people with disabilities.

People with disabilities:
1. Patients who will make a spontaneous full improvement over a short period of time: Mild stroke
2. Patients who will improve steadily and may or may not return to premorbid function: Moderate stroke or traumatic brain injury
3. Patients who will not improve greatly and can expect a residual level of disability, but some progress is possible: Severe stroke or traumatic brain injury
4. Patients who will deteriorate slowly over time: Multiple sclerosis or Parkinson's disease
5. Patients who will unfortunately progress steadily and rapidly: Motor neuron disease or malignant glioma

BOX 4 Prognostic variables that influence the survival, recovery, and ultimate outcome of an individual.

Prognostic variables:
- *Patient related*: Demographic variables and medical comorbidities
- *Lesion related*: Pathology, site and size of lesion, impairment characteristics, and coma at onset
- *Therapeutic interventions related*: Nature, timing and intensity of therapy, and psychosocial variables—premorbid personality, socioeconomic status, and role of family

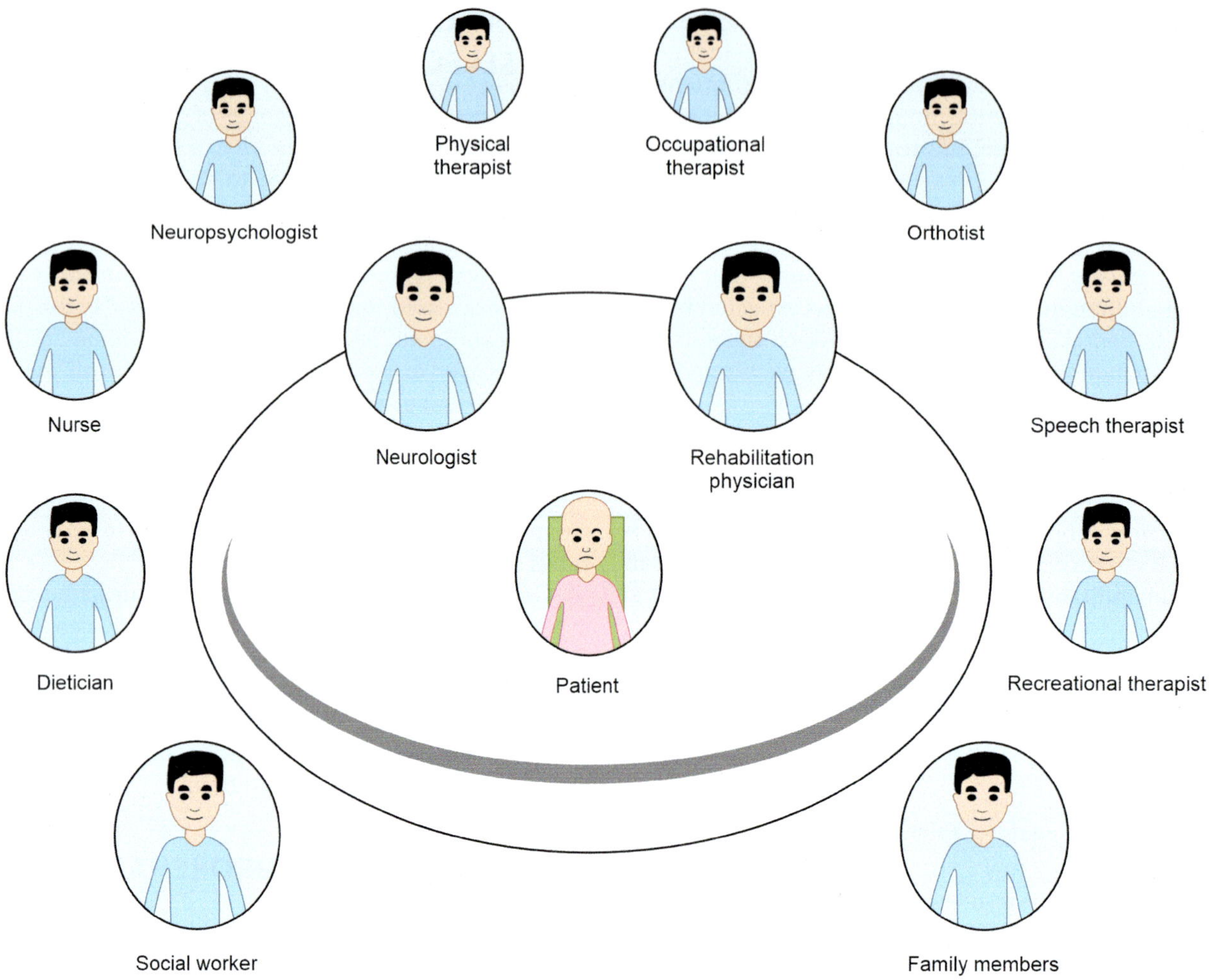

FIG. 1: Multidisciplinary team in patient-centered neurorehabilitation approach.

BOX 5 Features that define a rehabilitation team.

Features of rehabilitation team:
1. Shared commitment, a psychological attachment to the team
2. Shared team identity, the understanding of and meaning given to the team by other (external) healthcare professionals (and, presumably, the public and people in other organizations)
3. Shared and explicit team goals, giving the team a clear purpose
4. Agreed roles and responsibilities, delineating the unique and the shared areas of authority within the team
5. Interdependence between team members, both when making decisions and when undertaking actions
6. Integration of work, with team members focusing upon the team's goals generally and specifically

six features that define a rehabilitation service team are summarized in **Box 5**.

The three types of neurorehabilitation service delivery team models are:
1. *Multidisciplinary*: Work undertaken with other disciplines in parallel or sequentially.
2. *Interdisciplinary*: Work undertaken jointly with other disciplines.
3. *Transdisciplinary*: Work integrated across many disciplines, and undertaken collaboratively.

LEVELS OF REHABILITATION FROM HOSPITAL TO HOME

Rehabilitation is not a distinctly separate phase of care, beginning after acute medical intervention. Rather, it is an integral part of medical management and continues longitudinally through acute care, postacute care, and community reintegration. The rehabilitation program may be offered in different settings, such as in intensive care or high-dependency unit, an acute inpatient rehabilitation unit, a subacute rehabilitation inpatient unit, home care, or an outpatient center.

The acute rehabilitation setting is appropriate for those patients who meet the admission criteria and are able to tolerate 3 hours or more of active therapy per day. An acute setting is preferred if the patient requires close medical

BOX 6 Criteria for admission to a comprehensive acute inpatient rehabilitation program.

- Stable neurologic status
- Significant persisting neurologic deficit
- Identified disability affecting at least two of the following: Mobility, self-care activities, communication, swallowing, bowel or bladder control
- Adequate cognitive function to learn
- Sufficient communicative ability to engage with the therapist
- Reasonable physical ability and endurance to tolerate the active program
- Achievable therapeutic goals

and nursing monitoring of the medical status. Criteria for admission to a comprehensive acute inpatient rehabilitation program are summarized in **Box 6**.

If the patient's medical status is stable, but the patient is unable to tolerate more than 1 hour of therapy a day, a subacute rehabilitation setting is more appropriate. Other patients who require only minor degrees of assistance in self-care and mobility would be suitable for outpatient therapy or a home care program.

In developing countries, where the expertise is concentrated in urban areas, it becomes difficult on part of the patient and the family to sustain rehabilitation. Family-based rehabilitation helps to bridge the gap and support the patient with the necessary rehabilitation program. The practice of staying in a joint family reduces the caregiver burden and stress on a single person as multiple people help in rehabilitating the patient. The caregiver and providers in the family should be educated and counseled to provide physical, social, and economic support to the patient. The training of multiple family members in a family to provide rehabilitation reduces the fatigue to the caregiver. Family-based rehabilitation also reduces travel time and costs with improved economic viability.

NEUROREHABILITATION IN SPECIFIC NEUROLOGICAL DISORDERS

Stroke

The advances in the revascularization in stroke have evolved manifold and provide an opportunity to reverse the neurological deficit when performed in the window period. However, a significant proportion of up to two-thirds of patients have neurological deficits due to failed revascularization or are ineligible for revascularization including clinical presentation beyond the window period. Neurorehabilitation plays a critical role in the management of these stroke patients. The clinical improvement in stroke is mediated by restoration and compensation. These are executed by augmenting distant connectivity in the network and mapping the nearby areas (neural plasticity).[15]

The rehabilitation of motor, sensory, cognitive, speech, and swallowing is carried out by a multidisciplinary

BOX 7 Scales that are used in the measurement of clinical deficits in stroke patients.

Scales for measurement of clinical deficits in stroke patients:

- National Institute of Health Stroke Scale
- Barthel Index
- Modified Rankin Scale
- Fugl–Meyer Assessment
- Modified Ashworth Scale
- Berg Balance Scale
- Rivermead Mobility Index
- Frenchay Aphasia Screening Test
- Geriatric Depression Scale
- Medical Outcomes Study
- Montreal Cognitive Assessment

Source: https://ifnr.org/public/core/kar.php

team. The rehabilitation of patients with stroke should be formulated and tailored to the clinical deficit after assessment of the individual patient. The various scales that are useful in the assessment of clinical deficits in stroke patients are summarized in **Box 7**.

In motor rehabilitation, the use of passive and active stretches in limbs bilaterally may help to prime before the active training of the affected limbs. Strength training using resistive forces and electromyographic (EMG) biofeedback helps in the recovery of motor power. In constraint-induced movement therapy, patients who have partially preserved power are encouraged to use the affected limbs in conjunction with the restricted movements of the unaffected limbs. It improves motor power and reduces disability. The use of mirror box therapy is a useful therapeutic addition in the management of patients with severe arm paresis. Neuromuscular electrical stimulation of the nerves and muscles improves motor strength. The various forms of neuromuscular electrical stimulation include cyclical, EMG-triggered, contralateral limb movement-triggered, and functional electrical stimulation.[15-17]

The rehabilitation of sensory deficits improves sensory perception and aids in motor recovery. It is based on the sensory stimulation approach and sensory retraining approach. The sensory stimulation approach includes thermal stimulation using hot and cold packs, proprioceptive neuromuscular stimulation, peripheral magnetic stimulation, transcutaneous electrical stimulation, and intermittent pneumatic compression, which are effective in the clinical improvement of sensory deficits. The graded use of sensory restoration and mirror box therapy is based on the sensory restoration approach.[15-17]

Cognitive assessment of a patient following stroke is required for cognitive rehabilitation. Language deficit is common in patients with stroke affecting the dominant hemisphere. Cognitive rehabilitation of deficits is very essential for the recovery of the deficits and has been discussed under cognitive rehabilitation.[15-17]

Dysarthria, seen in half of the stroke patients, results from the paresis of the speech apparatus. Dysphagia that may occur in stroke patients produces significant morbidity by increasing the risk of aspiration. Patients with stroke should be assessed for swallowing dysfunction using a bedside swallowing test and should be initiated on oral feeds only after ensuring proper swallowing function.[15-17]

Traumatic Brain Injury

Traumatic brain injury (TBI) is an important cause of morbidity and mortality and is mostly caused by vehicle accidents. The importance of early rehabilitation has been emphasized to reduce hospital and ICU stay and reduce the incidence of complications including contractures, breakdown of skin, bladder and bowel dysfunction, sleep disturbances, and improved function. Patients with shorter post-traumatic amnesia (PTA) (<2 months), shorter duration of coma (<2 weeks), and high Glasgow Coma Scale (GCS) are associated with a favorable outcome. PTA more than 3 months, coma more than 3 months, low GCS, older age, presence of lesions in the brainstem in magnetic resonance imaging (MRI) brain, intracranial bleed, and midline shift in computed tomography (CT) brain are associated with poor outcome.[18]

In patients with severe limitation of function, passive movements and electrical stimulations are performed. In other patients, early rehabilitation is initiated carefully under monitoring and supervision with transfer to a chair, assisted performance of ADLs, and initiation of ambulation. In patients with disorders of consciousness **(Table 2)**, passive movement, stretching, and splinting play a major role. The use of neuromodulation, and stimulation of the thalamus, reticular formation in the midbrain may improve arousal. Recovery strategies are useful in the cognitive rehabilitation of patients—attention training, language therapy, internal and external compensatory strategies for memory, and training of metacognitive strategies. The goal of motor recovery includes augmenting endurance and strength and improving balance and walking which requires the active participation of the patient. The underlying principle to improve functional recovery includes performing task-oriented and repeated practice-based therapy. The use of task-specific constraint-induced movement therapy in which the patient performs specific tasks using the affected limb improves motor recovery. The compensatory strategies may require the use of assistive devices for the mobility of the patient. These include wheelchairs, walking aid, bracing, shower chair, and orthotics.

TABLE 2: Disorders of consciousness.

Disorder of consciousness	Definition
Coma	The state in which the patient is profoundly unaware and is unarousable
Unresponsive wakefulness syndrome	The state in which patient exhibits wakefulness but is unaware without any intentional behaviors
Minimally conscious state	The state in which the patient exhibits behaviors mediated cortically to external stimuli. It is not possible to establish functional communication. However, some patients may establish communication (MCS plus) and some may not show language processing behavior (MCS minus)
Conditions mimicking disorders of consciousness	
Locked-in syndrome	Patient is tetraplegic, anarthric, but can communicate through partially preserved communication
Functional locked syndrome	In these patients, the patient does not follow commands clinically. However, the corresponding brain activity may be elicited using fMRI/EEG

(fMRI: functional magnetic resonance imaging; EEG: electroencephalography)

Paroxysmal sympathetic hyperactivity, an important complication in severe traumatic injury, is characterized by tachycardia, tachypnea, increased blood pressure, increased sweating, temperature, and posturing of the limbs. It is necessary to minimize stimulation in these patients and provide supportive care. Heterotopic ossification, extraskeletal soft tissue lamellar bone formation, most commonly occurs in shoulders, elbows, and hips. It causes pain, swelling, redness, increasing spasticity, and triggers dysautonomia. Its formation is prevented by preventing trauma, improving the range of motion, reducing tone and muscle stretching.[18]

Spinal Cord Injury

The goals of rehabilitating a patient with spinal cord injury are improving quality of life (QoL) through creating independence in the ADLs and reinstating the patient at the community level. The strategies are restorative or compensatory. In the acute phase, the patient is assumed an upright posture using tilt table to encourage weight bearing and improve vascular tolerance, increasing mobility in the bed, passive stretching, and transferring the patient to the chair.[19]

Physical therapy for gait training can be performed using bodyweight-supported treadmill or robotics. Strength training for lower limbs muscles is performed using bicycles that are equipped with electrical stimulation. Occupational therapy focuses on achieving independence functionally in performing the ADLs, and providing the necessary modifications required in the home of the patient such as wheelchairs, ramps, shower chairs, and others. Bladder dysfunction begins with detrusor areflexia which sets in after 6–8 weeks. The treatment options depending on the phase of bladder dysfunction include indwelling catheter, clean intermittent catheterization, clean intermittent self-catheterization, and sacral neuromodulation. Other invasive strategies include augmented cystoplasty, dorsal rhizotomy, and sacral anterior root stimulation. Bowel dysfunction is a near universal complication. It is managed using digital stimulation, rectal evacuation, high-fiber diet, and drug therapy. Pain is a limiting clinical symptom in patients with spinal cord injury. It may be musculoskeletal pain, visceral pain, and neuropathic pain (segmental and diffuse pain). The treatment options include choosing the right pharmacotherapy or surgical options. Speech, language, and respiratory therapy focuses on improving the voice, reducing secretions and its clearance, resistance training of expiratory muscles, and use of assistive devices in communication.[19,20]

Rehabilitation in Parkinson's Disease

Rehabilitative strategies for Parkinson's disease and atypical parkinsonism are shown to improve motor and nonmotor symptoms. Multidisciplinary rehabilitation of Parkinson's disease is required to produce multidimensional improvement. The use of conventional physical training using active and passive interventions is shown to improve motor outcome, mobility, and balance. Aerobic training using cycling performed for 8 weeks at a low intensity is shown to improve Unified Parkinson's Disease Rating Scale (UPDRS) score. Strength and resistance training of upper limbs, lower limbs, and core improves strength, endurance, and motor symptoms. It is also beneficial in the improvement of cognitive scores. The impairment in gait produces a significant limitation in the ADLs. Gait training in Parkinson's disease using a treadmill is shown to improve gait metrics such as gait speed and stride length. After initial training and ensuring safety, a patient may continue to train independently under supervision.

Rehabilitation of nonmotor symptoms of Parkinson's disease is an essential component. Cue-based rehabilitation using visual cues (treadmill with transverse stripes), auditory cues (rhythmic auditory stimulation), or proprioceptive cues (vibrating wristband) can be delivered in an open loop (cues delivered in a predetermined manner) or closed loop (patient receives performance feedback that aids in improving response) that improves gait parameters. Speech disturbance in Parkinson's disease is difficult to treat using dopamine therapies. The use of Lee Silverman Voice Treatment - LOUD produces sustained improvement in speech parameters. The aquatic environment in hydrotherapy provides a safe environment for balance training and shows an improved balance score when compared to land-based aerobic rehabilitation. Occupational therapy helps the patient to adapt to the increasing demands in performing self-care activities, ADLs, mobility, safe home environment, and improving balance. Recent evidence has been emerging in the use of Yoga, dance, music singing, and martial arts (Tai-chi), exergaming in the rehabilitation of Parkinson's disease patients.[21,22]

Rehabilitation in Multiple Sclerosis

Despite the vast and fast-paced advances in treatment of multiple sclerosis (MS), a significant proportion of patients suffer disabilities affecting multiple neuroaxis requiring rehabilitation. A multidisciplinary team is required to address the various deficits that occur in MS. The rehabilitation improves neuroplasticity and offers neuroprotective effect. The rehabilitation of upper limb includes repetitive actions in the real or the virtual world, robotic rehabilitation for motor relearning, and constraint-induced movement therapy. The gait training and balance rehabilitation including aerobic physical exercise, robotic gait training, rhythmic auditory stimulation, exergaming, noninvasive brain stimulation, and task-oriented circuit training are shown to improve gait metrics. Aerobic training in hydrotherapy or on land helps to improve balance. Spasticity is disabling for the patient and significantly interferes with care and therapy. The management of spasticity is discussed in the following section. The aerobic personally tailored training program, aquatic training, is shown to improve fatigue in MS, which is a disabling symptom. Fatigue in MS is a disabling symptom. It includes cognitive and physical fatigue. Physical fatigue results from spasticity, ataxia, depression, and sleep disturbances. It is rehabilitated by a multidisciplinary team through exercise programs, counseling, and pharmacotherapy.[23]

DEFICIT-SPECIFIC REHABILITATION

Motor Rehabilitation

The rehabilitation of upper limbs deficit has been summarized under the section motor rehabilitation following stroke. The goal of gait rehabilitation is to restore gait in patients who are bedridden or have impaired gait. This can be established by performing repetitive gait cycles. A few hundred gait cycles are performed by the therapist with or without the assistance of exoskeleton. Patients with gait deficits who are ambulatory with or without support are trained on treadmill or the ground. Treadmill training is preferred in patients who require bodyweight support or specific targeted training such as endurance or speed training. Treadmill training with or without bodyweight support offers a subtle additional advantage over conventional physiotherapy approaches in improving gait parameters after stroke.[24]

Group therapy increases motivation and improves gait speed and distance. The use of functional electrical stimulation and virtual reality (VR) combined with treadmill training improves gait speed, endurance, and other metrics. It is feasible to conduct locomotor training programs for chronic stroke survivors with moderate disabilities. Improvements in ambulation provide the chronic stroke survivor with the opportunities to participate in the community and reduced burden on caregivers. Ankle foot orthoses are useful in the gait training of patients with foot drop.[17,25]

Spasticity may develop a few days or weeks following an insult to the upper motor neuron lesion. The spasticity may

TABLE 3: Management of spasticity.

Spasticity management	Drug/intervention
Nonpharmacological	• Stretching • Serial casting • Thermal stimulation • Electrical stimulation • Myogenic pressure • Biofeedback
Pharmacological—systemic	• Oral/intrathecal baclofen • Benzodiazepine • Tizanidine • Tolperisone • Dantrolene • Clonidine • Gabapentin • Nabilone
Pharmacological—locally injected	• Botulinum toxin injection • Phenol injection

TABLE 4: Treatment options for dysphagia.

Strategy		Intervention
Behavioral	Compensatory	• Adjustments of posture • Modification of diet • Modification of eating habits • Training the attender for Heimlich maneuver and swallow maneuver • Hygiene of the oral cavity
	Rehabilitative	• Strengthening of tongue and oropharyngeal musculature • Exercise for range of motion • Thermal stimulation • Neuromuscular electrical stimulation (Vital stim)
Medical and surgical treatment		• Cricopharyngeal botulinum toxin injection or myotomy or upper esophageal sphincter dilation • Percutaneous endoscopic gastrostomy

limit mobility, increase the risk of pressure sore, fracture, contracture, and heterotopic ossification, and interfere with the care of the patient. The tone of the muscle is assessed using Modified Ashworth Scale. Muscle charting for spasticity is useful in planning for the care of the patient and monitoring the response and progression. In a patient with acute worsening of spasticity infection, pain, deep vein thrombosis, and fracture should be considered.

The management of spasticity includes pharmacological (local and systemic) and nonpharmacological measures **(Table 3)**.[18]

Speech and Swallowing Rehabilitation

The speech training using phonatory, oromotor and respiratory exercises, Lee Silverman Voice Therapy, neuromodulation, constraint-induced dysarthria therapy improves poststroke dysarthria. Patients with swallowing dysfunction require evaluation by a swallowing therapist. Videofluoroscopy is the gold standard for instrumental evaluation of swallow to observe all three phases of swallowing. The treatment options for dysphagia include behavioral, medical, and surgical options. The behavioral options include compensatory and rehabilitative strategies **(Table 4)**.[16,17,26]

Cognitive and Behavioral Rehabilitation

Cognitive deficits can include problems in attention, concentration, memory, executive function, and hemineglect. The rare phenomenon of the persistent belief in the existence of an additional limb after a unilateral stroke is very unusual. When this phenomenon occurs in presence of a real limb, it is called a supernumerary phantom limb.[27]

In a patient with a language deficit following a neurological disorder, the screening test is performed and patients who test positive are evaluated formally using a Western aphasia battery or Boston diagnostic aphasia examination. The rehabilitative armamentarium in the management of language deficits includes constraint-induced aphasia therapy, augmentative communication, neurostimulation, articulatory cues, and repetitive phonemic practice. Cognitive training is useful in the improvement of attention and concentration. Memory deficits can be improved using compensatory or restorative strategies. Hemianopia is rehabilitated using visual restorative therapy or compensation using a normal visual field or prisms. Mirror therapy and galvanic stimulation of the vestibular nucleus are useful in the improvement of hemineglect.[16]

Poststroke mood disorders include depression, anxiety, and restlessness, which frequently affect participation in rehabilitation programs and lead to poor rehabilitation outcome. Depression was related primarily to demographic variables then to functional disability after stroke or lesion-related parameters.[28] Patients with neurological disorders requiring inpatient rehabilitation have impaired QoL that affects all domains of life. The social domain of QoL adversely affected functional abilities, but the correlation between patient parameters and functional abilities was insignificant.[29]

Visual Rehabilitation

The homonymous visual field deficit, which results from retrochiasmal lesion, recovers in the first few months and the recovery is insignificant beyond this period. The rehabilitation of visual field involves:[30]

- *Restorative approach*: The damaged neurons are reorganized with reformation of synapses by repeated training and focus on the recovery of lost vision using visual restoration therapy.
- *Compensatory approach*: The field defect is compensated using the normal visual field. This is achieved by visual search tasks or multisensory stimulation where the patient is trained to compensate using saccades directed toward the defective field.
- *Substitution therapy*: The environmental percept in the defective field is realigned to the intact visual field of the patient. This is achieved using optical prisms.

Vestibular and Balance Rehabilitation

Vestibular rehabilitation therapy is indicated in patients with stable vestibular deficits, psychogenic dizziness, central vertigo, mixed vertigo, elderly with dizziness, dizziness of uncertain etiology, and residual dizziness following repositioning maneuvers in benign paroxysmal positional vertigo (BPPV). It is not useful in episodic vertigo such as Ménière's disease. The components for vestibular rehabilitation therapy include exercises to enhance the stability of the gaze and posture, movements of the eye, ADLs, and exercises to reduce vertigo.

The use of balance and coordination training in the rehabilitation of ataxia patients is aimed at improving the QoL. Physical therapy should be initiated early in patients with ataxia. It reduces ataxia and improves motor performance. The balance exercises include static balance, dynamic balance, steps to prevent falling, and strategies to reduce injury while falling. The evidence in favor of physical exercise in ataxia has been demonstrated consistently. Balance training by force platform and visual feedback (FPVF) technique significantly improves balance and functional outcomes even in the chronic phase after stroke.[31]

The use of VR-based treadmill training and exergaming has also demonstrated benefits in patients with ataxia. However, further evidence is required to substantiate the finding.[32]

Bladder and Bowel Rehabilitation

Lower urinary tract dysfunction is commonly encountered in neurological disorders. Urodynamic study (UDS) is a useful tool to assess and manage the bladder following neurological diseases with urinary incontinence.[33]

The aim of management is continence, preventing upper urinary tract dysfunction and UTI and improving the QoL. The management of bladder dysfunction depends on the presence of voiding dysfunction or storage dysfunction. In patients with voiding dysfunction, the treatment options include intermittent or indwelling catheterization, botulinum toxin injection in external urethral sphincter, and sacral neuromodulation. In storage dysfunction, the options include behavioral therapy, pharmacotherapy, tibial neuromodulation, botulinum injection into detrusor muscle, sacral neuromodulation, and bladder augmentation surgery.[34]

The management of bowel dysfunction depends on if the patient has constipation or incontinence. The strategies include conservative strategies and alternative strategies. The conservative strategies include dietary modification, laxatives, abdominal massage in the clockwise direction, predetermined and planned evacuation of the bowel, suppositories, microenemas, and digital evacuation. The alternative strategies include biofeedback, anal plugs, transanal irrigation of colon, anterograde continence enema, percutaneous endoscopic colostomy, sacral anterior root stimulation, and surgical options (colostomy).[35]

ADVANCES IN NEUROREHABILITATION

The advances in neurorehabilitation have seen transformations that have augmented the clinical recovery of patients.

Pharmacotherapy in Neurorehabilitation

The role of pharmacotherapy in rehabilitation is useful in enhancing the recovery of clinical deficits. The European Academy of Neurology has recommended the use of cerebrolysin for motor recovery in the rehabilitation of moderate-to-severe stroke patients with National Institutes of Health Stroke Scale (NIHSS) ≥8. The use of piracetam may play a role in language recovery. However, the long-term sustained effect needs to be studied. Escitalopram may enhance memory and cognitive functioning beyond the antidepressant function. Rivastigmine as an add-on to rehabilitative strategies of hemineglect may aid in the recovery. Dopaminergic agents such as amantadine, levodopa, bromocriptine, and methylphenidate may improve cognitive recovery in TBI patients. GABAergic drugs such as zolpidem and baclofen may paradoxically improve arousal. Methylphenidate and cholinergic agonists (donepezil) improve attention and concentration and working memory respectively in patients with TBI **(Table 5)**.[15,36]

Neuromodulation

The neuromodulation techniques function by restoring the hemispheric imbalance created by lesion to a cortex that causes hypofunctioning of the lesioned cortex and hyperfunctioning of the contralesional cortex. It is mediated by altering the excitability of the cortex and improving neural plasticity. The neuromodulation can be performed by the use of magnetic stimulation [transcranial magnetic stimulation (TMS)], electrical stimulation [transcranial direct current stimulation (tDCS)], and central stimulation using rTMS in association with peripheral stimulation with an interstimulus interval. The use of neuromodulation is useful in the rehabilitation of motor and language deficits.[37]

TABLE 5: Benefits of pharmacotherapy in the neurorehabilitation.

Drug	Benefit
Cerebrolysin	Motor recovery in the rehabilitation of moderate-to-severe stroke
Piracetam	Language recovery
Levodopa	Motor recovery
Fluoxetine	Motor recovery
Escitalopram	Memory and cognitive functioning
Rivastigmine	Improves hemineglect
Dopaminergic agents (amantadine, levodopa, and bromocriptine)	Cognitive recovery
Methylphenidate	Cognitive recovery, attention, and concentration
Cholinergic agonist (donepezil)	Working memory

Robotics in Rehabilitation

Robotics has revolutionized the field of neurorehabilitation and has aided immensely in the management of patients in the current cyber age. The robot-assisted training is useful in performing repetitive actions in patients with severe paresis of arms and legs. It can be used to perform high doses of repetitive movements for up to 2 hours a day, 5 days a week, and up to 6 weeks. The use of robotic-assisted rehabilitation in the acute and subacute phases of stroke helps in the recovery of motor deficit and improves motor power. The use of multimodal rehabilitation such as VR with robotics can augment patient participation and hence recovery.[17]

The use of robotics in upper limb rehabilitation following stroke is beneficial, supported by moderate-quality evidence. However, further systematic analysis is required. The rehabilitation of lower limb deficit using robotics improves motor function, gait, and improves the ADL.[38,39]

Virtual Reality

The use of VR-based interventions using head-mounted displays has emerged providing experiences that are realistic, captivating, and motivating. The use of VR is useful to simulate a therapist in the virtual world motivating the patient to repeat the movement. The patient's limb movement can be tracked and hence can also be progressively monitored. The patient can also be provided with the feedback on his movement which is of utmost importance in providing clinical improvement. The augmentation of the motor activity directed toward a goal by the patient in the virtual world works akin to a mirror box therapy in improving neuroplasticity. It has also been evaluated in balance and postural control, lower limb gait training. VR as an adjuvant to conventional rehabilitation increases the overall time spent in therapy and improves the function of the upper limb and ADL. The research has also shown the modality to be relatively safe and no serious adverse events have been reported.[21,40]

Artificial Intelligence

The use of artificial intelligence (AI) has pervaded into all walks of life and neurorehabilitation. The types of machine learning are supervised learning, unsupervised learning, and reinforcement learning. Deep learning is a subset of machine learning with an input layer, hidden layers, and an output layer. The hidden layers provide weightage to the input layer that is required to provide the output. The use of AI has aided in the rehabilitation of various neurological domains. The use of AI therapists in robotic gait rehabilitation to provide verbal cues has been evaluated. The AI program receives information from the sensors loaded in the robotic exoskeleton. The verbal cues are incorporated into the AI program and data sets are provided for machine learning. The AI therapist was able to provide verbal cues like an experienced therapist in robotic gait rehabilitation.[15]

Brain–Computer Interface

It is useful in improving the disability of patients. The activity from the brain using EEG (slow cortical potentials, sensorimotor rhythms, P300 event-related potentials, steady state visual-evoked potential, and error-related negative evoked potential), fMRI (blood oxygenation levels), and near-infrared spectroscopy (changes in cerebral oxygenation) is fed into a computer interface where it is amplified, processed, decoded, and analyzed. In patients who have lost motor power and the ability to communicate, the decoded brain signal is useful to control a cursor to click on the commands or type a command on a screen. The use of decoded brain signal to control a prosthesis applied to the paralyzed arm can assist the patient in performing the ADLs and in the improved organization of the cortical network.[15]

Telerehabilitation

Telerehabilitation has emerged and become very active during the COVID-19 pandemic when social distancing was the norm.[41] Telerehabilitation is now widely used in the follow-up of patients from the comfort of their homes. It has resulted in improved patient compliance in rehabilitation due to ease of access. It also enables the availability of technical expertise in the rural areas.

The use of telerehabilitation has been used in the rehabilitation of Parkinson's disease to improve dynamic and static postural balance. The home-based telerehabilitation of upper limb provides clinical motor improvement that is comparable to the conventional training. The cognitive domains can be rehabilitated remotely using compensatory or restorative strategies. The telerehabilitation of MS patients is possible and results in improved motor outcomes.

The current pandemic implies the need for systematically developed tele-neurorehabilitation (TNR) interventions that are evaluated for their feasibility and acceptability and that is informed by available evidence from low- and middle-income countries. Given the lack of organized systems in place for the provision of neurorehabilitation services in general, there need to be sufficient budgetary allocations and a sector-wide approach to develop policies and systems for the provision of TNR services for persons with neurological disabilities.[42]

CONCLUSION

Rehabilitation of a patient with neurological deficit requires a multipronged approach with early initiation of therapy. An initial assessment of patient with individualized treatment tailored to the clinical deficits is of utmost importance. Prevention of secondary complications is essential in the rehabilitation of patient. Further, as the advancement in the techniques and evolution of equipment and robotics continue to expand, research with homogeneity of methodology is required in the field to establish the evidence.

REFERENCES

1. Johnson CO, Nguyen M, Roth GA, Nichols E, Alam T, Abate D, et al. Global, regional, and national burden of stroke, 1990–2016: a systematic analysis for the Global Burden of Disease Study 2016. Lancet Neurol. 2019;18(5):439-58.
2. Singh G, Sharma M, Kumar GA, Rao NG, Prasad K, Mathur P, et al. The burden of neurological disorders across the states of India: The Global Burden of Disease Study 1990–2019. Lancet Glob Health. 2021;9(8):e1129-44.
3. Mehndiratta MM, Aggarwal V. Neurological disorders in India: past, present, and next steps. Lancet Glob Health. 2021;9(8):e1043-4.
4. Barnes MP. Principles of neurological rehabilitation. J Neurol Neurosurg Psychiatry. 2003;74(suppl 4):iv3-7.
5. Brandstater ME. An overview of stroke rehabilitation. Stroke (1970). 1990;21(9):II-40.
6. Kotila M, Waltimo O, Niemi ML, Laaksonen RI, Lempinen M. The profile of recovery from stroke and factors influencing outcome. Stroke. 1984;15(6):1039-44.
7. Bach-y-Rita P. Recovery of function: Theoretical considerations for brain injury rehabilitation. Maryland: University Park Press;1980.
8. Bach-y-Rita P. Brain plasticity as a basis of the development of rehabilitation procedures for hemiplegia. Scand J Rehabil Med. 1981;13(2-3):73-83.
9. Kaplan MS. Plasticity after brain lesions: contemporary concepts. Arch Phys Med Rehab. 1988;69(11):984-91.
10. Illis LS. The effects of repetitive stimulation in recovery from damage to the central nervous system. Int Rehab Med. 1982;4(4):178-84.
11. Lehmann JF, DeLateur BJ, Fowler Jr RS, Warren CG, Arnhold R, Schertzer G, et al. Stroke: does rehabilitation affect outcome? Arch Phys Med Rehab. 1975;56(9):375-82.
12. Roth EJ. Medical rehabilitation of the stroke patient. Be stroke Smart. 1992;8:8.
13. Brandstater ME, Basmajian JV. Stroke Rehabilitation. Baltimore: Williams & Wilkins; 1987.
14. Brandstater ME. Prognostication in stroke rehabilitation. In: Chino N, Melvin JL (Eds). Functional evaluation of stroke patients. New York: Springer-Verlag; 1996. pp. 93-102.
15. Surya N, Srivastava A. Stroke rehabilitation. Reviews in Neurology, Stroke. New Delhi: Wolters Kluwer India (India) Pvt. Ltd.; 2019. pp. 295-310.
16. Platz T. Clinical pathways in stroke rehabilitation: Evidence-based clinical practice recommendations. Switzerland: Springer Nature; 2021.
17. Surya N, Someshwar H. (2020). Rehabilitation in Perceptual disorders in stroke patients. [online] Available from https://www.researchgate.net/publication/342338367_Rehabilitation_in_Perceptual_disorders_in_stroke_patients. [Last accessed February, 2023]
18. Iaccarino MA, Bhatnagar S, Zafonte R. Rehabilitation after traumatic brain injury. Handb Clin Neurol. 2015;127:411-22.
19. Mazwi NL, Adeletti K, Hirschberg RE. Traumatic spinal cord injury: recovery, rehabilitation, and prognosis. Current Trauma Reports. 2015;1(3):182-92.
20. Binder H. Traumatic spinal cord injury. Handb Clin Neurol. 2013;110:411-26.
21. Garcia-Agundez A, Folkerts AK, Konrad R, Caserman P, Tregel T, Goosses M, et al. Recent advances in rehabilitation for Parkinson's Disease with Exergames: A Systematic Review. J Neuroeng Rehabil. 2019;16(1):1-7.
22. Surya N, Srivastava A, Mohammed F, Someshwar H. Neuro-rehabilitation of movement disorders. In: Ranganathan LN (Ed). Reviews in Neurology 2020. New Delhi: Wolters Kluwer (India) Pvt Ltd.; 2020.
23. Surya N. Rehabilitation of multiple sclerosis patients in India. Ann Indian Acad Neurol. 2015;18(Suppl 1):S43.
24. Srivastava A, Taly AB, Gupta A, Murali T. Bodyweight supported treadmill training in chronic stroke survivors: A randomized control trial. Ann Phys Med Rehabil. 2016;59:234-41.
25. Srivastava A, Taly AB, Gupta A, Murali T. Rehabilitation interventions to improve locomotor outcome in chronic stroke survivors: A prospective, repeated measure study. Neurol India. 2015;63:347-52.
26. Barnes MP, Good DC. Neurological rehabilitation. Amsterdam: Elsevier; 2013.
27. Srivastava A, Taly AB, Gupta A, Noone ML, Murali T, Thirthahalli J, et al. Stroke with Supernumerary Phantom Limb: Case Study, Review of Literature and Pathogenesis. Acta Neuropsychiatrica. 2008;20:256-64.
28. Srivastava A, Taly AB, Gupta A, Murali T. Post-stroke depression: Prevalence and relationship with disability in chronic stroke survivors. Ann Indian Acad Neurol. 2010;13:123-7.
29. Gupta A, Taly AB, Srivastava A, Murali T. Quality of life & psychological problems in patients undergoing neurological rehabilitation at a tertiary center. Ann Indian Acad Neurol. 2008;11:225-30.
30. Dundon NM, Bertini C, Làdavas E, Sabel BA, Gall C. Visual rehabilitation: visual scanning, multisensory stimulation and vision restoration trainings. Front Behav Neurosci. 2015;9:192.
31. Srivastava A, Taly AB, Gupta A, Kumar S, Murali T. Post-stroke balance training: Role of force platform with visual feedback training. J Neurol Sci. 2009;287:89-93.
32. Chien HF, Zonta MB, Chen J, Diaferia G, Viana CF, Teive HA, et al. Rehabilitation in patients with cerebellar ataxias. Arq Neuropsiquiatr. 2022;80(3):306-15.

33. Gupta A, Taly AB, Srivastava A, Murali T. Urodynamics post-stroke in patients with urinary incontinence: Is there correlation between bladder type and site of lesion. Ann Indian Acad Neurol. 2009;12:104-7.
34. Panicker JN, De Sèze M, Fowler CJ. Neurogenic lower urinary tract dysfunction. Handb Clin Neurol. 2013;110:209-20.
35. Coggrave M, Norton C. Neurogenic bowel. Handb Clin Neurol. 2013;110:221-8.
36. Szelenberger R, Kostka J, Saluk-Bijak J, Miller E. Pharmacological interventions and rehabilitation approach for enhancing brain self-repair and stroke recovery. Curr Neuropharmacol. 2020;18(1): 51-64.
37. Hsu WY, Cheng CH, Liao KK, Lee IH, Lin YY. Effects of repetitive transcranial magnetic stimulation on motor functions in patients with stroke: a meta-analysis. Stroke. 2012;43(7):1849-57.
38. Pollock A, Farmer SE, Brady MC, Langhorne P, Mead GE, Mehrholz J, van Wijck F. Interventions for improving upper limb function after stroke. Cochrane Database Syst Rev. 2014;(11): CD010820.
39. Wu H, Gu XD, Fu JM, Yao YH, Li JH, Xu ZS. Effects of rehabilitation robot for lower-limb on motor function in hemiplegic patients after stroke. Zhonghua Yi Xue Za Zhi. 2012;92(37):2628-31.
40. Laver KE, Lange B, George S, Deutsch JE, Saposnik G, Crotty M. Virtual reality for stroke rehabilitation. Cochrane Database Syst Rev. 2017;(11):CD008349.
41. Surya N, Srivastava A, Nagda T, Palande D, Someshwar H. Education, training, and practices of neurorehabilitation in India during the COVID-19 pandemic. Front Neurol. 2021;12:626399.
42. Srivastava A, Swaminathan A, Chockalingam M, Srinivasan MK, Surya N, Ray P, et al. Tele-neurorehabilitation during the COVID-19 pandemic: Implications for practice in low- and middle-income countries. Front Neurol. 2021;12:667925.

126

CHAPTER

Neuropalliative Care

Rajinder K Dhamija, Roop Gursahani, Prafulla Shembalkar

INTRODUCTION

Palliative care (PC) is a modern and intersectional specialty that has evolved since its origin in the 1960s. Like intensive care and family medicine, its canvas is huge. It depends heavily on learnings from the social sciences, like public health. A significant evidence base has already emerged, especially for the management of physical symptoms. Since PC interventions tend to be complex, trial evidence is limited, especially for neuropalliative care (NpC). Multiple definitions of PC are available, which reflect its diverse priorities yet singular focus on disease-related suffering. PC's origins can be traced to two sources. The first, historical basis, was and is the pain and suffering endured by cancer patients at the end of life. The second, emerging basis, is the reorientation of medicine, away from paternalism to a patient-centered approach, more attuned to the needs of individuals with neurologic and other chronic nononcologic illnesses. Thus, PC is appropriate at all stages of serious illnesses and can be provided concurrently with curative or life-prolonging treatments. It can be provided in most care settings, e.g., home, hospitals, outpatient departments (OPDs), etc. Ideally, it should be provided by an interdisciplinary team to address different facets of the patient's care, i.e., physical by nurse or physician, psychologic by counselors or psychologists, spiritual by trained volunteers or chaplains, and social (including financial) by medical social workers **(Box 1)**.[1,2]

Neuropalliative care is the application of PC principles to the management of neurologic illness at all stages of life and disease. The cardinal principle is the relief of suffering in the patient and the ecosystem that she lives in: Family, significant others and the community. Total pain and suffering has four components: Physical, psychologic, social and spiritual. The PC process requires attention to multiple domains in addition to these four, such as structure of care and cultural aspects. This responsibility extends to the end of life and beyond, in the form of management of grief and bereavement. Communication is a foundational skill in PC and is needed for all aspects of management. Awareness of ethics and local legal constraints is essential since decision making is based on preference and has to be individualized. This differs from oncopalliative care, where cancer biology is the main driver of prognosis. Currently PC is largely rooted in oncology, but neurology is probably the specialty with the largest overall burden of PC needs. For neurologists in training and in practice, NpC requires a mental pivot that adds 'care' to 'cure' so that we can guide our patients through their entire journey from diagnosis to death and beyond.

BOX 1 Definitions[1,2] of palliative care, terminal illness, and end-of-life care.

- *Palliative care* (Indian Association of Palliative Care) is the active total care applicable from the time of diagnosis, aimed at improving the quality of life of patients and their families facing serious life-limiting illness, through the prevention and relief of suffering from pain and other physical symptoms as well as psychological, social, and spiritual distress through socially acceptable and affordable interventions
- *Terminal illness* is one from which recovery cannot be expected with the available treatment and death is considered to be unavoidable in the foreseeable future
- *End-of-life care* is an approach to a terminally ill patient that shifts the focus of care to symptom control, comfort, dignity, quality of life, and quality of dying rather than treatments aimed at cure or life prolongation

HISTORICAL BACKGROUND

Human rights, patient self-determination, and the end of life:[3] The patient–doctor relationship today is far different from what it was at the end of the 19th century. At that time, human equality was not given and medicine was no exception. The worst occurred in Germany, in the first half of the 20th century. The gas chambers were first used for involuntary active euthanasia for neurologically and psychiatrically disabled individuals. In the Nazi concentration camps, doctors set up ghastly human experiments that were meant to kill the subjects. The Nuremberg code on research with human subjects arose from this experience and this was hugely influential in aligning medicine with human rights. The Alma Ata declaration of the World Health Organization formally recognized universal healthcare as an absolute human right in 1979. Human equality and dignity are understood to be severely limited if everyone cannot access the same high standards of healthcare. By the 1960s, dramatic advances in medicine, especially in the advanced countries meant that many who would have died with severe illnesses, now recovered. But realizing that there will always be limits to medical technology, human rights campaigners began to highlight the rights of the dying to a peaceful death. The first living will, which limited medical care at the end of life, was released by a human rights lawyer in the late 1960s. These instruments became widespread in the USA through the 1970s and 1980s culminating in the Patient Self Determination Act passed by the US Congress in 1990. Subsequently, these Advance Medical Directives are widely used globally.[4,5] They were validated for use in India by the Supreme Court in 2018.

Palliative care began in the 1960s, thanks to one remarkable person. Cicely Saunders (1918–2005) can only be described as Gandhian in her thoughts and actions.[6] Starting her career as a nurse during World War II, she then trained as a social worker. During this period, she first encountered the painful sufferings of terminal cancer patients. She began to use morphine and systematized it by careful documentation. She then trained as a doctor because she was told that her work would not be respected if she remained a nurse! The first modern hospice for the dying, St Christopher's, started in 1967. This was followed by teaching and lecturing in the United States and Europe. The concept of total pain, where physical, psychosocial, and spiritual suffering merges and feeds into each other, is also her discovery. The Cicely Saunders Institute in London is the world leader in PC research. 50 years after she began work, the World Health Assembly in 2014 included PC as an essential human right.

Although Dame Cicely admitted and managed terminal amyotrophic lateral sclerosis (ALS) patients in her hospice soon after it started, PC remained largely limited to cancer. It was only in the early 2000s that neurologists in the USA began to appreciate that the PC approach had a lot to offer to neurology patients. Today, close to 200 American neurologists are doubly qualified in neurology and PC and NpC is fast becoming a recognized and shared subspecialty of Neurology and Palliative Medicine. The International Neuropalliative Care Society was formed in 2021.[7] Worldwide, neurologic disease is the second largest cause of mortality, but a study from Gadchiroli in rural Maharashtra showed that stroke was the leading cause of death there.[8] In any case, conditions that we manage are the leading causes of disability everywhere. These numbers make it obvious that neurology and PC are natural allies. In fact, when communities decide about PC needs, as in Malappuram in Kerala, dementia (19%) and stroke (17%) enrolments alone have already surpassed cancer (32%) **(Table 1)**.[9]

TABLE 1: Neurologic conditions for which palliative care is or may be applicable.

Chronic—adult	Chronic—pediatric	Acute
Dementia	Congenital malformations	Ischemic stroke
Parkinsonism	Perinatal brain injury	Intracranial hemorrhage
Motor neuron disease	Progressive neuromuscular disease	Severe encephalopathy or brain damage due to any cause
Stroke	Refractory epilepsy	Traumatic brain injury
Malignant brain tumors	Epileptic encephalopathy	Anoxic brain injury
	Metabolic brain disease	Quadriplegia: Any cause

PALLIATIVE CARE APPROACH: THE DOMAINS OF PC

As is obvious from the definition, PC has a very broad remit in its applications in disease, from diagnosis to death.[10] This is combined with a very sharp focus on relieving individual (hence the term person-centered) disease-related suffering. The primary aim is to identify what is most important to the patient and her family so that care is framed by their goals and preferences. For neurologists who choose to apply these principles and skills in their clinical work, the maxim is that cure and care must go together. And when a cure is not possible, care continues to be provided depending on patient needs, regardless of prognosis. Physician self-care too is part of the process and burnout is explicitly addressed **(Box 2)**.

Palliative care does this by addressing the needs of each patient under eight specific domains.[11] The focus may vary from patient to patient depending on the situation, but this helps in systematizing our work. The domains are as follows:

- *Structure and process of care*: PC management depends on making the best use of available resources. The following discussion is largely India specific:
    - *Care provider*: For neurologic patients, the first priority is to determine the care provider. This role evolves as the disease progresses. Initially, if the patient is reasonably independent and retains decision-making capacity, this will be a care partner (spouse, sibling, adult child, and significant other) who largely helps with support and logistics. With the decline in patient function, this role evolves into caregiver. The third role is that of paid caretaker and this may be occupied by a trained or untrained person. It is important to realize that the same

BOX 2 From a Guru of clinical neurology.

"The best test of a physician's suitability for the specialised practice of neurology is not his ability to memorise improbable syndromes but whether he can continue to support a case of motor neurone disease and keep the patient, his relatives and himself in a reasonably cheerful frame of mind."

—Professor WB Matthews, Practical Neurology, 1st Ed, 1963

caretaker may remain in that job for years, in which case they are often closer than their biological family.

- *Home care*: The terminal phase in neurology may stretch into years, unlike cancer where it is usually months. Thus, care has to be provided at home. The core member of the team is a nurse trained in PC. S/he may be joined by a nursing assistant ('compounder') and trained local community volunteers. Physicians provide supervision, focus on the medical treatment and prognosis, and formulate the care plan. In Kerala, this arrangement covers almost 60% of the population and is financed by community donations and panchayat/state government funds.[12] The Lancet Commission on Death and Dying[13] termed the Kerala system a "realistic utopia".
- *Hospital PC*: Teams are generally available in all cancer institutions but very few general hospitals have even a dedicated PC physician. Where available, they provide consultative services.
- *Primary and specialist PC*: Primary or generalist PC[14] is provided by neurologists who are trained in the basic principles of NpC and can (1) provide basic management of symptoms, depression, and anxiety; (2) discuss goals of care, prognosis, and advance care planning. Specialist PC manages refractory symptoms, complex psychologic issues, existential distress, issues of futility, and conflicts regarding goals/methods of treatment. It is led by physicians with training and qualifications in PC and is best provided by an interdisciplinary team.

- *Physical aspects of care*: The focus is on symptom management to improve functional status and quality of life (QoL). Validated tools are available for the assessment of symptoms and function but most of these were developed for oncology and are only now being adapted for neurology. IPOS-Neuro (available at *www.pos-pal.org*) has been developed for individuals with chronic neurologic conditions and focuses on symptoms and practical concerns. IPO-Dem[15] is meant for the systematic assessment of people with dementia and can be completed by family or unqualified staff. The distress thermometer[16] shows overall distress on a one-to-ten scale but has not been validated in nononcologic patients. One of these instruments can be filled out by the patient or caregiver at each clinic visit and helps the clinician to focus on the most relevant needs for that encounter. Evidence-based treatments are used as far as possible. Due process, as legislated for India, has to be followed for the use of controlled substances, i.e., opioids.
- *Psychologic and psychiatric aspects of care*: Regular screening is required for managing depression, anxiety, demoralization, and delirium.[17] Caregivers (and professional team members) need regular assessment for burnout, compassion fatigue, and moral distress.[18] It is important to have access to professionals who can handle these issues. Counselors who can handle these issues are being trained. It is important to remember that psychiatrists may not be oriented to handling end-of-life issues where counseling is more relevant than prescriptions. Disease-specific support groups are very valuable in this regard.[19,20] Members can provide emotional and moral support for each other because of their shared burdens and concerns. Information on coping strategies, available services, and experiences can be shared in a safe space and this builds community and enables advocacy. These groups can be either patient or professionally led (physician, social worker, etc.). Those impacted by uncommon diseases can connect online regardless of geographic separation and social media (WhatsApp) allows asynchronous participation. Participation has been shown to improve QoL by enhancing self-efficacy, empowerment, and adjustment and reducing anxiety and depression.
- *Social aspects of care*: A social history[21] includes ethnicity, marital status, children, occupation, and education. Tobacco, alcohol, and drugs also need to be included here as should other risks such as emotional health, seatbelt/helmet use, and exposure to violence (domestic or otherwise). Health-related behaviors, perceptions of and access to healthcare are also important (e.g., preference for alternative medicine, living in a rural area with no facilities, etc.). Social assessment allows the identification of family strengths and coping ability, availability of social support from relatives and community, and access to food, housing, and transportation. Ideally, a dedicated social worker or patient navigator helps with access to appointments, medications, nutrition, and other resources. However, all clinicians should be able to integrate awareness of social conditions into the care of seriously ill patients. This can easily be done in the usual neurologic clinic encounter and recorded with a simple genogram.
- *Spiritual, religious, and existential aspects*: Spirituality is distinct from religion and refers to the quest for meaning, purpose, and transcendence. It allows individuals to connect with family, community/society, and the sacred, and it is expressed in beliefs, values, and specific rites or practices. The simplest assessment is with a one-line question "Are you at peace?" (*"Aap ke man mein shanti hai kya?"*).[22] Sources of spiritual support and strength have to be identified and in neurology, this is usually a caregiver need. In the USA, secular chaplains provide this service, but this is nonexistent in India, partly because of

our misplaced confidence in our own spiritual traditions. As in psychology, this service too requires to be oriented to the needs of palliative and end-of-life care. Till then, this will have to be handled by the primary clinician with support from the clinical psychologist. One suggestion is to reach out to the local community to depute providers who are willing to be trained and can commit time.

- *Cultural aspects*: Patients and families have a right to identify cultural attributes that are important to them. This includes social class, ethnicity (caste/race), religion, and sexual identity (gender/orientation). The clinician needs to be aware that the biological family may not be the family of choice. Marginalized groups are typically unwilling to trust regular healthcare both because of poor health literacy as well as negative experiences such as disrespectful behavior. It is our responsibility to learn cultural humility and accept diversity.
- *End-of-life or terminal care* **(Box 1)**: In cancer, tumor biology determines the duration of the terminal phase. A patient spending >50% of his time in bed is unlikely to survive beyond 4 months. The duration of this transitional part of the terminal phase (preactive dying) in neurology depends both on prognosis and preference. In both neurology and oncology, intensive care can prolong the inevitable but much more so in neurology. A patient with motor neuron disease (MND) may choose to withdraw from or withhold ventilatory support. Feeding tubes and antibiotics may be withheld in dementia. Helping patients and families make these preference-based decisions is a key part of NpC. Transitioning to "comfort care" means that symptomatic management is prioritized. Common symptoms include pain, delirium, dyspnea, nausea–vomiting, constipation, urinary retention, gasping, death rattle, and seizures. All of these can be addressed, and it is important to anticipate them and keep medications handy. Status epilepticus is uncommon and can be managed with subcutaneous midazolam or phenobarbital. The onset of the dying process[23,24] can only be identified clinically, and the family needs to be prepared. Thus, for the clinician, knowledge of the dying process and the skill to communicate this information are both essential. Gasping is a prominent indicator of impending respiratory arrest. If death occurs at home, it is also important to designate a medical practitioner to confirm and certify death. It is good practice to reach out to the bereaved family and offer support if required for grief counseling **(Table 2)**.
- *Ethical and legal aspects*: The primary principles of ethical medical decision-making are universal and include autonomy (including substituted judgment), beneficence, nonmaleficence, and justice. Others that need to be considered include dignity, empathy/compassion, and honesty/fidelity/integrity. For clinical decision-making, if the institution has access, a clinical ethics consultation may be indicated.[25]

TABLE 2: Signs and symptoms of dying and the end of life.

Weeks to days before death	Days to hours before death
Active dying: • Delirium and increased drowsiness • Bedbound • Decreased oral intake • Reduced urine output (<4 discharges/day) • Incontinent • Hallucinations • Reduced or no communication/speech	*Imminent death*: • Deteriorating vital signs over hours • Sallow/pale, relaxed face with slack jaw • Cool/clammy, mottled extremities • Peripheral cyanosis • Cheyne–Stokes respiration • *Pooling of secretions*: "Death rattle" • *Mandibular movement*: Gasping

TABLE 3: Relevant issues and examples for application of Jonsen's four box model.

Medical indications: (Beneficence, nonmaleficence) *For example: PEG insertion in advanced leukodystrophy* • Medical problem • Goals of treatment • Possible outcomes and their probabilities	*Patient preference*: (Respect for autonomy) *For example: Respiratory support in a patient of ALS with features of frontal dementia* • Quality of information provided • Decision-making capacity • Appropriate surrogate decision maker
Quality of life: (Beneficence, nonmaleficence, autonomy) *For example: Decompressive hemicraniectomy in intracerebral hemorrhage* • Prognosis for recovery • Decision-making about acceptable QoL • Forgoing life-sustaining treatments	*Contextual features*: (Justice: Best interests decision-making) *For example: ICU admission for COVID infection in a nonverbal patient with dementia* • Who decides and why: conflicts of interest • Financial, legal, and public health issues • Resource allocation issues or triage

(ALS: amyotrophic lateral sclerosis; ICU: intensive care unit; PEG: percutaneous endoscopic gastrostomy; QoL: quality of life)

For the individual clinician, Jonsen's 4-box clinical model[26,27] combines the primary principles **(Table 3)** into four different relevant permutations. An alternate algorithmic approach has also been proposed[28] when patients and families request treatment that may be considered futile. Unlike ethics, legal considerations tend to be jurisdiction-specific and in India today we are in an evolving situation. Clinicians should be aware of the following medicolegal requirements in their area: surrogate hierarchy and possible roles of surrogate decision makers; advance care planning and valid advance medical directives; and requirements for death certification **(Table 3)**.

NEUROPALLIATIVE CARE SKILLS

As is obvious from the above, the PC approach goes far beyond traditional neurology with its limited focus on diagnosis and treatment.[29,30] Prognostication for instance takes on a far bigger role. But the real difference is in the way our didactic knowledge can be brought into full play by learning and deploying a panoply of soft skills, throughout the course of a patient's illness. This may seem intimidating for senior clinicians to unlearn and relearn. Residents and others, who are receptive, soon learn how to incorporate these techniques into routine practice. Unlike didactic knowledge, these qualities cannot be accessed from the internet and can never be replaced by artificial intelligence. Speaking personally, the authors feel that these attributes have sharply enhanced the joys and wonders of practicing neurology and medicine. They also seem to be a very effective burnout vaccine.

- Effective communication of prognosis (discussed in Chapter 129, Breaking Bad News: Communication Skills for Neurologists)
- *Navigate preference-sensitive decision making*: These are different from evidence-based decisions and will vary from patient to patient and condition to condition. Some examples are: (1) choosing between invasive and noninvasive ventilation or opting for only dyspnea management with opioids in MND; (2) clinically assisted nutrition and hydration (nasogastric or percutaneous endoscopic gastrotomy) versus hand feeding in advanced Parkinsonian syndromes and dementia; (3) antibiotic therapy for urosepsis in late-stage dementia; (4) intensive care versus comfort care for critical illnesses in any end-stage condition. These decisions are elaborated through goals of care discussions. Ideally, they should be recorded in advance medical directives (if made and communicated by the patient) or physician's orders for life-sustaining treatments (POLST) if made by either the patient or a surrogate. In India, the current POLST equivalent is the Do-Not-Attempt-Resuscitation (DNAR) form[31] released by the Indian Council of Medical Research. When communicating, DNAR is often replaced by the term AND (Allow Natural Death).
- *Manage shared decision-making*: It is unethical to take important decisions without patient concordance. To do this requires information that flows both ways.[32,33] The clinician must discuss options with benefits, uncertainties, and possible harms being clearly stated. The patient must tell their concerns and be prepared to be equal participants. Handling uncertainty is difficult on both sides, but transparency makes it possible. It is our responsibility to clarify the timeframe for taking decisions since most situations do not need immediate answers. Patients and families must be helped with access to resources that can help them to make decisions. It is too easy to blame them for googling their symptoms when we do not guide them to the correct literature (shared decision-making in neurocritical care will be covered in the Chapter 106 on Severe Acute Brain Injury).
- *Elicit total pain*: This is best addressed in an interdisciplinary clinic with a workflow that captures all aspects.[34] For instance, physical symptoms are substantially influenced by psychological distress. This in turn can be markedly affected by existential concerns and social difficulties. It is important to routinely elicit symptoms such as pain, sleep disturbance, sphincter control, constipation, nausea-vomiting, fatigue, and dyspnea. It is equally important to be aware that these can be influenced by psychosocial issues and existential concerns. Anxiety and depression must be assessed at each visit. A lead in question for social issues relates to difficulties with accessing healthcare (appointments, medication costs, etc.) and it is ideal to be able to refer to a social worker immediately. Existential issues (Why me? Why has God abandoned me?) are easy to miss in a busy clinic. These usually have to be addressed with compassion and presence, since patients also understand that their doctor does not have all the answers. Occasionally, a combination of existential and social (Who will take care of my family?) may need support from external agencies. The distress thermometer[16] is very useful for getting all relevant issues into one patient-filled document.
- *Administer end-of-life care*: Forgoing life support is the preferred term for withholding and withdrawal decisions since these are considered ethically and legally equivalent. This requires confirmation of medical futility or forecasts of how much neurologic recovery can be expected. The confirmation of brain death is often the responsibility of the neurology team. Once these situations are verified, due process requires careful documentation, the consensus within the treating team, and consent from the appropriate surrogate decision makers,[35] to proceed with palliative extubation or de-escalation with DNAR/AND orders. Palliative sedation refers to deep sedation to relieve intractable symptoms (e.g., severe dystonia,[36] pain unresponsive to opioids, etc.) with the acceptance that this may cause respiratory arrest.

THE ROADMAP MODEL OF NEUROPALLIATIVE CARE

Conceptual Models of Care

Traditional PC is rooted in oncology and hence follows the "Bow-tie" **(Fig. 1)** model,[37] where oncologic care dwindles and is replaced by supportive care which includes rehabilitation, PC, and bereavement support. This does not work for neurology, since diagnosis, management, and prognosis are intertwined and often uncertain and unclear throughout the course of the illness. A diagnosis of cancer

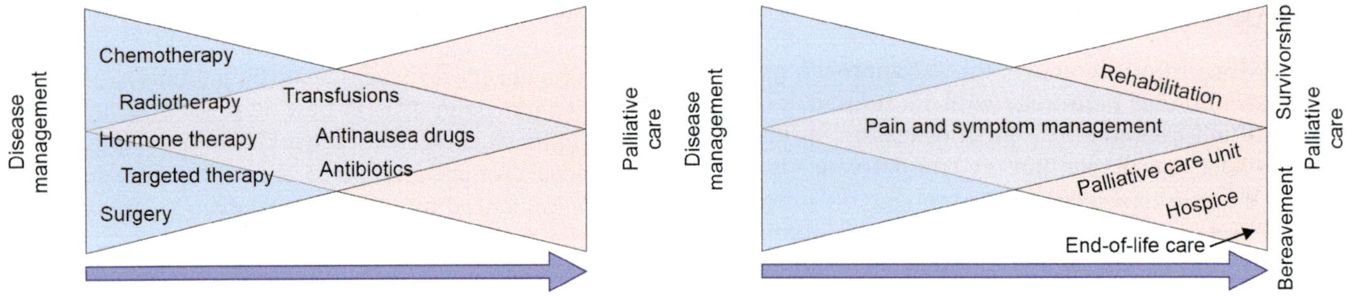

FIG. 1: Hawley's Bow-tie model of oncopalliative care.[35]

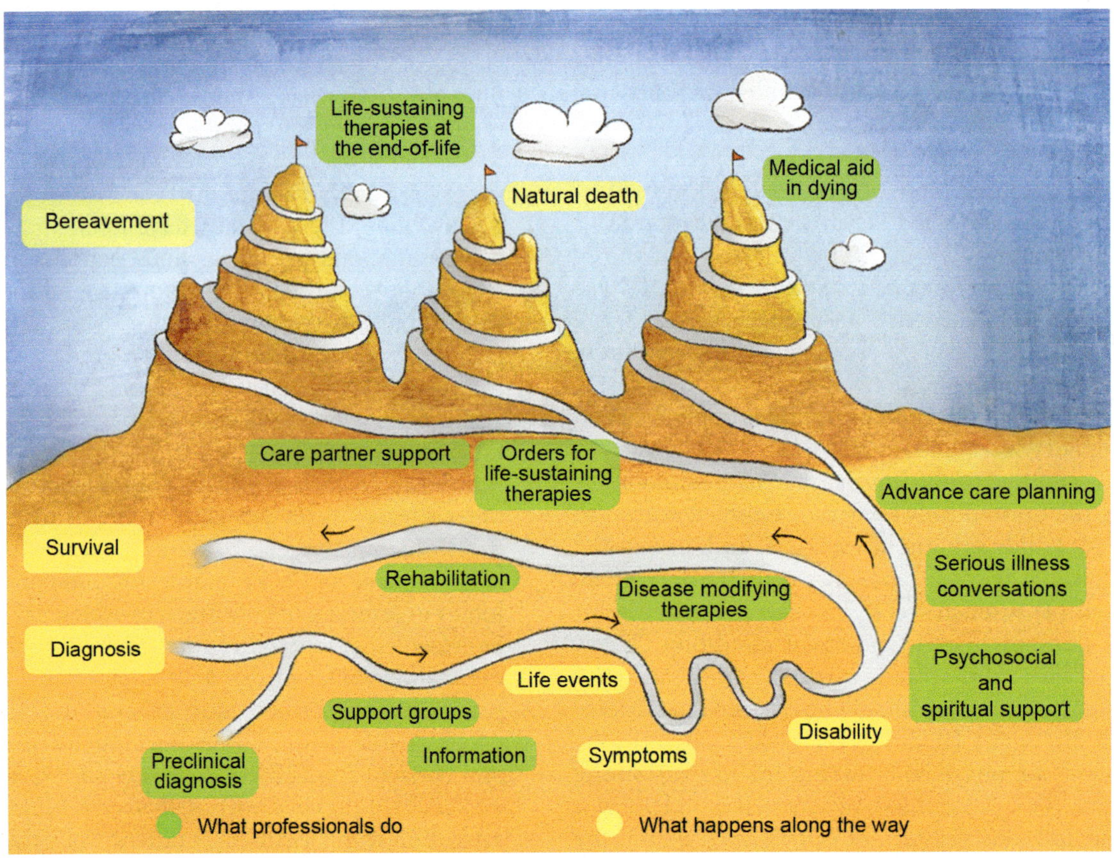

FIG. 2: The roadmap model of neuropalliative care.

Source: Gursahani R. Neuropalliative Care for India: Who, What, When, Where, Why, How. Natl Med J India. 2022;35:321-4.

simplifies communication requirements. Once cancer biology takes over, ethical and legal considerations also dwindle since there are only limited choices. This is not so in neurology and hence we prefer the roadmap model **(Fig. 2)**, which is based on narrative medicine.

Walking the Road with the Patient

Patients require support at diagnosis. Conveying a diagnosis such as Parkinsonism may seem simple to us since there are treatments available but for patients and families, it can be traumatic, and it has been described as a bombshell. Most practitioners understand the importance of giving a diagnosis of MND or glioblastoma but lacking the skills to do so with compassion leads to collusion with family to hide the diagnosis. This is unethical since this destroys the patient's autonomy. The correct information is a priority as is social support. Symptomatic management, disease-modifying treatments, life-prolonging interventions, and rehabilitation must all either proceed concurrently or must be looked at as integrated parts of a comprehensive plan. As the illness proceeds and the patient's condition deteriorates, communication skills take center stage. Serious illness conversations lead to goals of care discussions and advance care planning (see Chapter 129, Breaking Bad News: Communication Skills for Neurologists).

Caregiver Support

In neurologic illness, as the disease progresses, physical and cognitive decline increases the patient's dependence on the caregiver.[18] Eventually, this dependence is total, e.g., for feeding, cleaning, dressing, toileting, etc. This does not happen with cancer: decline to the point of total dependence if it occurs at all during the last few days or weeks of life. In chronic neurologic illness, this situation may last for years. As clinicians, we can only take care of the patient if we take care of the caregiver. The psychospiritual, physical, and financial burdens are substantial and must be explicitly recognized. Sleep deprivation and exhaustion are common and add to caregiver distress. Psychoeducational interventions have been used to improve coping. Simple things such as insisting on respite periods (when care is handed over to someone else) or preventive medical care (for the caregiver) or mindfulness therapy are all useful. At the very least, we must respect and recognize the caregiver explicitly and help them manage their own sense of loss.

End-of-life Pathways in Neurology

It is important to broach this topic with the patient (if possible) or family after asking their permission for this discussion. Three paths are possible and in the diagram, these are seen as flags on three separate peaks. (1) *Medical Aid in Dying* (MAiD), also termed Physician Assisted Suicide (PAS), is currently legal only in some jurisdictions in developed countries (Netherlands, Belgium, Canada, and some US states) and is clearly illegal in India. Traditional PC looks at patient requests for MAiD/PAS as a failure to provide adequate PC. But they see this from the perspective of oncopalliative care in which cancer biology does all the ethical decision-making. Our patients, faced with the loss of personhood, may see MAiD/PAS as an ultimate expression of human autonomy. This tension between the legal and the ethical needs to be settled by each country based on its capability to police and regulate this issue. Indian patients who can afford it currently access Dignitas in Switzerland. (2) *Natural death*: Till the 1960s, this was the default option everywhere but with increasing access to medical care, it needs to be selected from the menu. The final moments can be either at home or in the hospital and in most cases, it needs adequate palliation. If at home, certification must be arranged. (3) *Death on life support*: The ultimate expression is putting a clearly dying patient on a ventilator, as happened with Lata Mangeshkar. But life support treatment includes cardiopulmonary resuscitation, ventilation, extracorporeal membrane oxygenation, dialysis, clinically assisted nutrition and hydration (Ryle's tube and gastrostomy), intravenous fluids/antibiotics, and chemotherapy. Patients have a right to refuse any or all of these and doing so without consent is liable to legal action as per the Supreme Court judgment of 2018. In fact, in the US, most litigations related to the end of life are termed "Wrongful life" and are due to life support imposed in violation of clear advance directives.

PHYSICIAN SELF-CARE: BURNOUT, COMPASSION FATIGUE, AND MORAL DISTRESS

These are three interrelated issues that have been best studied in PC physicians and oncologists but are now recognized to be professional risks in all clinical specialties. We believe that neurologists with exposure and training in PC are better placed to understand, prevent, and mitigate these problems in themselves and their teams. Burnout is predominantly derived from stressors that arise within the work environment.[38] Compassion fatigue[39] is more specific to the doctor–patient relationship and is a form of traumatization that arises from exposure to the suffering of patients and families facing incurable illnesses. Moral distress[40] occurs when we know the ethically correct course of action but cannot follow it.

Burnout in neurologists has been recognized as a major problem in the USA.[38] It has three components: (1) emotional exhaustion: which results in cognitive and emotional distancing from one's work; (2) depersonalization (treating patients/families as objects, not individuals): this is usually the reason for callousness and negativity, manifesting as cynicism and desensitization; (3) lack of personal accomplishment: feeling ineffective and underachieving. This anhedonia (reduced ability to experience pleasure) is restricted to work only and thus differs from clinical depression. In one study, about 60% of practicing neurologists experience at least one symptom. This figure may be higher for overworked residents. Three types have been recognized: (1) frenetic (overinvested and hardworking), (2) underchallenged (indifferent perhaps because of insufficient challenge or meaning), and (3) worn-out (overwhelmed by work stress without emotional or other rewards). Burnout compromises patient care by making medical errors more likely. Maladaptive coping then leads to personal health and emotional consequences. It is a major factor in patient complaints and litigation, and it results in a reduction of healthcare system efficiency as senior and experienced clinicians withdraw from work.

Remedial measures have to be both organizational and personal. At the organizational level, resources should be available to ensure manageable schedules, work-life balance, and a conducive work environment. For US neurologists, the major issue seems to be the extensive documentation that is required by the electronic health record system. At the personal level, all of the followings have shown effectiveness but have not been studied comprehensively in neurologists: (1) communication skills training; (2) maintaining a high level of clinical competence; (3) updating oneself on current practice and guidelines; (4) availability of safe and nonjudgmental peer consultation; and (5) boundary setting, both personally and professionally. In addition, mindfulness and resilience are two learnable attributes that are often recommended. Mindfulness is a specific approach that teaches specific skills for observing sensations, thoughts, and feelings but with awareness and intention rather than emotion. It enhances the ability to focus on experience and learn from it. Resilience[41] refers to the ability to respond to crises with emotional and behavioral flexibility and to recover with minimal psychologic cost to oneself. This is particularly relevant at the level of residents who are just beginning to be exposed to the stress and demands of the workplace.

PALLIATIVE CARE CONSIDERATIONS IN SPECIFIC CATEGORIES

Dementia

Across dementia subtypes, it is important to recognize and to inform that this is a terminal disease, but the course stretches into years and occasionally decades. The trajectory of disease has been termed frailty, dementia, and even dwindling.[42] Priorities for PC interventions will change as the disease advances.[43] In early/mild dementia, it is important to nudge patients to complete both estate wills and advance care planning, especially nomination of substitute decision makers (healthcare proxy). Decision-making capacity is lost in moderate dementia and issues of safety such as falls, wandering, and abuse now arise. Behavioral and psychological symptoms lead to increasing caregiver distress.[44] It is important to screen for all of these during clinic visits. Dependence for basic activities of daily living marks the transition to severe dementia.[45,46] As communication is lost, it becomes important to prepare for swallowing dysfunction: feeding tubes are not recommended.[47] Pain assessment needs specific screening tools. As mobility gets limited, febrile episodes, pressure sores, dysphagia, and pneumonia become likely, and these identify 40–45% mortality in 6 months.[48] At this stage, PC has two specific responsibilities. One of these is deprescribing unnecessary medications, especially those that are effective only over prolonged periods (e.g., statins, antithrombotics, and vitamins) or those that have lost effect (anticholinesterases). The other is a discussion of goals of care with the family to avoid unnecessary hospitalization or intensive care unit (ICU) care at the end of life.

Parkinsonism and Related Disorders

Although mortality with Parkinson's disease and related disorders (PDRD) is higher than age-matched controls, most patients have many productive years with the disease. Yet most patients never forget the day when the diagnosis is delivered, and it is the clinician's responsibility to help them navigate the initial months and years.[49] There are significant information needs and support groups can be very helpful.[50] As disease advances, nonmotor symptoms significantly impact the QoL and must be monitored. Pain, psychosis, cognitive impairment, constipation, dysphagia, sialorrhea, and sleep disturbances all need to be systematically screened for and addressed with PD-specific screening tools. These issues may be significantly worse in patients with atypical PD syndromes.[51] Rivastigmine may be helpful for dementia and quetiapine and/or clozapine may be used for behavioral and psychiatric symptoms. Depression and demoralization are common and also affect the care partners who may also develop health problems. The terminal phase of the illness is marked by weight loss, rapid functional decline, and reducing medication benefit and must be explicitly recognized.[52,53] Whether or not to insert a feeding gastrostomy is a key issue in this phase and must be decided on an individual basis, unlike the clear recommendations in dementia and ALS.

Amyotrophic Lateral Sclerosis

The biggest palliative challenge for Indian neurologists is right in the beginning when the diagnosis has to be conveyed to the patient.[54] Doing so with compassion and clarity is a learnable skill (see Chapter 129, Breaking Bad News: Communication Skills for Neurologists) and is crucial in establishing trust. Indian patients are often younger and have a median survival duration of 9–10 years.[55] Older patients usually follow the terminal illness (also termed waterfall) trajectory. Therapeutic options (riluzole, edaravone, and "Relyvrio") have to be discussed and physical therapy[56-58] must be emphasized in the initial period. Range-of-motion and aerobic exercise are safe, but weight training requires supervision. Muscle symptoms such as cramps (quinine benzoate), spasticity (baclofen and tizanidine), and fasciculations (if bothersome: carbamazepine and phenytoin) can be treated pharmacologically. Hypersialorrhea and drooling may require anticholinergics (nortriptyline, local atropine eye drops) or even Botox or radiation of salivary glands. The pseudobulbar effect responds to antidepressants as well as a dextromethorphan–quinidine combination. In the terminal phase, early percutaneous endoscopic gastrostomy delays the need for ventilatory support.[59] Most patients choose noninvasive ventilation and dyspnea management with opioids for respiratory distress. Tracheostomy and invasive ventilation are more common when the patient has not been involved in the decision-making. A formal PC is essential for handling end-of-life issues, especially the withdrawal of ventilation.

Malignant Brain Tumors[60,61]

Wild-type isocitrate dehydrogenase glioblastoma is the most common primary malignant brain tumor and has a median survival of 12 months. Brain metastasis affects 20% of all systemic cancer and median survival ranges from 2 to 7 months. Seizures and headaches are common at diagnosis and at this stage, it is important to build trust and rapport. The information preferences and assimilative capacity of patients and caregivers must be assessed early since prognostic awareness is very common. Family and caregiver, if not the patient, must be made aware of the likelihood of loss of communication and cognition in the later stages. During the plateau phase after surgery and initial treatment, the key symptoms are iatrogenic—chemotherapy-related gastrointestinal distress and steroid toxicity. QoL is affected by neurologic deficits, behavioral symptoms, and existential distress. Urinary incontinence and gait impairment are key components of functional decline. Advance care planning conversations with the designation of surrogate/s should be initiated before decision-making capacity is lost. The end-of-life phase is dominated by seizures, delirium, and progressive swallowing impairment and a care plan for the dying process is essential. These are the only neurologic patients who are accepted in cancer hospices in India and early referral to specialist PC is recommended.

CONCLUSION

The past few decades have seen the flowering of PC globally. It now encompasses a comprehensive vision for high-quality person-centered care for all patients with life-limiting illnesses, from diagnosis to death. Neurologic patients are probably the largest single category for whom this service will be needed. Primary PC for neurologic illnesses will have to be provided by the neurologists caring for these patients. Ideally, a trained cadre of neuropalliative subspecialists will then provide specialist PC when needed.

REFERENCES

1. Indian Association of Palliative Care. What is Palliative Care? [online] Available from https://www.palliativecare.in. [Last accessed February, 2023]
2. Salins N, Gursahani R, Mathur R, Iyer S, Macaden S, Simha N, et al. Definition of terms used in limitation of treatment and providing palliative care at the end of life: The Indian Council of Medical Research Commission Report. Indian J Crit Care Med. 2018;22(4):249-62.
3. Gursahani R, Shembalkar P. What is neuropalliative care: making it work in India. Bombay Hosp J. 2021;63:213-7.
4. Lum HD, Sudore RL, Bekelman DB. Advance care planning in the elderly. Med Clin North Am. 2015;99(2):391-403.
5. Sabatino CP. The evolution of health care advance planning law and policy. Milbank Q. 2010;88(2):211-39.
6. Saunders C. The evolution of palliative care. J R Soc Med. 2001;94(9):430-2.
7. The Lancet Neurology. New hope for advancing neuropalliative care. Lancet Neurol. 2021;20(6):409.
8. Kalkonde Y, Deshmukh M, Kakarmath S, Puthran J, Agavane V, Sahane V, et al. A prospective study of causes of death in rural Gadchiroli, an underdeveloped district of India (2011-2013). J Glob Health Rep. 2019;3:e2019009.
9. Philip RR, Philip S, Tripathy JP, Manima A, Venables E. Twenty years of home-based palliative care in Malappuram, Kerala, India: a descriptive study of patients and their care-givers. BMC Palliat Care. 2018;17(1):26.
10. Simon J. Who needs palliative care? CMAJ. 2018;190(9):E234-5.
11. National Consensus Project for Quality Palliative Care. Clinical Practice Guidelines for Quality Palliative Care, 4th edition. Richmond, VA: National Coalition for Hospice and Palliative Care; 2018. [online] Available from https://www.nationalcoalitionhpc.org/wp-content/uploads/2020/07/NCHPC-NCPGuidelines_4thED_web_FINAL.pdf. [Last accessed February, 2023]
12. Azeez EPA, Anbuselvi G. Is the Kerala model of community-based palliative care operations sustainable? Evidence from the field. Indian J Palliat Care. 2021;27(1):18-22.
13. Sallnow L, Smith R, Ahmedzai SH, Bhadelia A, Chamberlain C, Cong Y, et al.; Lancet Commission on the Value of Death. Report of the Lancet Commission on the value of death: bringing death back into life. Lancet. 2022;399(10327):837-84.
14. Quill TE, Abernethy AP. Generalist plus specialist palliative care—creating a more sustainable model. N Engl J Med. 2013;368(13):1173-5.
15. Ellis-Smith C, Higginson IJ, Daveson BA, Henson LA, Evans CJ; BuildCARE. How can a measure improve assessment and management of symptoms and concerns for people with dementia in care homes? A mixed-methods feasibility and process evaluation of IPOS-Dem. PLoS One. 2018;13(7):e0200240.
16. Ownby KK. Use of the distress thermometer in clinical practice. J Adv Pract Oncol. 2019;10(2):175-9.
17. Brizzi K, Creutzfeldt CJ. Neuropalliative care: A practical guide for the neurologist. Semin Neurol. 2018;38(5):569-75.
18. Ransmayr G. Challenges of caregiving to neurological patients. Wien Med Wochenschr. 2021;171(11-12):282-8.
19. Bachmann P. Caregivers' experience of caring for a family member with Alzheimer's disease: A content analysis of longitudinal social media communication. Int J Environ Res Public Health. 2020;17(12):4412.
20. Soós MJ, Coulson NS, Davies EB. Exploring social support in an online support community for Tourette syndrome and Tic disorders: Analysis of postings. J Med Internet Res. 2022;24(10):e34403.
21. Behforouz HL, Drain PK, Rhatigan JJ. Rethinking the social history. N Engl J Med. 2014;371(14):1277-9.
22. Steinhauser KE, Voils CI, Clipp EC, Bosworth HB, Christakis NA, Tulsky JA. Are you at peace?: one item to probe spiritual concerns at the end of life. Arch Intern Med. 2006;166(1):101-5.
23. Iwashyna TJ. Recognizing a patient is acutely dying. Ann Am Thorac Soc. 2020;17(10):1195-8.
24. Shega J. (2021). What are the clinical signs of death? Vitas Healthcare. [online] Available from https://www.vitas.com/for-healthcare-professionals/making-the-rounds/2020/march/signs-of-active-dying. [Last accessed February, 2023]
25. Ilse B, Alt-Epping B, Günther A, Liman J, Simon A. Clinical ethics consultation in neurology—a case series. BMC Neurol. 2021;21(1):216.
26. Low JA, Ho E. Managing ethical dilemmas in end-stage neurodegenerative diseases. Geriatrics (Basel). 2017;2(1):8.
27. Cardenas D. Surgical ethics: a framework for surgeons, patients, and society. Rev Col Bras Cir. 2020;47:e20202519.
28. Winkler EC, Hiddemann W, Marckmann G. Evaluating a patient's request for life-prolonging treatment: an ethical framework. J Med Ethics. 2012;38(11):647-51.
29. Robinson MT, Holloway RG. Palliative care in neurology. Mayo Clin Proc. 2017;92(10):1592-601.
30. Sady ERR, Silva LMCJ, Veiga VC, Rojas SSO. Neuropalliative care: new perspectives of intensive care. Rev Bras Ter Intensiva. 2021;33(1):146-53.
31. Mathur R. ICMR Consensus Guidelines on 'Do Not Attempt Resuscitation'. Indian J Med Res. 2020;151(4):303-10.
32. Lapides DA. Shared decision-making in autoimmune neurology: making decisions in the face of uncertainty. Neurol Clin Pract. 2021;11(2):141-6.
33. Bernat JL, McQuillen MP. On shared decision-making and informed consent. Neurol Clin Pract. 2021;11(2):93-4.
34. Kluger BM, Persenaire MJ, Holden SK, Palmer LT, Redwine H, Berk J, et al. Implementation issues relevant to outpatient neurology palliative care. Ann Palliat Med. 2018;7(3):339-48.
35. Myatra SN, Salins N, Iyer S, Macaden SC, Divatia JV, Muckaden M, et al. End-of-life care policy: An integrated care plan for the dying:

A Joint Position Statement of the Indian Society of Critical Care Medicine (ISCCM) and the Indian Association of Palliative Care (IAPC). Indian J Crit Care Med. 2014;18(9):615-35.

36. Strand JJ, Feely MA, Kramer NM, Moeschler SM, Swetz KM. Palliative sedation and what constitutes active dying: A case of severe progressive dystonia and intractable pain. Am J Hosp Palliat Care. 2016;33(4):363-8.
37. Hawley PH. The bow tie model of 21st century palliative care. J Pain Symptom Manage. 2014;47(1):e2-5.
38. Busis NA, Shanafelt TD, Keran CM, Levin KH, Schwarz HB, Molano JR, et al. Burnout, career satisfaction, and well-being among US neurologists in 2016. Neurology. 2017;88(8):797-808.
39. Gallagher R. Compassion fatigue. Can Fam Physician. 2013;59(3):265-8.
40. Hildesheim H, Rogge A, Borzikowsky C, Witt VD, Schäffer E, Berg D. Moral distress among residents in neurology: a pilot study. Neurol Res Pract. 2021;3(1):6.
41. O'Dowd E, O'Connor P, Lydon S, Mongan O, Connolly F, Diskin C, et al. Stress, coping, and psychological resilience among physicians. BMC Health Serv Res. 2018;18(1):730.
42. Ballentine JM. (2018). The Five Trajectories: Supporting Patients during Serious Illness. [online] Available from https://csupalliativecare.org/wp-content/uploads/Five-Trajectories-eBook-02.21.2018.pdf. [Last accessed February, 2023]
43. van der Steen JT, Radbruch L, Hertogh CM, de Boer ME, Hughes JC, Larkin P, et al.; European Association for Palliative Care (EAPC). White paper defining optimal palliative care in older people with dementia: a Delphi study and recommendations from the European Association for Palliative Care. Palliat Med. 2014;28(3):197-209.
44. Harrison KL, Garrett SB, Halim M, Bernstein Sideman A, Allison TA, Dohan D, et al. "I Didn't Sign Up for This": Perspectives from Persons Living with Dementia and Care Partners on Challenges, Supports, and Opportunities to Add Geriatric Neuropalliative Care to Dementia Specialty Care. J Alzheimers Dis. 2022;90(3):1301-20.
45. Arcand M. End-of-life issues in advanced dementia: Part 1: goals of care, decision-making process, and family education. Can Fam Physician. 2015;61(4):330-4.
46. Arcand M. End-of-life issues in advanced dementia: Part 2: management of poor nutritional intake, dehydration, and pneumonia. Can Fam Physician. 2015;61(4):337-41.
47. Palecek EJ, Teno JM, Casarett DJ, Hanson LC, Rhodes RL, Mitchell SL. Comfort feeding only: a proposal to bring clarity to decision-making regarding difficulty with eating for persons with advanced dementia. J Am Geriatr Soc. 2010;58(3):580-4.
48. Mitchell SL, Teno JM, Kiely DK, Shaffer ML, Jones RN, Prigerson HG, et al. The clinical course of advanced dementia. N Engl J Med. 2009;361(16):1529-38.
49. Hall K, Sumrall M, Thelen G, Kluger BM; 2015 Parkinson's Disease Foundation sponsored "Palliative Care and Parkinson's Disease" Patient Advisory Council. Palliative care for Parkinson's disease: suggestions from a council of patient and carepartners. NPJ Parkinsons Dis. 2017;3:16.
50. Kluger BM, Dolhun R, Sumrall M, Hall K, Okun MS. Palliative care and Parkinson's disease: time to move beyond cancer. Mov Disord. 2021;36(6):1325-9.
51. Bluett B, Pantelyat AY, Litvan I, Ali F, Apetauerova D, Bega D, et al. Best practices in the clinical management of progressive supranuclear palsy and corticobasal syndrome: A Consensus Statement of the CurePSP Centers of Care. Front Neurol. 2021;12:694872.
52. Jordan SR, Kluger B, Ayele R, Brungardt A, Hall A, Jones J, et al. Optimizing future planning in Parkinson disease: suggestions for a comprehensive roadmap from patients and care partners. Ann Palliat Med. 2020;9(Suppl 1):S63-S74.
53. Lum HD, Kluger BM. Palliative Care for Parkinson Disease. Clin Geriatr Med. 2020;36(1):149-57.
54. Gursahani R. Communicating truth about serious illnesses in the Indian context. Natl Med J India. 2015;28(6):269-71.
55. Nalini A, Thennarasu K, Gourie-Devi M, Shenoy S, Kulshreshtha D. Clinical characteristics and survival pattern of 1,153 patients with amyotrophic lateral sclerosis: experience over 30 years from India. J Neurol Sci. 2008;272(1-2):60-70.
56. Karam CY, Paganoni S, Joyce N, Carter GT, Bedlack R. Palliative care issues in amyotrophic lateral sclerosis: An evidenced-based review. Am J Hosp Palliat Care. 2016;33(1):84-92.
57. Paganoni S, Karam C, Joyce N, Bedlack R, Carter GT. Comprehensive rehabilitative care across the spectrum of amyotrophic lateral sclerosis. Neuro Rehabilitation. 2015;37(1):53-68.
58. Danel-Brunaud V, Touzet L, Chevalier L, Moreau C, Devos D, Vandoolaeghe S, et al. Ethical considerations and palliative care in patients with amyotrophic lateral sclerosis: A review. Rev Neurol (Paris). 2017;173(5):300-7.
59. Miller RG, Jackson CE, Kasarskis EJ, England JD, Forshew D, Johnston W, et al.; Quality Standards Subcommittee of the American Academy of Neurology. Practice parameter update: the care of the patient with amyotrophic lateral sclerosis: drug, nutritional, and respiratory therapies (an evidence-based review): report of the Quality Standards Subcommittee of the American Academy of Neurology. Neurology. 2009;73(15):1218-26.
60. Pace A, Dirven L, Koekkoek JAF, Golla H, Fleming J, Rudà R, et al.; European Association of Neuro-Oncology Palliative Care Task Force. European Association for Neuro-Oncology (EANO) guidelines for palliative care in adults with glioma. Lancet Oncol. 2017;18(6):e330-40.
61. Philip J, Collins A, Brand C, Sundararajan V, Lethborg C, Gold M, et al. A proposed framework of supportive and palliative care for people with high-grade glioma. Neuro Oncol. 2018;20(3):391-9.

127
CHAPTER

Changing Approaches in Neurosurgery

Chandrashekhar E Deopujari, Chandan Mohanty, Milind Deogaonkar

INTRODUCTION

Like most other surgical branches, neurosurgery has evolved and considerably changed over the last few decades, with some new technical developments and the emergence of subspecialties. Though this is the most visible change for the patients and managers, other changes in the concepts of managing certain neurosurgical diseases, awareness of some new disease entities, and multidisciplinary management protocols have added further to patient safety with better outcomes.

The most important technical developments, which have influenced neurosurgery at the turn of the century, are—the development of minimally invasive techniques with the keyhole concept, intraoperative use of navigation systems, introduction of high-definition (HD) endoscopy in cranial procedures, and image enhancement in microscopic and endoscopic surgery. Endomicrosurgery has also become prevalent in degenerative spinal surgery with refined instrumentation. Neurointervention for cerebral as well as spinal vascular diseases has offered alternatives to surgery in many cases and its limitations are also better understood with wider use. The use of deep brain, spinal and peripheral nerve stimulation has brought about a big change in functional neurosurgery.

In this chapter, we have tried to enumerate most of the advances over the last quarter of a century in neurosurgery with several landmark trials, systemic reviews, and meta-analyses, which have shown us a way ahead for rationally treating our patients to the best of our ability for better outcomes.

BRAIN TUMORS

Imaging

Preoperative evaluation of tumors on new MRI (magnetic resonance imaging) sequences, viz., spectroscopy, diffusion, and perfusion imaging, has improved our understanding of tumors. In addition, diffusion tensor imaging (DTI) sequences have allowed us to see the displacement and infiltration of the important white matter tracts and given us a better idea of the invasive versus noninvasive nature of the tumors. This has given a much better idea of the resectability of the tumors and facilitated a safer way of approaching them by planning surgical approaches without disturbing these tracts.[1] Visualization of the lesser-known tracts such as SLF (superior longitudinal fasciculus), ILF (inferior longitudinal fasciculus), and arcuate fibers has allowed a better understanding of the problems related to their disturbances and helped in planning a surgical approach without traversing them **(Figs. 1A and B)**.[2] Blood-oxygen-level-dependent (BOLD) imaging method allows the identification of task activation areas thereby mapping the important functional motor areas, viz., speech, hand, foot, etc.[3] Further technological developments to identify areas of eloquence for intelligence, emotions, and personality by the MR software for parcellation to define connectomes have allowed surgeons to plan approaches to deeper lesions without impairment of higher functions.[4,5]

Adjuncts in Operative Planning

Image-guided Surgery

Image-guided surgery (IGS), as it was originally called, was introduced in neurosurgery in the 1990s[6,7] and has now become an integral part of surgery planning. The computer revolution entered the concept of stereotaxy (point stereotaxy) and made it possible to do "volume stereotaxy" with this magic wand. The externally applied fiducials were replaced by contouring for registration in the next-generation models, which have made it easier and less expensive to use this navigation technology. Preoperative computerized tomography (CT) as well as MRI can now be used in the operating room to localize the target (e.g., tumor) and find the most suitable point on the skull to enter

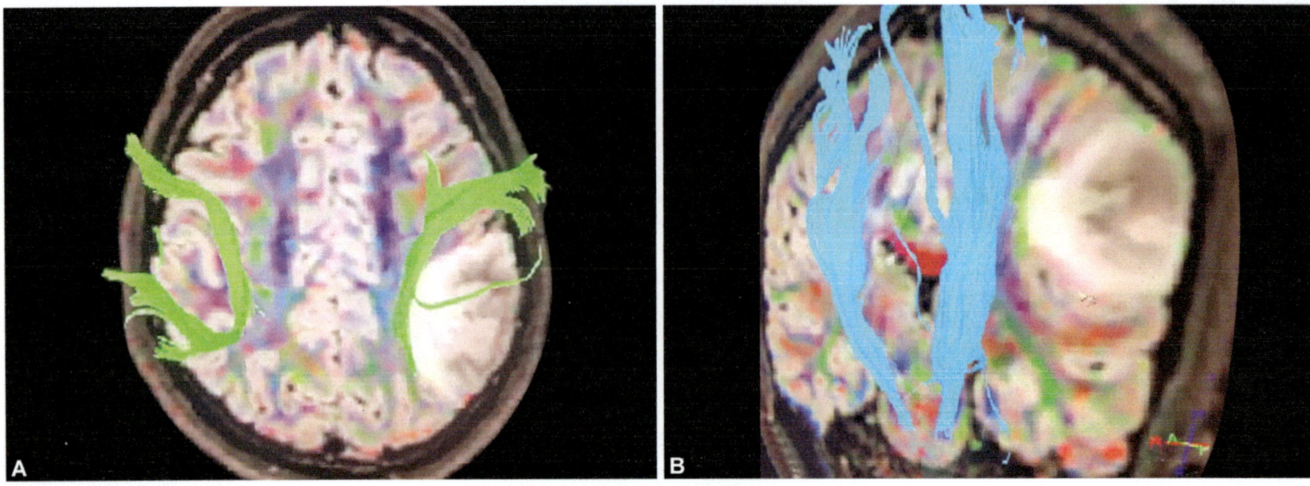

FIGS. 1A AND B: A 35-year-old female patient with seizures diagnosed to have low-grade glioma left parieto-occipital region. Diffuse tensor imaging identified important tracts. (A) It shows displaced superior longitudinal fasciculus (SLF), in green color, passing medially to the tumor on the left side; (B) It shows displaced pyramidal tract in blue color. Tumor was completely excised without any deficit.

safely with a proper trajectory to reach **(Figs. 2A to C)**. A precision biopsy could now be done and a more complete resection could be achieved. Shifts of the structures during the removal of the tumor and by the escape of cerebrospinal fluid (CSF) during the opening of the subarachnoid space or ventricle made this type of technique imprecise during the later stages of surgery. Other methods of surgical visualization then came to help. Some models of surgical navigation included an HD ultrasound to update the image during surgery.[8]

These systems depend on the optical coordination of signals from the hand-held pointer. However, microscope integration of the image and the use of dissecting instruments or suction as pointers improve their utility without stopping surgery from time to time. Electromagnetic (EM) systems have helped further by abolishing the interference caused by microscopes or other theater equipment or personnel blocking the optical signals and have also allowed us to use navigation without head fixation.[9] Malleable slim probes have helped in using these systems during endoscopic surgeries.

Intraoperative Visualization

Image enhancement during surgery with 5-Aminolevulinic acid (5-ALA), fluorescein, or indocyanine green (ICG) has improved the radicality of tumor excision without damage to eloquent areas and blood vessels and helps in the concept of supramaximal resection which is becoming popular in gliomas.[10] Image enhancement has now extended to endoscopic surgeries, in surgical loupes as well as headlights, widening its use to all methods of surgery. The use of 5-ALA has not only improved resection margins but has resulted in better progression-free survival in gliomas.[11]

Intraoperative MRI

Intraoperative MRI (iMRI) suites have allowed the evaluation of resection margins and removal of the residual lesion during the same procedure.[12] This has been particularly useful for low-grade gliomas, some childhood tumors, viz., ependymomas and large pituitary tumors.[13]

Functional Preservation in Tumors of Eloquent Areas

Functional preservation has further improved with the use of intraoperative neurophysiological monitoring (IONM). Evoked Potentials [somatosensory evoked potential (SSEP) and motor evoked potential (MEP)], EMG monitoring, as well as nerve and cortical stimulation methods have now been standardized and warn us before inflicting irreversible damage.[14] Re-emergence of "awake surgery" has further added safety in cases where speech preservation is the main goal.[15] All these developments have created a major interest in glioma surgery among neurosurgeons resulting in more radical resections of low- as well as high-grade gliomas.[16] A moderate increase in tumor-free survival and long-term survival in high-grade gliomas and a remarkable increase in both parameters in low-grade gliomas were seen in a large study by Berger and colleagues.[17] Since the availability of intraoperative imaging, awake surgery, and IONM, the concept of supramaximal resection is being practiced in many centers allowing for neuronal plasticity to aid functional recovery and achieving remarkable improvement in longevity in low-grade gliomas.[18]

Recent Developments in Neuropathology of Brain Tumors

Histopathology of CNS tumors has progressed with better and cheaper methods of immunohistochemistry and the application of molecular biology to understand tumor behavior. This has radically changed the classification of brain tumors after 2015 and has created a need for 3-step classification based on morphology, molecular markers, and histological grading.[19]

The differences between childhood gliomas and adults have been better defined. In adults, isocitrate dehydrogenase (IDH) mutation studies have significantly contributed to the understanding of primary and secondary malignant tumor behavior in diffuse gliomas, which directly influences the radicality of tumor excision during surgery as well as their prognosis. Tumors from the Oligodendroglia cell line seem to have much better prognosis, especially in the subgroup where codeletion of 1p and 19q is observed. On the other hand, the new entity of diffuse midline glioma with histone mutation of H3K27M seems to have a much worse prognosis.[20]

A childhood tumor, namely medulloblastoma of the posterior fossa, was the first tumor subjected to molecular stratification. The four groups thus described based on SHH, WNT, and other markers have improved the understanding of their behavior and response to therapy.[21] A similar trend is being seen with RELA fusion in dividing ependymomas into two separate entities.[22] Another posterior fossa tumor, brainstem glioma, has also been further classified for

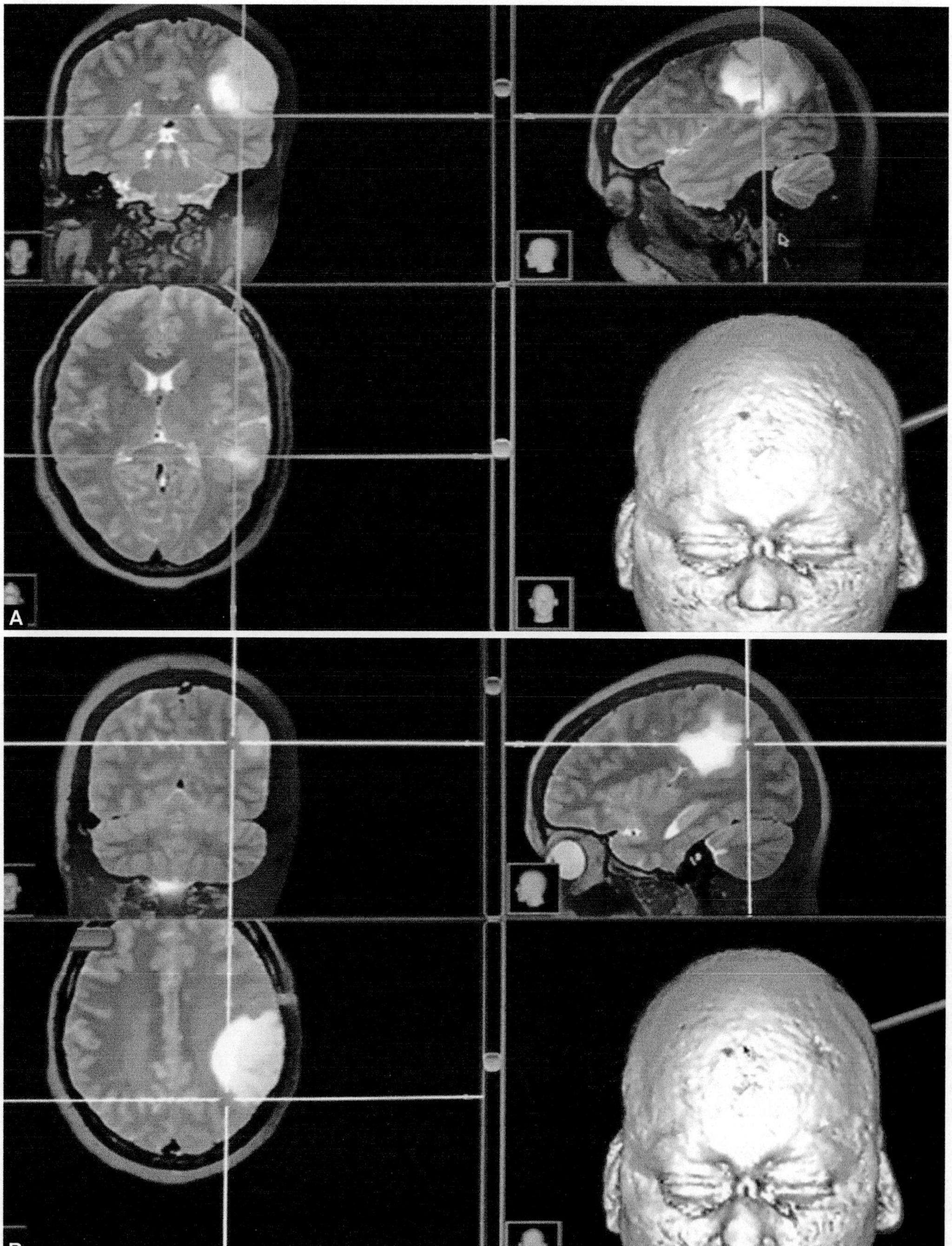

FIGS. 2A TO C: *Continued*

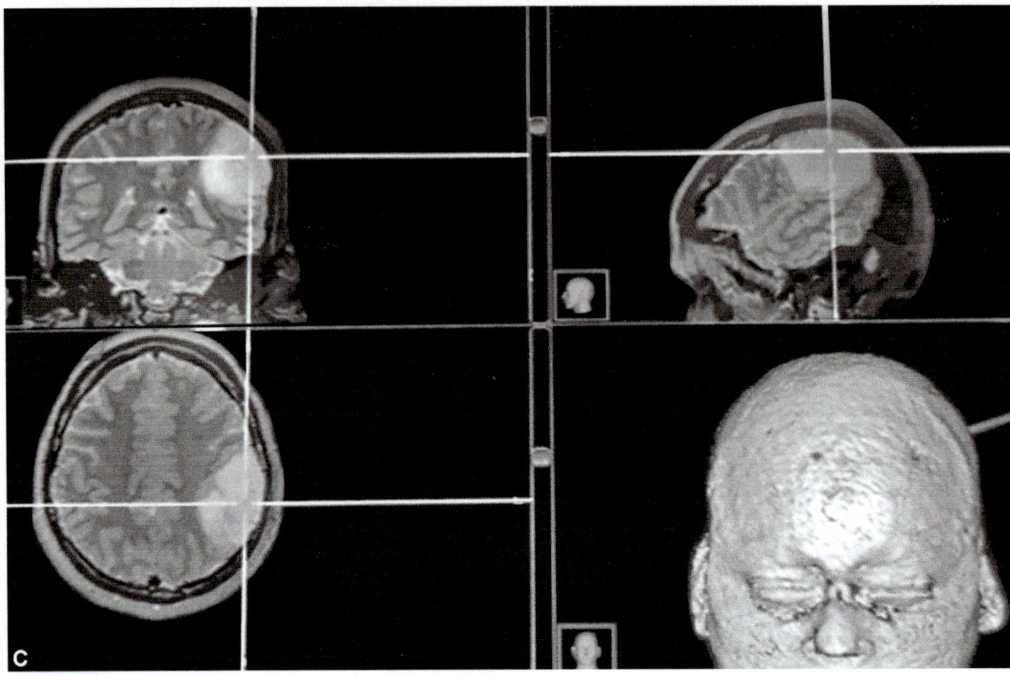

FIGS. 2A TO C: Intraoperative navigation was used for radical excision of the low-grade glioma patient. (A) Inferior extent of the tumor; (B) Posterior extend of the tumor; (C) Center of the tumor.

proper selection for biopsy or surgery and determining the outcome. This allows several low-grade tumors to be excised safely under neuromonitoring and also explains the dismal prognosis in diffuse pontine glioma (H3K27 mutated).[20]

Another childhood tumor (also seen occasionally in adults) that has shown the molecular difference between two subtypes is craniopharyngioma, where BRAF mutation is observed in the papillary type and β-catenin mutation is observed in the more common adamantinoma variety.[23] The pilocytic variety is the most benign of astrocytomas but has also occasionally shown more aggressive behavior which is now explained by their BRAF fusion or mutation status.[24]

Extra-axial Tumors

Surgery for extra-axial tumors, which are predominantly benign, and where more radical excision was proposed with newer extensive skull base approaches, has been tempered with the realization of preserving better functional status in these patients who have long-term survival, especially for preserving cranial nerves to avoid disabling pain, dysesthesias, facial disfigurement and hearing, swallowing and voice impairment, etc.[25,26]

The Role of Neuroendoscopy in Tumors

Though it was originally developed for surgery of hydrocephalus, neuroendoscopy has helped brain tumor surgery considerably in the last 25 years. A big change has come about with the endoscopy technique in the management of pituitary tumors with the endonasal approach. The panoramic view and the ability to take the surgical eye (vision) at the desired target have allowed us to reach areas beyond the microsurgical vision and removed the need for retractors with better preservation of nasal structures. The ability to look in many directions with 30°, 45°, and 70° scopes has allowed surgery to extend further in coronal and sagittal planes. It has changed the classification of pituitary tumors involving cavernous sinus (Knosp grading) and has allowed more complete removal of these tumors.[27] This is a very important factor in functioning tumors and influences long-term control rates and survival in acromegaly and Cushing's disease.[28]

The endoscopic endonasal approach has expanded further to skull base tumors by extended approaches for midline suprasellar tumors, viz., craniopharyngiomas and meningiomas, posteriorly to clival chordomas and foramen magnum pathology as well as laterally to pterygoid fossa and Meckel's cave **(Figs. 3A to D)**.[29,30] The suprasellar area may be reached, without disturbing the brain and even the pituitary, either in front or behind the stalk and future developments may allow this corridor safe clipping of the circle of Willis aneurysms.

Endoscopy has also influenced many transcranial microsurgical procedures which have become much less invasive with the use of endoscope assistance allowing looking around the corners, mainly in keyhole approaches.[31]

Apart from the surgical approach, the management of functioning pituitary tumors has undergone significant change with the availability and efficacy of medical treatment. This has virtually avoided surgery in most cases of prolactinomas which respond well to cabergoline.[32] Surgery in prolactinomas is now required only in cases resistant

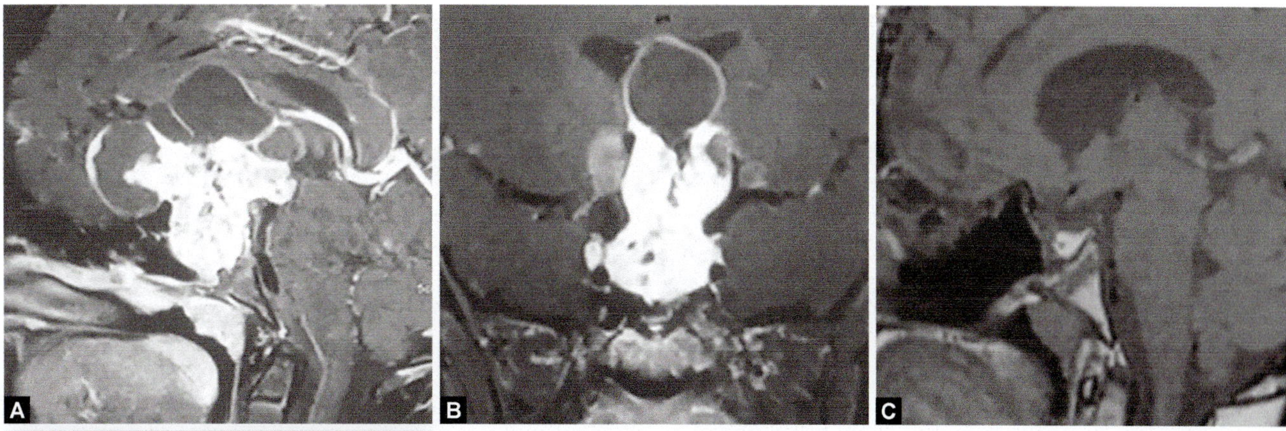

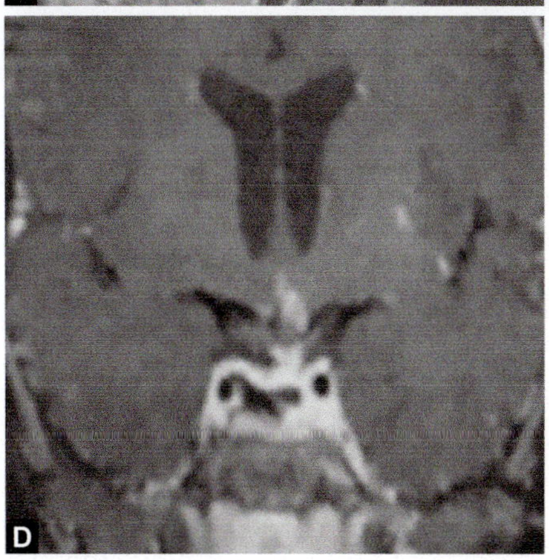

FIGS. 3A TO D: A 6-year-old male child presented with symptoms of raised increased intracranial tension (ICT). (A and B) show large seller–suprasellar lesion (craniopharyngioma) with complete obliteration of the third ventricle; (C and D) show postoperative scans with complete excision of the lesion with intact pituitary stalk achieved by combined endonasal transsphenoidal and frontal craniotomy for 2 staged excision of the tumor.

to cabergoline and rarely for impending visual failure. Somatostatin for HGH-secreting tumors has been very helpful but remains a complementary treatment to surgery due to limited efficacy and availability. The recent change in WHO classification of pituitary tumors has made us aware of their oncological potential but has not significantly changed their management.[33]

Endoscopy has also been applied regularly for the removal of intraventricular cysts and tumor biopsies. Neuroendoscopy is now practiced in many centers for the excision of colloid cysts and other avascular lesions with great success.[34] It has also significantly changed the algorithm of management of posterior third ventricular and pineal region tumors where endoscopic third ventriculostomy (ETV) and simultaneous biopsy are now proposed as the first-line surgical treatment.[35] This minimally invasive approach is especially important in younger patients, where further major surgery is not necessary as over two-thirds of patients can be satisfactorily managed with radiation and chemotherapy.[36]

Neuroendoscopy is playing an increasing role in the radical removal of tumors from inaccessible areas in the ventricular system as well **(Figs. 4A to C)**.[37,38] It has also been a useful adjunct to a microsurgical approach in larger tumors for devascularization, more complete excision, and confirming hemostasis.[39] More recently, several reports of its use in the parenchymal tumor have shown promise.[40,41]

Complementary Treatments in Brain Tumors

Complementary treatments have improved the prognosis of gliomas with more precise radiation in fractionated treatment with photons by micro-multileaf collimators in linear accelerator (LINAC)-based systems. The hippocampal sparing has also improved functional status in long-term survivors.[42] Concomitant therapy with Temozolomide (a radiation sensitizer) has now become the standard of care for high-grade gliomas.[43] Complementary use in follow-up treatment for six cycles has proved beneficial in a large trial while therapeutic use extending further to 1 year is under investigation, especially in the methylated group (for MGMT) which seems to be more sensitive to this treatment.[44]

Targeted therapies have become possible for certain tumors with known mutations, most notably for mTOR mutation in Subependymal giant cell astrocytoma (SEGA, usually associated with tuberous sclerosis) where surgery can be delayed or avoided in many cases and has also been found useful in reducing seizures.[45] Targeted therapy in BRAF-mutated pilocytic astrocytomas and craniopharyngiomas is under investigation.[46]

Stereotactic radiosurgery (SRS) has become a primary treatment option for small-to-medium benign skull base lesions, most remarkably for vestibular schwannomas. The control rates are over 90% with Gamma knife and more

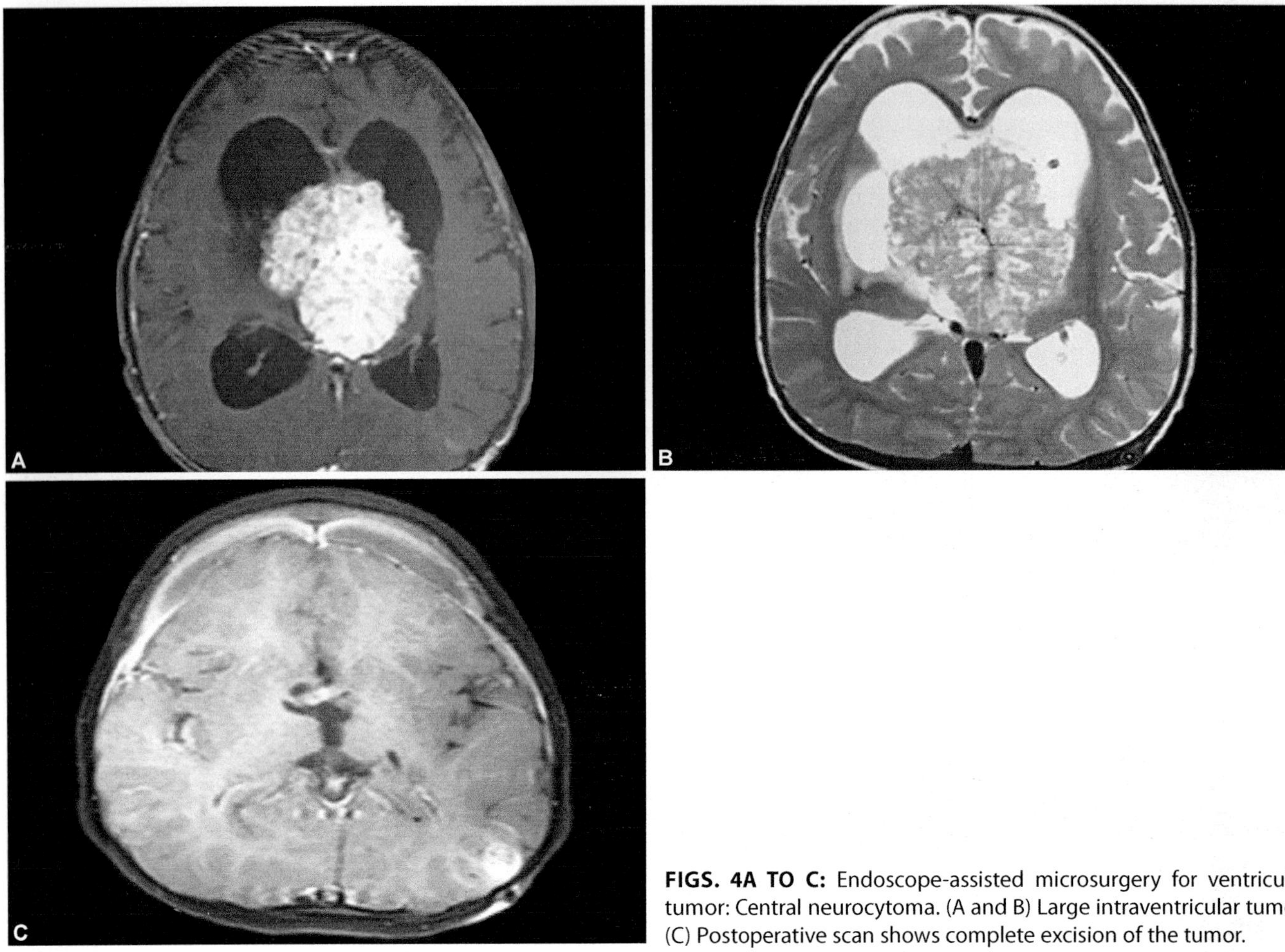

FIGS. 4A TO C: Endoscope-assisted microsurgery for ventricular tumor: Central neurocytoma. (A and B) Large intraventricular tumor; (C) Postoperative scan shows complete excision of the tumor.

recently with CyberKnife. For larger tumors, SRS has opened the option of being conservative during tumor surgery for dissection from the brainstem, nerves, etc. and using it as a complementary treatment to the small residual volume. Excellent control rates in the cavernous sinus, other skull base meningiomas, and schwannomas are encouraging and allow us to avoid the morbidity associated with these lesions.[25]

Proton beam therapy with pencil beams has acquired high precision in tumors requiring higher dose for control and is being recommended as a fractionated treatment in certain tumors, viz., chordomas with better results.[47]

HYDROCEPHALUS AND INTRAVENTRICULAR PATHOLOGY

Pediatric hydrocephalus treatment has also undergone a paradigm shift. ETV for obstructive hydrocephalus has become the standard of care with high success rates avoiding lifelong implantation of a shunt.[48] Though neuro-endoscopy started many years ago, the correct indications for ETV were understood with greater success in cases of congenital aqueduct stenosis.[49] The worry about the persistence of larger ventricular size compared to shunting has been addressed by similar developmental long-term outcomes for both modalities in patients treated during early childhood.[50]

The use of endoscopy in other varieties of hydrocephalus is finding more applications in tumoral hydrocephalus but has not proven to be superior in communicating a variety of hydrocephalus, viz., postinfective, posthemorrhagic or normal pressure hydrocephalus (NPH).[49] Secondary ETV is also being frequently performed with a fair degree of success in recent reports despite initial failure.[51-53]

Neuroendoscopy has also added to safer and less invasive ways of CSF diversion by other procedures, viz., septostomy and simplified multiloculated and complex hydrocephalus by creating a single cavity allowing a single shunt to drain thus avoiding the use of multiple shunts.[54]

VASCULAR NEUROSURGERY

Vascular neurosurgery has been greatly influenced by the proliferation of interventional methods, most notably for aneurysms. However, it has also tempered its use in arteriovenous malformation (AVM), with the realization of limited success, and SRS has found a major application in this area. The natural history of cavernous angiomas has been extensively studied with the rational use of surgery for bleeding as well as epilepsy.

Aneurysm Surgery

The ISAT (International Subarachnoid Aneurysm Trial) in the UK has started a big change in securing aneurysms presenting with subarachnoid hemorrhage (SAH) preferring coiling over clipping.[55] Several arguments about patients operated outside the study, anterior versus posterior circulation, young age versus old, and good grade versus bad, have all been answered by 5 and 10 years follow-ups of the same patient cohort,[56,57] and also by several other studies with a large volume of patients, most notably by the Barrow group in the US. Posterior circulation aneurysms are all being tackled by interventional techniques and the current indications for surgery for anterior circulation aneurysms mainly pertain to difficult-to-reach aneurysms, mainly of the middle cerebral artery (MCA). Surgery may still be required in cases of uncoilable or postcoiling recurrences **(Figs. 5A to E)**.[58]

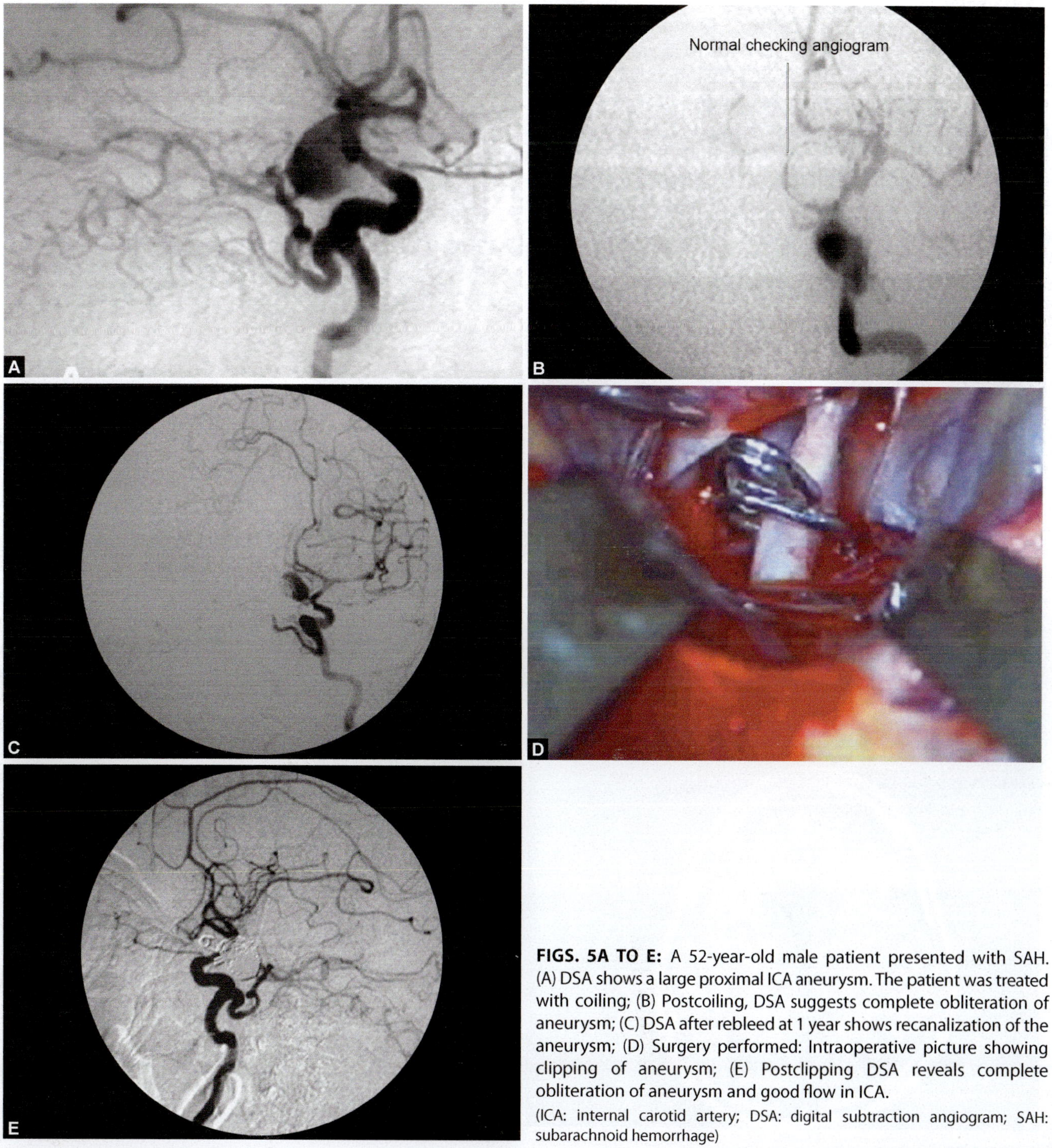

FIGS. 5A TO E: A 52-year-old male patient presented with SAH. (A) DSA shows a large proximal ICA aneurysm. The patient was treated with coiling; (B) Postcoiling, DSA suggests complete obliteration of aneurysm; (C) DSA after rebleed at 1 year shows recanalization of the aneurysm; (D) Surgery performed: Intraoperative picture showing clipping of aneurysm; (E) Postclipping DSA reveals complete obliteration of aneurysm and good flow in ICA.

(ICA: internal carotid artery; DSA: digital subtraction angiogram; SAH: subarachnoid hemorrhage)

Perioperative ICG or fluorescein angiography gives a much better idea about the complete obliteration of aneurysm, patency of distal vessels, and rapidity of distal flow. This has reduced the complication rate of incomplete clipping or inadvertent sacrifice of branches and reduced the need for postoperative angiography.[59]

Endovascular nimodipine injection for chemical angioplasty has become a standard treatment of postoperative vasospasm after SAH, especially in the situation of refractory cases to standard medical management.[60]

The wide neck aneurysms may be treated with stent assisted coiling and more recently by flow diverters. Flow diverters have now become the standard of care for proximal internal carotid artery (ICA) aneurysms, mainly involving the cavernous ICA, reducing the number of elective ICA occlusion and bypass procedures.[61]

Management of incidental detection of unruptured aneurysms has been well studied. The sizes over 5 mm and irregularity of the sac, especially near the tip, are statistically significant.[62] Some locations seem to be less prone to bleed, viz., proximal ICA. Hemodynamic aspects of the aneurysmal sac are being studied.[63]

Arteriovenous Malformations

Arteriovenous malformations have been studied for angioarchitecture to prognosticate their rupture. Several studies have shown the presence of intranidal aneurysms and stenosis on the venous drainage side to be related to the potential for hemorrhage.[64] The Spetzler Martin classification for risk stratification of treatment has been modified with the addition of age and previous hemorrhages (Lawton) for better prognostication.[65]

Comparative benefits of the three modalities of treatments have shown a clear advantage of surgery in grades I and II, followed by radiosurgery and only <30% of patients are cured by embolization despite improved agents. Grade 3–5 requires multimodality treatment **(Figs. 6A to G)**.[66] The same quantum of beneficial effects has been found in seizure control across the various treatment methods.[67] Seizure control with surgery as well as SRS has been satisfactory but not well studied for embolization alone.[68]

Neurointervention has been an important part of the management of brain AVMs, even when not curative, to reduce vascularity from inaccessible and deep feeders.

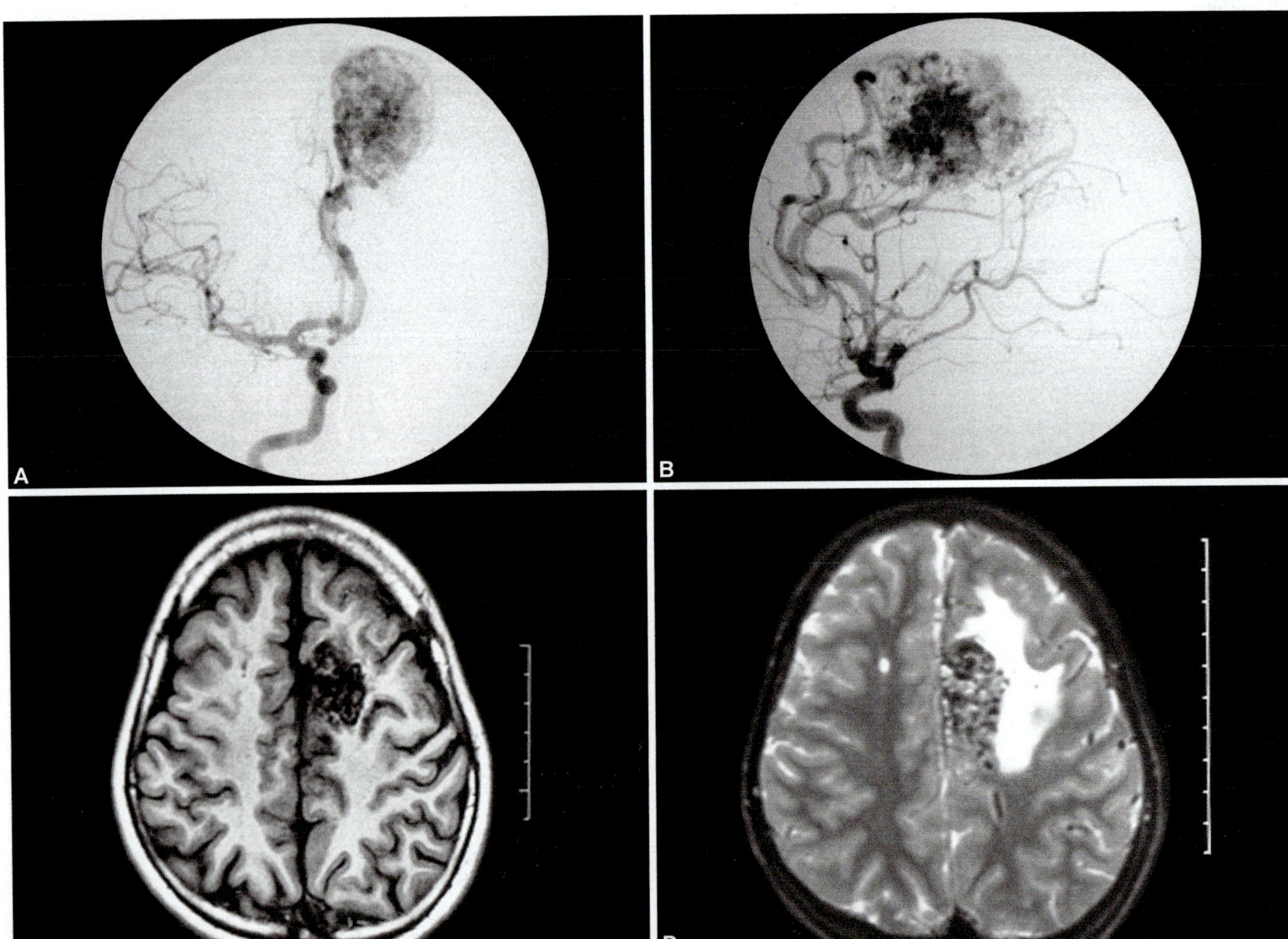

FIGS. 6A TO G: *Continued*

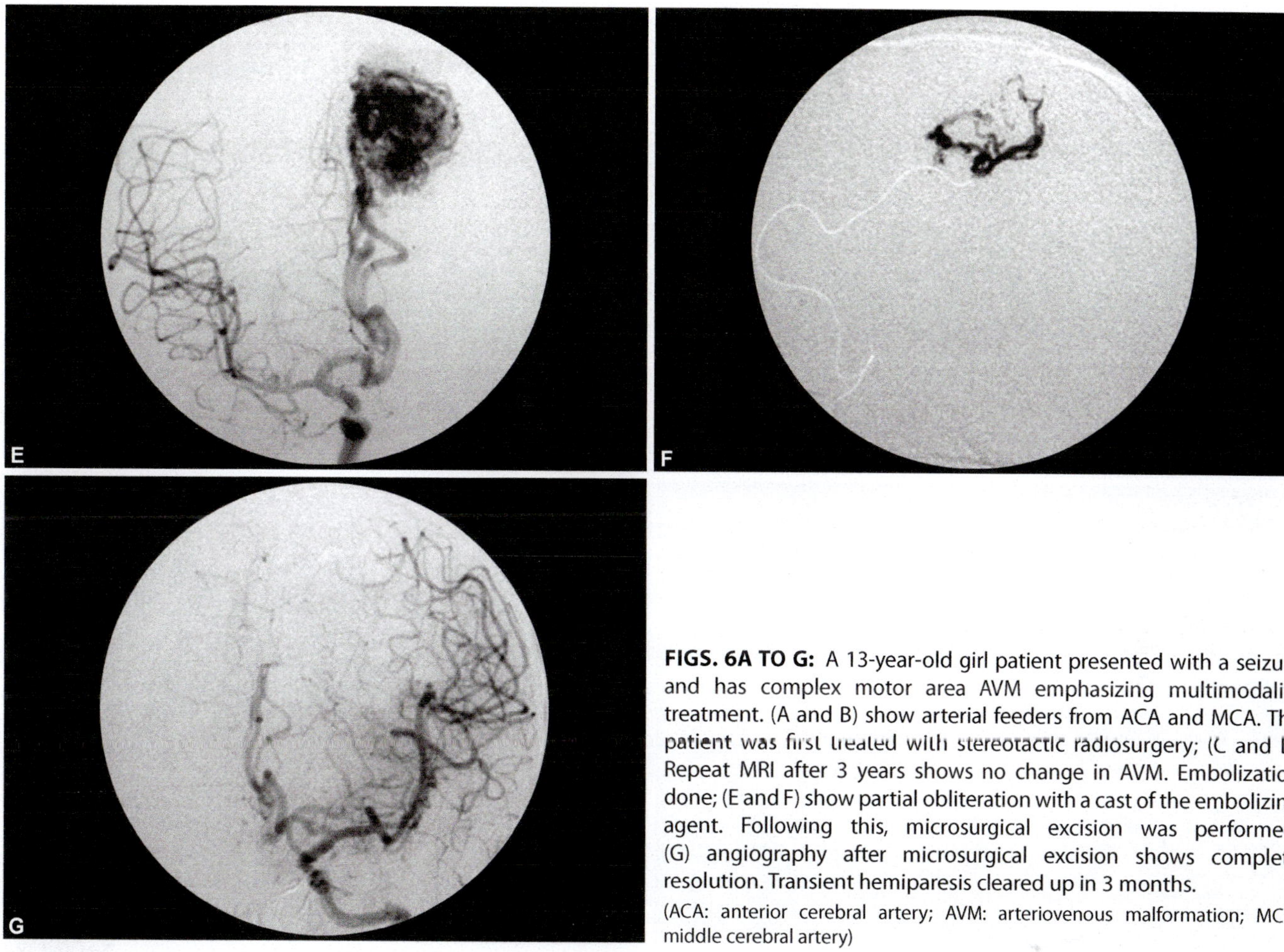

FIGS. 6A TO G: A 13-year-old girl patient presented with a seizure and has complex motor area AVM emphasizing multimodality treatment. (A and B) show arterial feeders from ACA and MCA. The patient was first treated with stereotactic radiosurgery; (C and D) Repeat MRI after 3 years shows no change in AVM. Embolization done; (E and F) show partial obliteration with a cast of the embolizing agent. Following this, microsurgical excision was performed; (G) angiography after microsurgical excision shows complete resolution. Transient hemiparesis cleared up in 3 months.

(ACA: anterior cerebral artery; AVM: arteriovenous malformation; MCA: middle cerebral artery)

However, its use to reduce the nidus before SRS has been questioned due to lower rates of obliteration observed in this group.[69]

Stereotactic radiosurgery forms an important modality of management in surgically inaccessible AVMs in eloquent areas with high cure rates in small-volume nidus.[70] For larger AVMs, fractionated radiosurgery has been tried with some success. Dose fractionation as well as volume fractionation protocols has been developed.[71]

For unruptured AVMs, the recent randomized controlled trial (ARUBA) suggested no active treatment superior to any treatment.[72] This has been contested by several groups for surgery as well as SRS. The benefits of surgery and SRS are better in studies outside of trial and the current consensus suggests surgery for grade I and II AVMs and not to interfere with higher grades unruptured AVMs.

Dural AVMs and arteriovenous fistulas (AVFs) are being increasingly recognized. These acquired lesions are seen in association with sinus thrombosis and may present with seizures, idiopathic intracranial hypertension (IIH), and rarely with hemorrhage.[73] The importance of a proper 6-vessel DSA cannot be overemphasized in these settings. Neurointerventional treatments can take care of these lesions efficiently.[74]

Cavernous Malformations of the Brain

Magnetic resonance imaging has allowed a large number of cavernous malformations to be diagnosed during investigations for headaches, strokes, and seizures. Several incidental lesions have also been found during investigations for other causes. Gradient echo and susceptibility-weighted imaging (SWI) techniques allow very small lesions to be picked up.[75] The natural history of these congenital malformations has become clearer with a large volume of patients being studied. Lancet published a long-term study of a large number of patients recently, which shows that previous hemorrhage and brainstem location has a much higher frequency of rehemorrhage resulting in morbidity and occasional mortality **(Figs. 7A to E)**.[76] Surgery remains the best way to remove these lesions and tackling them with preserved function has been the main challenge in recent times. The use of DTI to create a corridor and intraoperative monitoring to preserve the cranial nerve nuclei and major tracts has made it possible to accomplish these objectives.

The seizure potential of cavernous angiomas is another neurosurgical challenge. Supratentorial cavernomas presenting with seizures have shown over 90% Engel grade-1

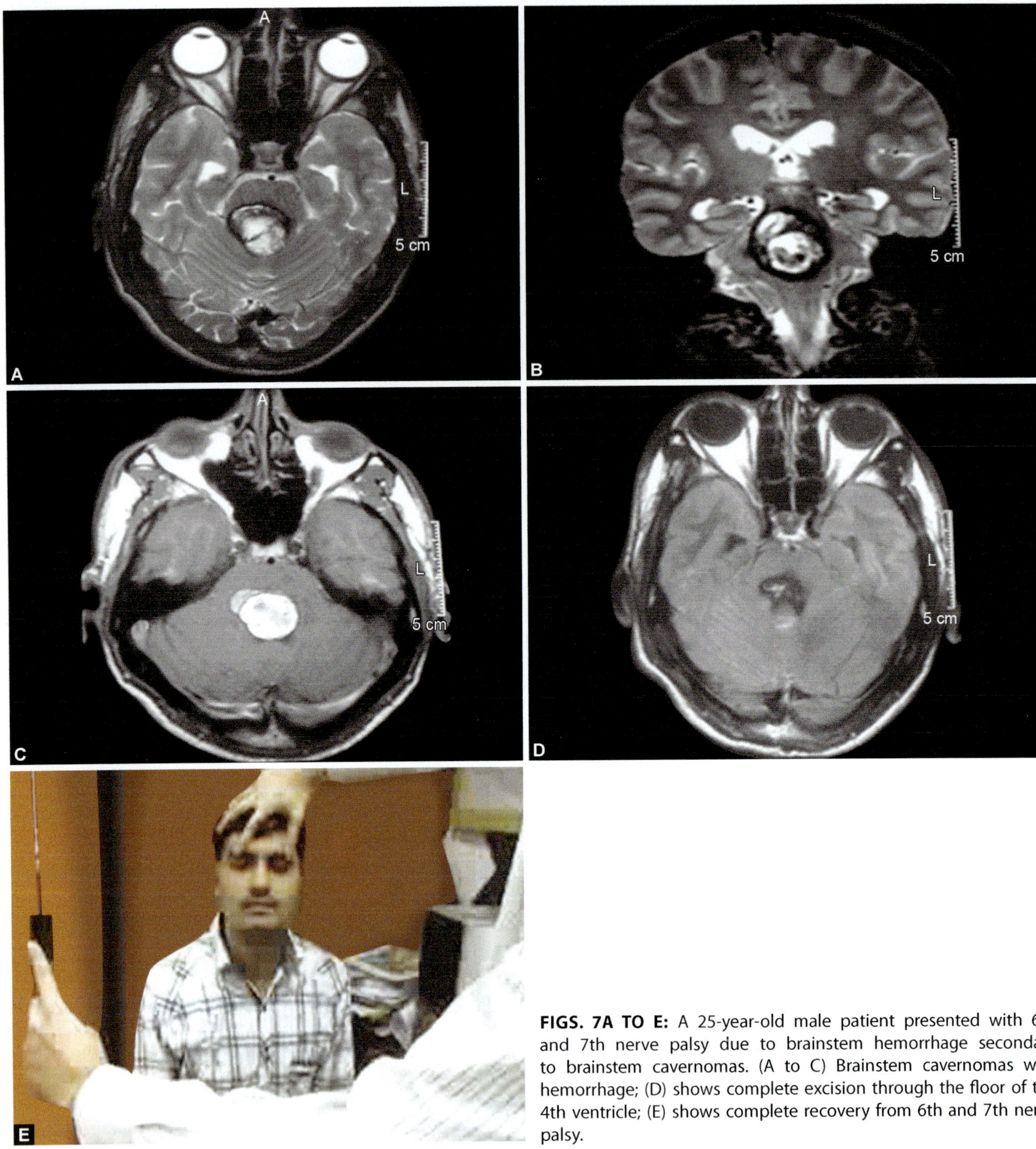

FIGS. 7A TO E: A 25-year-old male patient presented with 6th and 7th nerve palsy due to brainstem hemorrhage secondary to brainstem cavernomas. (A to C) Brainstem cavernomas with hemorrhage; (D) shows complete excision through the floor of the 4th ventricle; (E) shows complete recovery from 6th and 7th nerve palsy.

outcome with surgical excision including the surrounding rim of hemosiderin. The seizure rate is slightly lower in patients where the hemosiderin ring is not removed, viz., in eloquent areas. However, the most important factor in seizure control seems to be the duration of the seizure, with better results for surgery carried out within the first 2 years.[77,78]

The role of radiosurgery in cavernous angiomas, especially in eloquent and inaccessible areas, is being debated. Though some reports have shown a good outcome in reducing potential bleeds, its role is currently limited to inaccessible, residual, and recurrent lesions.[79]

Genetic predisposition for cavernous angiomas is not restricted to Hispanics and is also frequently recognized in

India. Unusual forms, viz., giant and cystic, are also being recognized and management strategies are discussed.[80]

Status of Bypass Surgery in Stroke and Other Indications

Superficial temporal artery (STA)-MCA bypass has seen a resurgence in ischemic strokes in the young related to Moyamoya disease. Though indirect anastomotic methods have an equally good outcome in the long term, it probably has a place in a setting of a cluster of strokes in a short period. Unfortunately, it is not possible to use it in very-small vessels, especially in children below 3 years, where the course of the disease is rapidly progressive.[81]

External carotid artery (ECA)/ICA bypass is being used more in the management of unclippable giant aneurysms and occasionally for skull base tumors when the ICA is permanently ligated or sacrificed.[82,83] High-flow bypasses are preferred while planning for sacrificing the carotid. The radial artery is favored for long-term patency rather than the traditional saphenous vein interposition.[84]

Spontaneous Intracerebral Hematoma

Many of these patients suffering from a ganglionic hemorrhage (mostly hypertensive) remain stable though hemiplegic with varying amounts of the clot. Though the volume of the clot has been used as an indicator for surgical evacuation, clinical deterioration under observation remains the most standard indication for surgical intervention. The practice of a conservative approach over several decades has been evaluated recently in two major trials, first on ganglionic and later on lobar hematomas have not shown a clear superiority of surgery in these patients.[85,86]

Minimally invasive approaches are being increasingly used for evacuation of hemorrhage to reduce collateral damage and endoscope-guided evacuation has found wide acceptance with or without a tubular retractor.[87-91]

Spinal AVMs and AVFs

Better resolution in spinal angiography has allowed a better classification of spinal AVMs. The more common lesion, viz., dural arteriovenous fistula (dAVF), typically arises at the radicular artery and creates ischemic neurological deficits due to venous hypertension. Embolization in expert hands is the best available treatment and has become the standard of care for these patients.[92] However, surgery can have equally good results by disconnecting the fistula at the nerve root and becomes the choice of treatment when the artery of Adamkiewicz is involved to avoid ischemic deficit, which may occur due to inadvertent blockage by embolizing material. Surgery has also become more precise through the use of ICG to confirm obliteration of the fistula and patency of the distal vessel.[93] Other varieties of spinal AVMs are usually more complex to treat and require a combined effort by the endovascular and surgical teams.

TRAUMATIC BRAIN INJURY

Management of neurotrauma has been rationalized with several trials, which have improved the understanding of the various mechanisms to prevent secondary injury. The idea that better ICU care and protocolized treatments reduced mortality in severe head injury received a severe jolt from the Chestnut study.[94] Several caveats in the study have been noted and the intracranial pressure (ICP) monitoring-based treatments have continued in several centers.[95] The consensus statement of a panel of experts continues to recommend that strong consideration should be given to provide pragmatic guidance and recommendations for monitoring even in absence of high-quality data.[96] Bioinformatics will probably play a big role in the management protocols of these critically ill patients and individualize their treatment in the future.[97]

Recent literature has recommended target values for various brain monitoring modalities **(Table 1)**. The experience in the use of ICP monitoring has rationalized the use of osmotic agents and stopped the use of steroids except for optic nerve injury. Mannitol is being replaced by hypertonic saline, especially in young patients, to avoid dehydration and renal toxicity.

Numerous biomarkers have been evaluated for prognostication and to detect ongoing injury to guide therapeutic interventions, though none of them has been used routinely in clinical practice. To date, only S100B has been used in limited centers to stratify patients with a mild head injury at presentation.

The place of decompressive craniotomy has been re-evaluated in diffuse brain injury and has been found to reduce mortality rates. However, severe and moderate morbidity in survivors has become a big challenge, especially for developing countries.[98] Decompression based on raised ICP has not shown much difference in outcome.[99] Timing of decompression and extent of surgical decompression are investigated further and various complications of decompressive craniotomy are being studied. Most notable complications include brain herniation through the defect or the trephine effect, contralateral development of subdural

TABLE 1: Therapeutic goals for neurocritical care in traumatic brain injuries.

Modality	Targeted values/thresholds
Intracranial pressure	20–25 mm Hg
Brain tissue oxygen tension	20 mm Hg
Cerebral microdialysis: • Lactate/pyruvate ratio • Brain glucose	 >25 (poor prognostic indicator) <0.8 mmol/L (poor prognostic indicator)
Optimum cerebral perfusion pressure	60–70 mm Hg
Pulse reactivity index	>0.25 (poor prognostic marker)

hematoma/hygroma, and delayed hydrocephalus. Early cranioplasty is useful in avoiding some of these issues.[100]

Therapeutic hypothermia though used for TBI at some centers has not been shown to reduce mortality and morbidity.[101,102]

Among the delayed complications, CSF leak is being more aggressively treated because of the possibility of disastrous infective complications; pneumococcal vaccine is recommended to reduce the subsequent possible meningitis.[103,104] Surgery is possible by endonasal endoscopic repair in the majority of cases and transcranial surgery is applied only for frontal sinus leaks, multiple fistulae, or accompanying high ICP states.

Nonsurgical treatment and steroids have found an important place in the management of chronic subdural hematoma (CSDH). This has been a very useful method to reduce inflammation of the dural membranes, reducing small rebleeds which are important for the progressive increase of the hematoma, and thereby delay or avoid surgery as many of these patients are on antiplatelet treatments.[105] Tranexamic acid has also been found to be an important agent for the conservative treatment of CSDH by reducing plasmin activity and lessening the osmotic gradient apart from reducing inflammation.[106] Surgery for evacuation usually remains restricted to burr-hole evacuation with the doubtful benefit of leaving a drain postoperatively. A craniotomy is, therefore, very rarely required for solid clots or very thick membranes.[107] The extent of craniotomy can be reduced by using endoscope assistance for more complete evacuation.[108] In refractory cases, middle meningeal artery embolization has shown great promise.[109,110]

EPILEPSY SURGERY

Localization of epileptic focus has become easier with newer MRI sequences, especially for focal cortical dysplasia. Apart from the standard video electroencephalography (EEG) recordings, magnetoencephalography (MEG) has given a better idea of concordance.[111] Invasive monitoring with ECOG has been further fortified by depth recordings with stereoelectroencephalography (SEEG) and robotic placements of electrodes have allowed greater use of the technique and also placement of more electrodes without additional burden to the patient or the surgeon.[112]

Epilepsy surgery has become less invasive and more precise in lesional surgery due to the availability of better navigation equipment and the incorporation of DTI and functional MRI (fMRI) in the planning.

For hemispheric epilepsies, standard hemispherotomy has been modified by several surgeons for avoiding hemosiderosis as well as leaving less dead space avoiding serious postoperative issues.[113] The periinsular technique is most commonly followed (Villemure, Spencer) and allows for a smaller incision and loss of brain tissue. Navigation allows a good disconnection even with this limited access, especially in patients with dilated ventricles.[114] More use of vertical hemispherotomy (Delalande) allows more complete resection in patients with small ventricles, viz., hemimegalencephaly.[115] This is being increasingly carried out with the endoscopic method, which minimizes the cranial opening and gives better visibility to disconnect at depth.[116,117]

A better definition of seizure focus on electrophysiology and MRI sequences is allowing limited disconnections, viz., temporo-parieto-occipital dissections without disturbance to motor tracts.[118] The use of IONM with mapping allows further safety to the sensory-motor cortex in a more precise manner. The availability of stimulators connected to surgical instruments, viz., suction during disconnection, also allows the preservation of subcortical structures and important tracts.

Corpus callosotomy is being performed much less frequently in the developed world with the availability of vagus nerve stimulation (VNS), which is giving equally good results in Lennox-Gastaut or similar disorders.[119]

Robotic or navigation-guided radiofrequency (RF) lesioning or LASER ablation is giving better results in conditions such as hypothalamic hamartoma (HH) and unreachable focus at depth in some cases.[120]

FUNCTIONAL NEUROSURGERY

The most important advance in functional neurosurgery in recent times is deep brain stimulation (DBS). Functional neuromodulation by using electrical stimulus is a relatively new concept. Bechtereva and colleagues in Russia[121] did the first implanted DBS. Benabid[122,123] published reports on the use of chronic electrical stimulation or DBS for the treatment of movement disorders early on. Due to its reversibility and adjustability, DBS has become the neurosurgical standard of care for movement disorders such as Parkinson's disease (PD), dystonia, and essential tremor over the past few decades.[124] It is also being increasingly used in conditions such as Tourette's syndrome, chronic pain, and psychiatric disorders such as depression and obsessive-compulsive disorder (OCD).[124]

Brain-computer interface (BCI) is another such recent advance that has provided hope for motor control.[125] Millions of people worldwide suffer from diseases that lead to paralysis through the disruption of signal pathways between the brain and the muscles. Neuroprosthetic devices are designed to restore lost function and could be used to form an electronic "neural bypass" to circumvent disconnected pathways in the nervous system. It has been shown that intracortically recorded signals can be decoded to extract information related to motion, allowing nonhuman primates and paralyzed humans to control computers and robotic arms through imagined movements as well as move parts of the body using functional electrical stimulation.[125]

The most recent use of virtual reality (VR) in neural augmentation is impressive. Immersive VR enables neural augmentation. It also helps to improve pain control[126] and can be used in motor and sensory augmentation. Neuromodulation-enhanced VR can be used in many such scenarios where available therapies fall short. The latest VR technology can be linked with the neuroscience of body perception and neuromodulation creating a new world of immersive digiceutical therapies.[126]

IDIOPATHIC INTRACRANIAL HYPERTENSION AND SPONTANEOUS INTRACRANIAL HYPOTENSION

Idiopathic intracranial hypertension affects the vision of obese females of the childbearing age group. Though the majority of patients can be treated with conservative management, CSF shunting and optic nerve sheath fenestration (ONSF) are being most commonly performed surgical procedures for resistant IIH. Lumboperitoneal shunting is preferred as ventricles are usually very small. ONSF is preferred when visual symptoms predominate or persist after shunting.[127] Recently, endoscopic endonasal ONSF is being done with good results.[128]

Spontaneous intracranial hypotension (SIH) is caused by spinal leakage of CSF and it is characterized by an orthostatic headache without a history of trauma or dural puncture. At present, epidural blood patch is the mainstay of treatment for SIH and occasionally associated subdural hematoma may require drainage.[129]

CONGENITAL ANOMALIES OF THE BRAIN

Among the various congenital anomalies of the brain in small children, craniosynostosis surgery has undergone a significant change with a better understanding of raised ICP, the role of venous congestion and hypertension associated, and the cosmetic aspect.[130] As is widely understood for craniofacial reconstructions, the forehead, nose, and face are better repaired at a later age. Many of the decompression procedures are, therefore, carried out by posterior decompression or distraction with temporary rods as the first step.[131,132]

Chiari malformation type II decompression for respiratory failure in a small group of meningomyelocele patients with a functioning shunt has not been found of much use.[133] Asymptomatic Chiari I with or without syringomyelia in small children is observed. Onsets of symptoms and increase in syrinx or ventricular size are evaluated at follow-up and treated accordingly.[134]

Arachnoid cysts of the middle fossa and suprasellar region are being increasingly treated with endoscopic fenestration and the role of shunt surgery and major craniotomy has considerably reduced in these patients.[135] Smaller arachnoid cysts of the middle fossa (Galassi type 1 and 2) frequently remain stable and do not require surgical treatment.[136]

CONGENITAL ANOMALIES OF THE SPINE

A better understanding of congenital anomalies of the spinal cord causing tethering has become a matter of major interest as it can develop neurological deficits during the growth period.[137] Better imaging and electrophysiology have allowed the rational use of preventive untethering surgery.

The concept of junctional neurulation[137] and the newer entities, viz., limited dorsal myeloschisis, has been described by Pang et al. **(Figs. 8A to C)**.[138] Lipomas have been classified further in a better way to allow proper use of surgery.[139,140] The uses of intraoperative monitoring including sphincters and stimulation methods have improved the safety of surgery.[141]

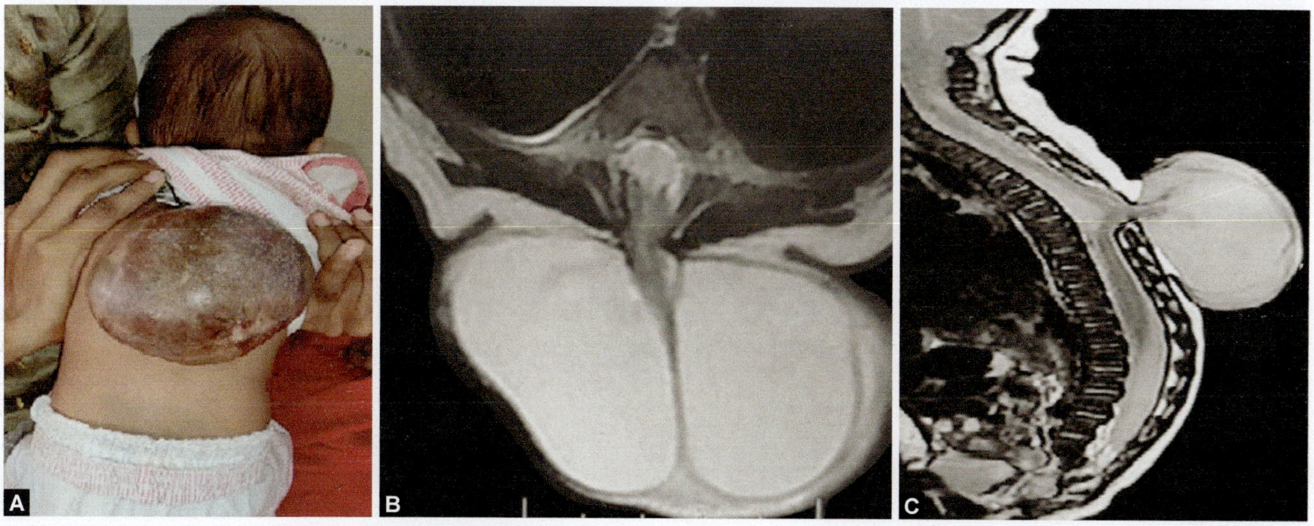

FIGS. 8A TO C: (A) A 6-month-old child presented with a large swelling on the dorsal back; (B and C) show cystic lesion without neural herniation, confirming limited dorsal myeloschisis (LDM).

CRANIOVERTEBRAL JUNCTION

Craniovertebral junction (CVJ) anomalies like basilar invagination have long been treated with transoral odontoidectomy followed by posterior wire-based instrumentation. Advancements in screw–rod constructs and a better understanding of biomechanics have helped in achieving excellent decompression and stability with purely posterior screw–rod instrumentation thus avoiding anterior surgery.[142,143] In addition, CVJ anomalies, which were previously thought to be "irreducible and fixed," can also be tackled safely and reduced with modern CVJ screw–rod constructs.[142,143] Multiple screw entry points and screw trajectories exist to achieve safe fixation in presence of anomalous vertebral artery anatomy. Though it is rarely required after a good distraction surgery, anterior decompression by odontectomy is being increasingly performed by endoscopic methods.[144,145]

SPINAL SURGERY

Recent advances in spine surgery have seen a trend toward minimally invasive approaches and better instrumentation, including robotics aided by better imaging. The conceptual changes in managing some congenital anomalies and spinal injuries are still evolving.

Minimally Invasive Spine Surgery

There have been rapid advances in the field of spine surgery. One of the most remarkable changes in spine surgery has been the rapid implementation and adoption of minimally invasive techniques in the management of spinal pathology. The era of minimally invasive spine surgery (MISS) techniques started in 1997 with the development of the tubular retractor by Foley et al.[146] This was followed by the widespread use of tubular retractor systems and endoscopes for the management of spinal diseases. Further refinement of spinal instrumentation such as the development of percutaneous pedicle screws, interbody cages, bone biologics like bone morphogenic protein, development of dural substitutes, etc. helped in popularizing the usage of MISS techniques. MISS techniques allow for the same procedure to be performed by minimizing injury to paraspinal muscles and reducing the access-related surgical trauma and thus reducing intraoperative blood loss, perioperative infection, perioperative pain, faster recovery, and early return to work than conventional open spine surgery **(Figs. 9A and B)**. Currently, it is possible to perform procedures like microendoscopic/endoscopic discectomy, spinal decompression, and transforaminal lumbar interbody fusion (TLIF) without general anesthesia thus making the procedure safer.[147]

Spinal Instrumentation

Modern spinal instrumentation using titanium screw–rod constructs replacing all wire-based instrumentation has helped in achieving rigid fixation, which in turn has allowed rapid postoperative mobilization techniques without long-term immobilization which was the norm with wire-based instrumentation. Modern spinal instrumentation is biomechanically stronger, achieves better spinal fusion, is compatible with MRI, and causes less tissue reaction and fewer artifacts in imaging. Standardization of spinal implants has made them easier to place and easier to revise. The widespread application of navigation-guided spinal surgery has immensely benefitted spine surgery by improving the accuracy of screw placement and also by potentially reducing radiation exposure.

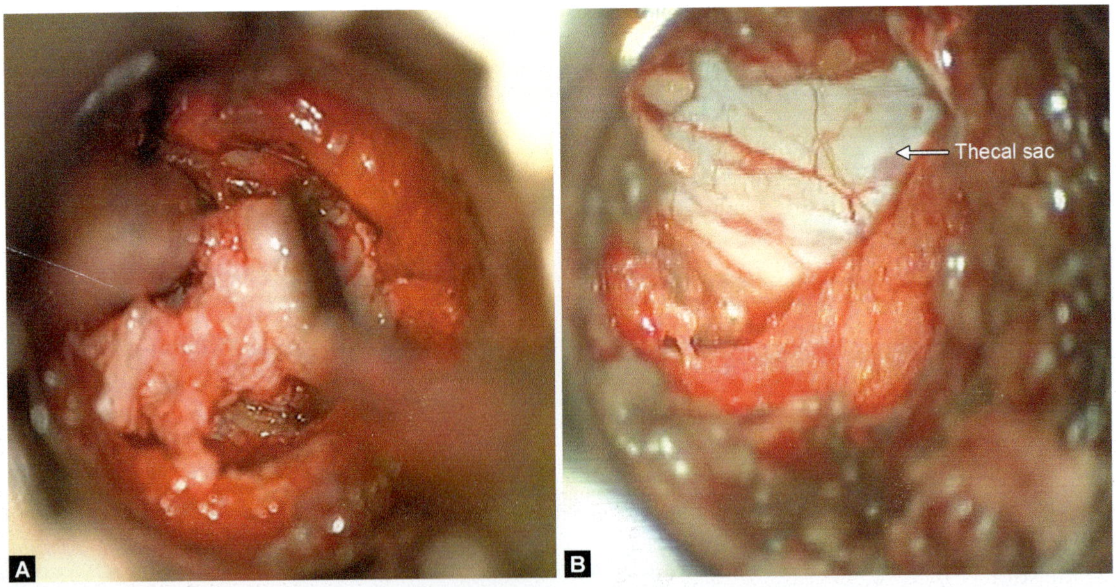

FIGS. 9A AND B: Minimally invasive spine surgery (MISS) discectomy using tubular retractor with minimal muscle trauma by dilation, without devascularization, with precise exposure: (A) Disk material; and (B) Thecal sac.

Pediatric spinal implants are also widely available now. 3D printing has opened newer avenues in the creation of patient-specific models for preoperative planning, guides for the placement of instrumentation, and eventually patient-specific spinal implants.[148] As further improvement in technology takes place, it is hoped that 3D printing will become cheaper and more widely available making the development of patient-specific implants a reality.

Application of Robotics in Spine Surgery

The use of robotics has become a reality in many surgical fields. In spine surgery, robotics works on a shared-control principle where both the surgeon and the robot control the surgical field simultaneously.[149] Currently, the use of the spine robot system is mainly for the placement of thoracolumbar pedicle screws. Multiple studies including randomized controlled trial (RCT) have shown that robot-assisted screw placement is more accurate than conventionally placed screws (97% *vs.* 95.4% accuracy).[150] Spine robotics is also useful in reducing the incidence of spinal revision surgery due to misplaced screws, reducing radiation exposure, helping in tumor excision, complex deformity surgery, etc.[149] The main limitations of spine robotics are the cost and availability.

Newer Imaging Modalities

Image acquisition techniques have undergone significant improvement in the past two decades. Low-dose weight-bearing X-ray (EOS) can take simultaneous AP and lateral radiographs producing a 2D or 3D with a lower dose of radiation than conventional imaging.[151] These imaging modalities have helped to understand the sagittal and coronal balance of the spine, as well as allowed the calculation of spinopelvic parameters to plan spinal deformity correction procedures.

Newer MRI modalities like SWI have helped in the identification of petechial hemorrhages in spinal cord injury (SCI). Diffusion-weighted imaging (DWI) and DTI have helped in understanding the microstructural changes of the spinal cord and the direction of demyelination or remyelination in patients with SCI and degenerative cervical myelopathy (DCM).[151,152] Functional connectivity of the spinal cord can be determined using resting state fMRI.[152] CT perfusion has been also been employed to differentiate between neoplastic and inflammatory diseases of the spine.[151]

Outcome Analysis

Better outcome parameters and patient-reported outcome measures have allowed the proper assessment of outcomes of various techniques.

There has been an incremental application of predictive analysis in spine surgery by using artificial intelligence with machine learning programs. This has led to better statistical models to predict patient outcomes and thus prognosticate patient outcomes. In a study of about 1 million patients undergoing spine surgery, the authors were able to predict a higher incidence of adverse events for patients requiring instrumentation, undergoing anterior and posterior fusion, presence of infection, and the presence of a neurological disorder using machine learning algorithms.[153] It is hoped in the future that several more outcome predictors will be found using "big data" analysis.

Landmark trials and results in the last two decades which have influenced the practice of spinal surgery are:

- *Lumbar degenerative disease*: SPORT was a landmark RCT that was first published in 2006, to compare the outcomes of surgery versus nonoperative management for treatment of lumbar disk herniation, lumbar canal stenosis, and lumbar stenosis with spondylolisthesis. The 4-year and 8-year follow-up data for lumbar disk patients revealed that the patients undergoing surgery had a consistently better outcome than patients not undergoing surgery. Interestingly, the 2-year follow-up data did not show any differences, most likely due to a high crossover to the surgery group.[154] The 2-year, 4-year, and 8-year follow-up data for degenerative lumbar spinal stenosis with spondylolisthesis patients revealed that the patients undergoing surgery had a consistently better outcome than patients not undergoing surgery, irrespective of the type of fusion surgery.[155] The 2-year, 4-year, and 8-year follow-up data for lumbar spinal stenosis patients revealed that the patients undergoing surgery had a consistently better outcome than patients not undergoing surgery.[156]
- *Degenerative cervical myelopathy*: DCM is the most common cause of spinal cord dysfunction worldwide. The role of surgery in moderate and severe DCM is firmly established. In mild DCM, the role of close clinical and radiological surveillance is warranted with an increasing role of surgery. The Cervical Spondylotic Myelopathy–International (CSM-I) trial showed that patients were more likely to achieve a good outcome if they had milder disease preoperatively, were younger in age, had no or minimal comorbidities, did not smoke, did not have gait disturbances, and had a shorter duration of symptoms.[157] CSM-S trial was an RCT to compare the outcomes of anterior surgery versus posterior surgery. The 1-year follow-up outcome data showed equivalence in the outcomes in both surgical groups.[158]
- *Spinal cord injury*: SCI is currently one of the most intensely researched conditions in the field of medicine. However, none of these interventions has made a successful transition from "bench to bedside." One of the controversial topics of the timing of surgery in SCI was answered in the STACSIS trial where it was shown that decompression surgery within 24 hours of injury not only was safe but also leads to better neurological outcomes.[159]

Since SCI and DCM share many pathophysiological processes, it is hoped that successful translational research in one field may lead to similar applications in the other.

NEUROANESTHESIA AND CRITICAL CARE

Brain and spine surgeries have become much safer with newer inhalational and intravenous agents, which are short-acting, less toxic anesthetic agents, and the emergence of better monitoring during surgery for hemodynamic parameters as well as the depth of anesthesia. Awake surgery for eloquent area tumors and epilepsy cases is being increasingly done in several centers.

Postoperative care has improved further with the advent of neuroanesthesia and neurocritical care as a specialty teaming with the new breed of specialist consultants. Neuroanesthesia and critical care training has also become formally available in India with accreditation. Traditionally, neurologists and neurosurgeons managing their ICU patients have changed in most academic units and taken over by neurocritical care consultants. Protocols have been developed for postoperative care with better patient outcomes.[160]

CONCLUSION

As can be seen from the above discussion, several advances have taken place in neurosurgical concepts, technology, and approaches to the management of most of neurosurgical diseases in the last few years. As a result, the procedures have become more precise, and respect for normal surrounding tissue is realized. Coupled with advances in the diagnostic armamentarium and improvement of perioperative specialized care, patient outcomes have been more satisfactory. The field is ever-changing and readers should use the information presented here as building blocks for their further reading.

REFERENCES

1. Nucifora RL, Melhem ER, Nucifora PG. DTI in neurosurgical planning. Wolf Diffusion Tensor Imaging: A Practical Handbook. Switzerland: Springer Nature; 2016. pp. 291-308.
2. Yagmurlu K, Middlebrooks EH, Tanriover N, Rhoton AL Jr. Fiber tracts of the dorsal language stream in the human brain. J Neurosurg. 2016;124(5):1396-405.
3. Vlieger EJ, Majoie CB, Leenstra S, Den Heeten GJ. Functional magnetic resonance imaging for neurosurgical planning in neurooncology. Eur Radiol. 2004;14(7):1143-53.
4. Henderson F Jr, Abdullah KG, Verma R, Brem S. Tractography and the connectome in neurosurgical treatment of gliomas: the premise, the progress, and the potential. Neurosurg Focus. 2020; 48(2):E6.
5. Doyen S, Nicholas P, Poologaindran A, Crawford L, Young IM, Romero-Garcia R, et al. Connectivity-based parcellation of normal and anatomically distorted human cerebral cortex. Hum Brain Mapp. 2022;43(4):1358-69.
6. Barnett GH, Kormos DW, Steiner CP, Weisenberger J. Intraoperative localization using an armless, frameless stereotactic wand. Technical note [technical note]. J Neurosurg. 1993;78(3):510-4.
7. Sandeman DR, Gill SS. The impact of interactive image guided surgery: the Bristol experience with the ISG/Elekta viewing Wand. Acta Neurochir Suppl. 1995;64:54-8.
8. Yeole U, Singh V, Mishra A, Shaikh S, Shetty P, Moiyadi A. Navigated intraoperative ultrasonography for brain tumors: a pictorial essay on the technique, its utility, and its benefits in neuro-oncology. Ultrasonography. 2020;39(4):394-406.
9. Hayhurst C, Byrne P, Eldridge PR, Mallucci CL. Application of electromagnetic technology to neuronavigation: a revolution in image-guided neurosurgery. J Neurol Surg. 2009;111(6):1179-84.
10. Teng CW, Huang V, Arguelles GR, Zhou C, Cho SS, Harmsen S, et al. Applications of indocyanine green in brain tumor surgery: review of clinical evidence and emerging technologies. Neurosurg Focus. 2021;50(1):E4.
11. Hadjipanayis CG, Widhalm G, Stummer W. What is the surgical benefit of utilizing 5-ALA for fluorescence-guided surgery of malignant gliomas? Neurosurgery. 2015;77(5):663-73.
12. Wirtz CR, Bonsanto MM, Knauth M, Tronnier VM, Albert FK, Staubert A, et al. Intraoperative magnetic resonance imaging to update interactive navigation in neurosurgery: method and preliminary experience. Comput Aided Surg. 1997;2(3-4):172-9.
13. Zaidi HA, De Los Reyes K, Barkhoudarian G, Litvack ZN, Bi WL, Rincon-Torroella J, et al. The utility of high-resolution intraoperative MRI in endoscopic transsphenoidal surgery for pituitary macroadenomas: early experience in the Advanced multimodality Image Guided Operating suite. Neurosurg Focus. 2016;40(3):E18.
14. Ringel F, Sala F. Intraoperative mapping and monitoring in supratentorial tumor surgery. J Neurosurg Sci. 2015;59(2):129-39.
15. Kanno A, Mikuni N. Evaluation of language function under awake craniotomy. Neurol Med Chir (Tokyo). 2015;55(5):367-73.
16. Hervey-Jumper SL, Berger MS. Maximizing safe resection of low- and high-grade glioma. J Neurooncol. 2016;130(2):269-82.
17. Sanai N, Berger MS. Glioma extent of resection and its impact on patient outcome. Neurosurgery. 2008;62(4):753-64; discussion 264-6.
18. Duffau H. Higher-order surgical questions for diffuse low-grade gliomas: supramaximal resection, neuroplasticity, and screening. Neurosurg Clin N Am. 2019;30(1):119-28.
19. Louis DN, Perry A, Reifenberger G, von Deimling A, Figarella-Branger D, Cavenee WK, et al. The 2016 World Health Organization Classification of Tumors of the central nervous system: a summary. Acta Neuropathol. 2016;131(6):803-20.
20. Louis DN, Perry A, Wesseling P, Brat DJ, Cree IA, Figarella-Branger D, et al. The 2021 WHO Classification of Tumors of the central nervous system: a summary. Neuro Oncol. 2021;23(8):1231-51.
21. Taylor MD, Northcott PA, Korshunov A, Remke M, Cho YJ, Clifford SC, et al. Molecular subgroups of medulloblastoma: the current consensus. Acta Neuropathol. 2012;123(4):465-72.
22. Witt H, Mack SC, Ryzhova M, Bender S, Sill M, Isserlin R, et al. Delineation of two clinically and molecularly distinct subgroups of posterior fossa ependymoma. Cancer Cell. 2011;20(2):143-57.
23. Fukuhara N, Iwata T, Inoshita N, Yoshimoto K, Kitagawa M, Fukuhara H, et al. Immunohistochemistry or molecular analysis: which method is better for subtyping craniopharyngioma? Endocr Pathol. 2021;32(2):262-8.
24. Sadighi Z, Slopis J. Pilocytic astrocytoma: a disease with evolving molecular heterogeneity. J Child Neurol. 2013;28(5):625-32.

25. Kondziolka D, Shin SM, Brunswick A, Kim I, Silverman JS. The biology of radiosurgery and its clinical applications for brain tumors. Neuro Oncol. 2015;17(1):29-44.
26. Sergi B, Settimi S, Federici G, Galloni C, Cantaffa C, De Corso E, et al. Factors influencing personalized management of vestibular schwannoma: A systematic review. J Pers Med. 2022;12(10):1616.
27. Micko AS, Wöhrer A, Wolfsberger S, Knosp E. Invasion of the cavernous sinus space in pituitary adenomas: endoscopic verification and its correlation with an MRI-based classification. J Neurosurg. 2015;122(4):803-11.
28. Shimon I, Melmed S. Management of pituitary tumors. Ann Intern Med. 1998;129(6):472-83.
29. Fatemi N, Dusick JR, de Paiva Neto MA, Kelly DF. The endonasal microscopic approach for pituitary adenomas and other parasellar tumors: a 10-year experience. Neurosurgery. 2008;63(4);(Suppl 2): 244-56; discussion 256.
30. Kassam AB, Snyderman C, Gardner P, Carrau R, Spiro R. The expanded endonasal approach: a fully endoscopic transnasal approach and resection of the odontoid process: technical case report. Neurosurgery. 2005;57(1);Suppl:E213; discussion E213.
31. Marx S, Clemens S, Schroeder HWS. The value of endoscope assistance during transcranial surgery for tuberculum sellae meningiomas. J Neurosurg. 2018;128(1):32-9.
32. Molitch ME, Drummond J, Korbonits M. Prolactinoma management. In: Feingold KR, Anawalt B, Boyce A (Eds). Endotext [internet]. South Dartmouth (MA): MDText.com, Inc.; 2000.
33. Nishioka H, Inoshita N. New WHO classification of pituitary adenomas (4th edition): assessment of pituitary transcription factors and the prognostic histological factors. Brain Tumor Pathol. 2018;35(2):57-61.
34. Stachura K, Grzywna E, Krzyżewski RM, Kwinta BM. Retrospective evaluation of endoscopic treatment in colloid cyst of the third ventricle. Wideochir Inne Tech Maloinwazyjne. 2021;16(3): 604-11.
35. Deopujari C, Shroff K, Karmarkar V, Mohanty C. Neuroendoscopy in the management of pineal region tumours in children. Child Nerv Syst. 2022. Online ahead of print.
36. Attri G, Gosal JS, Khatri D, Das KK, Bhaisora KS, Mehrotra A, et al. Endoscopic third ventriculostomy and simultaneous tumor biopsy in pineal region tumors using the "single burr hole" technique: an analysis of 34 cases. Asian J Neurosurg. 2020;15(4):976-82.
37. Deopujari CE, Karmarkar VS, Shaikh ST, Mohanty CB, Sharma V, Tadghare J, et al. Neuroendoscopy in the surgical management of lateral and third ventricular tumors: looking beyond microneurosurgery. Neurol India. 2021;69(6):1571-8.
38. Souweidane MM. Endoscopic surgery for intraventricular brain tumors in patients without hydrocephalus. Neurosurgery. 2008;62(6 Suppl 3):1042-8.
39. Oertel JM, Montibeller GR. Skull base endoscopic-assisted surgery. Endoscopy – innovative uses and emerging technologies. London: IntechOpen; 2015.
40. Plaha P, Livermore LJ, Voets N, Pereira E, Cudlip S. Minimally invasive endoscopic resection of intraparenchymal brain tumors. World Neurosurg. 2014;82(6):1198-208.
41. Bajaj J, Ratre S, Yadav YR. Endoscopic-assisted C2 transverse process mass excision. Neurol India. 2021;69(3):582-6.
42. Jalali R, Sudarsan RT. Advances in radiation therapy in malignant brain tumors. Int J Neurooncol. 2021;4(Suppl S1):208-16.
43. Stupp R, Mason WP, van den Bent MJ, Weller M, Fisher B, Taphoorn MJ, et al. Radiotherapy plus concomitant and adjuvant temozolomide for glioblastoma. N Engl J Med. 2005;352(10):987-96.
44. Chen S, Visintini S. Extended dosing (12 cycles) of adjuvant temozolomide in adults with newly diagnosed high grade gliomas: a review of clinical effectiveness, cost-effectiveness, and guidelines [internet]. Ottawa, (ON): Canadian Agency for Drugs and Technologies in Health; 2018.
45. Krueger DA, Care MM, Holland K, Agricola K, Tudor C, Mangeshkar P, et al. Everolimus for subependymal giant-cell astrocytomas in tuberous sclerosis. N Engl J Med. 2010;363(19):1801-11.
46. Kowalewski A, Durślewicz J, Zdrenka M, Grzanka D, Szylberg Ł. Clinical relevance of BRAF V600E mutation status in brain tumors with a Focus on a novel management algorithm. Target Oncol. 2020;15(4):531-40.
47. Alahmari M, Temel Y. Skull base chordoma treated with proton therapy: A systematic review. Surg Neurol Int. 2019;10:96.
48. Vogel TW, Bahuleyan B, Robinson S, Cohen AR. The role of endoscopic third ventriculostomy in the treatment of hydrocephalus. J Neurosurg Pediatr. 2013;12(1):54-61.
49. Kulkarni AV, Drake JM, Mallucci CL, Sgouros S, Roth J, Constantini S, et al. Endoscopic third ventriculostomy in the treatment of childhood hydrocephalus. J Pediatr. 2009;155(2):254-9.e1.
50. Kulkarni AV, Sgouros S, Leitner Y, Constantini S; International Infant Hydrocephalus Study Investigators. International Infant Hydrocephalus Study (IIHS): 5-year health outcome results of a prospective, multicenter comparison of endoscopic third ventriculostomy (ETV) and shunt for infant hydrocephalus. Child Nerv Syst. 2018;34(12):2391-7.
51. Linares Torres J, Ros López B, Iglesias Moroño S, Ros Sanjuán Á, Selfa Rodríguez A, Cerro Larrazábal L, et al. Re-Do endoscopic third ventriculostomy. Retrospective analysis of 13 patients. Neurocirugia (Astur: Engl Ed). 2021;2100026-9:S1130-1473(21)00026-9.
52. Yadav YR, Bajaj J, Ratre S, Yadav N, Parihar V, Swamy N, et al. Endoscopic third ventriculostomy - a review. Neurol India. 2021;69 (Suppl S2):502-13.
53. Shaikh S, Deopujari CE, Karmarkar V, Muley K, Mohanty C. Role of secondary endoscopic third ventriculostomy in children: review of an institutional experience. Pediatr Neurosurg;2019;54(3):188-195.
54. Oertel JM, Schroeder HW, Gaab MR. Endoscopic stomy of the septum pellucidum: indications, technique, and results. Neurosurgery. 2009;64(3):482-91; discussion 491.
55. Molyneux AJ, Kerr RS, Yu LM, Clarke M, Sneade M, Yarnold JA, et al. International Subarachnoid Aneurysm Trial (ISAT) of neurosurgical clipping versus endovascular coiling in 2143 patients with ruptured intracranial aneurysms: a randomised comparison of effects on survival, dependency, seizures, rebleeding, subgroups, and aneurysm occlusion. Lancet. 2005;366(9488):809-17.
56. Molyneux AJ, Kerr RS, Birks J, Ramzi N, Yarnold J, Sneade M, et al. Risk of recurrent subarachnoid haemorrhage, death, or dependence and standardised mortality ratios after clipping or coiling of an intracranial aneurysm in the International Subarachnoid Aneurysm Trial (ISAT): long-term follow-up. Lancet Neurol. 2009;8(5):427-33.
57. Molyneux AJ, Birks J, Clarke A, Sneade M, Kerr RSC. The durability of endovascular coiling versus neurosurgical clipping of ruptured cerebral aneurysms: 18 year follow-up of the UK cohort of the International Subarachnoid Aneurysm Trial (ISAT). Lancet. 2015;385(9969):691-7.
58. Spetzler RF, McDougall CG, Zabramski JM, Albuquerque FC, Hills NK, Russin JJ, et al. The Barrow Ruptured Aneurysm Trial: 6-year results. J Neurosurg. 2015;123(3):609-17.
59. Li J, Lan Z, He M, You C. Assessment of microscope-integrated indocyanine green angiography during intracranial aneurysm surgery: a retrospective study of 120 patients. Neurol India. 2009;57(4):453-9.
60. Park ES, Kim DW, Kang SD. Endovascular treatment of symptomatic vasospasm after aneurysmal subarachnoid hemorrhage: A three-year experience. J Cerebrovasc Endovasc Neurosurg. 2017;19(3):155-61.
61. Krishna C, Sonig A, Natarajan SK, Siddiqui AH. The expanding realm of endovascular neurosurgery: flow diversion for cerebral aneurysm management. Methodist Debakey Cardiovasc J. 2014;10 (4):214-9.

62. Wiebers DO, Whisnant JP, Huston J 3rd, Meissner I, Brown RD Jr., Piepgras DG, et al. Unruptured intracranial aneurysms: natural history, clinical outcome, and risks of surgical and endovascular treatment. Lancet. 2003;362(9378):103-10.
63. UCAS Japan Investigators, Morita A, Kirino T, Hashi K, Aoki N, Fukuhara S, et al. The natural course of unruptured cerebral aneurysms in a Japanese cohort. N Engl J Med. 2012;366(26):2474-82.
64. Kim H, Al-Shahi Salman R, McCulloch CE, Stapf C, Young WL, MARS Coinvestigators. Untreated brain arteriovenous malformation. Patient-level meta-analysis of haemorrhage predictors. Neurology. 2014;83(7):590-7.
65. Lawton MT, Kim H, McCulloch CE, Mikhak B, Young WL. A supplementary grading scale for selecting patients with brain arteriovenous malformations for surgery. Neurosurgery. 2010;66(4):702-13; discussion 713.
66. Van Beijnum J, van der Worp HB, Buis DR, Salman RA-S, Kappelle LJ, Rinkel GJE, et al. Treatment of brain arteriovenous malformations: a systematic review and meta-analysis. JAMA. 2011;306(18):2011-9.
67. Lak AM, Cerecedo-Lopez CD, Cha J, Aziz-Sultan MA, Frerichs KU, Gormley WB, et al. Seizure outcomes after interventional treatment in cerebral arteriovenous malformation–associated epilepsy: A systematic review and meta-Analysis. World Neurosurg. 2022;160:e9-e22.
68. Mamaril-Davis JC, Aguilar-Salinas P, Avila MJ, Nakaji P, Bina RW. Complete seizure-free rates following interventional treatment of intracranial arteriovenous malformations: a systematic review and meta-analysis. Neurosurg Rev. 2022;45(2):1313-26.
69. Peschillo S, Caporlingua A, Colonnese C, Guidetti G. Brain AVMs: an endovascular, surgical, and radiosurgical update. ScientificWorldJournal. 2014;2014:834931.
70. Kano H, Lunsford LD, Flickinger JC, Yang HC, Flannery TJ, Awan NR, et al. Stereotactic radiosurgery for arteriovenous malformations, Part 1: management of Spetzler-Martin grade I and II arteriovenous malformations. J Neurosurg. 2012;116(1):11-20.
71. Sirin S, Kondziolka D, Niranjan A, Flickinger JC, Maitz AH, Lunsford LD. Prospective staged volume radiosurgery for large arteriovenous malformations: indications and outcomes in otherwise untreatable patients. Neurosurgery. 2006;58(1):17-27.
72. Mohr JP, Parides MK, Stapf C, Moquete E, Moy CS, Overbey JR, et al. Medical management with or without interventional therapy for unruptured brain arteriovenous malformations (Aruba): a multicenter, non-blinded, randomized trial. Lancet. 2014;383(9917):614-21.
73. Satomi J, Satoh K. Epidemiology and etiology of dural arteriovenous fistula. Brain Nerve. 2008;60(8):883-6.
74. Cohen SD, Goins JL, Butler SG, Morris PP, Browne JD. Dural arteriovenous fistula: diagnosis, treatment, and outcomes. Laryngoscope. 2009;119(2):293-7.
75. Halefoglu AM, Yousem DM. Susceptibility weighted imaging: clinical applications and future directions. World J Radiol. 2018;10(4):30-45.
76. Horne MA, Flemming KD, Su IC, Stapf C, Jeon JP, Li D, et al. Clinical course of untreated cerebral cavernous malformations: a meta-analysis of individual patient data. Lancet Neurol. 2016;15(2):166-73.
77. Casazza M, Broggi G, Franzini A, Avanzini G, Spreafico R, Bracchi M, et al. Supratentorial cavernous angiomas and epileptic seizures: preoperative course and postoperative outcome. Neurosurgery. 1996;39(1):26-32; discussion 32.
78. Englot DJ, Han SJ, Lawton MT, Chang EF. Predictors of seizure freedom in the surgical treatment of supratentorial cavernous malformations. J Neurosurg. 2011;115(6):1169-74.
79. Kondziolka D, Lunsford LD, Flickinger JC, Kestle JRW. Reduction of hemorrhage risk after stereotactic radiosurgery for cavernous malformations. J Neurosurg. 1995;83(5):825-31.
80. Shroff K, Deopujari C, Karmarkar V, Mohanty C. Paediatric giant cavernomas: report of three cases with a review of the literature. Childs Nerv Syst. 2021;37(12):3835-45.
81. Matsushima T, Inoue T, Ikezaki K, Matsukado K, Natori Y, Inamura T, et al. Multiple combined indirect procedure for the surgical treatment of children with Moyamoya disease. A comparison with single indirect anastomosis with direct anastomosis. Neurosurg Focus. 1998;5(5):e4.
82. Ausman JI, Diaz FG, Sadasivan B, Gonzeles-Portillo M, Malik GM, Deopujari CE. Giant intracranial aneurysm surgery: the role of microvascular reconstruction. Surg Neurol. 1990;34(1):8-15.
83. Couldwell WT, Taussky P, Sivakumar W. Submandibular high-flow bypass in the treatment of skull base lesions: an analysis of long-term outcome. Neurosurgery. 2012;71(3):645-50; discussion 650.
84. Mohit AA, Sekhar LN, Natarajan SK, Britz GW, Ghodke B. High-flow bypass grafts in the management of complex intracranial aneurysms. Neurosurgery. 2007;60(2 Suppl 1):ONS105-22; discussion ONS122.
85. Mendelow AD, Gregson BA, Fernandes HM, Murray GD, Teasdale GM, Hope DT, et al. Early surgery versus initial conservative treatment in patients with spontaneous supratentorial intracerebral haematomas in the international surgical trial in intracerebral haemorrhage (STICH): A randomised trial. Lancet. 2005;365(9457):387-97.
86. Mendelow AD. Operation versus non-operative treatment for spontaneous supratentorial intracerebral haemorrhage: is a change in current clinical practice required? Neurol India. 2017;65(4): 759-60.
87. Yao Z, Hu X, You C, He M. Effect and feasibility of endoscopic surgery in spontaneous intracerebral hemorrhage: A systematic review and meta-analysis. World Neurosurg. 2018;113:348-356.e2.
88. Mould WA, Carhuapoma JR, Muschelli J, Lane K, Morgan TC, McBee NA, et al. Minimally invasive surgery plus recombinant tissue-type plasminogen activator for intracerebral hemorrhage evacuation decreases perihematomal edema. Stroke. 2013;44(3):627-34.
89. Hannah TC, Kellner R, Kellner CP. Minimally invasive intracerebral hemorrhage evacuation techniques: a review. Diagnostics (Basel). 2021;11(3):576.
90. Ratre S, Yadav N, Parihar VS, Dubey A, Yadav YR. Endoscopic surgery of spontaneous basal ganglionic hemorrhage. Neurol India. 2018;66(6):1694-703.
91. Deopujari C, Shaikh S. Spontaneous intracerebral hemorrhage. Neurol India. 2018;66(6):1704-5.
92. Sivakumar W, Zada G, Yashar P, Giannotta SL, Teitelbaum G, Larsen DW. Endovascular management of spinal dural arteriovenous fistulas. Neurosurg Focus. 2009;26(5):E15.
93. Thind H, Hardesty DA, Zabramski JM, Spetzler RF, Nakaji P. The role of microscope-integrated near-infrared indocyanine green videoangiography in the surgical treatment of intracranial dural arteriovenous fistulas. J Neurosurg. 2015;122(4):876-82.
94. Chesnut RM, Temkin N, Carney N, Dikmen S, Rondina C, Videtta W, et al. A trial of intracranial-pressure monitoring in traumatic brain injury. N Engl J Med. 2012;367(26):2471-81.
95. Dash HH, Chavali S. Management of traumatic brain injury patients. Korean J Anesthesiol. 2018;71(1):12-21.
96. Le Roux P, Menon DK, Citerio G, Vespa P, Bader MK, Brophy GM, et al. Consensus Summary Statement of the International Multidisciplinary Consensus Conference on multimodality Monitoring in Neurocritical Care: A statement for healthcare professionals from the Neurocritical Care Society and the European Society of Intensive Care Medicine. Neurocrit Care. 2014;21(S2): 1-26.
97. Hemphill JC, Andrews P, De Georgia M. Multimodal monitoring and neurocritical care bioinformatics. Nat Rev Neurol. 2011;7(8): 451-60.
98. Cooper DJ, Rosenfeld JV, Murray L, Arabi YM, Davies AR, D'Urso P, et al. Decompressive craniectomy in diffuse traumatic brain injury. N Engl J Med. 2011;364(16):1493-502.
99. Hutchinson PJ, Kolias AG, Timofeev IS, Corteen EA, Czosnyka M, Timothy J, et al. Trial of Decompressive Craniectomy for Traumatic Intracranial Hypertension. N Engl J Med. 2016;375(12):1119-30.

100. Gopalakrishnan MS, Shanbhag NC, Shukla DP, Konar SK, Bhat DI, Devi BI. Complications of decompressive craniectomy. Front Neurol. 2018;9:977.
101. Adelson PD. Hypothermia following pediatric traumatic brain injury. J Neurotrauma. 2009;26(3):429-36.
102. Hutchison JS, Ward RE, Lacroix J, Hébert PC, Barnes MA, Bohn DJ, et al. Hypothermia therapy after traumatic brain injury in children. N Engl J Med. 2008;358(23):2447-56.
103. Eljamel MS, Foy PM. Acute traumatic CSF fistulae: the risk of intracranial infection. Br J Neurosurg. 1990;4(5):381-5.
104. Rimmer J, Belk C, Lund VJ, Swift A, White P. Immunisations and antibiotics in patients with anterior skull base cerebrospinal fluid leaks. J Laryngol Otol. 2014;128(7):626-9.
105. Delgado-López PD, Martín-Velasco V, Castilla-Díez JM, Rodríguez-Salazar A, Galacho-Harriero AM, Fernández-Arconada O. Dexamethasone treatment in chronic subdural haematoma. Neurocirugia (Astur). 2009;20(4):346-59.
106. Kutty RK, Leela SK, Sreemathyamma SB, Sivanandapanicker JL, Asher P, Peethambaran A, et al. The outcome of medical management of chronic subdural hematoma with tranexamic acid - a prospective observational study. J Stroke Cerebrovasc Dis. 2020;29(11):105273.
107. Callovini GM, Bolognini A, Callovini G, Gammone V. Primary enlarged craniotomy in organized chronic subdural hematomas. Neurol Med Chir (Tokyo). 2014;54(5):349-56.
108. Singh H, Patir R, Vaishya S, Miglani R, Gupta A, Kaur A. Endoscopic evacuation of septated chronic subdural hemorrhage - Technical considerations, results, and outcome. Surg Neurol Int. 2022;13:8.
109. Srivatsan A, Mohanty A, Nascimento FA, Hafeez MU, Srinivasan VM, Thomas A, et al. Middle meningeal artery embolization for chronic subdural hematoma: meta-analysis and systematic review. World Neurosurg. 2019;122:613-9.
110. Ironside N, Nguyen C, Do Q, Ugiliweneza B, Chen CJ, Sieg EP, et al. Middle meningeal artery embolization for chronic subdural hematoma: a systematic review and meta-analysis. J Neurointerv Surg. 2021;13(10):951-7.
111. Alkawadri R, Burgess RC, Kakisaka Y, Mosher JC, Alexopoulos AV. Assessment of the utility of ictal magnetoencephalography in the localization of the epileptic seizure onset zone. JAMA Neurol. 2018;75(10):1264-72.
112. Mullin JP, Smithason S, Gonzalez-Martinez J. Stereo-electro-encephalo-graphy (SEEG) with robotic assistance in the presurgical evaluation of medical refractory epilepsy: A technical note. J Vis Exp. 2016;112(112):53206.
113. Lew SM. Hemispherectomy in the treatment of seizures: a review. Transl Pediatr. 2014;3(3):208-17.
114. Villemure JG, Daniel RT. Peri-insular hemispherotomy in paediatric epilepsy. Child Nerv Syst. 2006;22(8):967-81.
115. Delalande O, Bulteau C, Dellatolas G, Fohlen M, Jalin C, Buret V, et al. Vertical parasagittal hemispherotomy: surgical procedures and clinical long-term outcomes in a population of 83 children. Neurosurgery. 2007;60(2 Suppl 1):ONS19-32; discussion ONS32.
116. Chandra SP, Tripathi M. Endoscopic epilepsy surgery: emergence of a new procedure. Neurol India. 2015;63(4):571-82.
117. Bahuleyan B, Manjila S, Robinson S, Cohen AR. Minimally invasive endoscopic transventricular hemispherotomy for medically intractable epilepsy: a new approach and cadaveric demonstration. J Neurosurg Pediatr. 2010;6(6):536-40.
118. Mohamed AR, Freeman JL, Maixner W, Bailey CA, Wrennall JA, Harvey AS. Temporoparietooccipital disconnection in children with intractable epilepsy. J Neurosurg Pediatr. 2011;7(6):660-70.
119. Van Rijckevorsel K. Treatment of Lennox-Gastaut syndrome: overview and recent findings. Neuropsychiatr Dis Treat. 2008;4(6): 1001-19.
120. Tandon V, Chandra PS, Doddamani RS, Subianto H, Bajaj J, Garg A, et al. Stereotactic Radiofrequency Thermocoagulation of Hypothalamic Hamartoma Using Robotic Guidance (ROSA) Coregistered with O-arm Guidance. World Neurosurg. 2018;112:267-74.
121. Bechtereva NP, Bondartchuk AN, Smirnov VM, Meliutcheva LA, Shandurina AN. Method of electrostimulation of the deep brain structures in treatment of some chronic diseases. Confin Neurol. 1975;37(1-3):136-40.
122. Benabid AL, Pollak P, Louveau A, Henry S, de Rougemont J. Combined (thalamotomy and stimulation) stereotactic surgery of the VIM thalamic nucleus for bilateral Parkinson disease. Appl Neurophysiol. 1987;50(1-6):344-6.
123. Benabid AL, Pollak P, Gross C, Hoffmann D, Benazzouz A, Gao DM, et al. Acute and long-term effects of subthalamic nucleus stimulation in Parkinson's disease. Stereotact Funct Neurosurg. 1994;62(1-4):76-84.
124. Rezai AR, Machado AG, Deogaonkar M, Azmi H, Kubu C, Boulis NM. Surgery for movement disorders. Neurosurgery. 2008;62(Suppl 2): SHC-809.
125. Bouton CE, Shaikhouni A, Annetta NV, Bockbrader MA, Friedenberg DA, Nielson DM, et al. Restoring cortical control of functional movement in a human with quadriplegia. Nature. 2016;533(7602):247-50.
126. Solcà M, Krishna V, Young N, Deogaonkar M, Herbelin B, Orepic P, et al. Enhancing analgesic spinal cord stimulation for chronic pain with personalized immersive virtual reality. Pain. 2021;162(6): 1641-9.
127. Feldon SE. Visual outcomes comparing surgical techniques for management of severe idiopathic intracranial hypertension. Neurosurg Focus. 2007;23(5):E6.
128. Srivastava AK, Singh S, Khatri D, Jaiswal AK, Sankar R, Paliwal VK, et al. Endoscopic endonasal optic nerve decompression with durotomy: pis aller in the mind of a blind. Neurol India. 2020;68(1):54-60.
129. Upadhyaya P, Ailani J. A review of spontaneous intracranial hypotension. Curr Neurol Neurosci Rep. 2019;19(5):22.
130. Ghali GZ, Zaki Ghali MG, Ghali EZ, Srinivasan VM, Wagner KM, Rothermel A, et al. Intracranial venous hypertension in craniosynostosis: mechanistic underpinnings and therapeutic implications. World Neurosurg. 2019;127:549-58.
131. White N, Evans M, Dover MS, Noons P, Solanki G, Nishikawa H. Posterior calvarial vault expansion using distraction osteogenesis. Child Nerv Syst. 2009;25(2):231-6.
132. Goodrich JT. Skull base growth in craniosynostosis. Childs Nerv Syst. 2005;21(10):871-9.
133. Kim I, Hopson B, Aban I, Rizk EB, Dias MS, Bowman R, et al. Decompression for Chiari malformation type II in individuals with myelomeningocele in the National Spina Bifida Patient Registry. J Neurosurg Pediatr. 2018;22(6):652-8.
134. Spazzapan P, Bosnjak R, Prestor B, Velnar T. Chiari malformations in children: An overview. World J Clin Cases. 2021;9(4):764-773.
135. Deopujari CE, Shaikh ST, Karmarkar VS, Sudke AY, Mohanty CB, Biyani NK. Experience with management of intracranial arachnoid cysts. J Neurol Surg A Cent Eur Neurosurg. 2021;82(1):43-52.
136. Mustansir F, Bashir S, Darbar A. Management of arachnoid cysts: A comprehensive review. Cureus. 2018;10(4):e2458.
137. Eibach S, Moes G, Hou YJ, Zovickian J, Pang D. Unjoined primary and secondary neural tubes: junctional neural tube defect, a new form of spinal dysraphism caused by disturbance of junctional neurulation. Child Nerv Syst. 2017;33(10):1633-47.
138. Pang DMD, Zovickian JMD, Oviedo AMD, Moes GS. Limited dorsal myeloschisis: A distinctive clinicopathological entity. Neurosurgery. 2010;67(6):1555-79; discussion 1579.
139. Deopujari C, Mhatre M, Agrawal H. Non-dysraphic spinal lipomas. In: Alexiou G, Prodromou N (Eds). Pediatric neurosurgery for clinicians. Cham: Springer; 2022.
140. Morota N, Ihara S, Ogiwara H. New classification of spinal lipomas based on embryonic stage. J Neurosurg Pediatr. 2017;19(4): 428-39.

141. Hoving EW, Haitsma E, Oude Ophuis CM, Journée HL. The value of intraoperative neurophysiological monitoring in tethered cord surgery. Childs Nerv Syst. 2011;27(9):1445-52.
142. Goel A, Desai KI, Muzumdar DP. Atlantoaxial fixation using plate and screw method: a report of 160 treated patients. Neurosurgery. 2002;51(6):1351-6; discussion 1356.
143. Chandra PS, Prabhu M, Goyal N, Garg A, Chauhan A, Sharma BS. Distraction, compression, extension, and reduction combined with joint remodeling and extra-articular distraction: description of 2 new modifications for its application in basilar invagination and atlantoaxial dislocation: prospective study in 79 cases. Neurosurgery. 2015;77(1):67-80; discussion 80.
144. Deopujari CE, Karmarkar VS, Shah NJ. Endoscopic approaches to the craniovertebral junction and odontoid process. World Neurosurg. 2014;82(6 Suppl):S49-53.
145. Yadav YR, Parihar VS, Ratre S, Dubey A, Jindel S, Dubey MN. Endoscopic single stage trans-oral decompression and anterior C1 lateral mass and C2 pedicle stabilization for atlanto-axial dislocation. Neurol India. 2019;67(2):510-5.
146. Foley KT, Smith MM. Microendoscopic discectomy. Tech Neurosurg. 1997;3:301-7.
147. Kolcun JPG, Brusko GD, Wang MY. Endoscopic transforaminal lumbar interbody fusion without general anesthesia: technical innovations and outcomes. Ann Transl Med. 2019;7(Suppl 5): S167.
148. Sheha ED, Gandhi SD, Colman MW. 3D printing in spine surgery. Ann Transl Med. 2019;7(Suppl 5):S164.
149. Galetta MS, Leider JD, Divi SN, Goyal DKC, Schroeder GD. Robotics in spinal surgery. Ann Transl Med. 2019;7(Suppl 5):S165.
150. Tarawneh AM, Salem KM. A systematic review and meta-analysis of randomized controlled trials comparing the accuracy and clinical outcome of pedicle screw placement using robot-assisted technology and conventional freehand technique. Glob Spine J. 2021;11(4):575-86.
151. Nouh MR. Imaging of the spine: where do we stand? World J Radiol. 2019;11(4):55-61.
152. Martin AR, Tadokoro N, Tetreault L, Arocho-Quinones EV, Budde MD, Kurpad SN, et al. Imaging evaluation of degenerative cervical myelopathy: current state of the art and future directions. Neurosurg Clin N Am. 2018;29(1):33-45.
153. Han SS, Azad TD, Suarez PA, Ratliff JK. A machine learning approach for predictive models of adverse events following spine surgery. Spine J. 2019;19(11):1772-81.
154. Lurie JD, Tosteson TD, Tosteson A, Abdu WA, Zhao W, Morgan TS, et al. Long-term outcomes of lumbar spinal stenosis: eight-year results of the Spine Patient Outcomes Research Trial (SPORT). Spine (Phila Pa 1976). 2015;40(2):63-76.
155. Abdu WA, Sacks OA, Tosteson ANA, Zhao W, Tosteson TD, Morgan TS, et al. Long-term results of surgery compared with nonoperative treatment for lumbar degenerative spondylolisthesis in the spine patient outcomes research trial (SPORT). Spine (Phila Pa 1976). 2018;43(23):1619-30.
156. Lurie JD, Tosteson TD, Tosteson AN, Zhao W, Morgan TS, Abdu WA, et al. Surgical versus nonoperative treatment for lumbar disc herniation: eight-year results for the spine patient outcomes research trial. Spine (Phila Pa 1976). 2014;39(1):3-16.
157. Tetreault L, Kopjar B, Côté P, Arnold P, Fehlings MG. A clinical prediction rule for functional outcomes in patients undergoing surgery for degenerative cervical myelopathy: analysis of an international prospective multicenter data set of 757 subjects. J Bone Joint Surg Am. 2015;97(24):2038-46.
158. Ghogawala Z, Terrin N, Dunbar MR, Breeze JL, Freund KM, Kanter AS, et al. Effect of ventral vs dorsal spinal surgery on patient-reported physical functioning in patients with cervical spondylotic myelopathy: A randomized clinical trial. JAMA. 2021;325(10):942-51.
159. Fehlings MG, Vaccaro A, Wilson JR, Singh A, W Cadotte D, Harrop JS, et al. Early versus Delayed Decompression for traumatic Cervical Spinal Cord Injury: Results of the Surgical Timing in Acute Spinal Cord Injury Study (STASCIS). PLoS One. 2012;7(2):e32037.
160. Panda NB, Mahajan S, Chauhan R. Management of postoperative neurosurgical patients. J Neuroanaesthesiol Crit Care. 2019;6: 80-6.

7

SECTION

Counseling and Doctor–Patient Relationship

128

CHAPTER

Holistic Approach: The Art of Healing

Sudhir V Shah

INTRODUCTION

The World Health Organization defines health as a state of physical, mental, and social well-being. Health is the synchronization between the body, mind, and spirit.[1,2] According to Ayurveda, the old Indian healing system, Health is a state when the body, mind, and spirit are blissful (*Prasanna*) and that when all elements and all functions of the body are in order, and that when all perversions (*dosha and vikriti*) are balanced. Health is not merely the absence of the diseases. The unlimited and unrestricted free flow of life force energy across the body, mind, and spirit is defined as holistic health.[3]

Physical, mental, emotional, and spiritual well-being are all part of holistic health.[4] As a result, a person's holistic health can be achieved by the use of various treatments, including spirituality.[2]

Although proper diagnosis and medications are the most important aspects of patient and disease management, a holistic approach is required for total healing.[4,5] A holistic approach or medicine is a form of healing that takes into account the whole individual body, mind, spirit, and emotions in the pursuit of maximum health and wellness.[6] This concept of patient care has been part of the treatment since Hippocrates in Europe.[1]

ORIGIN

The word "Holistic" is derived from the word "Holism".[2]

The philosophical approach emphasizing that the whole is greater than the sum of its parts is known as holism. According to this, the whole cannot be comprehended by examining its constituent parts. The whole is made up of the elements that allow us to perceive and hear reality. When viewed from this aspect, the holistic approach can also be applied to medicine.[2]

While the term "holism" was coined in the 1890s, J Smut stated in his work "Holism and Evolution" in 1926 that "the world has been managed by a holistic process, in which the forms of substance increase continuously and new wholes are being formed," and went on to explain that "medical holism has individualistic, societal, and environmental aspects." Humans are regarded as being a part of the universe, nature, and supernature in which they live. In this view, disease and health are built into the spirit and body. The holistic approach to therapy and healing dates back over 5,000 years.[2]

"The natural healing power within us is the most significant source for recovery," Hippocrates, the Greek physician and founder of medical science, said.[1,2] Before administering a therapeutic drug, the doctor's job is to promote the body's natural healing abilities. "You cannot teach a guy anything; you can only help him find it inside himself," as said by Galileo.[2] Let "Food be our Medicine" and "a healthy mind in a healthy body," as Hippocrates (500 BCE) suggested. He centered his medical practice on a natural, holistic approach to disease treatment, emphasizing the necessity of knowing the patient's health, mental independence, and the need for harmony between the individual and the social and natural environment.[1]

Hippocrates highlighted the importance of a holistic approach, as well as taking into account the disease's spiritual repercussions. "It is more vital to know what kind of person has a disease than to know what kind of ailment a person has," he said.[2] Physical activity, art therapy, music, and drama were all important parts of his health promotion program.[1]

Ayurveda has also emphasized the importance of the holistic approach in great detail and has given characteristics of a good patient, a great physician and has drawn guidelines about the role of nursing staff, caretakers, and family members in the healing process. Also, the great philosopher Socrates (399 BCE) stated that "Just as it is impossible to treat the eye without thinking about the head, or to treat the head without thinking about the body, it is impossible to cure the body without curing the soul."[1]

As a result, healing is a much deeper process than simply relieving symptoms, diagnosing a disease, or even treating a condition. Healing guarantees that all of the body's systems are restored to their original state of balance and well-being.[4]

Every part of the human dimension is uniquely single as well as interconnected with each other, according to the holistic care philosophy, which focuses on individualism and accepts that there is a strong link between body, mind, and spirit.[2] Also, obtaining proper life balance is the key to achieving optimal health, which is the main goal of the treatment.[6]

HOLISTIC MEDICINE OR APPROACH

Holistic treatments treat the whole individual, taking into account mental and social elements rather than treating merely the symptoms of a disease.[7] It offers assistance that considers the whole individual, including its physical, emotional, social, and spiritual well-being.[8]

In many various aspects of holistic care, a holistic approach is considered.[2] This traditional approach not only focuses on the individual as a whole but also on how he or she interacts with his or her surroundings. It highlights the interrelationship between the mind, body, and spirit.[1] Because of people's nature, they should be assessed and treated holistically when necessary.[2] Holistic medicine is a kind of medicine that uses a combination of traditional and alternative therapies to prevent disease and promote optimal health.[3]

It can help to balance the immune system and hormone imbalances, as well as smoothen feelings of unrest, anxiety, and depression instantly and restore full, healthy function to various body systems, resulting in deep spiritual and emotional healing by breaking negative thoughts, and cycle patterns.[1] Holistic technique has the potential to improve mental and physical health while also being cost-effective.[7]

The physical and spiritual requirements should be prioritized in the idea of holism within the holistic care philosophy, without ignoring the medical therapeutic applications. It can be claimed that efficiently fulfilling psychosocial requirements among these demands contribute to the reduction of physical needs while also improving the effectiveness of medical treatment. The holistic treatment and care approaches, as well as the holistic diagnostic, must be examined together in the holistic care philosophy.[2]

Holistic medicine embraces all diagnostic and treatment approaches that are both safe and effective. Here, patient education and engagement in the healing process are important.[3] When treating the patient, it promises to combine traditional and complementary therapeutic approaches.[9] This approach, however, requires health practitioners to be able to analyze and view the patient as a whole "person," not just as a patient with an illness.[2]

What is the Difference between Holistic Medicine and Alternative Medicine?

Holistic medicine differs from alternative medicine in the following ways:

- It emphasizes overall health rather than treating a single ailment.
- It focuses on the individual rather than a specific ailment or condition.
- These systems regard the mind, body, and soul as a single unit.
- It is a way of life.
- Disharmony to mind, body, or spirit can lead to disease or injury.

Holistic medicine can be used ideally in conjunction with conventional medicine, not as a stand-alone treatment.[9]

When you consider modern medicine, developing technology, the inadequacy of healthcare systems, the rise in diseases, changes in climatic conditions, and the fact that healthcare professionals work long hours and under stress, it has become a complex system in which physicians are unable to devote enough time to their patients. Listening, inquiring, and checking are essential skills for providing a holistic service.[8] A health professional is supposed to be a good listener, a good speaker, a great thinker, comprehend and feel the emotions of others, and communicate effectively with good counseling skills to provide quality service in the field of health.[2]

CHARACTERISTICS OF HOLISTIC MEDICINE

Holistic medicine's cornerstone is the belief that each patient is a unique individual made up of body, mind, and spirit and that any healthcare must also take into account a person's surroundings.[10]

The holistic approach emphasizes each patient's uniqueness, the mutuality of the doctor–patient relationship, and each person's responsibility for his or her own health, as well as society's role in health promotion.[10]

PRINCIPLES OF HOLISTIC MEDICINE

It believes that unconditional love and support can heal all illnesses and injuries and that each person is ultimately responsible for his/her own health and well-being. The following are some more principles of holistic medicine:[6]

- A patient is a person, not a disease.
- Everyone has the ability to heal himself.[6]
- Illness is considered a sign of a dysfunction of the whole person, rather than an isolated organ event.
- It is best to look for the underlying causes of the disease rather than only treating the symptoms.[3]
- Treatment focuses on resolving the underlying cause of the ailment rather than just alleviating symptoms.[6]

- Holistic management includes lifestyle suggestions, self-care advice, and the avoidance of traditional medicines and procedures whenever possible.[9]
- Healing is a collaborative effort between the patient and the doctor, addressing all aspects of a person's life through a variety of healthcare approaches.[6]
- Holistic practitioners work closely with patients to have a better understanding of them.
- Holistic physicians use a variety of safe, effective diagnostic, and treatment alternatives, such as:[3]
    - Lifestyle adjustments and self-care education
    - Complementary alternatives
    - Conventional drugs and surgery
- Holistic doctors spend just as much time figuring out what kind of patient has a disease as they do figuring out what kind of ailment a patient has.
- The quality of the relationship developed between the physician and the patient, in which patient autonomy is promoted, is a major driver of healing outcomes.
- The ideal physician-patient interaction considers both the patient's and the physician's needs, desires, awareness, and understanding.
- Physicians have a big influence on their patients.
- Illness, pain, and the dying process can all be educational experiences for patients and doctors.
- Holistic physicians help patients to release the poisonous effects of hostility, shame, greed, despair, and prolonged fear, anger, and sadness by invoking the healing power of love, hope, laughter, and excitement.
- The most effective medication in life is unconditional love. Physicians try to treat patients, themselves, and other practitioners with unconditional love.
- Prevention is preferable to therapy because it is usually less expensive. The most cost-effective method involves invoking the patient's own natural healing skills.
- Optimal health entails a lot more than just avoiding illness. It is the deliberate pursuit of the best characteristics of the human experience's physical, environmental, mental, emotional, spiritual, and social elements.[3]

WHAT IS THE PURPOSE OF A HOLISTIC CARE PLAN?

For centuries, the medical profession has mostly relied on objective disease management, which consists solely of disease treatment. It has recently become clear that treating the sickness alone does not cure the patient as a whole. Treating the condition just alleviates the bodily symptoms, leaving the more complicated psychological, social, and spiritual issues unaffected. Medical practice should be much more than a "chemical game." It is a love-and-trust process. Unfortunately, in modern medicine, this principle is not given enough weight. A patient's quality of life is determined by the treatment of bodily symptoms as well as his psychological and spiritual well-being. As a result, for complete patient care, a holistic treatment approach is the need of the hour. In the framework of holistic cure, the caring attitude and friendliness of nursing and other paramedical staff are very critical.[11]

It is a type of healing based on the belief that diseases arise when the rhythm of the body, mind, soul, and emotions are out of balance. As per the American Holistic Health Association, practitioners must examine the following elements during diagnosis and therapy:[9]

- Physical factors
- Nutritional factors
- Environmental factors
- Emotional factors
- Spiritual factors
- Lifestyle factors[9]

Achieving well-being necessitates balancing the various components of the individual. These are the physical, emotional, mental, and spiritual aspects. This broader, holistic approach to health is an ongoing process that involves the integration of all of these factors.[12]

It can assist to think of yourself as a team with multiple members. Each member (each facet of yourself) must have their needs satisfied and must operate in unison with the other team members for the team to be effective. These characteristics of oneself are as follows:[12]

- Physical (your body)—your physical structure and the five senses that allow you to touch, see, hear, smell, and taste the world around you.
- Emotional (your feelings)—range of emotions, from fear and anger to love and joy
- Mental (your thoughts)—your knowledge, attitudes, and beliefs; your analytical self
- Spiritual (your spirit)—your relationship with yourself, your creativity, your life purpose, and your relationship with a Higher Power

All of these factors combine to make you a whole person. What occurs to one component can have an impact on the others. That is why being confined to bed with a sore back (physical) can cause depression (emotional), or repressing your anger (emotional) can cause headaches (both physical and emotional) (physical). The mind/body link is a term used to describe the relationship between your many components.

To improve your health, you must first become conscious of yourself. It will alert you if any component of your "self" is out of balance.[12]

HOLISTIC MEDICINE: TYPES OF TREATMENTS

Holistic practitioners employ a variety of therapeutic methods to assist their patients in taking charge of their own health and achieving optimal health. Depending on the practitioner's training, these are discussed here.[6,9]

Complementary and Alternative Therapies

- Homeopathy
- Naturopathy
- Acupuncture
- Physical therapy
- Chiropractic care
- Manual medicine
- Biomolecular therapies[6,9]

Note: It is important to remember that "natural remedies" do not automatically imply "safe." Acupuncture, e.g., has been known to induce infections if not performed correctly. Heavy metals are frequently found in herbal medications, which can harm the kidneys, liver, and heart. In cases of cancer or chronic disorders such as diabetes, holistic therapy cannot substitute traditional medication. When it comes to youngsters with autism or dyslexia, speech therapy and physiotherapy are better options than homeopathy.[9]

Ayurveda as a Holistic Complementary System of Healing: Charak and Sushrut

The term Ayurveda broadly refers to the ancient Hindu medical holistic profound system, recorded in texts dating back 3,000 years and divided into eight branches that correspond roughly to internal or general medicine, pediatrics, psychiatry, ear, nose and throat, surgery, toxicology, geriatrics, and rejuvenation.[13] Ayurvedic medicine proceeds from five bodily elements arranged according to three energies:

1. Space and air with the basic quality of movement
2. Fire with the basic quality of heat
3. Water and earth with the basic quality of fluidity

In diagnosing a patient, the physician will take pulses for these three energies on the nerves of the thumb, index, and middle fingers, and supplement this with careful examination of the fingernails, which indicate blood flow, and the eyes, which reflect disease and constitution. The intimate contact with each patient, from diagnosis through treatment, is underlined by a basic principle, as stated by Ayurvedic physician Brahmanand Swamigal, who insists that, "I do not treat diseases, I treat people."[13]

Achieving the balance between these basic *prakriti* elements *vata*, *pitta*, and *cough* through diet, exercise, lifestyle, herbal, and other medicines help get rid of diseases. There is a lot of insistence on lifestyle for the day and the season, the tailor-made diet for the person and there is a lot of emphasis on the prevention of the disease. In short, Ayurveda is more about the way of healthy life rather than about cure of the diseases. The basic difference between Ayurveda and Western allopathic medicine is important to understand. Western allopathic medicine currently tends to focus on symptomatology and disease, and primarily uses drugs and surgery to rid the body of pathogens or diseased tissue. Many lives have been saved by this approach. In fact, surgery is encompassed very well by Ayurveda. However, drugs, because of their toxicity, often weaken the body. Ayurveda does not focus on disease. Rather, Ayurveda maintains that all life must be supported by energy in balance. When there is minimal stress and the flow of energy within a person is balanced, the body's natural defense systems will be strong and can more easily defend against disease.[14]

It must be emphasized that Ayurveda is not always a substitute for Western allopathic medicine. There are many instances when the disease process and acute conditions can best be treated with drugs or surgery. Ayurveda can be used in conjunction with Western medicine to make a person stronger and less likely to be afflicted with disease and/or to rebuild the body after being treated with drugs or surgery.[14]

Patient Education on Lifestyle Changes and Self-care to Enhance Wellness

Some of the lifestyle adjustments one can make are:[6,9]

- Dietary changes
- Regular exercise
- Psychotherapy
- Relationship and spiritual counseling

Western Drugs and Surgical Treatments

The practitioners might also use western drugs and surgical treatments on occasion.[6,9]

How to Initiate Holistic Approaches?

Since all four aspects, namely the physical, emotional, mental, and spiritual, must work in harmony to obtain well-being, each part needs your attention and care to function optimally. When you are aware of your physical, emotional, mental, and spiritual well-being, you can take action swiftly to prevent illness if one or more of these components are out of balance.[12]

The following suggestions are some of the specific things you can do to enhance your health and promote your own wellness.

PHYSICAL WELLNESS

Good nutrition, a healthy weight, effective exercise, and proper relaxation are all essential for your physical well-being. Recognize what makes your body feel good and what makes it painful. When your body communicates, learn to listen to it. Some of the tips for good physical well-being are:[12]

- Consume nutritious, fresh foods.
- Sugar, salt, refined flour, and fatty foods should be avoided or limited.

- As far as possible, replace processed foods with fresh veggies and nutritious grains.
- Drink plenty of clean water. You may need to invest in a water filter system or consume bottled water in many areas where tap water is not pure.
- Make time for enjoyable physical activity. Joining a gym or lifting weights can be beneficial to certain people. Others enjoy and benefit from activities such as dancing, walking, bicycling, and skating. The most important thing is to get at least 20 minutes of such activity 3–5 days a week.
- Get enough rest. Many people are unaware that inattentiveness or a lack of motivation might be caused by a lack of sleep. Experiment to determine your natural rhythm and the amount of sleep you require to feel your best.[12]

By measuring the Healthy Eating Index or Healthy Diet Score, one may keep track of changes in diet quality in individuals and groups of people/patients and adjust interventions/dietary patterns as needed.[1]

EMOTIONAL WELLNESS

The emotion you require is forgiveness, love, and compassion; it also requires laughter and happiness, as well as joy with yourself and others. Recognize which individuals or activities make you feel happy, loving, and connected, and which make you feel angry, fearful, or depressed.[12] Emotional well-being is defined as the ability to control one's emotions. It refers to a person's ability to control their emotions and express the right emotions in the right situations. It enables us to notice, characterize, and label our emotions as well as the triggers that cause them.[15]

Role of Stress

Any encounter that generates tension, whether physical, psychological, or emotional, is commonly defined as "stress," especially if it triggers the "fight or flight reaction." Learning to handle stress can help you lessen its harmful effects on your body while also improving your mental well-being. This can be aided through mindfulness, which is a type of meditation that involves focusing on the present moment.[15]

A Guide to Mindfulness Practice

- Find a quiet location.
- Sit in a chair with your back supported and your feet on the ground, cross-legged, or in any other comfortable posture.
- Close your eyes or concentrate on a single point.
- Take a few deep breaths to clear your mind. Relax while you scan your entire body from head to toe.
- Next, pay attention to your breathing. In and out.
- If thoughts arise in your head, acknowledge them but do not follow them. As if they were fish in an aquarium, they drift by.
- If you have never meditated before, start with 5 minutes and work your way up to 20 minutes.
- If you do not have 20 minutes, do it four times a day for 5 minutes each time. This can be done daily.[15]

Some of the tips for good emotional well-being are:

- Laugh, play, and have a good time on a regular basis. Laughter is wonderful medicine, and the capacity to play is essential for maintaining a healthy lifestyle.
- Let others know how you are feeling. Spend time with the people you can confide in and offer them the gift of truly understanding you.
- Form warm, caring bonds with others. Allow yourself and others to be forgiven. If you have concerns or grievances with family or friends, confront them and reclaim the emotional intimacy you once had.[12]

MENTAL WELLNESS

Self-supportive attitudes, good ideas and opinions, and a positive self-image are all necessary for mental well-being. Recognize which thoughts make you smile and feel good, and which thoughts make you frown or tighten your muscles. Some of the tips for your mental well-being are:

- *Experiment with fresh concepts:* Find a pastime, enroll in a class, read a nonfiction book, or watch instructional programming on television.
- *Develop an optimistic mindset*: Instead of criticizing, focus on catching yourself and others doing something positive. Look for the positive aspects of a situation.
- *Take a look at your beliefs*: Listen to what other people have to say. Try to see things from their perspective when they disagree with you.[12]

Holistic health outcomes have shown to be improved with various psychological therapies such as:[7]

- Cognitive behavior therapy
- Behavioral therapies
- Problem solving therapies

They have been found to have an impact on a variety of things such as psychological distress, pain, physical health, medication adherence, as well as family outcomes.[7]

SPIRITUAL WELLNESS

In the spiritual, you need inner peace, openness to your creativity, and faith in your inner knowing. Be mindful of your spiritual state, what makes you experience inner calm, joy, and a sense that everything is in order. Be conscious of your intuitive thoughts, which will lead you to your highest good and provide you with the gift of creativity.[12]

However, raising awareness about the significance of spiritual health in providing holistic and global health remains critical. Poor spiritual health may raise the likelihood of poor mental and social health, and hence poor physical health, which can lead to diseases through the autonomic nervous system and other routes.[1]

Some of the tips to improve spiritual wellness are:

- *Spend some time alone with yourself*: Go fishing, meditate, or pray. In diverse ways, we connect with our inner selves or a higher power.
- *Allow yourself to be creative*: Learn to believe in your own creativity and intuition. Make your inner self known.
- *Appreciate the present moment*: Instead of reminiscing about the past or looking forward to the future, enjoy what you are doing right now.[12]

Spirituality must be incorporated into health applications.

Spirituality

Spirituality is an attempt to comprehend and acknowledge an individual's interactions with other humans, as well as their role in life and the meaning of life.[2] It is the process of learning and growing as a result of supreme power and personal relationships. If spirituality is defined in the context of a human's search for a relationship with a spirit, it is the human's expression of that search. Spiritualism is a metaphysical belief that the universe has a spiritual foundation and that the substance is separate from the spirit. It is characterized as a "unifying power" that is affected by both the body and the spirit and impacts both at the same time.[2]

Spirituality is one of the parts of a holistic approach that considers the notion of "social belonging." Individuals understanding of their own spirituality lead to increased internal calm and happiness.[2]

Spiritual care or approach is the incorporation of beliefs that are beneficial in coping with physical and spiritual challenges, particularly the emotional requirements of the individual, self-education, and self-actualization approach to the treatment process.[2]

In a study on spirituality, it was discovered that the majority of modern views fit into one of the three categories:

1. *God-centered spirituality*: Motivation for the idea and practice in theologies, and is envisioned to be broad or narrow.
2. *Earth-centered spirituality*: It emphasizes the relationship between an individual and ecology or nature.
3. *Humanistic (human-centered) spirituality*: Emphasizes the human's success or potential.[2]

Spirituality is thus viewed as a complex structure. The aspects of spirituality are a subject that focuses on wanting to be in harmony with the universe, seeking answers to infinity, and individual concentration on emotional anguish, physical ailment, or death.[2]

For many patients, religion and spiritual beliefs are quite significant. When a person's health, and may be his or her life, is in jeopardy, he or she is likely to seek medical help with both physical and spiritual symptoms. In the face of disease, people battle with common problems such as infirmity, suffering, loneliness, despair, and mortality, all while striving for hope, purpose, and personal value. Many doctors and nurses have intuitive and anecdotal perceptions that patients' religious beliefs and practices have a significant impact on their existential experiences with disease and death and this is supported by a recent study.[2]

TABLE 1: Studies reporting the effects of spirituality on health and wellness.[2]

Study details	Results
A study conducted by Dr Herbert Benson of the Mind/Body Medical Institute included 1,800 patients	There is a direct link between prayer and the cure of ailments
A study conducted in the United States and the United Kingdom	Praying decreases symptoms and speeds up the healing process
A study conducted by Michigan University	Religious people are less prone to experience depression and stress
A study conducted by Rush University of Chicago	Religious people have a 25% lower premature death rate than those who are not involved with religion
A study conducted by Duke University on 750 patients who had angiography	• The healing effect of "prayer" was scientifically proven • It was revealed that the cardiac patients who pray had a 30% less mortality rate a few years after the surgery

Religious and spiritual considerations have been proven to play a role in patients' coping methods and impact critical decisions when they are facing a terminal disease. In these situations, determining the required reassuring qualities for the patient to trust the higher power and cope with the current crisis is critical.[2]

Religion and spirituality were found to have favorable benefits on physical health in a study, and nurses tended to think of spirituality as a religious necessity. Many studies have demonstrated that spirituality has a direct impact on health, wellness, and quality of life **(Table 1)**.[2]

BENEFITS OF HOLISTIC THERAPY

Holistic treatment has the advantage of being a whole-body approach that treats mental, bodily, and spiritual well-being. It frequently enables people to better comprehend the relationships between these various parts of their lives and how they affect their health and wellness. Most of the holistic techniques are also strategies that people can use outside of treatment sessions to practice and accomplish on their own. This is especially useful in everyday life when people are confronted with events that can cause tension, anxiety, or mood swings.[16]

In addition to treatment, holistic approaches frequently emphasize prevention. Learning to use holistic remedies instead of waiting for a problem to arise may be beneficial in preventing problems that can impair a person's emotional, physical, social, or spiritual well-being.[16]

Wellness activities that are commonly used in holistic therapy are typically used to help people deal with tension and stress and increase overall well-being. People can better manage events that cause distress by employing techniques such as deep breathing, mindfulness, or meditation. Acupuncture, yoga, and deep breathing have all been shown to be useful for a variety of causes.[16]

Because of its approach to disease care, holistic medicine has various advantages, including:

- It claims to avoid many drugs' adverse effects.
- It claims to prevent relapse by focusing on the fundamental cause.
- It is frequently a whole lifestyle adjustment rather than a short remedy.
- It asserts that it prefers non-invasive procedures.
- More time with the practitioners for consultation.
- It allows people to have more control over their health and well-being.
- It increases the flow of life force energy in the patient and is patient-centered.[9]

According to a certain study, integrated, holistic care has several advantages:

- According to a 2017 article, holistic techniques provide both physical and emotional advantages while also being cost-effective.
- Mindfulness and meditation are effective in lowering anxiety and stress, and they may be customized for a variety of goals and situations, according to research.
- Guided imagery, which is commonly utilized in holistic approaches, can aid with sleep, mood, stress reduction, and relaxation.
- Deep breathing techniques have been demonstrated in studies to lower stress and increase relaxation, which can enhance both physical and mental health.[16]

Holistic therapy may be beneficial in the treatment of a variety of psychological issues including:[16]

- Addictions
- Anxiety
- Depression
- Problems with emotions
- Issues in the family
- Stress
- Trauma
- Work-related issues

Because this style of treatment aims to heal the whole person, it may be beneficial for issues that do not have a single, clear source or that influence several aspects of a person's life.[16]

If you are interested in trying holistic therapy, few things you should do to get started with, the first step is to locate an expert who specializes in holistic therapy.[16]

HOLISTIC PROVIDER

In the healing process, a kind, loving, and dedicated physician with good medical abilities and a strong compassionate nature is essential. Physicians must believe in the medicinal system they are using and that the treatment they are providing will benefit the patient.[4]

In certain circumstances, online treatment may be a possibility, but many more hands-on therapies (e.g., massage and Reiki) need in-person appointments. To begin your search, speak with your healthcare physician to see if they may recommend you to a holistic therapist in your area. Another option is to conduct a broad online search or browse a therapist directory.[16]

Medical doctors, osteopaths, naturopathic doctors, chiropractors, and homeopathic doctors are examples of holistic providers.[6] People who incorporate holistic techniques into their practices may go by other titles such as clinical psychologist or marriage and family therapist, so if there is a specific experience you want to try, you may need to ask about the techniques that they use.[16]

When looking for a holistic provider, keep the following things in mind:[6,9]

- Just do not go to anyone, randomly.
- Select a practitioner who is willing to devote sufficient time to get to know you.
- Get a recommendation from someone you trust or contact a reputable health group for a recommendation before choosing a holistic medicine practitioner.
- Finish your homework. Find out as much as you can about holistic doctor's training, experience, specialty, and affiliations with professional organizations and hospitals before choosing one. Are they certified by a reputable medical board in holistic medicine? Take into account the doctor's therapeutic philosophy as well. Is it in line with your own beliefs? Also make a proper description of your own ailments, in an organized manner.
- Look for a therapist who makes you feel at ease.
- Consider how at ease you are with the service provider. Do they make you feel at ease while you're around them? Is the provider considerate of your worries and convictions? Remember that holistic health is a collaborative effort including both you and the practitioner, so make sure you feel at ease and valued, and that you want to work with them.
- The time of your appointment. Choose a service provider who will spend enough time with you to fully comprehend your requirements.
- Seek the advice of a practitioner who prefers to get to know you by asking the proper questions. Prepare to answer a lot of questions about your food, exercise, sleep habits, how you feel emotionally, your religious beliefs and practices personal relationships, and more so that your doctor may understand you as a whole person and not just a sickness.
- Treatment alternatives. Does the wellness plan go beyond medicines when deciding on a treatment approach? Ascertain that the practitioner considers all lifestyle and medical aspects that may be contributing to your disease.[6,9]

Holistic health practitioners think that the entire person is made up of interdependent pieces and that if one portion fails, the rest of the body suffers. In this sense, having physical, emotional, or spiritual imbalances in one's life can hurt one's entire health.[6]

To treat a patient, a holistic doctor may use any type of healthcare, from conventional medication to alternative therapies. For example, when a person with migraine headaches visits a holistic doctor, the doctor will likely look at all of the potential factors that may be causing the person's headaches, such as other health problems, diet and sleep habits, stress, and personal problems, and preferred spiritual practices, rather than just prescribing medications. The treatment approach may include medications to alleviate symptoms, as well as lifestyle changes to help prevent headaches from returning.[6]

What to Expect?

During your initial appointment, your therapist will assess your current level of functioning and collaborate with you to set treatment goals. Because holistic therapy is adaptable, your needs can be assessed and your treatment plan adjusted as you proceed through therapy.[16]

Before you begin therapy, you should inquire about insurance and payment options. Your therapist may refuse to accept insurance as a method of payment because many holistic treatments are not covered by insurance. Before you begin therapy, check with your insurance provider to see what therapies are covered.[16]

CONCLUSION

In conclusion, the doctor and medical science must treat the patient as a whole as health is the synchronization between the body, mind, and spirit. A holistic approach is a form of healing that takes into account the whole individual, their body, mind, spirit, and emotions. It treats the whole individual rather than treating merely the symptoms of a disease. Also, a holistic approach has several advantages.

The main principle of the holistic approach is that it believes that unconditional love and support can heal all illnesses and injuries and that each person is ultimately responsible for their own health and well-being. All four aspects of an individual including the physical, emotional, mental, and spiritual must work in harmony to obtain well-being and each part needs your attention and care to function optimally.

Mutual trust and care between a patient and a physician can result in medical miracles. It is critical for a patient to have faith in the physician, develop a positive attitude toward the treatment and condition at hand, and follow a disciplined, simple lifestyle and diet, as well as proper rest and appropriate exercises, to allow the healing process to take place and ensure a quick and complete recovery. Yoga and meditation can aid in the restoration and maintenance of overall health.

Family members, friends, and relatives can help a patient heal by providing comfort and care. Prayers, affection, and a caring social environment are all essential components of the whole healing process. Patients, their family members, or caregivers must be given accurate and detailed information on the disease, diagnosis, treatment options, realistic disease outcomes, and updates on the patient's health.[5] This knowledge, according to medical studies, goes a long way and is significantly more effective in improving patient outcomes.

REFERENCES

1. Itharat A, Takahashi T, Singh RG, Singh RB, Krisentu K, Lobenberg L, et al. Holistic approaches for health education and health promotion. World Heart J. 2017;9(1):81-96.
2. Demirsoy N. Holistic Care Philosophy for Patient-Centered Approaches and Spirituality. In: Sayligil O (Ed). Patient-Centered Medicine. London: IntechOpen; 2017.
3. American Holistic Health Association. (2022). Principles of Holistic Medicine. [online] Available from https://ahha.org/selfhelp-articles/principles-of-holistic-medicine/ [Last accessed February, 2023].
4. Vagbhat. Astanga Hridaya Sutra Sthan. The Healing Process. [online] Available from https://www.planetayurveda.com/ayurveda-ebooks/astanga-hridaya-sutrasthan-handbook.pdf [Last accessed February, 2023].
5. WebMed. (2022). What Is Holistic Medicine? [online] Available from https://www.webmd.com/balance/guide/what-is-holistic-medicine [Last accessed February, 2023].
6. Shafran R, Bennett SD, McKenzie Smith M. Interventions to Support Integrated Psychological Care and Holistic Health Outcomes in Paediatrics. Healthcare (Basel). 2017;5(3):44.
7. NSW government. (2022). What is a holistic approach? [online[Available from https://www.health.nsw.gov.au/mentalhealth/psychosocial/principles/Pages/holistic.aspx [Last accessed February, 2023].
8. Jacob D, Uttekar PS. (2022). What Is Considered Holistic Medicine? [online] Available from https://www.medicinenet.com/what_is_considered_holistic_medicine/article.htm [Last accessed February, 2023].
9. Gordon JS. Holistic medicine: advances and shortcomings. West J Med. 1982;136(6):546-51.
10. Rathore P, Kumar S, Haokip N, Ratre BK, Bhatnagar S. CARE: A Holistic Approach Toward Patients During Pandemic: Through the Eyes of a Palliative Physician. Indian J Palliat Care. 2020;26 (Suppl 1):S95-8.
11. American Holistic Health Association. (2016). Wellness From Within: The First Step. [online] Available from https://ahha.org/wp-content/uploads/Ahhastep.htm [Last accessed February, 2023].
12. Progler Y. Ayurveda: The Art of Healing and Being in an Ancient Indian Tradition. JRMS. 2008;13(3):156-7.
13. Lad B. (2016). Ayurveda—A Brief Introduction and Guide. [online] Available from https://www.ayurveda.com/pdf/intro_ayurveda.pdf [Last accessed February, 2023].
14. Myasthenia Gravis Foundation of America. A Holistic Approach—A Guide for Patients/Family Members / Caregivers. [online] Available from https://s24.q4cdn.com/902352448/files/doc_downloads/mg_holistic_wellness_guide.pdf [Last accessed February, 2022].
15. Verywell mind. (2021). What Is Holistic Therapy. [online] Available from https://www.verywellmind.com/holistic-therapy-definition-types-techniques-and-efficacy-5196420#toc-types-of-holistic-therapy [Last accessed February, 2022].
16. Shah DV, Shah HS. Brain and neurological disorders, A Simplified Health Education Guide. Ann Indian Acad Neurol. 2017;20(1):84.

129

CHAPTER

Communication Skills for Neurologists: Breaking Bad News

Roop Gursahani, Rajinder K Dhamija, Prafulla Shembalkar

INTRODUCTION

Competence in medicine requires three sets of skills. Cognitive skills refer to the knowledge that is inherent to our practice (neuroanatomy, physiology, pharmacology, etc.). Practical and technical training emphasizes diagnosis, surgery, intervention, etc. Throughout our medical education, these are emphasized, learned, and assessed and we together with our colleagues, judge ourselves and each other by our mastery of both of these. But professional effectiveness depends heavily on a third skill which till now has rarely been taught formally. This is the skill of communicating effectively with our patients, colleagues, and society at large. Effective communication in medicine requires physicians to deploy goal-directed and situationally appropriate verbal messaging and nonverbal behaviors. These are social behaviors that can be learned (and taught). They are interrelated so that they can be carried out in sequence as part of preset protocols. As medicine moves out of its patriarchal traditions and internalizes human equality, these skills have become progressively more important and are at the core of person-centered medicine. The AETCOM (Attitude, Ethics and Communication) module course has introduced this in undergraduate MBBS education for Indian medical graduates.[1] This chapter is meant to guide the reader into the application of these techniques to clinical neurology. But didactic learning is no substitute for practical training and self-learning with experience. Readers of this textbook will need to access opportunities for this learning and it is important to recognize barriers within us that hold us back **(Table 1)**. Phrases and even scripts for these conversations are available but these are in English and we need to use our own words.[2] Those of us who are comfortable with these techniques soon begin to incorporate them into day-to-day clinical work. But in addition to these skills, we need knowledge about the prognosis of the specific illness in the patient and that leads us to the skill of prognostication.

TABLE 1: Difficult conversations: Self perceived barriers and their resolution.

Stressful; lack of confidence	Reduces with training, practice, and use of standardized protocols
Time consuming	Usually takes 15–20 minutes; if the initial conversation is done well, it reduces further questioning
Honesty destroys hope	Transparency reduces anxiety
Neurologic prognosis is uncertain, especially in the medium term	Signposts of decline can be identified; months-to-year prognostication allows preparation
Accepting our uncertainty will reduce their trust in our competence	Patients/families are willing to discuss prognostic uncertainty, since it allows for hope
Possible rejection of our diagnosis, prognosis	Recommend and facilitate second opinion
Accepting death is accepting failure	Accepting reality allows us to work with patients and families at maintaining quality of life till the very end

We then learn how to deploy our technical knowledge and sense of compassion to support both patient and caregiver/care partner throughout this journey.

PROGNOSTICATION IN NEUROLOGY AND CLINICAL MEDICINE

Foreseeing and Foretelling as Ethical Obligations

Till about 100 years ago, diagnosis, treatment, and prognosis were considered equally important skills for physicians.[3] Since then, with the rise of modern therapeutics, the significance of prognosis has been downgraded in both practice and research. This is a major loss to the intellectual content of clinical medicine. Physicians have been sociologically conditioned to avoid the burden of prognosis

BOX 1	From a sage of medicine.

"It appears to me a most excellent thing for the physician to cultivate Prognosis; for by **foreseeing** and **foretelling,** in the presence of the sick, the present, the past, and the future... he will be the more readily believed to be acquainted with the circumstances of the sick; so that men will have confidence to in trust themselves to such a physician."

The Book of Prognosis

—Hippocrates, 400 BC

because of a vague belief in the powers of self-fulfilling prophesies, both positive and negative ("if I say something bad will happen, it will!"). But prognostication is a core element of bioethics because without reasonably accurate information, the patient or family cannot really make independent decisions and autonomy is thus compromised. For example, at the end of life, it is not possible to discuss medical futility without talking about prognosis. If we have no idea of what lies ahead, the disease experience either is assumed to be random or predestined by fate. This then leads to magical thinking ("if one wishes for something, it does happen"), which is quite typical of childhood. Working logically toward the future is meaningless without knowing as much of it as possible. Hippocrates **(Box 1)** identified the two key elements of prognostication—(1) foreseeing and (2) foretelling. Both are essential. Foresight cannot be honed and tempered without a commitment to foretelling. To foretell effectively, we must be transparent about the limits of our accuracy. Communication skills (CS) are the vehicle for this enterprise, allowing us to convey realism with compassion. Goals for the future can then be identified and this gives patients and families some sense of control and optimism. Once we accept our moral and intellectual duty to prognosticate, it becomes easier to approach this process analytically. The key questions that we must endeavor to answer have been termed the five D's of prognosis—(1) *d*eath, (2) *d*isease progression, (3) *d*isability/*d*iscomfort, (4) *d*rug toxicity, and (5) *d*ollars (financial burden). In neurology, this can often be simplified to "how long" and "how well".

Disease Trajectories in Neurologic Illness

Five disease trajectories[4] (**Figs. 1A to E**) have been identified, when the functional status is plotted against time. These include:

1. *Sudden death*: This is proportionately more common under 50 years of age. After the age of 65, it accounts for <10% of all mortality.
2. *Waterfall trajectory*: Patients with disseminated cancer can maintain normal function for a certain period. Once the decline begins, the plot curves downward in a reasonably predictable manner, as tumor burden increases logarithmically, and biologic processes become unstoppable. This trajectory is also seen in motor neuron disease and possibly represents 20–25% of all deaths.
3. *Looping trajectory*: In about 15% of deaths, the initial decline is marked by crises and possible admissions to hospitals. Recovery is often incomplete, and these episodes of an entry-re-entry mask a downward course. This course is seen with organ failure (renal, hepatic, lung, and heart) but also with severe epilepsy and progressive multiple sclerosis.
4. *Frailty*: Together with dementia this probably accounts for 50% of all deaths. It is typically seen in octogenarians and older and the proportion is projected to rise as the population ages. This pattern shows a long, slow, and undulating decline. In neurologically impaired individuals, frailty may appear at earlier ages. It is best characterized as decreased physiologic reserve across multiple systems. The frail individual has an increased risk of falls, hospitalization, failure to thrive, and death.
5. *Fifth trajectory*[5]: This is an artifact of modern intensive care and proportions will vary depending on the medical system. Patients with primary or secondary brain involvement may not awaken and may transition to a chronic disorder of consciousness (unresponsive wakeful state, locked in syndrome, and minimally conscious state) with preserved brainstem reflexes and varying degrees of severe neurologic impairment.

It has been estimated that over 90% of all deaths can be predicted, with varying degrees of certainty, depending on the time frame. The most accurate is the short-term prediction of death (hours to days) once signs of active dying appear[6] (See Chapter 126 on Neuropalliative Care). In oncology, the prediction is still reasonably accurate in the medium term (days-weeks-months timeframe). For instance, in a patient with disseminated malignancy, once functional status declines to the Karnofsky scale of 40% or less (bedridden >50% of the time), survival is 3 months or less. Since this is largely biologically driven (i.e., by tumor burden), it cannot be altered. In nononcologic illnesses and in neurology in particular, this is much less predictable and decisional factors play a role. Life-saving treatments (e.g., feeding tubes, dialysis, and antibiotics) can alter medium-term prognosis and outweigh biologic factors. Prognostic predictability improves in the long term, i.e., months-to-years. Predictions of 1-year mortality in chronic neurologic illness are not available but we can extrapolate from those for frail older adults.[7] Of these, the Walter index **(Table 2)** on seniors over 70 years is based on gender; ability to perform five basic activities of daily living [ADL: (1) bathing, (2) dressing, (3) using the toilet, (4) transferring from bed to chair, and (5) eating]; two medical comorbidities [(1) malignancy and (2) congestive heart failure] and two laboratory values (creatinine and albumin). This index can predict 60–70% 1-year mortality. This is best conveyed to laypersons by giving them an idea of median durations

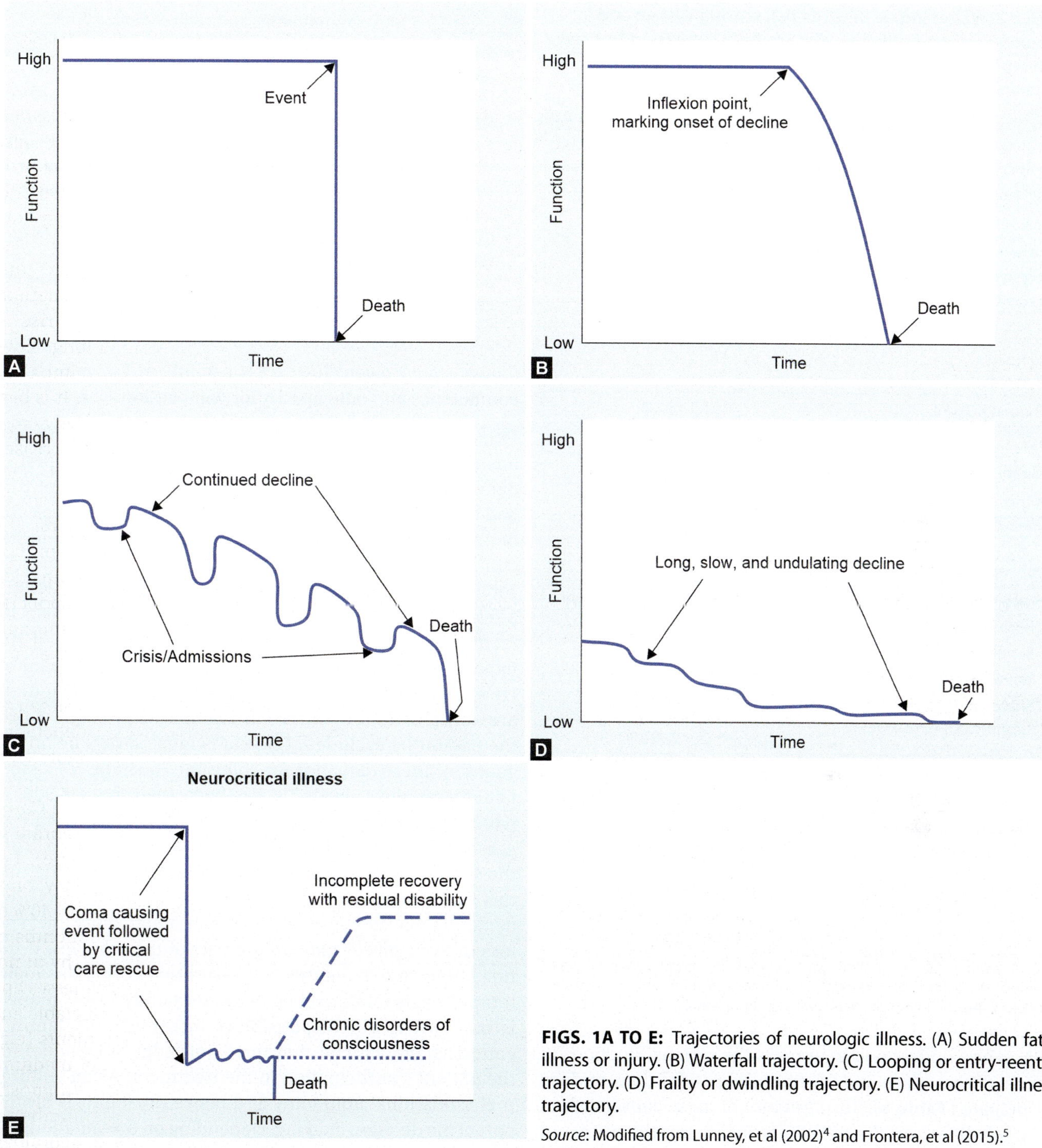

FIGS. 1A TO E: Trajectories of neurologic illness. (A) Sudden fatal illness or injury. (B) Waterfall trajectory. (C) Looping or entry-reentry trajectory. (D) Frailty or dwindling trajectory. (E) Neurocritical illness trajectory.

Source: Modified from Lunney, et al (2002)[4] and Frontera, et al (2015).[5]

with shorter and longer possibilities on a bell curve. Thus, average mortality of 60–70% in 1 year, translates to near 100% at the end of 3–4 years. This is discussed further in management of uncertainty below.

BREAKING BAD NEWS

Breaking bad news (BBN) is a key skill in neuropalliative care: Bad news is information that will negatively alter an individual's view of her future, evoking strong cognitive, behavioral, and emotional responses.[8] The usual examples of the BBN encounter include the diagnosis of motor neuron disease and malignant glioma. But even the diagnosis of multiple sclerosis, parkinsonism or dementia is life-altering and should never be done casually. It cannot be emphasized enough; how important it is to gain confidence and competence in CS. Our reluctance in this field stems from our failure to conceptualize and dissect the process.

TABLE 2: Walter index: Bedside risk scoring system and prediction of mortality in older adults (>70 years) admitted to hospital for acute illness, based on information at discharge.

Risk factor	Points	Cumulative points	Risk of death based on mortality in validation cohort (confidence intervals)
Male sex	1		
1–4 activities of daily living (ADL) dependent	2		
All ADL dependent	5		
Creatinine >3 mg/dL	2	0–1	4 (CI 2–6)
Albumin <3 g/dL	2	2–3	19 (CI 15–23)
CHF	2	4–6	34 (CI 29–39)
Solitary cancer	3	>6	64 (CI 58–70)
Metastatic cancer	8		

TABLE 3: A four-way matrix for communication tasks.

Participating patient, with DMC: • BBN: SPIKES protocol • Serious illness communication • Advance care planning • Shared decision making (full support vs. DNAR/POLST)	*Severe acute brain injury, patient without DMC:* • BBN, Identification of surrogate decision maker; ICU family meeting/SIC • Shared decision making (full support vs. DNAR/POLST)
Patient with DMC, but excluded: • Address collusion requests • BBN, SIC with surrogate decision maker • Shared decision making (full support vs. DNAR/POLST)	*Patient with impaired cognition and/or communication:* • Assess DMC • Identification of surrogate by patient • Goals of care, SIC; shared decision making (full support vs. DNAR/POLST)

(BBN: breaking bad news; DMC: decision making capacity; DNAR: do not attempt resuscitation; ICU: intensive care unit; POLST: Physician Orders for Life-Sustaining Treatment; SIC: serious illness conversation)

BBN is best understood in terms of the various situations in which it takes place and whether the patient does or does participate **(Table 3)**. The structure of these conversations is largely based on the SPIKES protocol, but the pace and content depend on the situation. The way we deploy verbal and body language and use silence are important. Training in CS depends heavily on role play and it is recommended that the interested reader take part in CS workshops that are run around the country as part of PallCare orientation. There is a wealth of guidance available online and it is important to access and use this material. In these conversations, compassion is the key attribute; empathy is less useful, and sympathy can often be rejected **(Box 2)**. The key outcome is trust between the patient and family on one side and the clinician and team on the other. Our stewardship of their illness is not a given. They are constantly assessing both our competence and our capacity for compassion.

BOX 2 Sympathy, empathy, and compassion.

- *Sympathy*: Pity-based response to a distressing situation; lacks relational understanding and focusses on self-preservation for the observer and her ego; generally considered unhelpful, demoralizing, and patronizing by the recipient
- *Empathy*: Affective response that acknowledges and attempts to understand the victim's suffering; emotional resonance and contagion means that the observer feels the pain; the recipient feels heard, understood, and validated
- *Compassion*: Virtuous, nonconditional, and altruistic response; seeks to address the suffering with an action-oriented response and emotional engagement; ameliorates distress and enhances caregiving

Preparing the ground: If the patient can participate and has decision-making capacity: S/he should be helped to decide the pace of the conversation. A warning shot that bad news is coming is essential. If it is possible, a break can be introduced at this point. Some ways of doing so in the clinic are to ask for additional investigations or prescribe some medications and then schedule a follow-up within a few days. A short time-out in the waiting room can be tactfully arranged. Depending on the seriousness, if the patient is alone, it may be necessary to ask for a companion. However, if the patient is insistent on an immediate answer, it must be delivered. Families may request that the patient be excluded. Clinicians must always be on the guard for these demands for collusion. In studies of cancer patient-caregiver dyads,[9] it has been seen that 80–90% of patients wanted to be told, while only 30–40% of caregivers agreed. The ostensible motive is always protection from the stress and depression of this knowledge, believing that this could negatively impact the course of the illness. Other dynamics may not be obvious, such as anticipatory grief and loss or even power play on the part of the relatives. If the first clinician making the diagnosis also accepts this logic, it rapidly gets reinforced by the wider family. If this request is made, it is our responsibility to explore the family's concerns and explain that this knowledge is essential for the patient's participation in the treatment. Asian cultures prefer relational autonomy and hence the family is always part of the decision-making. Depending on the situation, the immediate family often accepts the first clinician's offer to be the bearer of bad tidings, once we explain that this is our job and that we are trained to do so. If this is not done, patient anxiety compounds family stress and the situation becomes messy as second opinions are sought, and the cycle becomes self-perpetuating. Done well, these conversations reduce stress all around. As an ethical duty, the patient must at least be offered the option of participating. Up to a quarter of them may not want to do so and they can be asked to decide who is going to be the interlocutor. Ideally, this request for clarification, i.e., does the patient speak and if

BOX 3	From the most important person, the patient.
"I am glad I had a doctor like you during this diagnosis. It is not easy news to give anyone. I do not know how you do it everyday" —ALS patient, passed away in 2021	
(ALS: amyotrophic lateral sclerosis)	

not, who speaks for the patient, should be made during the initial or diagnostic consultation and the full discussion can happen subsequently. In Western medical practice, patient information is an ethical duty.[10] We believe that in India, the key barrier is the lack of physician knowledge and negative attitudes regarding CS.

Preparing the Clinician: These conversations are regularly considered to be stressful even for experienced clinicians. We fear the emotional components of these encounters, whether from patients or even from ourselves. No one likes to be the bearer of bad news, but if handled sensitively, this information is highly appreciated by patients **(Box 3)**. In terminal illnesses, this discussion has been documented to improve quality of life, reduce aggressive care, and contribute to a good death. In a landmark trial in lung cancer, adding palliative care (including BBN) to standard oncologic care, increased survival time. These discussions must be considered as much a procedure as is surgery and have to be approached as a learned skill.[11] Thus, CS training with mentorship, supervised work, assessment, and certification are followed by practice. Like any other skilled procedure, the performance of CS needs preparation before the procedure and reflection after it is done, to consider what went well and what did not. If done with colleagues, a debrief session is required. Because CS competence was never included in our curricula, clinicians are often afflicted by the Dunning–Kruger effect in which confidence and competence fluctuate substantially. Juniors are often over-confident. Bad experiences and stress then lead to despair, denial, and active avoidance. Training and self-learning finally lead to confident competence and stress then becomes manageable.

The conversation: Any one of the protocols mentioned in Berkey et al.[8] can be used. The discussion below is based on SPIKES (*S*etting, *P*erception, *I*nvitation, *K*nowledge, *E*motions, *S*ummary). An important rule is that the clinician should be speaking <50% of the time.

- *The setting is important*: A private area with both patient/family and clinician seated at the same level. To maintain eye contact, a distraction from notes and gadgets has to be avoided. Body language must be congruent (e.g., arms open and not folded, leaning forward, etc.). The patient has the right to decide who else needs to be there. If the patient cannot be part of the conversation, it is important to make sure that the key persons from the family are present, to avoid having to repeat the exercise. Finally, the clinician must also be prepared with clinical details and with a basic idea of what needs to be conveyed. It is useful to have reports available for visual impact, i.e., showing the lesion on the magnetic resonance imaging (MRI). If more than one provider is going to be present, then it is important to clarify who will lead the discussion and to have some consensus about the points to be conveyed.
- Check the patient/family's perception of the current situation, using open-ended questions. Identify misinformation, unrealistic expectations, and denial.
- Ask permission to continue and this is especially important if the patient is alone. If the patient cannot be present, as in an intensive care unit (ICU) family meeting, this step may be unnecessary. It is quite okay to break at this point and reconvene when convenient since these discussions should not be hurried unless required by the medical situation.
- Knowledge is then provided beginning with a summary of events thus far. A warning shot that bad news is coming may have been given before the meeting or as part of the setting up step. The initial statement by the clinician and team should not last >2–3 minutes. Not more than three chunks of simple information should be given since it is not easy to process more detail during emotion-laden situations. It is useful for clinicians to review these bullet points or headlines before the meeting to not lose focus. Use "ask-tell-ask" to recheck that they have understood.
- Emotions must be explicitly addressed, and the clinician must be prepared for this using the NURSE mnemonic. Emotion/s must be *n*amed, *u*nderstood, *r*espected, *s*upported, and *e*xplored. These are not sequential steps and flow into each other. It is acceptable to demonstrate one's own emotions but controllably and we learn detachment with experience. Compassion and empathy must be felt since fake emotions on our part are easily picked up.
- Summarizing with an explicit commitment to follow up is important. One can offer a mode of contact in case of further questions. This first conversation will be about the diagnosis, while prognosis is usually kept for a later discussion. So, in a progressive illness this sets the stage for subsequent serious illness conversations (SICs). If they ask, they can be told that further discussions will depend on how events and symptoms unfold. Never give the patient and family the impression that you have nothing more to offer. Symptom control and psychosocial support are always required. It is crucial to assess for suicidality at this point and if this conversation was held with the patient alone, every effort should be made to enlist a responsible companion for the next few hours or days.

SERIOUS ILLNESS CONVERSATION

Serious illnesses are health conditions that carry a significant risk of mortality. In addition, they deteriorate function in

ADL, impair quality of life, and/or excessively strain the caregivers. Most life-limiting neurologic illnesses satisfy this definition and include both acute (e.g., major stroke and traumatic brain injury) and chronic (refractory epilepsy, advanced dementia, or parkinsonism) conditions. The ICU family meeting is a variation of the same theme and is covered in greater detail in the Chapter 106 on Severe Acute Brain Injury. At this stage, the patient/family is usually aware of the diagnosis and may have some idea of what lies ahead (see below). Ideally, this is a dialogue with the patient hence the importance of initiating this conversation with the patient before they lose decision-making capacity. Unfortunately, in neurology it is too often held with the family/caregivers only late in the disease process or during a crisis. Identifying appropriate surrogate decision maker/s is thus an important intermediate step. If a cure is not possible, medical care must be anchored in patient and family preferences. To learn what these preferences require us to empower the patient/family by giving appropriate information and by being explicit, all this to be done with empathy and compassion.[12]

Dealing with life after BBN: Patients have described the BBN conversation as akin to having a bomb dropped on them[13] and it takes them some time to come to terms with this life-altering news. Even the diagnosis of treatable epilepsy in a child may leave the mother seriously traumatized. It is important to be aware so that we can meet patients at the point that they have reached in their journey as they grapple with the reality of a life-limiting illness. The immediate aftermath of the diagnosis has been termed guarded anticipation, reflecting the dynamic tension between acceptance of the diagnosis and anxiety about what lies ahead. This is the stage of second opinions and of hiding the diagnosis. The next stage is that of information seeking, either through public awareness material, support groups, or reading on the internet. Patients may shift doctors during this period, not for second opinions but for an empathetic physician who listens, answers, and validates concerns. The third stage is of understanding disease dynamics, symptoms, medications, treatment responses, and adverse effects and as physicians we must learn to respect this self-knowledge. Mr Google is an ally not a rival. The last stage is of incorporating this learning into daily life so that in effect the patient and family negotiate every day with the disease. These stages must also be understood as themes that may not always be sequential and may go back and forth in a patient living for decades with epilepsy, multiple sclerosis, or parkinsonism.

Spiritual issues: Discussion of spiritual issues is tricky because clinicians have no framework to identify and tackle these. In India, despite a rich spiritual heritage, no hospital has any access to secular chaplaincy services as is so prevalent in the USA. Patients and families have existential questions ("Why me..., Why is God punishing us..., I have been a good person...") and these need to be addressed. They understand that there are no answers but having their concerns validated by someone who understands the basic tenets of their faith is always helpful. Even the atheist and agnostic may want some discussion. The simple question "Are you at peace?" is an effective screening tool[14] for spiritual distress and should be used directly with every patient at least once while they can communicate.

Indications for SIC: SIC[15] can be initiated if any one of the following conditions are met and these indications often overlap in the same patient (**Table 4**).

- *Surprise question (SQ)*: The SQ is a prognostic tool that depends on our intuitive knowledge of our patient's overall situation. It takes into account clinical state, comorbidities, and social and other factors to give a whole picture of deterioration. It is considered applicable if you answer "No" to the following question "Would you be surprised if this patient were to die in the next year?". The SQ's accuracy ranges from 70% upward and can reach 80% in oncology.
- The occurrence of an event that may mark deterioration.
- Clinical triggers include symptoms that usually denote the progression of the disease.

TABLE 4: Triggers for serious illness conversations: Examples.

Event-based triggers	Clinical triggers	Intervention related	Wild card triggers
Any admission after the age of 80 years	Onset of behavioral and psychiatric symptoms in dementia or parkinsonism	Deciding about tracheostomy and PEG in patients with catastrophic brain injury	Surprise question
More than two admissions for the same condition within 6 months	Recurrence after completion of initial radiotherapy and chemotherapy for malignant glioma	Planning B-cell based therapy or autologous stem cell therapy for CNS demyelination	Patient/family request
Uncontrolled seizures or episode of status epilepticus in progressive conditions	Increasing dependence for basic activities of daily living	Consideration of surgery/ intervention for severe carotid disease after the age of 75 years	
Recurrent falls	Progressive dysphagia, weight loss	PEG placement in ALS or atypical parkinsonism	

(ALS: amyotrophic lateral sclerosis; CNS: central nervous system; PEG: percutaneous endoscopic gastrostomy)

- Planning a major treatment or intervention is a situation where we deploy the evidence base but patients/families use a preference-based approach.
- Patient or family request a discussion of the road map ahead.

Serious illness conversation protocol: Although this discussion largely follows the same sequence as the BBN protocols, it differs in explicitly discussing prognosis, eliciting values and comparing treatment options. Thus, unlike BBN which is largely unidirectional, i.e., from clinician to patient, SIC is necessarily a bidirectional dialogue. As in all palliative care, mnemonics abound. The REMAP strategy consists of reframe (explain the current situation), expect emotions (manage with NURSE as above), map (patient goals), align (with goals), and propose (a management plan). The PERSON mnemonic consists of P (perception of health status), E (exploration of the patient's earlier life when well), R (relating to medical reality), S (sources of worry), O (outline of options), and N (notify those who need to know). A simpler framework breaks it down into just three steps as given below.[16] The emphasis is on proceeding sequentially so that discussion of treatment plans is done only after the prognosis, values, and goals are clarified. This format is appropriate both for discussions involving the patient as well those with surrogates. As such it can be used in any situation where a major decision has to be made, e.g., discussing the option of targeted B cell therapies for secondary progressive multiple sclerosis.

1. *Sharing knowledge about the medical situation*: It is important to be mentally prepared with an estimate of the prognosis for the individual patient (see the section on prognostication above). The essential questions are "how long" and "how well". Clinicians understand that this has a high degree of unpredictability while patients and families abhor uncertainty. Participants for the discussion must be identified on the patient/family side. Depending on their health literacy we may offer soft copies of resources or trusted web links in advance. One simple way is to write down key terms in capitals if we do not have available literature for them. In India, we may be faced with someone who is barely literate and here we must do our best to use simple terms. But even illiterate seniors may have younger members of the family who are internet savvy and whom they can trust. The conversation itself begins with the first three steps of the SPIKES protocol—(1) arranging the setting, (2) understanding their perception, and (3) explicitly requesting permission/invitation to proceed. Explicit information is then provided, and this should include the time frame and expected functional status. "How long" is best answered without specific numbers but with a range, e.g., days-to-weeks, weeks-to-months, and so on. "How well" leads to a discussion of functional outcomes and signposts of decline. Unpredictability must be explained. Two frameworks for communicating uncertainty in exemplar patients are explained in **Table 5**. The only definitive clarification is for regaining normalcy ("I am sorry but that is not possible"), and that may need to be stated at the beginning. This statement should not last longer than 2–3 minutes and hence should ideally be thought through before beginning speaking, since we may have to deliver complex information chronologically. We should be prepared for and be able to respond to emotions that may be expressed.
2. *Identifying goals of care*: The ultimate aims of any healthcare intervention are one, two, or all of three—(1) longevity, (2) function, and (3) comfort.[17] With a serious illness, it may become necessary to prioritize between them, and trade-offs must be accepted. It is our responsibility to help explain this and then align our treatment plan to their choices. These choices will be based on the patient's beliefs, priorities, personal narrative, and hopes or fears. It is best to take cues from the earlier discussion on prognosis and ask questions like: "What is most important to you...", "what are you most afraid of...". Patient values and priorities as regard the three aims (longevity, function, and comfort) emerge from this dialogue (**Table 6**). Restating them "it seems

TABLE 5: Explaining uncertainty: How long and how well.

How long	How well
70/f, diagnosed ALS/MND 6 months ago, now developing dysarthria, discussing options of gastrostomy, ventilation	**70/f, hypertensive, right basal ganglionic intracerebral hematoma (75 cc volume), discussing decompressive craniectomy**
Rough estimate (for survival) is under 1 year	Most likely (my guess): will be bedridden with feeding tube and catheter, but will recognize and respond to family
Caveat: Impossible to predict with certainty, but I am worried time may be shorter	Worst case will have multiple medical complications and may never leave the hospital
Exceptions: It could be longer, and we hope our decisions (PEG/NIV) help her get some more time	Best case: Will speak, eat by mouth, may walk with support but will be dependent for most other ADL
Underwent PEG, later started NIV; passed away 8 months later, at home	Underwent craniectomy: Alive at 5 years, dependent for all ADL except eating

(ADL: activities of daily living; ALS: amyotrophic lateral sclerosis; MND: motor neuron disease; NIV: Noninvasive ventilation; PEG: percutaneous endoscopic gastrostomy)

TABLE 6: Goals of care.

	Longevity	Function	Comfort
Possible patient/family statements	"Her father lived to 90"	"I don't want to be dependent"	"We don't want him to suffer"
Values	Living as long as possible, not giving up	Maintaining physical and cognitive independence	Avoiding futile surgery, interventions, and life sustaining treatments
Wishes	Living till a specific event or milestone	Participating in relationships, social groups	Controlling pain, dyspnea, nausea, etc.
Preferences	Being able to decide when it is time to go	Staying at home, being with nature	Avoiding hospitalization, ICU
Duties	Avoiding becoming a burden	Performing a specific activity for meaning or joy	Spiritual: Conforming to religious requirements

the most important issue for you is..." allows us to clarify these goals of care. Multiple, contradictory goals may be expressed, and this reflects ambivalence and a continued grappling with loss. Goals may change and earlier goals may be sacrificed as the illness progresses.

3. *Treatment options*: The last phase begins with the understanding that the medical reality has changed from what they had experienced or expected, and the status quo cannot be continued. It may help to show a hand-drawn graph with an appropriate version of one of the trajectories above. With prior experience, the clinician can generate a menu of options for management plans (surgery, aggressive medical, watchful waiting, comfort care, etc.). Knowing that there are different choices is important and the benefits and burdens of different interventions can be weighed. Yes/no questions [e.g., "Do you want tracheostomy..., do you want to sign do not attempt resuscitation (DNAR)?"] should be avoided. We can then make recommendations that are aligned with the patient and family's goals. We can now circle back to the "How long", and "How well" questions[18] and perhaps put heuristic numerical estimates to our different outcome possibilities (e.g., "20% chance of surviving a full 12 months", "30% chance of being able to speak and eat by herself"). Even though we know these estimates carry significant risks of bias, these numbers do help people make up their minds. This is also the point at which our preceding values discussion now allows the patient/family and clinician to think of positive options for the last stages.

Although we have divided the SIC into phases, it usually flows in an iterative, circular fashion.

These stages are important for us conceptually, in that phases 1 and 2 have to be addressed before we can tackle decision-making. From the beginning we must make it clear that we are not just treating the disease but also managing the experience of living with it. The patient/family then understands that there are goals of comfort and that we can be trusted with addressing them. In neurodegenerative illnesses, goals of care discussions must start early, before cognitive, and communication problems. These have been shown to reduce depression and anxiety and do not reduce hope. We need to help patients and families discover nuggets of joy ("let uncle eat what he wants...").[19] In a long illness, this is preferable to a SIC in a crisis.

END-OF-LIFE CARE: DISCUSSION, DECISIONS, INSTRUMENTS

The discussions above culminate in end-of-life care planning. Because of the obvious implications, these should be covered by documented wishes and orders, which should be legally valid. In India, these are enabled by the common cause judgment of the Supreme Court, delivered in 2018.[20,21] According to this, "all adults with capacity to consent have the right of self-determination and autonomy... the right to refuse specific treatment or all treatment or opt for an alternative treatment, even if such decision entails a risk of death.... where a patient has already made a valid advance directive which is free from reasonable doubt and specifying that he/she does not wish to be treated, then such directive has to be given effect to...". This provides legal backing for advance medical directives (AMDs) and do-not-resuscitate (DNR) orders. However, it requires legislation to make these enforceable across the board. For instance, the relevant act in Taiwan specifies fines and disciplinary action for disregarding these documents. In the USA, the maximum medicolegal EoL litigation is for "wrongful life", i.e., resuscitation against the patient's or family's wishes.

Living wills, AMDs, and Advance Care Planning (ACP): Living wills were first propounded by human rights advocates in California in the late 1960s. The living will is so called because it comes into effect while the individual is still alive as against the standard estate will which applies only after the death of the individual. Over the next fourth to fifth decades, this has evolved into the system termed ACP, which is available in many countries globally. ACP is a process to guide decision-making about the individual's healthcare if and when she cannot decide for herself or to communicate her decisions.[22] This is activated through a quasi-legal instrument termed the AMD. The two major components of the AMD are: (1) Assignment of proxy (surrogate) decision maker/s (also termed Healthcare Power-of-Attorney): typically, one to three people can be included and the list is in order of priority. So if the first is not available, the second is called on and so on. (2) Guidance or instructions that specify the kind of treatment that this individual wants or does not want as life begins to end, when the patient is no longer able to communicate her wishes (living will). This includes the level of care, desired outcomes in terms of quality of life, etc. These documents vary substantially as regards the level of detail and this may or may not be specified in the legislation that sets up this system. The guidance in the document may be binding on proxy and medical team, in which case it is the proxies' responsibility to see that the patient's wishes are carried out. Alternatively, it may permit discretion on the part of the proxy so that discussion between proxies and doctors permits prognosis, outcomes, and values to be combined in the process termed shared decision making.[23] In countries with effective ACP systems, individuals are encouraged to avail of counseling to make these choices in their 60s or on the diagnosis of any major health condition or hospitalization. The AMD can then be revisited and updated as the health situation changes, with this being incorporated into the medical record. Younger individuals can make these AMDs if they are concerned about the possibility of catastrophic brain injury and the option of organ donation. Notably, Barack and Michelle Obama announced they had made their AMDs during his first presidential term, when he was in his 40s.

Advance Care Planning in neurology: In systemic cancer, the individual is usually able to specify her own wishes almost till the end, until the beginning of active dying. In contrast, in neurodegenerative illnesses such as dementia, decision-making capacity may be lost decades before death. The American Academy of Neurology, amongst other neurologic societies across the world, recommends its members begin discussing ACP as soon as feasible after diagnosis in patients with life-limiting neurologic illnesses.[24] This conversation has to be proactive, iterative, and integrated into routine medical care. Thus it evolves with the patient's medical situation as part of an ongoing medical relationship. In patients with diagnosed cognitive impairment [e.g., mini-mental state examination (MMSE) < 24], decision making capacity (DMC) has to be assessed and documented before finalizing the AMD. This is done by confirming[25] that the patient (1) understands the information being provided; (2) appreciates how this knowledge applies to herself; (3) can reason and infer consequences; and (4) can express or communicate her decision. Patients with moderate dementia may still be able to participate and at the very least they are often able to identify their preferred surrogate or proxy.

Do not attempt resuscitation, Allow Natural Death (AND), Physician Orders for Life-Sustaining Treatment (POLST): At the very end, it is necessary to have written orders that specify the level of care. The simplest is the DNAR/DNR or AND orders that prevent cardiopulmonary resuscitation (CPR) from being performed by default. The Indian Council of Medical Research (ICMR) has put together basic guide for Indian medical practitioners as an interim measure (after the 2018 judgment) till we have appropriate legislation.[26] Since the ICMR is a statutory body, in case of a dispute, courts are likely to recognize this to be part of standard medical practice. Medical Orders for Life-Sustaining Treatment (MOLST)/POLST are more elaborate documents that are used in many states in the USA. They include three levels of options: (1) CPR: yes or no; (2) full treatment (if CPR is chosen) versus selective treatments (without ICU/CPR) versus comfort-based care, and (3) medically assisted nutrition (yes, no, only for a trial period). These are brightly colored forms that are filled in when a terminal illness is identified or if the patient has a likely survival of 6 months or less. Multiple copies are made and put up everywhere, e.g., in all medical records, documents, on fridge doors at home, so that they are immediately visible in any emergency. The DNAR/AND and POLST documents must be signed by a doctor and the patient or proxy.[27]

CONCLUSION

This chapter gives a short introduction to the content of what we should be discussing with our patients when we diagnose significant neurologic conditions and illnesses. However, we all need to develop our scripts and nonverbal body language to manage these conversations. Ideally, this is an introduction to the necessary capability of CS and through this to the subspecialty of neuropalliative care.

REFERENCES

1. Lal S, Sehgal P. Integration of attitude, ethics, and communication competencies into competency-based UG curriculum. Indian J Community Med. 2022;47(1):4-7.
2. Ariadne Labs. (2015). Serious Illness Conversation Guide. [online] Available from https://www.ariadnelabs.org/wp-content/uploads/2017/05/SI-CG-2017-04-21_FINAL.pdf [Last accessed February, 2023].
3. Christakis NA. Prognostication and bioethics. Daedalus. 1999;128(4):197-214.
4. Lunney JR, Lynn J, Hogan C. Profiles of older medicare decedents. J Am Geriatr Soc. 2002;50(6):1108-12.
5. Frontera JA, Curtis JR, Nelson JE, Campbell M, Gabriel M, Mosenthal AC, et al; Improving Palliative Care in the ICU Project Advisory Board. Integrating palliative care into the care of neurocritically ill patients: A report from the improving palliative care in the ICU Project Advisory Board and the Center to Advance Palliative Care. Crit Care Med. 2015;43(9):1964-77.

6. Iwashyna TJ. Recognizing a patient is acutely dying. Ann Am Thorac Soc. 2020;17(10):1195-8.
7. Schneider C, Aubert CE, Del Giovane C, Donzé JD, Gastens V, Bauer DC, et al. Comparison of 6 mortality risk scores for prediction of 1-year mortality risk in older adults with multimorbidity. JAMA Netw Open. 2022;5(7):e2223911.
8. Berkey FJ, Wiedemer JP, Vithalani ND. Delivering bad or life-altering news. Am Fam Physician. 2018;98(2):99-104.
9. Ghoshal A, Salins N, Damani A, Chowdhury J, Chitre A, Muckaden MA, et al. To tell or not to tell: exploring the preferences and attitudes of patients and family caregivers on disclosure of a cancer-related diagnosis and prognosis. J Glob Oncol. 2019;5:1-12.
10. Raphael A, Hawkes CH, Bernat JL. To tell or not to tell? Revealing the diagnosis in multiple sclerosis. Mult Scler Relat Disord. 2013;2(3):247-51.
11. Nakagawa S. Communication—the most challenging procedure. JAMA Intern Med. 2015;175(8):1268-9.
12. Bernacki RE, Block SD; American College of Physicians High Value Care Task Force. Communication about serious illness care goals: A review and synthesis of best practices. JAMA Intern Med. 2014;174(12):1994-2003.
13. Phillips LJ. Dropping the bomb: the experience of being diagnosed with Parkinson's disease. Geriatr Nurs. 2006;27(6):362-9.
14. Steinhauser KE, Voils CI, Clipp EC, Bosworth HB, Christakis NA, Tulsky JA. "Are you at peace?": One item to probe spiritual concerns at the end of life. Arch Intern Med. 2006;166(1):101-5.
15. You JJ, Fowler RA, Heyland DK; Canadian Researchers at the End of Life Network (CARENET). Just ask: discussing goals of care with patients in hospital with serious illness. CMAJ. 2014;186(6):425-32.
16. Lu E, Nakagawa S. A "Three-Stage Protocol" for serious illness conversations: reframing communication in real time. Mayo Clin Proc. 2020;95(8):1589-93.
17. Briscoe J. The Goals of Care. Notes from a Family Meeting (Blogpost). [online] Available from https://familymeetingnotes.substack.com/p/notes-from-a-family-meeting-vol-1-f4a [Last accessed February, 2023].
18. Holloway RG, Gramling R, Kelly AG. Estimating and communicating prognosis in advanced neurologic disease. Neurology. 2013;80(8):764-72.
19. Kluger BM, Garvan CW, Holloway RG. Joy, suffering, and the goals of medicine. JAMA Neurol. 2021;78(3):265-6.
20. Supreme Court of India. (2018). Writ petition (civil) 215 of 2005; Common Cause vs Union of India. [online] Available from https://main.sci.gov.in/supremecourt/2005/9123/9123_2005_Judgement_09-Mar-2018.pdf [Last accessed February, 2023].
21. National Human Rights Commission. (2022). Press release: Important judgment of the Supreme Court of India. [online] Available from https://nhrc.nic.in/press-release/important-judgment-supreme-court-india-1#skipCont [Last accessed February, 2023].
22. Lum HD, Sudore RL, Bekelman DB. Advance care planning in the elderly. Med Clin North Am. 2015;99(2):391-403.
23. Elwyn G, Frosch D, Thomson R, Joseph-Williams N, Lloyd A, Kinnersley P, et al. Shared decision making: a model for clinical practice. J Gen Intern Med. 2012;27(10):1361-7.
24. Sokol LL, Young MJ, Paparian J, Kluger BM, Lum HD, Besbris J, et al. Advance care planning in Parkinson's disease: Ethical challenges and future directions. NPJ Parkinsons Dis. 2019;5:24.
25. Hegde S, Ellajosyula R. Capacity issues and decision-making in dementia. Ann Indian Acad Neurol. 2016;19(Suppl 1):S34-9.
26. Mathur R. ICMR Consensus Guidelines on 'Do Not Attempt Resuscitation'. Natl Med J India. 2020;33(2):107-12.
27. POLST. (2022). Honouring the wishes of those with serious illness and frailty. [online] Available from https://polst.org [Last accessed February, 2023].

INDEX

Page numbers followed by *b* refer to box, *f* refer to figure, *fc* refer to flowchart, and *t* refer to table.

A

C

D

E

G

H

I

J

K

L

N

O

P

S

T

W

X

Y

Z